Nadas'
PEDIATRIC
CARDIOLOGY

Nadas'
PEDIATRIC
CARDIOLOGY

THIRD EDITION

Edited by

Edward P. Walsh, MD

Associate Chair of Cardiology for Clinical Affairs
Cardiac Electrophysiology, Boston Children's Hospital
Professor of Pediatrics, Harvard Medical School

John E. Mayer Jr., MD

Senior Associate in Cardiac Surgery
Cardiac Surgery, Boston Children's Hospital
Professor of Surgery, Harvard Medical School

Sarah A. Teele, MD, MSHPEd

Medical Director, Cardiac Intensive Care Unit
Director, Senior Fellowship in Cardiac Intensive Care
Cardiac ICU and Inpatient Divisions, Boston Children's Hospital
Assistant Professor of Pediatrics, Harvard Medical School

David W. Brown, MD

Director of Cardiology Fellowship Training Program
Cardiac Imaging Division, Boston Children's Hospital
Associate Professor of Pediatrics, Harvard Medical School

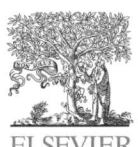

ELSEVIER

ELSEVIER
1600 John F. Kennedy Blvd.
Ste 1800
Philadelphia, PA 19103-2899

NADAS' PEDIATRIC CARDIOLOGY, THIRD EDITION   ISBN: 978-1-455-70599-3

Cover illustration: 3-dimensional cine MRI velocity mapping through the heart and great vessels (courtesy of Dr. Tal Geva).

Previous editions copyrighted 2006 and 1992.

Content Strategist: Melanie Tucker
Senior Content Development Specialist: Vaishali Singh
Publishing Services Manager: Shereen Jameel
Senior Project Manager: Manikandan Chandrasekaran
Design Direction: Patrick Ferguson

Printed in India

Last digit is the print number: 9 8 7 6 5 4 3 2

*Dedicated to the memories of Alexander S. Nadas (1913–2000)
and Aldo R. Castaneda (1930–2021), who were instrumental
in building the cardiovascular program at
Boston Children's Hospital and improving
the lives of countless young patients
with heart disease.*

Contributors

Dominic J. Abrams, MD
Co-Director, Center for Cardiovascular Genetics
Cardiac Electrophysiology Division, Boston Children's Hospital
Associate Professor of Pediatrics, Harvard Medical School
Chapter 20

Mark E. Alexander, MD
Director, Exercise Physiology
Cardiac Electrophysiology Division, Boston Children's Hospital
Associate Professor of Pediatrics, Harvard Medical School
Chapters 17, 52

Peta M.A. Alexander, MBBS
Director, Cardiac ECMO Program
Cardiac Critical Care Division, Boston Children's Hospital
Assistant Professor of Pediatrics, Harvard Medical School
Chapter 36

Catherine Allan, MD
Medical Director, Cardiac Critical Care Unit
Cardiac Critical Care Division, Boston Children's Hospital
Assistant Professor of Pediatrics, Harvard Medical School
Chapter 47

Christopher W. Baird, MD
Director, Heart Valve Program
Cardiac Surgery, Boston Children's Hospital
Associate Professor of Surgery, Harvard Medical School
Chapters 40, 43

Lisa Bergersen, MD, MPH
Cardiac Inpatient Division, Boston Children's Hospital
Associate Professor of Pediatrics, Harvard Medical School
Chapter 21

Rebecca Beroukhim, MD
Co-Director, Cardiac Tumor Program
Cardiac Imaging Division, Boston Children's Hospital
Assistant Professor of Pediatrics, Harvard Medical School
Chapters 42, 51, 61

Laura M. Bevilacqua, MD
Cardiac Electrophysiology Division, Boston Children's Hospital
Assistant Professor of Pediatrics, Harvard Medical School
Chapter 8

Vassilios Bezzerides, MD, PhD
Cardiac Electrophysiology and Cardiovascular Research Divisions, Boston Children's Hospital
Assistant Professor of Pediatrics, Harvard Medical School
Chapters 20, 66

Elizabeth D. Blume, MD
Chief, Advanced Cardiac Therapies Division, Boston Children's Hospital
Professor of Pediatrics, Harvard Medical School
Chapter 54

Roger E. Breitbart, MD
Chief, Inpatient Cardiology Division
Assistant Professor of Pediatrics, Harvard Medical School
Chapter 49

David W. Brown, MD
Director of Cardiology Fellowship Training Program
Cardiac Imaging Division, Boston Children's Hospital
Associate Professor of Pediatrics, Harvard Medical School
Chapters 4, 28, 29, 38, 39, 67

Ryan Callahan, MD
Attending Cardiologist (Invasive Cardiology), Children's Hospital of Philadelphia
Assistant Professor of Pediatrics, University of Pennsylvania Perelman School of Medicine
Chapters 16, 40

Chrystalle Katte Carreon, MD
Co-Director, Cardiac Registry
Department of Pathology, Boston Children's Hospital
Assistant Professor of Pathology, Harvard Medical School
Chapters 2, 3

Daniel A. Castellanos, MD
Cardiac Imaging Division, Boston Children's Hospital
Instructor of Pediatrics, Harvard Medical School
Chapter 10

Ming Hui Chen, MD, MMSc
Director, Stress Echocardiography Program
Cardiac Imaging Division, Boston Children's Hospital
Associate Professor of Pediatrics, Harvard Medical School
Chapter 11

Henry Cheng, MD
Director, Inpatient Transfer Team
Cardiac Critical Care Division, Boston Children's Hospital
Assistant Professor of Pediatrics, Harvard Medical School
Chapter 24

Steven D. Colan, MD
Director of Clinical Research
Cardiac Imaging Division, Boston Children's Hospital
Professor of Pediatrics, Harvard Medical School
Chapter 11

Kevin P. Daly, MD
Medical Director, Heart Transplant Program
Advanced Cardiac Therapies Division, Boston Children's Hospital
Assistant Professor of Pediatrics, Harvard Medical School
Chapter 30

Sarah D. de Ferranti, MD, MPH
Chief, Division of Ambulatory Cardiology, Boston Children's Hospital
Associate Professor of Pediatrics, Harvard Medical School
Chapters 44, 52

Pedro J. del Nido, MD
Chairman, Department of Cardiac Surgery
Cardiac Surgery, Boston Children's Hospital
William E. Ladd Professor of Child Surgery, Harvard Medical School
Chapters 34, 62

Elizabeth DeWitt, MD
Medical Director, Surgical Electrophysiology Program
Cardiac Electrophysiology Division, Boston Children's Hospital
Assistant Professor of Pediatrics, Harvard Medical School
Chapter 18

James DiNardo MD
Chief, Division of Cardiac Anesthesia, Boston Children's Hospital
Professor of Anesthesia, Harvard Medical School
Chapter 63

Audrey Dionne, MD
Cardiac Electrophysiology Division, Boston Children's Hospital
Assistant Professor of Pediatrics, Harvard Medical School
Chapters 46, 47

Sitaram M. Emani, MD
Director, Complex Biventricular Repair Program
Department of Cardiac Surgery, Boston Children's Hospital
Associate Professor of Surgery, Harvard Medical School
Chapters 32, 61

Jesse J. Esch, MD, MSc
Invasive Cardiology Division, Boston Children's Hospital
Assistant Professor of Pediatrics, Harvard Medical School
Chapter 15

Paul Esteso, MD, PhD
Co-Director, Cardiac Antithrombosis Management Program
Advanced Cardiac Therapies Division, Boston Children's Hospital
Instructor of Pediatrics, Harvard Medical School
Chapter 53

Eric N. Feins, MD
Surgical Director, Surgical Electrophysiology Program
Department of Cardiac Surgery, Boston Children's Hospital
Instructor of Surgery, Harvard Medical School
Chapters 40, 61

Michael D. Freed, MD
Ambulatory Cardiology Division, Boston Children's Hospital
Associate Professor of Pediatrics, Harvard Medical School
Chapter 4

Kevin Friedman, MD
Deputy Associate Chair of Cardiology for Clinical Affairs
Cardiac Imaging Division, Boston Children's Hospital
Associate Professor of Pediatrics, Harvard Medical School
Chapter 26

David R. Fulton, MD
Ambulatory Cardiology Division, Boston Children's Hospital
Associate Professor of Pediatrics, Harvard Medical School
Chapter 7

Francis Fynn-Thompson, MD
Surgical Director, Heart Transplant Program
Department of Cardiac Surgery, Boston Children's Hospital
Associate Professor of Surgery, Harvard Medical School
Chapter 54

Jessica C. Garbern, MD, PhD
Advanced Cardiac Therapies and Research Divisions, Boston Children's Hospital
Instructor of Pediatrics, Harvard Medical School
Chapter 48

Julia Garcia-Mancebo, MD
Post-Doctoral Research Associate
Cardiac Critical Care Division, Boston Children's Hospital
Chapter 23

Naomi Gauthier, MD
Director, Cardiac Fitness Program.
Ambulatory Cardiology Division, Boston Children's
    Hospital
Assistant Professor of Pediatrics, Harvard Medical School
    Chapter 12

Robert L. Geggel, MD
Ambulatory Cardiology Division, Boston Children's
    Hospital
Associate Professor of Pediatrics, Harvard Medical School
    Chapter 7

Diana L. Geisser, MD
Cardiac Critical Care Division, Boston Children's Hospital
Instructor of Pediatrics, Harvard Medical School
    Chapter 33

Laura Gellis, MD
Cardiac Imaging Division, Boston Children's Hospital
Instructor of Pediatrics, Harvard Medical School
    Chapter 38

Tal Geva, MD
Cardiologist-in-Chief
Cardiac Imaging Division, Boston Children's Hospital
Alexander S. Nadas Professor of Pediatrics, Harvard
    Medical School
    Chapters 3, 26, 51

Muhammad Bakr Ghbeis, MD
Cardiac Critical Care Division, Boston Children's Hospital
Instructor of Pediatrics, Harvard Medical School
    Chapter 41

Sunil J. Ghelani, MD
Cardiac Imaging Division, Boston Children's Hospital
Assistant Professor of Pediatrics, Harvard Medical School
    Chapter 31

Sarah W. Goldberg, MD, MPH
Cardiac Critical Care Division, Boston Children's Hospital
Instructor of Pediatrics, Harvard Medical School
    Chapter 41

Michelle Gurvitz, MD, MS
Boston Adult Congenital Heart Service, Boston Children's
    Hospital and Brigham & Women's Hospital
Associate Professor of Pediatrics, Harvard Medical School
    Chapter 55

Daniel L. Hames, MD
Cardiac Critical Care Division, Boston Children's Hospital
Instructor of Pediatrics, Harvard Medical School
    Chapter 27

David M. Harrild, MD, PhD
Cardiac Imaging Division, Boston Children's Hospital
Associate Professor of Pediatrics, Harvard Medical School
    Chapter 9

Jacob Hartz, MD, MPH
Director, Preventive Cardiology
Ambulatory Cardiology Division, Boston Children's
    Hospital
Instructor of Pediatrics, Harvard Medical School
    Chapter 44

Patricia Hickey, PhD, MBA, NEA-BC, FAAN
Senior Vice President and Associate Chief Nurse, Boston
    Children's Hospital
Assistant Professor of Pediatrics, Harvard Medical School
    Chapter 65

David Hoganson, MD
Director, Computational 3D Visualization Surgery
    Program
Department of Cardiac Surgery, Boston Children's
    Hospital
Instructor of Surgery, Harvard Medical School
    Chapter 62

Kathy Jenkins, MD, MPH
Cardiac Inpatient and Ambulatory Divisions, Boston
    Children's Hospital
Professor of Pediatrics, Harvard Medical School
    Chapter 40

David Kane, MD
Associate Director of Cardiology Fellowship Training
    Program
Cardiac Inpatient Division, Boston Children's Hospital
Assistant Professor of Pediatrics, Harvard Medical School
    Chapter 49

Aditya K. Kaza, MD, MBA
Director, Neonatal Cardiac Surgery
Department of Cardiac Surgery, Boston Children's
    Hospital
Associate Professor of Surgery, Harvard Medical School
    Chapters 27, 28, 62

John N. Kheir, MD
Cardiac Critical Care Division, Boston Children's Hospital
Associate Professor of Pediatrics, Harvard Medical School
    Chapter 23

R. Krishna Kumar, MD, DM
Clinical Professor and Head, Pediatric Cardiology
Amrita Institute of Medical Sciences and Research Centre
    Chapter 45

Michael H. Kwon, MD
Department of Cardiac Surgery, Boston Children's
    Hospital
Instructor of Surgery, Harvard Medical School
    Chapter 60

Ronald V. Lacro, MD
Director, Cardiovascular Genetics Clinic
Cardiac Genetics Program, Boston Children's Hospital
Associate Professor of Pediatrics, Harvard Medical School
    Chapters 5, 6

Michael J. Landzberg, MD
Boston Adult Congenital Heart Service, Boston Children's
    Hospital and Brigham & Women's Hospital
Associate Professor of Medicine, Harvard Medical School
    Chapters 25, 57

Peter Lang, MD
Director Cardiology Fellowship Training Program (1996–
    2011)
Cardiac Critical Care Division (1978–1988, 1996–2015),
    Boston Children's Hospital
    Chapter 35

Joan M. LaRovere, MD
Cardiac Critical Care Division, Boston Children's Hospital
Assistant Professor of Pediatrics, Harvard Medical School
    Chapter 64

Jami Levine, MS, MD
Director for Education in Cardiac Imaging
Cardiac Imaging Division, Boston Children's Hospital
Assistant Professor of Pediatrics, Harvard Medical School
    Chapters 22, 37

James Ernest Lock, MD
Cardiologist-in-Chief (1993–2016)
Invasive Cardiology Division (1984–2016), Boston
    Children's Hospital
    Foreword

Shannon Lyon, DO, MSCR
Ambulatory Cardiology Division, Boston Children's
    Hospital
Instructor of Pediatrics, Harvard Medical School
    Chapters 44, 52

Douglas Y. Mah, MD
Director, Pacemaker and ICD Program
Cardiac Electrophysiology Division, Boston Children's
    Hospital
Associate Professor of Pediatrics, Harvard Medical School
    Chapter 19

Gerald R. Marx, MD
Director, Ultrasound Imaging Research
Cardiac Imaging Division, Boston Children's Hospital
Associate Professor of Pediatrics, Harvard Medical School
    Chapter 34

Nicola Maschietto, MD, PhD
Invasive Cardiology Division, Boston Children's Hospital
Assistant Professor of Pediatrics, Harvard Medical School
    Chapter 14

Gregory S. Matte, CCP, LP, FPP
Chief Perfusionist and Manager of Cardiac Perfusion
Department of Cardiac Surgery, Boston Children's
    Hospital
    Chapter 60

John E. Mayer Jr., MD
Senior Associate in Cardiac Surgery
Cardiac Surgery, Boston Children's Hospital
Professor of Surgery, Harvard Medical School
    Chapters 1, 4, 29, 30, 31, 36, 37, 59, 60, 67

Kimberly I. Mills, MD
Cardiac Critical Care Division, Boston Children's Hospital
Assistant Professor of Pediatrics, Harvard Medical School
    Chapter 29

Kshitij Mistry, MD, MMSc
Director, Quality and Outcomes Program in Cardiology
Cardiac Critical Care Division, Boston Children's Hospital
Assistant Professor of Pediatrics, Harvard Medical School
    Chapter 28

Mary P. Mullen, MD, PhD
Director, Pulmonary Hypertension Service, Boston
    Children's Hospital
Assistant Professor of Pediatrics, Harvard Medical School
    Chapter 56

Viviane G. Nasr, MD, MPH
Division of Cardiac Anesthesia, Boston Children's Hospital
Associate Professor of Anesthesia, Harvard Medical School
    Chapter 63

Meena Nathan, MD, MPH
Director, Cardiac Surgery Clinical Research
Department of Cardiac Surgery, Boston Children's
    Hospital
Assistant Professor of Surgery, Harvard Medical School
    Chapter 51, 61

Jane W. Newburger, MD, MPH
Associate Chair of Cardiology for Academic Affairs
Commonwealth Professor of Pediatrics, Harvard Medical
  School
Chapters 42, 46, 55

Patricia O'Brien, MSN, CPNP-AC/PC
Cardiac Nurse Practitioner, Boston Children's Hospital
Chapter 65

Sharon E. O'Brien, MD
Chief of Pediatric Cardiology
Associate Professor of Pediatrics, Boston University School
  of Medicine
Chapter 50

Edward T. O'Leary, MD
Cardiac Electrophysiology Division, Boston Children's
  Hospital
Assistant Professor of Pediatrics, Harvard Medical School
Chapter 19

Diego Porras, MD
Chief, Invasive Cardiology Division, Boston Children's
  Hospital
Associate Professor of Pediatrics, Harvard Medical School
Chapters 13, 14

Andrew J. Powell, MD
Chief, Cardiac Imaging Division, Boston Children's
  Hospital
Professor of Pediatrics, Harvard Medical School
Chapters 9, 43

Ashwin Prakash, MD
Director, Cardiac MRI and CT
Cardiac Imaging Division, Boston Children's Hospital
Associate Professor of Pediatrics, Harvard Medical School
Chapter 10

William T. Pu, MD
Associate Chair of Cardiology for Basic and Translational
  Research
Cardiovascular Research Division, Boston Children's
  Hospital
Aldo R. Castaneda Professor of Pediatrics, Harvard
  Medical School
Chapter 66

Daniel Quiat, MD, PhD
Cardiac Genetics Program, Boston Children's Hospital
Instructor of Pediatrics, Harvard Medical School
Chapters 48

Brian Quinn, MD
Invasive Cardiology Division, Boston Children's Hospital
Instructor of Pediatrics, Harvard Medical School
Chapter 13

Luis Quinonez, MD
Director, Surgical Coronary Artery Program
Department of Cardiac Surgery, Boston Children's
  Hospital
Instructor of Surgery, Harvard Medical School
Chapter 42

Rahul H. Rathod, MD
Associate Chair of Cardiology for Finance and Business
  Operations
Cardiac Imaging Division, Boston Children's Hospital
Associate Professor of Pediatrics, Harvard Medical School
Chapter 59

Jonathan Rhodes, MD*
Director, Exercise Physiology (2002–2022)
Chapter 12

Amy E. Roberts, MD
Co-Director, Center for Cardiovascular Genetics
Cardiac Genetics Program, Boston Children's Hospital
Associate Professor of Pediatrics, Harvard Medical School
Chapters 5, 6

Carla P. Rodriguez-Monserrate, MD
Boston Adult Congenital Heart Service, Boston Children's
  Hospital and Brigham & Women's Hospital
Instructor of Pediatrics, Harvard Medical School
Chapter 58

Christina Ronai, MD, MSEd
Cardiac Imaging Division, Boston Children's Hospital
Assistant Professor of Pediatrics, Harvard Medical School
Chapter 39

Theresa Saia, DNP, APRN, CPNP
Director of Ambulatory Cardiac Nursing
Cardiac Nurse Practitioner, Boston Children's Hospital.
Chapter 65

Susan F. Saleeb, MD
Ambulatory Cardiology Division, Boston Children's
  Hospital
Assistant Professor of Pediatrics, Harvard Medical School
Chapter 50

---

* We sadly note the passing of our friend and colleague, Jonathan Rhodes,
in 2022 after a long illness.

Joshua W. Salvin, MD, MPH
Cardiac Critical Care Division, Boston Children's Hospital
Associate Professor of Pediatrics, Harvard Medical School
Chapter 35

Stephen P. Sanders, MD
Director, Cardiac Registry
Department of Cardiology, Boston Children's Hospital
Professor of Pediatrics (Part-Time), Harvard Medical School
Chapters 2, 3, 43

David Schidlow, MD, MMus
Director, Heterotaxy Program
Cardiac Imaging Division, Boston Children's Hospital
Assistant Professor of Pediatrics, Harvard Medical School
Chapter 32

Keri M. Shafer, MD
Boston Adult Congenital Heart Service, Boston Children's Hospital and Brigham & Women's Hospital
Assistant Professor of Pediatrics, Harvard Medical School
Chapter 57

Bryan D. Siegel, MD
Cardiac Critical Care Division, Boston Children's Hospital
Instructor of Pediatrics, Harvard Medical School
Chapter 56

Michael N. Singh, MD
Inpatient Director, Adult Congenital Heart / Pulmonary Hypertension Program
Boston Adult Congenital Heart Service, Boston Children's Hospital and Brigham & Women's Hospital
Assistant Professor of Pediatrics and Medicine, Harvard Medical School
Chapter 33

Tajinder Singh, MD, MSc
Advanced Cardiac Therapies Division, Boston Children's Hospital
Associate Professor of Pediatrics, Harvard Medical School
Chapter 53

Sarah A. Teele, MD, MSHPEd
Medical Director, Cardiac Intensive Care Unit
Director, Senior Fellowship in Cardiac Intensive Care
Cardiac ICU and Inpatient Divisions, Boston Children's Hospital
Assistant Professor of Pediatrics, Harvard Medical School
Chapters 31, 32, 64, 67

Ravi R. Thiagarajan, MD, MPH
Chief, Division of Cardiac Critical Care, Boston Children's Hospital
Professor of Pediatrics, Harvard Medical School
Chapter 64

John K. Triedman, MD
Chief, Cardiac Electrophysiology Division, Boston Children's Hospital
Professor of Pediatrics, Harvard Medical School
Chapter 18

Wayne Tworetzky, MD
Director, Fetal Cardiology Program
Cardiac Imaging Division, Boston Children's Hospital
Associate Professor of Pediatrics, Harvard Medical School
Chapter 16

Anne Marie Valente, MD
Chief, Adult Congenital Heart / Pulmonary Hypertension Program
Boston Adult Congenital Heart Service, Boston Children's Hospital and Brigham & Women's Hospital
Professor of Medicine and Pediatrics, Harvard Medical School
Chapter 58

Christina VanderPluym, MD
Medical Director, Cardiac Antithrombosis Management and Monitoring Program
Advanced Cardiac Therapies Division, Boston Children's Hospital
Associate Professor of Pediatrics, Harvard Medical School
Chapter 54

Edward P. Walsh, MD
Associate Chair of Cardiology for Clinical Affairs
Cardiac Electrophysiology, Boston Children's Hospital
Professor of Pediatrics, Harvard Medical School
Chapters 1, 8, 17, 26, 34, 51, 67

Fred Ming-Chieh Wu, MD
Boston Adult Congenital Heart Service, Boston Children's Hospital and Brigham & Women's Hospital
Assistant Professor of Pediatrics, Harvard Medical School
Chapter 59

Suellen Yin, MD
Ambulatory Cardiology Division, Boston Children's Hospital
Instructor of Pediatrics, Harvard Medical School
Chapter 12

Foreword

In 1956, Alexander Sandor Nadas traveled from Boston to Groningen in the Netherlands for a 1-year sabbatical. He had a singular goal: to write his seminal textbook, *Pediatric Cardiology*. This endeavor was not without risk. The field was tiny, the body of knowledge sparse and often incorrect, and the therapeutic successes rare and, even then, mostly incomplete.

Everyone who reads these words will know what came next: an explosion of understanding and successes almost unparalleled in any medical field. Examine the body of basic knowledge, the diagnostic tools, the therapeutic options, and (that most essential end-product) the catalog of healthy survival for various lesions. Then compare the original Nadas' text with the current version, and one's expectations for the future of our field will be strengthened.

Did Dr. Nadas envision this future when he labored in his Dutch study 65 years ago to finish that first slender volume? Can any of the 101 contributors to this magnificent new volume see ahead another 65 years? Perhaps not. But they have captured their time and place with thoughtful clarity and precision. If future professionals caring for children with heart disease continue a relentless, self-critical, and data-driven approach to build the field, one cannot hope for better.

James Ernest Lock
Little Compton, Rhode Island
Cardiologist-in-Chief (1993–2016)
Boston Children's Hospital

Preface

In the preface to the first edition of his pediatric cardiology textbook published in 1957, Alexander S. Nadas stated: *"I do not intend to write a reference book.....I hope to put proper emphasis on clinical recognition and management."* Subsequent editions in 1964, 1972, 1994, and 2006 by Dr. Nadas and his successors at Boston Children's Hospital remained true to this theme by providing a solid clinical foundation without trying to be encyclopedic. We upheld the tradition for this new volume by including enough material to orient the reader to the modern complexities of pediatric cardiology and cardiac surgery while still ensuring the most important take-home messages for each chapter could be fully digested after a single reading. Likewise, the number of references has been kept deliberately short to better focus our audience on landmark articles and useful reviews. If we have done our job correctly, this should whet the reader's appetite for more in-depth information to be acquired by studying contemporary journals and caring for actual patients. The latter activity, after all, will always be the undisputed gold standard in medical education.

In addition to providing a general update on diagnosis and treatment, this new edition incorporates several changes to enhance the learning experience. First, most chapters open with five key teaching points highlighting critical content. Second, our cardiac surgeons have taken an active role as coauthors on multiple chapters to provide a more comprehensive view of patient management. Third, new chapters have been added focusing on timely topics such as the failing Fontan circulation, pregnancy in women with congenital heart disease, novel surgical approaches to single ventricle, and evolving transcatheter interventions for hemodynamic lesions and arrhythmias. Finally, our publishing partners at Elsevier have kindly agreed to provide a companion e-book version (complete with video loops) that can be accessed from personal electronic devices. We hope such refinements will prove valuable to our readers at all stages of their careers. It should also be noted that we have refrained from making firm recommendations on medication dosages in this new addition, since textbooks are by nature too static to keep up with evolving data. Readers are referred to web-based or hospital-based formularies that are continuously updated with best-practice dosage guidelines.

As was the custom in previous editions, authors have been drawn primarily from the faculty within our own program. While this introduces a certain degree of institutional bias into management recommendations, we do not mean to suggest our approach is the exclusive way to treat heart disease in the young, but only that it has proven effective in our center's experience. Reference lists have been constructed carefully to ensure that alternate approaches are suitably recognized.

Well over 60 years have passed since Dr. Nadas' original textbook was published. To appreciate how far we have come over that time span, just consider his 1957 description of the prognosis for transposition of the great arteries: *"The clinical course is a grim one. Of our 36 patients, 12 died in the first month, 13 between one and four months, and only 3 lived beyond one year. Death approaches with catastrophic rapidity."* We are grateful to Dr. Nadas and the generations of clinicians who followed in his footsteps that such is no longer the case.

Edward P. Walsh
Boston, Massachusetts

Contents

Video Contents

Historical Notes

1

A Brief History of Pediatric Cardiology and Congenital Heart Surgery

EDWARD P. WALSH AND JOHN E. MAYER JR.

"The further backward you can look, the further forward you are likely to see."

Winston Churchill

The history of our subspecialty can be traced back more than 500 years to the early pathologic descriptions of congenital heart defects in humans. Perhaps it is not surprising that Leonardo da Vinci was the first to report on the subject when he discovered an atrial septal defect during a heart dissection in 1513.[1] Subsequent milestones include Stensen's initial description in 1671 of what was later labeled as Fallot's tetralogy, a case of single ventricle reported by Chemineau in 1699, pulmonary atresia as described by Hunter in 1784, transposition of the great arteries as noted in a compendium of defects published by Thomas Peacock in 1858, and a host of other pathologic observations on septal defects and valve abnormalities throughout the 1800s, including Ebstein's eponymous condition in 1866.[2,3] But it was not until the early 1900s that a clinical approach to congenital heart disease arose, heralded by Maude Abbott's classic atlas, and aided by new diagnostic tools such as the electrocardiogram, chest fluoroscopy, and cardiac catheterization. The chronology in Table 1.1 highlights some of the major accomplishments during the 20th century that are highly relevant to our field.[4-8]

Exciting progress continues in the 21st century as described throughout the remainder of this textbook, but

TABLE 1.1	Important 20th Century Events in Cardiology and Cardiac Surgery	
1902	Electrocardiogram	Einthoven; Leiden, The Netherlands
1907	Atlas of CHD	Abbott; Montreal, Canada
1929	Cardiac catheterization	Forssmann; Eberswalde, Germany
1930	Cardiology program established at Harriet Lane Home	Taussig; Baltimore, USA
1930	WPW syndrome described	Wolff & White; Boston, USA and Parkinson; London, UK
1938	PDA ligation	Gross; Boston, USA
1939	Cardiac angiography	Castellanos; Havana, Cuba
1941	Hemodynamic cardiac catheterization	Richards & Cournand; New York, USA
1944	Jones' criteria for rheumatic fever	Jones; Boston, USA
1944	Blalock-Taussig-Thomas shunt	Blalock & Taussig & Thomas; Baltimore, USA
1944	Coarctation repair	Crafood & Nylin; Stockholm, Sweden
1946	Potts shunt	Potts; Chicago, USA
1947	First clinical pediatric cardiology textbook	Taussig; Baltimore, USA

TABLE 1.1	Important 20th Century Events in Cardiology and Cardiac Surgery—cont'd	
1948	Mitral valvotomy	Harken; Boston, USA
1948	Pulmonary valvotomy	Brock; London, UK
1949	Cardiology program established at Boston Children's Hospital	Nadas; Boston, USA
1950	Blalock-Hanlon operation	Blalock & Hanlon; Baltimore, USA
1952	ASD closure under hypothermic circulatory arrest	Lewis & Varco; Minneapolis, USA
1952	ASD closure using cardiopulmonary bypass	Gibbon; Philadelphia, USA
1953	M-mode echocardiography	Edler & Hertz; Lund, Germany
1954	Repair of VSD using cross-circulation	Lillehei & Varco; Minneapolis, USA
1955	Repair of VSD & tetralogy of Fallot using DeWall oxygenator	Lillehei; Minneapolis, USA
1956	Pulmonary artery banding	Muller & Dammann; Charlottesville, USA
1957	First edition of this textbook	Nadas; Boston, USA
1957	Long QT syndrome described	Jervell & Lange-Nielsen; Oslo, Norway
1958	Glenn shunt	Glenn; New Haven, USA
1958	First implantable pacemaker	Senning; Stockholm, Sweden
1959	Successful atrial-level switch for TGA	Senning; Stockholm, Sweden
1960	Transseptal catheterization	Brockenbrough; Bethesda, USA
1961	Pediatric cardiology subboard established	American Board of Pediatrics; Chapel Hill, USA
1962	Waterston shunt	Waterston; London, UK
1964	Alternate atrial-level switch for TGA	Mustard; Toronto, Canada
1966	Balloon atrial septostomy	Rashkind; Philadelphia, USA
1967	Programmed stimulation for electrophysiology studies	Durrer; Amsterdam, Netherlands
1967	Kawasaki disease described	Kawasaki; Tokyo, Japan
1968	Surgery for WPW syndrome	Sealy; Durham, USA
1968	Atrio-pulmonary connection for tricuspid atresia	Fontan; Bourdeaux, France
1969	His bundle recording catheter	Scherlag; New York, USA
1972	First fully dedicated pediatric cardiac ICU	Williams & Castaneda; Boston, USA
1974	Infant primary repair for CHD	Castaneda; Boston, USA
1976	Successful arterial switch for TGA	Jatene; Sao Paulo, Brazil
1976	Prostaglandins to maintain ductal patency	Olly; Toronto, Canada
1977	Maternal lupus linked to congenital complete heart block	Chameides; Hartford, USA
1977	First natural history study of CHD	(multicenter)
1978	2-D echocardiography	Eggleton; Indianapolis, USA
1979	Doppler flow analysis	Hatle; Trondheim, Norway
1979	Transcatheter closure PDA	Rashkind; Philadelphia, USA
1979	Intraoperative mapping of conduction tissues in CHD	Dick; Boston, USA
1980	Transesophageal echo	Hisanaga; Nagoya, Japan
1980	Implantable cardioverter defibrillator developed	Mirowski; Baltimore, USA
1980	Cardiac MRI	Ingwall & Pohost; Boston, USA

Continued

TABLE 1.1	Important 20th Century Events in Cardiology and Cardiac Surgery—cont'd	
1980	Fetal echocardiography	Kleinman; New Haven, USA / Allan; London, UK
1981	Indomethacin for PDA closure	(multicenter)
1981	Surgery for HLHS	Norwood & Lang & Hansen; Boston, USA
1982	Transcatheter dilation of pulmonary valve stenosis	Kan; Baltimore, USA
1983	DC catheter ablation for arrhythmias in pediatrics	Gillette; Houston, USA
1983	Transcatheter ASD closure	Rashkind; Philadelphia, USA
1983	Neonatal arterial switch operation for TGA	Castaneda & Norwood, Boston, USA
1983	Adenosine for supraventricular tachycardia	DiMarco; Charlottesville, USA
1984	Color Doppler	Omoto; Saitama, Japan
1984	Successful pediatric heart transplant for CHD	Rose; New York, USA
1985	Transcatheter dilation of branch pulmonary artery stenosis	Lock; Boston, USA
1985	Bidirectional cavopulmonary shunt	Hopkins & Oldham, Durham, USA
1985	Pediatric ECMO	Bartlett; Ann Arbor, USA
1985	Transcatheter dilation of mitral stenosis	Lock; Boston, USA
1989	Mutation of fibrillin gene linked to Marfan syndrome	Dietz; Baltimore, USA
1990	3-D echocardiography	von Ramm; Durham, USA
1990	RF catheter ablation for arrhythmias in pediatrics	Van Hare; San Francisco, USA
1990	Transcatheter dilation of congenital aortic stenosis	Keane; Boston, USA
1990	Modification of Fontan procedure with atrial fenestration	Bridges & Lock & Castaneda; Boston, USA
1991	Bethesda conference on adult CHD	Perloff; Los Angeles, USA
1991	First gene abnormality in long QT syndrome identified	Keating; Salt Lake City, USA
1991	Transcatheter VSD closure	Lock; Boston, USA
1992	Inhaled NO for pulmonary hypertension in CHD	Haydar; Paris, France
1993	22q11 deletion linked to CHD	Kelly; London, UK
1993	Neurologic outcomes after hypothermic circulatory arrest	Newburger & Jonas, Boston, USA
1993	Second natural history study of CHD	(multicenter)
1993	Arrhythmia ablation in complex CHD	Triedman & Walsh; Boston, USA
1995	3-D electroanatomic arrhythmia mapping	Ben-Haim; Tal Aviv, Israel
1997	TBX5 mutation linked to Holt-Oram syndrome	Basson; Boston MA / Yi Li; Nottingham, UK
1998	Neurodevelopmental outcomes after surgery for CHD	Rappaport & Newburger; Boston, USA

Note: Dates in most cases reflect first event, while some reflect year of first manuscript publication.
ASD, Atrial septal defect; CHD, congenital heart disease; DC, direct current energy; ECMO, extracorporeal membrane oxygenation; HLHS, hypoplastic left heart syndrome; MRI, magnetic resonance imaging; NO, nitric oxide; PDA, patent ductus arteriosus; RF, radiofrequency energy; TGA, transposition of the great arteries; VSD, ventricular septal defect; WPW, Wolff-Parkinson-White.

with each advance comes new challenges. A prime example is the nearly exponential increase in adult survivors of congenital heart disease who require a new breed of cardiologist and novel care models to provide optimal long-term management.[9] Similarly, modern diagnostic tests (e.g., cardiac MRI) and evolving therapies (e.g., fetal catheter interventions) have become more technically demanding and labor-intensive. As a consequence, the cardiac workforce at all major institutions has expanded dramatically since the early days of our subspecialty (Fig. 1.1).

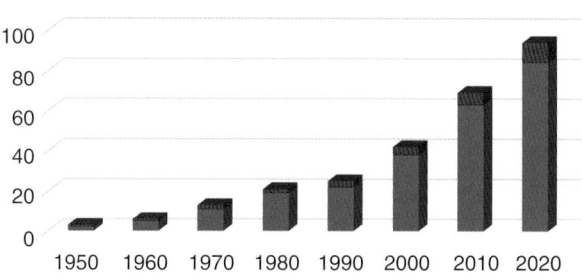

Full-time cardiologists and cardiac surgeons
Boston Children's Hospital

• **Fig. 1.1** Number of full-time cardiologists and cardiac surgeons at Boston Children's Hospital (1950–2020).

Progress in our field, whether it involves clinical care or bench research, is an iterative process built upon the accomplishments of those who came before. Furthermore, it is highly dependent upon cross-disciplinary collaboration between cardiologists, cardiac surgeons, cardiac anesthesiologists, and cardiac nursing. Unless we understand and appreciate the contributions of others, our ability to innovate for the future is hampered. We hope this brief historical survey orients the reader to the brilliant work done by past generations so that today's state-of-the-art is not taken for granted.

References

1. Rashkind WJ. Pediatric cardiology: a brief historical perspective. Pediatr Cardiol. 1979;1:63-71.
2. Noonan JA. A history of pediatric specialties: the development of pediatric cardiology. Pediatr Res. 2004;56:298-306.
3. Schiebler GL, Gravenstein JS, Van Mierop LH. Ebstein's anomaly of the tricuspid valve. Translation of original description with comments. Am J Cardiol. 1968;22:867-873.
4. Westaby S. Landmarks in Cardiac Surgery. Oxford, UK: Mosby-Year Book and Oxford University Press; 1997.
5. Mormile R, Quadrini I, Squarcia U. Milestones in pediatric cardiology: making possible the impossible. Clin Cardiol. 2013;36: 74-76.
6. Mahle WT, John JB, Silverman NH. The history of the development of paediatric echocardiography. Cardiol Young. 2009;19(suppl 2): 26-34.
7. Walsh EP, Dick M II. History of research accomplishments in pediatric electrophysiology. Congenit Heart Dis. 2013;8: 362-369.
8. Freedom RM, Lock JE, Bricker JT. Pediatric cardiology and cardiovascular surgery: 1950-2000. Circulation. 2000;102(20 suppl 4): IV58-IV68.
9. Thakkar AN, Chinnadurai P, Lin CH. Adult congenital heart disease: magnitude of the problem. Curr Opin Cardiol. 2017; 32:467-474.

SECTION II

Developmental Anatomy and Physiology

2

Cardiac Embryology

STEPHEN P. SANDERS AND CHRYSTALLE KATTE CARREON

"The transformation of an epithelial sheet of cells into a functional heart is one of the most intriguing morphogenetic processes of embryonic development."

Kelly and Buckingham, 2002[1]

KEY LEARNING POINTS

- Recognize the molecular and anatomic complexity of cardiac development and the contributions of various tissue sources to the heart.
- Understand how deviations from normal development could result in structural heart defects.

- Identify how the molecular biology of cardiac development offers potential opportunity for non-surgical treatment of some congenital heart defects.

The normal heart is a complex structure composed of multiple parts—the result of an intricate developmental program. A basic knowledge of cardiac development facilitates understanding the origins of the myriad congenital defects that affect the human heart. Since the last edition of this book (2006), a great deal has been learned about cardiac development. This chapter presents an overview of cardiac embryology highlighting some of the newer findings from the last about 20 years. The emphasis is on anatomy, integrated with basic elements of molecular and cellular developmental biology. Where appropriate, we will point out how failure of normal developmental processes could result in congenital heart defects. As a supplement to the text, a video (video link) created using 3D models, derived from human embryos at various Carnegie stages (CS) in the Carnegie collection, accompanies this chapter. Be aware that the models were created from embryo sections prepared with standard histology stains without molecular markers. Consequently, segmentation of the models is based on our interpretation of the anatomy with the limitations of that approach.

Early Human Development

In the first 2 weeks (Fig. 2.1), the zygote undergoes asynchronous cell division to form totipotent blastomeres organized in a solid sphere, the morula. Cells subsequently differentiate and reorganize to form the hollow blastocyst. The inner cell mass of the blastocyst flattens to form the embryonic disc.[2] Implantation in the uterine wall is completed during the second week. Formation of the placenta is well underway. The dorsal-ventral and the rostral-caudal axes are determined by the end of the second week—processes not well understood in the human embryo.[2] From this point on, we will describe only events with direct bearing on the cardiovascular system, as much as possible in temporal sequence.

Week 3

The main events of the third week (CS 6–10) include gastrulation, establishment of the heart-forming fields, establishment of left-right axis, and formation of the primitive heart tube.

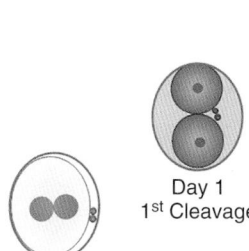
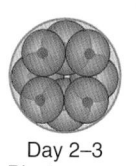
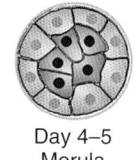
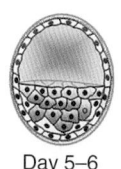
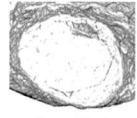

Zygote

Day 1
1st Cleavage

Day 2–3
Blastomeres

Day 4–5
Morula

Day 5–6
Blastocyst

Day 7–9
Implantation

• **Fig. 2.1** Early human development. The zygote is formed at fertilization with completion of the second meiotic division of the ovum and formation of the female and male pronuclei. Soon after, the zygote undergoes the first cleavage. Blastomeres continue to divide about once per 24 hours. At about 16- to 32-cell stage, the blastomeres compact to form the morula. Cells begin to differentiate into inner and outer cell masses, and fluid begins to collect at one end of the morula as it becomes the blastocyst. Implantation into the uterine wall occurs early in the second week.

At the beginning of the third week, the embryo consists of a bilaminar disc with the dorsal epiblast, a pseudostratified columnar epithelium, and the ventral primitive endoderm or hypoblast (Fig. 2.2). The primitive streak develops at the caudal end of the disc as an elongating groove in the epiblast progressing toward the center of the embryo.[3] Cells on each side undergo an epithelial-to-mesenchymal transition (EMT) and ingress through the streak to form the mesoderm (Fig. 2.2). Heart-forming cells come from about the middle one-third of the streak and express mesoderm posterior 1 and 2 (MESP-1 and MESP-2), which are necessary for normal migration of these cells to the anterior lateral plates where they assemble as bilateral heart-forming fields.[4]

The first or primary heart field lies ventral and lateral, while the second or secondary heart field is dorsal and medial[4] (Fig. 2.3A). The designations *first heart field* and *second heart field* reflect the spatial distribution, temporal diversity in differentiation, and differences in the molecular developmental program rather than separate origins. All heart precursors derive from cells expressing, at least transiently, islet 1 (ISL1) and NKX2-5.[5] The lateral plate mesoderm is divided into somatic and splanchnic portions by the coalescing intraembryonic coelom that will become the pericardial, pleural, and peritoneal cavities[6] (Fig. 2.4). The first heart field begins to differentiate almost immediately in response to inductive signals from the underlying endoderm[7] (Fig. 2.4). Endocardial and myocardial precursors segregate out from the heart field mesenchyme.[8] The spatial extent of heart cell differentiation is limited by inhibitory signals from the notochord medially, and neural tissue and head mesenchyme dorsally and laterally.[9] The second heart field cells remain undifferentiated and proliferating, possibly because they are more distant from the endoderm.[10] These cells express ISL1[10] and a subset express T-box transcription factor 1 (TBX1),[4] the gene in the DiGeorge critical region linked to conotruncal heart defects.[11] The second heart field cells will be added to both ends of the heart tube over the next 1–2 weeks,[4] contributing primarily to the atria, right ventricle, and outflow (Fig. 2.3B).

Transmission of left-right axis information to the lateral plates is accomplished at the end of gastrulation in the node, a bowl-shaped structure at the rostral end of the primitive streak (Fig. 2.5). The currently accepted model (2-cilia model)[12] involves motile cilia in the pit of the node and sensory cilia around the periphery. The motile cilia spin clockwise, generating flow of fluid from right to left across the node. The sensory cilia on the left side of the node, but not the right side, are deformed by the fluid flow (and possibly respond to agents from filipodia carried by the fluid), opening a calcium channel. The calcium current stimulates a transcription cascade beginning with NODAL (expressed by cells around the node and in the left lateral plate) and culminating in expression of PITX2, which confers left-sided character to the left lateral plate. The right lateral plate appears to develop by default. The gene regulatory network involves several ciliary proteins, transcription factors, and receptors. Mutations of genes encoding some of these proteins have been implicated in heterotaxy syndrome.[13]

The lateral edges of the embryo approach the midline ventrally at the end of the third week and fuse together, converting the flat, disc-shaped embryo into a tube[6] (Fig. 2.6A). This action brings the heart fields together in the midline, ventral to the forming foregut and rostral to the advancing anterior intestinal portal (Fig. 2.6B). Rapid neural growth results in head flexion, bringing the heart fields from rostral to the stomodeum (future mouth) and developing brain, to caudal and ventral to the forming pharynx. At first, the myocardium forms a trough open dorsally toward the foregut and enclosing bilateral vascular channels in continuity with the primitive arch arteries and dorsal aortae rostrally and caudally with inflow vessels draining the yolk sac[10] (Fig. 2.7A).

Outside the heart-forming area, signals from structures such as the notochord induce capillaries in the network that has formed throughout the embryo to coalesce in

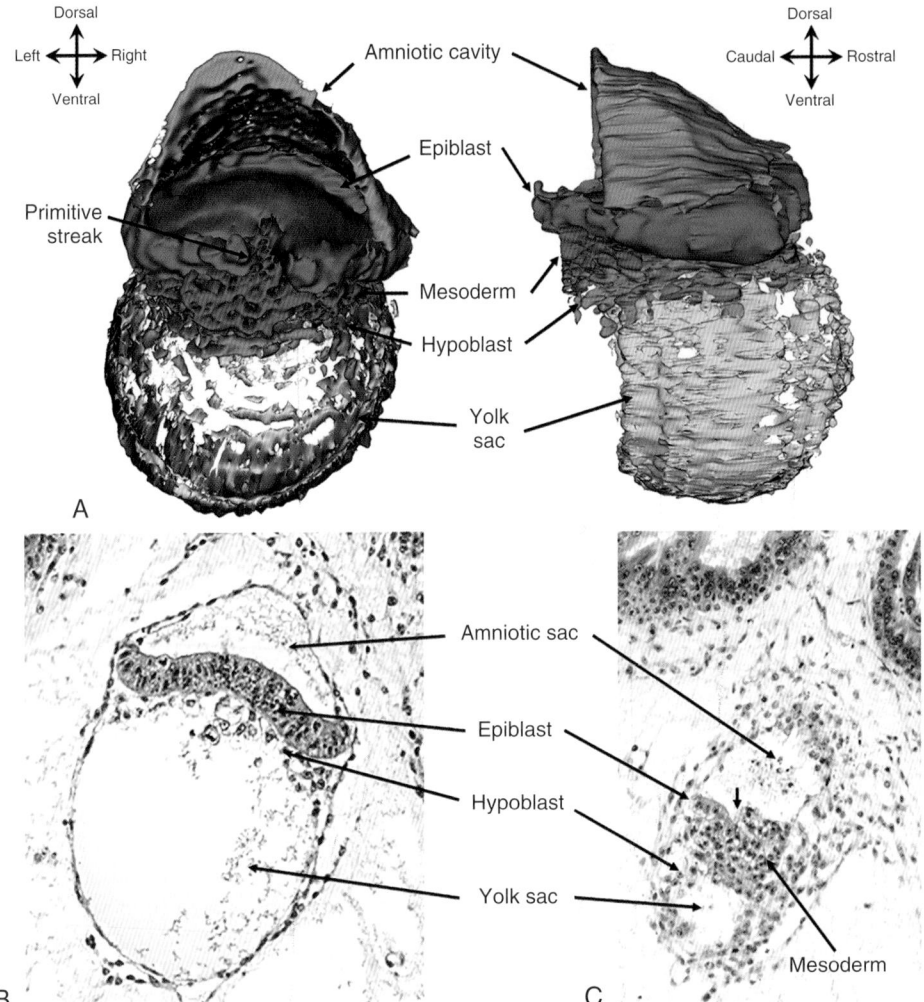

• **Fig. 2.2** (A) 3D reconstruction of the disc embryo from caudal and lateral aspects at CS 6 (mid-third week) during early gastrulation. Mesoderm *(red)* has collected between the epiblast *(brown)* dorsally and the hypoblast *(green)* ventrally at the caudal end of the embryo disc where the primitive streak has developed. (B) Rostral section through the embryo showing apposition of the hypoblast or primitive endoderm to the epiblast with no mesoderm at this level because gastrulation has just begun. (C) A more caudal section showing the primitive streak (⇓) and ingressing mesodermal cells.

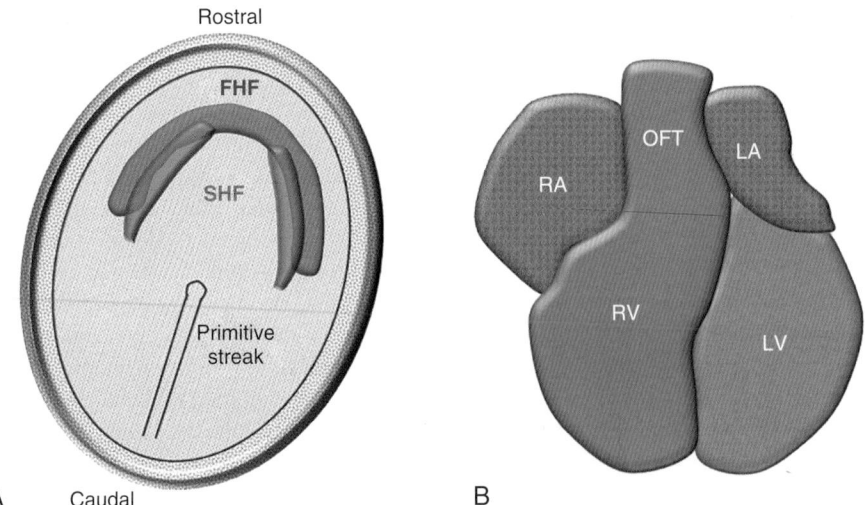

• **Fig. 2.3** (A) Cartoon of a dorsal view of post-gastrulation disc embryo showing ventral and lateral first *(FHF, blue)* and dorsal and medial second *(SHF, orange)* heart fields in the anterior lateral plates. (B) Cartoon of mature heart showing contributions of FHF *(blue)* and SHF *(orange)*. *LA,* Left atrium; *LV,* left ventricle; *OFT,* outflow tract; *RA,* right atrium; *RV,* right ventricle.

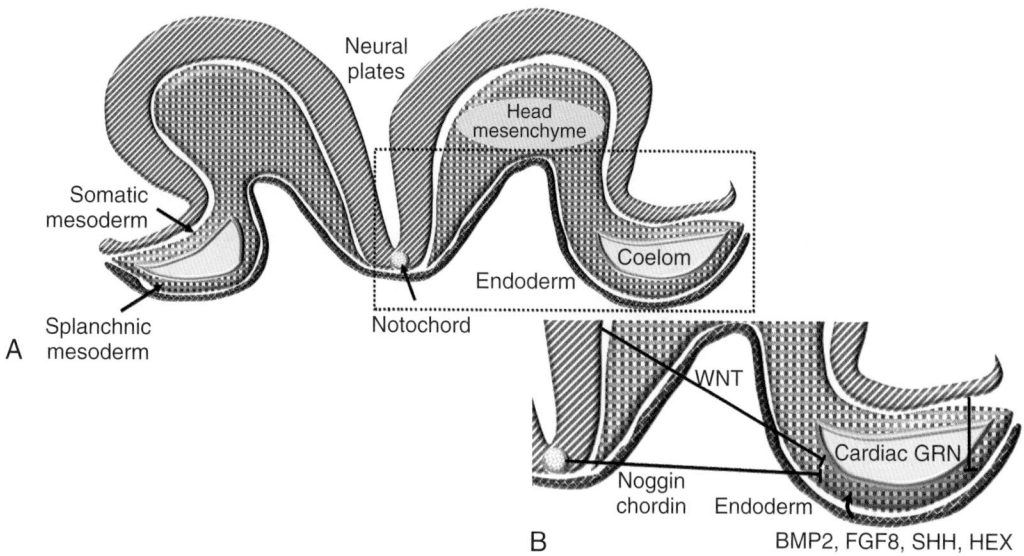

• **Fig. 2.4** (A) Cartoon of a section through a CS 7 embryo in late third week showing the division of the lateral plates by the intraembryonic coelom forming somatic mesoderm dorsally and splanchnic mesoderm, that is the source of the heart, ventrally. (B) Blow-up of the lateral plate *(dashed box in A)* showing induction of heart cells (endocardium and myocardium, *violet*) by signals from the endoderm (BMP2, FGF8, SHH, HEX), which induce expression of the cardiac gene regulatory network (GRN) including NKX2-5, GATA factors, TBX5, TBX20, myocardin, and others. Inhibitory factors from the notochord (Noggin, Chordin), neural tissue, and head mesenchyme (WNT signaling) limit the size of the heart-forming field.

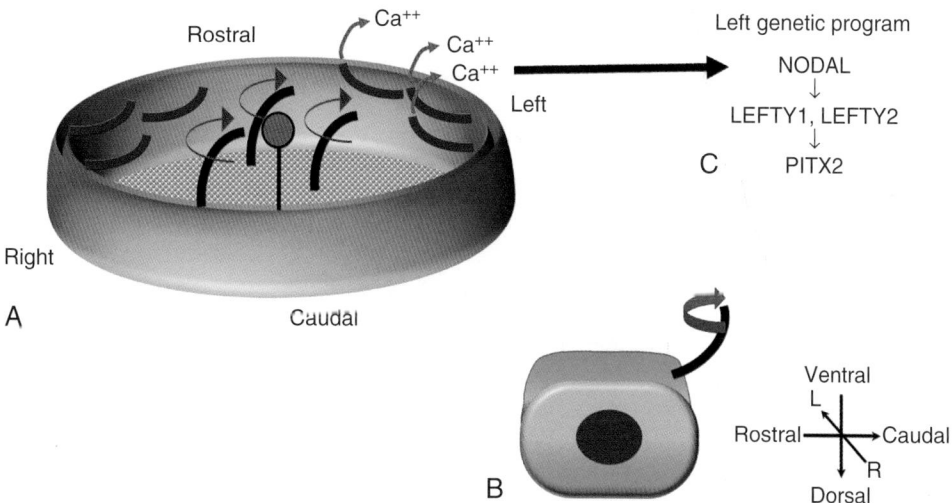

• **Fig. 2.5** (A) Cartoon of a ventral view of the node, a bowl-shaped structure at the rostral end of the primitive streak. Motile cilia *(black)* generate left-to-right fluid flow that deforms sensory cilia *(red)*, opening calcium channels. There are also filopodia on the floor of the node with active substances within the vesicles *(orange)*. (B) Motile cilia form on the caudal aspect of the convex nodal cells. Because they are at an acute angle to the surface, only the part of the stroke away from the surface directed leftward is effective in moving fluid. The leftward flow of fluid and possibly active agents carried by the fluid stimulate sensory cilia only on the left side of the node initiating the left genetic program (C), which confers left-sided character to the left lateral plate. The right side seems to develop by default.

specific locations forming larger vessels such as the dorsal aortae.[14] As ventral closure proceeds, the two endocardium-lined vascular channels within the myocardial trough fuse to form a single channel, and the myocardium closes dorsally around the channel to form the primitive heart tube[15] (Fig. 2.7B). The tube is composed of a 1- or 2-cell-thick outer myocardium, a thick layer of ground substance (cardiac jelly), and an inner 1-cell-thick endocardium (Figs. 2.6B and 2.7B).

Week 4

During the fourth week (CS 11–12) the newly formed heart tube begins peristaltic contraction, undergoes looping, begins chamber formation, initiates ventricular septation, and adds the epicardium and the myocardium of the sinus venosus. Neural crest cells arrive in the pharyngeal arches, and remodeling of the early pharyngeal arch arteries begins.

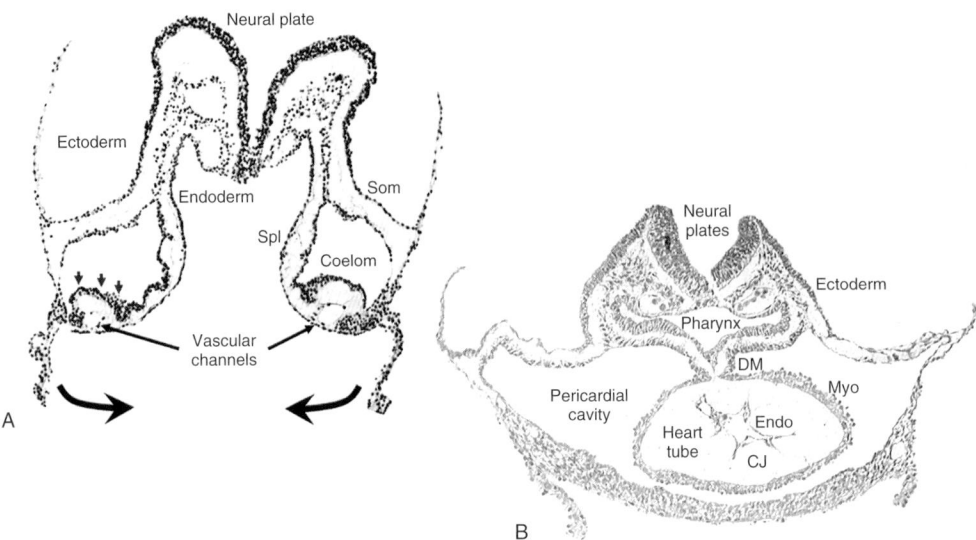

• **Fig. 2.6** (A) A section through a CS 9 embryo at the end of the third week beginning to close ventrally *(curved arrows)*. The coelom separates the somatic *(Som)* and splanchnic *(Spl)* mesoderm. The myocardium has begun to differentiate *(red arrows)* bilaterally, and bilateral vascular channels have formed. (B) A section from a CS 10 embryo at the beginning of the fourth week. The somatic mesoderm and ectoderm have enclosed the pericardial cavity and the single heart tube formed by fusion of the bilateral channels, with a 1- to 2-cell layer of myocardium (Myo) externally, a thick layer of ground substance called cardiac jelly *(CJ)*, and a 1-cell thick endocardium *(Endo)* internally. The pharynx or foregut is dorsal to the heart tube and its suspending dorsal mesocardium *(DM)*. The neural plates are closing dorsally to form the neural tube.

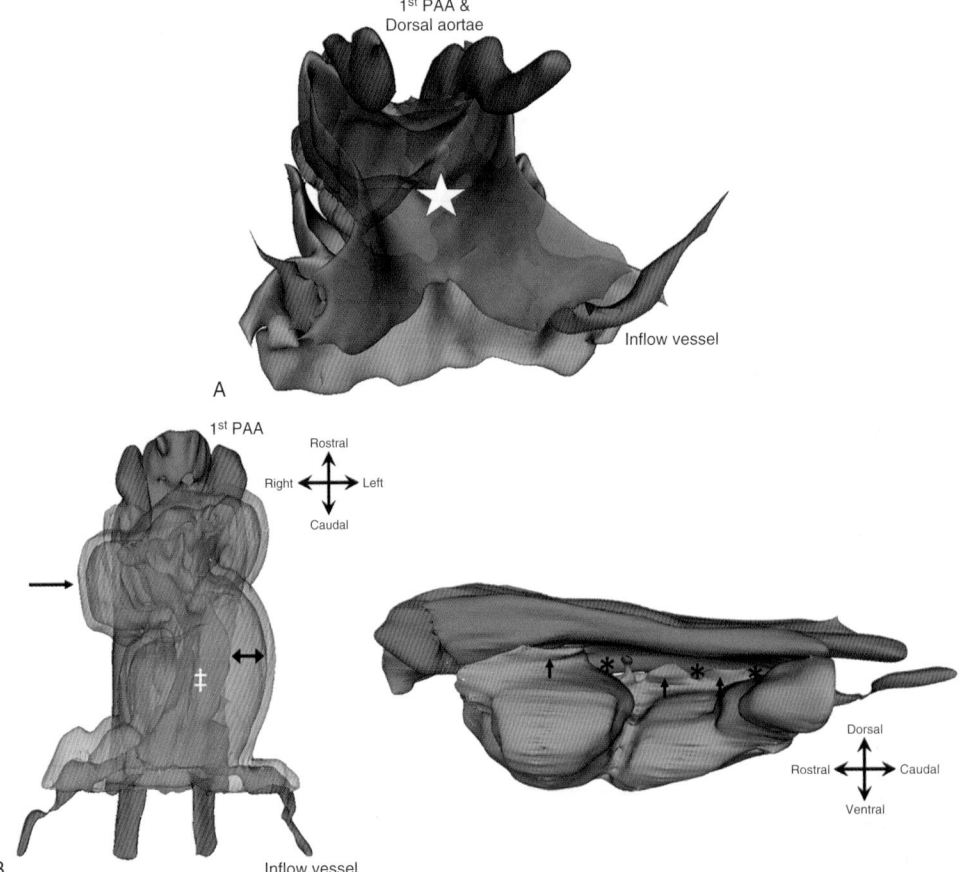

• **Fig. 2.7** A series of 3D reconstruction showing heart tube formation and looping. (A) Caudal view of a CS 9 embryo at beginning of the fourth week showing the trough-shaped sheet of myocardium *(green)* rostral to the anterior intestine portal *(star)* and open dorsally to the pharynx *(brown)*. Bilateral vascular channels *(orange)* are between the myocardium and pharynx with inflow vessels caudal and the first or primitive pharyngeal arch arteries *(PAA)* and dorsal aortae rostral. (B) Ventral *(left)* and lateral *(right)* views of a CS 10 embryo in early fourth week. There is a single endocardium-lined lumen *(‡)* within the myocardial tube *(green)* surrounded by a thick layer of cardiac jelly *(double-headed arrow)* and a thin layer of myocardium. The inflow vessels join to form the single lumen which splits rostrally to form the 1st PAA which are continuous with the dorsal aortae. Dextral or D looping is beginning near the outflow *(arrow)*. Left lateral view shows the dorsal mesocardium *(arrows)* (DM) connecting the heart tube to the prepharyngeal mesoderm. The DM is beginning to break down in places *(*)* as the heart tube begins to loop.

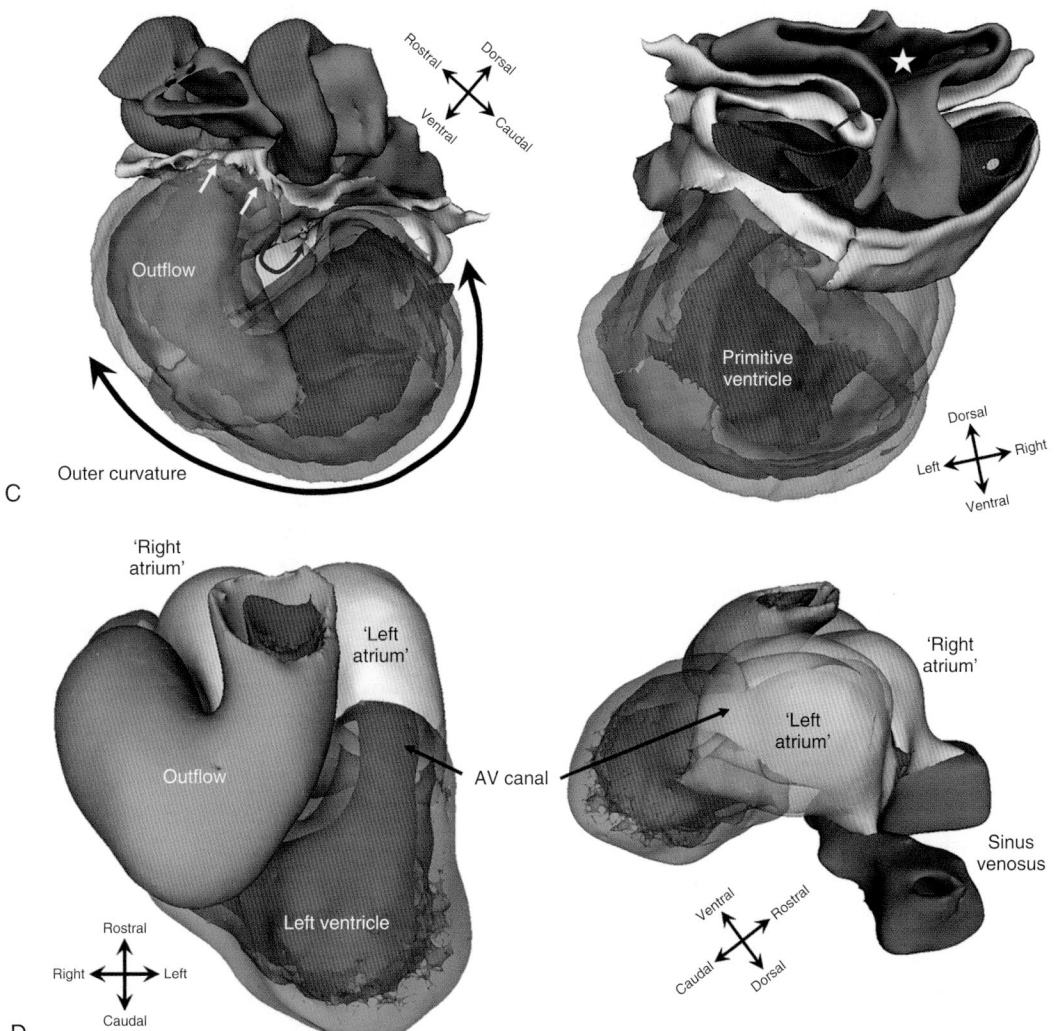

• **Fig. 2.7, cont'd** (C) Left anterior *(left)* and posterior *(right)* oblique views of a CS 11 embryo at mid-fourth week. Anterior oblique view shows the looping heart tube with the outflow far rightward. The presumptive right *(gold)* and left *(white)* atria are to the left of the outflow. The DM has broken down except at the outflow end where the outflow myocardium is continuous with the anterior second heart field in the dorsal pericardial wall *(white arrows)* and at the inflow end where the atrial myocardium is continuous with the posterior second heart field *(red arrow)*. Chambers will begin to balloon out of the outer curvature *(curved black double-headed arrow)*, while the small inner curvature *(double-headed red arrow)* grows very little. Posterior oblique view shows the primitive ventricle descending below the inflow (presumptive atria). *Star* indicates anterior intestinal portal. (D) Ventral *(left)* and lateral *(right)* views of a CS 12 embryo in late fourth week. Ventral view shows the onset of ballooning expansion of the left ventricle from the primitive ventricle at the outer curvature. The outflow has elongated and developed the characteristic bend. The distal part of the outflow has moved medially between the presumptive right and left atria. The atrioventricular *(AV)* canal is apparent as an elongated narrow connection between the presumptive left atrium and left ventricle. The lateral view shows the AV canal and the sinus venosus.

The heart tube is suspended along its length by the dorsal mesocardium from the prepharyngeal mesoderm[16] that contains the ISL1+ proliferating second heart field cells[10] (Fig. 2.7B). The second heart field cells enter the enlarging heart tube at both ends through the dorsal mesocardium.[17] At this stage, enlargement of the heart tube is almost exclusively due to addition of second heart field cells, with little cell division occurring within the heart tube.[10] The heart tube grows faster than the pericardial cavity, resulting in buckling or bending of the heart tube called looping[18] (Fig. 2.7B and C). There might be an active looping mechanism as well.[18] A poorly understood biasing mechanism normally results in rightward or dextral bending (D-loop).[4]

Leftward bending (L-loop) results in ventricular inversion and can be seen in complete situs inversus (as in Kartagener syndrome) or in several congenital heart defects (e.g., congenitally physiologically corrected transposition and heterotaxy syndrome).

As looping progresses, the dorsal mesocardium breaks down, leaving connections with the prepharyngeal mesoderm only at the inflow and outflow ends of the tube[16] (Fig. 2.7C). From this point, second heart field cells are added only at the inflow and outflow ends. Cells from the level of the first pharyngeal arch are added to the outflow first and will contribute to the right ventricle.[19] As the heart tube descends, cells from around the second pharyngeal arch are added in sequence and will become the outflow of the primitive heart. The same ISL1+ and TBX1+ mesodermal fields that supply cells to the forming heart also contribute to branchiomeric muscles of the face, pharynx, and larynx,[19] explaining the occurrence of cardiofacial syndromes. The caudal aspect of the second heart field contributes mainly to the myocardium of the atria, the superior venae cavae, and the pulmonary veins.[20] Interestingly, the left side of the caudal second heart field also contributes myocardium under the pulmonary valve (subpulmonary infundibulum).[4,20] Since the atrial septation complex derives from caudal second heart field, this might explain the known association of some conotruncal anomalies (tetralogy of Fallot, truncus arteriosus) with atrioventricular canal defects.

Looping introduces the equivalent of one complete helical turn in the heart tube.[21] Because the heart tube is anchored to the pericardium at each end, a complete helical turn cannot be introduced without distorting the heart tube. The result is a helical perversion, two opposite-handed half helical turns. This is analogous to what happens to old-fashioned telephone cords when twisted. This might explain the opposite chirality of the two ventricles. Further elongation allows the primitive ventricle to descend below the inflow (Fig. 2.7C). At this stage, the primitive outflow lies far to the right of the inflow. Further elongation pushes the outflow back centrally so that the developing atria are on either side of the outflow[21] (Fig. 2.7D). Failure of centralization of the outflow is the likely mechanism for left juxtaposition of the atrial appendages and probably explains its invariant association with an abnormal outflow (mostly, transposition of the great arteries).[22]

During looping, the heart chambers begin to expand or balloon out from specified sites on the outer curvature of the heart tube[23] (Fig. 2.7D). The left ventricle begins first from the primitive ventricle, followed by the right ventricle from under the outflow and the atria from each side of the common atrial chamber. Chamber development results from re-initiation of cell division at these specified sites. In contrast, the small, inner curvature remains as primitive heart tube myocardium with minimal proliferation. Consequently, the slowly growing segments between the chambers become apparent as constrictions: the atrioventricular canal between the developing left atrium and left ventricle; the primary foramen between the developing ventricles; and the outflow above the right ventricle.[23]

Signaling from the endocardium via NOTCH, neuregulin, and bone morphogenic protein 10 (BMP10) initiates proliferation within the basal or outer myocardial layer.[24] Trabecular myocardium accumulates in the chamber-forming regions as cardiac jelly disappears with approximation of endocardium and myocardium. As the chamber wall expands outward, the accumulating cells push into the cavity as a complex trabecular meshwork of 1–3 cells in thickness[25]

(Fig. 2.8). Myocardial mass increases while still being supplied with nutrients and oxygen by diffusion from chamber blood.

The right ventricle is derived from the second heart field, while the left ventricle develops from first heart field cells[4] (Fig. 2.3B). The genetic programs operative in the two heart fields differ but have some factors in common.[26] The left side of the ventricular septum and the apex of the left ventricle develop from the primitive ventricle, a derivative of the first heart field. The left ventricular free wall develops from TBX2– expressing atrioventricular canal myocardium, also a derivative of the first heart field, which differentiates into working ventricular myocardium by an unknown process.[27] Failure of proliferation and incorporation of this myocardial contribution is a potential mechanism for left heart hypoplasia.

The interventricular septum accrues between the ballooning ventricles because of the limited growth potential of the primary foramen at the base of the ventricles[28] (Figs. 2.8 and 2.14B). The trabeculae in the inferior and apical wall between the ventricles condense to form a solid septum.[25] Myocardium from each ventricle contributes to the ipsilateral side of the septum, with the left ventricle contributing about two-thirds of the mass of the septum and the right ventricle one-third.[28]

Near the end of the fourth week, the confluence of the venous channels entering the common atrial chamber dilates forming the sinus venosus, which is initially connected

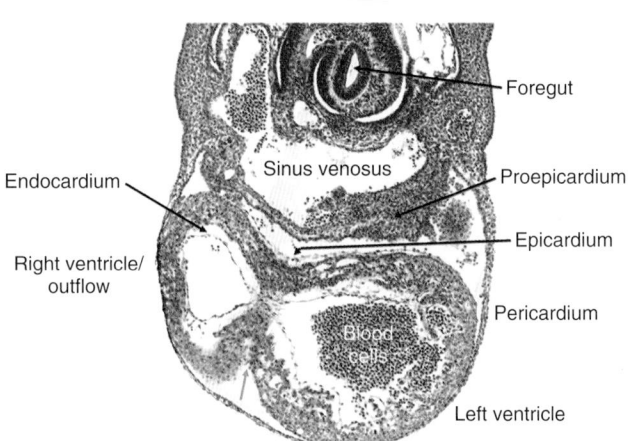

• **Fig. 2.8** Section through the sinus venosus and developing ventricles in a CS 13 embryo at the beginning of the fifth week. A trabecular network is beginning to form in the ballooning left ventricle where the cardiac jelly is disappearing and the endocardium is closely apposed to the myocardium. In contrast, the right ventricle, a day or two behind the left ventricle, has minimal trabecular myocardium and the endocardium is still separated from the myocardium by cardiac jelly. As the ventricles expand outward, the ventricular septum (green arrow) begins to accrue between them because the crest of the septum, the primitive foramen, has little growth potential. Compare with Fig. 2.14B at CS 15. The proepicardium is seen adjacent to the sinus venosus and epicardium has begun to cover the myocardium dorsally but not ventrally. The heart is enclosed within the pericardium.

symmetrically to both sides of the common atrium[29] (Figs. 2.7D and 2.8). The sinus venosus is initially mesenchymal, developing from tissue at the caudal-lateral margin of the heart fields that expresses TBX18 and hyperpolarization-activated cyclic nucleotide-gated potassium channel 4 (HCN4), but not NKX2-5.[30] As the atria develop, the connection to the left side of the common atrium (future left atrium) is lost, so the sinus venosus connects solely to the future right atrium. A little later the tissue of the sinus venosus transforms into myocardium, the source of the sinoatrial node. The right horn of sinus venosus eventually becomes incorporated into the right atrium as the smooth intercaval portion, and the left horn forms the coronary sinus. Coronary sinus defects (communications between the coronary sinus and the left atrium) could represent persistent connections of the left horn of the sinus venosus to the left side of the common atrium. Alternatively, these uncommon defects could develop later by dissolution of the walls separating the two structures.

As the sinus venosus is developing, the final layer is added to the heart—the epicardium (Fig. 2.8). The epicardium derives from the proepicardium, a diverse collection of cells near the inflow end of the heart tube[31] that express a variety of markers including TBX18, Wilms tumor 1 (WT1), scleraxis (SCX), and Semaphorin 3D (SEMA3D).[32] These cells originate from the same caudal-lateral region of the heart-forming fields as the sinus venosus myocardium.[30] The proepicardium is like bunches of grapes or cauliflower that break off, float across the pericardial cavity, and attach to the surface of the developing heart. There is also direct spread from the proepicardium. The epicardial cells form a single cell layer over the myocardium completely covering the atria and ventricles by the end of week 6.[17] A thin layer of ground substance forms between the epicardium and myocardium. Some epicardial cells undergo EMT and enter the subepicardial space and the myocardium. Epicardium-derived cells give rise to cardiac fibroblasts, a few endothelial cells of epicardial coronary arteries, most coronary artery smooth muscle, atrioventricular sulcus mesenchyme, and some atrioventricular valve interstitial cells.[33] The epicardium of the outflow derives from splanchnic mesoderm near the arterial end of the heart tube, expresses different molecular markers, and does not undergo EMT or form other cell types.[34]

By CS 12, neural crest cells have populated the pharyngeal arches. These cells are essential for normal patterning of the pharyngeal arch arteries and provide the smooth muscle layer of these vessels.[35] The neural crest cells also interact with second heart field cells in the prepharyngeal mesoderm, modulating the competing influences of fibroblast growth factor signaling that favors proliferation and bone morphogenic protein signaling that promotes differentiation into cardiomyocytes.[35] An improper balance of these competing influences appears be a cause of conotruncal anomalies.

The first or primitive arch artery has involuted to form the maxillary artery, and the second pharyngeal arch artery is diminishing and will form the stapedial artery[36] (Fig. 2.9A). The third pharyngeal arch artery is forming and will soon become the dominant artery. The cardinal venous system has formed but is still small (Fig. 2.10A). The omphalomesenteric veins, future hepatocardiac channel and portal vein (Fig. 2.11), drain the omphalomesenteric sac and developing gut. The umbilical veins are the dominant venous channels entering the sinus venosus.

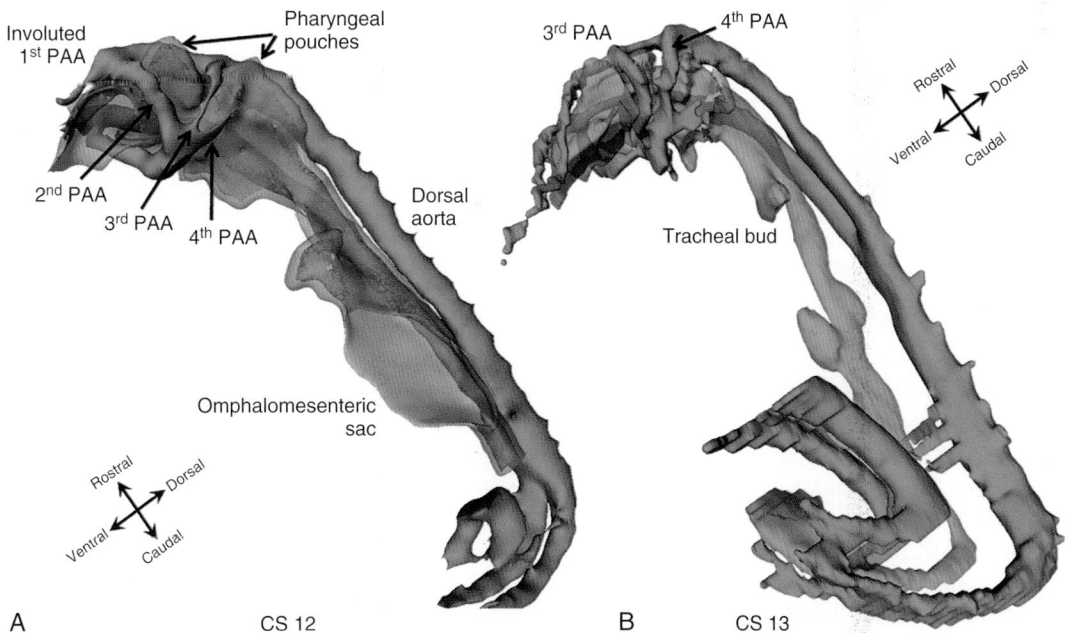

• Fig. 2.9 A series of 3D reconstructions illustrating formation of the systemic arterial system. (A) A CS 12 embryo at the end of the fourth week. The primitive or 1st pharyngeal arch artery (PAA) has involuted and the 2nd PAA is dominant. The dorsal aortae have fused together distally forming the descending aorta. The 3rd and 4th PAA are developing. (B) A CS 13 embryo, early fifth week. The 2nd PAA has involuted and the 3rd and 4th PAAs are dominant. The bilateral branch pulmonary arteries (left is shown, *red arrow*) extend toward the tracheal-lung bud which has grown out from the ventral aspect of the foregut. The 6th PAAs *(green arrows)* are beginning to sprout from the branch pulmonary arteries and dorsal aortae.

Continued

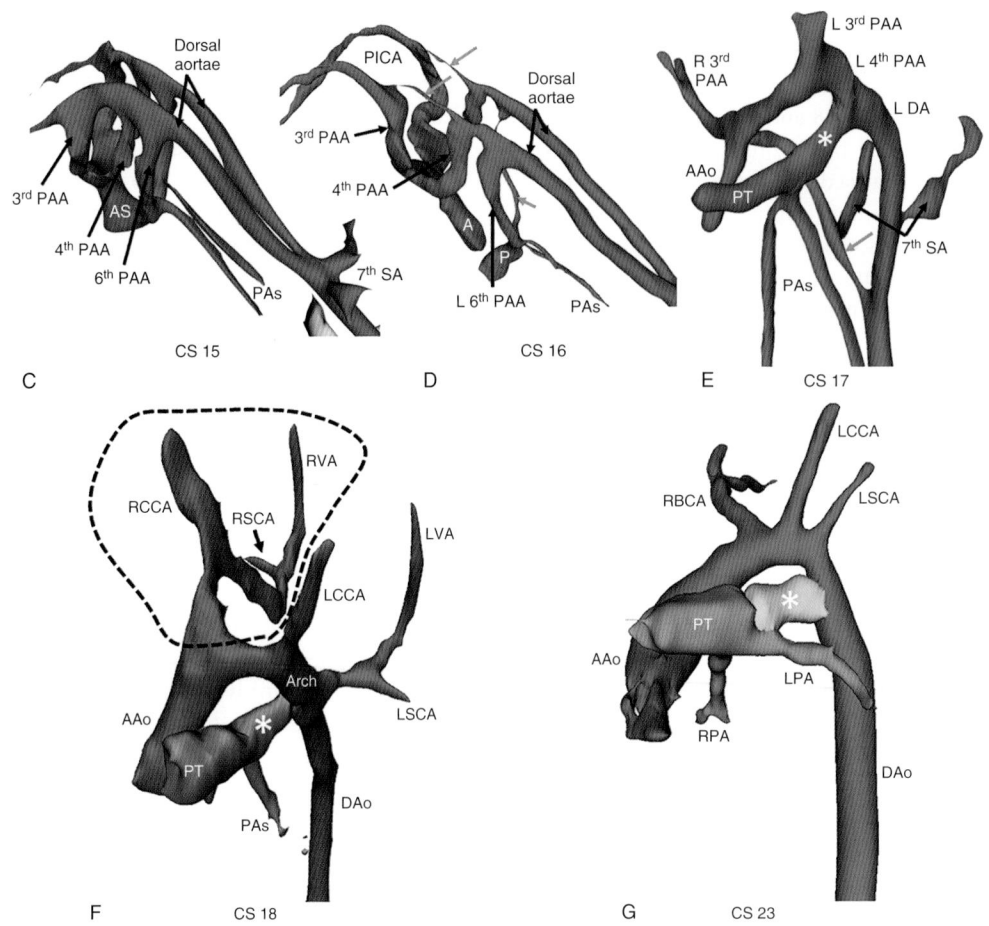

• **Fig. 2.9, cont'd** (C) A CS 15 embryo, early sixth week, viewed from the left side. The third, fourth, and sixth PAAs are bilaterally symmetrical and connect the aortic sac *(AS)* with the ipsilateral dorsal aorta. The 6th PAAs have grown out of the branch pulmonary arteries *(PAs)*. The dorsal aortae join to form the descending aorta from which arise the seventh segmental arteries *(seventh SA)*, the presumptive subclavian arteries. (D) Similar view of the arch system of a CS 16 embryo, end sixth week. The segment of dorsal aorta between the 3rd and 4th PAAs, the carotid duct *(blue arrows)*, is involuting and will soon disappear. The cranial part of each dorsal aorta, the presumptive internal carotid artery *(PICA)*, is then connected only to the third PAA, the presumptive common carotid artery. The right 6th PAA *(green arrow)* is involuting and will disappear, leaving only the left 6th PAA, the presumptive ductus arteriosus. The aortic sac has divided into separate aortic *(A)* and pulmonary *(P)* channels. (E) Left anterior view of the arch system of a CS 17 embryo, early seventh week. The 3rd PAAs have become the common carotid arteries. The left 4th PAA is now forming the definitive left aortic arch along with the left dorsal aorta *(LDA)*. Note that the 7th SA have migrated proximally, from distal to the junction of the dorsal aortae to proximal to it. The left 6th PAA has formed the left ductus arteriosus *(*)*. The segment of the right dorsal aorta distal to the right 7th segmental artery *(green arrow)* is involuting and will soon disappear, forming the right brachiocephalic (innominate) artery. *AAo,* Ascending aorta; *PT,* Pulmonart trunk. (F) Similar view of a CS 18 embryo, mid-seventh week. The right dorsal aorta distal to the 7th segmental artery has involuted creating the brachiocephalic artery *(inside dashed line)* that will remodel to the adult morphology as shown in G. The definitive aortic arch *(Arch)* is the derivative of the left fourth arch. *DAo,* Descending aorta; *LCCA,* left common carotid artery; *LSCA,* left subclavian artery; *LVA,* left vertebral artery; *RCCA,* right common carotid artery; *RSCA,* right subclavian artery; *RVA,* right vertebral artery. (G) By CS 23, end eighth week, the aortic arch system has remodeled to essentially the adult pattern. *LPA,* Left pulmonary artery; *RBCA,* right brachiocephalic artery; *RPA,* right pulmonary artery.

Week 5

During the fifth week (CS 13–14), the atrioventricular and outflow cushions form, atrial septation begins, and the pulmonary vein canalizes, forming a luminal connection with the left atrium. The atrioventricular canal begins to expand rightward, creating the connection between the right atrium and right ventricle, and neural crest cells begin to invade the outflow cushions. Myocardial growth and proliferation shift from forming trabecular myocardium to compact myocardium. The coronary vascular plexus begins forming in the subepicardial space. Pharyngeal arch artery remodeling continues with further development of the third, fourth, and sixth arches.

In contrast to chamber-forming regions of the heart tube, in the atrioventricular canal and outflow, cardiac jelly increases in thickness in response to bone morphogenic protein signaling from the underlying myocardium.[37] Two swellings form first in the atrioventricular canal, the superior and inferior endocardial cushions (Fig. 2.12 A). Endocardial cells on the surface of the cushions undergo EMT and ingress into the cushions to form valve interstitial cells. A day or two later, a similar process occurs in the outflow, forming two elongated cushions or outflow ridges (Fig. 2.13A) The outflow cushions are populated by EMT of endocardial cells as well as by direct invasion of second heart field cells that enter from the end of the outflow.[38]

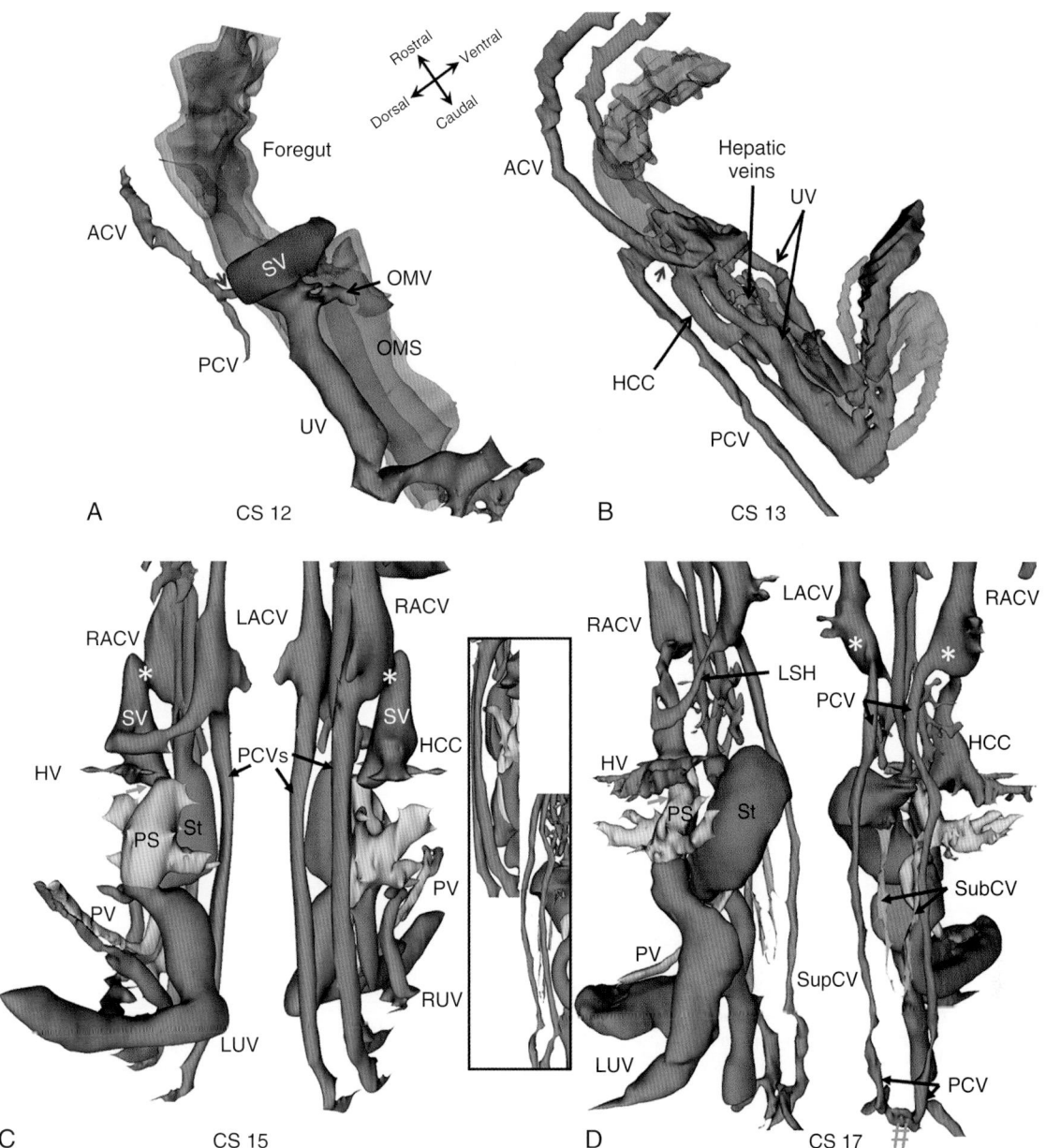

• **Fig. 2.10** A series of 3D reconstructions illustrating formation of the systemic venous system. (A) A CS 12 embryo at the end of the fourth week. The anterior *(ACV)* and posterior *(PCV)* cardinal veins are newly formed and connect via the common cardinal vein (red arrow) with the sinus venosus *(SV)*. The omphalomesenteric veins *(OMV)* drain the omphalomesenteric sac. *(OMS)* The umbilical veins *(UV)* are the largest venous channels. Anastomoses are forming between the UVs and the hepatic circulation. (B) At CS 13, early fifth week, the cardinal venous system has enlarged. The distal OMVs are remodeling to form the portal venous system, and the hepatocardiac channel *(HCC)* has formed from the proximal right OMV. (C) Left anterior view *(left)* and right posterior view *(right)* of a CS 15 embryo, early sixth week. The cardinal venous system is predominant. The right *(RACV)* and left *(LACV)* anterior cardinal veins join the PCVs and drain to the SV via the common cardinal veins (*). The left *(LUV)* and right *(RUV)* umbilical veins formed anastomoses with the hepatic venous system and lost their direct connection with the SV. The RUV has started to involute and is now much smaller than the LUV which connects with the portal sinus *(PS)*. The ductus venosus *(green arrow)* has developed from the proximal part of the right OMV and connects the PS and LUV with the HCC. The HCC drains the hepatic veins *(HV)* and ductus venosus to the SV. The portal vein *(gold) (PV)* has developed from the distal portions of the OMVs. (D) Similar views of a CS 17 embryo, early seventh week. The ACVs remain the dominant anterior venous channel. The left horn of sinus venosus (LSH), draining the left cardinal system, has begun to involute. The PCVs have largely been replaced by the supracardinal veins *(SupCV)*, except proximally at the junction with the common cardinal vein (*) and distally at the iliac bifurcation (#). Initially anastomoses formed between these systems proximally and distally after which the central part of the PCVs involuted. The insets between C and D show the difference in course of the PCV *(upper left)* at CS 15 and of the SupCV *(lower right)* at CS 17. The SupCV is more ventral and lateral resulting in the bent course of the composite venous pathway. The subcardinal venous system *(SubCV)*, seen in main figure, has formed around the site of the developing kidney. Anastomoses develop between the paired SubCVs as well as between the SubCVs and SupCVs.

Continued

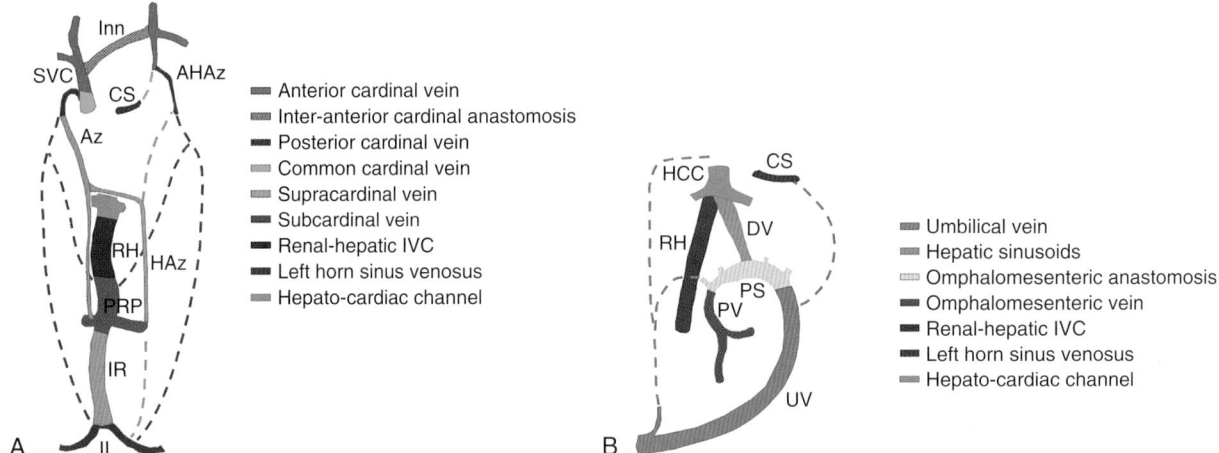

• **Fig. 2.10, cont'd** (E) Similar views in a CS 18 embryo, late seventh week. The connection of the LACV to the SV is more tenuous. The renal-to-hepatic inferior vena cava *(R-H IVC)* has developed asymmetrically on the right between the right SubCV and the HCC. The infrarenal IVC *(InfR IVC)* has developed from the right SubCV and probably a segment of the right SupCV. A portion of the left SubCV is still present. (F) Similar views in a CS 23 embryo, end of eighth week. An anastomosis has formed between the RACV and LACV, the left innominate vein *(LInnV)*, and the direct connection of the LACV with the SV has disappeared. The definitive IVC has developed from the HCC, the asymmetric renal-hepatic IVC, the right SubCV and probably part of the right SupCV. The azygos and hemiazygos veins derive from the SupCVs, with the azygos arch formed by the right PCV. The ductus venosus *(red arrow)* has elongated and developed the characteristic constriction important for regulating placental blood flow.

• **Fig. 2.11** Representation showing the embryologic origins of the components of the systemic (A) and portal (B) venous systems. *AHAz,* Accessory Hemi-Azygos Vein; *Az,* Azygos Vein; *CS,* Coronary Sinus; *DV,* Ductus Venosus; *HAz,* Hemi-Azygos Vein; *HCC,* Hepato-Cardiac Channel; *Il,* Iliac Veins; *Inn,* Innominate Vein; *IR,* Infrarenal Inferior Vena Cava (After Patten BM. Human Embryology. 2nd ed. New York, NY: McGraw–Hill; 1953:637–681, with permission.)

Toward the end of the fifth week, a subpopulation of neural crest cells that entered the pharyngeal arches continues migrating and invades the outflow ridges.[38] These cells are essential for fusion of the septal and parietal outflow ridges to septate the common outflow into aortic and pulmonary channels. A few days later, two additional atrioventricular cushions form,[39] the left and right lateral cushions, as well as two small additional outflow cushions,[38] the aortic and pulmonary intercalated cushions.

By the beginning of the fifth week, the edges of the attachments of the dorsal mesocardium to the common atrial chamber have become prominent on the posterior common atrial wall as the left and right pulmonary ridges[39] (Fig. 2.12A). Between the ridges, in the pulmonary pit, a strand of endothelial cells extends through the dorsal mesocardium and continues with endothelial strands that run rostral and caudal, ventral to the developing foregut—the mid-pharyngeal endothelial strands (Fig 2.14A). As the trachea buds out from the ventral aspect of the foregut into mesenchyme continuous with the dorsal mesocardium,[39] these endothelial strands form a capillary plexus around the developing airway and lung buds. The endothelial strand traversing the dorsal mesocardium lumenizes to form the common pulmonary vein, establishing continuity between the vascular plexus of the lung buds and the left atrium (Fig. 2.14B). During the fifth and sixth weeks, pulmonary vein myocardium, derived from NKX2-5+, PITX2c+, and TBX18– second heart field cells,[20] invests the pulmonary veins out to the second- and third- order branches. The common pulmonary vein will become incorporated into the left atrium as the smooth posterior and superior walls. Failure of expansion and incorporation of the common pulmonary vein is a likely mechanism for cor triatriatum.

At the superior part of the right pulmonary ridge, a small swelling develops, and overlying endocardial cells undergo EMT to populate it with mesenchymal cells.[39] The thin

sheet of tissue formed by downward and anterior growth of this mesenchymal cap is the septum primum, or primary atrial septum (Fig. 2.12B). The inferior aspect of the right pulmonary ridge begins to protrude into the common atrial cavity under the septum primum because of an advancing column (or spine) of posterior second heart field cells.[39] Known as the dorsal mesenchymal protrusion or spina vestibuli or vestibular spine, this prominence will be instrumental in closing the ostium primum or the first interatrial communication.[40] The mesenchymal tissue eventually muscularizes, forming the muscular base of the atrial septum, except for the core of the structure which remains fibrous as the tendon of Todaro.[40]

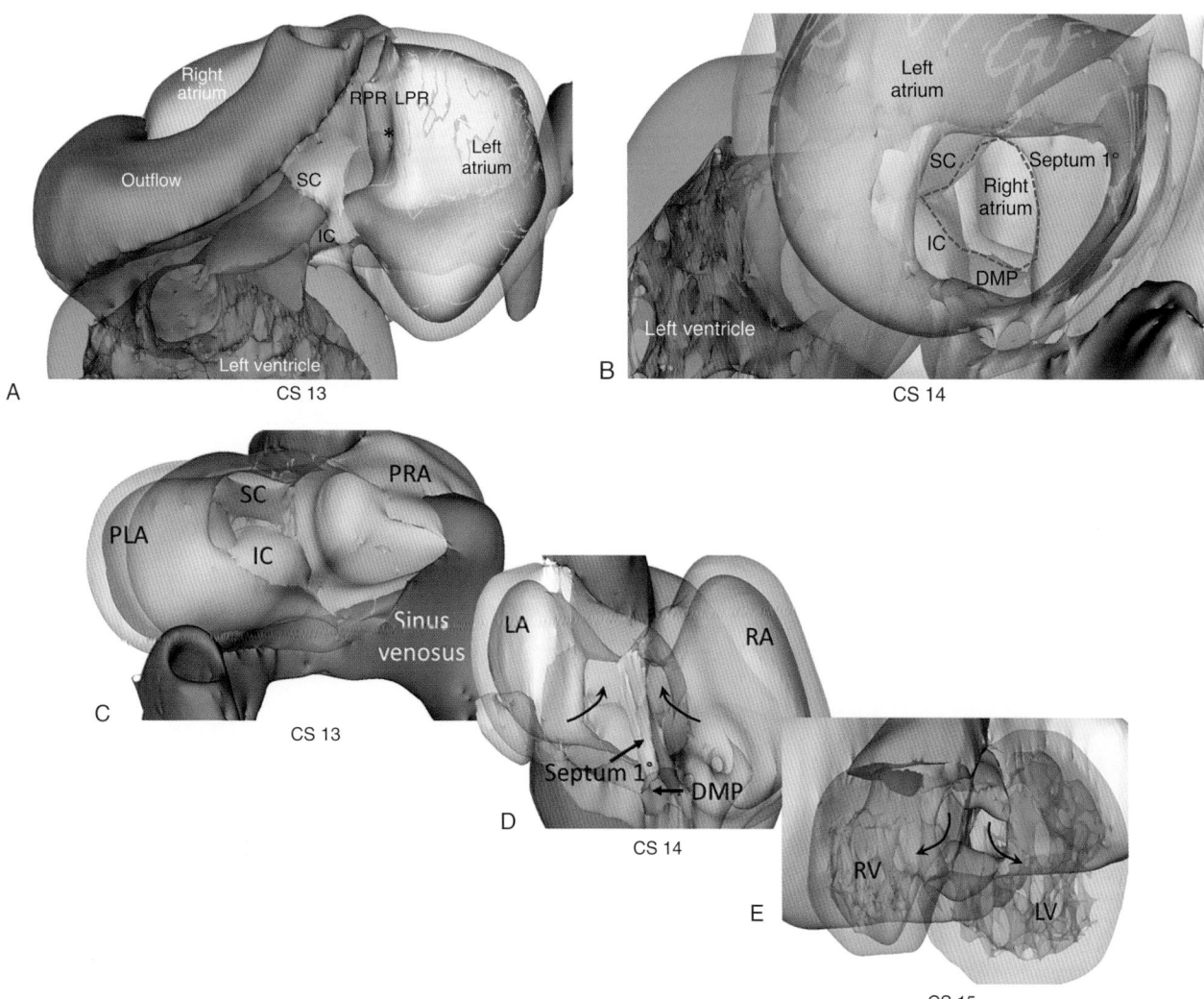

• **Fig. 2.12** A series of 3D reconstructions illustrating septation of the common atrium and atrioventricular canal. (A) A CS 13 embryo viewed from the left side. The superior *(SC)* and inferior *(IC)* atrioventricular endocardial cushions have developed in the atrioventricular canal. The right *(RPR)* and left *(LPR)* pulmonary ridges on the posterior wall of the left atrium mark the lateral edges of the attachments of the dorsal mesocardium. The pulmonary pit *(*)* is the point where the endothelial strand traversing the dorsal mesocardium will lumenize to form the common pulmonary vein (Fig. 2.14A). (B) A CS 14 (mid-fifth week) embryo viewed from the left side. The septum primum *(Septum 1°)* has begun to grow down from the posterior-superior part of the RPR and the dorsal mesenchymal protrusion *(DMP)* is protruding into the atrial cavity at the posterior-inferior aspect of the RPR, making up the atrial septation complex. These structures are extending toward the *SC* and *IC* encroaching on the ostium primum or first interatrial communication *(dashed red line)*. (C) A CS 13 embryo (early fifth week) viewed from the back of the atria. The atrioventricular canal, marked by the *SC* and *IC*, connects only the presumptive left atrium *(PLA)* with the left ventricle and does not drain the presumptive right atrium *(PRA)* directly. (D) Similar view of a CS 14 embryo (late fifth week). The atrioventricular canal has expanded under the right atrium, draining both atria *(LA and RA)* into the left ventricle, as the atrial septation complex (septum primum and DMP) divides the common atrium. (E) A CS 15 embryo (early sixth week) viewed from the ventricular apices. The atrioventricular canal has now expanded through the primitive foramen and over the right ventricle *(RV)*, establishing direct communication between the right atrium and RV.

Continued

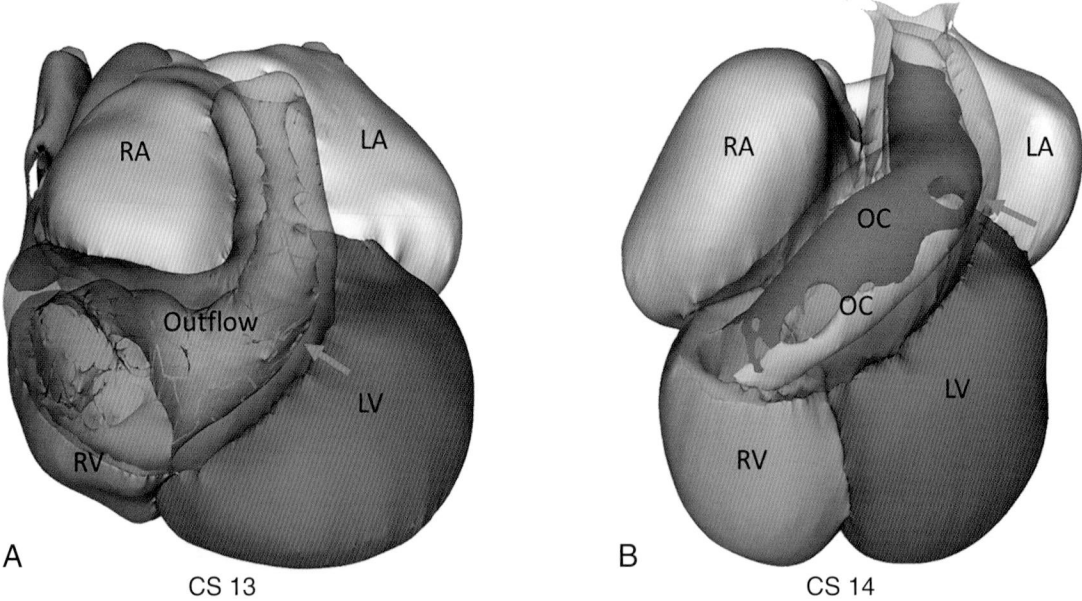

• **Fig. 2.12, cont'd** (F) A CS 15 embryo (early sixth week) viewed from the left side. The septum primum and the DMP continued to grow toward the atrioventricular cushions, encroaching on ostium primum *(dashed red line)*. Before closure of ostium primum, the septum primum breaks down at its origin from the atrial wall, creating ostium secundum *(Ostium 2´)*, the second interatrial opening, which will become the foramen ovale. (G) Posterior view of a CS 17 embryo after completion of septation of the atria and atrioventricular canal showing the separate left *(LAVO)* and right *(RAVO)* atrioventricular orifices and the foramen ovale with right-to-left flow *(black curved arrow)*.

• **Fig. 2.13** A series of 3D reconstructions illustrating outflow development. (A) Anterior view of a 3D reconstruction of a CS 13 embryo (early fifth week) with outflow myocardium semitransparent. The outflow is a single myocardial tube connecting the developing right ventricle *(RV)* with the extrapericardial aortic sac (not shown). The outflow has lengthened and moved to a central position between the developing left *(LA)* and right *(RA)* atria (compare with Fig. 2.7C and D). The bend in the outflow *(blue arrow)* marks the future location of the sinotubular junction of the semilunar valves. The part distal to the bend will become the intrapericardial great arteries, and the part proximal will become the semilunar roots and valves and the ventricular outflows. (B) Similar view of a CS 14 embryo (end fifth week). The outflow has shortened as the proximal part has been incorporated into the enlarging RV. A pair of outflow cushions or ridges (OC) have developed on opposite walls of the outflow. The outflow is still aligned solely with the RV, the left ventricle (LV) still ejecting through the primitive foramen. The blue arrow marks the future sinotubular junction.

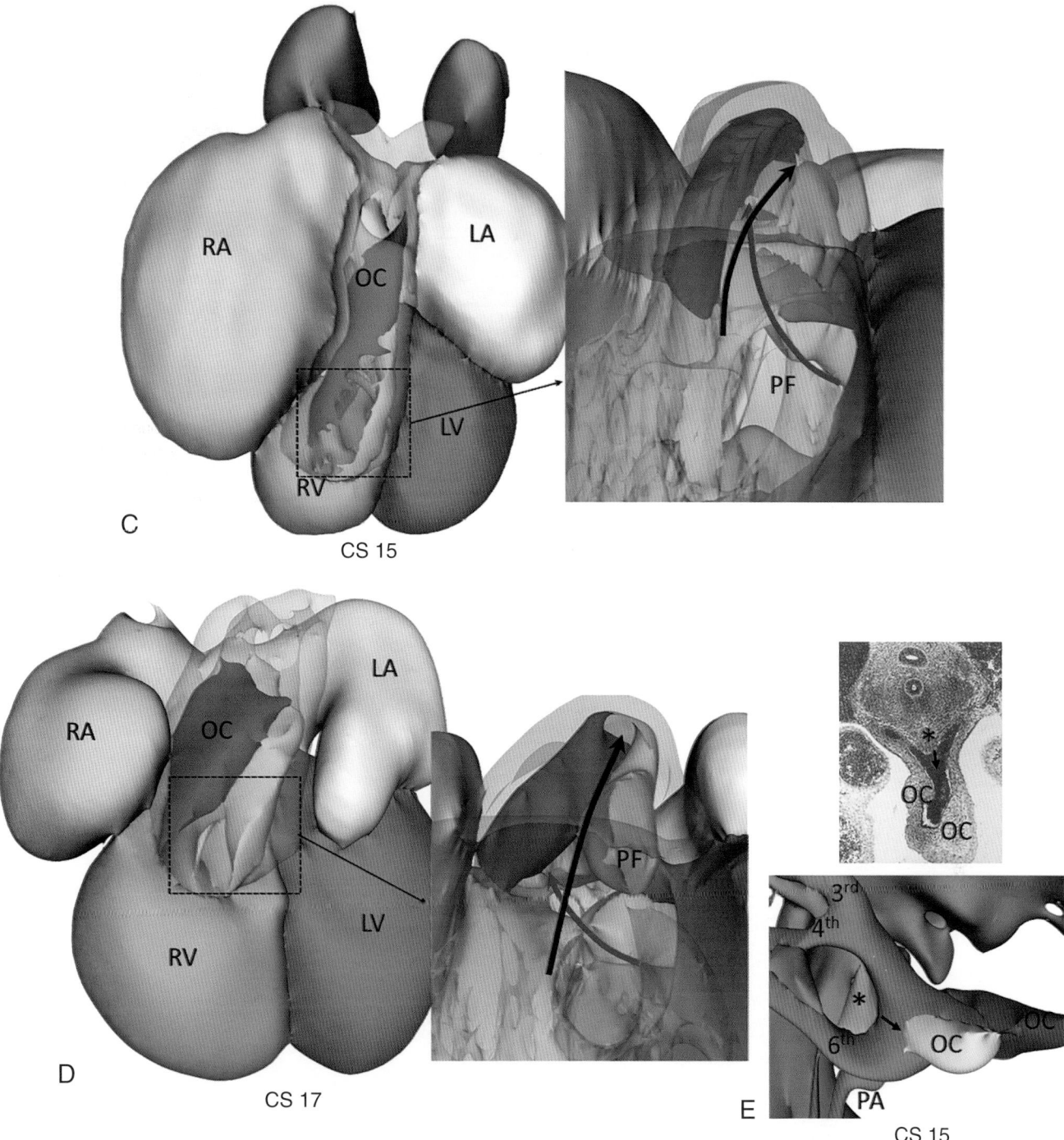

• **Fig. 2.13, cont'd** (C) Similar view of a CS 15 embryo (early sixth week). The outflow has shortened further and straightened as the proximal part continues to be incorporated into the RV and outflow myocardium is lost by apoptosis. The OCs have begun to spiral around each other as the proximal outflow rotates counterclockwise (viewed from the RV). The inset to the right shows the OCs fusing distally to form separate aortic *(red arrow)* and pulmonary *(black arrow)* channels. (D) Similar view of a CS 17 embryo (early seventh week). Fusion of the OCs has proceeded proximally and the outflow has shortened further. The inset to the right shows the posterior aortic channel aligned with the PF *(red arrow)* and the anterior pulmonary channel aligned with the body of the RV *(black arrow)*. (E) Right lateral view of a (histological section and 3D reconstruction of distal outflow and aortic sac in a CS 15 embryo. The fusing OCs are dividing the distal outflow into aortic (with third and fourth arch arteries) and pulmonary (with sixth arch arteries and pulmonary arteries [PA] components). The OCs will fuse with a triangular ingrowth of tissue from the dorsal wall of the aortic sac *(*)* to complete distal outflow division. *Continued*

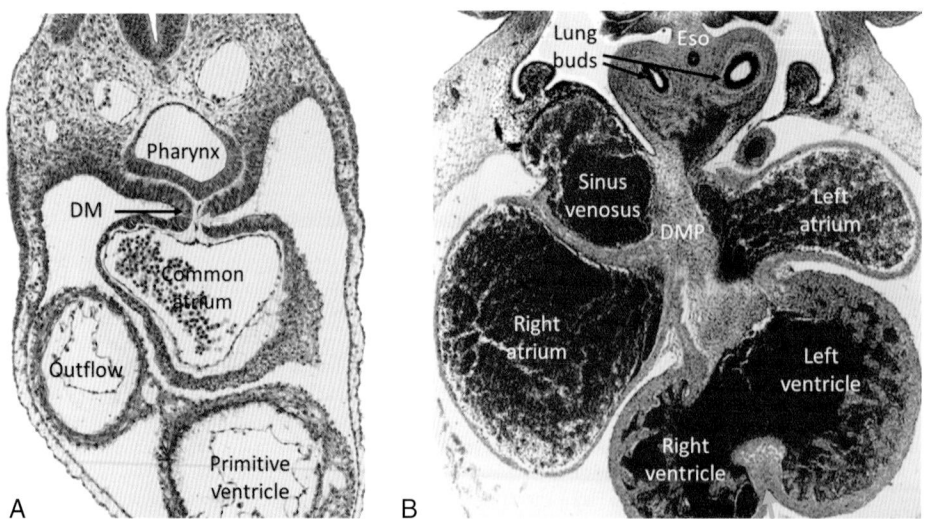

• **Fig. 2.13, cont'd** (F) A CS 19 embryo (end seventh week) viewed from the semitransparent RV with the RA removed. The left corner inset is the reference view for both upper and lower panels. Upper panel: View of the outflow showing the anterior PA and posterior aorta *(Ao)* separated by the fusing proximal OCs *(curved yellow arrows)* that are forming the infundibular or outlet septum *(IS)*. The superior atrioventricular endocardial cushion *(SC)* is draped over the inferior rim of the primitive foramen. The residual communication between the ventricular outflows is between the fusing limbs of the IS and the SC. Lower panel: The same anatomy viewed from the right side showing the outflow paths that will be formed as the limbs of the OCs fuse together and join the SC. The pulmonary outflow *(black curved arrow)* is anterior to the developing outflow septum, and the aortic outflow *(curved blue arrow)* is posterior through the primitive foramen. (G) Same CS 19 embryo viewed through the semitransparent LV with the LA removed. The right corner inset is the reference view for both panels. Upper panel: View from left and posterior showing the residual communication between the outflows *(*)*. Lower panel: View from left and anterior showing the alignment of the Ao with the LV through the primitive foramen *(dashed ellipse)*.

• **Fig. 2.14** (A) A section through a CS 12 embryo (end of fourth week) showing the endothelial strand *(orange arrow)* extending from the endocardium of the common atrial chamber through the dorsal mesocardium *(DM)*. Endothelial strands continue rostral and caudal, ventral to the developing pharynx. As the trachea and lungs bud out of the ventral aspect of the pharynx/foregut, these strands lumenize to form a vascular plexus supplying it. The strand running in the DM will become the common pulmonary vein. (B) A section through an embryo at CS 15 (early sixth week) showing the common pulmonary vein *(orange arrow)* entering the medial aspect of the left atrium, draining the vascular plexus around the developing lung buds. The dorsal mesenchymal protrusion *(DMP)*, part of the atrial septation complex, is to the right of the common pulmonary vein, marking the location of the right pulmonary ridge. Note the ventricular septum *(green arrow)* is continuing to develop as the ventricles balloon out more at the outer curvature. *Eso,* Esophagus.

As atrial septation is proceeding as described above, the annulus of the atrioventricular canal begins to expand to the right.[41] Until this point, the atrioventricular canal connected only the developing left atrium with the developing left ventricle (Fig. 2.12C). Systemic venous blood entering the developing right atrium crossed into the left atrium to pass through the atrioventricular canal. During normal development, the canal expands rightward, first under the right atrium so that both atria transiently drain through the canal into the developing left ventricle[41] (Fig. 2.12D). Continued rightward expansion establishes direct connection of the developing right atrium and right ventricle[41] (Fig. 2.12E). Disorders of this process result in congenital heart disease. It is likely that typical tricuspid atresia (absent connection type with no element of the tricuspid valve) results from failure of expansion of the atrioventricular canal with completion of atrial septation to the rightward aspect of the superior and inferior atrioventricular cushions. Double-inlet left ventricle likely results from failed expansion of the ventricular end of the canal through the primary foramen and over the developing right ventricle, so both right and left atria drain into the developing left ventricle.

To this point, myocardial proliferation in the developing chambers has yielded an extensive network of trabecular myocardium driven partly by NOTCH1 activation by a Delta-like ligand expressed in endocardium.[42] A shift to NOTCH1 activation by a Jagged ligand changes the pattern of myocardial proliferation from trabecular to compact myocardium[42] (Fig. 2.15). The increase in compact myocardium does not appear to be due to fusion or compaction of the trabecular myocardial layer (which does not change much in thickness during embryogenesis), but rather to accrual of new, solid or compact, myocardium due to a shift in signaling pathways.[42]

An intact epicardium, a source of retinoic acid, erythropoietin, and insulin-like growth factor 2 signaling, as well as epicardium-derived cardiac fibroblasts, is also necessary for production of normal compact myocardium.

Concomitant with the shift in the growth pattern of the cardiac chambers, coronary artery formation begins (Fig. 2.16A). Vessels sprout from the sinus venosus onto the dorsal surface of the heart and spread by angiogenesis to form a plexus in the subepicardial space, branching perpendicular to the surface as well to form intramyocardial vessels.[43] In addition, the endocardium sends buds that further contribute to coronary vessels.[44]

The endocardium appears to be essentially the sole source of coronary endothelial cells for vessels in the ventricular septum[44] and inner layers of the ventricular free walls (Fig. 2.16B). A subgroup of epicardium-derived cells that express SCX and SEMA3D also yield a few coronary endothelial cells.[32] Over the fifth and sixth weeks, the coronary vascular plexus expands to cover the surface of the heart. During its development, the coronary plexus is not connected to the aorta and there is no significant flow of blood in the developing coronary vessels.

The second pharyngeal arch artery involutes forming the stapedial artery.[36] The third, fourth, and sixth pharyngeal arch arteries form sequentially (Fig. 2.9B). The paired third and fourth arches develop directly between the aortic sac and the ipsilateral dorsal aorta. By this point, the tracheal bud has developed from the ventral aspect of the pharynx with initiation of lung development. The right and left branch pulmonary arteries have formed by coalescence of capillaries from the posterior aspect of the aortic sac supplying the ventral foregut around the site of the tracheal bud.[36] It appears that

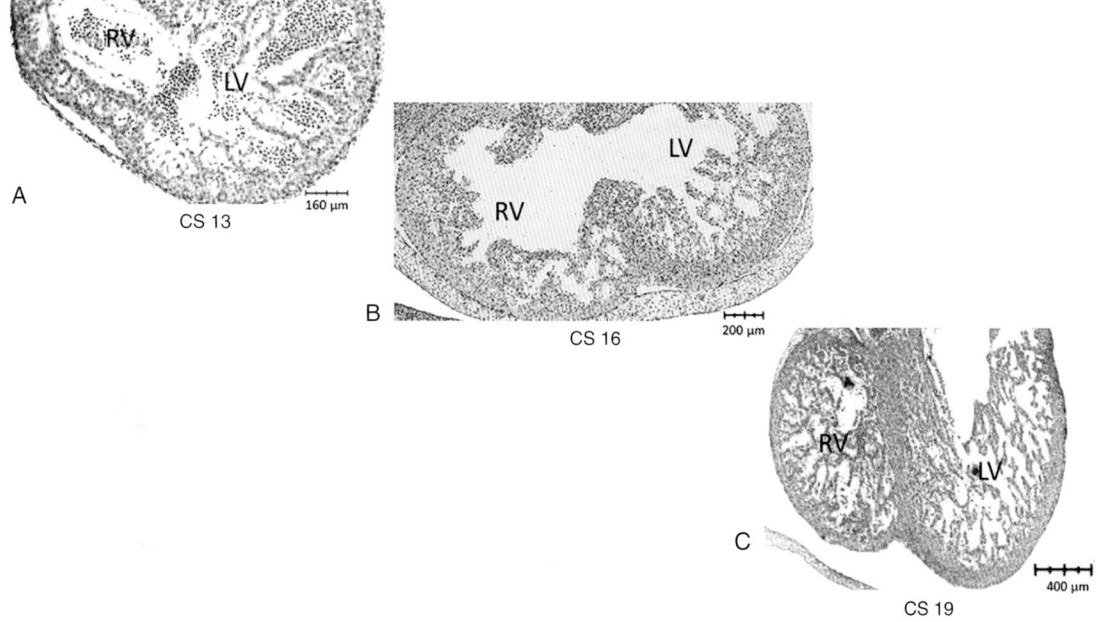

• **Fig. 2.15** (A) A section of the ventricles of a CS 13 embryo (early fifth week) showing the trabecular growth pattern of the left ventricle *(LV)* with a thin rim of the compact myocardium. (B) Similar view of a CS 16 embryo (end sixth week) showing that the trabecular myocardium has not reduced in thickness, but the compact myocardium has more than doubled. (C) Similar view of a CS 19 embryo (end seventh week) showing extensive trabecular myocardium while the compact myocardium has increased about 50% compared with B.

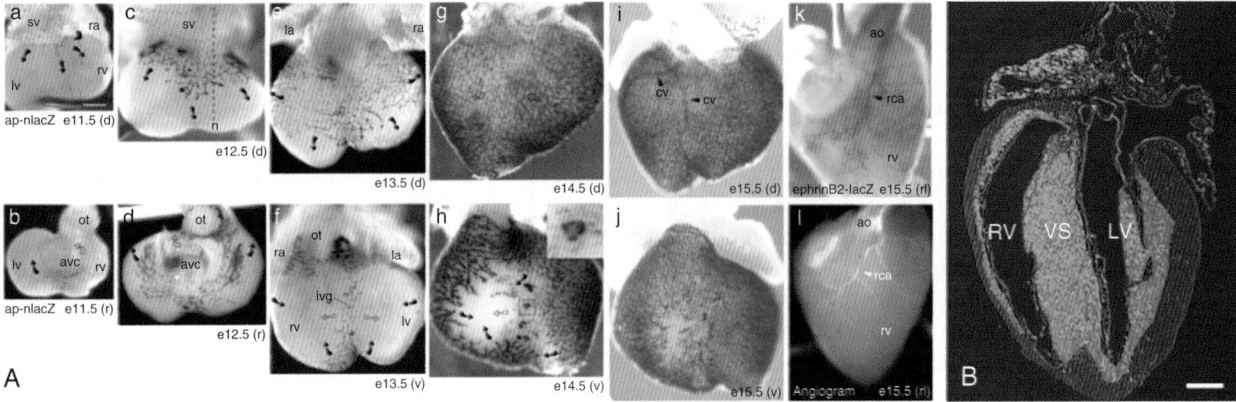

• **Fig. 2.16** (A) A staged series of whole mount mouse embryo hearts stained for a marker for vascular endothelium, but not endocardium, showing sprouts appearing from the sinus venosus at e11.5 (comparable to late sixth week in human) and progressively spreading over the dorsal, lateral, and ventral surfaces of the myocardium, covering the heart by e15.5 (comparable to mid-eighth week in human). (B) A four-chamber section of adult mouse heart stained to show coronary vessels derived from early coronary development *(red)* on the outer ventricular walls, which appear to derive mostly from sinus venosus. However, in the ventricular septum and the inner ventricular walls *(green)*, coronary endothelium appears to derive mostly from endocardial cells that have transitioned in these areas. In rodents, this later wave of coronary artery development extends into the neonatal period. It is unclear how this applies to human development. *ao,* aorta; *avc,* atrioventricular canal; *ivg,* interventricular groove; *LV,* left ventricle; *ot,* outflow tract; *ra,* right atrium; *rca,* right coronary artery; *RV/rv,* right ventricle; *sv,* sinus venosus; *VS,* ventricular septum (*A,* With permission from Red-Horse K, Ueno H, Weissman IL, Krasnow MA. Coronary arteries form by developmental reprogramming of venous cells. *Nature.* 2010;464(7288):549–553; *B,* With permission from Tian X, Pu WT, Zhou B. Cellular origin and developmental program of coronary angiogenesis. *Circ Res.* 2015;116:515–530.)

the paired sixth pharyngeal arch arteries (future ductus arteriosi) sprout out of the ipsilateral branch pulmonary artery and connect with the ipsilateral dorsal aorta.[36] This explains why the ductus arteriosus—the derivative of the sixth arch artery—typically connects with the proximal part of the ipsilateral branch pulmonary artery. Further, if the proximal portion of the branch pulmonary artery actually developed from the sixth arch artery as has been suggested, one would expect this part of the branch pulmonary artery to become stenotic or atretic when the ductus arteriosus closes postnatally, even in the normal heart. However, branch pulmonary artery stenosis is seen essentially only in cases in which ductal flow was reduced or reversed *in utero* (e.g., tetralogy of Fallot). The fifth arch artery either does not usually develop in humans or is transient. Persistence of this vessel explains some anomalies of the aortic arch.[45] The right umbilical vein is involuting and the omphalomesenteric veins are remodeling to form the portal venous system (Figs. 2.10B, 2.10C, and 2.11). The left umbilical vein has formed a connection to the developing portal circulation and has lost the direct connection with the sinus venosus. The ductus venosus now connects the portal sinus with the hepatocardiac channel, directing umbilical venous blood into the right atrium.

Week 6

During the sixth week (CS 15–16), ostium secundum or the second interatrial communication (foramen ovale) opens; ostium primum or the first interatrial communication closes; the superior and inferior atrioventricular endocardial cushions fuse centrally, dividing the atrioventricular canal into two channels; and the common outflow divides distally into aortic and pulmonary channels. The atrioventricular and

semilunar valves begin remodeling from the respective cushions, and the epicardium completes coverage of the heart. Coronary artery development and pharyngeal arch artery remodeling continue.

Before closure of the ostium primum, septum primum begins to break down at its origin from the posterior-superior wall of the atrium by a process of apoptosis and matrix metalloproteinase activity.[39] This creates ostium secundum or the second interatrial communication—the foramen ovale (Fig. 2.12F). Excessive removal of septum primum (or ectopic removal) results in a secundum atrial septal defect (called that because it is abnormal persistence of the ostium secundum).[46]

By this time, the atrioventricular canal has expanded over the right ventricle, establishing direct communication between the right atrium and the right ventricle.[41] The septum primum continues to grow down toward the superior atrioventricular cushion, encroaching on the primary interatrial foramen or ostium primum. Simultaneously, the dorsal mesenchymal protrusion projects into the inferior part of the atrium, also approaching the cushions.[40] As the dorsal mesenchymal protrusion advances toward the superior and inferior cushions, it closes ostium primum and fills the space between the cushions as they fuse together centrally[40] (Fig. 2.12G). The septum primum, in contact with the superior aspect of the dorsal mesenchymal protrusion, joins the superior cushion, completing septation of the common atrium into the left and right atria. Atrioventricular canal defects (atrioventricular septal defects), either partial (primum atrial septal defect) or complete, appear to be due, at least in part, to hypoplasia and underdevelopment of the dorsal mesenchymal protrusion.[40] Fusion of the superior and inferior cushions divides the atrioventricular canal into separate left and right channels, aligning and connecting the ipsilateral atrium and ventricle (Fig. 2.12G). Remodeling of the atrioventricular cushions, including the left and right lateral cushions, begins formation of the leaflets of the atrioventricular valves and the central fibrous body[47] (Fig. 2.17A). Although epicardium-derived sulcus mesenchyme is collecting at the atrioventricular groove, the myocardium remains continuous from atria through the atrioventricular canal to ventricles[48] (Fig. 2.17A).

The definitive outflow of the embryonic heart began to develop as an endocardially lined and myocardially covered tube during the fourth and fifth weeks by addition of cells from the second heart field at its junction with the aortic sac in the dorsal pericardial wall. The outflow was far to the right initially but moved leftward between the developing atria and formed a prominent bend in its midportion in association with elongation[22] (Fig. 2.13A). The portion between the bend and the pericardial reflection will become the intrapericardial parts of the aorta and pulmonary trunk, the portion at and just proximal to the bend the semilunar roots and valves, and the most proximal portion, the subvalvar arterial outflows.[49] During the sixth week, the outflow shortens (Fig. 2.13B and C) due to incorporation of the most proximal part into the free wall of the right ventricle[50] and due to apoptosis of the myocardial outer layer distally.[51] The two cushions or ridges (septal and parietal cushions) that have formed in the outflow begin to fuse together under the influence of cardiac neural crest cells that have invaded the cushions.[38,52] The fusing outflow cushions septate the common outflow into separate aortic and pulmonary channels.

As the distal ends of the cushions fuse, they join a triangular shelf composed of second heart field and cardiac neural crest cells protruding from the dorsal wall of the aortic sac between the fourth arch arteries ventrally and the 6th arch arteries and branch pulmonary arteries dorsally, completing distal septation of the outflow[38,52] (Fig. 2.13E). Concomitant with septation, the proximal outflow undergoes counterclockwise rotation (viewed from the right ventricle), resulting in spiral orientation of the fusing cushions and bringing the proximal aortic channel dorsal and rightward and the pulmonary channel ventral and

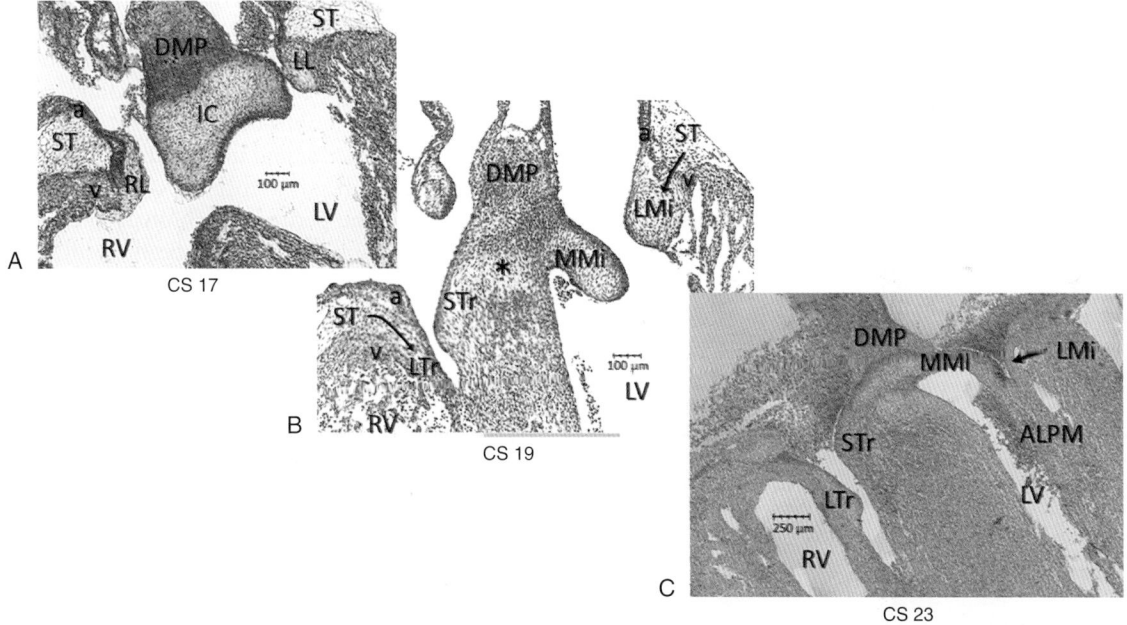

• **Fig. 2.17** (A) A section through the atrioventricular junction of a CS 17 embryo (early seventh week). The inferior *(IC)* and superior (not shown) atrioventricular cushions have fused, dividing the atrioventricular canal into right and left channels, aligned with the ipsilateral ventricle. The dorsal mesenchymal protrusion *(DMP)* has fused with the cushions closing the ostium primum. Right *(RL)* and left *(LL)* lateral atrioventricular cushions have formed at the lateral walls of the atrioventricular junction. Although sulcus tissue *(ST)* has accumulated at the epicardial side of the atrioventricular junction, the atrial *(a)* and ventricular *(v)* myocardium remain continuous across the atrioventricular junction. (B) Similar section of a CS 19 embryo (end seventh week) showing remodeling of the cushions and atrioventricular junctions. The fused superior and inferior cushions *(*)* are draped over the crest of the ventricular septum. The left side of the fused cushions has elongated, extending into the cavity of the left ventricle *(LV)* unsupported by ventricular myocardium and will form the medial mitral leaflet *(MMi)*. In contrast, the rightward part of the fused cushions is densely attached to the right side of the ventricular septum and will form the septal tricuspid leaflet *(STr)*. The lateral mitral leaflet *(LMi)*, developing from the LL cushion, and lateral tricuspid leaflets *(LTr)*, developing from the RL cushion, have lengthened and extended into the respective ventricular cavity supported by ventricular myocardium. The ST has invaded between the atrial and ventricular myocardium *(curved black arrows)* becoming continuous with the developing lateral atrioventricular leaflets and forming part of the annulus of the atrioventricular valves and the fibrous insulation between atrial *(a)* and ventricular *(v)* myocardium. Epicardially derived cells of the ST contribute to the population of valve interstitial cells of the lateral leaflets but not the medial leaflets. (C) Similar section from a CS 23 embryo (end eighth week). The MMi has thinned and elongated further and is connected with the antero-lateral papillary muscle *(ALPM)* that has formed by coalescence of trabecular myocardium on the free wall (see B). The LMi is connected to the ALPM as well. The STr leaflet remains densely attached to the septum and will not be freed until 10–12 weeks. The LTr continues to be supported by ventricular myocardium that is forming a papillary muscle in the RV. The myocardium on the ventricular surface of the leaflet will undergo apoptosis leaving the fibrous leaflet except at the leaflet tip which will become the myotendinous junction.

leftward[53] (Fig. 2.13C and D). Failure of normal counter-clockwise rotation is associated with a variety of conotruncal anomalies including tetralogy of Fallot, truncus arteriosus, and double-outlet right ventricle.[53]

The semilunar valves form from the fused outflow cushions and intercalated cushions by a process of apoptosis and excavation to form the pocket-like valve cusps[54] (Fig. 2.18A–C) coordinated by a complex gene regulatory network,[37] some elements of which have been implicated in congenital valve abnormalities. For example, NOTCH1 mutations have been implicated in congenital bicommissural aortic valve[55] and gain-of-function mutations in PTPN11 are associated with pulmonary valve dysplasia in Noonan syndrome.[56] The fused septal and parietal cushions give rise to the two facing aortic and pulmonary leaflets and sinuses, while the intercalated cushions on the opposite wall yield the non-facing leaflets and sinuses. Both cardiac neural crest and endocardium-derived mesenchyme participate in formation of the facing valvar components, although few neural crest derivatives remain in the mature valve.[38] In contrast, the intercalated cushions seem to contain only second heart field cells.[38] Like the atrioventricular valves, the semilunar valves continue to remodel and mature postnatally.[57]

At the beginning of the sixth week, the aortic arch system is symmetrical, composed of the third, fourth, and sixth arches connecting the remodeled aortic sac to the dorsal aorta on each side (Fig. 2.9C). The seventh segmental branches of the descending aorta, the future subclavian arteries, arise distal to the junction of the two dorsal aortae. During the sixth and seventh weeks, the aortic arch system remodels extensively.[36] As described above, a shelf of tissue protrudes between the fourth and sixth arches and fuses with the distal ends of the septal and parietal outflow cushions, dividing the aortic sac into aortic and pulmonary channels. The right sixth arch

(right ductus arteriosus) involutes progressively and disappears by about the end of the sixth week (Fig. 2.9D). The dorsal aorta between its junctions with the third and fourth arches bilaterally (carotid duct) begins to involute and will disappear entirely by the end of the sixth week or early in the seventh week (Fig. 2.9D). This leaves the third aortic arch on each side as the only connection to the cranial part of the dorsal aorta, the presumptive internal carotid artery. The external carotid artery develops as a branch of the cranial dorsal aorta. This is how the third arch becomes the common carotid artery. By a poorly understood mechanism, probably involving differential growth of parts of the aorta, the seventh segmental arteries (presumptive subclavian arteries) migrate proximally from the descending aorta onto the dorsal aortae[36] (Fig. 2.9E). The supracardinal and subcardinal venous systems have formed and the posterior cardinal veins have involuted (Fig. 2.10D).

Week 7

During the seventh week (CS 17–19), the intrapericardial great arteries remodel into separate arterial vessels, the proximal outflow is divided separating the left and right ventricular outflows, the atrioventricular and semilunar valves continue to thin and elongate, atrioventricular fibrous insulation begins to form, the sinus node becomes detectable in the sinus venosus myocardium, and the septum secundum or limbus begins to form as an infolding of the atrial wall posterior and inferior to the dividing outflow. Papillary muscles begin to form by coalescence of ventricular trabeculae. The peritruncal coronary plexus forms and endothelial strands begin to invade the wall of the newly formed aortic root. Pharyngeal arch arteries and the systemic venous system continue to remodel.

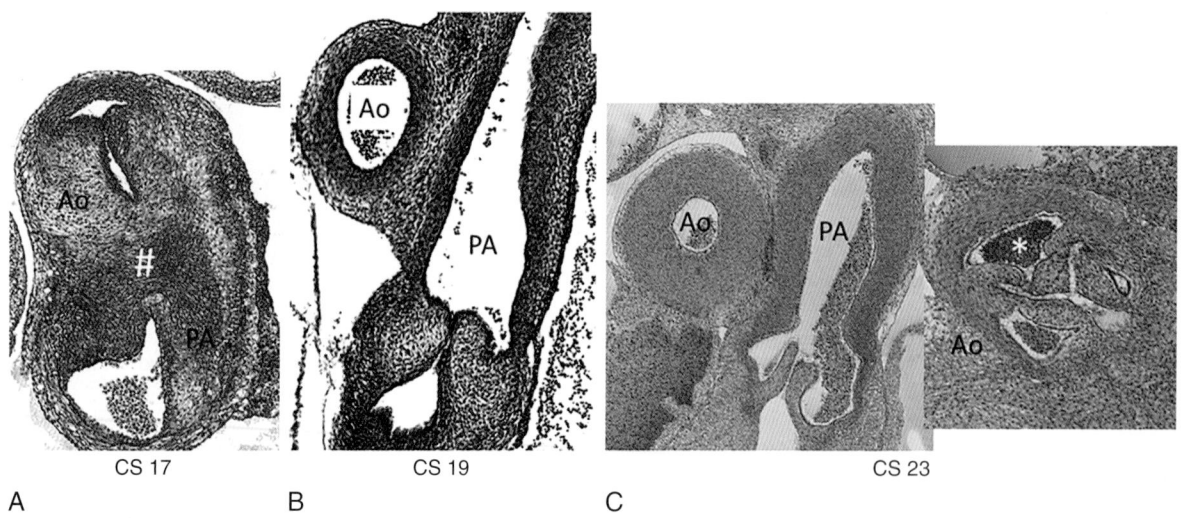

CS 17   CS 19   CS 23

A   B   C

• **Fig. 2.18** (A) A section through the recently divided outflow in a CS 17 embryo (early seventh week). The two main outflow cushions have fused centrally *(#)* dividing the outflow into aortic *(Ao)* and pulmonary *(PA)* channels. The facing semilunar cusps are starting to develop from the fused cushions. The intercalated cushions are not seen in this cut. (B) A section through the divided outflow in a CS 19 embryo (end seventh week). Pulmonary semilunar leaflets are being sculpted from the outflow cushions by apoptosis and action of matrix metalloproteinases. The intrapericardial ascending aorta *(Ao)* and pulmonary artery *(PA)* are rapidly remodeling into separate vessels. (C) Sections of the outflow vessels in a CS 23 embryo (end eighth week). Longitudinal section through the pulmonary root *(left panel)* showing further sculpting of the pulmonary root and thinning of the pulmonary leaflets. The Ao and PA have remodeled into separate vessels. The right panel shows a cross-section through the developing aortic valve. The non-facing leaflet and sinus *(*)* have developed from the intercalated cushion.

Soon after division of the outflow into separate aortic and pulmonary channels, the intrapericardial vessels distal to the developing semilunar valves rapidly remodel into separate spiraling arteries (Fig. 2.18B and C). There is little evidence for transdifferentiation of myocardium into smooth muscle or fibrous tissue. The free walls of the great arteries and arterial roots develop from second heart field mesenchyme, while the facing walls develop from the fused outflow cushions containing both second heart field mesenchyme and neural crest cells.[58] The myocardium under the pulmonary valve remains as a sleeve of infundibular muscle, while the myocardium under the aortic valve appears to undergo apoptosis so that the developing aortic valve becomes continuous with the superior endocardial cushion component of the developing medial mitral leaflet.[59]

The outflow cushions proximal to the developing semilunar valves continue to fuse together (Fig. 2.13F and G). The parts of the cushions immediately below the valves contain neural crest cells as well as second heart field cells.[16,59] In contrast, the most proximal part of the cushions that will form the muscular outflow septum is populated by EMT of outflow endothelium (second heart field–derived endothelium).[16] The mesenchymal outflow septum fuses with the superior endocardial cushion to form the membranous septum.[59] The outflow septum joins the rightward aspect of the inferior and leftward rims of the primary foramen, aligning the aortic root with the left ventricle through the primary foramen and the pulmonary trunk with the right ventricle (Fig. 2.13F and G). Myocardial cells from the adjacent walls of the outflow grow into the initially mesenchymal outflow septum converting it to muscle.[60] Perhaps the different origin of this structure explains why it can behave independently of the rest of the outflow septum, for example, failing

to form in doubly committed subarterial defects or being malpositioned in other conotruncal anomalies (e.g., tetralogy of Fallot, double-outlet ventricle).

The coronary vascular plexus forms a ring of vessels around the developing outflow (a corona or crown of vessels, hence the name coronary arteries). Endothelial sprouts from this peritruncal plexus begin to invade the developing aortic root.[43,44] How sprouts are guided to the aorta and not the pulmonary trunk and why generally only sprouts entering the facing aortic sinuses are stabilized and persist as the coronary trunks is unclear but seems to involve myocardial cells in the aortic wall at the site of entry into the aorta, epicardium-derived cells important for apoptosis at the site of entry, and preotic neural crest cells that contribute smooth muscle for the coronary stems. The coronary plexus that has developed over the heart has undergone extensive remodeling to create the typical large epicardial vessels. As soon as the invading endothelial strands lumenize to form the coronary trunks, blood begins to flow within the coronary system.

The sinus node develops in TBX18+ and NKX2-5– sinus venosus myocardium under the influence of TBX3 at the superior vena cava–right atrial junction. The remainder of the sinus venosus myocardium begins to express NKX2-5 and develops into working atrial myocardium.

The superior limbus or septum secundum begins to develop in the roof at the junction of the left and right atria by infolding of the wall, possibly as the atrial chambers expand outward around the outflow (Fig. 2.19). This process will continue into the fetal period.

Trabeculae on the ventricular walls to which the atrioventricular endocardial cushions are joined begin to coalesce into papillary muscles (Fig. 2.17C). The remodeling cushions continue to elongate and thin, and chordae begin to become

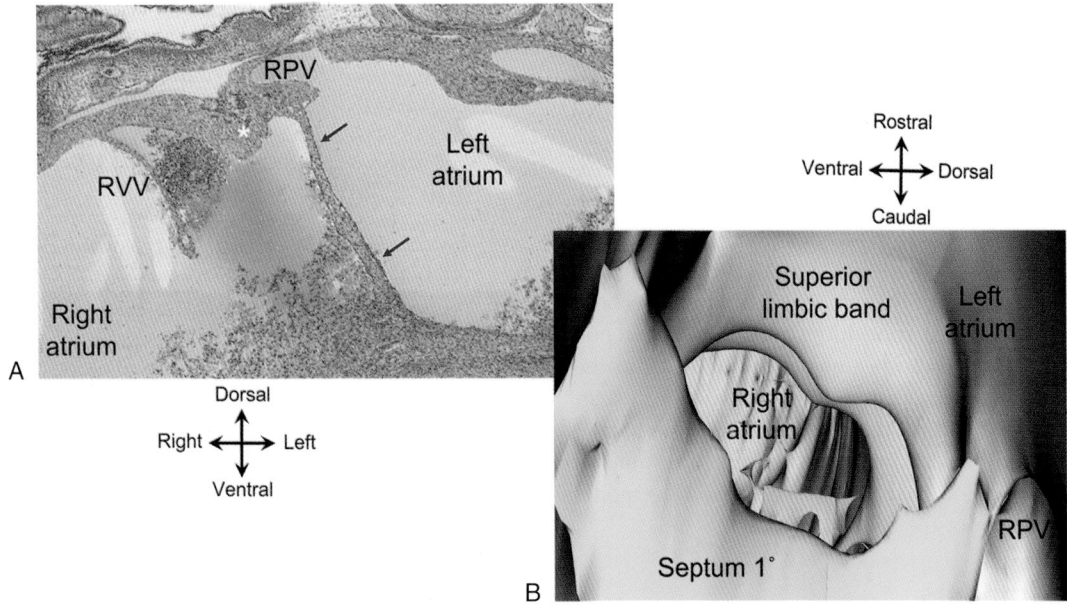

• **Fig. 2.19** (A) A section through the superior aspect of the atrial septum in a CS 23 embryo (end eighth week). The superior limbic band or septum secundum is developing as an infolding in the roof of the atrium (*) to the right of the insertion of septum primum *(red arrows)* and the entrance of the right upper pulmonary vein *(RPV)*. The right venous valve *(RVV)* is seen in the right atrium. (B) A 3D reconstruction of the atrial septum as viewed from within the left atrium in the same CS 23 embryo. The section in A is through the posterior attachment of septum primum *(septum 1')*, near the RPV.

apparent as fenestrations develop in the distal leaflets.[57] Epicardium-derived cells in the atrioventricular sulcus begin to invade between the atrioventricular canal myocardium and ventricular myocardium[61] (Fig. 2.17B and C). These mesenchymal cells join the atrioventricular endocardial cushions, which are forming valve leaflets, to create the fibrous insulation between the atria and ventricles. The epicardium-derived cells contribute to the atrioventricular fibrous annulus as well as the mural leaflets of the atrioventricular valves.[61] This process continues into fetal life and is essential to avoid pre-excitation syndromes. Fibrous separation occurs everywhere except posteriorly where the atrioventricular node and penetrating bundle form from atrioventricular canal myocardium and ventricular myocardium, respectively.[62]

The part of the right dorsal aorta between the seventh segmental artery and the descending aorta involutes leaving the left fourth arch and left dorsal aorta as the definitive left aortic arch[36] (Fig. 2.9F). Failure of involution of this segment of dorsal aorta results in a vascular ring—double aortic arch. The right brachiocephalic or innominate artery is formed from the right horn of the aortic sac. The right third arch becomes the common carotid artery. The right subclavian artery is formed from the right fourth arch proximally, a part of right dorsal aorta and the right seventh segmental artery distally. Intersubcardinal anastomoses form between the subcardinal veins at the site of entrance of the renal veins (perirenal plexus) (Fig. 2.10E). The renal-to-hepatic segment of the inferior vena cava develops from the rightward aspect of the perirenal plexus to the hepatocardiac channel, the only part of the venous system that is asymmetrical from its inception (Fig. 2.11). The infrarenal inferior vena cava develops from the right supracardinal vein below its anastomosis with the perirenal plexus, while the iliac veins are derived from the posterior cardinal veins. The azygos and hemiazygos veins are derived from the supracardinal veins above their anastomoses with the perirenal plexus. The right supracardinal vein also makes an anastomosis with the proximal posterior cardinal vein. While the bulk of the azygos vein derives from supracardinal vein, the arch and connection to the superior vena cava is from the posterior cardinal vein.

Week 8

During the eighth week (CS 20–23), atrioventricular and semilunar valves continue to remodel with thinning and elongation, a process that continues postnatally. The septal leaflet of the tricuspid valve begins delamination from the septum. Failure of this process appears to result in Ebstein anomaly. Development of the fibrous insulation at the atrioventricular groove continues with completion not before weeks 10–12. Coronary arteries continue to remodel and expand. Growth of the heart continues.

Acknowledgments

We thank William Pu, MD, for his thoughtful review of this chapter and his very helpful suggestions. Human embryo sections used for 3D reconstructions were obtained from the Virtual Human Embryo Project (VHE) (http://virtualhumanembryo.lsuhsc.edu/default.htm). The 3D reconstructions were created using 3D Slicer 4.5.0-1(https://www.slicer.org/).

References

1. Kelly RG, Buckingham ME. The anterior heart-forming field: voyage to the arterial pole of the heart. *Trends Genet.* 2002; 18:210-216.
2. Molè, MA, Weberling A, Zernicka-Goetz M. Comparative analysis of human and mouse development: from zygote to pre-gastrulation. *Curr Top Dev Biol.* 2020;136:113-138.
3. Ghimire, S, Mantziou V, Moris N, Arias AM. Human gastrulation: the embryo and its models. *Dev Biol.* 2021;474:100-108.
4. Kelly RG, Buckingham ME, Moorman AF. Heart fields and cardiac morphogenesis. *Cold Spring Harb Perspect Med.* 2014;4:a015750.
5. Ma Q, Zhou B, Pu WT. Reassessment of Isl1 and Nkx2–5 cardiac fate maps using a Gata4-based reporter of Cre activity. *Dev Biol.* 2008;323:98-104.
6. Sadler TW. *Langman's Medical Embryology.* 14th ed. Philadelphia, PA: Lippincott Williams & Wilkins; 2018:80-88.
7. Lopez-Sanchez C, Garcia-Martinez V. Molecular determinants of cardiac specification. *Cardiovasc Res.* 2011;91:185-195.
8. Sugi Y, Markwald RR. Endodermal growth factors promote endocardial precursor cell formation from precardiac mesoderm. *Dev Biol.* 2003;263:35-49.
9. Rana MS, Christoffels VM, Moorman AF. A molecular and genetic outline of cardiac morphogenesis. *Acta Physiol.* 2013;207:588-615.
10. Sizarov A, Ya J, de Boer BA, et al. Formation of the building plan of the human heart: morphogenesis, growth, and differentiation. *Circulation.* 2011;123:1125-1135.
11. Yagi H, Furutani Y, Hamada H, et al. Role of TBX1 in human del22q11.2 syndrome. *Lancet.* 2003;62:1366-1373.
12. Hirokawa N, Tanaka Y, Okada Y. Cilia, KIF3 molecular motor and nodal flow. *Curr Opin Cell Biol.* 2012;24:31-39.
13. Zhu, L, Belmont JW, Ware SM. Genetics of human heterotaxias. *Eur J Hum Genet.* 2006;14:17-25.
14. Drake CJ, Fleming PA. Vasculogenesis in the day 6.5 to 9.5 mouse embryo. *Blood.* 2000;95:1671-1679.
15. DeRuiter MC, Poelmann RE, VanderPlas-de Vries I, et al. The development of the myocardium and endocardium in mouse embryos. Fusion of two heart tubes? *Anat Embryol (Berl).* 1992;185:461-473.
16. Snarr BS, Kern CB, Wessels A. Origin and fate of cardiac mesenchyme. *Dev Dyn.* 2008;237:2804-2819.
17. Sylva M, van den Hoff MJB, Moorman AFM. Development of the human heart. *Am J Med Genet A.* 2014;164A:1347-1371.
18. Bayraktar M, Männer J. Cardiac looping may be driven by compressive loads resulting from unequal growth of the heart and pericardial cavity. Observations on a physical simulation model. *Front Physiol.* 2014;5:112.
19. Lescroart F, Hamoua W, Francou A, et al. Clonal analysis reveals a common origin between nonsomite-derived neck muscles and heart myocardium. *Proc Natl Acad Sci U S A.* 2015;112:1446-1451.
20. Lescroart F, Mohun T, Meilhac SM. Lineage tree for the venous pole of the heart clonal analysis clarifies controversial genealogy based on genetic tracing. *Circ Res.* 2012;111:1313-1322.
21. Männer J. On the form problem of embryonic heart loops, its geometrical solutions, and a new biophysical concept of cardiac looping. *Ann Anat.* 2013;195:312-323.
22. Männer J, Heinicke F. A model for left juxtaposition of the atrial appendages in the chick. *Cardiol Young.* 2003;13:152-160.

23. Moorman AFM, Christoffels VM. Cardiac chamber formation: development, genes and evolution. *Physiol Rev.* 2003;83:1223-1267.

24. Wilsbacher L, McNally EM. Genetics of cardiac developmental disorders: cardiomyocyte proliferation and growth and relevance to heart failure. *Annu Rev Pathol.* 2016;11:395-419.

25. Captur G, Wilson R, Bennett MF. Morphogenesis of myocardial trabeculae in the mouse embryo. *J Anat.* 2016;229:314-325.

26. Srivastava D. Making or breaking the heart: from lineage determination to morphogenesis. *Cell.* 2006;126:1037-1048.

27. Aanhaanen WT, Brons JF, Domínguez JN, et al. The Tbx2+ primary myocardium of the atrioventricular canal forms the atrioventricular node and the base of the left ventricle. *Circ Res.* 2009;104:1267-1274.

28. Franco D, Meilhac SM, Christoffels VM. Left and right ventricular contributions to the formation of the interventricular septum in the mouse heart. *Dev Biol.* 2006;294:366-375.

29. Sizarov A, Anderson RH, Christoffels VM, Moorman AF. Three-dimensional and molecular analysis of the venous pole of the developing human heart. *Circulation.* 2010;122:798-807.

30. Mommersteeg MTM, Domínguez JN, Wiese C, et al. The sinus venosus progenitors separate and diversify from the first and second heart fields early in development. *Cardiovasc Res.* 2010;87:92-101.

31. Manner J, Perez-Pomares JM, Macias D, Munoz-Chapuli R. The origin, formation and developmental significance of the epicardium: a review. *Cells Tissues Organs.* 2001;169:89-103.

32. Katz TC, Singh MK, Degenhardt K, et al. Distinct compartments of the proepicardial organ give rise to coronary vascular endothelial cells. *Dev Cell.* 2012;22:639-650.

33. Winter EM, Gittenberger-de Groot AC. Epicardium-derived cells in cardiogenesis and cardiac regeneration. *Cell Mol Life Sci.* 2007;64:692-703.

34. Perez-Pomares JM, Phelps A, Sedmerova M, Wessels A. Epicardial-like cells on the distal arterial end of the cardiac outflow tract do not derive from the proepicardium but are derivatives of the cephalic pericardium. *Dev Biol.* 2003;227:56-68.

35. Hutson MR, Kirby ML. Role of cardiac neural crest in the development of the caudal pharyngeal arches, the cardiac outflow and disease. In: Rosenthal N, Harvey RP, eds. *Heart Development and Regeneration.* Amsterdam, NY: Academic Press; 2010:143-169, 441-463.

36. Rana MS, Sizarov A, Christoffels VM, Moorman AF. Development of the human aortic arch system captured in an interactive three-dimensional reference model. *Am J Med Genet.* 2014;164A:1372-1383.

37. Combs MD, Yutzey KE. Heart valve development: regulatory networks in development and disease. *Circ Res.* 2009;105:408-421.

38. Sizarov A, Lamers WH, Mohun TJ, Brown NA, Anderson RH, Moorman AF. Three-dimensional and molecular analysis of the arterial pole of the developing human heart. *J Anat.* 2012;220:336-349.

39. Wessels A, Anderson RH, Markwald RR, et al. Atrial development in the human heart: an immunohistochemical study with emphasis on the role of mesenchymal tissues. *Anat Rec.* 2000;259:288-300.

40. Snarr BS, Wirrig EE, Phelps AL, Trusk TC, Wessels A. A spatiotemporal evaluation of the contribution of the dorsal mesenchymal protrusion to cardiac development. *Dev Dyn.* 2007;236:1287-1294.

41. Wessels A, Vermeulen JL, Verbeek FJ, et al. Spatial distribution of "tissue-specific" antigens in the developing human heart and skeletal muscle. III. An immunohistochemical analysis of the distribution of the neural tissue antigen G1N2 in the embryonic heart; implications for the development of the atrioventricular conduction system. *Anat Rec.* 1992;232:97-111.

42. D'Amato G, Luxán G, del Monte-Nieto G, et al. Sequential Notch activation regulates ventricular chamber development. *Nat Cell Biol.* 2016;18:7-20.

43. Sharma B, Chang A, Red-Horse K. Coronary artery development: progenitor cells and differentiation pathways. *Annu Rev Physiol.* 2017;79:1-19.

44. Tian X, Pu WT, Zhou B. Cellular origin and developmental program of coronary angiogenesis. *Circ Res.* 2015;116:515-530.

45. Bamforth SD, Chaudhry B, Bennett M, et al. Clarification of the identity of the mammalian fifth pharyngeal arch artery. *Clin Anat.* 2013;26:173-182.

46. Nadeau M, Georges RO, Laforest B, et al. An endocardial pathway involving Tbx5, Gata4, and Nos3 required for atrial septum formation. *Proc Natl Acad Sci U S A.* 2010;107:19356-19361.

47. de Lange FJ, Moorman AFM, Anderson RH, et al. Lineage and morphogenetic analysis of the cardiac valves. *Circ Res.* 2004;95:645-654.

48. Lockhart MM, Phelps AL, van den Hoff MJ, Wessels A. The epicardium and the development of the atrioventricular junction in the murine heart. *J Dev Biol.* 2014;2:1-17.

49. Anderson RH, Webb S, Brown NA, et al. Development of the heart: (3) formation of the ventricular outflow tracts, arterial valves, and intrapericardial arterial trunks. *Heart.* 2003;89:1110-1118.

50. Rana MS, Horsten NCA, Tesink-Taekema S, et al. Trabeculated right ventricular free wall in the chicken heart forms by ventricularization of the myocardium initially forming the outflow tract. *Circ Res.* 2007;100:1000-1007.

51. Watanabe M, Choudhry A, Berlan M, et al. Developmental remodeling and shortening of the cardiac outflow tract involves myocyte programmed cell death. *Development.* 1998;125:3809-3820.

52. Anderson RH, Chaudhry B, Mohun TJ, et al. Normal and abnormal development of the intrapericardial arterial trunks in man and mouse. *Cardiovasc Res.* 2012;95:108-115.

53. Bajolle F, Zaffran S, Kelly RG, et al. Rotation of the myocardial wall of the outflow tract is implicated in the normal positioning of the great arteries. *Circ Res.* 2006;98:421-428.

54. Maron BJ, Hutchins GM. The development of the semilunar valves in the human heart. *Am J Pathol.* 1974;74:331-344.

55. Garg V, Muth AN, Ransom JF, et al. Mutations in NOTCH1 cause aortic valve disease. *Nature.* 2005;437:270-274.

56. Tartaglia M, Kalidas K, Shaw A, et al. PTPN11 mutations in Noonan syndrome: molecular spectrum, genotype-phenotype correlation, and phenotypic heterogeneity. *Am J Hum Genet.* 2002;70:1555-1563.

57. Aikawa E, Whittaker P, Farber M, et al. Human semilunar cardiac valve remodeling by activated cells from fetus to adult: implications for postnatal adaptation, pathology, and tissue engineering. *Circulation.* 2006;113:1344-1352.

58. Richardson R, Eley L, Donald-Wilson C, et al. Development and maturation of the fibrous components of the arterial roots in the mouse heart. *J Anat.* 2018;232:554-567.

59. Watanabe M, Jafri A, Fisher SA. Apoptosis is required for the proper formation of the ventriculo-arterial connections. *Dev Biol.* 2001;240:274-288.

60. van den Hoff MJB, Moorman AFM, Ruijter JM, et al. Myocardialization of the cardiac outflow tract. *Dev Biol.* 1999;212:477-490.

61. Lockhart MM, Phelps AL, van den Hoff MJ, Wessels A. The epicardium and the development of the atrioventricular junction in the murine heart. *J Dev Biol.* 2014;2:1-17.

62. Aanhaanen WTJ, Mommersteeg MTM, Norden J, et al. Developmental origin, growth, and three-dimensional architecture of the atrioventricular conduction axis of the mouse heart. *Circ Res.* 2010;107:728-736.

3

Morphologic-Anatomic Diagnosis: Normal and Pathologic Cardiac Morphology

STEPHEN P. SANDERS, CHRYSTALLE KATTE CARREON, AND TAL GEVA

"This method and its terminology have stood the test of time, apply conveniently in all situations (no matter how complex), and have not required any significant changes over the past decade or more..."

Richard Van Praagh, 1984[1]

KEY LEARNING POINTS

- The heart is a complex organ composed of segments.
- The segments have characteristic morphology which is the basis of their identity.
- Segmental analysis involves determining the location of the heart and the situs, alignments, and connections of the segments.
- The variety of segmental combinations results in many basic types of human hearts.

- Each segment has specific associated anomalies that contribute to the overall physiology.
- A comprehensive diagnosis includes heart location, segmental analysis, and compilation of segment-specific diagnoses, which allows deduction of the physiology.

The normal human heart is a complex structure, the congenitally malformed heart even more so. A systematic and comprehensive method for analyzing the heart is essential for effective communication among caregivers and for data archiving and extraction. We use the morphologic-anatomic diagnostic method,[1] also known as segmental analysis.[2,3] This method provides a way of describing the heart that is structured, specific, and inclusive, but also succinct.[4,5] In this chapter, we will describe the morphologic-anatomic method[1,3] and the cardiac morphology[6-8] that is the basis for the method.

Cardiac Structure

The normal human heart comprises a consistent set of components or segments, each with characteristic morphology.[4,9] The main cardiac segments are the atria, the ventricles, and the great arteries. The main segments are connected in sequence by two connecting segments, the atrioventricular canal or junction and the conus or infundibulum. The atrial segment is the only clearly lateralized segment, being closely correlated with the venous and visceral anatomy.[10]

The ventricles develop in sequence along the linear heart tube with much less clear relationship to the genes controlling lateralization.[11] The great arteries develop from an initially common outflow and a symmetrical system of aortic sac rami, pharyngeal arch arteries, and dorsal aortae, again with unclear relationship to lateralization.[12] The atrioventricular canal includes the fibrous insulation between atrial and ventricular myocardium, the penetrating (His) bundle of the conduction system, and the atrioventricular valves, the morphology of which is largely determined by the ventricle with which they connect.[13] The conus or infundibulum is the muscular sleeve that connects the developing semilunar valves with the ventricular mass in the embryonic heart, remaining in complete form only under the pulmonary valve in the normal heart.[14]

Each main segment has characteristic morphology (described below), which is the basis for its identity, not its position in space.[4,6,7] For example, "right atrium" or "left ventricle" is the name of a specific chamber based on morphology and not its position. Consequently, use of "morphologic right atrium" or the like is superfluous. The atrioventricular valves also have characteristic morphology in the great majority of cases justifying the use of the names of the valves, mitral and tricuspid, in most situations. However, in some abnormal hearts in which morphologic features of the valves are insufficient (e.g., double-inlet right ventricle [DIRV]), use of left or right atrioventricular valve might be more accurate. The infundibulum or conus is simply a sleeve of muscle supporting one or both semilunar valves and separating it (them) from the atrioventricular canal. In the embryonic heart, the infundibulum or conus has a free wall, the circumferential ring of muscle under the developing semilunar valves, and a septum, the sheet of muscle extending toward the ventricles from the junction of the semilunar valves and dividing the infundibulum or conus into subaortic and subpulmonary portions. In the normal heart, a complete infundibulum or conus is present only under the pulmonary valve because most of the subaortic infundibular free wall disappears late in embryogenesis and only a small part of the infundibular septum remains in a septal position, but the conal anatomy can be highly variable in abnormal hearts.

Heart Location

The position and orientation of the heart in the body must be understood for physical diagnosis, imaging studies, and anatomical dissection[3] (Fig. 3.1). Most often the heart is in the left chest with the apex directed leftward (levocardia). In subjects with situs inversus totalis, and in some congenital abnormalities, the heart is predominantly in the right chest (dextrocardia). When the apex is pointed to the right, more or less mirror image of levocardia, this is known as primary dextrocardia. The orientation of the heart is very different from levocardia, so that different imaging planes must be used to study the heart. In addition, some complex heart diseases, such as heterotaxy syndrome and congenitally physiologically corrected transposition, are often associated with primary dextrocardia.

Sometimes the heart is in the right chest, but the orientation of the heart is similar to levocardia, the apex to the left or somewhat inferior. This is called secondary dextrocardia, or dextroposition, because it is usually associated with hypoplasia of the right lung or a space-occupying lesion in the left chest such as congenital diaphragmatic hernia. Here, similar imaging planes to those used in levocardia, but centered over the right chest, are appropriate. Further, the types of heart defects seen are usually simpler, such as partially anomalous pulmonary venous connection[15] or anomalous origin of the left pulmonary artery from the right pulmonary artery.[16]

In some cases, the heart is midline with the apices directed inferiorly and anteriorly (mesocardia). This is also associated with complex heart defects and must be studied using unusual imaging planes.

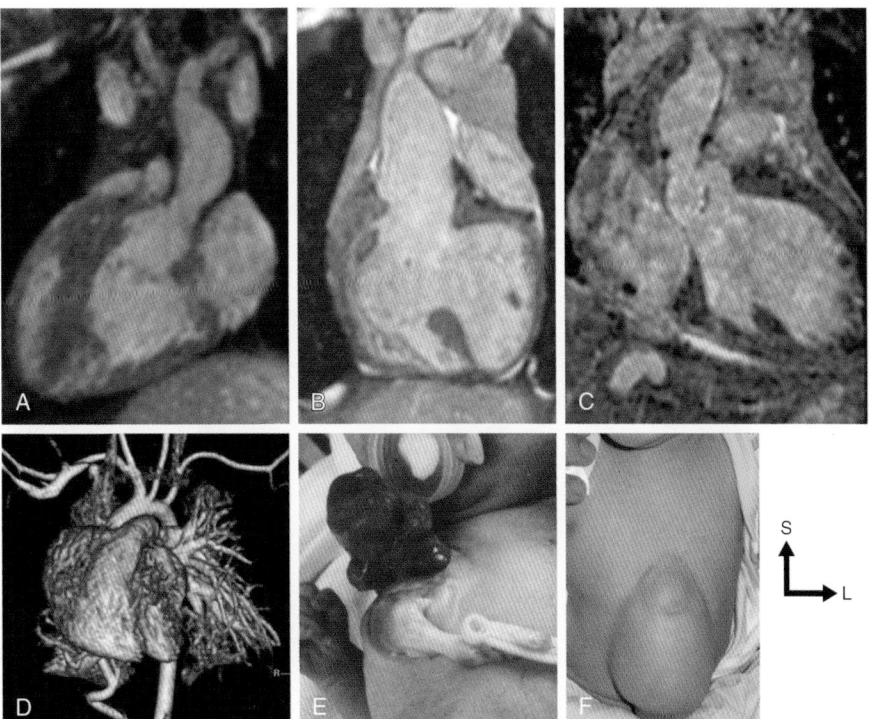

• **Fig. 3.1** Location of the heart. **(A)** Primary dextrocardia, apex to the right. **(B)** Mesocardia, apex anterior/ inferior. **(C)** Levocardia, apex to the left. **(D)** Secondary dextrocardia, heart in the right chest due to another abnormality, but oriented like levocardia. **(E)** Complete ectopia cordis with omphalocele and umbilical cord below the heart. **(F)** Abdominal ectopia cordis. *L,* Left; *S,* superior. (A-C: FIGURE 105-2 Used with permission from Sabiston and Spencer Surgery of the Chest by Frank Sellke, Pedro del Nido, Scott Swanson, 9th edition, Elsevier, 2015; **D:** FIGURE 105-3 Used with permission from Sabiston and Spencer Surgery of the Chest by Frank Sellke, Pedro del Nido, Scott Swanson, 9th edition, Elsevier, 2015; **F:** Figure 1 from Chia HL, Rasheed MZ, Ong KK, et al. Repair of ectopia cordis using a resorbable poly-L-lactic polyglycolic acid plate in a patient with pentalogy of Cantrell. J Pediatr Surg 2012; 47:e1–e4. Reprinted with permission.).

Finally, rarely the heart is outside the thorax, called ectopia cordis. In most such cases, the heart is partially or completely outside the body through a thoracoabdominal midline closure defect.[17,18] Rarely the heart can be in the upper abdomen through a diaphragmatic defect.[18]

Segmental Morphology

Familiarity with the morphology (anatomy) of the various segments is necessary to make accurate and complete diagnoses. Each main segmental component comes in two forms that are approximately mirror images or stereoisomers.[4,9] In this section, we will describe the morphologic characteristics of each component and demonstrate its two isomers.

Veins and Atria

The *systemic veins* comprise: (1) the superior vena cava, which receives an innominate or brachiocephalic vein draining the opposite side of the head, shoulder, and arm, and an azygos vein that connects with a perirenal venous plexus; (2) the inferior vena cava, which receives a variable number of hepatic veins; and (3) the coronary sinus, which receives a number of cardiac veins. The systemic veins normally drain into the right atrium (Fig. 3.2).

A variable number of *pulmonary veins* (2–6) connect to the posterior aspect of the left atrium (Fig. 3.2). The atria are composed of three parts: the appendage, which derives from the atrial portion of the primitive heart tube; the venous component, a smooth-walled intercaval part of the right atrium from sinus venosus and the dome and posterior wall of the left atrium from common pulmonary vein; and the flange of myocardium surrounding the atrioventricular valves, the vestibule, that develops from atrioventricular canal myocardium.[19]

The *right atrium*, the systemic venous atrium, receives the systemic veins, has a broad-based appendage with pectinate muscles that extend out onto the vestibule of the atrioventricular valve, and has the fossa ovalis as a prominent feature on its septal surface (Fig. 3.3). The fossa is bounded superiorly by the septum secundum or limbus and inferiorly and leftward by the muscular base of the atrial septum. The floor of the fossa is formed by the septum primum or primary atrial septum. The sinoatrial node is located in the crista terminalis at the junction of the superior vena cava and right atrium[20,21] (Fig. 3.4). The atrioventricular node is located in the atrial septum near the atrioventricular junction and just below the apex of the triangle of Koch[21] (Fig. 3.3). The solitus or usual right atrium is organized with the superior vena cava entering superior and rightward of the fossa, the coronary sinus ostium inferior and leftward of the fossa, and the atrioventricular valve leftward of the fossa (Fig. 3.3A). The inverted or mirror image right atrium is organized oppositely (Fig. 3.3B).

The *left atrium*, the pulmonary venous atrium, receives two to six pulmonary veins, is smooth-walled, has a small, finger-like appendage with pectinate muscles confined to it, and displays septum primum as a hammock-like structure on its septal surface (Fig. 3.5). In the solitus or usual left atrium viewed from the back (Fig. 3.5A), the right pulmonary veins enter to the right of the septum primum and adjacent to the atrial septum, the small appendage is superior and to the left of septum primum, and the atrioventricular valve is to the left. The inverted or mirror image left atrium is organized oppositely (Fig. 3.5B).

As noted above, the atria are the only segment that lateralizes in clear coordination with left-right lateralization of the body. With viscero-atrial situs solitus, the right atrium is right-sided and the left atrium left-sided, and the opposite in viscero-atrial situs inversus. When the left-right organization

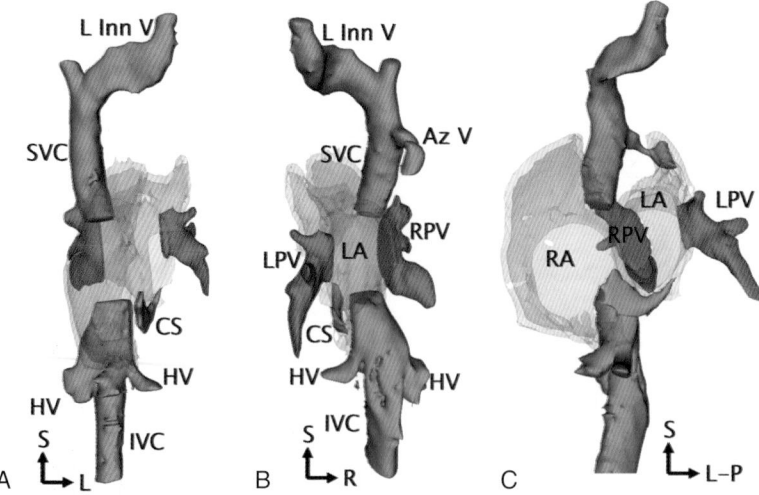

• **Fig. 3.2** Systemic and pulmonary veins. 3D reconstruction from an Magnetic Resonance Image Steady-State Free Precession (MRI SSFP) data set. **(A)** Anterior or frontal view showing left innominate vein *(L Inn V)*, superior vena cava *(SVC)*, inferior vena cava *(IVC)* with hepatic veins *(HV)*, and the coronary sinus *(CS)*. **(B)** Posterior view showing the azygos vein *(Az V)* joining the SVC posteriorly. The left *(LPV)* and right *(RPV)* pulmonary veins join the left atrium *(LA)*. **(C)** View toward the atria showing the systemic veins joining the right atrium *(RA)* and pulmonary veins the LA.

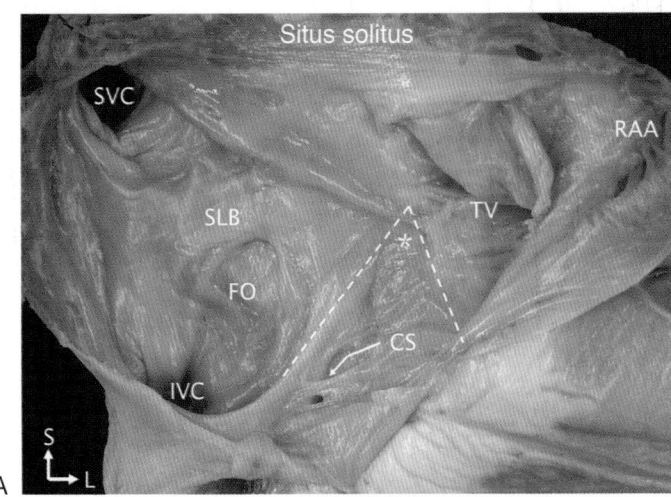
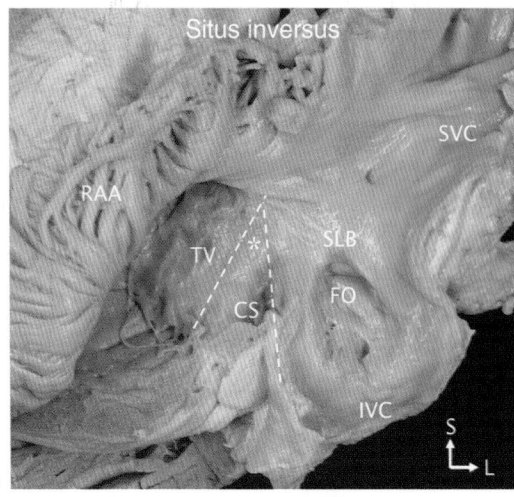

• **Fig. 3.3** Right atrium. An opened solitus right atrium (RA) **(A)** and inversus RA **(B)** illustrating their mirror-image relationship. In both, the fossa ovalis *(FO)* occupies the central part of the atrial septum with the superior limbic band *(SLB)* or septum secundum forming its superior border. The superior vena cava *(SVC)* enters from right and superior in the solitus RA but left and superior in the inversus RA. The inferior vena cava *(IVC)* enters inferiorly, to the right of the Eustachian valve in the solitus RA but to the left in the inversus RA. The coronary sinus *(CS)* and tricuspid valve *(TV)* are to the left of the FO in the solitus RA and to the right in the inversus RA. The opened right atrial appendage *(RAA)* is adjacent to the TV. The atrioventricular node (*) is near the apex of the triangle of Koch *(dashed white lines)* formed by the Eustachian ridge to the right in solitus and to the left in inversus, the annulus of the TV, and the CS inferiorly. *L,* Left; *S,* superior.

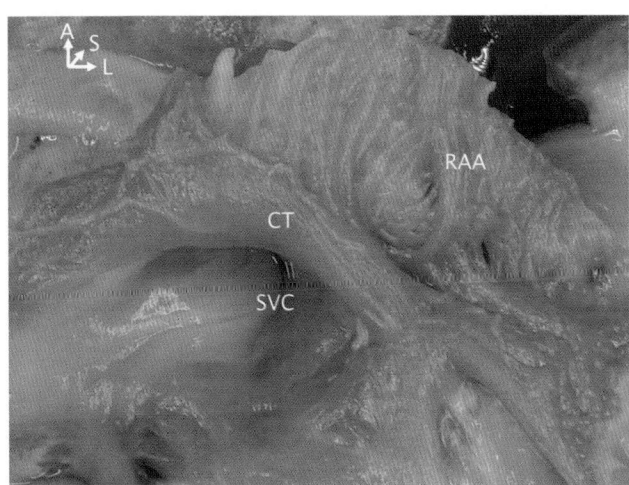

• **Fig. 3.4** The opened solitus right atrium showing the crista terminalis *(CT),* the location of the sinoatrial node, between the superior vena cava *(SVC)* and the right atrial appendage *(RAA).* The pectinate muscles of the RAA end in the CT.

of the body is disturbed (heterotaxy syndrome), the atria often do not follow either the solitus or inversus pattern, a condition called situs ambiguus[9] (Fig. 3.6). The atrial septum may be rudimentary, pectinate muscle morphology is often symmetrical, characteristic structures may be missing or inapparent (e.g., coronary sinus), and venous connections are atypical. Although this has also been called atrial appendage isomerism,[22] true isomerism of the atrial appendages is rare in heterotaxy syndromes.

Ventricles

The ventricles have an inflow portion or body with a trabecular apex, and an outflow. Variably located papillary muscles receive chordal attachments of the atrioventricular valves.

The *right ventricle* is a triangular or trapezoidal chamber with coarse trabeculations, septal attachments of the tricuspid valve, and a muscular outflow, the infundibulum or conus, that separates the semilunar valve from the tricuspid valve[8] (Fig. 3.7). The inflow (sinus) portion that receives attachments of the tricuspid valve is demarcated from the outflow (infundibulum) by a muscular ridge, the crista supraventricularis, composed of the parietal band—infundibular septum continuum, septal band, and moderator band. These structures surround the proximal os infundibuli, the communication between the inflow and outflow portions. The axes of the inflow and outflow portions are approximately perpendicular. The solitus, D-loop, or usual right ventricle, is organized with inflow from the right and outflow to the left as viewed from the free wall. It can be described using the right hand with the thumb in the tricuspid valve, fingers toward the outflow, and palm against the septum[4] (Fig. 3.7A). The inverted or L-loop right ventricle is organized oppositely and can be described using a left hand (Fig. 3.7B).

The *tricuspid valve* typically has three leaflets, the superior (anterior), inferior (posterior), and medial or septal leaflets, although the superior and inferior leaflets are sometimes fused[23] (Fig. 3.8). The commissures between leaflets are at the main papillary muscles: the superior-septal commissure is at the medial papillary muscle or papillary muscle of the

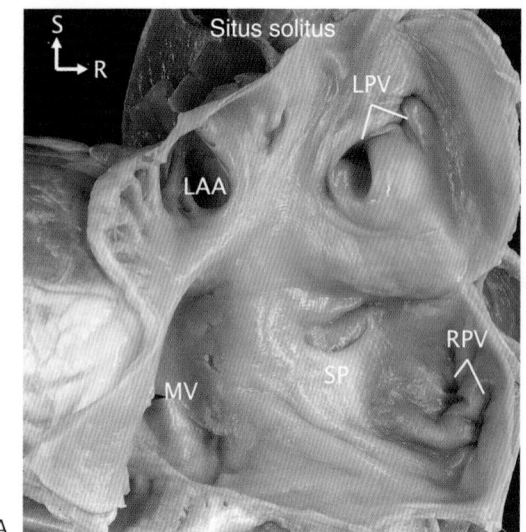
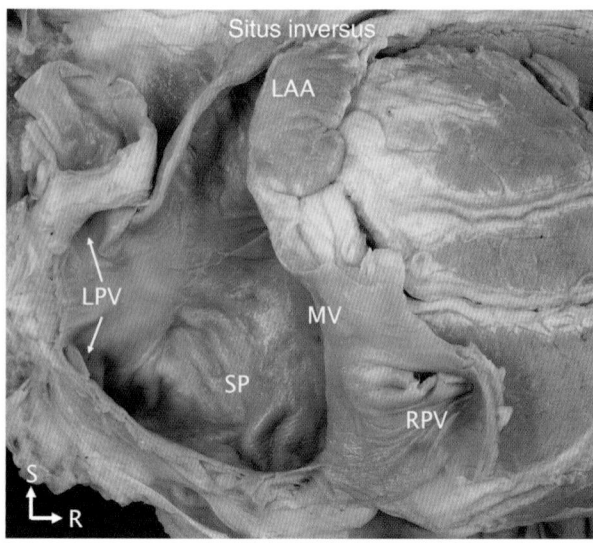

• **Fig. 3.5** Left atrium. An opened solitus left atrium (LA) **(A)** and inversus left atrium **(B)** viewed from the back. Septum primum *(SP)* is in the central part of the septum and the walls of the LA are smooth. In the solitus atrium, the small appendage *(LAA)* with pectinate muscles confined to it, is superior and to the left and the right pulmonary veins *(RPV)* are adjacent to the atrial septum. In contrast, in the inversus LA, the LAA is superior and rightward and the left pulmonary veins *(LPV)* are adjacent to the septum. *MV,* Mitral valve.

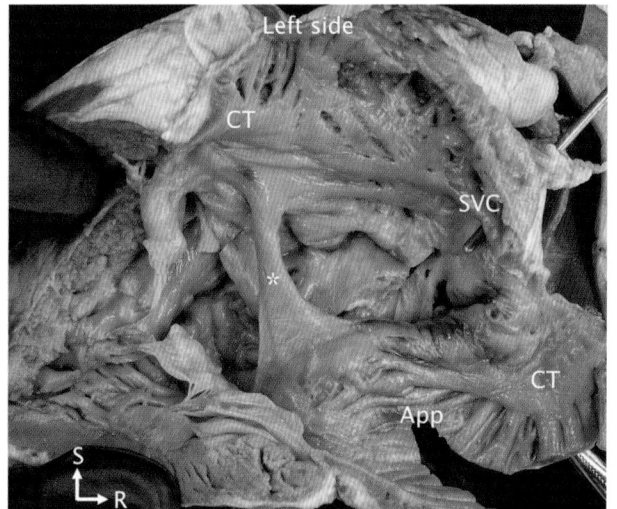
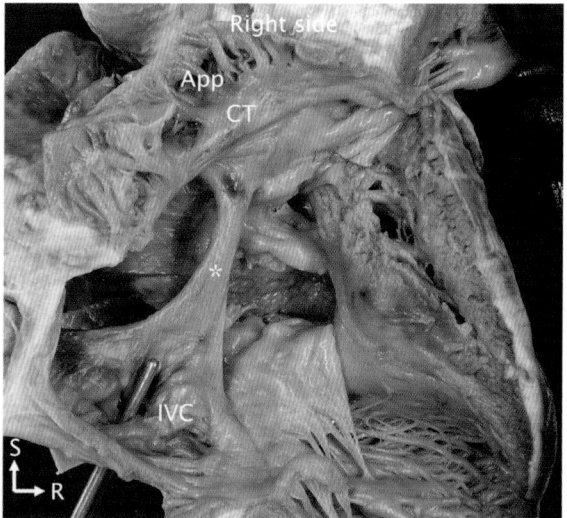

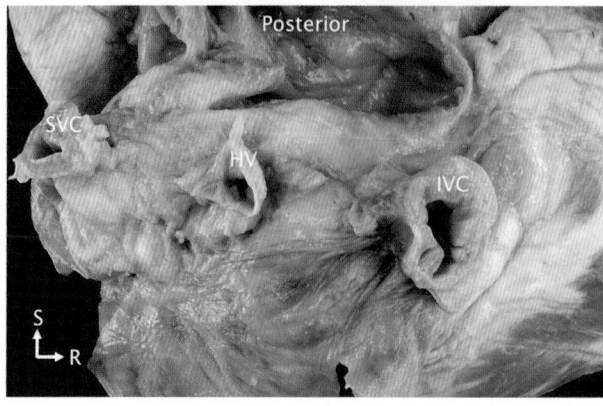

• **Fig. 3.6** Situs ambiguus. **(A)** Left side of the atrium showing an appendage *(App)* with right atrial pectinate muscle architecture, a crista terminalis *(CT)*, and a left superior vena cava *(SVC)*. There is only a strand of atrial septum *(*)* present. **(B)** Right side of the atrium showing entrance of IVC, an appendage similar to the left side and a CT. There is a common atrioventricular canal defect as well. **(C)** Back of the atrium showing entrance of SVC, a hepatic vein *(HV)*, and an inferior vena cava *(IVC)*.

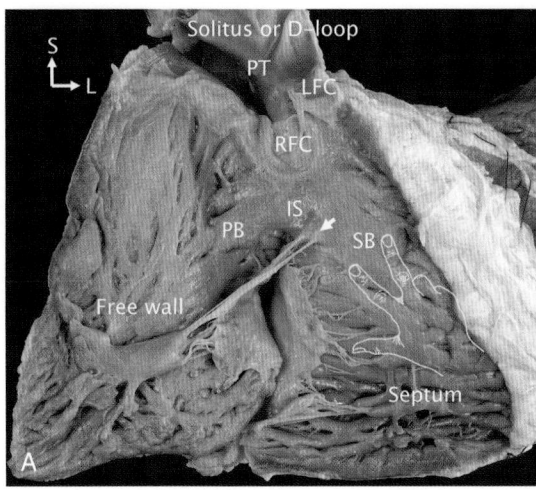
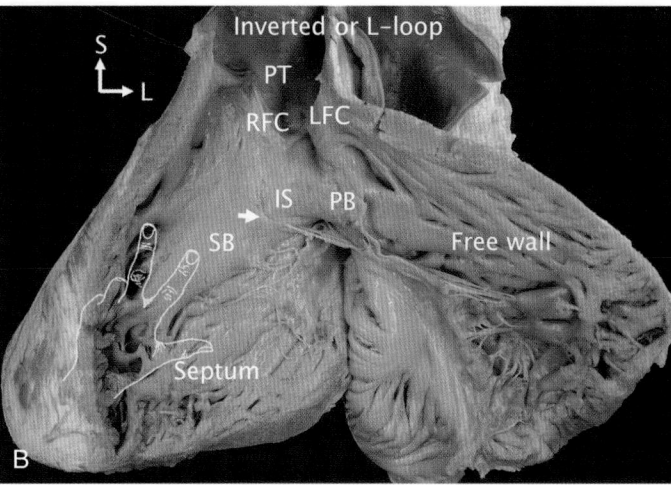

• **Fig. 3.7** Right ventricle. An opened solitus or D-loop right ventricle (RV) **(A)** and an inverted or L-loop RV **(B)**. The inflow portion is below the papillary muscle of the conus or medial papillary muscle *(white arrow)* and receives the attachments of the tricuspid valve. The infundibular septum *(IS)* joins the limbs of the septal band *(SB)* at the medial papillary muscle and continues to the free wall as the parietal band *(PB)*. The muscular sleeve above the medial papillary muscle is the infundibulum or conus and supports the pulmonary valve. The solitus RV is described using a right hand, with thumb in the tricuspid valve, fingers toward the outflow, and palm against the septum. In contrast, the inverted RV requires a left hand. *L*, Left; *LFC*, left-facing cusp of pulmonary valve; *PT*, pulmonary trunk; *RFC*, right-facing cusp of pulmonary valve; *S*, superior.

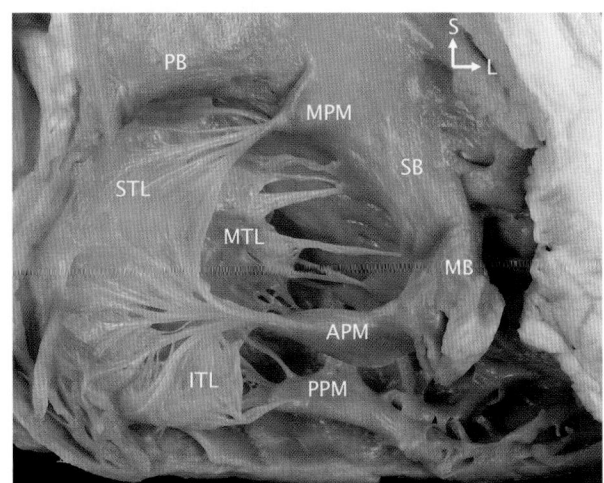

• **Fig. 3.8** The tricuspid valve. The medial or septal leaflet *(MTL)*, between the medial papillary muscle *(MPM)* or papillary muscle of the conus and the posterior (inferior) papillary muscle *(PPM)*, has numerous direct attachments to the ventricular septum, characteristic of the valve and the right ventricle. The superior (anterior) leaflet *(STL)* attaches to the MPM and the anterior (superior) papillary muscle *(APM)*. The inferior (posterior) leaflet *(ITL)* is between the APM and PPM. At the commissures associated with the APM and PPM, frond chords from both leaflets attach to the same papillary muscle, facilitating co-aptation of leaflets. However, usually only the STL has attachments to the MPM while the MTL attaches to the septum, putting this commissure at risk for regurgitation with annular dilation. *ITL*, Inferior tricuspid leaflet; *MB*, moderator band; *PB*, parietal band; *SB*, septal band.

conus (also known as the papillary muscle of Lancisi, named after the Italian anatomist Giovanni Maria Lancisi); the superior-inferior commissure is at the anterior papillary muscle; the inferior-septal commissure is at the posterior or inferior papillary muscle. At the superior-septal commissure,

the leaflets do not usually share a papillary muscle making this commissure at risk for regurgitation due to splaying as the valve annulus dilates. At the other commissures, frond chords connect adjacent leaflets to the same papillary muscle. The septal leaflet is typically attached directly to the septal surface by chords with few or no septal papillary muscles.

The *left ventricle* is bullet shaped and has fine apical trabeculations and a smooth basal septal surface, a pair of free wall papillary muscles (Fig. 3.9), and parallel inflow and outflow portions separated by the medial leaflet of the mitral valve with the outflow between the medial mitral leaflet and the septum[8] (Fig. 3.10). The medial mitral leaflet is in fibrous continuity with the semilunar valve because the subsemilunar conal or infundibular free wall has involuted (Fig. 3.10). The solitus or D-loop left ventricle is left-handed, with the thumb in the mitral valve, fingers toward the outflow, and palm against the septum[4] (Fig. 3.9A). The inverted or L-loop left ventricle is described by a right hand (Fig. 3.9B).

The *mitral valve* is a bi-leaflet valve with a deep medial leaflet occupying about one-third of the annulus and a shorter mural or lateral leaflet occupying about two-thirds of the annulus[24] (Fig. 3.11). The commissures between leaflets are aligned with the two papillary muscle groups, with chordal insertions from both leaflets onto each papillary muscle. The papillary muscle heads form a "U" or horseshoe shape.

The *interventricular septum* is a muscular wall, contributed by both ventricles during development,[25] that separates the bodies and outflows of the ventricles (Fig. 3.12). The septum can be subdivided based on developmental origin and/or location.[26] The septum between the bodies of the ventricles is the muscular septum plus the membranous septum, which is located at the septal-superior commissure

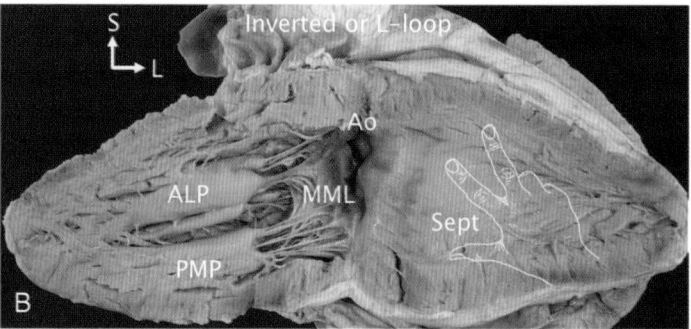

• **Fig. 3.9** The left ventricle. Opened solitus or D-loop left ventricle (LV) **(A)** and an inverted or L-loop LV **(B)**. The smooth basal septal surface *(Sept)* is characteristic of the LV as are the pair of free wall papillary muscles, the anterolateral *(ALP)* and posteromedial *(PMP)* papillary muscles. The mitral valve has no direct chordal attachments to the septum. The solitus or D-loop LV is left-handed, while the inverted or L-loop LV is right-handed. *Ao,* Aortic valve; *MML,* medial mitral leaflet.

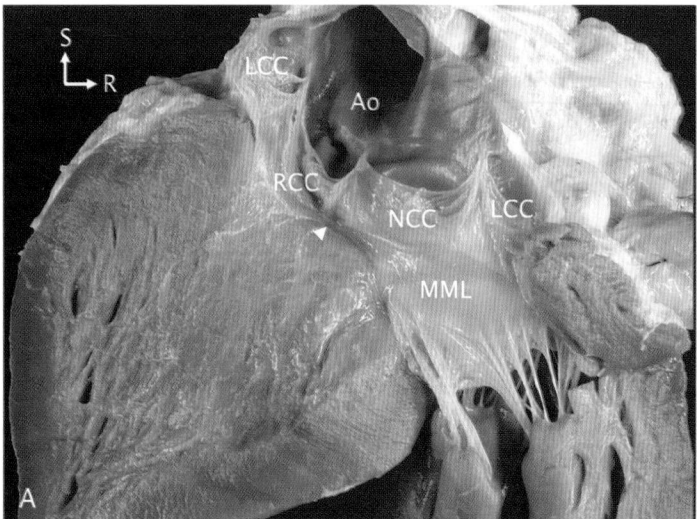
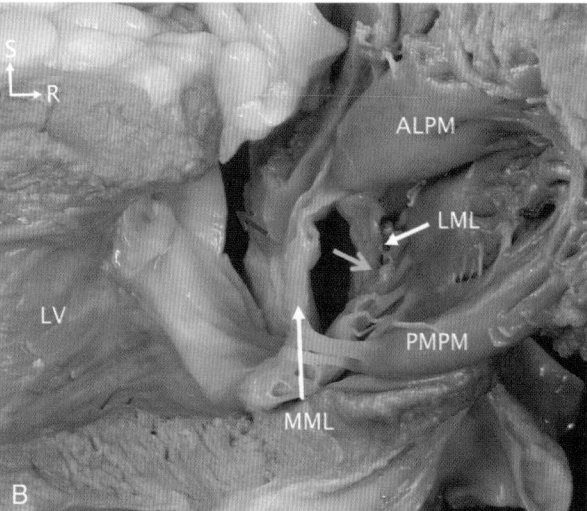

• **Fig. 3.10** The left ventricle. **(A)** An opened solitus or D-loop left ventricle (LV) showing the fibrous continuity between the medial mitral leaflet *(MML)* and all of the noncoronary cusp *(NCC)* and about half of the left coronary cusp *(LCC)* of the aortic valve (note that the LCC has been divided). The membranous septum *(white arrowhead)* is below the commissure between the NCC and the right coronary cusp *(RCC)* and the infundibular or outlet septum is superior to it, mostly below the RCC and partly the LCC. **(B)** Solitus of D-loop LV viewed from apex toward base showing the anterolateral *(ALPM)* and posteromedial *(PMPM)* on the free wall with attachments of medial *(MML)* and lateral *(LML)* mitral leaflets to both. The LV outflow *(red arrow)* is between the MML and the septum and is parallel to the LV inflow *(green arrow). Ao,* Aorta; *R,* right; *S,* superior.

of the tricuspid valve (Figs. 3.10 and 3.12). The muscular septum can be divided into basal or inlet (behind the septal leaflet of tricuspid valve), mid (between free edge of tricuspid valve and moderator band) and apical (apical to the moderator band) segments. The outlet or infundibular septum is the part superior to the medial papillary muscle or the papillary muscle of the conus and between the limbs of the septal band (Fig. 3.12).

Great Arteries

The great arteries are each composed of a root with semilunar valve cusps and sinuses of Valsalva and an elastic tubular portion with branches.[14]

The *aortic valve* has three approximately equal cusps separated by commissures (Fig. 3.10). Two cusps and sinuses of Valsalva are adjacent to the pulmonary valve (facing or septal cusps and sinuses), the left and right coronary cusps and sinuses. The respective coronary ostia are in these facing sinuses and can be multiple, especially on the right. The nonfacing cusp and sinus are on the opposite side. The tubular portion extends superiorly from the sino-tubular junction sequentially as the intrapericardial ascending aorta, aortic arch, and descending thoracic aorta. The brachiocephalic arteries arise from the aortic arch as the innominate artery, the left common carotid artery, and finally the left subclavian artery. The ligamentum arteriosum, the remnant of the ductus arteriosus, joins the descending aorta just distal to

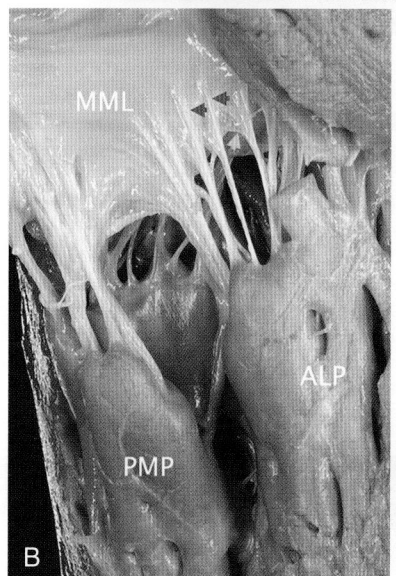
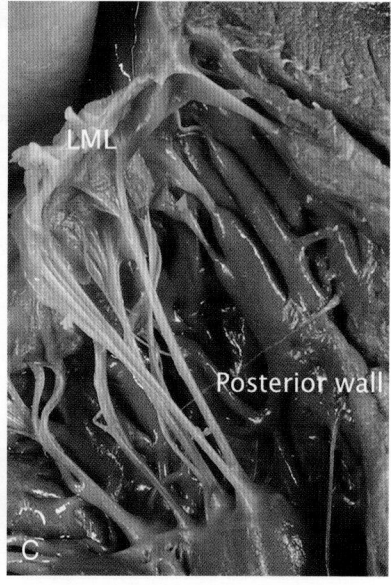

• **Fig. 3.11** The mitral valve. **(A)** Opened mitral valve showing the atrial surface. The lateral mitral leaflet *(LML)* has been divided so that a part is on each side of the medial mitral leaflet *(MML)*. The commissures between the leaflets *(white arrows)* are over the anterolateral *(ALP)* and posteromedial *(PMP)* papillary muscles. The MML is longer from annulus to free edge but occupies only about one-third of the annulus, whereas the shorter LML occupies about two-thirds of the annulus. The papillary muscle heads are U shaped and receive chordae from both leaflets. **(B)** The ventricular surface of the MML showing primary or edge chords *(yellow arrows)* attaching to the free edge of the leaflet and secondary or strut chords *(red arrows)* that attach onto the body of the leaflet. **(C)** A view of the LML from the ventricle showing primary or edge *(yellow arrow)*, secondary or strut *(red arrow)*, and tertiary *(green arrow)* chords. Primary or edge chords prevent leaflet edge prolapse and regurgitation. Secondary or strut chords transmit force from the papillary muscles to the valve structure and maintain leaflet shape. Tertiary chords attach to the base of the leaflet and the posterior wall and are peculiar to the LML. The function is unknown.

the left subclavian artery. The solitus or usual aorta has its valve posterior and rightward, and courses anterior to the right of the pulmonary trunk (Fig. 3.13A). The inverted normal aorta is positioned oppositely (Fig. 3.13B).

The *pulmonary valve* is similar to the aortic valve, but the sinuses of Valsalva tend to be shallower and do not normally contain coronary artery ostia (Fig. 3.7). The tubular portion, the pulmonary trunk, is short and intrapericardial. It bifurcates at the pericardial reflection into right and left branch pulmonary arteries. The ligamentum arteriosum joins either the proximal part of the ipsilateral branch pulmonary artery or the distal part of the pulmonary trunk.

The solitus pulmonary trunk has its valve anterior and leftward relative to the aortic valve, with the trunk coursing posteriorly to the left of the ascending aorta reaching the left-sided bifurcation (Fig. 3.13A). The right pulmonary artery passes posterior to the ascending aorta and the left pulmonary artery anterior to the descending thoracic aorta. The inverted normal pulmonary trunk is organized oppositely (Fig. 3.13B).

The coronary arteries arise from the aortic root from the sinuses of Valsalva facing the pulmonary trunk except in rare cases.[27] The branching pattern is largely determined by the ventricle that the artery supplies.[8] In the solitus

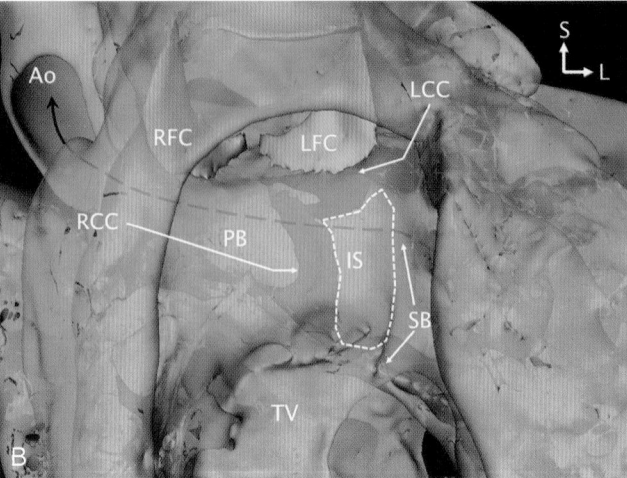

• **Fig. 3.12** **(A)** Opened right ventricle showing components of the ventricular septum. The muscular septum is the largest part. The septal band *(white line with double arrows)* with superior and inferior limbs is a prominent feature, with anterior muscular septum above and inflow muscular septum below. Basal inflow muscular defects are behind the medial tricuspid leaflet *(MTL)*, mid muscular defects between the edge of the MTL and the moderator band *(*)*, and apical defects apical of moderator band. The membranous septum *(white single arrow)* is at the commissure between MTL and the superior tricuspid leaflet *(STL)*. The infundibular septum *(IS)* is between the limbs of septal band *(double arrows)*. **(B)** A 3D reconstruction of a wax-infiltrated heart with the myocardium semitransparent to show internal features. The IS is between the limbs of septal band *(SB)* and below the right *(RCC)* and left *(LCC)* coronary cusps of the aortic valve. The left ventricular outflow and ascending aorta *(Ao, dashed black line)* is seen through the infundibular muscle. The IS maintains a septal position while the parietal band *(PB)* now forms the posterior infundibular wall because of involution of the subaortic conus or infundibulum. *LFC,* Left-facing cusp of pulmonary valve; *RFC,* right-facing cusp of pulmonary valve; *TV,* tricuspid valve.

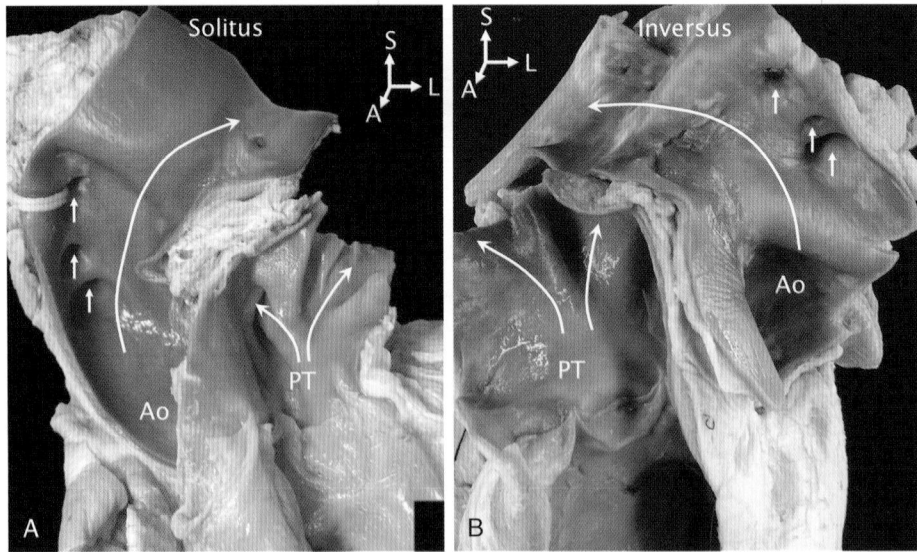

• **Fig. 3.13** Great arteries. Opened aorta *(Ao)* and pulmonary trunk *(PT)* in situs solitus **(A)** and situs inversus **(B)**. The Ao is posterior and rightward in situs solitus but posterior and leftward in situs inversus. The pulmonary bifurcation is to the left of the Ao in situs solitus but to the right in situs inversus. The brachiocephalic arteries *(straight arrows)* arise from the aortic arch.

normal heart the left coronary ostium is in the left posterior sinus, the left main coronary artery is short and bifurcates into an anterior descending or interventricular artery and a circumflex artery (Fig. 3.14). Branches of the anterior descending artery include one or more diagonal arteries that cross the left ventricular free wall and several perforating arteries that supply the anterior portion of the interventricular septum. The circumflex artery gives off one or more obtuse marginal branches before rounding the left atrioventricular junction to supply a variable amount of the posterior left ventricle and, in about 10% of subjects, the posterior descending artery. The right coronary artery arises

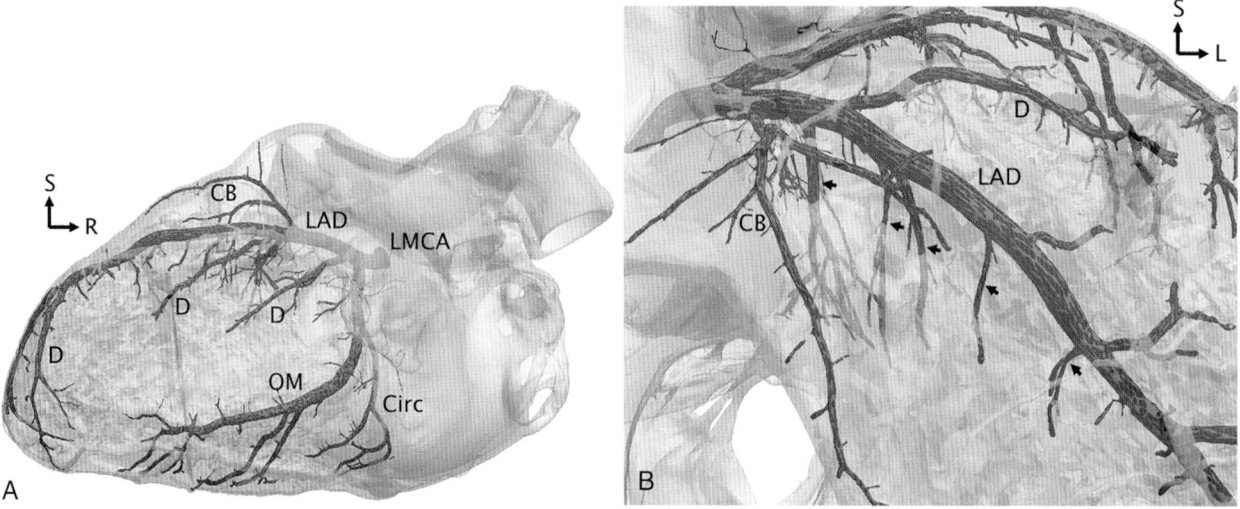

• **Fig. 3.14** Left coronary artery. Two views of a 3D reconstruction of a wax-infiltrated normal heart with the left main coronary artery *(LMCA)* and branches shown in red. **(A)** Posterior view shows the bifurcation of the LMCA into the left anterior descending *(LAD)* or anterior interventricular groove artery with several diagonal branches *(D)*, and the left circumflex artery *(Circ)* with a large obtuse marginal branch *(OM)*. A conus branch *(CB)* arises from the LAD in this heart. **(B)** Anterior view of the LAD with several septal perforating branches *(black arrows)*. *L,* Left; *R,* right; *S,* superior.

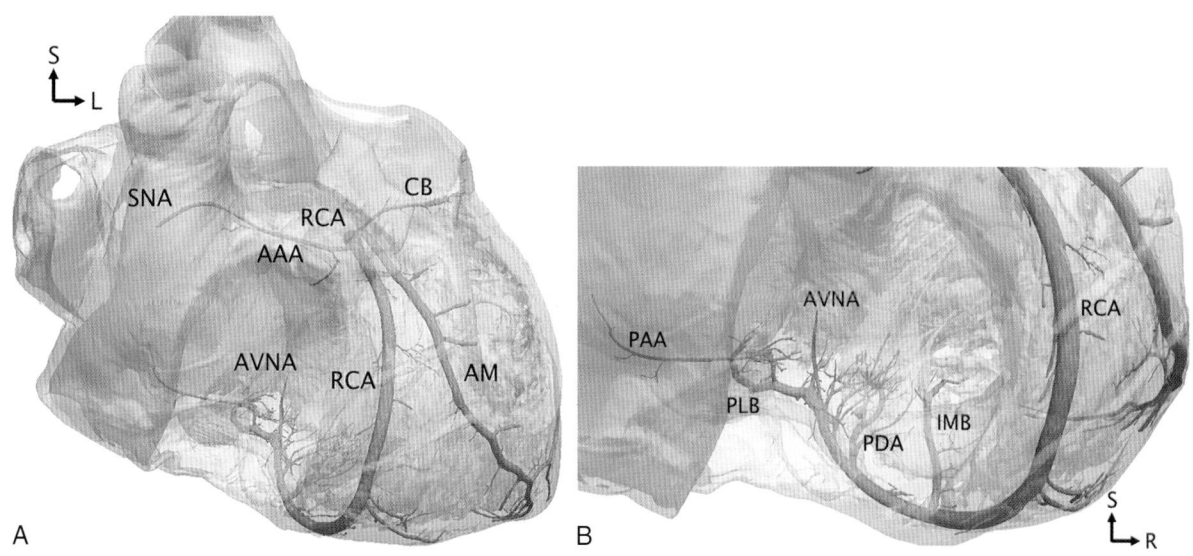

• **Fig. 3.15** Right coronary artery. **(A)** Anterior view of the right coronary artery *(RCA)* and branches—a conus branch *(CB)*, a large acute marginal artery *(AM)*, and the anterior atrial artery *(AAA)*, which supplies the sinus node artery *(SNA)*. **(B)** A posterior-inferior view showing the inferior marginal branch *(IMB)*, the posterior descending artery *(PDA)* or posterior interventricular artery with several septal perforating arteries, the posterior lateral branch *(PLB)* and the posterior atrial artery *(PAA)*. The AV nodal artery *(AVNA)* is supplied by the RCA. *L,* Left; *R,* right; *S,* superior.

from the right anterior sinus, courses in the right atrioventricular groove, and gives rise to the posterior descending artery in about 90% of subjects (Fig. 3.15). Coronary dominance is determined by which artery gives rise to the posterior descending artery. The first branch of the right coronary artery in about 60% of subjects is the anterior atrial artery, which usually supplies the sinoatrial node. In the remainder,

the anterior atrial artery arises from the left circumflex artery. Subsequent branches of the right coronary artery are a series of preventricular arteries that supply the infundibulum and anterior free wall, the acute marginal artery, and posterior atrial arteries. The atrioventricular node artery is a branch of the posterior descending artery, as are a series of perforating arteries that supply the posterior interventricular septum.

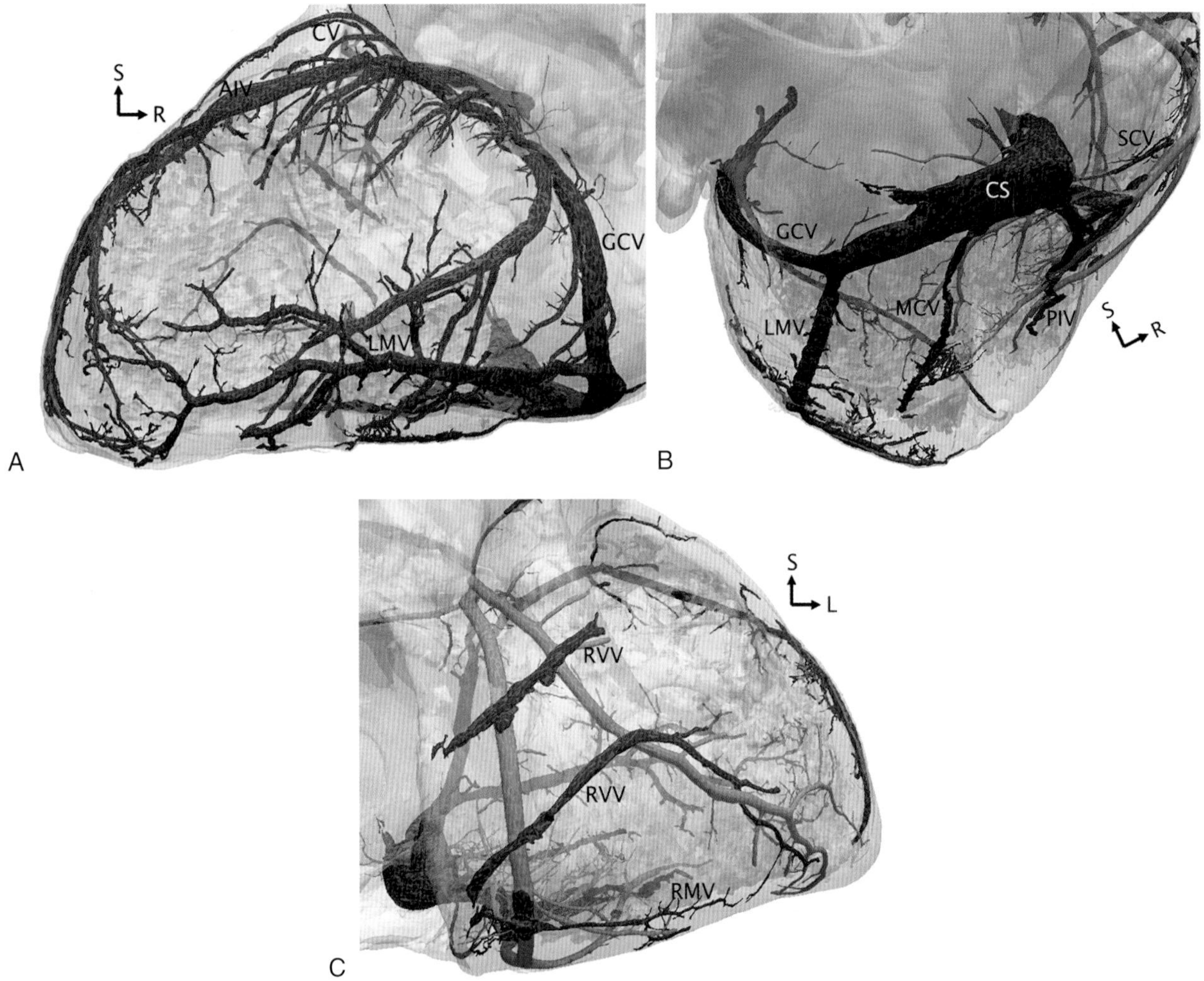

• **Fig. 3.16** Cardiac veins. **(A)** Posterior view of the left ventricle showing the anterior interventricular vein *(AIV)* that becomes the great cardiac vein *(GCV)* in the left AV groove, the conal vein *(CV)*, and the left marginal vein *(LMV)*. **(B)** Inferior view showing the coronary sinus *(CS)*, which receives the GCV, the middle cardiac vein *(MCV)*, the posterior interventricular vein *(PIV)*, and the small cardiac vein *(SCV)*. **(C)** A right anterior view showing the right ventricular veins *(RVV)* and the right marginal vein *(RMV)* that drain directly into the right atrium. *L,* Left; *R,* right; *S,* superior.

The *cardiac veins* course with the principal epicardial arteries (Fig. 3.16). The anterior interventricular vein parallels the anterior descending artery, becomes the great cardiac vein in the left atrioventricular groove, receives the marginal, left lateral, and medial veins, before joining the coronary sinus at the junction with the ligament of Marshall. The posterior interventricular vein, middle vein, and small cardiac vein join the coronary sinus directly. The infundibulum and anterior right ventricular wall are drained directly to the right atrium by the infundibular vein, right anterior vein, and right marginal vein, respectively.

Segmental Analysis

The cardiac segments are identified and characterized using the morphologic criteria described above. The situs or internal organization of each segment, the segmental alignments (what drains into what), and the segmental connections (how the cardiac segments are physically joined to each other) are determined.

The *situs* or *organization* of the three main segments is recorded using set notation.[1,4,9] The set contains three elements as {1, 2, 3} surrounded by braces and demarcated by commas (Fig. 3.17). The first element describes the visceroatrial situs which can be solitus (S), inversus (I), or ambiguus (A). The second element describes the ventricular situs or

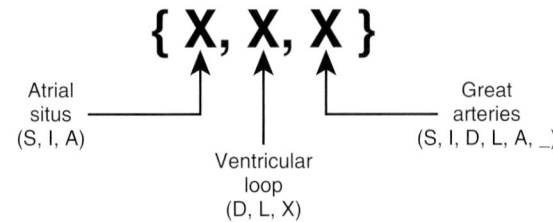

• **Fig. 3.17** Set notation shorthand for indicating situs of the main cardiac segments.

loop. Solitus or usual ventricles result from a dextral or D-loop (D) during development, while inverted or mirror-image ventricles result from a levo or L-loop (L). Rarely it is impossible to discern the ventricular situs or loop, which is indicated by X for unknown. The third element is the situs or position of the great arteries and is indicated by the position of the aortic valve relative to the pulmonary valve. The syntax for this segment is more complicated because there are more possibilities. Solitus or inversus normally related great arteries are indicated by S or I, respectively. These letters are used only if three criteria are met: the great arteries are normally related to each other (aortic valve posterior and rightward and pulmonary valve anterior and leftward for solitus, and the opposite for inversus); the great arteries are concordantly aligned with the ventricles (aorta with the left ventricle, pulmonary trunk with the right ventricle); and the great arteries are normally connected to the ventricles (aorta connected to the left ventricle by aortic-mitral fibrous continuity and the pulmonary trunk to the right ventricle by a complete conus or infundibulum). Any other arrangement with two great arteries is considered malposed great arteries, described using D when the aorta is to the right, L when the aorta is to the left, and A when the aorta is

directly anterior. If there is a single arterial root (almost always an aorta), we use either an X or leave the third position blank because there is nothing with which to compare the position of the aorta, so the other letters do not make sense. By convention, we have considered tetralogy of Fallot with pulmonary atresia and truncus arteriosus, two anomalies with a single arterial root, as forms of normally related great arteries because of the resemblance of the outflow to tetralogy of Fallot.[28] There is not universal agreement regarding the criteria for normally related great arteries. Some would consider cases in which the arterial roots are normally related to each other with only subpulmonary conus as normally related great arteries regardless of the ventriculo-arterial alignment (e.g., posterior, rightward aorta in continuity with the tricuspid valve and both great arteries aligned with the right ventricle).

The *segmental alignments* are determined by the blood flow—what drains into what.[9] The atrioventricular alignments are concordant when blood flows as in the normal heart (e.g., right atrium to right ventricle, left atrium to left ventricle), and discordant when blood flow is opposite (right atrium to left ventricle and left atrium to right ventricle) (Fig. 3.18). Other possible atrioventricular alignments

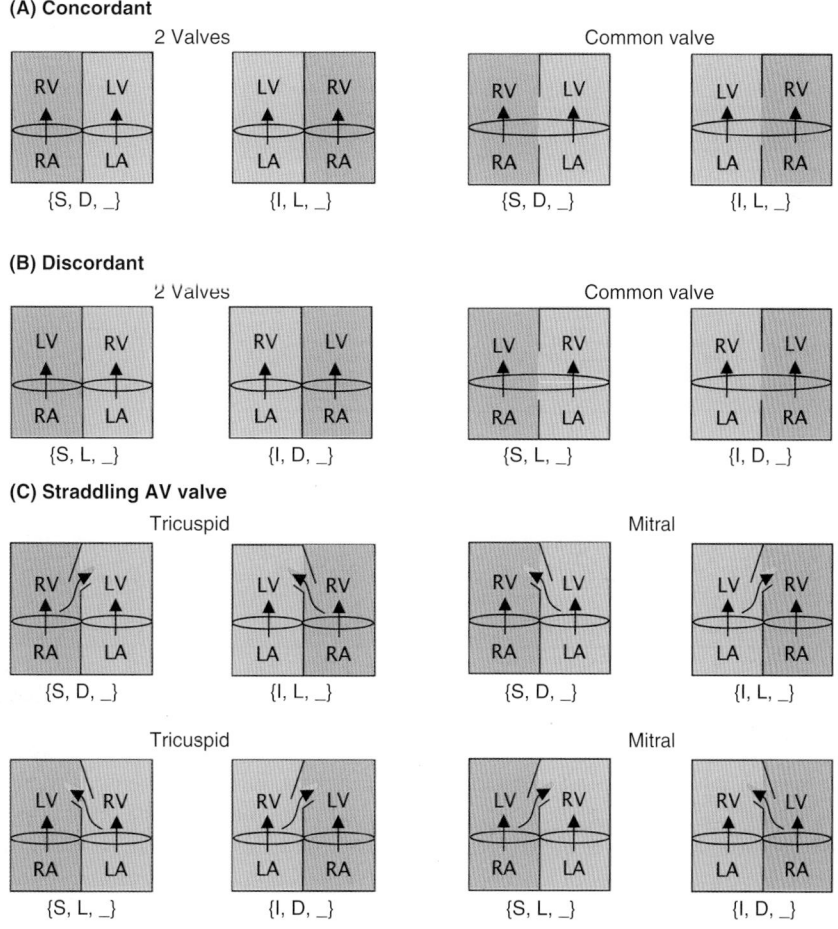

• **Fig. 3.18** Atrioventricular alignments and connections. *DILV,* Double-inlet left ventricle; *DIRV,* double-inlet right ventricle; *LA,* left atrium; *LV,* left ventricle; *OFC,* outflow chamber; *RA,* right atrium; *RV,* right ventricle.

Continued

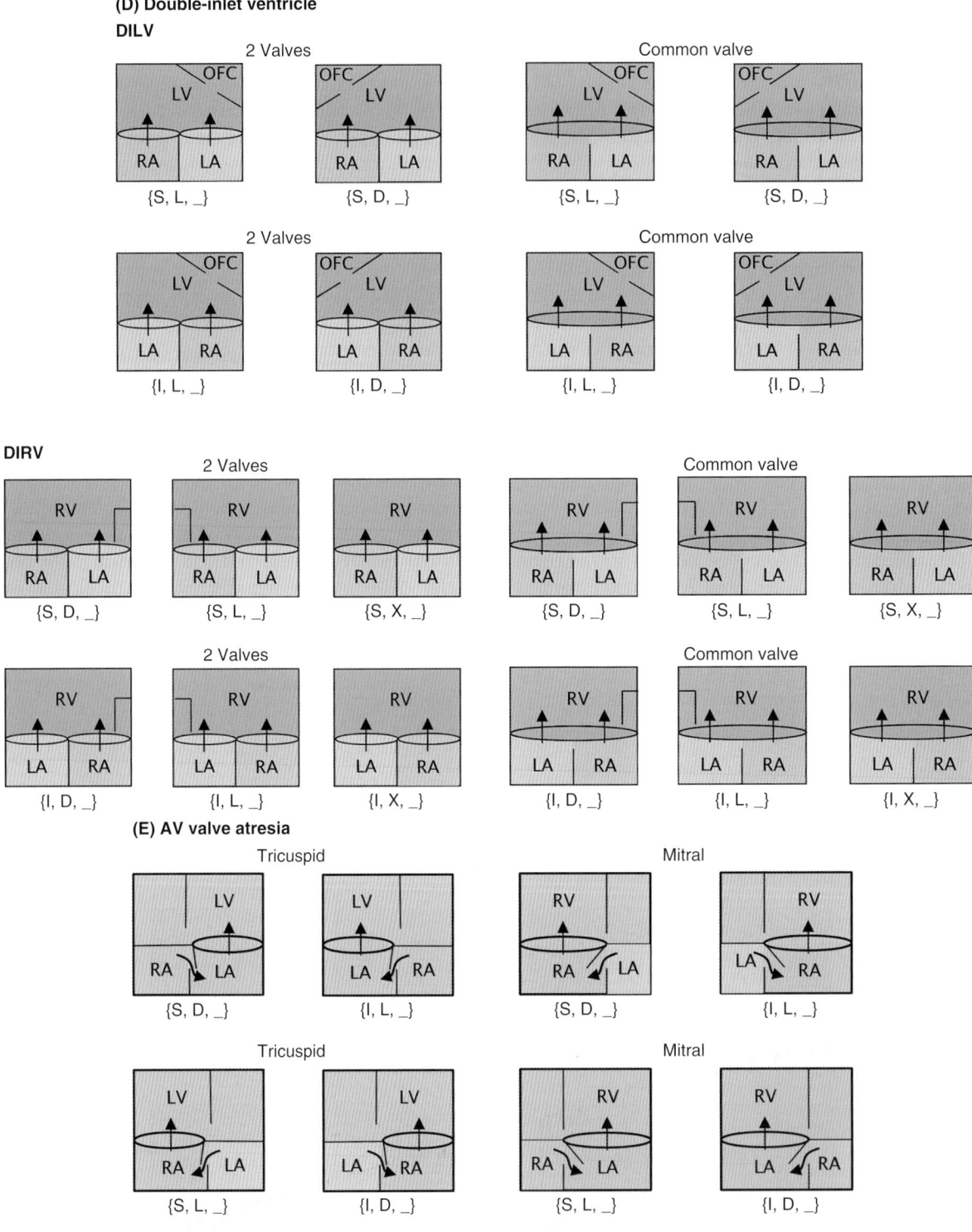

• **Fig. 3.18, cont'd**

include straddling atrioventricular valve, double-inlet ventricle, and atrioventricular valve atresia.

In the great majority of hearts, the atrioventricular segmental situs and alignments are concordant, or in harmony; i.e., if there is atrioventricular situs concordance there is also alignment concordance and vice versa.[29,30] Consequently, most of the time atrioventricular situs correctly predicts alignment. However, in rare hearts, atrioventricular situs

wrongly predicts alignment. All such hearts reported to date have juxtaposition of the atrial appendages and some have crisscross atrioventricular valves. In such cases, the presence of situs-alignment disharmony should be stated in the diagnosis, otherwise situs-alignment harmony can be assumed.

Concordant and discordant ventriculo-arterial alignments are defined in the same way as atrioventricular alignments, based on blood flow in the normal heart (Fig. 3.19).

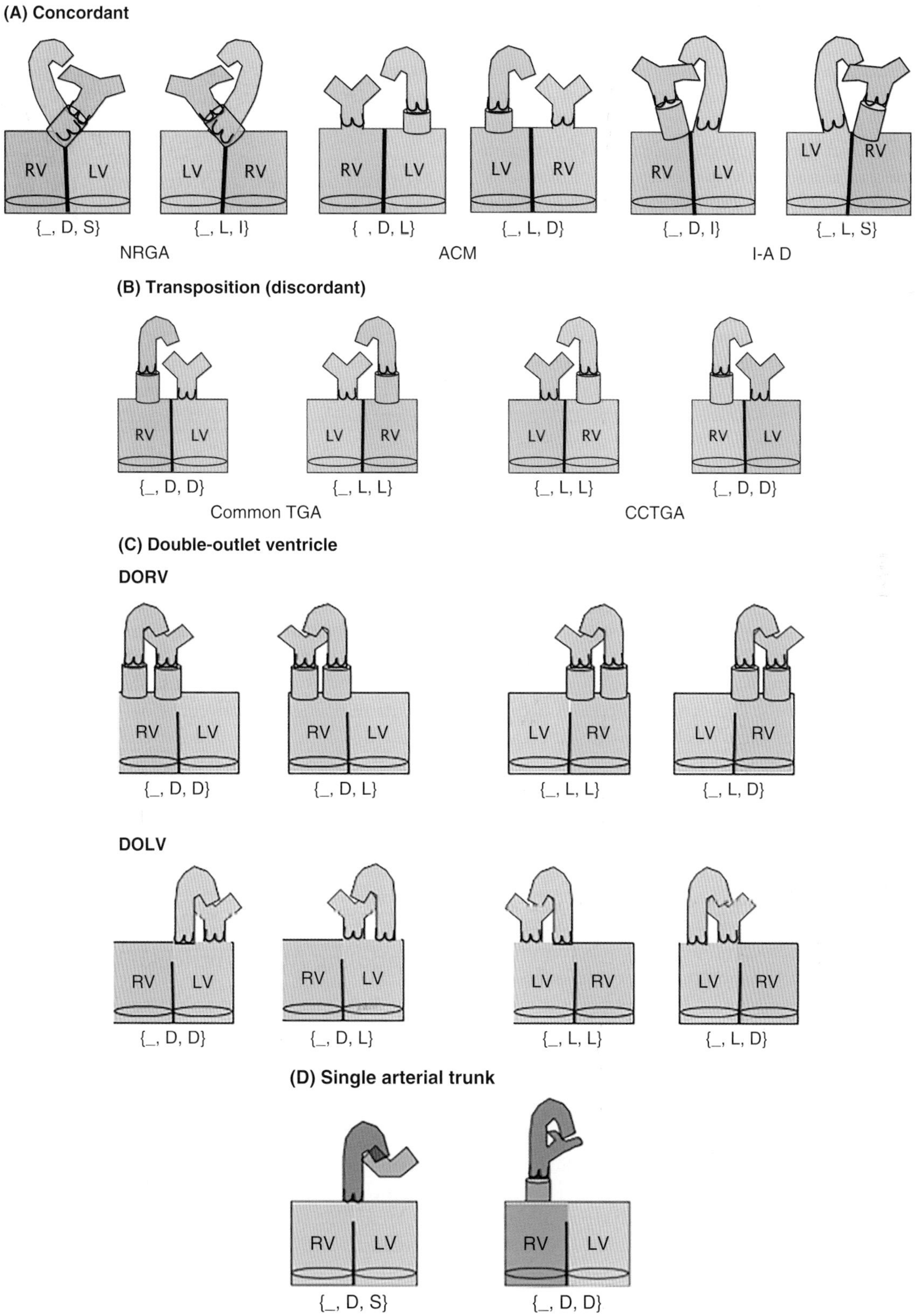

(A) Concordant

{_, D, S}   {_, L, I}   { , D, L}   {_, L, D}   {_, D, I}   {_, L, S}

NRGA   ACM   I-A D

(B) Transposition (discordant)

{_, D, D}   {_, L, L}   {_, L, L}   {_, D, D}

Common TGA   CCTGA

(C) Double-outlet ventricle

DORV

{_, D, D}   {_, D, L}   {_, L, L}   {_, L, D}

DOLV

{_, D, D}   {_, D, L}   {_, L, L}   {_, L, D}

(D) Single arterial trunk

{_, D, S}   {_, D, D}

• **Fig. 3.19** Ventriculoarterial alignments and connections. **(A)** Concordant alignments include normally related great arteries *(NRGA)*, anatomically corrected malposition *(ACM)* (only situs solitus shown with atrioventricular concordance and discordance), and infundibulo-arterial discordance *(I-A D)*. **(B)** Ventriculo-arterial discordance is another term for transposition. Common and congenitally physiologically corrected transposition *(CCTGA)* are shown in both atrial situs solitus and inversus. **(C)** Double-outlet right ventricle *(DORV)* and double-outlet left ventricle *(DOLV)* are shown in situs solitus and inversus. **(D)** Single arterial trunk is shown with an overriding trunk as a form of NRGA (tetralogy of Fallot with pulmonary atresia and as a right ventricular truncus arteriosus with complete subsemilunar conus. This could also be a right ventricular aorta with pulmonary atresia. *LV,* Left ventricle; *RV,* right ventricle.

Concordant alignments include solitus and inversus normally related great arteries, anatomically corrected malposition, and isolated ventriculo-arterial discordance. Discordant ventriculo-arterial alignment is known as transposition of the great arteries. Other possible alignments include double-outlet ventricle and single arterial root with right ventricular aorta. With the exception of normally related great arteries (S or I), ventriculo-arterial situs is not predictive of alignment; i.e., the set {_,D,D} could apply to any arterial malposition with two great arteries in which the aorta is to the right of the pulmonary trunk. Consequently, the ventriculo-arterial alignment is stated first in the diagnosis, followed by the segmental set, followed by other important diagnostic features (e.g., transposition of the great arteries {S,D,D} with straddling tricuspid valve and pulmonary stenosis).[1]

The *segmental connections* describe the manner in which segments are joined one to the other.[9] The atria and ventricles are connected by the atrioventricular canal or junction. Consequently, atrioventricular connections mirror atrioventricular canal anatomy and alignments (Fig. 3.18). The possible connections are separate valves into separate ventricles, common valve into two ventricles, straddling atrioventricular valve, double-inlet ventricle, common-inlet ventricle, atrioventricular valve atresia with imperforate valve, and atrioventricular valve atresia with absent atrioventricular connection. We separate the latter two connections because the anatomy and developmental mechanisms are different,[31] and the outcomes might be as well.

Ventriculo-arterial connections depend on conal or infundibular anatomy[4] (Fig. 3.19). Unlike at the atrioventricular junction, ventriculo-arterial alignments and connections are much more loosely correlated. In solitus and inversus normally related great arteries, there is complete subpulmonary conus only with absence of the subaortic conal free wall resulting in aortic-mitral fibrous continuity. Other ventriculo-arterial connections include subaortic conus only (typical of common or D-loop transposition of the great arteries), bilateral subarterial conus (typical of double-outlet right ventricle [DORV]), and bilaterally absent subarterial conus (rare, but seen in a variety of conotruncal anomalies).[32] This information may be stated in the main diagnosis when atypical, e.g., transposition of the great arteries {S,D,D} with bilaterally absent subarterial conus and outlet ventricular septal defect.

Segment-specific diagnoses such as atrial septal defects, ventricular septal defects, valve abnormalities, and aortic arch or pulmonary artery abnormalities are compiled and listed in the final diagnosis in segmental order.[1]

Types of Human Hearts

There are several broad categories of human hearts based on segmental analysis.[9] Segment-specific associated diagnoses may vary within each category. The following is necessarily somewhat complicated because congenital heart disease is highly variable. We have attempted to follow Einstein's advice (possibly apocryphal but no less fitting) to make things as simple as possible, but no simpler. Further simplification leaves out rare but important categories of hearts and is detrimental for clinical management and for understanding the morphogenesis of congenital heart defects.

Normal Segmental Situs, Alignments, and Connections

The normal heart comes in two varieties: solitus normally related great arteries {S,D,S} and inversus normally related great arteries {I,L,I} (Figs. 3.18A and 3.19A). The alignments are all concordant and the ventriculo-arterial connections are subpulmonary conus only with aortic-mitral fibrous continuity in both. Segment-specific diagnoses such as septal defects, valvar dysfunction, and aortic arch abnormalities might be present, but the basic architecture of the heart is normal.

Isolated Atrial Discordance

This type of heart has two forms: solitus normally related great arteries {I,D,S} with isolated atrial inversion and inversus normally related great arteries {S,L,I} with isolated atrial non-inversion[33,34] (Figs. 3.18B and 3.19A). The situs of the atria is discordant with the situs of the other segments resulting in atrioventricular alignment discordance. By definition, the ventriculo-arterial alignments are concordant and connections normal. A single segmental alignment discordance results in cyanosis, in this case due to systemic venous blood from the right atrium entering the left ventricle and aorta. The treatment is an atrial switch operation because the alignment discordance is between atria and ventricles.[35]

Straddling Atrioventricular Valve

Straddling means that an atrioventricular valve has chordal insertions on both sides of the ventricular septum. There are several variants of this category (Fig. 3.18C). Either atrioventricular valve can straddle with either atrioventricular situs concordance or discordance.[1] Here the concept of alignment concordance and discordance does not work because one atrioventricular valve is aligned with both ventricles.

Straddling tricuspid valve with atrioventricular situs concordance, {S,D,_} or {I,L,_}, allows some systemic venous blood to enter both ventricles. Straddling tricuspid valve with atrioventricular situs discordance, {S,L,_} or {I,D,_}, allows some pulmonary venous blood to enter both ventricles. The ventriculo-arterial alignment can be concordant (normal), discordant (transposition), or rarely double-outlet ventricle (Fig. 3.19A–C).

Straddling mitral valve with atrioventricular situs concordance {S,D,_} or {I,L,_} allows some pulmonary venous blood to enter both ventricles but with atrioventricular situs discordance, {S,L,_} or {I,D,_}, allows some systemic venous blood into both ventricles. Straddling mitral valve is essentially always associated with DORV (Fig. 3.19C) or occasionally transposition of the great arteries (Fig. 3.19B).

The ventriculo-arterial connection is either bilateral sub-arterial conus or subaortic conus with fibrous continuity between the pulmonary valve and the straddling part of the mitral valve.

Double-Inlet Ventricle

Both atria are aligned with the same ventricle, a left ventricle in most cases, with DIRV accounting for < 2% of cases (Fig. 3.18D). There is atrioventricular situs discordance in about 50% of double-inlet left ventricles (DILV), {S,L,_}, and concordance in about 50%, {S,D,_}. In either case, there is usually common mixing of systemic and pulmonary venous blood in the ventricle, although remarkable streaming has been reported in rare cases.[36] The atrioventricular connection is either double-inlet or common-inlet, the latter mostly in heterotaxy syndrome. The ventriculo-arterial alignment is usually discordant (transposition of the great arteries) (Fig. 3.19B) or double-outlet (Fig. 3.19C), but concordant (normally related great arteries) (Fig. 3.19A) in a few cases of DILV. In DIRV, the ventriculo-arterial alignment is always DORV (Fig. 3.19C). Ventriculo-arterial connections are usually subaortic conus only in DILV and bilateral conus in DIRV, but other types of connection occur as well.

Atrioventricular Valve Atresia

Either atrioventricular valve can be atretic, but the mechanisms seem to be different (Fig. 3.18E). Only one atrium is aligned with a ventricle, so that atrioventricular alignment concordance/discordance is not applicable. Tricuspid atresia occurs with atrioventricular situs concordance, {S,D,_} or {I,L,_}, outlet atresia of the systemic venous atrium, or in atrioventricular situs discordance, {S,L,_} or {I,D,_}, outlet atresia of the pulmonary venous atrium. The atrioventricular connection can be either absent connection, typical of tricuspid atresia with no evidence that the valve ever formed, or imperforate valve, valve elements present with fused leaflets, seen with defects that prevent normal opening of the tricuspid valve such as congenital pulmonary regurgitation with intact septum.[37] The ventriculo-arterial alignment is concordant in more than half of cases and discordant (transposition) in most of the rest (Fig. 3.19A and B).

Mitral atresia also occurs with atrioventricular situs concordance, {S,D,_} or {I,L,_}, outlet atresia of the pulmonary venous atrium, and atrioventricular situs discordance, {S,L,_} or {I,D,_}, systemic venous atrial outlet obstruction. The atrioventricular connection is much more often imperforate valve, absent connection being rare.[31] This suggests that the mitral valve usually forms, and that atresia is due to growth failure. The ventriculo-arterial alignment is usually concordant, but DORV is not rare (Fig. 3.19A and C). Even in the latter case, the ventriculo-arterial connection is often subpulmonary conus only.

Isolated Ventricular Discordance

As the name implies, there is situs discordance between the ventricular segment and the other segments, solitus normally related great arteries {S,L,S} with isolated ventricular inversion or inversus normally related great arteries {I,D,I} with isolated ventricular non-inversion[34,38] (Figs. 3.18B and 3.19A). However, there is only atrioventricular alignment discordance, resulting in cyanosis. Despite ventriculo-arterial situs discordance, there is alignment concordance because the aorta is aligned with and normally connected to the ipsilateral left ventricle and the pulmonary trunk to the ipsilateral right ventricle. As with isolated atrial discordance, the treatment is an atrial switch operation.[35] The left ventricle and mitral valve are already in the systemic circuit and the right ventricle and tricuspid valve in the pulmonary circuit.

Isolated Infundibulo-Arterial Discordance

In this rare type of heart, there is ventriculo-arterial situs discordance, solitus or inversus normally related great arteries, {S,D,I} or {I,L,S}, respectively, with isolated infundibulo-arterial discordance[39,40] (Figs. 3.18A and 3.19A). Nonetheless, ventriculo-arterial alignment is concordant and connections normal. In the absence of other significant abnormalities, the physiology is normal and the ventricles function in their usual role.[41] However, most reported cases have a ventricular septal defect and pulmonary stenosis (tetralogy of Fallot-like outflow).

Transposition of the Great Arteries

Transposition derives from the Latin verb transponere meaning to place across, in this case to place the great arteries across the ventricular septum, aorta from right ventricle and pulmonary trunk from left ventricle.[42] The ventriculo-arterial alignment discordance defines transposition, not the position of the great arteries or even the ventriculo-arterial connections. There are two broad categories of transposition, common transposition with only ventriculo-arterial alignment discordance, and congenitally physiologically corrected transposition with both atrioventricular and ventriculo-arterial alignment discordance (Figs. 3.18A, B and 3.19B).

The most frequent cardiotypes for common transposition are {S,D,D} and {I,L,L} although the position of the aorta can be variable, directly anterior (A) or even posterior (P) in rare cases.[42] Ventriculo-arterial situs discordance, in addition to alignment discordance (e.g., {S,D,L}) is a rare syndrome often associated with right ventricular hypoplasia.[43] The most common ventriculo-arterial connection in common transposition is subaortic conus only, but any type of connection is possible.[32] Common transposition causes cyanosis because there is a single segmental alignment discordance, in this case at the ventriculo-arterial level, and can be corrected with an arterial switch operation.

Congenitally physiologically corrected transposition occurs in situs solitus, {S,L,L}, as well as situs inversus {I,D,D}. Atrioventricular and ventriculo-arterial (double) discordance, in isolation, do not cause cyanosis, but the right ventricle functions as the systemic ventricle. Most cases are associated with ventricular septal defect, tricuspid valve abnormalities, and pulmonary outflow obstruction.[44] The most common ventriculo-arterial connection is subaortic conus only. Surgical correction usually involves an atrial and an arterial switch operation or intraventricular baffle to direct the left ventricle to the aorta because of the double discordance.[45] A switch operation at two levels is required to establish the left ventricle as the systemic ventricular chamber and to prevent cyanosis.

Double-Outlet Ventricle

Double-outlet ventricle means that both great arteries are aligned completely or nearly completely with one ventricle. We do not find the "50% rule"[46] useful because it is not clinically meaningful. It makes no difference to the patient or the surgeon if the aorta in tetralogy of Fallot is 50% or 60%—or even 70%—above the right ventricle. The physiology is the same and correction will be performed the same way. When the aorta is completely aligned with the right ventricle, however, the ventricular septal defect can become restrictive, aligning the left ventricle with the aorta becomes more difficult and requires commandeering right ventricular real estate, shrinking its size. As with several other categories of hearts, ventriculo-arterial concordance/discordance is not applicable.

DORV accounts for > 99% of double-outlet ventricles, double-outlet left ventricle being very rare (Fig. 3.19C). DORV is an extremely heterogenous category with essentially any cardiotype possible.[47] There are three main groups: DORV as an isolated conotruncal anomaly without other major anomalies; DORV with significant atrioventricular valve abnormalities (e.g., common atrioventricular canal, atrioventricular valve atresia, straddling valve); and DORV associated with heterotaxy syndrome (Figs. 3.18A, B, C, and E). While the most common ventriculo-arterial connection is bilateral subarterial conus, others are possible, especially subpulmonary conus only.

Double-outlet left ventricle is also quite heterogenous.[48] The variety with cardiotype {S,D,D} and pulmonary stenosis resembling tetralogy of Fallot is probably most frequent. Bilaterally deficient or absent subarterial conus is a frequent type of ventriculo-arterial connection, but others are possible as well.

Anatomically Corrected Malposition

This type of heart probably best illustrates the difference between alignment and connection. The characteristic feature is normal ventriculo-arterial alignment but abnormal connection[49,50] (Figs. 3.18A, 3.18B, and 3.19A). The most frequent type is anatomically corrected malposition {S,D,L}, with concordant atrioventricular and ventriculo-arterial alignments. However, the ventriculo-arterial connection is left-sided subaortic conus aligned with the left ventricle and either absent or deficient right-sided subpulmonary conus aligned with the right ventricle. Ventriculo-arterial situs discordance (D-loop ventricles but L-positioned aorta) is also characteristic. In the absence of associated defects, the physiology is normal. However, ventricular septal defects, usually two, are almost invariably present plus or minus pulmonary stenosis, resulting in the physiology of a large ventricular septal defect or tetralogy of Fallot. The ventricular septal defects include the typical outflow defect between the limbs of septal band and an anterior muscular defect between the subaortic infundibulum and the anterior right ventricle. Correction involves closure of the ventricular septal defects and relief of pulmonary stenosis if present. Typically, the right coronary artery crosses the pulmonary outflow tract, complicating relief of pulmonary stenosis.[51]

The less common type is anatomically corrected malposition {S,L,D}, with atrioventricular situs and alignment discordance, resulting in cyanosis even in the absence of associated defects.[52] Here the right-sided aorta with subaortic conus is aligned concordantly with the right-sided left ventricle and the left-sided pulmonary trunk, with deficient or no conus, is aligned with the left-sided right ventricle. Surgical correction here involves an atrial switch operation in addition to correction of associated defects.[35]

Both types have been reported extremely rarely in situs inversus, cardiotypes {I,L,D} and {I,D,L}.[53] Of note, the long muscular subaortic conus present in all types is at risk for dynamic, and eventually fixed, subaortic stenosis.

Single Arterial Trunk From Right Ventricle

A single arterial trunk is almost invariably an aorta or truncus arteriosus (Figs. 3.18A and B and 3.19D). If the trunk arises from the right ventricle, it cannot be considered an example of normally related great arteries, as one would the overriding aorta in tetralogy of Fallot with pulmonary atresia or truncal root in usual truncus arteriosus (see above). It also does not fit the definition of the other categories of hearts with arterial malposition described above because there is only one arterial root. The set notation for arterial malposition described above does not work because there is no other root with which to compare the position of the aorta. Consequently, the last element of the segmental set can be left blank or denoted with an X, {A,D,_} or {A,D,X}. This type of heart is seen in heterotaxy syndrome with long-segment pulmonary atresia or in rare cases of truncus arteriosus with complete subtruncal conus, usually truncus type IV.[54] The connection is subaortic or subtruncal conus only.

Summary

A comprehensive anatomic diagnosis of congenital heart defects involves the following elements:
1. Spatial position of the heart.
2. Identification of cardiac components based on morphology.

3. Analysis of segmental situs, alignments, and connections.
4. Compilation of associated defects segment by segment.

Once a complete anatomic diagnosis is established, the physiology can be deduced based on hemodynamic principles. As Dr. Richard Van Praagh often said, "Physiology is like the first derivative of anatomy, various anatomic arrangements can produce similar physiology."

Acknowledgments

We would like to express our great appreciation to Dr. Richard Van Praagh, the author of the previous edition of this chapter, as well as our mentor and colleague over many years. We also acknowledge Keito Mori, MD Candidate, Mie University Graduate School of Medicine, Mie, Japan, for creating the 3D reconstructions of coronary arteries and cardiac veins.

References

1. Van Praagh R. Diagnosis of complex congenital heart disease: morphologic-anatomic method and terminology. *Cardiovasc Intervent Radiol.* 1984;7:115-120.
2. Van Praagh R. The segmental approach to diagnosis of congenital heart disease. The cardiovascular system. *Birth Defects Orig Artic Ser.* 1972;8:4-23.
3. Van Praagh R, Vlad P. Dextrocardia, mesocardia, and levocardia: the segmental approach to diagnosis in congenital heart disease. In: Keith JD, Rowe RD, Vlad P, eds. *Heart Disease in Infancy and Childhood.* New York: Macmillan; 1978:638-695.
4. Van Praagh R, Weinberg PM, Van Praagh S. Malposition of the heart. In: Moss AJ, Adams FH, Emmanouilides GC, eds. *Heart Disease in Infants, Children and Adolescents.* 2nd ed. Baltimore: Williams and Wilkins; 1977:394-417.
5. Van Praagh R. Terminology of congenital heart disease, glossary and commentary. *Circulation.* 1977;56:139-143.
6. Lev M. Pathologic diagnosis of positional variations in cardiac chambers in congenital heart disease. *Lab Invest.* 1954;3:71-82.
7. Van Praagh R, David I, Gordon D, Wright GB, Van Praagh S. Ventricular diagnosis and designation. In: Godman MJ, ed. *Paediatric Cardiology, World Congress, London, 1980, vol. 4.* Edinburgh: Churchill Livingstone; 1981:153-168.
8. Van Praagh R, Plett JA, Van Praagh S. Single ventricle: pathology, embryology, terminology and classification. *Herz.* 1979;4:113-150.
9. Van Praagh R. The importance of segmental situs in the diagnosis of congenital heart disease. *Semin Roentgenol.* 1985;20:254-271.
10. Galli D, Domínguez JN, Zaffran S, et al. Atrial myocardium derives from the posterior region of the second heart field, which acquires left-right identity as Pitx2c is expressed. *Development.* 2008;135:1157-1167.
11. Thomas T, Yamagishi H, Overbeek PA, Olson EN, Srivastava D. The bHLH factors, dHAND and eHAND, specify pulmonary and systemic cardiac ventricles independent of left-right sidedness. *Dev Biol.* 1998;196:228-236.
12. Sizarov A, Lamers WH, Mohun TJ, Brown NA, Anderson RH, Moorman AF. Three-dimensional and molecular analysis of the arterial pole of the developing human heart. *J Anat.* 2012;220:336-349.
13. Ho SY. Anatomy of the atrioventricular junction, atrioventricular grooves, and accessory pathways. *Card Electrophysiol Clin.* 2020;12:437-445.
14. Merrick AF, Yacoub MH, Ho SY, Anderson RH. Anatomy of the muscular subpulmonary infundibulum with regard to the Ross procedure. *Ann Thorac Surg.* 2000;69:556-561.
15. Çiçek S, Arslan AH, Ugurlucan M, Yildiz Y, Ay S. Scimitar syndrome: the curved Turkish sabre. *Semin Thorac Cardiovasc Surg Pediatr Card Surg Annu.* 2014;17:56-61.
16. Chen SJ, Lee WJ, Lin MT, et al. Left pulmonary artery sling complex: computed tomography and hypothesis of embryogenesis. *Ann Thorac Surg.* 2007;84:1645-1650.
17. Gabriel A, Donnelly J, Kuc A, et al. Ectopia cordis: a rare congenital anomaly. *Clin Anat.* 2014;27:1193-1199.
18. Escobar-Diaz MC, Sunderji S, Tworetzky W, Moon-Grady AJ. The fetus with ectopia cordis: experience and expectations from two centers. *Pediatr Cardiol.* 2017;38:531-538.
19. Anderson RH, Brown NA, Moorman AFM. Development and structures of the venous pole of the heart. *Dev Dyn.* 2006;235:2-9.
20. Ho SY, Sánchez-Quintana D. Anatomy and pathology of the sinus node. *J Interv Card Electrophysiol.* 2016;46:3-8.
21. Ho SY. Clinical pathology of the cardiac conduction system. *Novartis Found Symp.* 2003;250:210-221.
22. Frescura C, Ho SY, Giordano M, Thiene G. Isomerism of the atrial appendages: morphology and terminology. *Cardiovasc Pathol.* 2020;47:107205.
23. Sanders SP, Pluchinotta FR. Tricuspid valve: embryology and anatomy. In: Giamberti A, Chessa M, eds. *The Tricuspid Valve in Congenital Heart Disease.* 1st ed. Milano: Springer; 2014:1-11.
24. Silbiger JJ, Bazaz R. Contemporary insights into the functional anatomy of the mitral valve. *Am Heart J.* 2009;158:887-895.
25. Franco D, Meilhac SM, Christoffels VM, et al. Left and right ventricular contributions to the formation of the interventricular septum in the mouse heart. *Dev Biol.* 2006;294:366-375.
26. Lopez L, Houyel L, Colan SD, et al. Classification of ventricular septal defects for the eleventh iteration of the international classification of diseases - striving for consensus: a report from the International Society for Nomenclature of Paediatric and Congenital Heart Disease. *Ann Thorac Surg.* 2018;106:1578-1589.
27. Loukas M, Groat C, Khangura R, Owens DG, Anderson RH. The normal and abnormal anatomy of the coronary arteries. *Clin Anat.* 2009;22:114-128.
28. Van Praagh R. Truncus arteriosus: what is it really and how should it be classified? *Eur J Cardiothorac Surg.* 1987;1:65-70.
29. Anderson RH, Smith A, Wilkinson JL. Disharmony between atrio-ventricular connections and segmental combination. unusual variants of "crisscross" hearts. *J Am Coll Cardiol.* 1987;10:1273-1276.
30. Van Praagh R. When concordant or discordant atrioventricular alignments predict the ventricular situs wrongly. I. Solitus atria, concordant alignments, and l-loop ventricles. II. Solitus atria, discordant alignments, and d-loop ventricles. *J Am Coll Cardiol.* 1987;10:1278-1279.
31. Ando M, Satomi G, Takao A. Atresia of tricuspid or mitral orifice: anatomic spectrum and morphogenetic hypothesis. In: Van Praagh R, Takao A, eds. *Etiology and Morphogenesis of Congenital Heart Disease.* Mt. Kisco: Futura; 1980:421-487.
32. Pasquini L, Sanders SP, Parness IA, et al. Conal anatomy in 119 patients with d-loop transposition of the great arteries and ventricular septal defect: an echocardiographic and pathologic study. *J Am Coll Cardiol.* 1993;21:1712-1721.
33. Clarkson PM, Brandt PWT, Barratt-Boyes BG, Neutze JM. Isolated atrial inversion. *Am J Cardiol.* 1972;29:877-881.

34. Pasquini L, Sanders SP, Parness I, et al. Echocardiographic and anatomic findings in atrioventricular discordance and ventriculoarterial concordance. *Am J Cardiol.* 1988;62:1256-1262.

35. Konstantinov IE, Lai L, Colan SD, et al. Atrioventricular discordance with ventriculoarterial concordance: a remaining indication for the atrial switch operation. *J Thorac Cardiovasc Surg.* 2004;128:944-945.

36. Macartney FJ, Partridge JB, Scott O, Deverall PB. Common or single ventricle. An angiocardiographic and hemodynamic study of 42 patient. *Circulation.* 1976;53:543-554.

37. Weinberg PM. Anatomy of tricuspid atresia and its relevance to current forms of surgical therapy. *Ann Thorac Surg.* 1980;29: 306-311.

38. Van Praagh R, Van Praagh S. Isolated ventricular inversion: a consideration of morphogenesis, definition and diagnosis of nontransposed and transposed great arteries. *Am J Cardiol.* 1966;17:395-406.

39. Foran RB, Belcourt C, Nanton MA, et al. Isolated infundibulo-arterial inversion {S,D,I}: A newly recognized form of congenital heart disease. *Am Heart J.* 1988;116:1337-1350.

40. Santini F, Jonas RA, Sanders SP, Van Praagh R. Tetralogy of Fallot {S,D,I}: successful repair without a conduit. *Ann Thorac Surg.* 1995;59:747-749.

41. Liske MR, Kavanaugh-McHugh AL, Parra DA. Isolated infundibuloarterial inversion. *Pediatr Cardiol.* 2006;27:289-292.

42. Van Praagh R, Perez-Trevino C, Lopez-Cuellar M, et al. Transposition of the great arteries with posterior aorta, anterior pulmonary artery, sub-pulmonary conus and fibrous continuity between aortic and atrioventricular valves. *Am J Cardiol.* 1971;28:621-631.

43. Houyel L, Van Praagh R, Lacour-Gayet F, et al. Transposition of the great arteries {S,D,L}. Pathologic anatomy, diagnosis, and surgical management of a newly recognized complex. *J Thorac Cardiovasc Surg.* 1995;110:613-624.

44. Graham Jr TP, Bernard YD, Mellen BG, et al. Long-term outcome in congenitally corrected transposition of the great arteries. *Am Coll Cardiol.* 2000;36:255-261.

45. Karl TR, Weintraub RG, Brizard CP, Cochrane AD, Mee RB. Senning plus arterial switch operation for discordant (congenitally corrected) transposition. *Ann Thorac Surg.* 1997;64: 495-502.

46. Anderson RH, Becker AE, Wilcox BR, Macartney FJ, Wilkinson JL. Surgical anatomy of double-outlet right ventricle - a reappraisal. *Am J Cardiol.* 1983;52:555-559.

47. Van Praagh S, Davidoff A, Chin A, et al. Double outlet right ventricle - anatomic types and developmental implications based on a study of 101 autopsied cases. *Coeur.* 1982;13:389-440.

48. Van Praagh R, Weinberg PM, Srebro JP. Double-outlet left ventricle. In: Adams FH, Emmanouilides GC, Riemenschneider TA, eds. *Moss' Heart Disease in Infants, Children, and Adolescents.* Baltimore: Williams & Wilkins; 1989:461-485.

49. Van Praagh R, Durnin RE, Jockin H, et al. Anatomically corrected malposition of the great arteries {S, D, L}. *Circulation.* 1975;51:20-31.

50. Anderson RH, Becker AE, Losekoot TG, Gerlis LM. Anatomically corrected malposition of great arteries. *Br Heart J.* 1975;37:993-1013.

51. Huang SC, Chiu IS, Lee ML, et al. Coronary artery anatomy in anatomically corrected malposition of the great arteries and their surgical implications. *Eur J Cardiothorac Surg.* 2011;39:705-710.

52. Zakheim R, Mattioli L, Vaseenon T, Edwards W. Anatomically corrected malposition of the great arteries {S,L,D}. *Chest.* 1976;69:101-104.

53. Anderson RH, Arnold R, Jones RS. D-bulboventricular loop with l-transposition in situs inversus. *Circulation.* 1972;46: 173-179.

54. Matsuoka R, Van Praagh S, Van Praagh R. Rare types of truncus arteriosus communis. *Circulation.* 1982;66:II–359.

4

Fetal and Transitional Circulation

DAVID W. BROWN, MICHAEL D. FREED, AND JOHN E. MAYER JR.

KEY LEARNING POINTS

- The fetal circulation is a parallel circulation rather than a circulation in series, facilitated by the key fetal shunts—the ductus venosus, foramen ovale, and ductus arteriosus.
- The right ventricle performs about two-thirds of the cardiac work *in utero* and is at systemic pressure, reflected in chamber size and thickness, which may explain why right-sided defects are generally better tolerated than left-sided defects after birth.
- The preferential right-to-left shunting of umbilical venous blood across the foramen ovale to the left heart allows for the most oxygenated, nutrient-rich blood from the placenta to be directed to the developing myocardium and fetal brain.
- Right-to-left shunting at the ductus arteriosus allows most right ventricular blood to bypass the high-resistance lung vasculature and return to the descending aorta and the placenta.
- The parallel fetal circulation facilitated by these fetal shunts allows for continued adequate *in utero* tissue and placental

blood flow even in the setting of a wide variety of complex cardiac malformations.
- At birth, the transition to a circulation in series is remarkable for a dramatic drop in pulmonary vascular resistance, increase in pulmonary blood flow, and thus left heart filling, and simultaneous dramatic increase in systemic vascular resistance with removal of the low-resistance placenta with clamping of the umbilical cord. Flow across the three fetal shunts typically becomes negligible as each transitions toward closure over subsequent hours to days of life.
- Disturbances in normal fetal circulatory flow patterns from congenital malformations can affect the normal growth of cardiac chambers, valves, and vascular structures with the result that many congenital cardiac defects occur in association with hypoplasia of other structures in the same fetal flow pathway.

Fetal Circulation

Most of our modern understanding of the circulation before birth comes from more than 40 years of research on fetal lambs.[1-4] More recently, some of this data have been largely corroborated by phase-contrast cardiac magnetic imaging studies in near-term human fetuses.[5] The fetal circulation is arranged in parallel, rather than in a series, the right ventricle delivering the majority of its output to the placenta for oxygenation, and the left ventricle delivering the majority of its output to the heart, brain, and upper part of the body (Fig. 4.1). However, there is mixing of the streams at the atrial level that sends more highly saturated blood to the fetal myocardium and brain, and shunting at the great vessel level that diverts blood from the immature lungs to the placenta for oxygen exchange. This parallel circulation permits fetal survival despite a wide variety of complex cardiac lesions.

Key to understanding the fetal circulatory physiology is appreciating crucial aspects of the placenta and the fetal lungs. The placenta is a unique and remarkable low-resistance organ that is responsible for a number of functions, including oxygen and carbon dioxide gas exchange, elimination of waste

products such as urea and bilirubin, synthesis of glycogen and fatty acids, production of a variety of hormones, and transfer of crucial nutrients including glucose, amino acids, and immunoglobulins and other proteins to the fetus. The fetal lungs are relatively collapsed and filled with fetal lung fluid secreted by the developing fetal lungs, with the saccular and (very late in gestation) alveolar spaces deflated; the pulmonary circulation *in utero* is a high-resistance circuit. Thus, in broad strokes, the fetal circulation is designed to maximize flow to the placenta while minimizing flow through the lung circulation.

Fetal Circulatory Blood Flows

Due to the parallel nature of the fetal circulation, flow in various components of the system is often expressed as a percentage of combined ventricular output (Fig. 4.1). Normally, blood returning from the placenta via the umbilical vein courses through the fetal liver, draining via the **ductus venosus** into the distal left hepatic vein or directly into the inferior vena cava near its junction with the right atrium. The ductus venosus allows the majority of oxygen and nutrient-rich venous blood from the placenta to bypass the

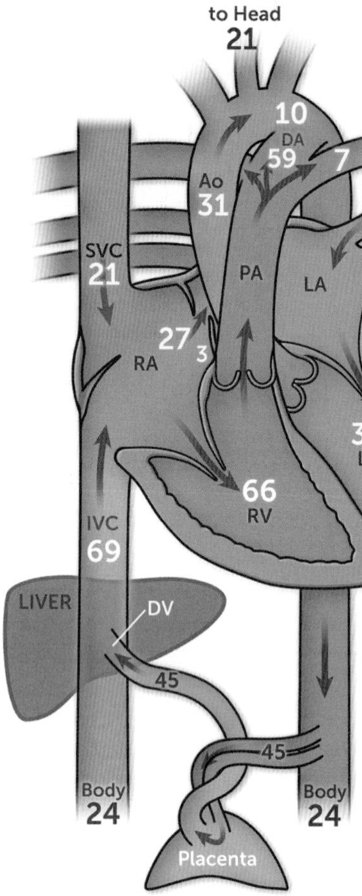

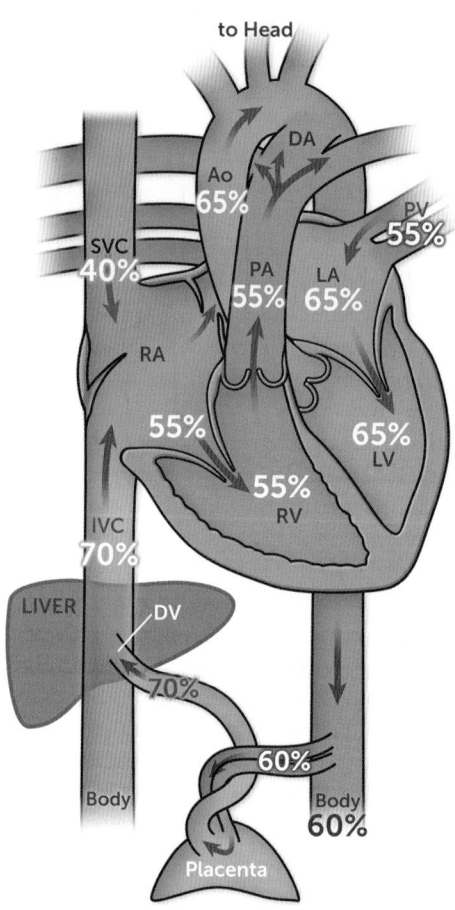

• **Fig. 4.1** Fetal circulatory blood flow. The course of the circulation in the late-gestation fetal lamb. The numbers represent the percentages of combined ventricular outputs. Blood returning from the placenta passes through the liver, with the majority passing through the ductus venosus *(DV)* to the inferior vena cava *(IVC)*. Some of the return from the IVC is diverted by the crista dividens and Eustachian valve in the right atrium *(RA)* through the foramen ovale into the left atrium *(LA)*, where it meets the pulmonary venous return *(PV)* and passes into the left ventricle *(LV)* and is pumped into the ascending aorta. Most of the ascending aortic flow goes to the coronary, subclavian, and carotid arteries, with only 10% of combined ventricular output passing through the aortic arch (indicated by the narrowed point in the aorta) into the descending aorta *(Ao)*. The remainder of the IVC flow mixes with return from the superior vena cava *(SVC)* and coronary veins (3%) and passes into the RA and right ventricle *(RV)* and is pumped into the pulmonary artery *(PA)*. Because of the high pulmonary resistance, only 7%–10% passes through the lungs (PV), with the rest going into the ductus arteriosus *(DA)* and then to the Ao, to the placenta and lower half of the body. (Data modified from Rudolph AM. The changes in the circulation after birth. Their importance in congenital heart disease. *Circulation.* 1970;41:343–359.)

• **Fig. 4.2** The fetal hypoxemic environment. The numbers indicate the percentage of oxygen saturation in the late-gestation lamb. The oxygen saturation is the highest in the inferior vena cava *(IVC)*, representing flow that is primarily from the placenta. The saturation of the blood in the heart is slightly higher on the left side than on the right side due to the higher saturated placental return diverted through the PFO to the left side of the heart. *Ao,* Aorta; *DA,* ductus arteriosus; *DV,* ductus venosus; *LA,* left atrium; *LV,* left ventricle; *PA,* pulmonary artery; *PV,* pulmonary venous; *RA,* right atrium; *RV,* right ventricle; *SVC,* superior vena cava. (Data modified from Rudolph AM. The changes in the circulation after birth. Their importance in congenital heart disease. *Circulation.* 1970;41:343–359.)

hepatic sinusoidal circulation. The ductus venosus also has a sphincter-like function that prevents excessive venous return to the right atrium; in rare cases of congenital absence of the ductus venosus, cardiac congestion with dilated atria and atrioventricular valve regurgitation is noted.

In the right atrium, the blood from the inferior vena cava is divided into two streams by the crista dividens and the Eustachian valve, fetal structures that direct some of the umbilical venous blood across the atrial septum; about

40% of the blood returning from the inferior vena cava (27% of the combined ventricular output) passes across the **foramen ovale** into the left atrium, where it joins with the pulmonary venous return from the fetal lungs, passing through the mitral valve into the left ventricle. This blood is then pumped out the ascending aorta where it supplies the coronary, carotid, and subclavian arteries. The nature of shunting at the foramen ovale allows the most oxygen- and nutrient-rich blood to be supplied to the developing myocardium and fetal brain. The remaining third of ascending aorta flow (10% of combined ventricular output) passes across the distal aortic arch (the aortic isthmus) into the descending aorta.

The majority of blood returning from the inferior vena cava joins the superior vena caval drainage and coronary sinus return before passing through the tricuspid valve into the right ventricle and pulmonary artery. Because the fluid-filled lungs and constricted pulmonary arterioles offer a high resistance to flow, most of the blood, almost 90%, passes not to the lungs but through the open **ductus arteriosus** into the descending aorta and the low-resistance placenta.

There is animal experimental evidence and inferential clinical evidence that disturbances in these normal fetal blood flow patterns have effects on the development of the cardiac chambers, valves, and vasculature. Most commonly decreased *in utero* flow through a developing cardiovascular structure is associated with hypoplasia of that structure.[6]

Fetal Hypoxemic Environment

The oxygen saturation and content of the blood are considerably lower in the fetus than in the neonate or child, because of the lower efficiency of the placenta compared with the lung as an organ for oxygen exchange (Fig. 4.2). The fetus compensates for this hypoxemic environment by at least three important adaptations. First, the fetal kidneys respond by increasing erythropoietin, which increases red blood cell production and red cell mass, improving oxygen-carrying capacity of fetal blood; the hematocrit at birth is typically in the 45%–60% range. Second, fetal red blood cells contain fetal hemoglobin, which has a higher affinity for oxygen than other forms of hemoglobin. This results in a leftward shift of the oxyhemoglobin curve, allowing for increased oxygen uptake in low-oxygen environments such as the placenta. Third, the fetus has reduced oxygen consumption relative to the newborn due to maternal and placental supports, including less energy expenditure for thermoregulation, respiration, digestion, and renal resorption.

Blood returning from the placenta via the umbilical veins has the highest Po_2 (32–35 mm Hg; oxygen saturation, 70%). The blood that passes into the right atrium is diverted through the foramen ovale into the left atrium and mixes with the less saturated pulmonary venous return, lowering the Po_2 slightly to 26–28 mm Hg (oxygen saturation about 65%) in the left ventricle before its distribution to the ascending aorta and upper half of the body.

The umbilical venous return destined for the right ventricle mixes with the superior vena caval return (Po_2 12–14 mm Hg; oxygen saturation, 40%), reducing the oxygen tension of blood passing into the right ventricle, main pulmonary artery, and descending aorta to about 20–22 mm Hg (oxygen saturation, 50%–55%). Thus, blood with the highest oxygen content is diverted to the coronary arteries and brain, and that with the lowest oxygen content is diverted to the placenta, increasing the efficiency of fetal circulatory oxygen uptake in the low-oxygen environment.

Fetal Hemodynamics, Myocardium, and Circulatory Responses

The wide communication between the atria allows for near equalization of pressures in the atria (Fig. 4.3). Similarly, the patency and large size of the ductus arteriosus results in equalization of pressures in the aorta and pulmonary artery.

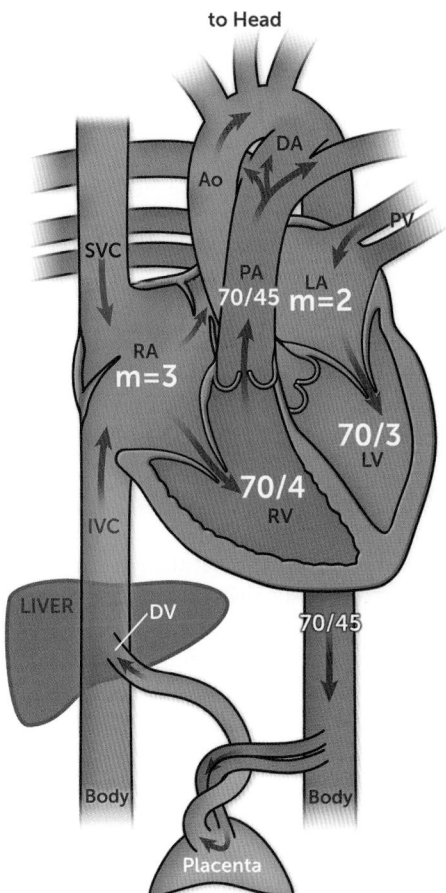

• **Fig. 4.3** Fetal hemodynamics. The numbers indicate the pressures observed in late-gestation lambs. Because large communications between the atrium and great vessels are present, the pressures on both sides of the heart are virtually identical. *Ao,* Aorta; *DA,* ductus arteriosus; *DV,* ductus venosus; *IVC,* inferior vena cava; *LA,* left atrium; *LV,* left ventricle; *PA,* pulmonary artery; *PV,* pulmonary venous; *RA,* right atrium; *RV,* right ventricle; *SVC,* superior vena cava. (Data modified from Rudolph AM. The changes in the circulation after birth. Their importance in congenital heart disease. *Circulation.* 1970;41:343–359.)

Because atrial and great vessel pressures are equal, in the absence of pulmonic or aortic stenosis, the ventricular pressures are also equal, with a late gestation systolic pressure of approximately 70 mm Hg, using amniotic pressure as zero.

The fetus has a limited ability to adjust cardiac output. The primary determinants of cardiac output are heart rate, filling pressure (preload), resistance against which the ventricles eject (afterload), and myocardial contractility. The most important fetal circulatory response to adjust fetal cardiac output is in changing heart rate. Spontaneous changes in heart rate are associated with electrocortical activity as well as with the sleep rate and fetal activity. Using continuous measurements of left and right ventricular output, utilizing electromagnetic flow probes, Rudolph and Heymann[7] have shown that spontaneous increases in heart rate are associated with increasing ventricular output, whereas decreases in heart rate result in a considerable fall of both right and left ventricular output. By electrically pacing the right atrium above the resting level of 160–180 beats/minute, the left ventricular output eventually increases to about 15% above resting levels. Decreasing the heart rate by 50% by vagal stimulation caused a fall in output of approximately 30%.

Contrary to the significant effects of increasing or decreasing heart rate on fetal cardiac output, increasing preload (even to levels as high as a right atrial pressure of 20 mm Hg) produces only relatively small increases in the ventricular output, suggesting that the fetal ventricle normally functions near the top of its Starling function curve and has little reserve to increase cardiac output. Increasing the work of the heart by increasing afterload (by inflating a balloon in the fetal descending aorta or by methoxamine)[8] produces a dramatic fall in right ventricular output, suggesting that the fetal heart is very sensitive to increases in afterload.

Morphometric studies on the fetal myocardium have demonstrated a significant decrease in myofibrillar content per tissue volume, suggesting that the fetal myocardium has much less contractile tissue than the adult. The active tension produced in excised strips of fetal myocardium was less than that produced by adult myocardium, possibly because of the myofibrillar content, a reduced content of sarcoplasmic reticulum, and/or the T-tubule system.[9]

All of the above data suggest that the fetal myocardium is structurally and functionally immature compared with an older child or adult. The fetal heart appears to work at the peak of its ventricular function curve, with increases in preload causing little or no change in the cardiac output, and increases in afterload resulting in a marked depression. The limited ability of the fetal heart to respond to stress seems to be mediated primarily through increasing the heart rate.

Fetal Circulatory Consequences With Congenital Heart Disease

The structure, hemodynamics, and myocardial function of the fetal circulation have significant consequences in the neonate with congenital heart disease:

- The parallel circulation, with connections at the atrial and great vessel level, allows a wide variety of cardiac malformations (even severe forms, with valvar atresia and anatomic variations of single ventricle) to provide adequate transport of blood to the placenta to pick up oxygen and deliver it to the tissues.
- The right ventricle performs approximately two-thirds of the cardiac work before birth. This is reflected in the size and thickness of the right ventricle before and after birth and may explain why left-sided defects are poorly tolerated after birth compared with right-sided lesions.
- Because the normal flow across the aortic isthmus is small (10% of ventricular output), the aortic isthmus is especially vulnerable to small changes in intracardiac flow from various congenital defects. This may account for the relatively high incidence of narrowing (coarctation of the aorta) or atresia (interrupted aortic arch) in this region as the ductus arteriosus closes in the setting of lesions like mitral valve disease, bicuspid aortic valve

or subaortic stenosis or other congenital lesions that may decrease left ventricular flow.
- Because pulmonary blood flow *in utero* is very small compared with that immediately after birth, anomalies preventing normal pulmonary return (total anomalous pulmonary return, cor triatriatum, etc.) may be well tolerated but difficult to detect *in utero* when pulmonary venous return is normally low. This small amount of flow is nevertheless critical to the normal development of pulmonary vasculature.
- Fetal adaptations to the low levels of circulating oxygen before birth, including increased hematocrit, may account for the relative comfort of newborn infants with cyanotic heart disease who may be active and feed well with an arterial Po_2 of 20–25 mm Hg, a level that would lead to cerebral and cardiac anoxia, acidosis, and death within a few minutes for the older child or adult.
- The limited ability of the fetal circulation to respond to stress, including immature myocardium and relative dependence on heart rate alone for augmenting cardiac output, makes the hemodynamic consequences of congenital heart disease after birth that much more difficult to tolerate.
- Birth is a time of stress for the left ventricle. With the switch from parallel to an in-series circulation, there is an increased amount of left heart blood to pump and higher systemic vascular resistance with removal of the placenta from the circulation. In addition, there is increased fetal oxygen demand with assumption of the work of thermal regulation, respiration, and digestion that was previously done by the placenta.

Transitional Circulation

Within a few moments of birth, profound changes must occur as the newborn rapidly switches from the placenta to the lung as the organ of respiration.[10] Failure of any one of a complex series of pulmonary or cardiac events that take place within minutes of birth can lead to generalized hypoxemia and brain damage or death.

Soon after the onset of spontaneous respiration, the placenta is removed from the circulation, either by clamping the umbilical cord or, more naturally, by constriction of the umbilical arteries. This suddenly increases the systemic resistance as the low-resistance placenta is excluded from the circulation. At approximately the same time, the onset of spontaneous respiration expands the lungs and brings oxygen to the pulmonary alveoli. Reduction in the pulmonary vascular resistance results from simple physical expansion of the vessels and from the chemo-reflex vasodilation of the pulmonary arteries caused by the high level of oxygen in the alveolar gas.

This sudden increase in systemic vascular resistance and drop in pulmonary vascular resistance causes a reversal of the flow through the ductus arteriosus from right-to-left to left-to-right. Before birth, the relative pulmonary and systemic resistances cause 90% of the right ventricular output to go through the ductus arteriosus into the descending aorta; by a few minutes after birth, 90% of right ventricular output goes to the pulmonary arteries, with the pulmonary blood flow increasing from 35 mL/kg/minute to 160–200 mL/kg/minute.

The rapid drop in systemic venous return to the inferior vena cava as the umbilical venous flow is cut off, as well as the increase in pulmonary venous return as the pulmonary blood flow increases, causes the left atrial pressure to rise and the right atrial pressure to fall. When left atrial pressure exceeds right atrial pressure, the flap valve of the foramen ovale closes against the edge of the crista dividens, eliminating left-to-right or right-to-left shunting.

There have been questions in the past regarding how much these marked circulatory changes are influenced by the mechanical changes in the lung parenchyma due to the onset of ventilation, how much by the vasodilatory effects of oxygen, and how much by the increase in systemic vascular resistance, with constriction of the umbilical vessels removing low-resistance placenta from the circulation. Teitel et al.,[11] using monitored fetal sheep near term, found that ventilation alone caused dramatic changes in the central flow patterns, attributable to a large decrease in pulmonary vascular resistance and an associated increase in pulmonary blood flow. Ventilation alone increased the pulmonary venous return from 8% of combined ventricular output to 31%, whereas right ventricular output (which had formerly ejected 90% to the ductus arteriosus) was reduced to less than 50%. Oxygenation further changed the flow patterns, so that more than 90% of the flow from the main pulmonary artery went to the lungs rather than through the ductus arteriosus. Umbilical cord occlusion had few additional effects.

Usually, the ductus arteriosus remains patent for several hours or days after birth. Initially, the pulmonary vascular resistance exceeds systemic vascular resistance, so that there is a small right-to-left (pulmonary artery-to-aorta) shunt with some systemic desaturation to the lower half of the body. Anything that increases the pulmonary vascular resistance, such as acidosis, hypoxemia, polycythemia, or lung disease, may exacerbate or prolong the normal transient left-to-right shunt. Within a few hours of birth, however, in the normal child, the pulmonary vascular resistance has fallen below systemic vascular resistance, resulting in a small "physiologic" left-to-right (aorta-to-pulmonary artery) shunt with slightly increased pulmonary flow but no arterial desaturation. Normally, within 10–15 hours of birth, the ductus arteriosus has closed eliminating shunting, although permanent structural closure (represented in the ligamentum arteriosum) may not take place for another 2 to 3 weeks.

The mechanism of closure of the ductus arteriosus is not completely understood, although it is generally characterized by two phases: functional closure with ductal constriction; and anatomical closure with vascular remodeling. During intrauterine life, low levels of circulating oxygen and high levels of prostaglandin E_2[12] (PGE_2) produced by the placenta and the ductus arteriosus help maintain ductal patency. After birth, the placenta is removed from the circulation, PGE_2 is metabolized in the pulmonary circulation, and there is further decline of signaling by downregulation of ductal PGE_2 receptors, resulting in ductal constriction.[13] The administration of exogenous PGE_1, which acts via receptors to increase intracellular levels of cyclic AMP and cause vasodilation, has been demonstrated to keep the ductus arteriosus open for days, weeks, or months in infants with congenital heart disease.[14] For more than 40 years, intravenous PGE_1 has been the mainstay of therapy for the clinical stabilization of infants with ductal-dependent congenital heart disease prior to more definitive surgical or transcatheter intervention. Furthermore, inhibitors of the prostaglandin production pathway such as indomethacin,[15] ibuprofen,[16] and, more recently, acetaminophin[17] have been demonstrated to cause ductal constriction in premature infants with patent ductus arteriosus; the effectiveness/side-effect profile currently favors ibuprofen in these infants, although further investigation for the optimal strategy is ongoing.

The vascular remodeling phase of ductal closure is more complex and less well understood but involves multiple histologic changes including disruption of the vascular elastic lamina layer of the ductus, ingrowth of endothelial cells, increased extracellular matrix production, and migration and proliferation of smooth muscle cells into the subendothelial space.[18] These changes all bring about a cushion of tissue that helps obliterate the vessel lumen, along with the adhesion of blood cellular components such as mononuclear cells,[19] activated by local vascular wall ischemia pathways, and platelets that form a platelet plug.[20] There is some evidence that thrombocytopenia can be associated with increased prevalence of patent ductus arteriosus, further evidence of the importance of blood cellular components in this process.[21]

Although some hypoxemia is present soon after birth, because of right-to-left shunting through the ductus arteriosus over the first few hours of life, with continued vasodilation and improved ventilation/perfusion ratios, the normal arterial Po_2 gradually increases from 50 mm Hg at 10 minutes to 62 at 1 hour and 75–83 between 3 hours and 2 days of age. With continued vasodilation, the pulmonary pressure gradually falls to about 30 mm Hg within approximately 48 hours. Although further falls in the pulmonary vascular resistance continue for several weeks, the transition to adult circulation is virtually completed within the first few days of life.

References

1. Rudolph AM. The effects of postnatal circulatory adjustments in congenital heart disease. *Pediatrics*. 1965;36:763-772.
2. Rudolph AM, Heymann MA. The circulation of the fetus in utero. Methods for studying distribution of blood flow, cardiac output and organ blood flow. *Circ Res*. 1967;21:163-184.
3. Rudolph AM, Heymann MA. The fetal circulation. *Annu Rev Med*. 1968;19:195-206.

4. Rudolph AM. Congenital cardiovascular malformations and the fetal circulation. *Arch Dis Child Fetal Neonatal Ed.* 2010;95: F132-F136.

5. Prsa M, Sun L, van Amerom J, et al. Reference ranges of blood flow in the major vessels of the normal human fetal circulation at term by phase-contrast magnetic resonance imaging. *Circ Cardiovasc Imaging.* 2014;7:663-670.

6. Poelmann RE, Gittenberger-de Groot AC. Hemodynamics in cardiac development. *J Cardiovasc Dev Dis.* 2018;5:54.

7. Rudolph AM, Heymann MA. Cardiac output in the fetal lamb: the effects of spontaneous and induced changes of heart rate on right and left ventricular output. *Am J Obstet Gynecol.* 1976;124: 183-192.

8. Gilbert RD. Effects of afterload and baroreceptors on cardiac function in fetal sheep. *J Dev Physiol.* 1982;4:299-309.

9. Hoerter J, Mazet F, Vassort G. Perinatal growth of the rabbit cardiac cell: possible implications for the mechanism of relaxation. *J Mol Cell Cardiol.* 1981;13:725-740.

10. Rudolph AM. The changes in the circulation after birth. Their importance in congenital heart disease. *Circulation.* 1970;41: 343-359.

11. Teitel DF, Iwamoto HS, Rudolph AM. Effects of birth-related events on central blood flow patterns. *Pediatr Res.* 1987;22: 557-566.

12. Coceani F, Olley PM. The response of the ductus arteriosus to prostaglandins. *Can J Physiol Pharmacol.* 1973;51:220-225.

13. Bouayad A, Kajino H, Waleh N, et al. Characterization of PGE2 receptors in fetal and newborn lamb ductus arteriosus. *Am J Physiol Heart Circ Physiol.* 2001;280:H2342-H2349.

14. Freed MD, Heymann MA, Lewis AB, Roehl SL, Kensey RC. Prostaglandin E1 infants with ductus arteriosus-dependent congenital heart disease. *Circulation.* 1981;64:899-905.

15. Gersony WM, Peckham GJ, Ellison RC, Miettinen OS, Nadas AS. Effects of indomethacin in premature infants with patent ductus arteriosus: results of a national collaborative study. *J Pediatr.* 1983;102:895-906.

16. Ohlsson A, Walia R, Shah SS. Ibuprofen for the treatment of patent ductus arteriosus in preterm or low birth weight (or both) infants. *Cochrane Database Syst Rev.* 2015;(2):CD003481.

17. Hammerman C, Bin-Nun A, Markovitch E, Schimmel MS, Kaplan M, Fink D. Ductal closure with paracetamol: a surprising new approach to patent ductus arteriosus treatment. *Pediatrics.* 2011;128:e1618-e1621.

18. Gittenberger-de Groot AC, van Ertbruggen I, Moulaert AJ, Harinck E. The ductus arteriosus in the preterm infant: histologic and clinical observations. *J Pediatr.* 1980;96:88-93.

19. Waleh N, Seidner S, McCurnin D, et al. Anatomic closure of the premature patent ductus arteriosus: the role of CD14+/CD163+ mononuclear cells and VEGF in neointimal mound formation. *Pediatr Res.* 2011;70:332-338.

20. Echtler K, Stark K, Lorenz M, et al. Platelets contribute to postnatal occlusion of the ductus arteriosus. *Nat Med.* 2010;16: 75-82.

21. Dani C, Poggi C, Fontanelli G. Relationship between platelet count and volume and spontaneous and pharmacological closure of ductus arteriosus in preterm infants. *Am J Perinatol.* 2013; 30:359-364.

SECTION III

Cardiac Genetics

5

Genetics of Congenital Heart Disease

AMY E. ROBERTS AND RONALD V. LACRO

KEY LEARNING POINTS

- Genetic causes likely contribute to the vast majority of cases of CHD, yet current technologies identify the genetic etiology in only about 45% of cases.
- Determining the genetic etiology of CHD is increasingly possible with readily available diagnostic testing.
- Discoveries of the genetic controls of normal heart development have led to the identification of a large number of genes that, when altered, cause CHD.

- There is both locus heterogeneity (the same phenotype caused by different genetic abnormalities) and phenotypic heterogeneity (a specific genetic abnormality can cause different phenotypes) in CHD.
- Understanding the genetic etiology for an individual's CHD gives insight into prognosis, the chance of extra-cardiac complications, and recurrence risk estimates for the individual and his/her family.

Introduction

The incidence of congenital heart disease (CHD) is estimated at 6–12 per 1000 live births, but the true prevalence is likely higher because mild CHD (e.g., bicuspid aortic valve [BAV]) may not be diagnosed until after childhood. Genetic causes contribute to an estimated 90% of CHD cases. The advent of genomic techniques and increased understanding of the genetic control of cardiovascular development have greatly increased the ability to identify a genetic cause for many cases of CHD. Exact figures vary depending upon methods used and inclusion/exclusion criteria, but it is currently estimated that a genetic etiology is positively identifiable in up to 45% of cases of CHD.[1] The genetic etiology of the unexplained cases is likely not monogenic but due to gene-gene interactions, gene-environment interactions, and/or polygenic inheritance.[2] The observed significant intrafamilial variability in penetrance and expression for a given single gene cause also provides evidence for the importance of epigenetic factors.

Cardiac Development

The traditional nomenclature for classifying structural heart defects is based on presumed embryologic events or on anatomic characteristics and location. Although helpful in naming complex cardiac defects, earlier classification systems may have obscured important pathogenetic relationships. The understanding of the genetic underpinning of the stages of cardiac development including heart fields, cardiac looping, chamber morphogenesis, non-chamber myocardium, and the cardiac conduction system has advanced quickly since the completion of the Human Genome Project in 2003 and, along with it, our ability to identify specific genetic causes of CHD.

Heart Fields

The chambers of the heart are known to be derived from two different progenitor populations: the first heart field, which gives rise to the future atria and left ventricle; and the second heart field, which gives rise to the outflow tract and the right ventricle. The first heart field originates from the lateral plate mesoderm bilaterally, thought to be induced by signaling pathways including bone morphogenic protein and fibroblast growth factor from the anterior endoderm. The size of the first heart field is restricted by retinoic acid signaling. Excess exposure in humans to vitamin A or its analogs, the retinoids, can cause embryonic defects and CHD, including conotruncal and great artery malformations such as transposition of the great vessels, double-outlet right ventricle, and tetralogy of Fallot. Expression of *NKX2-5* from the cardiac progenitor fields begins early. Heterozygous mutations in the *NKX2.5*, which encodes a DNA transcription factor, were among the first evidence of a genetic cause for CHD and were initially found in pedigrees with autosomal dominant transmission of cardiac septal defects and atrioventricular conduction abnormalities. *NKX2.5* pathogenic variants have subsequently been identified in individuals with atrial septal defect (ASD), ventricular septal defect (VSD), Ebstein malformation, tetralogy of Fallot, truncus arteriosus, double-outlet right ventricle, L-transposition of the great arteries, interrupted aortic arch, subvalvar aortic stenosis, hypoplastic left heart syndrome (HLHS), and coarctation of the aorta (CoA)[3] (Table 5.1).

Cardiac Looping

One of the earliest events in cardiac morphogenesis is the formation of the normal D (dextral)-cardiac loop from the previously symmetric, midline cardiac tube. The left-right axis of the heart is set up by a highly conserved set of genes including Wnt signaling pathway genes *NODAL*, *LEFTY-1/2*, and *SOUTHPAW*. Chamber identity of the left ventricle is associated with *HAND1* expression and identity of the right ventricle with *HAND2* expression.[3] Abnormalities at this stage of cardiac development frequently lead to complex CHD and associated visceral malformations. In humans, situs abnormalities (heterotaxy syndrome) have been observed in pedigrees consistent with autosomal dominant, autosomal recessive, and X-linked recessive inheritance, suggesting that multiple genes regulate cardiac looping and determine cardiac and visceral situs. Heterotaxy may also be caused by teratogenic exposures, especially maternal diabetes. Isolated CHD resulting from isomerism and disturbed looping may be caused by mutations in genes that control early left-right patterning and the earliest steps in cardiogenesis. Genes currently implicated in human heterotaxy include *ZIC3*, *LEFTYA*, *CFC1*, *ACVR2B*, *CFAP53*, *MMP21*, *NODAL*, *MNS1*, and *PKD1L1*.[4] Humans with immotile cilia syndrome (Kartagener syndrome, primary ciliary dyskinesia [PCD]), an autosomal recessive disorder, have ciliary dynein defects and laterality defects, as well as respiratory problems and male infertility. The coexistence of ciliary abnormalities, CHD, and/or dextrocardia and polysplenia has been reported, and heterotaxy is present in approximately 12% of individuals with PCD.[5] The pathogenesis of dextro

TABLE 5.1 Single Gene Causes of Isolated Congenital Heart Disease (CHD) by Lesion and Functional Class

CHD Lesion	Genes Implicated in Non-Syndromic Disease
Aortic valve stenosis	*NOTCH1**, NR2F2*, SMAD6**, TAB2***
Atrial septal defect	*ACTC1***, CITED2*, CRELD1**, GATA4*, GATA5*, MEIS2*, MYH6***, NOTCH1**, NKX2-5*, SMAD2*, TBX1*, TBX5*, TBX20**
Atrioventricular septal defect	*ACVR1**, CRELD1**, GATA4*, GATA6*, GJA1**, NR2F2*, TBX5**
Bicuspid aortic valve	*GATA5*, NOTCH1**, SMAD6**, TAB2**,*
Coarctation of the aorta	*MEIS2*, NOTCH1**, NR2F2*, SMAD6***
Double-outlet right ventricle	*GATA5*, NODAL**, NOTCH1**, NR2F2*, SMAD2*, ZFPM2**
Ebstein anomaly	*MYH7****
Hypoplastic left heart syndrome	*GJA1**, HAND1*, MYH6***, NKX2-5*, NOTCH1**, NR2F2**
Interrupted aortic arch	*TBX1**
Mitral valve stenosis	*TBX20**
Pulmonary atresia	*GJA1***
Pulmonary artery stenosis	*JAG1***
Patent ductus arteriosus	*MYH11***, SMAD2**
Pulmonary valve stenosis	*GATA4*, HAND2**
Pulmonary vein stenosis	*GATA4*, NOTCH1***
Supravalvar aortic stenosis	*ELN****
Tetralogy of Fallot	*FLT4, GATA4*, GATA5*, GATA6*, HAND2*, JAG1**, KDR, NKX2-5*, NODAL**, NOTCH1**, NR2F2*, TAB2**, TBX1*, ZFPM2**
Total anomalous pulmonary venous return	*PDGFRA***
Transposition of great arteries	*MED13L*, NODAL***
Truncus arteriosus	*GATA6*, NKX2.6**
Ventricular septal defect	*CITED2*, GATA4*, GATA5*, GJA1**, HAND1*, HAND2*, MEIS2*, NODAL**, NOTCH1**, NR2F2*, SMAD2*, TBX1*, TBX5*, TBX20**

*Transcription factor; **cell signaling and adhesion protein; ***structural protein.

(D)-transposition of the great vessels is thought to involve failure of the conotruncal cushions to spiral. Patients with non-syndromic CHD and damaging variants in cilia-related genes generally have transposition of the great arteries.[6]

Anomalous Pulmonary Venous Return

Anomalous pulmonary venous connections are believed to arise from abnormalities in targeted growth, either as an isolated CHD or as part of heterotaxy. The pulmonary veins form as an outpouching of endothelial-lined mesenchymal tissue from the lung buds, and coalesce into the common pulmonary vein, which bridges across the splanchnic space and fuses with the posterior wall of the primitive left atrium at 5 weeks' gestation. By further remodeling, the common pulmonary vein is gradually absorbed into the posterior wall of the left atrium such that the four pulmonary veins enter the heart individually by 8 weeks' gestation. The mechanism is undefined but likely involves an attraction between the pulmonary veins and the left atrium. If connection of the common pulmonary vein to the left atrium does not occur, primitive venous drainage to systemic veins persists (totally anomalous pulmonary venous connection). If absorption of the common pulmonary vein into the left atrium is incomplete, a membrane may persist between the pulmonary veins and the left atrium (cor triatriatum). Recent studies have implicated variants in *PDGFRA*, *ANKRD1/CARP*, as well as genes in the retinoic acid signaling pathway including *RBP5*, *NODAL*, and *RDH10* to confer susceptibility to TAPVR.[7]

Chamber Morphogenesis

The chambers are specified by spatially restricted patterns of gene expression. During mouse heart development, basic helix-loop-helix (bHLH) transcription factors are expressed in a complementary fashion and are restricted to segments of the heart tube fated to form the right and left ventricles. The early ventricular chamber is formed by ballooning of the outer curvature of the heart tube which proceeds by asymmetric growth of the myocardium primarily on the outer curvature of the primitive ventricle. *GATA4* expression leads to decreased cardiomyocyte proliferation which may be why mutations in *GATA4* are seen with ASD, atrioventricular canal (AVC) defect, VSD, pulmonary vein stenosis, and tetralogy of Fallot[8] (Table 5.1). *GATA4* encodes a transcription factor known to play a critical role in cardiogenesis. Studies of large kindreds inheriting a fully penetrant autosomal dominant disorder in which all affected individuals had secundum ASDs, several also with additional CHDs, including VSDs, AVC defects, and pulmonary valve stenosis, have been found to have pathogenic *GATA4* variants. It has been shown that three core cardiac transcription factors during embryonic heart development, *GATA4*, *TBX5*, and *NKX2-5*, which have been associated with secundum ASDs, are now known to produce proteins that form complexes with one another.[9]

Non-Chamber Myocardium

Non-chamber myocardium includes the AVC and outflow tract. Normal development requires suppression of the expression of chamber specific genes. *TBX2/3* and *BMP2/4* repress *ANF* and other chamber-specific genes. The endocardial cushions are the valve forming tissue of the heart that form between the atrium and ventricle from the non-chamber myocardium of the AVC. Normal development is dependent upon vascular endothelial growth factor (VEGF). Polymorphisms in VEGF pathway genes are associated with valvuloseptal CHD. The high frequency of AVC defects in Down (trisomy 21) syndrome is a clue to the genetic mechanism(s) involved in cushion morphogenesis. Increased adhesion of trisomy 21 cells is the basis of a long-standing model for abnormal AVC development. Fetal trisomy 21 fibroblasts explanted from endocardial-cushion–derived structures appear more adhesive *in vitro* than those explanted from normal control fetuses. If the fusion of the atrioventricular cushions is time and location dependent, and the migration of cells in the trisomic embryo is delayed, then there is a greater chance of the process not occurring.[10] Type VI collagen may have a role in the pathogenesis of AVC defects in trisomy 21 syndrome. The COL6A1/COL6A2 gene cluster, which encodes the alpha-1 and alpha-2 chains for type VI collagen, respectively, fall within the CHD-critical region on chromosome 21. Differences in adhesion to type VI collagen between cultured skin fibroblasts isolated from people with and without trisomy 21 suggest a potential mechanism for developmental defects.[11] Because half of individuals with trisomy 21 have structurally normal hearts, researchers have looked for genetic factors within and outside of the trisomic region that may modify the penetrance of AVC defects. An overrepresentation of deleterious variants has been detected in VEGF-A pathway genes, *COL6A1*, *CRELD1*, *FBLN1*, *FRZB*, *GATA5*, *NOTCH4*, and *CEP290* in individuals with Down syndrome and AVC defects versus those without CHD.[12]

Multiple families have been reported to have autosomal-dominant AVC defects with incomplete penetrance, demonstrating that AVC defects can be inherited as a single gene defect. There are five established genetic loci for isolated AVC defects, also known as atrioventricular septal defects (AVSDs), designated AVSD1 through AVSD5. An AVSD susceptibility locus (AVSD1) maps to chromosome 1p31-p21; AVSD2 is caused by pathogenic variants in *CRELD1* on chromosome 3p25; AVSD3 is caused by pathogenic variants in *GJA1* on chromosome 6q22; AVSD4 is caused by pathogenic variants in *GATA4* on chromosome 8p23.1; and AVSD5 is caused by pathogenic variants in *GATA6* on chromosome 18q11.[13] The CRELD family consists of two matricellular proteins thought to be involved in cell adhesion processes. In a study of 52 people with non–trisomy 21–related AVC defects, approximately 6% of the subjects had missense mutations in the coding region of *CRELD1*. *GJA1* encodes a gap junction protein known as connexin 43 (Cx43), an abundantly expressed protein in the ventricular myocardium and in cardiac neural crest cells. Compound heterozygous variants have been reported in several individuals with AVSD.[13] GATA factors constitute a family of transcriptional regulatory proteins expressed with distinct developmental and tissue-specific profiles and are thought to regulate cell-restricted programs of gene expression. Neural crest cells migrate from the cranial neural crest to the developing heart and are critical for proper outflow tract septation. Ectomesenchymal cells from neural crest are essential for expression of tissue derivatives of each branchial arch and pouch. In addition, neural crest cells course through arches 4, 6, and probably 3 to participate in septation of the conotruncus and aortic sac. Mechanical ablation of small amounts of preotic neural crest in animal models produces a spectrum of conotruncal malformations including truncus arteriosus and subarterial VSD.[3] Conotruncal malformations, particularly type B interruption of the aortic arch, truncus arteriosus, and tetralogy of Fallot, are overrepresented in patients with 22q11.2 deletion syndrome, where they are seen in association with hypoplasia or aplasia of the thymus and parathyroid gland, which are derivatives of pharyngeal pouches III and IV. Pathogenic variants in *TBX1*, one of the genes in the 22q11.2 critical region, are associated with isolated and syndromic conotruncal abnormalities and are thought to be due to abnormal neural crest cell migration.[14] Other human neural crest/branchial arch syndromes that have an overrepresentation of conotruncal malformations and that are associated with abnormalities of branchial arch derivatives include the facio-auriculo-vertebral spectrum (oculo-auriculo-vertebral dysplasia, hemifacial microsomia, Goldenhar syndrome), CHARGE syndrome due to pathogenic variants in *CHD7*, thalidomide embryopathy, and retinoic acid embryopathy.

Ebstein Anomaly

The tricuspid valve cusps are almost exclusively derived from the interior of the embryonic right ventricular myocardium by a process of undermining of the right ventricular wall. Abnormalities of this process of reabsorption of ventricular myocardium may lead to the Ebstein anomaly (EA) with displacement of the functional tricuspid valve annulus into the right ventricle. EA is a genetically heterogeneous CHD, in which microdeletions in 1p36 and 8p23.1, and a missense mutation in the actin-binding protein Filamin A (FLNA), have been described. Differences in micro RNA and messenger RNA abundance levels in patients with EA and age and sex-matched healthy volunteers have been shown in pathways that are mostly involved in signal transduction and cellular interaction.[15]

Cardiac Conduction System

Many transcription factors are needed for development of the cardiac conduction system. *TBX3* is expressed in the sinoatrial node and deletion leads to node dysfunction. The AV node derives from the primitive AV canal of non-chamber myocardium. *TBX2* is expressed in the AV canal and then in the AV node. There is highly enriched expression of the MAP kinase-dependent transcription factor *ETV1* in the proximal and distal ventricular conducting system, including cardiac Purkinje cells. A phenome-wide association study identified a link between *ETV1* and bundle branch block and heart block in humans.[16] Pathogenic variants in *NKX2-5* that impair the ability of the transcription factor to bind DNA often result in AV block, with or without CHD. The knowledge that *NKX2-5* is the etiology is clinically relevant as the associated risk of progressive conduction disease and sudden cardiac death impacts decision-making regarding pacemakers and implantable defibrillators.[2]

Clinical Considerations

Dysmorphic features, extracardiac malformations, and developmental delay are commonly associated with congenital heart defects (25%–30%) and should prompt an evaluation for a possible syndrome (see Chapter 6 for a discussion of syndromic forms of CHD).

Allelic and Non-allelic Heterogeneity

Genetic heterogeneity has been documented or is suspected for a number of conditions. In other words, there can be different causes for the same disease or phenotype. Genetic heterogeneity can be allelic (different mutations at the same gene locus) or non-allelic (mutations at different gene loci causing similar phenotypes), and can explain, at least in part, the variability in clinical phenotype (pattern and severity of expression). For example, many different mutations of the fibrillin gene have been identified in Marfan syndrome (allelic heterogeneity). In contrast, mutations for several different genes encoding myocardial structural proteins (e.g., *MYH7*, *TPM3*, *TNNT2*) are associated with hypertrophic cardiomyopathy (HCM; non-allelic heterogeneity). Similarly, mutations for several different genes encoding cardiac ion channels are associated with long QT syndrome. For HCM and long QT syndrome, the severity of clinical manifestations and risk for complications such as sudden death depend on the nature of the genetic mutation. Some mutations are associated with mild disease, whereas others are associated with a severe clinical phenotype. Genetic testing and gene pathway-specific therapies are now available for some cardiomyopathies and inherited arrhythmias,[17,18] and gene therapy is an active area of research.[19]

The etiology of CHD is currently the focus of intense research. In the past, genetic counseling for isolated congenital CHD (i.e., without extracardiac malformations or syndromic diagnosis) was transmitted as generalized advice, with the use of an overall recurrence risk for first-degree relatives of 2% to 5%. These malformations were said to be multifactorial, which refers to defects caused by the combined effects of one or more alleles at a number of loci interacting with stochastic and/or environmental factors. However, the familial (apparent mendelian or single gene) occurrence of virtually all forms of CHD has been noted. In the past, the study of familial CHD in humans has been hindered by a number of factors including reduced penetrance, variable expressivity, genetic heterogeneity, small family size, and decreased survival and reproductive capability especially in those individuals with complex defects. Recent epidemiologic and familial studies[20] suggest that specific genetic influences may be more important than previously recognized, and that certain malformations are more likely to have a stronger genetic component.

Clinical and echocardiographic studies of first-degree relatives of patients with complete common AVC have detected previously unsuspected congenital heart defects that were clinically less significant than the proband's CHD but were part of the same mechanistic spectrum (e.g., atrioventricular type of septal defects and left-axis deviation). The incidence of CHD in first-degree relatives of apparently non-syndromic children with congenital aortic valve stenosis (AVS), CoA, and HLHS is about 20% for mothers, 15% for fathers, and 5%–20% for siblings.[21] This increased recognition of the importance of family history and family screening for BAV and left ventricular outflow tract obstruction (LVOTO) defects is reflected by the recommendation by the American College of Cardiology and the American Heart Association (ACC/AHA) that first-degree family members of patients with BAV should be screened for BAV and LVOTO defects as well.[22]

Genetic Testing in CHD

An accurate genetic evaluation will aid in guidance of medical, surgical, and palliative management; it will allow for early screening for associated anomalies and neurodevelopmental complications; it will inform prognostic information given to families; it can be used to test at-risk family members; and it will allow for recurrence risk estimates and family planning with perinatal diagnostic testing options. Prior to genetic testing, a thorough three-generation pedigree review, evaluation for extra-cardiac anomalies, detailed cardiac phenotyping, and dysmorphic features can aid in choosing the best diagnostic test and in interpreting variants of uncertain significance. Additionally, individuals or their guardians should provide informed consent for testing, and when genome-wide sequencing is offered, for opting in or out of receiving secondary findings. Secondary findings are pathogenic findings in genes unrelated to the primary purpose of the testing.

With comprehensive genomic analysis, an estimated 20%–45% of cases will have an identifiable damaging coding variant in definitive genes for CHD (variants that significantly co-segregate in families with CHD, are enriched in unrelated individuals with CHD versus controls, or account for CHD in those with syndromic CHD) or in candidate genes for CHD (similar properties to definitive genes but without statistical significance to allow for a "definitive" classification).[3] Syndromic CHD with neurodevelopmental delay or extracardiac anomalies makes up 30% of all CHD cases and about 50% have a genetic diagnosis.[23]

The techniques of molecular genetics are becoming increasingly useful for the study of familial CHD. Copy number variants (CNVs) are diagnosed by chromosomal microarray (CMA), a high-resolution method for detecting copy number changes (gains or losses) across the entire genome in a single assay at a resolution of 20–400 kb. These CNVs range in size from single genes to large segmental gains or losses. Almost 10% of cases of CHD will have a CNV typically including known cardiac genes, left-right patterning genes, or deletions of genes in the Wnt signaling pathway.[21] Specific forms of CHD including interrupted aortic arch type B, isolated aortic arch anomaly, truncus arteriosus, tetralogy of Fallot, or VSD with aortic arch anomaly are more commonly due to a CNV than other forms of CHD.[3] Examination of recurrent syndromic CNVs has provided a window into finding individual CHD genes. For example, the recurrent 7q11.23 chromosomal deletion causes Williams syndrome, characterized by distinctive facies, intellectual disability, growth and endocrine abnormalities, peripheral pulmonary artery stenosis, and supravalvar aortic stenosis. Pathogenic variants or intragenic deletions in *ELN*, a gene within the Williams syndrome critical region, have been detected in familial autosomal dominant supravalvar aortic stenosis without the other features of Williams syndrome. Identification of a CNV in syndromic CHD allows for the identification of potential non-cardiac complications that can inform perioperative management, required screening studies, and anticipatory guidance. Identification of a causative CNV in isolated CHD can also provide prognostic information. An analysis of outcomes in 422 cases of isolated CHD found decreased transplant-free survival, 2.6-fold increased risk of death or transplant, worse linear growth, and worse neurocognitive outcomes in those with CHD and a pathogenic CNV versus those with CHD without a pathogenic CNV.[24]

Sanger sequencing and next-generation sequencing are utilized to identify damaging variants in individual genes. Gene panels are available to interrogate genes associated with a particular form of CHD (e.g., tetralogy of Fallot) or associated with a particular diagnostic category (e.g., heterotaxy). Complex presentations not consistent with a known syndromic diagnosis or individuals with non-diagnostic CMA and/or gene panel testing may benefit from a genome-wide analysis.

Whole exome sequencing (WES), also known as exome sequencing, is a two-step process of first selecting only the subset of DNA that encodes proteins (the exome, ~2% of the genome), and second, sequencing that exonic DNA using high-throughput DNA sequencing technology. Analysis is enhanced by including samples from family members to identify *de novo* variants in sporadic CHD or to look for segregation in familial CHD. WES enables a genome-wide analysis that may be superior to single gene or gene panel analysis for the ability to identify mutations in genes that were not tested due to an atypical clinical presentation and the ability to identify pathogenic variants in more than one gene that together contribute to a complex phenotype in an individual patient. Recent research, accelerated through the Human Genome Project, has resulted in the rapid identification of disease genes causing congenital heart defects using this method. The NHLBI Pediatric Cardiac Genomics Consortium (PCGC) has collected > 10,000 CHD probands, including > 5000 parent-offspring trios. WES of 1213 trios from this cohort showed that ~10% of cases are attributable to *de novo* variants in > 400 target genes, including dramatic enrichment for damaging pathogenic variants in genes encoding chromatin modifiers (23665959 and 26785492). Whole exome analysis also has been shown to be of high yield when applied to kindreds with familial CHD where a causative variant can be identified in about one-third of families.[25] Syndromic CHD cases are more likely to have *de novo* truncating variants in known CHD genes, and isolated CHD cases are more likely to have protein truncating variants in known CHD genes inherited from an unaffected parent, implying incomplete penetrance or an oligogenic etiology.[26]

Whole genome sequencing (WGS) enables the sequencing of the entire genome in a single assay. WGS includes both the protein-coding and non-coding (promoter, intronic, and untranslated) regions of the human genome, allowing for the potential detection of characterized/pathogenic variants in regions that are not assessed by WES. While much of the data generated from WGS is not well understood at this time, it may provide more reliable coverage of the exonic regions than WES and simultaneously can detect CNVs. As costs decrease, WGS may become a first-line diagnostic test in CHD because it provides CNV analysis without needing a separate CMA and exome sequencing without requiring a separate WES and with the added non-coding region analysis. Because any genomic testing has the potential to uncover unanticipated results, soliciting informed consent and providing pre and post-test genetic counseling are essential.

In addition to the lengthening list of genes that cause syndromic CHD, an increasing number of specific genes are now implicated in the pathogenesis of isolated (non-syndromic) CHD. These genes are summarized in Table 5.1 by CHD lesion, but such a list is constantly evolving and never complete. Some of the genes listed are relatively well characterized, whereas others have only been described in a few probands or families but the precise mechanism of disease remains unknown. While some testing labs offer gene panel testing by CHD lesion, because many individuals have more than one form of CHD that would implicate more than one panel, because it can be difficult to appreciate dysmorphic features, cognitive delays, and extracardiac anomalies in infants, and because gene discovery is often ahead of developed gene panels in clinical laboratories, WES or, ideally, WGS, is of higher yield in identifying causative variants. Having WES or WGS data has the added benefit of being available to be re-analyzed in the future to look for variants in newly discovered genes.

Although the general principles of multifactorial inheritance may still apply in many situations, the recurrence risk

TABLE 5.2 Recurrence Risks for Congenital Heart Defects in Siblings

Defect	Percentage at Risk	
	One Sibling Affected	Two Siblings Affected
Ventricular septal defect	3	10
Patent ductus arteriosus	3	10
Atrial septal defect	2.5	8
Tetralogy of Fallot	2.5	8
Pulmonary stenosis	2	6
Coarctation of aorta	2	6
Aortic stenosis	2	6
Transposition	1.5	5
Endocardial cushion defects	3	10
Fibroelastosis	4	12
Hypoplastic left heart	2	6
Tricuspid atresia	1	3
Ebstein anomaly	1	3
Truncus arteriosus	1	3
Pulmonary atresia	1	3

From Nora JJ, Nora AH. Update on counseling the family with a first-degree relative with a congenital heart defect. *Am J Med Genet.* 1988;29:137. Reprinted with permission of John Wiley & Sons, Inc.

may be underestimated in other situations. Therefore, when a specific genetic etiology cannot be found, risk projections should be based on the specific congenital heart defect involved as well as the genetic and teratogenic history in an individual family or pregnancy. The recurrence risks for siblings (Table 5.2) and offspring (Table 5.3) are for isolated, non-syndromic malformations and are based on combined data published during the 1960's-1980's from European and North American populations.

Familial Cardiomyopathy and Arrhythmias

Cardiomyopathies can be divided into five subgroups according to structural and functional changes of the myocardium: (1) HCM, (2) dilated cardiomyopathy (DCM), (3) arrhythmogenic right ventricular cardiomyopathy (ARVC), (4) restrictive cardiomyopathy (RCM), and (5) non-classified cardiomyopathies such as isolated left ventricular non-compaction cardiomyopathy (LVNC).[27] Genetic mutations in multiple genes encoding sarcomeric proteins have been associated with HCM. Mutations in the gene encoding dystrophin not only cause Duchenne and Becker muscular dystrophy but also cause familial X-linked

TABLE
5.3 **Recurrence Risks for Congenital Heart Defects in Offspring Given One Affected Parent**

	Percentage at Risk	
Defect	Mother Affected	Father Affected
Aortic stenosis	13–18	3
Atrial septal defect	4–4.5	1.5
Atrioventricular canal	14	1
Coarctation of aorta	4	2
Patent ductus arteriosus	3.5–4	2.5
Pulmonary stenosis	4–6.5	2
Tetralogy of Fallot	2.5	1.5
Ventricular septal defect	6–10	2

From Nora JJ, Nora AH. Update on counseling the family with a first-degree relative with a congenital heart defect. *Am J Med Genet.* 1988;29:137. Reprinted with permission of John Wiley & Sons, Inc.

DCM (see Chapter 48). Thousands of causative cardiomyopathy mutations have been characterized from hundreds of genes to date, and there are clinically available cardiomyopathy gene panels that include more than 200 genes encompassing all cardiomyopathy subtypes in isolated and non-isolated forms.[28-32] These genes encode proteins making up the structure of the sarcomere, cytoskeleton, desmosome, ion channels or nuclear lamina, and proteins participating in Ca^{21} handling during the contraction phase of action potential or affecting cardiac energy metabolism. Abnormalities in genes encoding cardiac potassium and sodium channels have been linked to long QT syndrome and other inherited arrhythmias (see Chapter 20).

Mitochondrial disorders

Cardiomyopathy is a common clinical feature of several well-known mitochondrial syndromes (MELAS [mitochondrial myopathy, encephalopathy, lactic acidosis, stroke] syndrome, MERRF [myoclonic epilepsy and ragged-red fibers] syndrome, NADH-coenzyme Q reductase deficiency, Kearns-Sayre syndrome, MIMyCA [maternally inherited myopathy and cardiomyopathy]). Mitochondrial cardiomyopathy, which is usually accompanied by skeletal and neuromuscular abnormalities, has been attributed to missense mutations, point mutations, and deletion mutations. In addition, isolated DCM has been reportedly associated with myocardial mitochondrial DNA deletions or mutations.[33]

Conclusions

Advances in technology have fueled the discovery of the genetic underpinnings of CHD including germline variants, CNVs, and variants in non-coding sequences. However, the genetic etiology remains unknown in more than half of individuals with CHD, so there is still much to learn. Future directions of analysis include expression profiling from affected cardiac tissue, oligogenetic analysis, cohort enhanced assessment of non-coding sequences, and better evaluation of the effects of environmental exposures. This work requires large, collaborative studies with a sufficient number of cases to allow for robust analyses. Each discovery benefits both our understanding of the developmental biology and the care and outcomes of individuals and their families.

References

1. Diab NS, Barish S, Dong W, et al. Molecular genetics and complex inheritance of congenital heart disease. *Genes (Basel).* 2021; 12:1020.
2. Nees SN, Chung WK. The genetics of isolated congenital heart disease. *Am J Med Genet C Semin Med Genet.* 2020;184:97-106.
3. Jerves T, Beaton A, Kruszka P. The genetic workup for structural congenital heart disease. *Am J Med Genet C Semin Med Genet.* 2020;184:178-186.
4. Li AH, Hanchard NA, Azamian M, et al. Genetic architecture of laterality defects revealed by whole exome sequencing. *Eur J Hum Genet.* 2019;27:563-573.
5. Shapiro AJ, Davis SD, Ferkol T, et al. Laterality defects other than situs inversus totalis in primary ciliary dyskinesia: insights into situs ambiguus and heterotaxy. *Chest.* 2014;146:1176-1186.
6. Liu X, Chen W, Li W, et al. Exome-based case-control analysis highlights the pathogenic role of ciliary genes in transposition of the great arteries. *Circ Res.* 2020;126:811-821.
7. Nash D, Arrington CB, Kennedy BJ, et al. Shared segment analysis and next-generation sequencing implicates the retinoic acid signaling pathway in total anomalous pulmonary venous return (TAPVR). *PLoS One.* 2015;10:e0131514.
8. Rajagopal SK, Ma Q, Obler D, et al. Spectrum of heart disease associated with murine and human GATA4 mutation. *J Mol Cell Cardiol.* 2007;43:677-685.
9. Robbe ZL, Shi W, Wasson LK, et al. CHD4 is recruited by GATA4 and NKX2-5 to repress noncardiac gene programs in the developing heart. *Genes Dev.* 2022;36:468-482.
10. Pelleri MC, Gennari E, Locatelli C, et al. Genotype-phenotype correlation for congenital heart disease in Down syndrome through analysis of partial trisomy 21 cases. *Genomics.* 2017;109:391-400.
11. Gittenberger-de Groot AC, Bartram U, Oosthoek PW, et al. Collagen type VI expression during cardiac development and in human fetuses with trisomy 21. *Anat Rec A Discov Mol Cell Evol Biol.* 2003;275:1109-1116.
12. Trevino CE, Holleman AM, Corbitt H, et al. Identifying genetic factors that contribute to the increased risk of congenital heart defects in infants with Down syndrome [published correction appears in Sci Rep. 2021;11:15164]. *Sci Rep.* 2020;10:18051.
13. Pugnaloni F, Digilio MC, Putotto C, De Luca E, Marino B, Versacci P. Genetics of atrioventricular canal defects. *Ital J Pediatr.* 2020;46:61.
14. Morgenthau A, Frishman WH. Genetic origins of tetralogy of fallot. *Cardiol Rev.* 2018;26:86-92.
15. Abu-Halima M, Wagner V, Becker LS, et al. Integrated microRNA and mRNA expression profiling identifies novel targets and networks associated with Ebstein's anomaly. *Cells.* 2021;10:1066.

16. Fishman GI. Transcriptional regulation of the cardiac conduction system. *Trans Am Clin Climatol Assoc.* 2020;131:48-54.

17. Morelli C, Ingrasciotta G, Jacoby D, Masri A, Olivotto I. Sarcomere protein modulation: the new frontier in cardiovascular medicine and beyond. *Eur J Intern Med.* 2022;102:1-7.

18. Andelfinger G, Marquis C, Raboisson MJ, et al. Hypertrophic cardiomyopathy in Noonan Syndrome treated by MEK-Inhibition. *J Am Coll Cardiol.* 2019;73:2237-2239.

19. Kawajiri K, Ihara K, Sasano T. Gene therapy to terminate tachyarrhythmias. *Expert Rev Cardiovasc Ther.* 2022;20:431-442.

20. Hinton RB Jr. Martin LJ, Tabangin ME, Mazwi ML, Cripe LH, Benson DW. Hypoplastic left heart syndrome is heritable. *J Am Coll Cardiol.* 2007;50(16):1590-1595.

21. Pierpont ME, Brueckner M, Chung WK, et al. Genetic basis for congenital heart disease: revisited: a scientific statement from the American Heart Association [published correction appears in Circulation. 2018;138:e713]. *Circulation.* 2018;138:e653-e711.

22. Hiratzka LF, Bakris GL, Beckman JA, et al. 2010 ACCF/AHA/AATS/ACR/ASA/SCA/SCAI/SIR/STS/SVM guidelines for the diagnosis and management of patients with Thoracic Aortic Disease: a report of the American College of Cardiology Foundation/American Heart Association Task Force on Practice Guidelines, American Association for Thoracic Surgery, American College of Radiology, American Stroke Association, Society of Cardiovascular Anesthesiologists, Society for Cardiovascular Angiography and Interventions, Society of Interventional Radiology, Society of Thoracic Surgeons, and Society for Vascular Medicine [published correction appears in Circulation. 2010;122:e410]. *Circulation.* 2010;121:e266-e369.

23. Blue GM, Kirk EP, Giannoulatou E, et al. Advances in the genetics of congenital heart disease: a clinician's guide. *J Am Coll Cardiol.* 2017;69:859-870.

24. Kim DS, Kim JH, Burt AA, et al. Burden of potentially pathologic copy number variants is higher in children with isolated congenital heart disease and significantly impairs covariate-adjusted transplant-free survival. *J Thorac Cardiovasc Surg.* 2016;151:1147-1151.e4.

25. LaHaye S, Corsmeier D, Basu M, et al. Utilization of whole exome sequencing to identify causative mutations in familial congenital heart disease. *Circ Cardiovasc Genet.* 2016;9:320-329.

26. Sifrim A, Hitz MP, Wilsdon A, et al. Distinct genetic architectures for syndromic and nonsyndromic congenital heart defects identified by exome sequencing. *Nat Genet.* 2016;48:1060-1065.

27. Charron P, Arad M, Arbustini E, et al. Genetic counselling and testing in cardiomyopathies: a position statement of the European Society of Cardiology Working Group on Myocardial and Pericardial Diseases. *Eur Heart J.* 2010;31:2715-2726.

28. Brodehl A, Gerull B. Genetic insights into primary restrictive cardiomyopathy. *J Clin Med.* 2022;11:2094.

29. Krahn AD, Wilde AAM, Calkins H, et al. Arrhythmogenic right ventricular cardiomyopathy. *JACC Clin Electrophysiol.* 2022;8:533-553.

30. Ušaj M, Moretto L, Månsson A. Critical evaluation of current hypotheses for the pathogenesis of hypertrophic cardiomyopathy. *Int J Mol Sci.* 2022;23:2195.

31. Hershberger RE, Jordan E. Dilated cardiomyopathy overview. In: Adam MP, Everman DB, Mirzaa GM, et al., eds. *GeneReviews®.* Seattle, WA: University of Washington, Seattle; July 27, 2007.

32. Cannie D, Elliott P. The genetics of left ventricular noncompaction. *Curr Opin Cardiol.* 2021;36:301-308.

33. Mazzaccara C, Mirra B, Barretta F, et al. Molecular epidemiology of mitochondrial cardiomyopathy: a search among mitochondrial and nuclear genes. *Int J Mol Sci.* 2021;22:5742.

6

Dysmorphology and Syndromes

RONALD V. LACRO AND AMY E. ROBERTS

KEY LEARNING POINTS

- Syndromes can be caused by teratogens, chromosomal aberrations, copy number variations including contiguous gene deletion disorders, and single gene disorders.
- Congenital heart defects are commonly associated with malformation syndromes.
- Individuals suspected or confirmed to have a syndrome should be screened for heart disease based on the specific diagnosis.

- Detection of a congenital heart defect should prompt a search for associated extracardiac malformations and identification of a possible syndrome. The specific congenital heart defect can sometimes be helpful in leading to a specific syndrome diagnosis.
- Prognosis and recurrence risk for the heart defect depends heavily on the underlying syndrome diagnosis.

Introduction

Congenital heart defects are common in malformation syndromes. Approximately 70% of spontaneous abortuses and stillborn fetuses with a congenital heart defect and 25% of children with a congenital heart defect have associated extracardiac malformations, often as part of a multiple malformation syndrome. Such syndromes are caused by chromosomal aberrations, other genetic abnormalities such as single gene disorders and copy number variants (deletions and duplications), teratogens, and unknown causes. For multiple malformation syndromes, the prognosis and recurrence risk for congenital heart disease depend largely on the underlying syndrome. Detection of a congenital heart defect should prompt a search for associated extracardiac malformations and identification of a possible syndrome. Similarly, individuals with malformation syndromes associated with congenital heart disease should be evaluated for the presence of a cardiovascular defect. This discussion will be limited to the more common multiple malformation syndromes and those less common ones in which congenital heart defects are either frequent or distinctive. The genetic basis of congenital heart disease, including heart disease in the setting of syndromes, is reviewed in detail in a scientific statement from the American Heart Association.[1]

Patterns of Syndromic Congenital Cardiac Malformations

Since there is a large number of malformation syndromes with cardiovascular involvement, it is helpful to discuss these syndromes by the patterns of cardiovascular defects associated with them.

Nonspecific Increased Risk

For many malformation syndromes, there is a nonspecific increased risk for congenital cardiovascular malformations (i.e., the overall risk for cardiac defects is higher than the general population risk, but the distribution of types of defects is similar to the general population). In these syndromes, defects that are common are those that are also common in the general population, such as atrial septal defect, ventricular septal defect, and patent ductus arteriosus.

Increased Risk for Specific Defect(s)

For some syndromes, there is an increased risk for a specific congenital heart defect. For example, in Noonan syndrome, valvar pulmonary stenosis due to a dysplastic pulmonary valve is very common, whereas aortic stenosis is very rare.

Hypertrophic cardiomyopathy is seen in approximately 20% of individuals with Noonan syndrome. In such syndromes, the nature of the cardiovascular malformation can support or contradict the proposed syndrome diagnosis.

Increased Risk for a Specific Family or Spectrum of Defects

For some syndromes, there is an increased risk for a pathogenetic family or spectrum of related defects. For example, in Turner syndrome, the entire spectrum of left heart obstructive/hypoplastic lesions is observed. Although coarctation is the most common defect requiring intervention, the spectrum of defects associated with Turner syndrome ranges from a bicuspid or bicommissural aortic valve without stenosis/regurgitation to hypoplastic left heart syndrome. Similarly, the full spectrum of atrioventricular canal defects is observed in individuals with trisomy 21 syndrome, and conotruncal and aortic arch malformations are overrepresented in the chromosome 22q11.2 deletion syndrome.

Defect Pathognomonic for a Specific Syndrome

Occasionally, a specific cardiovascular malformation is virtually pathognomonic for the syndrome. For example, supravalvar aortic stenosis (SVAS) and the associated elastin arteriopathy are uncommon in the general population but are very common in Williams syndrome. When SVAS is diagnosed in a child with dysmorphic features, growth delay, and/or developmental delay, the diagnosis is likely to be Williams syndrome. Testing for a deletion or pathogenic missense variant of the *ELN* gene at 7q11.23 can differentiate Williams syndrome from familial SVAS (see discussion on Williams syndrome and familial SVAS).

Defect Required for Diagnosis of Syndrome

Finally, for some syndromes, the cardiovascular malformation is highly suggestive of the syndrome or is part of the diagnostic criteria for the syndrome. For example, aortic root dilation and lens dislocation are major criteria for the diagnosis of Marfan syndrome. The presence of aortic root dilation should lead to a differential diagnosis that includes Marfan syndrome. Similarly, the combination of upper limb and cardiac malformations should lead to a differential diagnosis that includes Holt-Oram syndrome.

Teratogens

Teratogens are chemical, physical, and biologic agents capable of inducing congenital anomalies. Table 6.1 summarizes the known or potential teratogens that involve the cardiovascular system. Some teratogens produce distinct clinical syndromes or recognizable patterns of malformation, the most common of which is the fetal alcohol syndrome, whereas other agents cause an increased incidence of single or multiple malformations without a specific syndrome pattern (e.g., maternal

TABLE 6.1 Cardiovascular Abnormalities Caused by Teratogens

Chemical Teratogens	
Fetal alcohol syndrome	VSD, ASD, TOF, coarct Ao
Fetal hydantoin syndrome	VSD, ASD, TOF, coarct Ao, PS, PDA
Fetal trimethadione syndrome	Combined defects
Fetal valproate syndrome	Nonspecific
Fetal carbamazepine syndrome	VSD, TOF
Retinoic acid embryopathy	Conotruncal abnormalities
Thalidomide embryopathy	Conotruncal abnormalities
Fetal warfarin syndrome	PDA, peripheral PS
Fetal lithium exposure	Ebstein anomaly, ASD, tricuspid atresia
Biological Teratogens	
Maternal PKU fetal effects	VSD, TOF, coarct Ao
Maternal lupus/Sjögren syndrome	Complete AV block, cardiomyopathy, L-TGA
Fetal rubella syndrome	VSD, ASD, PDA, peripheral PS and other arterial defects
Maternal diabetes	VSD, coarct Ao, D-TGA, hypertrophic cardiomyopathy

ASD, Atrial septal defect; *AV,* atrioventricular; *coarct Ao,* coarctation of aorta; *D-TGA,* D-looped transposition of the great arteries; *L-TGA,* L-looped transposition of the great arteries; *PDA,* patent ductus arteriosus; *PKU,* phenylketonuria; *PS,* pulmonary stenosis; *TOF,* tetralogy of Fallot; *VSD,* ventricular septal defect.

ingestion of lithium or maternal diabetes). Biologic teratogens include maternal illnesses (e.g., maternal phenylketonuria or maternal lupus erythematosus) or maternal-fetal infections (e.g., rubella) that can cause birth defects.

Fetal Alcohol Syndrome

General Clinical Characteristics

One of the most common malformation syndromes, with an estimated frequency greater than 1 in 1000 live births, fetal alcohol syndrome (Fig. 6.1) is also one of the most common identifiable causes of intellectual disability.

Genetic Considerations

The most serious consequence of prenatal alcohol exposure is its effects on brain development and function.

Cardiovascular Considerations

About half of all individuals with fetal alcohol syndrome have congenital cardiovascular malformations. By far the most common defect is ventricular septal defect, followed by atrial septal defect and tetralogy of Fallot. Less commonly reported lesions include atrioventricular canal defect,

hypoplasia or absence of one pulmonary artery, subaortic stenosis, and complex defects.

Chromosomal Syndromes

Given the large number of chromosomal syndromes, this review will be limited to the most common disorders. The incidence of chromosomal abnormalities is about 1 in 200 at birth and much higher among spontaneous abortions and stillborn fetuses. In a series of spontaneous abortuses and stillborn fetuses with congenital heart defects, a chromosomal abnormality was confirmed in 19% and suspected in up to 36%. Studies using high-resolution chromosomal analysis have shown that as many as 13% of all infants with congenital cardiovascular malformations have chromosomal abnormalities. The vast majority of these infants have trisomy 21 syndrome (Down syndrome), which accounts for about 10% of all live born infants with congenital cardiovascular malformations diagnosed in the first year of life.

Trisomy 21 Syndrome (Down Syndrome)

General Clinical Characteristics

Trisomy 21 syndrome (Fig. 6.2) is the most frequent chromosomal aberration affecting live born infants, with an

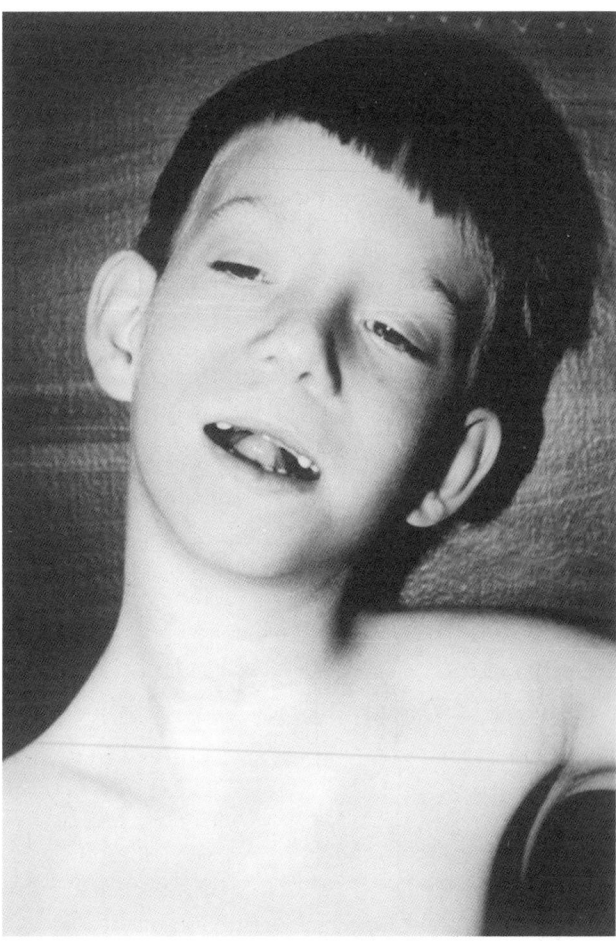

• **Fig. 6.1** Fetal alcohol syndrome. Typical facies in a child with severe manifestations of prenatal alcohol exposure. Note the short, down-slanting palpebral fissures, short upturned nose, long smooth philtrum, and thin upper lip.

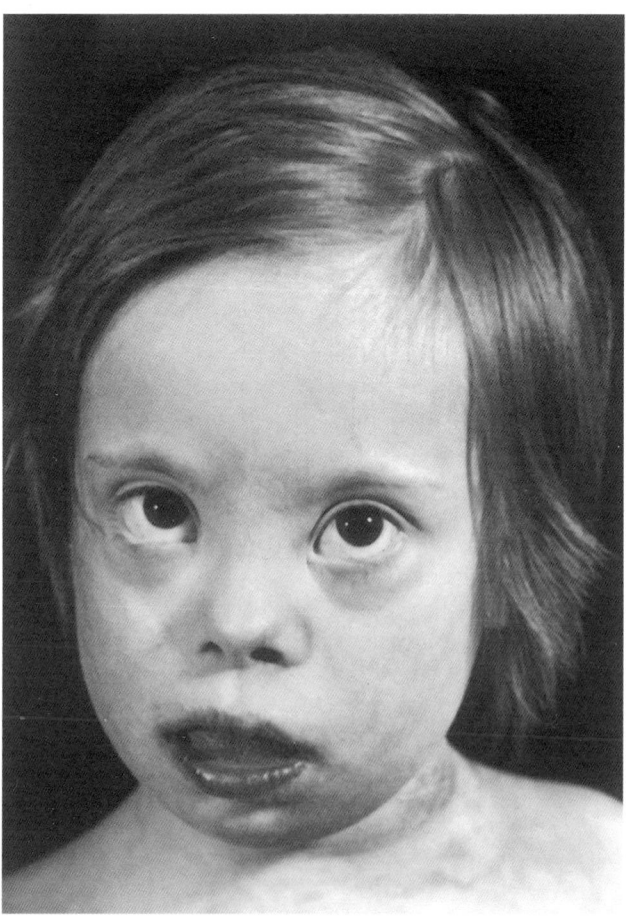

• **Fig. 6.2** Trisomy 21 (Down) syndrome. Note the flat, expressionless face, small nose, low nasal bridge, bilateral epicanthal folds, and protrusion of the tongue.

incidence of 1 in 660 live births. The phenotype of trisomy 21 syndrome is well recognized.

Genetic Considerations

This syndrome is associated with advanced maternal age: 94% are due to non-disjunction, which results in three full copies of chromosome 21 in each cell; about 3% are due to parental translocation; and 3% are due to mosaicism. The risk of recurrence for Down syndrome is about 1%, except in rare cases of a parent who is a translocation carrier, when the risk for recurrence will depend on the type of translocation and the sex of the parent that carries it.

Prenatally, trisomy 21 is most often identified when there is advanced maternal age or when fetal sonographic findings indicate an increased risk. Prenatal detection of a common atrioventricular canal defect should raise suspicion for Down syndrome, particularly when seen with other sonographic findings suggestive of the syndrome, such as increased nuchal thickness and echogenic foci.

Cardiovascular Considerations

Cardiovascular malformations are found in 40–50% of individuals with Down syndrome. There is a distinctive spectrum of cardiac defects with an overrepresentation of endocardial cushion defects (atrioventricular canal defects) compared with the general population. The most common abnormalities (in decreasing order of frequency) include common atrioventricular canal, ventricular septal defect, tetralogy of Fallot, and patent ductus arteriosus. Left-sided obstructive defects such as coarctation and valvar aortic stenosis are rare.

Trisomy 18 Syndrome

General Clinical Characteristics

Trisomy 18 syndrome (Fig. 6.3) is the second most common autosomal chromosomal aberration in humans, with an incidence of 1 in 3500 newborns. The major features found in virtually all affected individuals include intrauterine growth retardation, microcephaly, characteristic craniofacial features (prominent occiput, short palpebral fissures, malformed and low-set ears, small mouth, narrow palate, and micrognathia), clenched hands, a short sternum, a low arch pattern of the dermal ridges on the fingertips, and severe cardiac malformations.

Most infants with trisomy 18 syndrome have severe perinatal difficulties attributable to severe brain dysfunction and severe cardiac defects. Most die within a week of birth, most commonly because of apneic spells. Cardiovascular failure and aspiration pneumonia are common. Survival into the teens and adult age has been reported and is more common in those offered palliative or corrective surgical repair of their CHD, but all have had severe intellectual disability and were completely dependent on care.

Genetic Considerations

The risk of recurrence for trisomy 18 syndrome is estimated to be less than 1%.

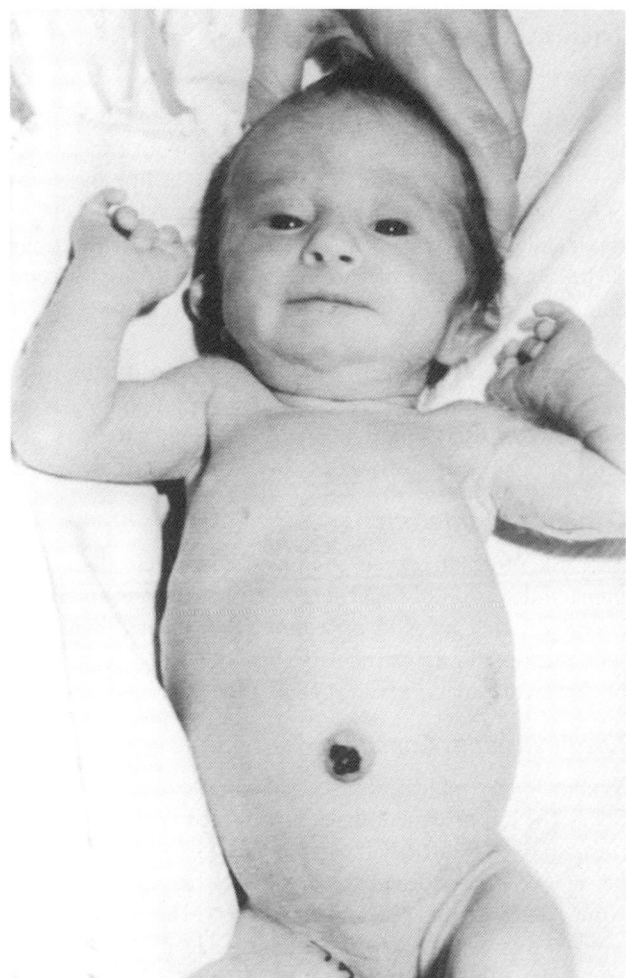

• **Fig. 6.3** Trisomy 18 syndrome in a newborn infant with complex cardiac defects. Note petite facial features, clenched hands, and short sternum.

Prenatal detection of intrauterine growth retardation, decreased fetal activity, and clenched fists, accompanied by visceral, cardiac, and limb malformations suggests trisomy 18 syndrome.

Cardiovascular Considerations

Cardiovascular defects are found in virtually all liveborn infants with trisomy 18 syndrome. Characteristic cardiac malformations in a series of 41 karyotyped and autopsied cases of trisomy 18 syndrome included a ventricular septal defect in all cases, polyvalvular disease (malformations of more than one valve) in 93%, a subpulmonary infundibulum in 98%, and a striking absence of transposition of the great arteries and inversion at any level (cardiac or visceral), findings which appear to be characteristic of all autosomal trisomies. The ventricular septal defect was associated with anterosuperior conal septal malalignment in 61% of cases. The malformations of the atrioventricular and semilunar valves were characterized by redundant or thick myxomatous leaflets, long chordae tendineae, and hypoplastic or absent papillary muscles. Other defects included double-outlet right ventricle (10%), all with mitral atresia, and tetralogy of Fallot (15%).

Trisomy 13 Syndrome

General Clinical Characteristics

Trisomy 13 syndrome has an incidence of about 1 in 5000 live births. The major features include cleft lip and palate; holoprosencephalic defects of the eye, nose, lip, and forebrain; postaxial polydactyly; and localized skin defects of the scalp at the vertex (cutis aplasia congenita). Microphthalmia, colobomata of the iris, and retinal dysplasia are common. Apneic spells, seizures, and severe intellectual disability are hallmarks.

Infants with trisomy 13 syndrome have a dismally poor prognosis, as in trisomy 18 syndrome. Although long-term survival has been reported occasionally, all survivors are profoundly impaired.

Genetic Considerations

The risk of recurrence is presumed to be less than 1%. Prenatal detection of facial abnormalities, such as holoprosencephaly, cleft lip with or without cleft palate, hand and foot malformations, particularly postaxial polydactyly, and cardiovascular malformations suggests trisomy 13 syndrome.

Cardiovascular Considerations

The incidence of cardiovascular malformations is about 80%. The most frequent defects include patent ductus arteriosus (63%), ventricular septal defect (48%), atrial septal defect (40%), abnormal valves (22%), coarctation of the aorta (10%), and dextrocardia (6%). The majority of affected infants (75%) have complex defects.

Trisomy or Tetrasomy 22p (Cat Eye Syndrome)

General Clinical Characteristics

The classic pattern of malformations includes mild intellectual disability, hypertelorism, down-slanting palpebral fissures, iris coloboma, preauricular pits or tags, and anal and renal malformations, but there is wide variability of phenotypic expression.

Genetic Considerations

The small marker chromosome in the cat eye syndrome is either a tandem duplication of proximal 22q or an isodicentric (22)(pter-q11).

Cardiovascular Considerations

Cardiovascular malformations have been reported in about 40%, and the occurrence of totally anomalous pulmonary venous connection has been observed in several studies. Additional defects include tetralogy of Fallot, ventricular septal defect, persistent left superior vena cava, interruption of the inferior vena cava, and tricuspid atresia.

Turner Syndrome

General Clinical Characteristics

The major features of Turner syndrome (Fig. 6.4) include short stature, primary amenorrhea due to ovarian dysgenesis, webbed neck, congenital lymphedema, and cubitus valgus. The incidence of Turner syndrome is 1 in 5000 live born female infants.

Genetic Considerations

Although common in the first trimester, most 45,X conceptuses are spontaneously aborted. They constitute 25% of spontaneous abortions during the first trimester of pregnancy. More than half of live born individuals have a 45,X karyotype without evidence of mosaicism. The remainder show mosaicism and/or more complex rearrangements involving the X chromosome (ring, deletion, isochromosome Xq, isodicentric X, etc.) and/or Y chromosome.

Prenatal recognition of coarctation of the aorta, left-sided hypoplasia, or hypoplastic left heart syndrome in a female infant with hydrops fetalis or cystic hygroma and renal malformation suggests Turner syndrome.

Cardiovascular Considerations

Between 20% and 40% of girls with Turner syndrome have significant cardiovascular malformations, most commonly coarctation of the aorta (70%), often bicommissural aortic valve, and aortic stenosis—defects typically not common in girls. In fact, girls with Turner syndrome are prone to a spectrum of left-sided obstructive/hypoplastic defects ranging in severity from asymptomatic bicommissural aortic valve to hypoplastic left heart syndrome. Aortic dilation, dissection, and rupture also have been reported, but the incidence and risk factors for these complications are unclear. Systemic hypertension is more common in Turner syndrome than the general population, and should be treated aggressively.

Contiguous Gene Deletion Syndromes

Contiguous gene deletion syndromes result from the loss of multiple contiguous genes from a particular chromosomal segment. Typical clinical features include growth deficiency, developmental delay and intellectual disability, and congenital anomalies. The deletion can present *de novo* with a negative family history or can be inherited in an autosomal dominant fashion.

Chromosome 22q11.2 Deletion Syndrome, Also Encompassing the Following: DiGeorge Syndrome, Velocardiofacial Syndrome, Conotruncal Anomaly Face Syndrome

General Clinical Characteristics

The chromosome 22q11.2 deletion syndrome (Fig. 6.5) is common, with an estimated incidence of at least 1 in 4000. A broad spectrum of clinical manifestations is associated with 22q11.2 deletions, and phenotypic expression is highly variable. Multiple system involvement includes immune deficiency; hypocalcemia and hypoparathyroidism; palatal, laryngotracheal, gastrointestinal, musculoskeletal, ophthalmologic, craniofacial, and central nervous system anomalies; developmental delay/learning disability, and psychiatric illness.

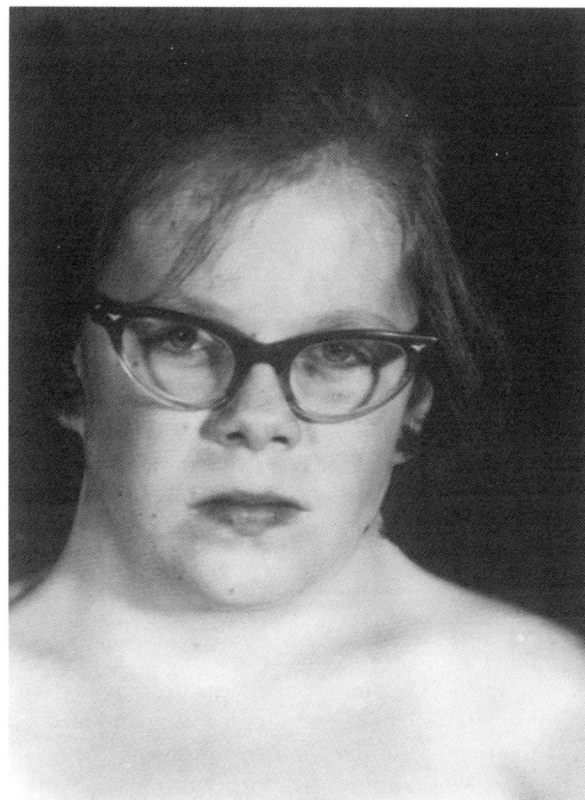
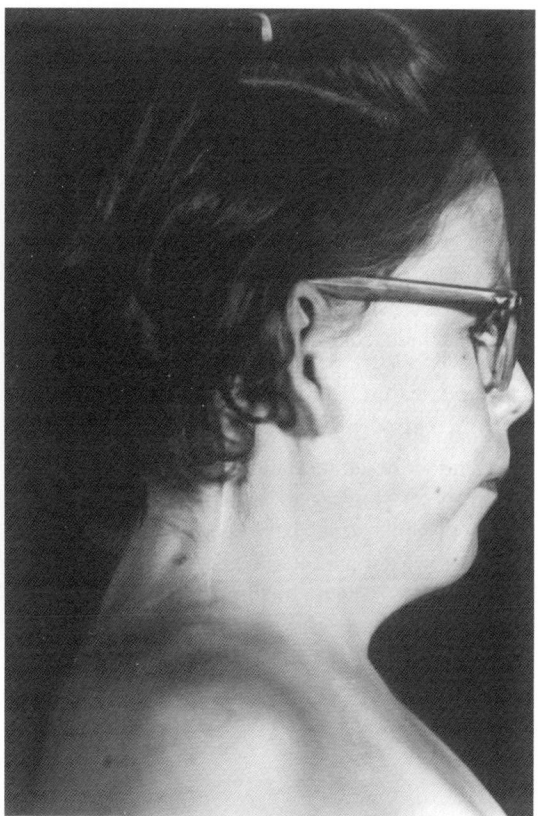

• **Fig. 6.4** Turner syndrome. Turner syndrome in a young woman with coarctation of the aorta. Note the webbed neck, broad chest, prominent ears, and multiple pigmented nevi.

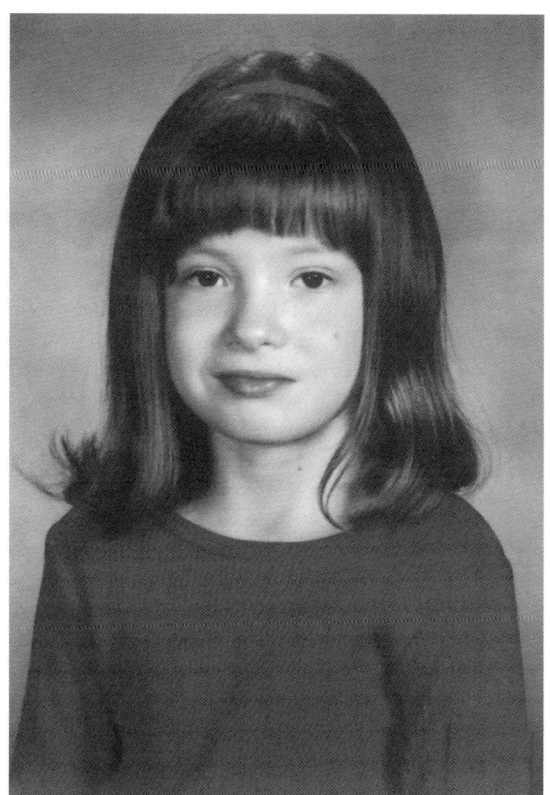

• **Fig. 6.5** Chromosome 22q11.2 deletion syndrome. Facial features are characteristic but can be relatively subtle especially in infants. Note the tubular nose, bulbous nasal tip, and short philtrum.

Genetic Considerations

Rarely, an abnormality is detected by standard karyotype. In most cases (approximately 80%), a microdeletion can be demonstrated by chromosomal microarray or FISH (fluorescence *in situ* hybridization) testing of the critical region. In the remainder of cases, there is a mutation within the *TBX1* gene (one of the genes in the critical region) or presumably a small deletion not detectable by chromosomal microarray. Deletions involving chromosome 10p also have been associated with the 22q11.2 deletion phenotype but are far less common.

Cardiovascular Considerations

Cardiovascular anomalies are present in 75%–80% of patients with a 22q11.2 deletion, and conotruncal malformations account for 70% of the heart defects associated with a 22q11.2 deletion. When a conotruncal malformation is detected either prenatally or postnatally (tetralogy of Fallot, truncus arteriosus, type B interrupted aortic arch), a chromosomal microarray is recommended to detect a 22q11.2 deletion.

The most common congenital heart defects include tetralogy of Fallot, truncus arteriosus, conoventricular ventricular septal defect, type B interruption of the aortic arch, and other aortic arch anomalies. Anatomic features that are associated with higher likelihood of a 22q11.2 deletion include right aortic arch (abnormal arch sidedness), abnormal aortic arch branching pattern (e.g., aberrant subclavian artery on either side), and discontinuous pulmonary arteries. Other heart defects, including atrial septal defect, pulmonary valve stenosis, hypoplastic left heart syndrome, double-outlet right ventricle, transposition of the great arteries, vascular rings, heterotaxy syndrome, and isolated aortic dilation have been reported less commonly.

Williams Syndrome/Elastin Arteriopathy

General Clinical Characteristics

Williams syndrome (Fig. 6.6) is a contiguous gene deletion syndrome caused by deletion at 7q11.23. Common clinical manifestations include characteristic facial features, typical cardiovascular defects (vascular stenoses, elastin arteriopathy), a specific cognitive profile and unique personality characteristics ("social personality"), connective tissue and skeletal abnormalities, and endocrine abnormalities. Infants generally are colicky (sometimes secondary to hypercalcemia) and show poor weight gain, while adults have short stature and a tendency toward overweight and obesity, with increased risk for systemic hypertension, diabetes mellitus, and diverticulosis.

Genetic Considerations

Williams syndrome is a contiguous gene deletion syndrome associated with a 1- to 2-megabase deletion on the long arm

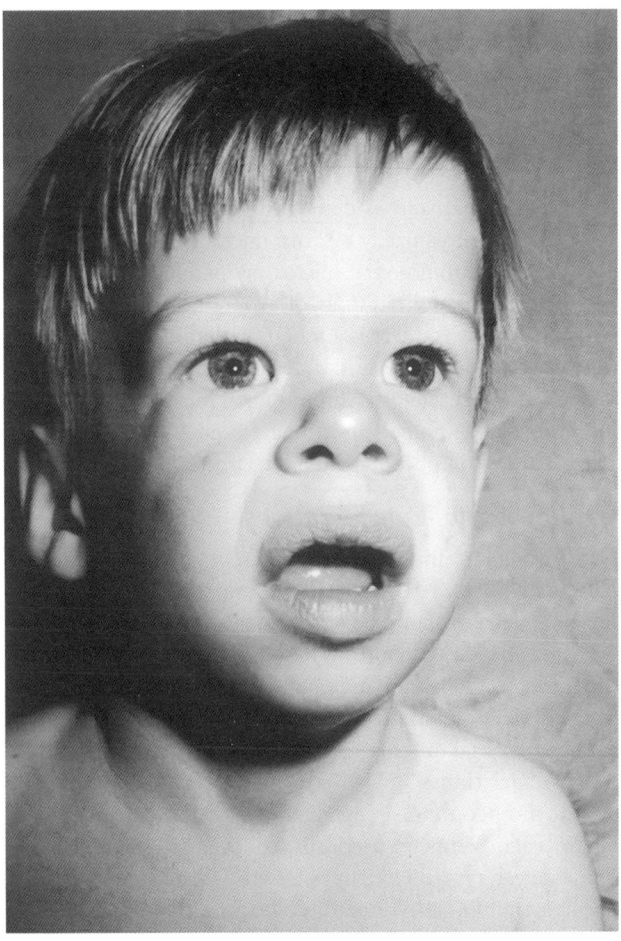

• **Fig. 6.6** Williams syndrome in a 2-year-old boy with supravalvar aortic stenosis. Note the typical facies including a stellate pattern of the iris, short anteverted nose, long philtrum, prominent lips, and large, open mouth.

of chromosome 7, including the entire elastin gene (*ELN*) and over 20 additional genes. The loss of these additional genes account for the non-elastin-related manifestations of Williams syndrome.

In contrast, familial (non-syndromic) SVAS is caused by mutations in *ELN*. A translocation disrupting the elastin gene as well as intragenic deletions and mutations involving the elastin gene have been identified in non-syndromic SVAS. Individuals with familial SVAS typically do not show evidence of a complete deletion of *ELN* (negative chromosomal microarray).

Cardiovascular Considerations

At least half of individuals with Williams syndrome have cardiovascular defects consisting most commonly of thickening of the aortic or arterial wall and narrowing of the lumen. SVAS is the most frequent single defect, but any of the systemic and pulmonary arteries can be affected. Narrowing at the sinotubular ridge can be detected by echocardiography and angiography postnatally, but may be difficult to detect prenatally.

The SVAS complex or elastin arteriopathy can occur as part of Williams syndrome or as an isolated autosomal dominant disorder (non-syndromic SVAS). The SVAS complex is a diffuse arteriopathy which can affect all segments of the aorta; any of its branches including the coronary arteries, the brachiocephalic vessels, the mesenteric and the renal arteries, as well as the pulmonary and cerebral arteries. Abnormalities in elastin production are thought to be responsible for the cardiovascular phenotype in both Williams syndrome and non-syndromic SVAS, so the similarity in vascular abnormalities is predictable.

Jacobsen Syndrome (11q Terminal Deletion Disorder)

General Clinical Characteristics

Jacobsen syndrome is a rare contiguous gene syndrome caused by partial deletion of the long arm of chromosome 11. The prevalence is estimated to be 1 in 50,000 to 100,000 live births. The most common clinical features include characteristic facial dysmorphism, prenatal and postnatal growth deficiency, developmental delay, thrombocytopenia, and pancytopenia.

Genetic and Prenatal Considerations

The type and size of the deletion on the long arm of chromosome 11 vary.

Cardiovascular Considerations

Congenital heart defects occur in more than half of affected individuals: about one-third with membranous ventricular septal defect, about one-third with left ventricular outflow tract defects ranging in severity from bicuspid aortic valve to hypoplastic left heart syndrome, and the remaining third with a wide variety of other congenital heart defects.

Hypoplastic left heart syndrome is highly overrepresented in patients with Jacobsen syndrome (5–10%), an estimated frequency that is 1000 to 2000 times that of the general population.

Single Gene Disorders

Alagille Syndrome

General Clinical Characteristics

The typical manifestations of Alagille syndrome (arteriohepatic dysplasia), an autosomal dominant disorder, include peripheral pulmonary artery stenosis, intrahepatic cholestasis due to bile duct paucity, distinctive facies (prominent forehead and chin, deep-set eyes, long nose), anterior chamber abnormalities of the eye, especially posterior embryotoxon, and butterfly hemivertebrae.

Genetic and Prenatal Considerations

This syndrome is caused by mutations or deletions of the *JAG1* gene, which encodes for Jagged 1, a ligand in the Notch intercellular signaling pathway, or the *NOTCH2* gene which encodes a NOTCH receptor transmembrane protein.

Cardiovascular Considerations

Cardiac abnormalities are present in > 90% of affected individuals. Peripheral pulmonary artery stenosis is most common, although other defects including tetralogy of Fallot, pulmonary valve stenosis, atrial septal defect, ventricular septal defect, aortic stenosis, and coarctation of the aorta have also been observed.

Char Syndrome

General Clinical Characteristics

Char syndrome is characterized by the triad of typical facial features (wide-set eyes, down-slanting palpebral fissures, thick lips), patent ductus arteriosus, and hand anomalies (aplasia or hypoplasia of the middle phalanges of the fifth fingers).

Genetic and Prenatal Considerations

Autosomal dominant inheritance, associated with mutations in *TFAP2B*.

Cardiovascular Considerations

Patent ductus arteriosus is most common. Other heart defects including muscular ventricular septal defects and complex congenital defects have also been observed.

CHARGE Syndrome

General Clinical Characteristics

CHARGE stands for *c*oloboma, *h*eart defect, choanal *a*tresia, *r*etarded growth and development, *g*enital hypoplasia, and *e*ar anomalies including hearing loss. The phenotypic spectrum also includes cranial nerve anomalies, vestibular defects, cleft lip and/or palate, hypothyroidism, tracheoesophageal, renal and brain anomalies, and seizures. Prognosis is highly variable and depends on the severity of manifestations.

Genetic and Prenatal Considerations

CHARGE is an autosomal dominant syndrome associated with mutations and deletions involving the *CHD7* gene.

Cardiovascular Considerations

Congenital heart defects are common (50%–70%), especially conotruncal malformations and aortic arch anomalies. Other defects include patent ductus arteriosus, atrioventricular canal, ventricular septal defect, and atrial septal defect.

Ellis–van Creveld Syndrome (Chondroectodermal Dysplasia)

General Clinical Characteristics

Ellis–van Creveld syndrome is a rare, autosomal recessive disorder associated with short stature of prenatal onset (short limbs), ectodermal dysplasia manifested by hypoplastic nails and dental anomalies (neonatal teeth, partial anodontia, small teeth, and/or delayed eruption), postaxial polydactyly, narrow thorax, and cardiac defects. Most survivors have normal intelligence. Adult stature is in the range of 43–60 inches. Dental problems are frequent.

Genetic Considerations

The syndrome is associated with mutations of two nonhomologous genes at chromosome 4p16 (*EVC1* and *EVC2*). For couples with at least one affected child, the recurrence risk is 25% for each subsequent pregnancy (autosomal recessive). The incidence is as high as 5 in 1000 in the Old Order Amish community of Lancaster County, PA.

Cardiovascular Considerations

About 50% of patients have congenital heart defects. Atrial septal defect or common atrium occurs in about half of patients with congenital heart disease. Other less frequent defects include patent ductus arteriosus, persistent left superior vena cava, hypoplastic left heart syndrome, coarctation of the aorta, totally anomalous pulmonary venous connection, and transposition of the great arteries.

Holt-Oram Syndrome

General Clinical Characteristics

Holt-Oram syndrome (Fig. 6.7) is characterized by the combination of upper limb and cardiovascular malformations. Affected individuals may have isolated upper limb defects, isolated heart defects, or a combination. All gradations of skeletal defects involving the upper limb and shoulder girdle, ranging from mild hypoplasia of the thumb to phocomelia, can occur even within the same family. All patients with involvement of the upper limbs have defects involving the thumb. There is no correlation between the

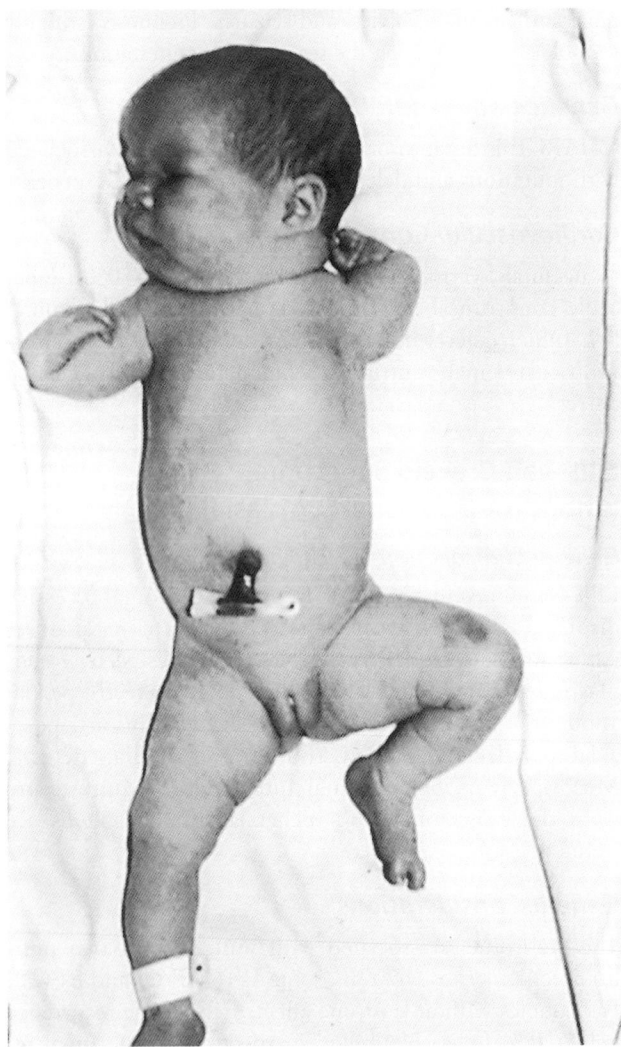

• **Fig. 6.7** Holt-Oram syndrome in a newborn infant with an atrial septal defect. Note the bilateral deficiency of the upper limbs.

severity of the defect of the limb and the cardiac defect. Prognosis is dependent on the degree of skeletal deformity and the nature of the cardiac anomaly. Intelligence is normal, and there are no associated visceral malformations.

Genetic Considerations

This is an autosomal dominant disorder with variable expression, but complete or near-complete penetrance. The gene for Holt-Oram, *TBX5*, encodes a DNA transcription factor. Other families do not have *TBX5* mutations, consistent with genetic heterogeneity.

Cardiovascular Considerations

Congenital heart defects are observed in at least half of affected individuals, although there may be an ascertainment bias toward cardiac defects. Atrial septal defect and ventricular septal defect are the most common defects, but a number of cardiac phenotypes have been reported including normal, first-degree atrioventricular block, ostium primum atrial septal defects, isolated ventricular septal defects, and hypoplastic left heart syndrome.

Kabuki Syndrome

General Clinical Characteristics

Kabuki syndrome is characterized by typical facial features (particularly the long palpebral fissures with eversion of the lateral third of the lower eyelid, arched and broad eyebrows, short columella with depressed nasal tip, and large, prominent, or cupped ears), minor skeletal anomalies, persistence of fetal fingertip pads, postnatal growth deficiency, and intellectual disability.

Genetic Considerations

The genes associated with Kabuki syndrome include *KMT2D* (chromosome 12) and *KDM6A* (X chromosome). Inheritance is autosomal dominant for *KMT2D* and X-linked for *KDM6A*.

Cardiovascular Considerations

Approximately 70% of individuals with Kabuki syndrome have a congenital heart defect. Left-sided obstructive lesions, especially coarctation of the aorta are the most common. Other defects include septal defects, bicuspid aortic valve, mitral valve anomalies, conotruncal malformations, and hypoplastic left heart syndrome. Hypertrophic cardiomyopathy and aortic root dilation have been reported occasionally.

Loeys-Dietz Syndrome

General Clinical Characteristics

Loeys-Dietz syndrome is an autosomal dominant connective tissue disorder associated with vascular findings (aortic and arterial aneurysms and dissections), skeletal manifestations, craniofacial features including widely spaced eyes, bifid uvula/cleft palate, and craniosynostosis, skin findings including translucent skin, easy bruising, and dystrophic scars. Other findings include a predisposition for allergic/inflammatory disease including asthma, eczema, and food or environmental allergies, as well as an increased incidence of gastrointestinal inflammation including eosinophilic esophagitis, gastritis, and inflammatory bowel disease. There is wide variability in the distribution and severity of clinical features, even within the same family, ranging from severe vascular and extravascular involvement in one individual to very subtle systemic features in the presence of severe vascular involvement in another.

Genetic and Prenatal Considerations

Loeys-Dietz syndrome is associated with mutations and deletions involving the following genes: *SMAD2*, *SMAD3*, *TGFB2*, *TGFB3*, *TGFBR1*, and *TGFBR2*.

Cardiovascular Considerations

The major sources of morbidity and early mortality associated with Loeys-Dietz syndrome are dilatation of the aortic root and ascending aorta with a predisposition for aortic dissection and rupture, mitral valve prolapse with or without regurgitation. Individuals with Loeys-Dietz syndrome generally have a more aggressive vascular course with routine involvement of the distal aorta and peripheral arterial tree (e.g., vertebral and carotid arteries), especially when compared with Marfan syndrome. In contrast to Marfan syndrome, vascular dissection can occur in early childhood and at aortic dimensions that are not usually associated with risk for dissection. Arterial tortuosity is common, and the degree of arterial tortuosity correlates with risk for vascular complications. Congenital heart defects, especially bicuspid aortic valve, patent ductus arteriosus, and atrial septal defect, are more common in Loeys-Dietz syndrome, compared with Marfan syndrome and the general population.

Marfan Syndrome

General Clinical Characteristics

Marfan syndrome, with an incidence of about 1 in 5,000, is the most common and best characterized of the connective tissue disorders with serious cardiovascular manifestations. This condition is an autosomal dominant, multisystem disorder with a wide variability of phenotypic expression involving the skeletal, ocular, cardiovascular, and other systems.

Genetic Considerations

Mutations or deletions involving *FBN1*, the gene encoding the connective tissue protein fibrillin-1, have been found in the vast majority of cases. There is a severe early-onset form of Marfan syndrome, also associated with mutations or deletions in *FBN1*, typically but not exclusively in exons 23-32.

Cardiovascular Considerations

Nearly all patients have some cardiovascular involvement, most commonly mitral valve prolapse and aortic root dilation. The risk for aortic regurgitation, dissection, and rupture increases with progressive enlargement of the aortic root. Beta-blockers and angiotensin receptor blockers retard the rate of dilatation of the aortic root and ascending aorta. In adults, replacement of the root is generally recommended when the aortic root diameter is greater than 5.0 cm of if the growth rate exceeds 5–10 mm/year. Surgical options include valve-sparing aortic root replacement or composite valve graft repair with a prosthetic aortic valve. Because of the relatively low risk of prophylactic aortic root replacement in Marfan syndrome and the devastating effects on short- and long-term survival after aortic dissection, some are now advocating surgery when the aortic root diameter exceeds 45 mm, especially if there is a family history of aortic dissection.

Noonan Syndrome and Other RASopathies (Noonan Syndrome with Multiple Lentigines, Cardiofaciocutaneous Syndrome, Costello Syndrome)

General Clinical Characteristics

Noonan syndrome (Fig. 6.8) is the most common of the RASopathies, which are a group of predominantly autosomal dominant conditions with overlapping cardiac, growth,

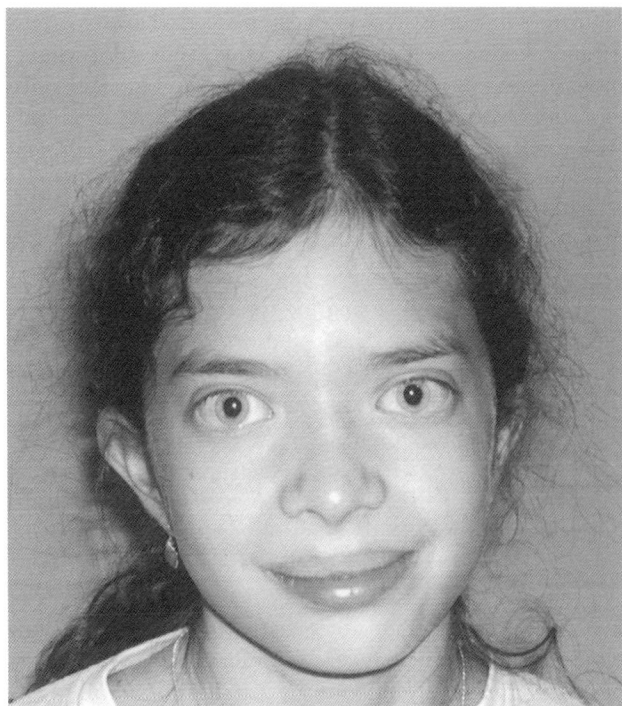

• **Fig. 6.8** Noonan syndrome. Note widely spaced eyes, bulbous nasal tip, and low-set ears.

craniofacial, and neurodevelopmental phenotypes. They are caused by pathogenic variants in genes that encode proteins involved in the RAS/mitogen-activated protein kinase pathway which plays an important role in cellular function.

Noonan syndrome is characterized by recognizable facial features, short stature, and variable involvement of the eye and ear, as well as the gastrointestinal, endocrine, hematologic, lymphatic, neurological, behavioral, orthopedic, renal, and genitourinary systems.

Genetic Considerations

The genes associated with Noonan syndrome include *PTPN11, SOS1, RAF1, KRAS, LZTR1, MRAS, NRAS, RIT1, SHOC2, SOS2, BRAF, RASA2, and RRAS2.* Causative pathogenic variants activate the Ras MAP Kinase pathway with downstream activation of MEK and ERK. As such, MEK-inhibiting drugs, developed to treat melanoma and other cancers that cause similar pathway activation, are being offered to infants with severe cardiac and lymphatic disease. *PTPN11* is more likely to cause pulmonary valve stenosis and less likely to cause hypertrophic cardiomyopathy. Septal defects are more commonly associated with *SOS1* mutations. Although overall only about 20% of individuals with Noonan syndrome have hypertrophic cardiomyopathy, 95% of individuals with *RAF1* mutation and 75% with *RIT1* mutation have HCM.

Cardiovascular Considerations

Cardiac involvement is seen in 80% to 90% of affected individuals, including congenital heart defects and hypertrophic cardiomyopathy. At least 50% of individuals with

Noonan syndrome have congenital heart defects. About 75% of those with congenital heart defects have valvar pulmonary stenosis secondary to a dysplastic pulmonary valve with thickened valve leaflets which can be resistant to balloon valvotomy. Other defects reported include atrial septal defect, mitral valve anomalies, aortic coarctation, and tetralogy of Fallot. Hypertrophic cardiomyopathy, which can involve both ventricles, is observed in 10% to 20% of cases. The cardiomyopathy is often mild, but can present as a severe, rapidly progressive and life-threatening form in early infancy. The 1-year survival in those with HCM and heart failure before 6 months of age is 34%. Aortic and arterial dilatation/aneurysm and coronary atresia also have been reported less commonly.

Other RASopathies

Noonan syndrome with multiple lentigines (*PTPN11, RAF1, BRAF, MAP2K1*), Costello syndrome (*HRAS*), and cardiofaciocutaneous syndrome (*BRAF, MAP2K1, MAP2K2, KRAS*) are other RASopathies that share common phenotypic features including facial appearance, developmental delay, short stature, and cardiac defects in 75% of cases. Pulmonary valve stenosis, atrial septal defect, and hypertrophic cardiomyopathy are the most common cardiac abnormalities in all of the RASopathies. Those with Noonan syndrome with multiple lentigines have a much higher incidence of hypertrophic cardiomyopathy than those with Noonan syndrome. Those with Costello syndrome can be complicated by arrhythmia, most typically a chaotic atrial rhythm/multifocal atrial tachycardia. This atrial tachycardia has also been reported in other RASopathies but much less frequently than with Costello syndrome.

VACTERL/VATER Association

General Clinical Characteristics

An association is a non-random occurrence of multiple anomalies. A given association, such as the VACTERL association, can occur in isolation or as part of a broader pattern of malformation, such as in trisomy 18 syndrome or infants born to mothers with diabetes.

The VACTERL association includes vertebral defects, anal atresia, cardiac defects, tracheoesophageal fistula, and renal anomalies, radial and thumb defects, single umbilical artery, and prenatal-onset growth deficiency. Generally, it has occurred sporadically in an otherwise unaffected family. Identification of VACTERL association defects in a particular individual does not, in itself, imply a diagnosis. Rather, the presence of one or more VACTERL-associated malformations should alert the clinician to the presence of other VACTERL defects.

Genetic Considerations

The etiology of this pattern of malformation is not fully delineated but likely heterogeneous.

Cardiovascular Considerations

Although ventricular septal defects are most common, a wide variety of cardiac lesions has been seen.

Reference

1. Pierpont ME, Brueckner M, Chung WK, et al. Genetic basis for congenital heart disease: revisited: a scientific statement from the American Heart Association. *Circulation*. 2018;138:e653-e711.

SECTION IV

Noninvasive Tools of Diagnosis

7

History, Physical Examination, Oximetry, Chest Radiograph, and Other Baseline Testing

ROBERT L. GEGGEL AND DAVID R. FULTON

"Listen to your patients; they are telling you the diagnosis."

Adapted from Sir William Osler

KEY LEARNING POINTS

- A thorough and informed patient history and physical exam is critical to the diagnosis and management of patients with suspected or documented congenital heart disease.
- A complete cardiac examination includes inspection, palpation, and auscultation.

- The chest radiograph provides information on the cardiac, pulmonary, and skeletal status. An example of a structured approach to interpretation is the "Rule of Six."

While the specialty of pediatric cardiology has made remarkable advances in imaging and therapy over the past half century, the bedrock of patient evaluation remains the history and physical examination. Details obtained from these basic methods enable the physician to compile an appropriate differential diagnosis, order tests in a logical manner, and efficiently care for the patient.

Patient History

The pediatric history requires obtaining information from the care providers, and, after early childhood, also from the patient. It is important to establish a trusting and empathetic relationship with the family. As outlined in a previous edition of this book,[1] it is helpful to conduct the interview in a relaxed manner so that information can be recalled and shared with the physician.

Pertinent issues to be addressed in the history depend on the age of the patient and the clinical concern. The following topics need to be considered.

1. Prenatal testing: The results of fetal ultrasound studies performed during pregnancy can identify structural

disease before birth. Of neonates treated for cyanotic congenital heart disease at Boston Children's Hospital in 2013, 99% of those born at nearby tertiary care medical centers and 32% delivered at community-based hospitals were diagnosed prenatally.[2]

2. Pregnancy history: Maternal use of some medications can influence the likelihood of congenital heart disease (CHD) developing in the fetus (see Chapter 6). Maternal diabetes mellitus is associated with an increased incidence of transposition of the great arteries (TGA), hypertrophic cardiomyopathy, coarctation, and ventricular septal defect (VSD). Maternal systemic lupus erythematosus is associated with fetal complete atrioventricular block.[3] Maternal exposure to infectious agents can contribute to cardiac defects in the neonate: for example, rubella with peripheral pulmonary stenosis; patent ductus arteriosus (PDA), or VSD; and Coxsackie virus with myocarditis.

3. Perinatal history: Maternal history of premature rupture of membranes, fever, or use of sedatives or anesthetics raises concern about sepsis and decreased respiratory effort. For infants with cyanosis, gestational age, Apgar score, and history of meconium aspiration are useful to

determine the likelihood of hyaline membrane disease, perinatal asphyxia, persistent pulmonary hypertension of the newborn, or pneumonia. The response to oxygen helps to distinguish a cardiac from pulmonary basis for cyanosis (see Routine Laboratory Tests section later in this chapter).[4]

4. Neonatal pulse oximetry screening for critical CHD: In 2011 the Department of Health and Human Services and the American Academy of Pediatrics recommended pulse oximetry screening to aid in the detection of seven cyanotic heart lesions including hypoplastic left heart syndrome, pulmonary atresia with intact ventricular septum, tetralogy of Fallot (TOF), tricuspid atresia, total anomalous pulmonary venous return, D-loop TGA, and truncus arteriosus. The protocol involves testing between 24 and 48 hours of age in the well-infant nursery and is judged to be positive if the oxygen saturation in the right hand or foot is < 90% at any time, if the oxygen saturations in the right hand and foot are between 90% and < 95%, or if there is > 3% difference between values in the right hand and foot on three occasions measured 1 hour apart.[5] The protocol has been adopted across the United States. A failed test prompts obtaining an echocardiogram. A passed test does not rule out CHD, so early follow-up evaluation after hospital discharge is still needed. The protocol can also identify some patients with coarctation of the aorta although a minority of patients with this condition are detected.[6]

5. Other birth defects: A variety of syndromes are associated with CHD[7] (see Chapter 6). Commonly encountered syndromes and the frequency and most common type of CHD include trisomy 21 (45%; atrioventricular canal defect, VSD, TOF), VACTERL syndrome (vertebral defects, anal atresia, cardiac defect, tracheoesophageal fistula, renal anomaly, limb anomaly) (50%; VSD, TOF), trisomy 13 or 18 (more than 80%; VSD), Noonan syndrome (50%; pulmonary stenosis, hypertrophic cardiomyopathy), Turner syndrome (35%; aortic stenosis, cardiomyopathy, coarctation), Williams syndrome (50%; supravalvar aortic stenosis, coarctation, peripheral pulmonary stenosis), and Marfan syndrome (nearly all patients; aortic dilation, mitral valve prolapse, mitral regurgitation, aortic regurgitation).

6. Family history: CHD affecting a previous child or a parent increases the risk for structural heart disease in the infant.[8] Early myocardial infarction in first-degree relatives (younger than 50 years for men, younger than 60 years for women) merits screening for hyperlipidemia (see Chapter 44). Sudden death is associated with various genetic diseases, including cardiomyopathy, prolonged QT interval, Brugada syndrome, Marfan syndrome, and arrhythmogenic right ventricular dysplasia.[9] Hypertension in the extended family should lead to close monitoring of this variable, especially in adolescence when essential hypertension may initially develop.

7. Initial detection of murmur: Knowledge of the time a murmur was initially detected leads a clinician to consider different categories of cardiac disease. For neonates, murmurs detected in the first 6 hours of life typically involve valve regurgitation (e.g., tricuspid valve from perinatal stress, mitral valve from cardiac dysfunction) or valve stenosis, whereas murmurs detected after 6 hours of age can also represent shunt lesions that present as pulmonary vascular resistance falls (e.g., atrial septal defect [ASD]) or VSD, PDA, peripheral pulmonary stenosis). It is important to note that some neonates may only be examined initially by a physician after 6 hours of age, and others may have both valve stenosis and septal defects (e.g., TOF). Systolic murmurs detected initially at 2–4 years of age frequently are innocent but can represent structural heart disease if the patient was uncooperative for earlier examinations, had progression in the severity of the lesion, or developed an acquired condition. During childhood, a new murmur of mitral or aortic regurgitation raises the possibility of rheumatic heart disease and inquiry should be made about a history of streptococcal pharyngitis, unexplained fever, arthritis, chorea, and rashes.

8. Growth and development: The normal infant gradually eats a larger volume of food at increasing intervals. This pattern is not observed in infants with lesions associated with poor cardiac function, pulmonary edema, or significant left-to-right shunting (ratio of pulmonary to systemic flow greater than 2:1). Lesions associated with large shunts gradually become symptomatic as pulmonary vascular resistance decreases over the first 2–8 weeks of life. Infants with lesions associated with shunting at the ventricular or great vessel level are generally more symptomatic than those with only atrial level shunting. Symptoms consist of tachypnea, diaphoresis, and feeding difficulties of early fatigue and decreased oral intake. Such infants can have failure to thrive and delays in developmental milestones.

9. Cyanosis: Cyanosis can have a cardiac, pulmonary, central nervous system, or hematologic basis.[4] Cyanosis is often initially detected by experienced nurses in the newborn unit. The characteristics of fetal hemoglobin and the presence of darker skin pigmentation make the detection of mild cyanosis more difficult.

   Infants with TOF can have cyanotic spells (see Chapter 26). A single well-documented episode is an indication to proceed with surgical repair or palliation. In regions of the world where screening or infant surgery is not available, older children without prior intervention can have squatting episodes to relieve these cyanotic spells.

   A common occurrence, especially in fair-skinned infants, is the transient development of peripheral cyanosis involving the distal extremities and perioral region. This appearance often occurs with cold exposure, such as after a bath, and represents vasomotor instability, a normal finding in infancy.

10. Common issues evaluated in childhood and adolescence: Although a variety of symptoms lead to cardiac consultation, several issues are frequently encountered.

    a. *Endurance:* Parents, teachers, coaches or the patient may note decreased exercise tolerance compared with peers. Activity limitations may have a cardiac basis or be caused by poor general conditioning, obesity, exercise-induced reactive airway disease, other pulmonary disease, or neuromuscular disease. Determining the severity, duration, and progression of limitations and associated symptoms distinguishes among these possibilities.

    b. *Chest pain:* Chest pain is a frequent symptom in children and has a cardiac basis in only 1–6% of patients.[10] Heart conditions include structural heart disease, such as left ventricular outflow obstruction, aortic dissection, ruptured sinus of Valsalva aneurysm, coronary artery anomalies, arrhythmia or acquired heart diseases including pericarditis, myocarditis, or Kawasaki disease.

       In children, chest pain typically has a musculoskeletal or idiopathic basis and is self-resolving. Musculoskeletal issues include costochondritis, myodynia, rib fracture, or slipping rib syndrome. Slipping rib syndrome involves the 8th, 9th, and 10th ribs, whose costal cartilages do not attach to the sternum; these ribs are attached to each other by fibrous tissue that is susceptible to trauma. If these fibrous connections are weakened, the ribs can rub together, irritating the intercostal nerve and producing pain. Patients can describe "something slipping or giving away," "a popping sensation," or "hearing a clicking sound." Musculoskeletal pain typically is sharp in quality, is located at the costochondral junction or insertion site of the pectoralis major muscle group, and frequently increases during inspiration. There often is a history of activity that can lead to muscle injury, such as sports, weight lifting, use of a heavy backpack, or direct trauma.

       Other causes of chest pain include hyperventilation; psychiatric disorders; breast disease; respiratory disease, including pneumonia, pneumothorax, pneumomediastinum, or reactive airway disease; pulmonary hypertension; pulmonary embolism; gastrointestinal disorders; and exposure to toxins (e.g., cocaine, cannabis, cigarettes). A full discussion can be found in Chapter 52. In the absence of associated symptoms of illness, positive physical examination findings related to the cardiac or respiratory systems, or symptoms during exertion, a serious organic cause is unlikely.

    c. *Syncope:* Syncope is more common during adolescence than in childhood and frequently has a vasovagal or orthostatic basis. These episodes are often preceded by symptoms of diaphoresis, nausea, or development of tunnel vision. Consciousness is usually regained quickly upon becoming supine. There often is a history of dehydration, exposure to a warm environment (crowded auditorium, hot summer day, warm shower), or standing for prolonged periods of time. Syncope can be precipitated by hair combing, cough, painful stimulation, fear, hyperventilation, micturition, or defecation. Orthostatic changes in blood pressure can be exacerbated by a variety of medications, including diuretics or vasoactive agent. Primary cardiac causes include right or left ventricular obstructive heart disease, pulmonary hypertension, and arrhythmia, including prolonged QT syndrome, bradyarrhythmia, or tachyarrhythmia. The occurrence of symptoms during or shortly after exercise can be associated with a vasovagal mechanism but increases the risk for an underlying cardiac basis.[11] Syncope can also be caused by neurologic disorders, including seizures, breath-holding spells, or migraine headaches. Seizures can be associated with tonic-clonic movements and post episode fatigue. Breath-holding spells often occur with sudden fright, pain, or frustration in children between 18 months and 5 years of age. A review of syncope can be found in Chapter 52.

    d. *Palpitations:* Awareness of palpitations may represent an abnormality in rate or rhythm. Sinus tachycardia associated with anxiety or activity usually has a gradual onset and resolution. Supraventricular tachycardia typically has a sudden onset and end as the circuit responsible for supporting the arrhythmia opens and closes. Other tachyarrhythmias (e.g., atrial flutter, atrial fibrillation, ventricular tachycardia) can have a similar pattern. Prolonged episodes of these arrhythmias can be associated with dizziness or syncope. Tachyarrhythmia occurring with exercise may represent catecholamine-sensitive ventricular tachycardia. Irregular rhythms can represent atrial, junctional, or ventricular premature beats. Some patients with rare premature beats note every single one, whereas others with thousands of daily premature beats only come to medical attention when an irregular rhythm is noted on physical examination. Detailed review of arrhythmia can be found in Chapters 17–20.

Physical Examination

The physical examination needs to be thorough because heart disease can affect multiple organ systems. The order of the examination will vary depending on the age of the patient. For infants and toddlers, it is often best to perform auscultation first when the patient is more likely to be quiet. Many portions of the physical examination can be performed with the infant or toddler in the parent's lap, which can aid in the level of patient cooperation. Infants can be fed or given a pacifier to achieve a quiet state.

General Examination

General inspection of the child will give clues to the state of health, cyanosis, or anemia. Height and weight measurements plotted on growth curves aid in determining the presence of failure to thrive. Heart disease associated with large left-to-right shunts, pulmonary edema, or ventricular dysfunction can impair growth. In such patients, weight typically is affected before height. Infants should gain at least 20 g/day; weight gain less than this amount caused by heart disease is an indication for medication (e.g., diuretics, correction of anemia if present) and use of caloric-supplemented food. If these methods are insufficient, surgical intervention is necessary. A normal infant can grow while receiving 100 calories/kg/day; infants whose growth is impaired by heart disease typically require 130–140 calories/kg/day. Expressed breast milk or formula contains 20 calories/ounce; each can be supplemented in stages with carbohydrate or fat to provide 30 calories/ounce so that caloric needs are fulfilled even if the infant has reduced volume of intake. For the mother interested in maintaining breast-feeding and depending on the degree of failure-to-thrive, some feedings can occur at the breast, whereas others can consist of supplemented expressed breast milk. An approach to caloric supplementation is outlined in Table 7.1.

General inspection also gives clues to the presence of syndromes that frequently are associated with specific heart disease. Extracardiac anomalies occur in about 20% of patients with CHD.[12] Multiple syndromes have characteristic facies (see Chapter 6). A webbed neck and short stature are seen in Turner syndrome. Arachnodactyly, pectus deformity, scoliosis, and arm span exceeding height are features of Marfan syndrome. Radial dysplasia is a component of Holt-Oram syndrome. A large-for-gestational-age neonate can be associated with maternal diabetes mellitus.

TABLE 7.1	Breast Milk: Increased Calorie Recipes	

24 calories per ounce
3 ounces breast milk
1 teaspoon infant formula
  powder
	26 calories per ounce
	3 ounces breast milk
	1½ teaspoons infant
	  formula powder

28 calories per ounce
3 ounces breast milk
1½ teaspoons infant
  formula powder
½ teaspoon Duocal®
  powder **or**
0.8 mL vegetable oil
	30 calories per ounce
	3 ounces breast milk
	1½ teaspoons infant
	  formula powder
	1 teaspoon Duocal®
	  powder or
	1.5 mL vegetable oil

If tolerated, the caloric concentration can be advanced every 3–4 days. For non-nursing mothers using commercial formula, consult nutritionist for individual formula recommendations.

Vital Signs

Review of vital signs enables the clinician to form a general appraisal of the patient and consider certain diagnostic possibilities.

Pulse

The pulse is examined with respect to rate, rhythm, prominence, and variation.

Rate

Sinus tachycardia occurs in a variety of conditions, including anxiety, fever, pain, anemia, large left-to-right shunts, decreased cardiac contractility, cardiac tamponade, sepsis, pulmonary disease, or hyperthyroidism. Supraventricular tachycardia in infants or children typically occurs at a rate that is too rapid to count by an observer (more than 180-200 beats/minute). Bradycardia occurs in high-level athletes and in children with eating disorders (anorexia nervosa, bulimia), hypothyroidism, or heart block. The average resting heart rate in the first week of life is 125 beats/minute, at 1 year is 120 beats/minute, at 5 to 8 years is 100 beats/minute, and at 12–16 years is 85 beats/minute.[13]

Rhythm

A phasic variation related to the respiratory cycle (faster during inspiration) is characteristic of sinus arrhythmia. This pattern is more common in young children than in adults and is a normal variation. The variation in heart rate occasionally can be profound, but review of an electrocardiogram leads to the diagnosis. Occasional premature beats can represent atrial, ventricular, or junctional premature beats. Non-conducted atrial premature beats are the most common cause of a "pause" in the well-newborn nursery and typically resolve during the first month of life. Isolated ventricular premature beats are common in adolescence; resolution with exercise performed in the examination room (jumping jacks) suggests a benign etiology.

Prominence

Bounding pulses are present in febrile states, hyperthyroidism, exercise, anxiety, severe anemia, complete heart block, and with aortic runoff lesions that produce increased pulse pressure (e.g., aortic regurgitation, PDA, arteriovenous malformations, aortopulmonary window, truncus arteriosus). The prominent pulse classically associated with aortic regurgitation has been termed *Corrigan's pulse* or *water hammer pulse*. Such prominent pulses also produce visible ebbing and flowing of the capillary pulse that can be observed by partially compressing the nail bed, a phenomenon termed *Quincke's pulse*.

Generalized decreased pulses are associated with low cardiac output. This can be caused by acquired heart disease such as myocarditis, with CHD such as obstructive lesions or cardiomyopathy, and with pericardial tamponade or constrictive pericarditis. A rare form of vasculitis affecting the large arteries, Takayasu's arteritis, can be associated with decreased pulses and is termed *pulseless disease*.[14]

Differential prominence of pulses is present in several conditions. The most common is coarctation of the aorta, which usually is associated with easily palpable upper extremity pulses (if left ventricular function is normal) and reduced or absent femoral pulses. If there is a large coexisting PDA and right-to-left ductal shunting, the lower extremity pulses may be normal, although in such circumstances, there may be differential oxygen saturation levels between the upper and lower body. In infants with large thighs, the femoral pulse occasionally can be difficult to locate. The leg should be abducted; the femoral artery is located in the groin region along the line that joins the knee with the umbilicus. Coarctation usually occurs in the aortic isthmus just distal to the origin of the left subclavian artery. In some infants, the origin of the left subclavian artery can be involved, so the pulse in the left arm is weaker than the pulse in the right arm. In rare cases, there can be anomalous origin of the right subclavian artery from the descending aorta in an infant with coarctation, so pulses in all four extremities are reduced; in such patients, the carotid pulse will be more prominent. In patients with supravalvar aortic stenosis, a lesion often present in Williams syndrome, the pulse in the right arm can be more prominent than the pulse in the left arm; this discrepancy is produced by the Coanda effect, which increases flow to the innominate artery. Finally, Takayasu's arteritis can preferentially affect individual brachiocephalic arteries or portions of the aorta with resultant differences in extremity pulses.[14]

Variation

Variable pulse impulse in the same location occurs in several conditions. Pulsus paradoxus involves an exaggerated decrease in inspiratory systolic pressure of more than 10 mm Hg and is associated with pericardial tamponade or severe respiratory distress (see discussion of blood pressure below). Pulsus alternans consists of a decrease in systolic pressure on alternate beats and indicates severe left ventricular dysfunction. This variation is more easily appreciated when observing intravascular blood pressure recordings than by palpating the pulse.[1] Pulsus bisferiens consists of a pulse with two peaks separated by a plateau and can occur in patients with either obstructive left ventricular cardiomyopathy or large left ventricular stroke volumes.

Blood Pressure

While four extremity blood pressures are often obtained, with the rare exceptions of aortitis or aberrant origin of the subclavian artery in a patient with coarctation, obtaining the blood pressure in the right arm and one leg provides sufficient screening. The right arm is preferred because the origin of the left subclavian artery can be stenosed in some patients with coarctation. Unless a femoral artery was injured in a previous catheterization, the pressure should be similar in each leg.

Accuracy of blood pressure measurement depends on selection of a properly sized cuff, in infants and toddlers on a quiet and cooperative state, and in older children and adolescents on assessment of the presence of anxiety (white-coat hypertension). The inflatable bladder should have a length sufficient to fully encircle the circumference of the extremity and a width to cover about 75% of the distance between the joints on either end of the portion of the extremity around which the cuff is placed.[15] If the cuff is too small, artificially high values are obtained. The cuff needs to be applied snugly around the extremity because a loose-fitting cuff needs higher pressure to occlude the artery. Agitation leads to elevation in blood pressure. A coarctation can be missed if the infant is quiet while the arm pressure is obtained and crying during measurement of the leg pressure. In many clinics, the blood pressure is measured in triage, and note is not made of patient behavior. If the femoral pulses are diminished and the blood pressure values demonstrate no arm–leg discrepancy, the physician should repeat the measurements when the infant is observed to be cooperative to confirm the values. If hypertension is noted in children or adolescents who are anxious, it is helpful to repeat the measurements at the end of the examination when the patient may be more relaxed.

There are several techniques available to measure blood pressure, including palpation and the Doppler method, each of which estimates systolic pressure; auscultation, which is technically difficult in an infant or toddler; and the oscillometric method, which is the most commonly used technique in clinics and medical wards. Another method, the flush technique, is rarely used and yields values closer to the mean pressure. The techniques are reviewed in Chapter 44. The lower extremity systolic pressure can be 5–10 mm Hg greater than the upper extremity value because of the standing wave effect, with successive heart beats adding to the pressure downstream. Systolic pressure in the upper extremity that is more than 10 mm Hg higher than that in the lower extremity is a sign of coarctation of the aorta.

The pulse pressure is the difference between systolic and diastolic values. The pulse pressure is increased in conditions associated with bounding pulses and decreased in states associated with diminished pulses.

When checking for pulsus paradoxus, the auscultation method must be used. Initially, the systolic pressure is estimated by quickly deflating the inflated cuff. The cuff is then reinflated about 20 mm Hg above this value and slowly deflated (1–2 mm Hg/beat). The systolic pressures at which the Korotkoff sound is initially auscultated intermittently and then consistently are noted; the difference in these values is the pulsus paradoxus. A pulsus paradoxus greater than 10 mm Hg is abnormal and is a feature of pericardial tamponade or severe respiratory disease.

Respirations

Tachypnea is present with pulmonary parenchymal disease, pulmonary edema, large left-to-right shunts, and conditions causing metabolic acidosis. In infants at rest, persistent respiratory rates of more than 60 breaths/minute are abnormal; transient increases can occur after eating or agitation. Tachypnea can be accompanied by intercostal or subcostal retractions, flaring of the alae nasi, or audible wheezing. Orthopnea is a sign of left ventricular dysfunction or severe elevation in pulmonary venous pressure.

Venous Pressure

In the cooperative child or adolescent, venous pressure can be estimated by examination of the jugular vein. When the patient is sitting or reclining at a 45-degree angle, the jugular vein should not be visible above the level of the clavicle. Measuring the difference in the height of the jugular vein with a parallel line drawn through the level of the manubrium yields central venous pressure (Fig. 7.1).

The venous pulsation is undulating and non-palpable, decreases with inspiration, and changes in height with patient position. Distinguishing the various components (a, c, and v waves; x and y descents) is difficult in children, both because of neck size and the presence of tachycardia. Prominent jugular venous waves are present in a variety of conditions, including atrial contraction into a stiff right ventricle or against a closed tricuspid valve (e.g., tricuspid atresia; complete heart block, in which case prominent pulsation is intermittent), tricuspid regurgitation, pericardial disease (pericardial tamponade, constrictive pericarditis), vein of Galen malformation, or superior vena cava obstruction.

Cardiac Examination

The cardiac examination includes inspection, palpation, and auscultation. The classic description by Osler also included percussion of the cardiac border, which is currently rarely done and is not as reliable in detecting cardiomegaly as the readily available imaging techniques of radiography or echocardiography.

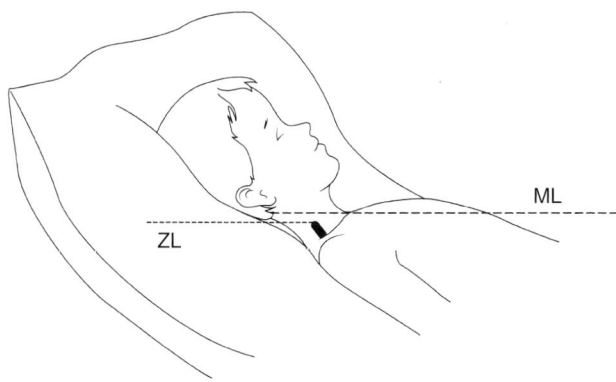

• **Fig. 7.1** Clinical estimation of venous pressure. With the patient lying at approximately 45 degrees, the pressure *(ZL)* in the right atrium does not rise above the manubrium *(ML)*. (From Lewis T. Diseases of the Heart Described for Practitioners and Students, 2nd ed. New York: Macmillan, 1937.)

Inspection

A visible apical impulse is present in left ventricular volume overload lesions, including significant mitral or aortic regurgitation, or lesions associated with large left-to-right shunts at the ventricular or great artery level. A visible parasternal impulse is associated with right ventricular volume overload lesions: for example, TOF absent pulmonary valve associated with severe pulmonary regurgitation, severe tricuspid regurgitation associated with Ebstein anomaly, and large arteriovenous malformations.

Palpation

Palpation involves evaluation of ventricular impulses, thrills, and heart sounds. The apical impulse is detected using the tips of the index and middle fingers and is normally located in the left midclavicular line in the fourth or fifth intercostal space. The apical impulse is displaced laterally and is more prominent in left ventricular overload lesions such as severe aortic or mitral regurgitation or lesions associated with large left-to-right shunts at the ventricular or great vessel level. The apical impulse is right-sided in dextrocardia or displaced in a rightward direction in conditions including left-sided congenital diaphragmatic hernia, left lobar emphysema, or scimitar syndrome. The right ventricular impulse is detected by placing the hand on the chest with the heads of the metacarpals along the left costochondral junctions. A prominent lift indicates right ventricular hypertension or right ventricular volume overload. The right ventricular impulse can also be assessed in the epigastric area. The palm of the right hand is placed on the abdomen so that the index and middle fingers can slide under the xiphoid process; the tips of the fingers can palpate the right ventricular impulse.

Precordial thrills indicate the presence of a murmur of at least grade 4. The timing and location of thrills should be noted. Systolic thrills at the left lower sternal border usually are caused by VSDs that may be small and associated with a high interventricular systolic pressure gradient or large and associated with a large left-to-right shunt. Occasionally, a thrill in this region is caused by tricuspid regurgitation if there is right ventricular hypertension. Mitral, aortic, and pulmonary thrills are located at the apex, right upper sternal border, or left upper sternal border, respectively. Aortic valve thrills can sometimes also be detected over the carotid artery or in the suprasternal notch. A suprasternal notch thrill is rarely associated with pulmonary stenosis, so a palpable thrill in this area distinguishes aortic stenosis from pulmonary stenosis. Precordial thrills associated with aortic or pulmonary stenosis indicate significant degrees of obstruction. Diastolic thrills can occur at the apex with mitral stenosis, or along the left sternal border with aortic or pulmonary regurgitation.

A palpable second heart sound (S_2) usually indicates severe pulmonary hypertension but can also occur when the aorta has an anterior location, such as in TGA. A palpable first heart sound (S_1) can be present in hyperdynamic states.

Auscultation

Thorough auscultation requires the examiner to follow a simple rule: listen to one sound at a time. Components to be evaluated or assessed to be present include S_1, S_2, S_3, S_4, ejection click, opening snap, pericardial rub, and murmurs (systolic, diastolic, continuous). Some congenital cardiac lesions produce multiple abnormal sounds and murmurs, so all available data must be identified to make a correct diagnosis. For example, a soft systolic murmur at the left upper sternal border may represent an innocent flow murmur. If there is also a widely fixed split S_2, the murmur may represent an atrial septal defect (ASD). If there is a variable systolic ejection click in the same region, the murmur may represent valvar pulmonary stenosis.

For auscultation to be completed, the proper environment and tools must be used. The examination room should be quiet without extraneous noises from the patient, relatives, or ventilation system. The stethoscope should have a bell to detect low-frequency sounds and a diaphragm for high-frequency sounds. In infants, an adult-sized diaphragm covers most of the precordium, so a pediatric-sized version aids in localizing sounds. The tubing should be no longer than 16–18 inches with a bore of 1/8 inch. There should be no leak from the chest piece to ear piece so that sound transmission is optimized.[16] The patient should be evaluated in more than one position, including supine, sitting, and standing, depending on the diagnosis, because some heart sounds change or are more easily appreciated with different patient posture. A comprehensive set of recordings of heart sounds and murmurs is available in Geggel.[17]

First Heart Sound

S_1 is produced by mitral and tricuspid valve closure and is coincident with the QRS complex on the electrocardiogram (Fig. 7.2). S_1 is usually perceived as a single sound because the mitral and tricuspid valve components are nearly simultaneous.[18] In the pediatric age range, some patients can have a split S_1 that is typically most easily detected over the tricuspid area at the left lower sternal border. If the split is detected at the apex, consideration must be given to an early systolic ejection click associated with a bicuspid aortic valve, and echocardiography may be needed for differentiation. S_1 also can be split in right bundle branch block due to delay in tricuspid valve closure.

The intensity of S_1 is increased in high cardiac output states because of greater velocity of leaflet closure and in conditions associated with greater mitral valve excursion during closure, including short PR interval and mild mitral stenosis because the elevated left atrial pressure maintains the valve in a more open position. The intensity of S_1 is decreased in conditions associated with low cardiac output, elevated ventricular end-diastolic pressure, mitral regurgitation due to failure of valve coaptation, or decreased valve excursion associated with prolonged PR interval or severe

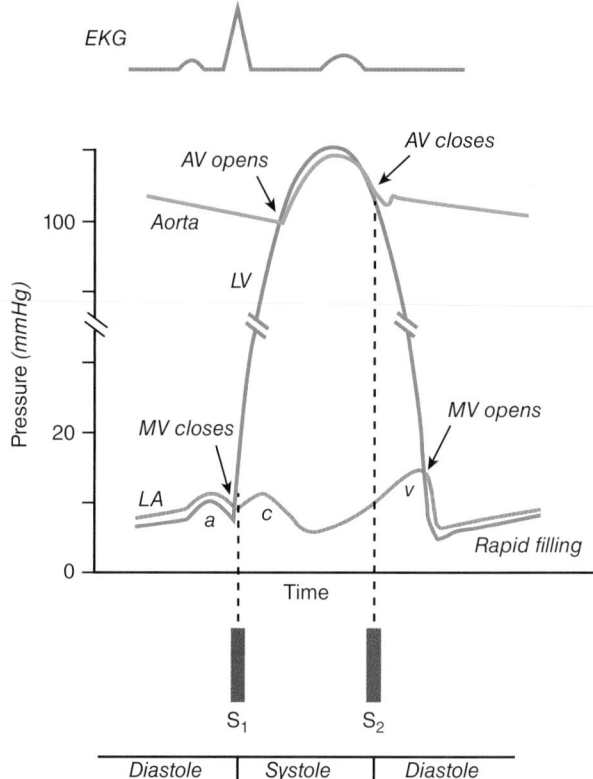

• **Fig. 7.2** The normal cardiac cycle depicted for left-sided chambers. Similar relationships exist for the right-sided chambers. Substitute right atrium for left atrium *(LA)*, right ventricle for left ventricle *(LV)*, and pulmonary artery for aorta. The *a* wave of the atrial pulse coincides with the P wave on the electrocardiogram *(EKG)*. The mitral valve *(MV)* closes as LV pressure exceeds atrial pressure and produces the first heart sound *(S$_1$)*. This coincides with the QRS complex on the EKG. MV closure increases atrial pressure and produces the *c* wave on the atrial pressure curve. The aortic valve *(AV)* subsequently opens as ventricular pressure exceeds aortic pressure. The AV closes during ventricular relaxation and produces the second heart sound *(S$_2$)*. This roughly coincides with the end of the T wave on the EKG. Atrial pressure rises (*v* wave) owing to filling of the atria while the MV is closed. The MV opens as left ventricular pressure falls below left atrial pressure. (From Marino BS, Goldblatt A. Heart sounds and murmurs. In: Lilly LS [ed]. *Pathophysiology of Heart Disease.* Philadelphia: Lea & Febiger, 1992:18.)

mitral stenosis.[18] Patients with complete heart block have variable intensity of S_1.[1]

Second Heart Sound

S_2 is produced by closure of the semilunar valves and is typically best appreciated at the left upper sternal border. The quality of S_2 yields important information on cardiac physiology. The pulmonary valve normally closes after the aortic valve because of relative delayed electrical activation of the right ventricle and lower pulmonary impedance. The respiratory cycle has different effects on the pulmonary and systemic circulations. Inspiration increases venous return to the right heart and lowers pulmonary impedance, which prolongs right ventricular systole, and reduces pulmonary venous return to the left heart, which shortens left ventricular systole. During inspiration, the aortic and pulmonary valve components of S_2 split by about 0.05 seconds. These effects are reversed in expiration, so S_2 typically becomes single.[18] Detecting splitting of S_2 is always challenging. If the split is easily detected, the split is often wide. In infants with tachycardia and tachypnea, correlating S_2 with the respiratory cycle is impossible. The best the examiner can do is to detect variability with a split present in some beats and not in others.

A widely fixed split S_2 occurs with right ventricular volume overload lesions, the most common of which is ASD.[17] Less common conditions of total or partial anomalous pulmonary venous connection or large arteriovenous malformation can produce a similar feature. In these conditions, the persistent right ventricular volume overload delays pulmonary valve closure so that the split is greater than 0.05 seconds, often as long as 0.10 seconds. Wide inspiratory splitting with respiratory variation occurs with right bundle branch block, pulmonary stenosis, or idiopathic dilation of the main pulmonary artery due to delayed activation or prolonged contraction of the right ventricle. As pulmonary stenosis progresses, splitting becomes difficult to detect due to a softer pulmonary closure sound and prolongation of the murmur beyond the aortic component. Wide splitting can also occur with significant mitral regurgitation due to shortened left ventricular ejection time and earlier closure of the aortic valve. Paradoxical splitting is uncommon in children and involves detecting two components to S_2 in expiration and a single sound in inspiration; this can occur with delayed or prolonged left ventricular contraction in patients with left bundle branch block, aortic stenosis, or some forms of Wolff-Parkinson-White syndrome.

The intensity of S_2 depends on the pressure closing the semilunar valves and the anterior-posterior position of the great arteries. The most common cause of a loud S_2 is pulmonary hypertension, which can arise from a variety of causes (see Chapter 56).[17,18] Pulmonary hypertension can be caused by increased pulmonary flow or elevated pulmonary vascular resistance; evaluation of murmurs often helps to distinguish between these two mechanisms, with the former being associated with diastolic rumbles across the atrioventricular valve that receives increased flow. Increased intensity of S_2 is also present in patients with TGA because of the anterior location of the aorta, and often in TOF.

Mild or moderate pulmonary hypertension is associated with a narrowly split S_2. S_2 is single in patients with severe pulmonary hypertension because the elevated diastolic pressure in the pulmonary circulation closes the pulmonary valve sooner. S_2 is also single when there is atresia of one semilunar valve.

Third Heart Sound

The third heart sound (S_3) is produced during the rapid filling phase of the ventricle in early diastole and is best heard with the bell of the stethoscope. This sound produces a gallop rhythm that has the cadence of the syllables of "Ken-tuc-ky." The last component of this sequence represents the third heart sound.[17,18] This sound can be detected

in some normal children, although this is not very common. Cardiac diseases associated with S_3 include myocardial dysfunction or volume overload conditions, especially those created by large left-to-right shunts. In the latter, the sound is followed by a diastolic murmur created by increased flow across the affected atrioventricular valve. S_3 produced by the left ventricle is detected in the apical region, whereas that from the right ventricle is noted at the left lower sternal border.

Fourth Heart Sound

The fourth heart sound (S_4) is produced by atrial contraction in late diastole and is also best heard with the bell of the stethoscope. This sound produces a gallop rhythm that has the cadence of the syllables of "Ten-nes-see." The first component of this sequence represents the S_4.[17,18] This sound is abnormal and is seen in conditions associated with decreased ventricular compliance, so that increased atrial contractile force is required to fill the ventricle. These conditions include those produced by myocardial ischemia or ventricular hypertrophy such as hypertrophic cardiomyopathy, systemic hypertension, and valvar aortic or pulmonary stenosis. An S_4 is not produced if there is coexisting atrial fibrillation or junctional tachycardia because of absent atrial contraction.[1]

When both S_3 and S_4 are present, there is a quadruple rhythm. In such a situation, if there is tachycardia and resulting shortening of diastole, the two extra sounds may become superimposed and create a summation gallop.[18]

Opening Snap

An opening snap is a high-frequency sound associated with mitral stenosis.[17] As the degree of mitral stenosis progresses, the opening snap occurs earlier in diastole because of elevated atrial pressures and becomes softer because of decreased leaflet mobility.

Clicks

Ejection clicks are brief, high-frequency, sharp sounds that have a quality distinct from S_1 and S_2. They usually are associated with abnormal valve structure. Evaluation of location, timing (early versus mid-systolic), and nature (constant versus variable) enables the examiner to determine the affected valve (Table 7.2). In patients with mitral valve prolapse, the click may be associated with a murmur of mitral regurgitation that is only present or louder in the standing than supine position because of reduced left ventricular volume that produces a greater degree of prolapse.

The click associated with aortic stenosis or bicuspid aortic valve is best detected at the apex rather than the aortic valve region at the right upper sternal border.[17] The click associated with pulmonary stenosis is located at the left upper sternal border and is variable and louder in expiration because of greater systolic valve excursion in this phase of the respiratory cycle.[17,18] Clicks associated with semilunar valve stenosis become softer as the degree of obstruction progresses, because of reduced valve mobility. Ebstein

TABLE 7.2 **Qualities of Clicks Associated With Valve Disorders**

Valve	Location	Timing in Systole	Nature
Mitral	Apex	Mid to late	Constant
Aortic	Apex	Early	Constant
Pulmonary	LUSB	Early	Variable
Tricuspid	LLSB	Mid to late	Constant

LLSB, Left lower sternal border; *LUSB,* left upper sternal border.

TABLE 7.3 **Grading of Intensity of Heart Murmurs**

Grade 1: Faintest sound that can be detected; often detected by cardiologists but not by general physicians
Grade 2: Soft murmur that is readily detectable
Grade 3: Louder than grade 2 but not associated with a palpable precordial thrill
Grade 4: Easily detected murmur associated with a palpable precordial thrill
Grade 5: Very loud murmur audible with the stethoscope placed lightly on the chest
Grade 6: Extremely loud murmur audible with the stethoscope off the chest

From: Marino BS, Goldblatt A. Heart sounds and murmurs. In: Lilly LS (ed): *Pathophysiology of Heart Disease.* Philadelphia: Lea & Febiger, 1992: 18–29; Freeman AR, Levine SA. The clinical significance of the systolic murmur: A study of 1,000 consecutive "non-cardiac" cases. *Ann Intern Med.* 1933;6:1371.

anomaly of the tricuspid valve can be associated with a systolic click at the left lower sternal border.

Clicks occasionally occur in conditions associated with dilation of the aorta or pulmonary artery. The latter can occur with pulmonary hypertension, PDA, or idiopathic dilation of the main pulmonary artery. In neonates with left-to-right shunting across a PDA, there may be multiple systolic clicks at the left upper sternal border that sound like rolling a pair of dice in one's hand. This sound may be produced by wavelike expansion of the pulmonary artery.[17] Clicks can also be produced by membranous VSDs associated with aneurysm of the ventricular septum and are located at the left lower sternal border.

Pericardial Friction Rub

A pericardial friction rub is created when inflamed visceral and parietal pericardial surfaces contact each other. The sound is similar to rubbing two pieces of sandpaper together and has a grating quality. The rub may be auscultated in systole, diastole, or continuously and is best heard with the diaphragm.[17] The rub is typically loudest along the left sternal border with the patient sitting and leaning forward and often has inspiratory accentuation. It commonly is present after surgery involving entry into the pericardial space and in pericarditis. The sound is not present if there is a moderate to large pericardial effusion because the two surfaces of the pericardium cannot rub together.

Murmurs

Various features of a murmur need to be evaluated.

Intensity. The intensity of a murmur is graded on a scale of 1–6 (Table 7.3).[19] Murmurs grade 4 or greater are associated with a palpable precordial thrill; an isolated thrill in the suprasternal notch does not qualify for a grade 4 murmur. The loudness depends on both the pressure gradient and the volume of blood flowing across the site creating the murmur. For example, the murmur associated with moderate neonatal pulmonary stenosis or large VSD increases in the first few weeks of life as pulmonary vascular resistance decreases, producing a larger pressure gradient in the former and an increased left-to-right shunt in the latter.

Timing. Systolic murmurs are created by flow through stenotic semilunar valves or regurgitant atrioventricular valves, other stenotic regions (coarctation, double chamber right ventricle, subvalvar or supravalvar semilunar valve obstruction, peripheral pulmonary stenosis), or increased cardiac output across normal semilunar valves associated with tachycardia or anemia. The innocent Still's murmur is discussed separately in Chapter 52.

Diastolic murmurs are caused by regurgitant flow across semilunar valves or turbulent flow across atrioventricular valves.[17] The latter can represent true stenosis, as in mitral stenosis, or relative stenosis that is seen in patients with large left-to-right shunt lesions or significant atrioventricular valve regurgitation. The normal atrioventricular valve can accommodate twice normal stroke volume non-turbulently. Larger blood flows create a murmur. Left-to-right shunt lesions associated with pulmonary-to-systemic flow ratio greater than 2:1 in patients with an ASD will produce a diastolic murmur across the tricuspid valve at the left lower sternal border[17] and in patients with a VSD will create a diastolic murmur across the mitral valve at the apex; similar murmurs are present with moderate to severe tricuspid and mitral regurgitation, respectively. Such murmurs are low velocity, best heard with the bell of the stethoscope, and usually of low intensity (grade 1 or 2).

Continuous murmurs begin in systole and persist through S_2 into early, mid, or all of diastole. Such murmurs often are audible throughout the cardiac cycle but can have phasic variation in intensity depending on the pressure gradient in systole and diastole. They are produced when there are connections between the following:

1. Systemic and pulmonary arterial circulations: surgically created Blalock-Taussig, Waterston, Potts, or central shunts, PDA, aortopulmonary collateral artery, aortopulmonary window, anomalous left coronary artery arising from the main pulmonary artery.
2. Systemic arteries and veins: arteriovenous malformation.
3. Systemic arteries and cardiac chambers: coronary arteriovenous fistula, ruptured sinus of Valsalva aneurysm.
4. Disturbed flow in arteries: collateral circulation associated with severe coarctation.
5. Disturbed flow in veins: venous hum.

A continuous murmur is distinguished from a to-and-fro murmur, which consists of two murmurs, one that occurs in systole and the other that occurs in diastole. A to-and-fro murmur does not continue through S_2 but instead has peak intensity earlier in systole. Examples include patients with combined aortic stenosis and aortic regurgitation, combined pulmonary stenosis and pulmonary regurgitation, or VSD associated with prolapsed aortic cusp and aortic regurgitation.

Timing also includes whether the murmur occurs in early, mid, or late systole or diastole. An early systolic murmur at the left lower sternal border is characteristic of a small muscular VSD; in this condition, as the ventricle contracts, the septal defect closes so that the murmur is not holosystolic.[17] A mid to late systolic murmur at the apex is characteristic of mild mitral regurgitation associated with mitral valve prolapse; as the ventricle decreases in size during systole, a mitral valve with either redundant valve tissue or lengthened chordae tendineae can become incompetent.

Location and radiation. The region where a murmur is loudest and direction of radiation provide additional clues to the diagnosis. Aortic valve stenosis has maximal intensity at the right upper sternal border and may radiate to the suprasternal notch and carotid arteries. Aortic valve regurgitation is most easily detected at the left upper sternal border with the patient sitting, leaning forward, in expiration. Pulmonary stenosis and regurgitation are maximal at the left upper sternal border. The severity of aortic or pulmonary regurgitation correlates with the amount of radiation: mild limited to the left upper sternal border, moderate being audible also at the left midsternal border, and severe radiating to the left lower sternal border. The systolic murmur of peripheral pulmonary stenosis common in infancy is maximal at the left or right upper sternal border and radiates to the infraclavicular and axillary regions and to the back. Systolic murmurs at the left lower sternal border usually represent a VSD but can be associated with tricuspid regurgitation. The murmur of tricuspid regurgitation usually increases during inspiration. Mitral valve disease is best heard at the apex with the patient in the lateral decubitus position. Mitral regurgitation typically radiates to the axilla.

Sites other than the precordium need to be auscultated as well. Coarctation is best heard in the intrascapular region on the back. Long-standing severe coarctation can produce collateral circulation audible as continuous murmur over the ribs where the intercostals arteries course. Arteriovenous malformations may be audible over the affected body region, for example, the cranium for vein of Galen malformations or right upper quadrant for hepatic source.

Shape. Diamond-shaped murmurs occur with ventricular obstructive lesions (semilunar valvar, subvalvar, or supravalvar stenosis, coarctation) or hyperdynamic states (anemia, hyperthyroidism, fever). These murmurs begin after S_1 and end before the component of S_2 (aortic or pulmonary) associated with the side of the heart from which the murmur originates. Holosystolic murmurs have a plateau shape and are characteristic of VSDs other than small muscular defects or with atrioventricular valve regurgitation. These murmurs begin with S_1 and end with the aortic or pulmonary component of S_2, depending on whether they are left- or right-sided in origin. Decrescendo murmurs decrease in intensity during the cardiac cycle and include the diastolic murmurs of aortic regurgitation and pulmonary regurgitation.

Quality. Harsh murmurs are characteristic of murmurs caused by ventricular outflow tract obstruction or hyperdynamic states. Blowing murmurs are typical of valve regurgitation. A rumbling quality is a feature of diastolic turbulence across atrioventricular valves. A vibratory, musical, or humming property is associated with the innocent Still's murmur (see Chapter 52).

Chest Examination

Chest Deformity

CHD associated with cardiomegaly can produce prominence of the left chest due to the effects of cardiac contraction against an elastic rib cage.[1] Pectus carinatum is a feature of Marfan syndrome. Pectus excavatum is associated with mitral valve prolapse, which often improves after surgical correction of the chest wall deformity.[20]

Chest Wall Examination

Chest pain in children frequently has a musculoskeletal basis, including costochondritis, slipping rib syndrome, or myodynia. The diagnosis of musculoskeletal pain can be confirmed if a similar quality of discomfort is reproduced by palpation of the chest. The examination should include palpation of the costochondral junctions, the insertion site of the pectoralis major muscle group by grasping the head of the muscle between the examiner's fingers and thumb, the inframammary area, and other regions of the chest where pain is reported. In patients with slipping rib syndrome, the examiner can perform the "hooking" maneuver by placing fingers around the lower costal margin and lifting anteriorly to elicit a click and reproduce pain.[10] The demonstration of pain reproduction and an explanation of the anatomic basis are reassuring to the family and patient and help allay concerns about the heart.

Pulmonary Auscultation

Lesions associated with excessive pulmonary flow or left-sided dysfunction or obstruction can be associated with inspiratory rales or expiratory wheezing. These features are also present in patients with reactive airway disease or pneumonia.

Abdomen Examination

Palpation of the liver yields information about visceral situs and central venous pressure. A right-sided liver indicates normal situs of the abdominal viscera, a left-sided liver indicates situs inversus, and a midline liver indicates the presence of situs ambiguous and heterotaxy. Hepatomegaly is present in conditions associated with elevated central venous pressure. Percussion of the liver size helps to distinguish patients with "false" hepatomegaly caused by inferior displacement by a flattened diaphragm caused by hyperinflation. Palpation of the liver is easier when the abdomen is soft. Flexing the knees can relax the abdominal musculature. In infants, the liver can normally be palpated about 2 cm below the costal margin in the mid-clavicular line. In children, the liver can be palpated 1 cm below the right costal margin. An engorged liver is usually tender to palpation. A pulsatile liver is palpated in patients with elevated right atrial pressure, most commonly associated with significant tricuspid regurgitation.

In infants, a spleen tip can occasionally be palpated under the costal margin. Location of the spleen also aids in determination of visceral situs. Elevated central venous pressure usually does not produce splenomegaly. An enlarged spleen is a feature of bacterial endocarditis, and in a known cardiac patient with fever or new regurgitant murmur, this physical finding should prompt thorough evaluation of that complication.

Ascites is an uncommon feature of CHD. Placing one hand in each flank and detecting a fluid wave with one hand created by pressure applied by the other can determine its presence.

Extremities examination

Edema

Pitting edema in infants generally has a renal rather than cardiac basis. In children and adolescents, edema can be caused by cardiac dysfunction. In patients with a modified Fontan procedure, edema can be caused by protein-losing enteropathy, a complication that occurs with high venous pressure. Swelling of the face, neck, and arms can occur with superior vena cava obstruction that occasionally is seen after Senning or Mustard repair for TGA, bidirectional Glenn shunt for palliation of functional single ventricle, after Warden procedure (anastomosis of the superior vena cava to the right atrial appendage) for repair of superior sinus venosus defect, intravascular thrombosis associated with an indwelling central venous catheter, or obstructing mediastinal mass. Obstruction of the inferior vena cava or iliac or femoral veins occasionally occurs secondary to *in utero* thrombosis or as a complication of catheterization and can produce edema of the abdomen and lower extremities. Doughy, non-pitting swelling of the hands and feet represents lymphedema that is seen in some infants with Turner syndrome.

Clubbing

Clubbing is a feature of chronic cyanosis and is uncommon in early infancy. The change in appearance of the distal portion of the digit consists of rounding or convexity of the nail bed and thickening and shining of the skin at the base of the nail (Fig. 7.3). With marked clubbing, the terminal phalange becomes bulbous.

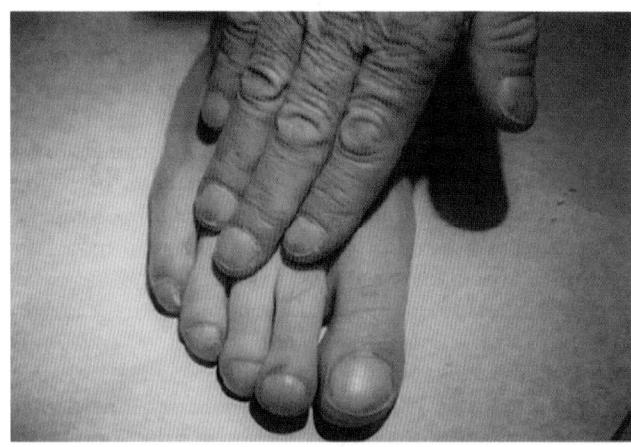

• **Fig. 7.3** A 55-year-old man with unrepaired large patent ductus arteriosus, Eisenmenger's syndrome, and right-to-left shunting at the ductal level producing differential cyanosis. The transcutaneous oxygen saturation was 92% in the fingers and 84% in the toes. The central hematocrit was 65%. Clubbing is more apparent in the toes than in the fingers. (From OPENPediatrics.org, Geggel's Congenital Heart Disease Library, edited by Robert Geggel, MD, Boston Children's Hospital.)

Differential Cyanosis

Certain congenital heart defects create differential cyanosis in which the upper half of the body is pink and the lower half blue, or vice versa. Systemic-level pulmonary vascular resistance and a PDA need to be present for this phenomenon to occur. The oxygen saturation is higher in the upper extremity in patients with normally related great arteries if there is right-to-left shunting at the level of the ductus arteriosus. This can occur in infants with persistent pulmonary hypertension of the newborn, severe coarctation of the aorta, or interrupted aortic arch. The differential effect is reduced if there is also right-to-left shunting at the level of the foramen ovale, or if there is left-to-right shunting across a coexisting VSD. The lower portion of the body can be more cyanotic than the upper segment in older patients with Eisenmenger syndrome caused by a persistent large PDA (Fig. 7.3). In patients with TGA associated with either coarctation or pulmonary hypertension, differential cyanosis can be reversed with lower levels of oxygen saturation in the upper extremity.

Routine Laboratory Tests

A variety of laboratory tests may be required for appropriate management of children with CHD. Selective aspects of these tests are mentioned below.

Hematology Tests

Leukocytosis

The white blood cell count may be elevated in infectious diseases (acute rheumatic fever, bacterial endocarditis, pericarditis), airway disease associated with excessive pulmonary flow or pulmonary venous congestion, or inflammatory conditions (aortitis, collagen vascular disease). Leukocytosis can also occur in patients with urinary tract infections, common in those with renal anomalies, or in patients with sinusitis, which can be a complication of chronic use of nasotracheal intubation or a nasogastric tube for nutritional support.

Hematocrit

The hematocrit is elevated in patients with cyanotic heart disease. In such patients, it is important to also check the mean corpuscular volume (MCV) to rule out relative anemia. Patients with microcytic anemia (MCV < 80) are at increased risk for thrombotic complications, including cerebrovascular accidents.[21] The normal red blood cell has a biconcave surface membrane structure; the microcytic red blood cell has a less redundant membrane and is more likely to lodge in rather than pass through the capillary bed. In such patients, low-dose iron therapy should be instituted and the hematocrit response carefully monitored to avoid excessive polycythemia. Hematocrit levels greater than 70% are associated with exponential increases in blood viscosity and decreased cardiac output that can produce symptoms of decreased exercise tolerance, headache, cerebrovascular accident, and chest pain.[22] If such symptoms are present in patients with this degree of polycythemia, partial erythropheresis should be performed. The amount of whole blood to remove can be calculated from the following formula:

$$\text{Blood volume to remove (mL)} = \text{Estimated blood volume (mL)} \times (\text{Hct}_i - \text{Hct}_d)/\text{Hct}_i,$$

where Hct_i is the initial venous hematocrit and Hct_d is the desired venous hematocrit.

The blood volume is 85 mL/kg in a neonate, 70 mL/kg in a child, and 65 mL/kg in an adult. The hematocrit should not be reduced by more than 10%, because such patients require increased oxygen-carrying capacity for adequate oxygen delivery to the tissues. It is safest to do an isovolumetric exchange, replacing blood withdrawn with an equal volume of normal saline, fresh frozen plasma, or 5% salt-poor albumin.

Platelets

Polycythemia is frequently associated with thrombocytopenia (platelet levels, 50,000–80,000/mm³) because megakaryocytes are "crowded out" by red blood cell precursors in the bone marrow. Thrombocytosis is a feature of Kawasaki disease, with platelet counts occasionally exceeding 1 million/mm.

Howell-Jolly Bodies

Patients with heterotaxy syndrome can have asplenia. In such patients, microscopic evaluation of the peripheral blood smear will demonstrate Howell-Jolly bodies, red blood cells that contain small purple staining inclusions containing DNA and which are normally removed from the circulation in patients with a functioning spleen. Howell-Jolly bodies can normally be present in the first few weeks of life. A liver-spleen scan with technetium-99m

or abdominal ultrasound can confirm the absence of a spleen.

Inflammatory Markers

The erythrocyte sedimentation rate (ESR) and C-reactive protein (CRP) are elevated in inflammatory conditions and in bacterial endocarditis. The CRP rises faster during the acute phase of the illness and falls faster during recovery than the ESR.

Urinalysis

Hematuria can be a feature of bacterial endocarditis. The specific gravity yields information on fluid status. Pyuria can be associated with urinary tract infections or inflammatory conditions such as Kawasaki disease.

Blood Chemistries

Serum levels of sodium, potassium, chloride, calcium, magnesium, and phosphorous are monitored for patients receiving diuretics or those presenting with arrhythmias, especially if ventricular in origin. Dosing for anticoagulation can be monitored by determining plasma heparin levels if unfractionated heparin is used or anti-factor Xa levels in those receiving enoxaparin. The loading dose varies with age and risk of bleeding, so that a formulary should be consulted. For those receiving warfarin sodium, the international normalized ratio (INR) is monitored. The goal for the INR value varies with indication for use (mechanical prosthetic valve, cerebrovascular accident prophylaxis, cardiomyopathy, atrial fibrillation, or right-to-left shunting).[23] Special precautions are required for obtaining an INR in patients with polycythemia and hematocrit greater than 55–60%. The typical tubes used for the assay contain a set amount of diluent that assumes a normal plasma volume. Patients with significant polycythemia need some of the diluent removed or else an artificially elevated INR value will be obtained. The laboratory should be contacted to determine the amount of diluent to remove for a given hematocrit level.

Blood Cultures

Blood cultures for bacterial and fungal pathogens are required for evaluation of endocarditis. Ideally, a minimum of three cultures from separate venipunctures are obtained on the first day to definitively evaluate this condition; if there is no growth by the second day, an additional two cultures may be obtained (see Chapter 50).[23]

Level of Oxygenation

Transcutaneous oxygen saturation from preductal and postductal sites identifies patients with cyanosis, including those with differential cyanosis, and is also useful in establishing the response to prostaglandin E_1 infusion. The oxygen-hemoglobin dissociation curve is steep for oxygen tension values less than 70 mm Hg; thus, for lower levels, small decreases in oxygen tension are associated with large decreases in oxygen saturation.

Additional information is obtained from arterial blood gas measurement. An elevated arterial P_{CO_2} value may reflect the presence of pulmonary disease. A reduced pH level raises concern about poor cardiac output. The combination of severe hypoxemia, metabolic acidosis, and marked hypercarbia can also occur in patients with D-loop TGA when there is inadequate mixing at the atrial, ventricular, and great vessel level. A combination of low oxygen saturation and normal oxygen tension is present in methemoglobinemia. In this uncommon condition, blood has a chocolate-brown color and does not become red when exposed to air.

The hyperoxia test is useful in distinguishing cardiac from pulmonary causes of cyanosis. In cyanotic heart disease associated with intracardiac right-to-left shunting, blood in the pulmonary veins is fully saturated with oxygen in ambient air. Administering higher concentrations of inspired oxygen increases the amount of dissolved oxygen but has minimal effect on systemic oxygen saturation or oxygen tension levels. Conversely, patients with pulmonary disease have pulmonary venous desaturation. Administering supplemental oxygen typically increases pulmonary venous oxygen levels and improves systemic oxygenation. The hyperoxia test is performed by placing the patient in 100% oxygen for 10 minutes either using an Oxyhood or endotracheal tube if already intubated. An arterial blood gas should be obtained from a preductal source (right arm); alternatively, transcutaneous P_{O_2} monitors can be used. Patients with cyanotic heart disease rarely have preductal oxygen tension exceed 150 mm Hg, whereas patients with pulmonary disease usually exceed this value.[24] The level of arterial P_{O_2} in 100% oxygen helps to distinguish the various types of cyanotic heart disease (Table 7.4).

The interpretation of the hyperoxia test requires determination of both the arterial P_{O_2} and oxygen saturation. Because of the characteristics of the oxygen dissociation curve, a patient receiving a fractional inspired oxygen concentration of 1.0 could have 100% oxygen saturation associated with an arterial P_{O_2} of 75, a value that is abnormal. It is important to note that systemic oxygen tension can increase in some patients with cyanotic heart disease if there is coexisting airway disease (e.g., pulmonary edema or pneumonia) or mixing lesions involving both right-to-left and left-to-right shunting. In the latter situation (e.g., truncus arteriosus or single ventricle with PDA), supplemental oxygen may decrease pulmonary vascular resistance, thereby increasing pulmonary flow, which, when mixing with a fixed amount of systemic venous return, produces a higher level of aortic oxygenation. For such patients, the chest radiograph typically demonstrates cardiomegaly and prominent pulmonary vascularity. Even though the preductal oxygen tension may increase over ambient air levels in these conditions, the value rarely exceeds 150 mm Hg.[24] Some patients with severe lung disease may have minimal improvement with supplemental oxygen. In these patients, however, the chest radiograph and arterial P_{CO_2} level aid in establishing the underlying disorder.

TABLE 7.4   Typical Results of Hyperoxia Test

	FiO$_2$ = 0.21 PaO$_2$ (% saturation)		FiO$_2$ = 1 PaO$_2$ (% saturation)	PaCO$_2$
Normal	>70 (>95)		>300 (100)	35
Pulmonary disease	50 (85)		>150 (100)	50
Neurologic disease	50 (85)		>150 (100)	50
Methemoglobinemia	>70 (<85)		>200 (<85)	35
Cardiac Disease				
Parallel circulation*	<40 (<75)		<50 (<85)	35
Mixing with reduced PBF†	<40 (<75)		<50 (<85)	35
Mixing without restricted PBF‡	40-60 (75–93)		<150 (<100)	35
	Preductal	Postductal		
Differential cyanosis§	70 (95)	<40 (<75)	variable	35–50
Reverse differential cyanosis¶	<40 (<75)	>50 (>90)	variable	35–50

*D-loop transposition of the great arteries with or without ventricular septal defect.
†Tricuspid atresia with pulmonary stenosis or pulmonary atresia, pulmonary atresia or critical pulmonary stenosis with intact ventricular septum, tetralogy of Fallot.
‡Truncus arteriosus, total anomalous pulmonary venous connection without obstruction, hypoplastic left heart syndrome, single ventricle without pulmonary stenosis or pulmonary atresia.
§Persistent pulmonary hypertension of newborn, interrupted aortic arch, severe coarctation of aorta.
¶D-loop transposition of the great arteries associated with either coarctation or suprasystemic pulmonary artery pressure.
Adapted from Marino BS, Bird GL, Wernovsky G. Diagnosis and management of the newborn with suspected congenital heart disease. *Clin Perinatology.* 2001;28:91–136.

Chest Radiograph

The chest radiograph provides information on the cardiac, pulmonary, and skeletal status. A structured approach to interpretation is the "Rule of Six."

1. Size of heart: The normal heart size is less than 50% of the cardiothoracic diameter. In infants, a large overlying anterior thymus can give the impression of cardiomegaly. The thymus has a non-smooth undulating border that distinguishes it from a cardiac chamber (Fig. 7.4D). Massive cardiomegaly in a neonate most commonly is associated with marked enlargement of the right atrium that can occur in Ebstein anomaly (Fig. 7.4F) or pulmonary atresia with intact atrial septum.

2. Shape of heart: Patients with D-loop TGA can have an "egg-on-side" appearance due to anterior-posterior relationship of the great arteries creating a narrow mediastinum (Fig. 7.4G). Infants with TOF can have a boot-shaped heart (Fig. 7.4E). Cardiomegaly associated with a large pericardial effusion often has a "water-bottle" appearance that resolves once the

effusion is drained (Fig. 7.4K). Unrepaired supracardiac total anomalous pulmonary venous connection beyond childhood has a "snowman" appearance created by an enlarged heart, dilated vertical vein, innominate vein, and superior vena cava (Fig. 7.4I).

3. Symmetry/status of pulmonary vasculature: Left-to-right shunt lesions have increased pulmonary arterial markings (Fig. 7.4A, B, and D), whereas cyanotic lesions with obstructive right-sided lesions typically have oligemic lung fields (Fig. 7.4E). Chronic pulmonary hypertension, as occurs in Eisenmenger's syndrome, produces prominent central pulmonary arteries that taper rapidly creating a pruning effect (Fig. 7.4L). Patients with scimitar syndrome have a curvilinear structure in the right chest representing the pulmonary vein draining anomalously to the inferior vena cava and variable degrees of right lung hypoplasia (Fig. 7.4J). Some patients with D-loop TGA have more prominent markings in the right lung because the long axis of the

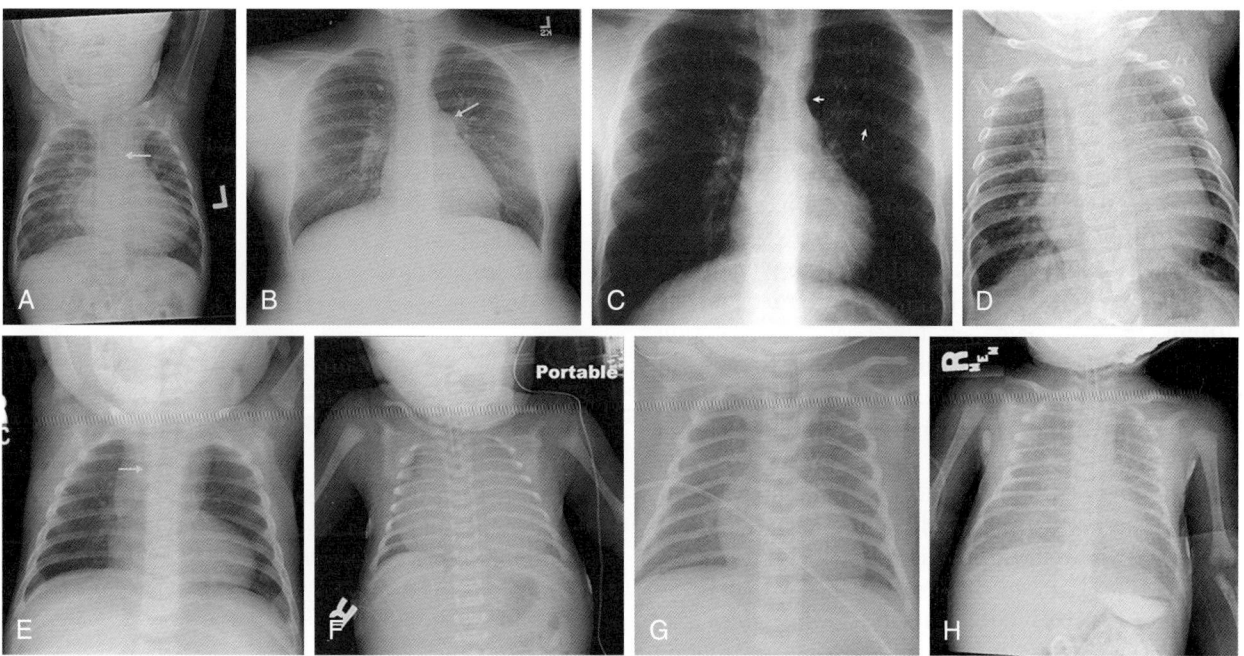

• **Fig. 7.4** Anterior-posterior chest radiographs of a variety of congenital heart lesions. **(A)** A 4-month-old with large membranous ventricular septal defect showing moderate cardiomegaly, symmetrically increased pulmonary blood flow, hyperinflation, and a left aortic arch (arrow points to slight indentation in the left side of trachea by the aortic arch). **(B)** Adolescent with large secundum atrial septal defect showing prominent main pulmonary artery (arrow) and pulmonary vascular markings. **(C)** A 14-year-old with coarctation of the aorta with indentation of the aorta in the region of the coarctation (horizontal arrow) and rib notching of the inferior rib margin (vertical arrow). **(D)** A 3-month-old with large patent ductus arteriosus and one-half systemic pulmonary artery pressure showing cardiomegaly, increased pulmonary artery flow, and hyperinflation. There is an overlying thymic shadow with an undulating border in the left upper lung region. **(E)** A 3-month-old infant with tetralogy of Fallot showing a boot-shaped heart, decreased pulmonary vascularity and right aortic arch (arrow). **(F)** A neonate with Ebstein anomaly of the tricuspid valve, large patent ductus arteriosus, decreased right ventricular contractility and severe tricuspid and pulmonary regurgitation showing severe cardiomegaly; an endotracheal tube is positioned in the trachea. **(G)** A 1-day-old with D-loop transposition of the great arteries showing a narrow mediastinum caused by anterior-posterior orientation of the aorta and pulmonary artery creating a narrow vascular pedicle and an appearance of an "egg-on-a-string" or an egg lying on its side. There is an endotracheal tube and a nasogastric feeding tube. **(H)** A neonate with infradiaphragmatic total anomalous pulmonary venous return showing normal heart size, pulmonary edema, and hyperinflation. There is contrast in the gastrointestinal system from a previously performed upper gastrointestinal series.

Continued

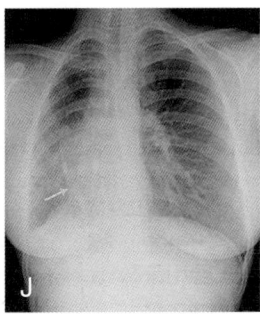
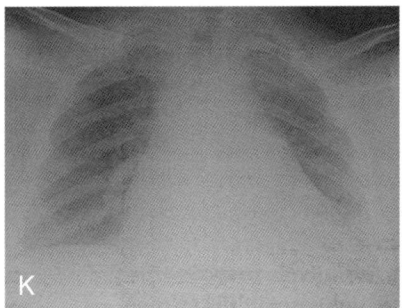
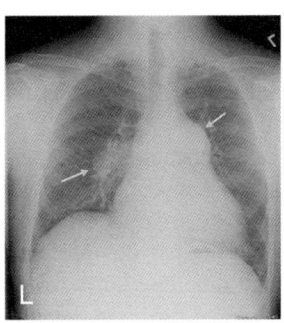

• **Fig. 7.4, cont'd** **(I)** An adult with unrepaired supracardiac total anomalous pulmonary venous connection to the innominate vein showing a "snowman" image with the lower portion represented by moderate cardiomegaly and the upper portion represented by the dilated vertical vein along the left mediastinum *(arrow)*, dilated innominate vein in the superior mediastinum, and dilated right superior vena cava along the right mediastinum *(arrow)*. There is a prominent main pulmonary artery in the superior portion of the left cardiac contour. At catheterization, the ratio of pulmonary to system flow was 4:1 and main pulmonary artery pressure 47/20, mean 32 mm Hg. **(J)** A 14-year-old with scimitar syndrome showing mesocardia, hypoplasia of the right lung, and a prominent scimitar vein in the right chest *(arrow)*. **(K)** A 15-year-old with viral pericarditis and large pericardial effusion showing cardiomegaly in a "water-bottle" shape and decreased lung volumes. At the time of pericardiocentesis, 390 mL of fluid was removed. **(L)** An adult with unrepaired large ventricular septal defect and Eisenmenger syndrome showing cardiomegaly, dilated main pulmonary artery *(arrow in left chest)* and prominent central pulmonary arteries with rapid tapering of distal pulmonary arteries *(arrow in right chest)*. (All images From OPENPediatrics.org, Geggel's Congenital Heart Disease Library, edited by Robert Geggel, MD, Boston Children's Hospital.)

left ventricle is more in line with the right than left pulmonary artery. Infants with obstructive infradiaphragmatic pulmonary venous return have normal heart size and pulmonary edema, a pattern specific for this diagnosis (Fig. 7.4H). Because of the relationship of the bronchi with the pulmonary arteries and left atrium, the left main, left upper, and right middle bronchi are more susceptible to compression by enlarged vessels or chambers (Fig. 7.5). Depending on the degree of obstruction, emphysema or atelectasis is produced.[25]

4. Side of aortic arch: The tracheal air shadow has an indentation on the side of the aortic arch (Fig. 7.4A and E). A right aortic arch is present in 25% of patients with TOF and 30% of patients with truncus arteriosus. Patients with coarctation of the aorta may have the figure-of-3 sign caused by focal indentation in the isthmus region, and if long-standing, inferior rib notching produced by prominent collateral arteries (Fig. 7.4C).

5. Situs: The heart is usually in the left chest (levocardia), but in some patients can be located centrally (mesocardia) or in the right chest (dextrocardia).

6. Skeletal anomalies: Skeletal anomalies are associated with some syndromes.

Radioisotope Scans

Nuclear pulmonary perfusion scans are helpful in determining the percentage of perfusion to the right and left lungs and aid in determining the effect of intervention (surgical or catheterization) for peripheral pulmonary stenosis. Quantitative nuclear angiography can also estimate

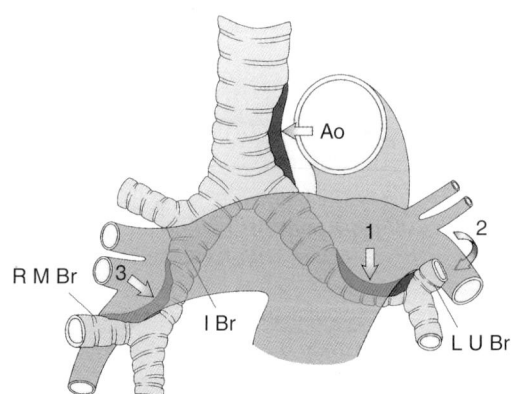

• **Fig. 7.5** Portions of the tracheobronchial tree at increased risk for compression from enlarged pulmonary arteries or left atrium. The left pulmonary artery courses superior to the left main bronchus *(1)* and hooks around the left upper bronchus *(LU Br) (2)*. The distended left pulmonary artery pushes the aorta *(Ao)* medially and accentuates the indentation of the trachea made by a left aortic arch. The left recurrent laryngeal nerve lies in this area and can be compressed. The branch of the right pulmonary artery that supplies the right lower lobe *(3)* crosses the junction of the intermediate bronchus *(I Br.)* and right middle bronchus *(RM Br)*. The left atrium lies below the tracheal bifurcation. Enlargement of the left atrium increases the angle of the tracheal bifurcation mainly by upward deflection of the left main bronchus. (From Stranger P, Lucas RV Jr, Edward JE. Anatomic factors causing respiratory distress in acyanotic congenital heart disease. *Pediatrics.* 1969;43:760.)

the degree of left-to-right shunting; this noninvasive measurement assists the clinician in determining whether a significant-sized shunt is present. Myocardial perfusion scans evaluate ventricular function and are discussed in Chapter 11.

Arrhythmia Evaluation

A variety of recording devices are available for cardiac rhythm surveillance. A full discussion is presented in Chapter 8.

Acknowledgments

Dr. Rita Teele, a long-time member of the medical center's Department of Radiology, instructed generations of trainees in the "Rule of Six" approach to interpretation of the chest radiograph.

References

1. Geggel RL, Fyler DC. History, growth, nutrition, physical examination, and routine laboratory tests. In: Keane JF, Lock JE, Fyler DC, eds. *Nadas' Pediatric Cardiology*. 2nd ed. Philadelphia: Elsevier; 2006:697-714.

2. Johnson LC, Lieberman E, O'Leary E, Geggel RL. Prenatal and newborn screening for critical congenital heart disease: findings from a nursery. *Pediatrics*. 2014;134:916-922.

3. Frohn-Mulder IM, Meilof JF, Szatmari A, Stewart PA, Swaak TJ, Hess J. Clinical significance of maternal anti-RO/SS-A antibodies in children with isolated heart block. *J Am Coll Cardiol*. 1994; 23:1677-1681.

4. Geggel RL. *Diagnosis and Initial Management of Cyanotic Heart Disease in the Newborn*. UpToDate; 2022. Available at: http://www.uptodate.com.

5. Kemper AR, Mahle WT, Martin GR, et al. Strategies for implementing screening for critical congenital heart disease. *Pediatrics*. 2011;128:e1259-e1267.

6. Geggel RL. Coarctation of the aorta: delay in diagnosis and referral basis from infancy to adulthood. *J Pediatr*. 2022;242:57-62.

7. Marino BS, Bird GL, Wernovsky G. Diagnosis and management of the newborn with suspected congenital heart disease. *Clin Perinatol*. 2001;28:91.

8. Whittemore R, Wells JA, Castellsague X. A second-generation study of 427 probands with congenital heart defects and their 837 children. *J Am Coll Cardiol*. 1994;23:1459.

9. Bagnall RD, Weintraub RG, Ingles J, et al. A prospective study of sudden cardiac death among children and young adults. *N Engl J Med*. 2016;374:2441-2452.

10. Geggel RL, Endom EE. *Nontraumatic Chest Pain in Children and Adolescents: Approach and Initial Management*. UpToDate; 2022. Available at: http://www.uptodate.com.

11. Friedman KG, Alexander ME. Chest pain and syncope in children: a practical approach to the diagnosis of cardiac disease. *J Pediatr*. 2013;163:896-901.

12. Greenwood RD, Rosenthal A, Parisi L, et al. Extracardiac anomalies in children with congenital heart disease. *Pediatrics*. 1975; 55:485-492.

13. Davignon A. Percentile charts: ECG standards for children. *Pediatr Cardiol*. 1980;1:133-152.

14. Saadoun D, Vautier M, Cacoub P. Medium- and large-vessel vasculitis. *Circulation*. 2021;143:267-282.

15. Flynn JT, Kaelber DC, Baker-Smith CM, et al. Clinical practice guideline for screening and management of high blood pressure in children and adolescents. *Pediatrics*. 2017;140:e20171904.

16. Rappaport MB, Sprague HB. Physiologic and physical laws that govern auscultation, and their clinical application. *Am Heart J*. 1941;21:257.

17. Geggel RL. *Approach to the Infant or Child with A Cardiac Murmur*. UpToDate; 2022. Available at: http://www.uptodate.com.

18. Marino BS, Goldblatt A. Heart sounds and murmurs. In: Lilly LS, ed. *Pathophysiology of Heart Disease*. Philadelphia: Lea & Febiger; 1992:18-29.

19. Freeman AR, Levine SA. The clinical significance of the systolic murmur: a study of 1,000 consecutive "non-cardiac" cases. *Ann Intern Med*. 1933;6:1371-1385.

20. Shamberger RC, Welch KJ, Sanders SP. Mitral valve prolapse associated with pectus excavatum. *J Pediatr*. 1987;111:404.

21. Phornphutkul C, Rosenthal A, Nadas AS, et al. Cerebrovascular accidents in infants and children with cyanotic congenital heart disease. *Am J Cardiol*. 1973;32:329.

22. Ammash N, Warnes CA. Cerebrovascular events in adult patients with cyanotic congenital heart disease. *J Am Coll Cardiol*. 1996;28:768.

23. Otto CM, Nishimura RA, Bonow RO, et al. 2020 ACC/AHA guideline for the management of patients with valvular heart disease: executive summary. *Circulation*. 2021;143:e35-e71.

24. Jones RWA, Baumer JH, Joseph MC, et al. Arterial oxygen tension and response to oxygen breathing in differential diagnosis of congenital heart disease in infancy. *Arch Dis Child*. 1976;51:667.

25. Stanger P, Lucas Jr RV, Edwards JE. Anatomic factors causing respiratory distress in acyanotic congenital cardiac disease. *Pediatrics*. 1969;43:760.

8

Electrocardiography

EDWARD P. WALSH AND LAURA M. BEVILACQUA

KEY LEARNING POINTS

- There are two types of cardiac action potential. Working atrial and ventricular myocardium have the "fast response" type (dependent on sodium influx for initial depolarization). Cells of the sinus node and atrioventricular node have the "slow response" type (dependent primarily on calcium for depolarization). The latter is most notable for spontaneous automaticity.
- The electrocardiogram (ECG) needs to be interpreted in the context of clinical history and physical examination. "Blind" reading is hazardous. This is

especially true for interpretation of ST-segment and T-wave abnormalities.
- There is wide age-related variation in normal ECG values for children. Tables of normal data must be consulted for proper interpretation (Table 8.1).
- A normal-appearing ECG does not rule out serious underlying heart disease, particularly in neonates.
- Every cardiologist needs to be familiar with the "Top-10 Don't Miss" ECG findings in young patients (Table 8.2), the identification of which can be life-saving.

Although cardiac structure and function are best evaluated with more sophisticated imaging techniques in the current era, the electrocardiogram (ECG) is not, and never will be, obsolete. For well over a century it has remained the quickest, safest, and least expensive diagnostic test in cardiology, and is unparalleled in its ability to register arrhythmias and conduction defects. With proper interpretation, the ECG also offers critical information regarding cardiac position, chamber enlargement, myocardial damage, and certain metabolic disorders. Mastery of the ECG is an essential skill for all cardiologists.

Cardiac Electrical Activity

The Cellular Action Potential

The ECG is several steps removed from electrical activity at the cellular level, but the two are intimately related. Cellular events need to be recorded directly using microelectrodes with tips that are small enough to record across or through an individual cell membrane. Once the microelectrode connects with the cytoplasm, it encounters a field of net negative charge relative to the extracellular environment. This is the *diastolic resting potential* of the cell, which is maintained by the selective permeability of membrane channels to certain ions, as well as the operation of membrane ion pumps. If the cell interior becomes slightly depolarized (i.e., less

negatively charged), it may reach a critical value referred to as the *threshold potential*. At this point, voltage-sensitive membrane ion channels open to allow a rush of positive ions to enter the cell and an *action potential* develops.

Two types of cardiac action potentials are recognized. The first, known as the *fast response* or *sodium channel type*, occurs in cells of atrial and ventricular muscle, His-Purkinje tissue, and (presumably) accessory atrioventricular pathways. These cells register a resting potential around –90 mV and rely on sodium ions as the positive charge carrier for their initial phase 0 depolarization (Fig. 8.1). Immediately following phase 0, there is a complex sequence of opening and closing for the various ion channels involved with potassium, sodium, and calcium flux. This proceeds in an orderly fashion beginning with return of the phase 0 voltage overshoot back to an equilibrium voltage with the extracellular environment (phase 1), which is then maintained for a period known as the phase 2 plateau. The transit of calcium, in particular, during this extended plateau phase is critical for *excitation-contraction coupling* and mechanical function of the heart. Eventually the cell undergoes phase 3 repolarization to restore conditions back to the phase 4 resting state.

The second variety, referred to as the *slow response* or *calcium channel* type, occurs in cells of the sinoatrial (SA) node and the atrioventricular (AV) node. It is distinguished by a resting potential of about –60 mV and has a less acute

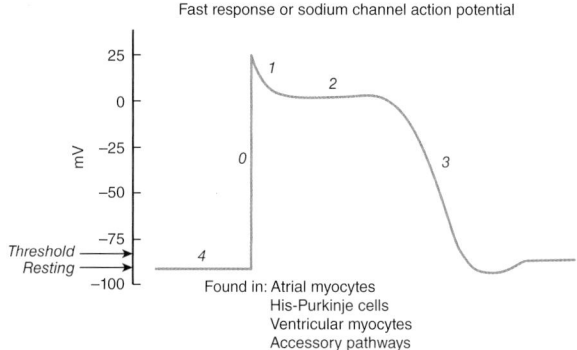

• **Fig. 8.1** Diagrammatic action potential of a "fast response" cardiac cell. The rapid depolarization during phase 0 is caused by sodium influx.

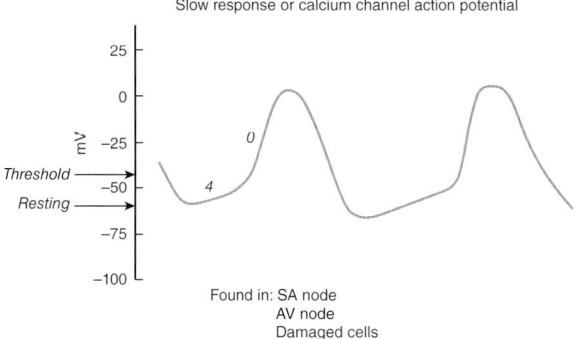

• **Fig. 8.2** Diagrammatic action potential of a "slow response" cardiac cell. The depolarization during phase 0 is predominantly due to calcium influx. Note gradual spontaneous depolarization during phase 4 which imparts the property of automaticity to such cells. *AV,* Atrioventricular; *SA,* sinoatrial.

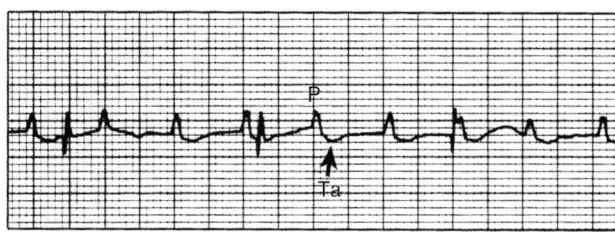

• **Fig. 8.3** The Ta wave of atrial repolarization seen in a patient with complete heart block and atrial enlargement.

a prior stimulus is known as the *refractory period*, which lasts until cells have nearly completed their repolarization process (late phase 3 or early phase 4).

Intracardiac Conduction

Spontaneous depolarization of the SA node activates adjacent atrial muscle cells so that a wave of depolarization spreads from the high right atrium to reach the low right atrium after about 25 msec, and finishes up at the lateral left atrium after about 80 msec. Electrical activity from the SA node cannot be recorded from the body surface, but atrial muscle depolarization is clearly registered as the P wave. The P wave corresponds to phase 0 of the action potentials from atrial myocytes and reflects the leading edge of the depolarization wavefront as it travels from cell to cell. Once all atrial cells have undergone their initial rapid depolarization and enter the phase 2 plateau, the P wave is complete. Phase 3 repolarization of atrial cells causes a very subtle deflection on the surface ECG referred to as the T_A wave. This wave is rarely seen since it is usually obscured by the QRS complex, but under special conditions such as AV block, atrial repolarization may be appreciated (Fig. 8.3).

As the atrial activation wavefront passes through the low right atrium, depolarization of the AV node is initiated. The AV node is a complex interface consisting predominantly of slow-response cells located in *Koch's triangle* (Fig. 8.4). Conduction velocity within the AV node is relatively slow and varies according to the timing of atrial impulses. Premature beats or accelerated atrial rhythm can exaggerate AV nodal delay in a manner described as *decremental conduction*, which ultimately can produce the stereotypic pattern of *Wenckebach periodicity* (Fig. 8.5). This pattern is rather specific to slow response cells. In contrast, conduction through fast response cells tends to be all-or-none with a fairly fixed conduction velocity.

Electrical activity within the AV node is not registered directly on the surface ECG. One must rely on upstream events (P wave) and downstream events (QRS complex) as an indirect reflection of the process. On the surface ECG, the PR interval provides a rough estimate of AV node conduction, but there is more to this interval than AV node activity alone. To be precise, the PR interval includes conduction times: (a) from high to low in the right atrium, (b) through the AV node proper, and (c) within the His-Purkinje system. To dissect the PR interval into individual components, a transvenous electrode catheter

upstroke for phase 0 depolarization. These cells utilize predominately calcium to provide the inward ionic current during phase 0, and inscribe an action potential contour that is more dome shaped without a discrete phase 1 or phase 2 (Fig. 8.2). The most important feature of slow response cells is the property of *automaticity*. Spontaneous upward drift of the diastolic potential during phase 4, driven by the so-called *funny current*, enables such cells to reach threshold of their own accord and thereby act as the natural pacemaker for the heart.

Healthy fast response cells may also achieve spontaneous depolarization, albeit at very slow rates that only appear as escape rhythms in the setting of sinus node dysfunction or heart block. Diseased fast response cells, in contrast, might begin to depolarize rapidly and repetitively if membrane damage results in either a higher resting potential, a lower threshold potential, or other derangements in transmembrane ion kinetics (see Chapter 17).

Whenever a cardiac cell depolarizes, the voltage change stimulates neighboring cells via *gap junctions* so activation is transmitted rapidly from cell to cell. For this process to repeat smoothly, cells must have sufficient time to repolarize and recover between stimuli. If the initiating impulse is premature, the cells may be unprepared, or only partially prepared, for reactivation. The time needed to recover from

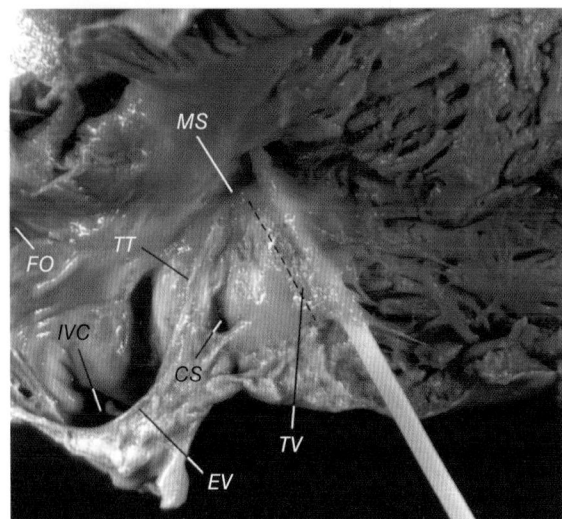

• **Fig. 8.4** View of the interior of the right atrium emphasizing the landmarks of the Koch's triangle. A probe has been positioned under the tricuspid valve leaflet *(TV)* to help localize its edge *(dotted line)*. The apex of Koch's triangle is the membranous septum *(MS)*, with its long sides marked by the tendon of Todaro *(TT)* and the edge of the TV. Its base is at the coronary sinus *(CS)*. The compact atrioventricular node is located in the apical third of the triangle. The foramen ovale *(FO)*, inferior vena cava *(IVC)*, and eustachian valve *(EV)* are labeled for anatomic orientation.

can be positioned near the His bundle as part of an electrophysiologic study. This recording reveals localized low right atrial activation, followed by a sharp deflection from the bundle of His, and finally ventricular activation. An index of true AV node conduction time can be obtained by measuring the interval between low right atrial depolarization and the His bundle signal, referred to as the *AH interval* (Fig. 8.6).

The excitation process next enters the common bundle of His. Cells of the His-Purkinje system have fast response action potentials and rapid conduction velocity. The propagated impulse traverses the common bundle, splits into right and left bundle branches, and exits from terminal Purkinje fibers to begin activation of ventricular myocytes, all in about 40 msec. On the His bundle catheter recording, the time from the initial His deflection to the beginning of ventricular activation (*HV interval*) provides a measure of His-Purkinje conduction time.

Conduction in the His-Purkinje network occurs as cells are depolarizing. Repolarization occurs well after the excitation wavefront has already passed on to ventricular muscle. His-Purkinje cells exhibit the longest plateau phase of any cardiac tissue; hence, their repolarization tends to be one of the last electrical events during a cardiac cycle and can contribute to a small terminal U wave on the normal ECG.

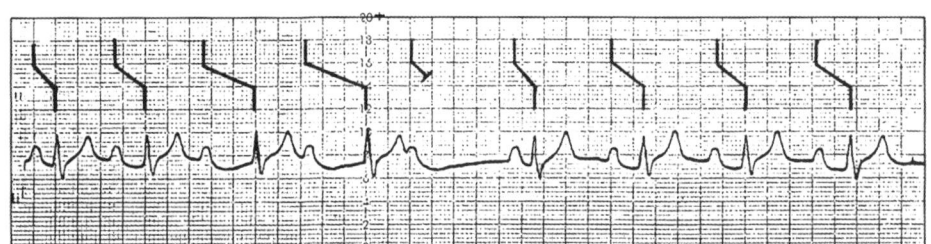

• **Fig. 8.5** Lead II rhythm strip and laddergram demonstrating atrioventricular (AV) nodal Wenckebach phenomenon. This decremental conduction pattern is typical for slow response cells in the AV node.

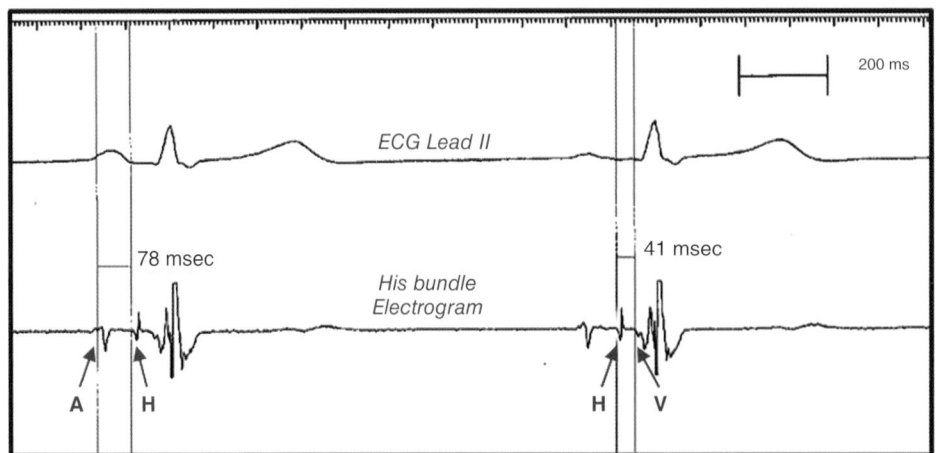

• **Fig. 8.6** Simultaneous surface ECG lead II and the His bundle electrogram. The A-H interval (normal at 78 msec in this case) is measured from the beginning of the "A" deflection to the beginning of the "H" deflection. The H-V interval (normal at 41 msec in this case) is measured from the beginning of the "H" deflection to the earliest onset of ventricular activation.

As the excitation wavefront exits Purkinje fibers, phase 0 of ventricular myocyte depolarization begins. The Purkinje system is highly arborized at its terminal portion, and its multiple exit points activate several different ventricular regions in rapid succession, beginning with left-to-right septal activation, followed by activation of the left and right apex, the endocardium of the right and left ventricular free walls, the free wall epicardium, the base of the left ventricle and, finally, the right ventricular outflow tract. The advancing wavefronts in each region combine to generate the QRS complex.

The QRS is complete once all ventricular cells have depolarized (usually within 90 msec). The ST segment is registered while the cells are at their phase 2 plateau. At the onset of phase 3 repolarization, inscription of the T wave begins. Repolarization is far less homogeneous than depolarization; hence, there is a very protracted duration for the T wave compared with the sharp QRS. Once all ventricular myocytes are back to phase 4, the T wave is complete.

Registration of Cardiac Electrical Activity From the Body Surface

It should be apparent from the preceding discussion that signals registered by the ECG reflect abrupt changes in cellular conditions, with the P wave and QRS complex marking the acute phase 0 transition from resting potential to the fully depolarized state, and the T_A, T, and U waves marking phase 3 repolarization back to the diastolic resting potential. In fact, when all cells in a given cardiac chamber are fully depolarized (phases 1 and 2) or fully repolarized (phase 4), the signal recorded from the body surface has the same isoelectric appearance even though intracellular conditions differ dramatically. Thus, what is measured with an ECG is not cellular voltage, but rather the current that arises at the boundary between depolarized and repolarized cells as activation and deactivation wavefronts move through a cardiac chamber. This boundary acts as a dipole, which generates current because of the presence of opposing charges in front and behind. Movement of this dipole relative to an ECG recording electrode produces the electrocardiographic signal. In addition to direction of wavefront propagation, ECG signals can be further qualified by amplitude (which is largely proportional to the number of cells being stimulated at a given time by the wavefront) and duration (which reflects regional conduction velocity). The basic principles of cardiac excitation and recording are summarized in Fig. 8.7. The interested reader is referred to several comprehensive reviews for further details.[1,2]

The Electrocardiogram

Lead Systems and Technique

The standard ECG evolved from a three-lead system introduced by Einthoven to a 12- or 15-lead tracing used for pediatric recording. The two major lead groupings include the

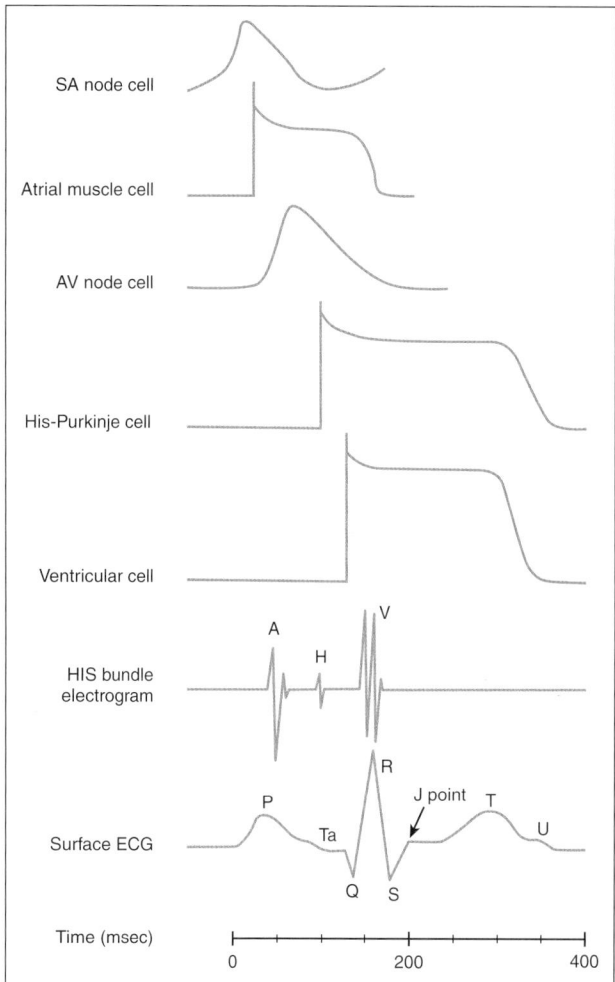

• **Fig. 8.7** Timing of cellular action potentials, intracardiac electrograms from the bundle of His, and the surface ECG. *AV,* Atrioventricular; *SA,* sinoatrial.

limb leads and the precordial leads. The limb leads can be further subdivided into Einthoven's traditional bipolar system (I, II, and III), and the "augmented" unipolar lead system (aVR, aVL, and aVF) developed by Wilson and Goldberger. Einthoven's leads record potentials between electrode pairs: right arm–left arm (lead I), right arm–left leg (lead II), and left arm–left leg (lead III). The augmented unipolar leads record from a single limb in reference to a zero potential central terminal: right arm (aVR), left arm (aVL), and left leg (aVF). A depolarization wavefront moving toward the positive terminal of one of these leads registers a positive deflection on the ECG. These leads form a compass around the frontal plane divided into 360 degrees, with lead positions and degree coordinates as shown in Fig. 8.8.

The precordial leads (V4R through V7) view the electrical activity in the horizontal plane. They are all unipolar and referenced to a zero potential central terminal, but without augmentation (Fig. 8.9).

Routine recordings are made with a chart speed of 25 mm/second and an amplitude response of 1 mV/10 mm. If a patient's ventricular voltages are exceptionally large, the amplitude response might be reduced to 1 mV/5 mm or

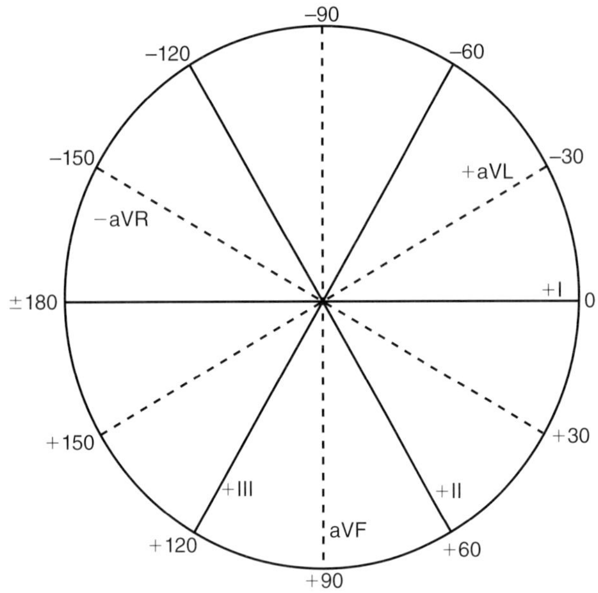

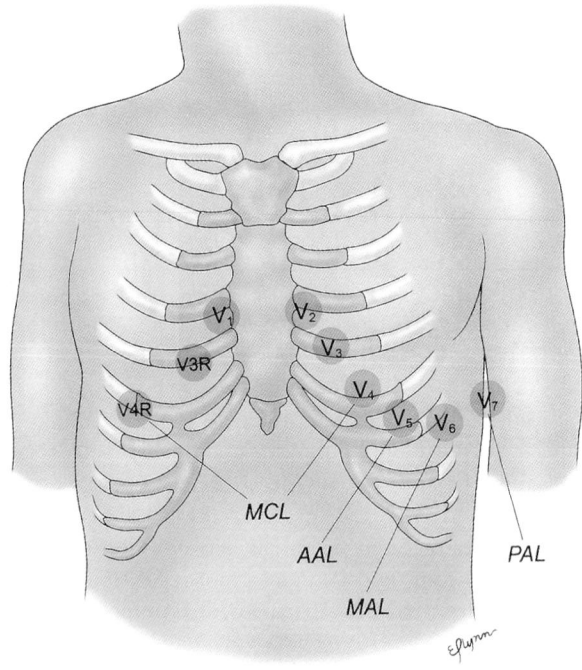

• **Fig. 8.8** Degree coordinates and positive pole of the limb ECG leads in the frontal plane.

• **Fig. 8.9** Proper location of the precordial leads for pediatric ECG recording. Landmarks for proper positioning include midclavicular line (*MCL*), anterior axillary line (*AAL*), midaxillary line (*MAL*), and posterior axillary line (*PAL*). Careless positioning can result erroneous voltage recordings.

even 1 mV/2.5 mm to avoid signal overlap. Whenever non-standard amplification is used for ECG display, the appropriate calibration mark must be highlighted.

The Normal Electrocardiogram

The normal values referred to in this discussion have been drawn from our experience at Boston Children's Hospital,

the classic publication of Davignon,[3] and a recent update in normal voltage data from Saarel et al.[4] Selected values are abstracted for quick reference in Table 8.1. The ECG should be read in a systemic fashion, beginning with rhythm analysis and measurements of axes and intervals, followed by waveform analysis, all of which must be synthesized into a final impression based on history and physical examination. Owing to the wide variation in age-adjusted normal values, as well as numerous benign variants, a firm diagnosis of "normal" on a pediatric ECG tracing can actually be one of the hardest conclusions to reach, especially if one is forced to read a tracing without full knowledge of the patient's clinical condition. It is often said that an ideal ECG interpretation should be accompanied by a medical history and hands-on physical exam to guarantee proper clinical context.

Axis

Axis refers to the predominant direction of a waveform in the frontal plane. By identifying the limb lead with the largest positive deflection for the waveform in question, and remembering the coordinates for this lead on the frontal compass face, one can assign a value in degrees for the mean axis. The easiest example involves the P wave. Because normal atrial activation begins at the SA node and spreads through the atrium high-to-low and right-to-left, the wavefront of depolarization flows southeast in the frontal plane. Lead II (+60 degrees) best records this area and usually registers the largest positive P wave. The P-wave axis for a normal heart in sinus rhythm should be between 0 degrees and +90 degrees regardless of the patient's age.

The mean QRS axis is calculated in a similar fashion by identifying the limb lead with the largest positive R wave and assigning the corresponding degree value. The normal QRS axis has age-dependent variation. For neonates in whom the right ventricle is relatively hypertrophied by virtue of its intrauterine workload, the axis is directed rightward at about 120 degrees. As the left ventricle becomes dominant during the first 6 months of life, the axis shifts toward +60 degrees and should remain between +5 degrees and +110 degrees thereafter.

The T-wave axis in the frontal plane is usually concordant with the QRS. There may be some discrepancy in the early months of life, but by the time the child is 6 months old, the QRS and T axes should not differ by more than 60 degrees.

Rhythm and Rate

Cardiac excitation arising from the SA node generates a P wave with a normal axis at physiologic rates for age. Rate determination is a straightforward exercise (Fig. 8.10). *Respirophasic sinus arrhythmia* is a normal finding in healthy children, as is *wandering atrial pacemaker* where a subsidiary P wave with a different axis may emerge during episodic SA node slowing.

P Wave

The contour and amplitude of the P wave are an indirect measure of atrial size. The normal P wave should have a smooth

TABLE 8.1	Normal Range for Selected ECG Measurements in Children*							
Age	0–7 days	1 wk–1 mo	1 mo–6 mo	6 mo–1 yr	1 yr–5 yr	5–10 yr	10–15 yr	>15 yr
QRS axis (degrees)	70–180 (120)	45–160 (100)	10–120 (80)	5–110 (60)	5–110 (60)	5–110 (60)	5–110 (60)	5–110 (60)
PR lead II (msec)	80–150 (100)	80–150 (100)	80–150 (100)	80–150 (100)	80–150 (120)	80–150 (120)	90–180 (140)	100–190 (160)
QRS duration (msec)	50–80 (65)	50–80 (65)	50–80 (65)	50–80 (70)	55–85 (70)	55–85 (70)	60–90 (75)	60–90 (80)
QTc† (msec)	(variable)	≤ 450 male ≤ 460 female						
R-wave V_1 (mm)	5–25 (15)	3–22 (10)	3–20 (10)	2–20 (9)	2–18 (8)	1–15 (5)	1–12 (5)	1–6 (2)
R-wave V_5 (mm)	2–20 (10)	3–25 (12)	5–30 (17)	10–30 (20)	10–35 (23)	13–38 (25)	10–35 (20)	7–21 (13)
R-wave V_6 (mm)	1–12 (5)	1–17 (7)	3–20 (10)	5–22 (12)	6–22 (14)	8–25 (16)	8–24 (15)	5–18 (10)
T wave V_1 (direction)	upright or +	negative					(variable)	upright or +

*Values reported as 2nd–98th percentile (mean), except for QTc (maximum value) and T wave (gross direction).
†QTc as corrected by Bazett's formula (QTc = QT/square root of RR interval)

Major division = 0.20 second
Minor division = 0.04 second

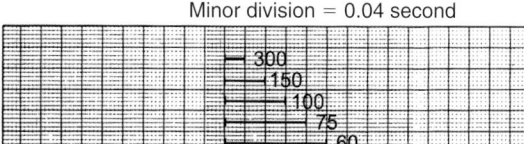
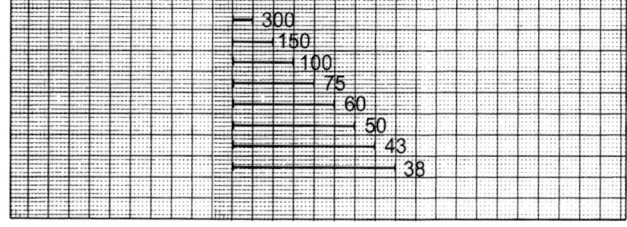

• **Fig. 8.10** At chart paper speed of 25 mm/second, each major division = 0.20 second, and each minor division = 0.04 second. Heart rate in beats per minute can quickly be determined from the number of large divisions between the QRS.

dome shape in lead II and should not be taller than 0.3 mV or wider than 120 msec in duration. Occasionally, there may be a small notch in the P wave of lead II, but this is acceptable if amplitude and duration fall within the normal range.

PR Interval

The PR interval is measured from the beginning of the P wave to the initial deflection of ventricular activation (it is a PQ interval to be more precise). As noted earlier, the PR includes several electrical events, with AV node conduction accounting for the major portion. The normal PR interval is < 150 msec in young children and < 180 msec in adolescents and adults. A prolonged PR interval can be due to enhanced vagal tone, atrial muscle disease, certain medications, or disease involving the AV node and/or the His-Purkinje system. A short PR interval (<100 msec) is observed in *Wolff-Parkinson-White (WPW)* syndrome.

QRS Complex

The QRS complex is evaluated for its morphology, amplitude, and duration. The QRS morphology is dictated by the

sequence of regional ventricular activation, and the balance (right versus left) of ventricular muscle mass. The normal heart leaves a characteristic QRS shape in each lead of the ECG, which may vary because of distorted activation sequence, cardiac malposition, hypertrophy, or preexcitation. Beyond infancy, the normal pattern is one of a small Q wave, followed by a large R and a small S wave in left-sided leads (I, II, aVL, V3–V6), while right-sided leads (aVR, III, V4R–V2) typically register a small R followed by a S wave.

QRS amplitude offers a semi-quantitative measure of ventricular mass. Normal age-related values are established for R wave amplitude, as well as for Q and S wave amplitudes, in each individual lead. Tables of normal data should be on hand during review of all pediatric ECGs. Modern software for computerized ECG reading often has normal age-specific data imbedded within its program.

The duration of the QRS complex relates to speed of conduction within the His-Purkinje system and through ventricular muscle. Duration increases slightly with age. The QRS width is usually < 70 msec in neonates and < 90 msec in those older than 6 months. Prolongation of the QRS may be seen with block of His-Purkinje conduction (bundle branch block), slow myocyte conduction (due to muscle injury, drugs, or electrolyte disturbances), severe ventricular hypertrophy, and some cases of preexcitation.

ST Segment

Ventricular muscle cells are in the plateau phase of their action potential (phase 2) during the ST segment. Because no electrical wavefronts are advancing or retreating through the ventricles, the body surface recording is normally isoelectric. The *J point* at the termination of the S wave marks the beginning of the ST segment and normally does not deviate more than 1 mm from the baseline. One normal variant is the *early repolarization* pattern, seen occasionally in healthy adolescent patients where the J point can be elevated 2–4 mm. Usually, this elevation is observed in the lateral (V4–V6) and inferior (II, III, aVF) leads and is accompanied by tall T waves in the same leads. The diagnosis of benign early repolarization should not be made if the elevation is more than 4 mm and/or the T wave is of low amplitude.

T Wave

The T wave corresponds to phase 3 repolarization of ventricular myocytes. The normal T-wave amplitude is variable and is not routinely quantitated. The direction of the T wave, however, deserves attention. As mentioned, discordance of the frontal plane QRS and T axis by more than 60 degrees may suggest pathology. The precordial leads follow somewhat different rules for T-wave direction. Over the left chest, the T wave is still normally concordant with the QRS, but there are important age-dependent variations in the rightward leads. From birth to about 7 days of age, the T wave is upright in all precordial leads. After this, the T wave becomes negative over the right chest (V4R–V2), while remaining positive in the left chest leads. This pattern persists until early adolescence, when the T waves tend to resume an upright direction in V1. This sequence is critical to remember during analysis of ECGs in children, since an upright T wave in the right precordial leads between the age of 7 days and early adolescence is a potential indicator of right ventricular hypertrophy (RVH).

QT Interval

The QT interval is a reflection of the action potential duration for ventricular myocytes. It is measured from the onset of the QRS to the point of T-wave termination. Because the normal QT varies with heart rate (longer at slow rates, shorter at fast rates), the measurement is adjusted with Bazett's formula (QT/square root R-R = rate-corrected QTc). Some transient QTc prolongation can be seen as a normal variant during the first week of life, but thereafter should be ≤ 450 msec in males and ≤ 460 msec in females.[5] A prolonged QTc should raise concern. The hereditary *long QT syndromes* are potentially fatal disorders, and early detection on an ECG is imperative. The QTc is also prolonged by certain drugs, hypothermia, Williams syndrome, and some electrolyte imbalances. Most modern ECG recording equipment will measure the QT and calculate a QTc automatically, though it must be emphasized that machine errors are not rare and manual confirmation is recommended, especially when evaluating a patient with worrisome symptoms or a concerning family history.

U Wave

The U wave is thought to reflect the relatively late repolarization process of His-Purkinje cells and some mid-layer left ventricular myocytes. It is not always apparent on the ECG of normal patients. When present, a normal U wave is of low amplitude (less than one-fourth the height of the T wave) and has the same polarity as its T wave. When the U wave is abnormally prominent (more than half the height of the T wave), it should be included in the measurement of the QT interval. The amplitude of the U wave may become accentuated secondary to hypokalemia, antiarrhythmic drugs, and some channelopathies.

The Abnormal Electrocardiogram

The ECG should never be interpreted in isolation. There should be specific questions to answer when the test is ordered regarding rhythm, intervals, hypertrophy, myocardial injury, etc. Additionally, one should constantly bear in mind that a child can have serious heart disease with a normal-appearing ECG, particularly in the first few days of life.

Rate and Rhythm

Cardiac rhythm should be the first item scrutinized on the ECG tracing. If the rhythm is abnormal, assumptions regarding axis, intervals, and ST/T appearance may become invalid. To evaluate these issues accurately, the ECG needs to be repeated after sinus rhythm is restored. Detailed discussion of arrhythmias will be found in Chapter 17.

Cardiac Malpositions

Chamber orientation is reflected on the ECG by the axis and the morphology of the P wave and the QRS complex. Atrial situs is determined with reasonable accuracy by deciding which side of the atrium contains the SA node. In normal situs solitus, the SA node generates a P wave axis of about +60 degrees, whereas in situs inversus the activation emanates from high in the left-sided atrium, so the P axis is about +120 degrees (Fig. 8.11). Variable patterns may be seen in the heterotaxy syndromes. For example, some patients with heterotaxy syndrome may have bilateral SA nodes, and the P wave axis may alternate or fuse between +60 degrees and +120 degrees. In other patients with heterotaxy, the SA node may be absent altogether, resulting in a slow subsidiary atrial pacemaker with variable location or junctional escape rhythm.

Gross ventricular orientation is best estimated from the precordial leads. Normal levocardia has a characteristic pattern of relatively low (or predominately negative) voltage in the right chest leads (V4R to V2) with positive forces of higher amplitude in the mid and left chest leads. In *dextrocardia*, the pattern is reversed. Further insight into ventricular anatomy may be gained by determining the ventricular looping. In *L-loop* ventricles, the normal left-right relationship is inverted and the septal activation wavefront travels right-to-left. This changes the QRS morphology to one of initial Q waves in right-sided leads, with small initial R waves on the left side (Fig. 8.12).

Atrial Enlargement

The ECG is a fairly good indicator of atrial enlargement. Because the right atrium is the first to depolarize, indicators of right-sided enlargement are found in the early portions of the P wave. The diagnostic criterion for isolated right

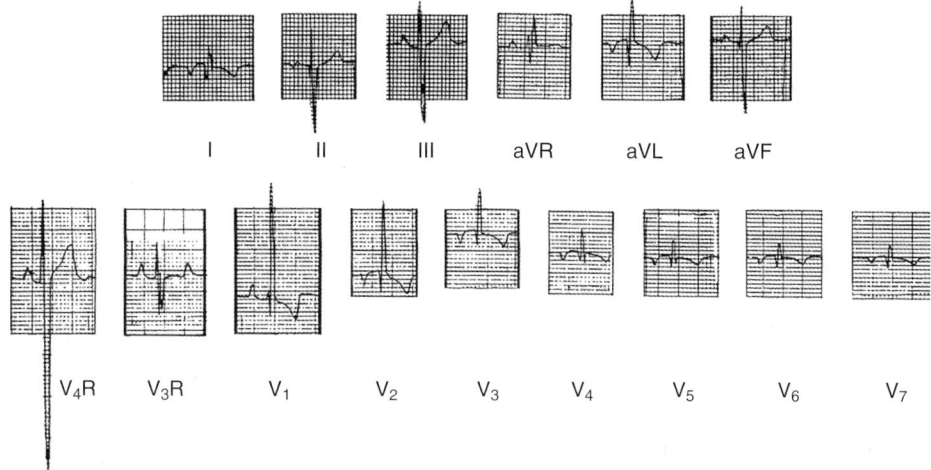

• **Fig. 8.11** Electrocardiogram from a 6-year-old patient with documented situs inversus and a P-wave axis of + 150 degrees. Dextrocardia is also present.

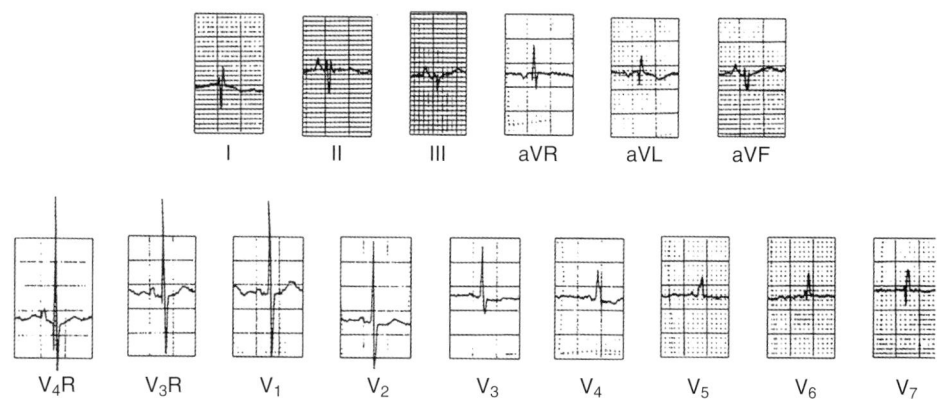

• **Fig. 8.12** The ECG in a patient with L-looped ventricles (note the RSR pattern in V4–V7, and the Q wave in V4R and V3R) and dextrocardia (note prominent voltage over the right chest).

atrial enlargement is the presence in lead II of a peaked narrow P wave greater than 0.30 mV in amplitude, accompanied by either a tall P wave or a biphasic P wave with an early deep negative deflection in lead V1 (Fig. 8.13). Left atrial enlargement is reflected in the terminal portion of the P wave. The classic findings include a broad, notched P wave in lead II (duration greater than 120 msec), or a deep slurred terminal portion of a biphasic P wave in V1 (Fig. 8.14). Many patients with complex congenital heart defects (especially single ventricle) can demonstrate a combination of both patterns (Fig. 8.15).

Right Ventricular Hypertrophy

Screening for RVH is important in pediatric practice because so many congenital defects impose an increased work load on this chamber. Fortunately, the criteria that have emerged are fairly sensitive (Fig. 8.16).

R Wave Amplitude in V1 Higher Than the 98th Percentile for Age

This finding is specific outside of the neonatal period. The height of the R wave in this lead correlates well with right

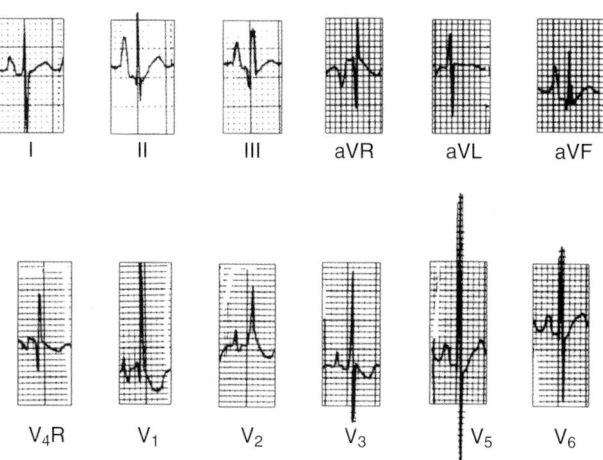

• **Fig. 8.13** Electrocardiogram showing right atrial enlargement.

ventricular systolic pressure and is sufficiently quantitative to allow prediction of right ventricular pressure for isolated pulmonary valve stenosis in older children using the formula: R wave height (in millimeters) × 5 = peak systolic pressure (mm Hg).

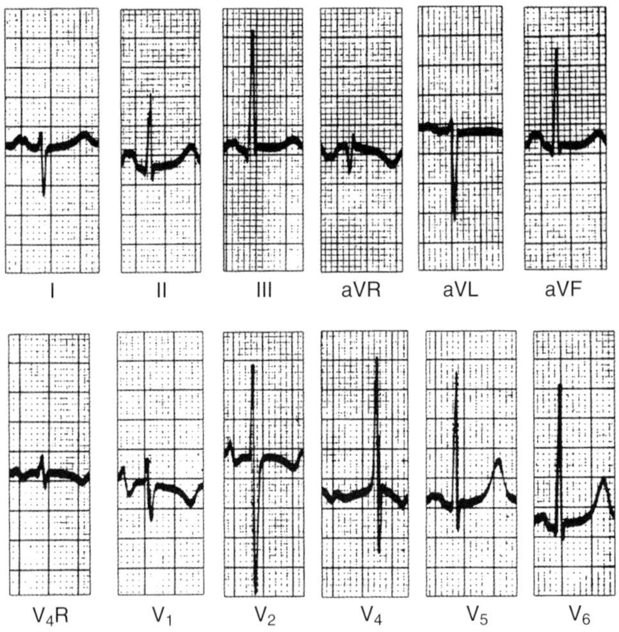

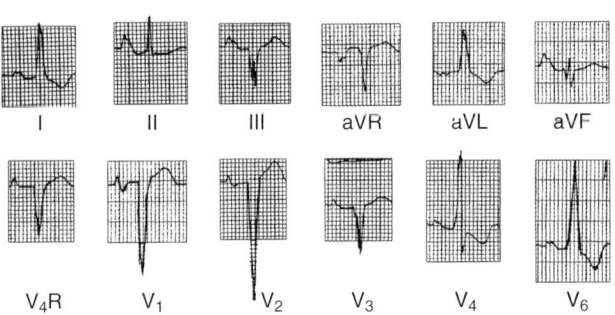

• **Fig. 8.14** Electrocardiogram showing left atrial enlargement.

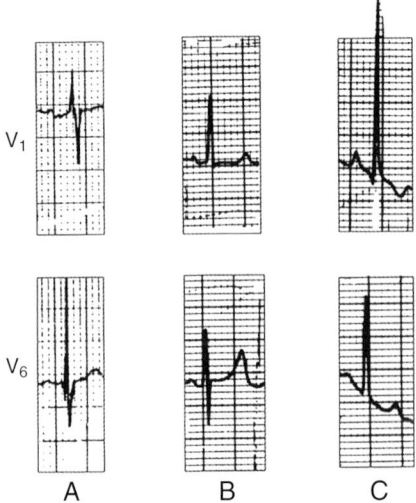

• **Fig. 8.15** Electrocardiogram showing biatrial enlargement.

• **Fig. 8.16** Electrocardiogram patterns with varying degrees of right ventricular pressure load hypertrophy. **(A)** Mild right ventricular hypertrophy (RVH) in a 9-month-old suggested by an upright T wave in V1, but without excess R wave voltage. **(B)** Moderate RVH in a 4-year-old with an upright T wave and excess R wave voltage in V1. **(C)** Marked RVH in a 7-year-old showing a very tall R wave with an inverted T wave in V1.

Abnormal T Wave Direction in V1

As mentioned, the T-wave direction in lead V1 changes with time: upright in newborns, negative beyond the age of 7 days, and positive again in adolescents and adults. A persistently upright T wave after the seventh day of life can be an indicator of elevated right ventricular pressure, and when combined with R-wave amplitude, even greater precision is possible.

S Wave Depth in V6 Greater Than the 98th Percentile for Age

This measurement is useful in patients with increased right ventricular pressure secondary to chronic lung disease. Respiratory disorders such as cystic fibrosis can lower the voltage pattern recorded from the right chest because of heart rotation and hyperexpansion of the lungs. Despite low anterior forces, RVH can still be diagnosed when the lateral S wave is very deep. This pattern of RVH, when associated with right atrial enlargement in a patient with severe pulmonary disease, is often referred to as a *cor pulmonale* pattern (Fig. 8.17).

Right Axis Deviation

Isolated right-axis deviation is not specific for RVH. When present in conjunction with other RVH criteria, it lends additional support for the diagnosis.

RSR' Pattern in V1

It is important to understand the significance and limitations of this finding in the pediatric population.[6] Increased right ventricular volume loads imposed by common lesions such as an atrial septal defect may create a pattern in V1 of an initial R wave followed by an S wave and terminating with a tall R' wave. A diagnosis of RVH should be made only when the secondary R' wave is large in amplitude (Fig. 8.18). Many normal children may have a similar pattern with a lower-amplitude R' wave. It is also useful to examine the distribution of the RSR' pattern in multiple precordial leads since large right ventricular volume loads may cause the RSR' pattern to extend from V4R all the way across to V4, whereas the pattern does not extend beyond V2 in normal children.

Left Ventricular Hypertrophy

Identification of left ventricular hypertrophy (LVH) from the ECG is an imperfect exercise.[7] The diagnosis can be

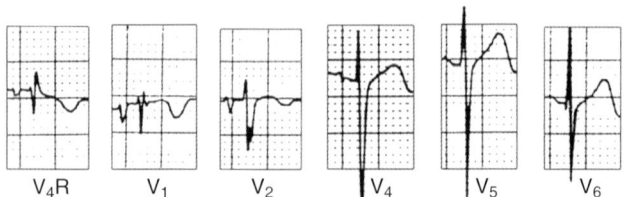

• **Fig. 8.17** The pattern of right ventricular hypertrophy seen in chronic lung disease (cystic fibrosis in this case), characterized by deep, lateral S waves but normal voltages in the right chest due to hyperinflation of the lungs.

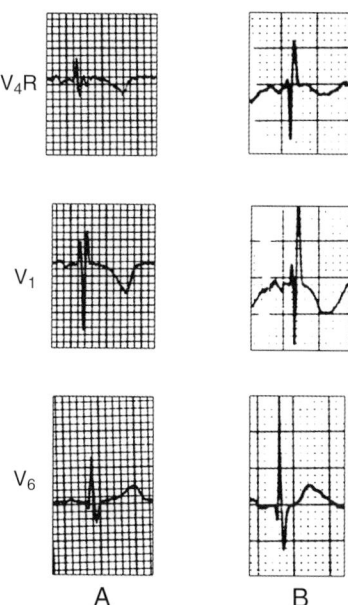

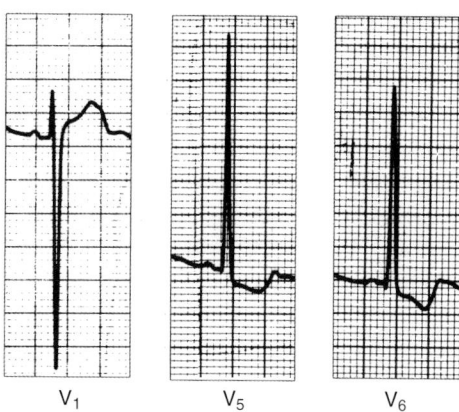

• **Fig. 8.20** The typical ECG pattern for left ventricular hypertrophy (LVH) due to increased pressure load in a patient with aortic stenosis, showing minimal Q waves in V5 and V6. The R-wave amplitude is only slightly above normal, but the T-wave inversion supports LVH.

• **Fig. 8.18** The RSR' pattern in lead V1. **(A)** Normal patient without heart disease. **(B)** Patient with increased right ventricular volume load due to large atrial septal defect (note the taller R' wave).

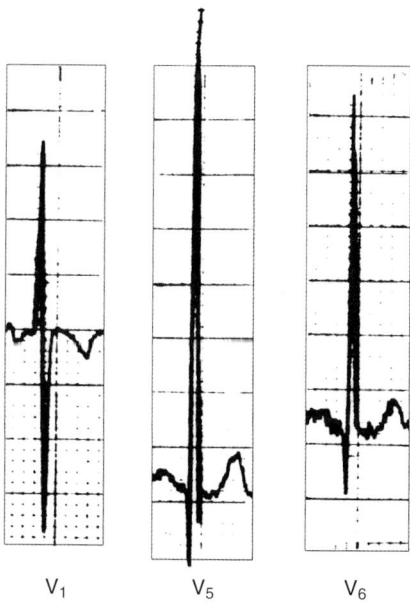

• **Fig. 8.19** The typical ECG pattern for left ventricular hypertrophy due to a large volume load, with deep Q waves in V5 and V6 in an infant with a large ventricular septal defect.

difficult until the process is advanced, and is best entertained when multiple criteria are fulfilled.

R Wave Amplitude in V5–V6 Greater Than the 98th Percentile for Age

The voltage criteria for LVH are not very exact and are best applied when excessive voltage is present in both V5 and V6 (Fig. 8.19). Hypertrophy may be present with normal left precordial forces, and in some normal children (particularly athletic teenagers) the R wave amplitude may exceed

the 98th percentile. Voltages can also appear artifactually excessive if the precordial leads were positioned carelessly.

Lateral T-Wave Inversion

In studies of aortic stenosis, T-wave abnormalities were identified as the most specific indications of LVH. LVH can cause a pattern of inverted T waves in the inferior limb leads (II, III, aVF) and left precordial leads (V5 and V6), sometimes associated with depression of the ST segment. There may or may not be voltage indications of LVH (Fig. 8.20). Although the presence of these T wave changes usually suggests advanced degrees of hypertrophy, the presence of ischemia or myocardial inflammation must be excluded before this criterion can be applied with certainty.

Left Axis Deviation

An abnormal leftward axis is supportive evidence for LVH. The utility of this criterion is best appreciated in the neonate, where the QRS axis is normally directed rightward. The presence of a *mature* axis in the 0-degree to +90-degree range, or a *superior* axis in the 0-degree to –90-degree range in early infancy strongly suggests a cardiac abnormality.

Abnormal Lateral Q Wave

The Q wave in leads V5 and V6 (septal depolarization) may be distorted if the left ventricle is very dilated or markedly thick. There can be deviation and rotation of septal position, and increased competition from left apex and left free-wall depolarization. As a broad generalization, a dilated volume-loaded left ventricle tends to have an abnormally deep Q wave in the leftward leads in lesions such as aortic regurgitation, patent ductus, or ventricular septal defect. Concentric hypertrophy from a pressure load such as aortic stenosis is more likely to be associated with a small or absent Q wave. The pattern in septal hypertrophy due to hypertrophic myopathy is quite variable, but most often involves prominent sharp Q waves in V5 and V6.

Single Ventricle Hypertrophy

There are no firm criteria to apply for hypertrophy of a single ventricle in complex congenital anomalies. What is most surprising is that an ECG in such conditions can look deceptively normal at times, at least for the newborn. However, voltage criteria for single ventricles generally exceed those for either RVH or LVH in some precordial leads as the children age. The exact QRS morphology is highly variable, depending on the presence and location of ventricular septal tissue, ventricular looping pattern, which anatomic ventricle is dominant, and the orientation of the heart within the thorax. One may be able to predict which ventricle is absent by noting which side of the precordium has deficient positive voltage. Hypoplastic ventricle may also be suspected if a septal Q wave is absent in all precordial leads.

Intraventricular Conduction Abnormalities

Below the common His bundle, intraventricular conduction tissue divides into the right and left bundle branches. The left bundle fans out over much of the left ventricular septal surface, but may be considered to split into two major divisions directed toward the respective papillary muscles: the left anterior and left posterior fascicles. Partial or complete block at any one of these sites creates regional delay in ventricular activation and a characteristic change in the QRS pattern. Likewise, the presence of an accessory conduction pathway distorts the regional activation pattern by stimulating a ventricular segment ahead of schedule.

Incomplete Right Bundle Branch Block

An RSR' pattern in the right precordial leads with normal QRS duration (Fig. 8.18) may indicate an incomplete conduction disturbance in the right ventricle. However, an identical pattern may be seen in healthy normal individuals, or in patients with right ventricular volume overload as previously discussed.[6] The diagnosis of incomplete block should be reserved for situations in which RSR' is associated with a slightly prolonged QRS duration in the absence of a left-to-right shunt at the atrial level.

Complete Right Bundle Branch Block

When transmission is interrupted in the right bundle branch, the septum and left ventricle can activate normally, but the right ventricle depends upon slower cell-to-cell activation spreading left-to-right. The resultant QRS complex has a prolonged duration (>100 msec for infants, >120 msec for older patients) and a characteristic morphology that reflects the slow activation wavefront spreading toward the right heart (Fig. 8.21). The initial portion of the QRS is generated by the usual septal and initial left ventricular depolarization and thus, is quite similar to normal (small R wave in V1, QR in V6). The subsequent slow wavefront traveling toward the right heart inscribes a tall slurred R' wave in V1 and an equally sluggish S wave in V6. A pattern of complete right bundle branch block is a frequent observation following surgical repair of ventricular septal defects.

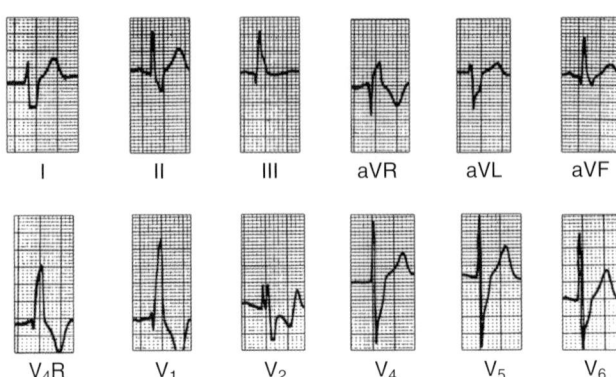

• **Fig. 8.21** Electrocardiographic pattern of complete right bundle branch block.

Diagnosing ventricular hypertrophy on the ECG is difficult in the presence of complete right bundle branch block. Attempts to correlate right ventricular pressure and/or volume with the height of the R' wave, QRS duration, or the extent of RSR' distribution across the precordium have met with only partial success. Likewise, bundle branch block results in diffuse changes in the ST segment, T wave, and QT interval, so the usual electrocardiographic markers of ischemia and prolonged QTc are lost.

Left Anterior Hemiblock

Conduction block in the left anterior fascicle produces a shift in QRS axis to the range of –60 degrees, without prolongation of QRS duration. Whereas the anterior-superior and posterior-inferior portions of the normal left ventricle are usually depolarized simultaneously by their respective fascicles, block in the anterior limb changes the sequence. The inferior regions activate normally, but the depolarization wavefront must then spread upward, producing a superiorly directed vector in the frontal plane. Isolated block in the anterior fascicle is rare in children but may occur with myocardial inflammation, ischemia, and surgical or catheter trauma.

Certain congenital cardiac anomalies, notably endocardial cushion defects and tricuspid atresia, present with electrocardiographic patterns of a leftward *superior QRS axis* that mimic left anterior hemiblock (Fig. 8.22). The abnormal axis is not due to true conduction defects in these cases, but instead results from the abnormal anatomic location of the conduction fibers in cushion defects or the unusual left ventricular shape and orientation in tricuspid atresia.

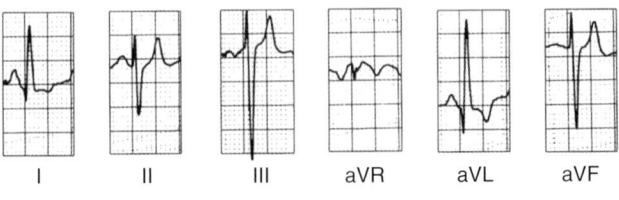

• **Fig. 8.22** Superior axis (–60 degrees) in a patient with tricuspid atresia.

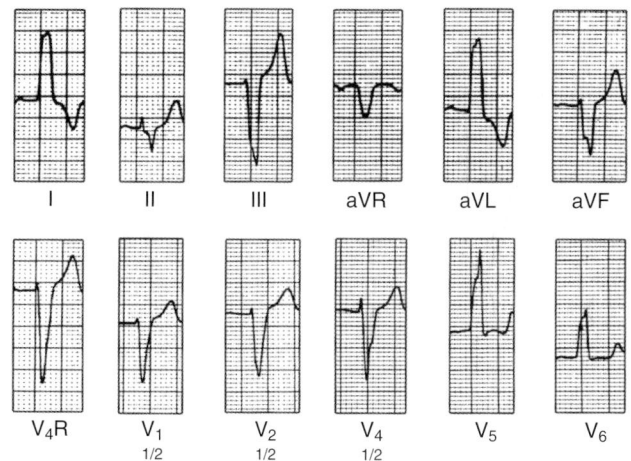

• **Fig. 8.23** Electrocardiographic pattern of complete left bundle branch block.

Left Posterior Hemiblock

The QRS duration remains normal, but the axis is shifted right and inferior to about +120 degrees when the posterior fascicle is interrupted. The activation pattern in the left ventricle is just the reverse of anterior hemiblock. Because right-axis deviation is seen commonly in infants and children with RVH, the label of posterior hemiblock should be reserved for instances when an abrupt axis shift has occurred between serial ECGs. True posterior hemiblock is exceptionally rare in young patients.

Complete Left Bundle Branch Block

When the main left bundle branch is damaged or interrupted, ventricular activation begins primarily via the right bundle. The septum must now depolarize right to left, and the left ventricle must rely on late transmission of the activation wavefront which is directed leftward and posterior (Fig. 8.23). The QRS is prolonged, slurred, and directed away from the right chest leads (mostly negative in V1) and toward the lateral precordial leads (positive in V5–V7). As with complete right bundle branch block, ventricular hypertrophy, ischemic changes, and QT prolongation cannot be interpreted from ECGs. Advanced LVH can produce an electrocardiographic pattern identical to that of complete left bundle branch block.

Preexcitation

Preexcitation implies that a portion of ventricular tissue is being activated ahead of schedule relative to normal His-Purkinje conduction. In WPW syndrome, this early activation occurs over a small accessory connection between atrial and ventricular muscle located anywhere along the right or left atrioventricular grooves. As an atrial depolarization wavefront approaches the ventricles, it may advance over the accessory pathway, the normal AV node, or both. Normal AV nodal conduction normally involves a brief delay, but accessory pathways transmit rapid activation to a focal ventricular segment. The region of early activation generates a *delta wave* (Fig. 8.24) on the ECG with a short

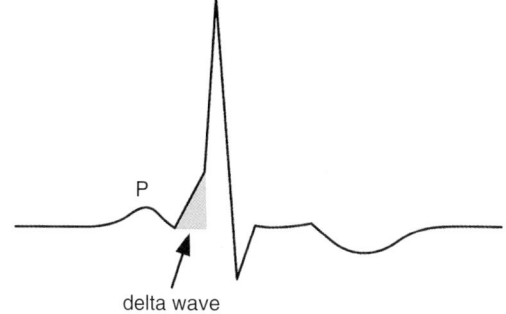

• **Fig. 8.24** Short P-R interval and the delta wave of ventricular preexcitation.

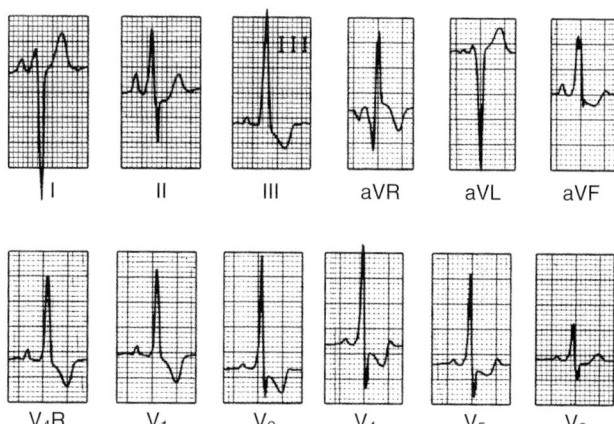

• **Fig. 8.25** Electrocardiogram showing Wolff-Parkinson-White syndrome in a patient with a left-sided accessory pathway. The precordial pattern is akin to right bundle branch block.

PR interval (to be precise, a P-delta interval). Because some portion of ventricular activation still occurs over the normal His pathway, there is fusion between preexcitation and the normal depolarization sequence.

The electrocardiographic patterns in the WPW syndrome are variable, depending on the accessory pathway location and its conduction characteristics. At the most simplistic level, left-sided accessory pathways can be expected to produce negative delta waves in the left-sided ECG leads (I, aVL, V5, V6) and positive delta waves in the right-sided leads (aVR, V4R–V1), generating a gross QRS morphology reminiscent of right bundle branch block (Fig. 8.25). Right-sided and septal accessory pathways are usually associated with positive delta waves in the left-sided leads and a QRS pattern more closely resembling left bundle branch block (Fig. 8.26). Several ECG algorithms have been developed[8] that provide more exacting estimates of accessory pathway location based on delta wave polarity and QRS shape in multiple leads (see Chapters 17 and 18). In the presence of preexcitation, the ability to use the ECG for evaluation of hypertrophy, changes in the ST and T wave, and QT measurement is lost (similar to bundle branch block).

ST Segment and T-Wave Abnormalities

No other aspect of ECG interpretation is as dependent on clinical history as the evaluation of abnormalities of the ST

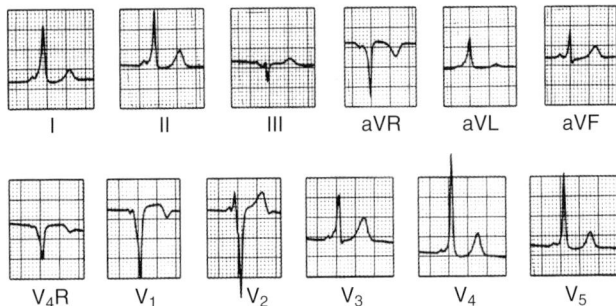

• **Fig. 8.26** Electrocardiogram showing Wolff-Parkinson-White syndrome in a patient with a right-sided accessory pathway. The precordial pattern is akin to left bundle branch block.

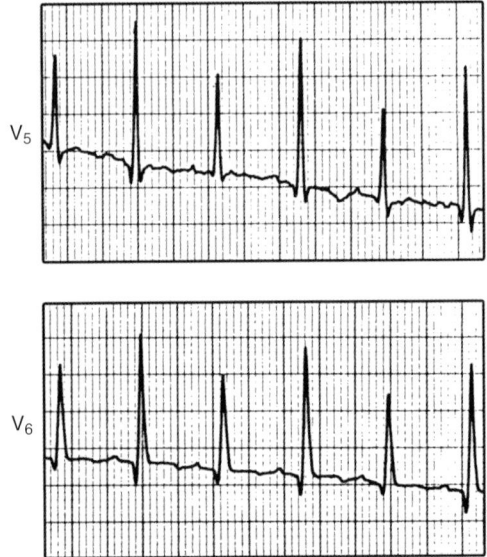

• **Fig. 8.27** Electrical alternans in a teenage boy with large pericardial effusion. Note also the nonspecific flattening of the T wave in V5 and V6.

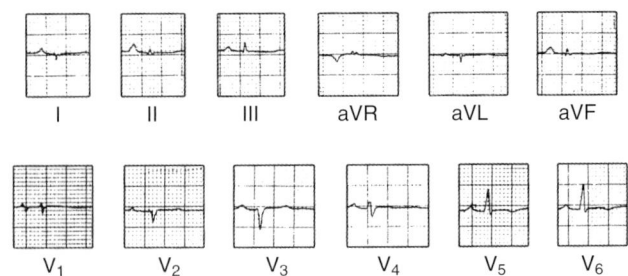

• **Fig. 8.28** Dramatically low QRS voltage in a patient with dilated myopathy from myocarditis. (From Fyler DC, Hanley & Belfus, eds. Nadas' Pediatric Cardiology, Philadelphia, 1992.)

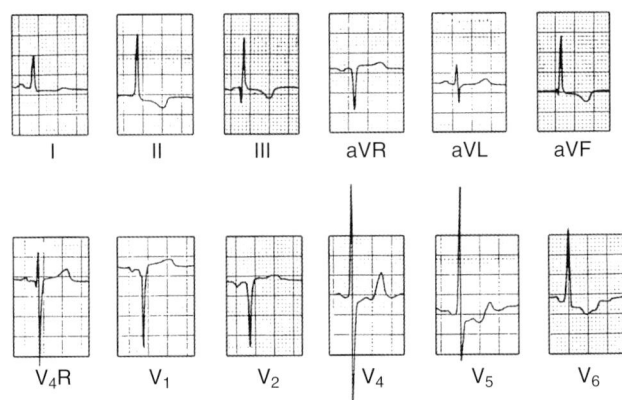

• **Fig. 8.29** Electrocardiogram from a patient with hypertrophic obstructive cardiomyopathy showing left ventricular hypertrophy by voltage criteria along with T-wave inversion.

segment and T wave. Pathologic changes are often non-specific. Elevation or depression of the J point and changes in the T wave can be seen in mostly any condition involving myocyte injury, pericardial inflammation, abnormal ion channel function, or certain electrolyte disturbances.

Pericarditis and Pericardial Effusion

Pericardial inflammation produces changes in the ST segment and T wave that evolve as the disorder progresses.[9] The earliest finding is elevation of the ST segment with preservation of normal T-wave amplitude and direction. Later, the T wave becomes flattened. As opposed to the focal changes in the ST segment and T wave that are seen under ischemic conditions, the electrocardiographic findings in pericarditis are diffuse and involve most leads. The presence of a large effusion in the pericardial space can also result in diminished ventricular voltages and/or a pattern of QRS amplitude variation known as *QRS alternans* (Fig. 8.27).

Myocarditis

The electrocardiographic findings in myocarditis are variable but usually involved diminished ventricular voltages

(Fig. 8.28) and T-wave inversion during the acute illness. Atrioventricular and intraventricular conduction disturbances, along with ventricular arrhythmias, are common.

Hypertrophic Cardiomyopathy

The changes in the ST segment and T wave seen in hypertrophic cardiomyopathy are similar to advanced hypertrophy from any cause. The lateral T waves are inverted and the J point may be depressed. Voltage criteria for LVH are usually present (Fig. 8.29). About 30% of patients also have prominent sharp Q waves in the lateral and inferior leads and may display left axis deviation.[10] Some patients with hypertrophic myopathy may also have preexcitation from accessory atrioventricular pathways, but the PR interval may appear short in hypertrophic myopathy even when such pathways are absent. A formal electrophysiology study is sometimes needed to distinguish *pseudopreexcitation*[11] from a true WPW pattern in this disease.

Arrhythmogenic Ventricular Dysplasia

This hereditary disease involves dilated myopathy (usually right ventricular, but can involve the septum and left ventricle as well) and recurrent ventricular tachycardia. The classic ECG findings[12] include variable degrees of right ventricular conduction delay, a pattern of inverted precordial T waves extending from V4R out to V4 or beyond, accompanied by ventricular ectopy. In advanced cases, a

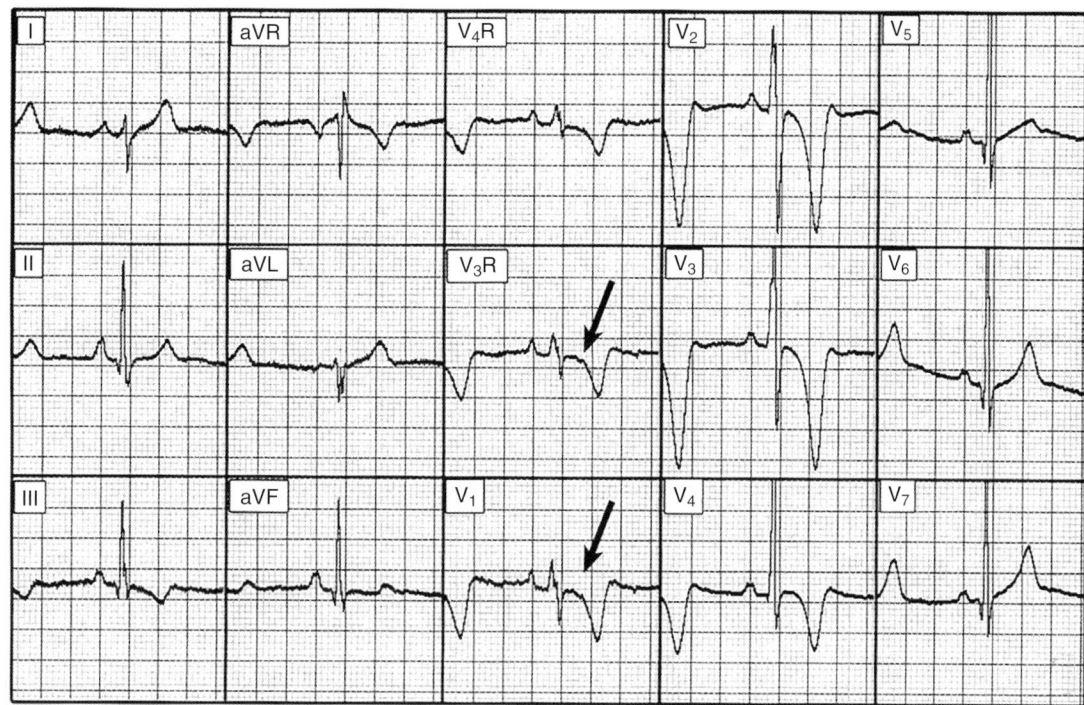

• **Fig. 8.30** Electrocardiogram from a teenage patient with familial arrhythmogenic right ventricular (RV) dysplasia who had documented ventricular tachycardia, as well as a dilated RV on echocardiogram. Note the deeply negative precordial T waves, and the subtle epsilon wave in the right chest leads (arrow).

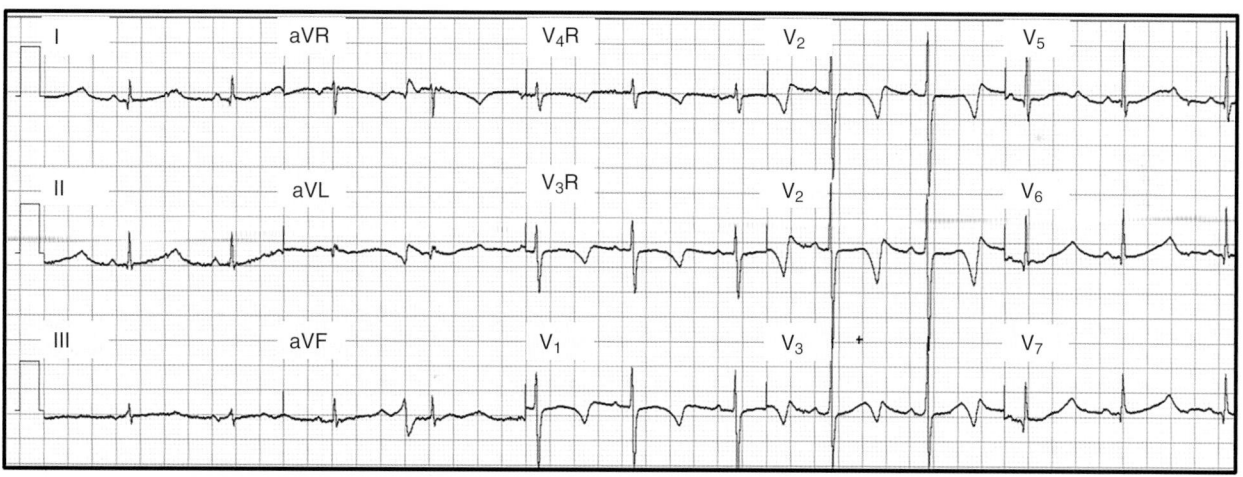

• **Fig. 8.31** Marked QT prolongation in a patient with congenital deafness and compound heterozygous mutations for long QT syndrome. This patient required aggressive therapy with medications, sympathectomy, and implantable defibrillator.

so-called *epsilon wave* can sometimes be detected in the right precordial leads as a small high-frequency spike during the early portion of ST segment (Fig. 8.30).

Long QT Syndrome

A prolonged QTc may indicate a membrane channelopathy associated with one of the heredity long QT syndromes (see Chapter 20). Because of the serious prognosis attached to this disorder,[13] it is imperative that the QT interval be scrutinized carefully on all ECG recordings. Leads II, V5, and V6 are usually the most reliable for this purpose (Fig. 8.31). In addition to prolonged duration, long QT syndrome can also produce abnormal contours for repolarization signals, such as *notched T waves* and gross alterations in T wave direction known as *T wave alternans* (Fig. 8.32).

Short QT Syndrome

Short QT syndrome is a very rare hereditary channelopathy associated with ventricular arrhythmias and a strikingly short QTc value of < 0.34 sec (Fig. 8.33), usually with tall peaked T waves.[14]

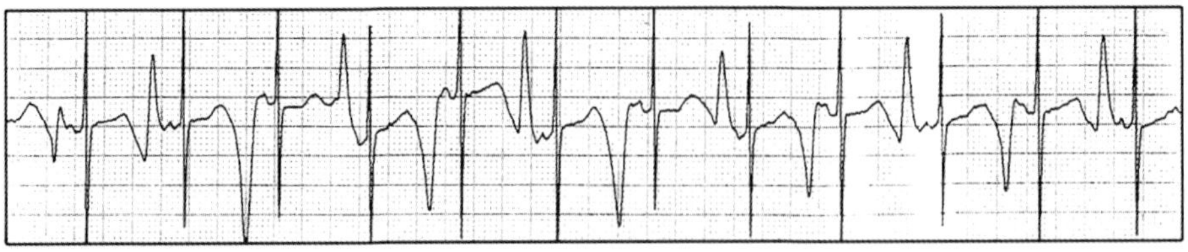

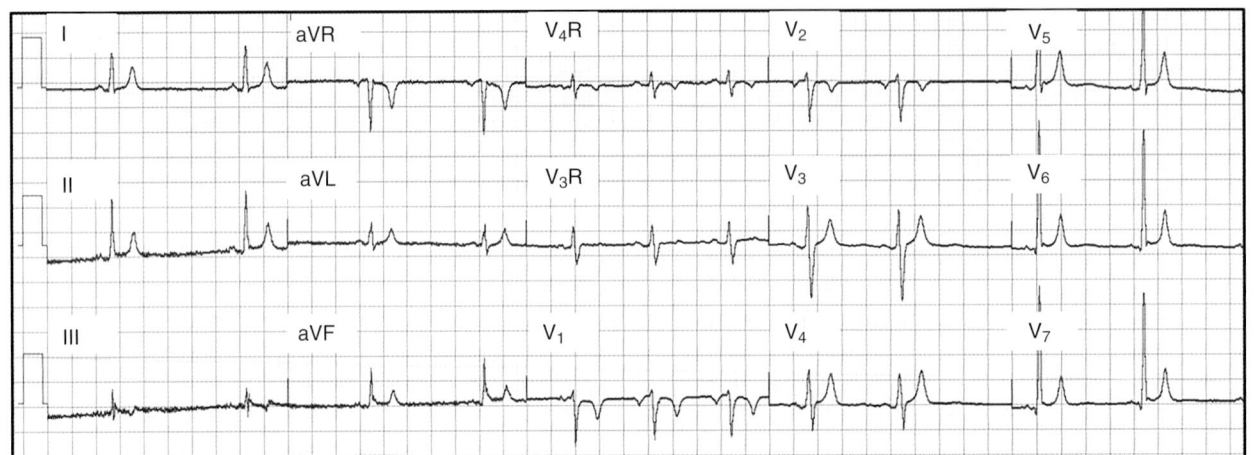

• **Fig. 8.32** Dramatic T-wave alternans in a patient with a severe form of long QT syndrome.

• **Fig. 8.33** Electrocardiogram from a patient with familial short QT syndrome. The QTc in this case is as short as 300 msec. Note tall peaked T waves.

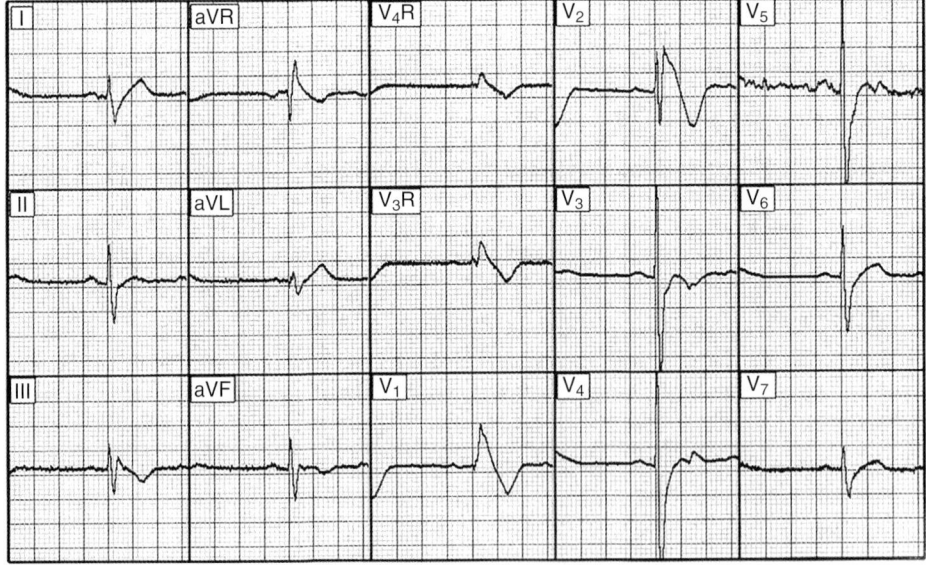

• **Fig. 8.34** Electrocardiogram from a young boy with recurrent ventricular tachycardia due to Brugada syndrome. Note unusual appearance of the ST segment and T waves in the right precordium.

Brugada Syndrome

Brugada syndrome is associated with right ventricular conduction delay, noticeable ST elevation in leads V1 through V3 (Fig. 8.34), and ventricular arrhythmias.[15] The QTc tends to be normal. These findings can wax and wane in a given patient, so the ECG appears rather normal at times, but the abnormalities can become especially pronounced whenever the patient is febrile.

Ischemia and Infarction

Myocardial ischemia is a rare problem in pediatric practice, but it may occur with certain congenital anomalies or acquired injury to the coronary vasculature.[16] Hypoxic insults result in an evolution of electrocardiographic findings which tend to parallel cellular events. During the initial *ischemic phase,* T waves can become peaked in leads that record near the affected myocardial segment, and if the

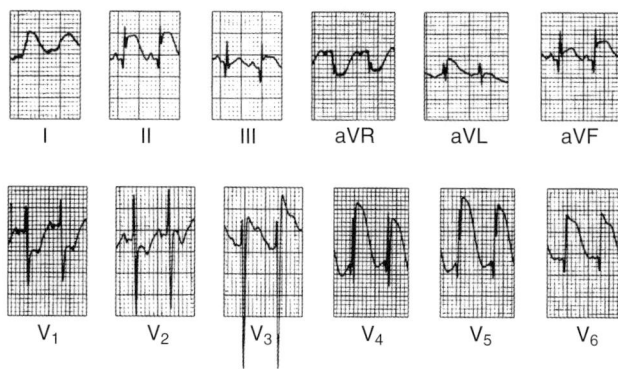

• **Fig. 8.35** Electrocardiogram showing acute ischemia with lateral (V4–V6) and inferior (aVF) elevation of the ST segment.

insult is transmural, this is accompanied by elevation of the ST segment. If the insult is restricted to subendocardial muscle, ST depression is more commonly seen. If the pathologic process is promptly reversed, these changes can resolve. However, if the insult persists, the *injury phase* commences, reflected on the ECG as a more dramatic shift in the ST segment into a so-called *tombstone* pattern (Fig. 8.35). During the injury phase, correction of the underlying cause may still permit myocardial salvage, but when the injury persists, cell death *(infarction)* follows, reflected on the ECG as a diminution of R wave voltage and the appearance of broad pathologic Q waves in those leads facing the infarcted segment.

Electrolyte Abnormalities

Significant changes may occur on the surface ECG with electrolyte disturbances, most notably potassium, calcium, and magnesium imbalance. With *hyperkalemia*, the electrocardiographic findings are quite specific for anything more than mild abnormalities. Moderate elevation of serum potassium concentration (>5.5 mEq/L) causes tall, peaked T waves, along with some widening of the QRS complex. Marked elevation (>7.0 mEq/L) causes profound widening of the P wave and QRS complex, resulting in a pattern for sinus rhythm resembling a sine wave that mimics ventricular tachycardia (Fig. 8.36). Fibrillation and asystole can result from severe elevations of serum potassium. *Hypokalemia* (<3.0 mEq/L) results in a low-amplitude,

flattened T wave, with the appearance of prominent U waves, and likewise puts patients at risk for ventricular arrhythmias. *Calcium* and *magnesium* predominantly influence the speed of cellular repolarization. Low levels of either ion prolong the QT interval, whereas high serum levels may shorten the QT slightly.

The Top-10 "Don't Miss" Electrocardiographic Patterns

Certain high-risk cardiac conditions have specific ECG findings in sinus rhythm that are critical for pediatric cardiologists to recognize. These disorders are discussed individually elsewhere throughout this text, but are listed in Table 8.2 to stress the importance of prompt (and potentially life-saving) recognition.

Ambulatory ECG Monitoring

A standard ECG captures only 10 seconds of data, but some clinical questions need to be addressed by longer-term recording with the patient engaged in their daily activities. The most common indication for ambulatory ECG monitoring

TABLE 8.2	Top-10 "Don't Miss" ECG Patterns for Pediatric Patients
Long QT syndrome	QTc > 450 msec (male) or > 460 msec (female) without identifiable cause
Short QT syndrome	QTc < 340 msec (either sex)
WPW syndrome	Short PR and "delta wave"
Brugada syndrome	J point elevation > 2 mm V1 and V2 with "coved type" ST segment and terminal negative T wave
Superior QRS axis (−30 to −90 degrees)	Consider AV canal defect or tricuspid atresia
Arrhythmogenic cardiomyopathy	T wave inversion V1–V5, RVCD, possible "epsilon wave"
Hypertrophic cardiomyopathy	Variable, but usually tall R-waves with deep sharp Q waves V5 & V6, and/or T wave inversion V5 & V6
Unexplained bundle branch block	Consider intrinsic conduction system disease (e.g., Kearns-Sayre syndrome)
Anomalous left coronary from PA	Deep sharp Q waves leads I, aVL, V5 & V6; ST ischemic changes; variable loss of R wave voltages V3–V6
Severe hyperkalemia	QRS widening and "sine wave" appearance

AV, Atrioventricular; *PA,* pulmonary artery; *RVCD,* right ventricular conduction delay; *WPW,* Wolff-Parkinson-White syndrome.

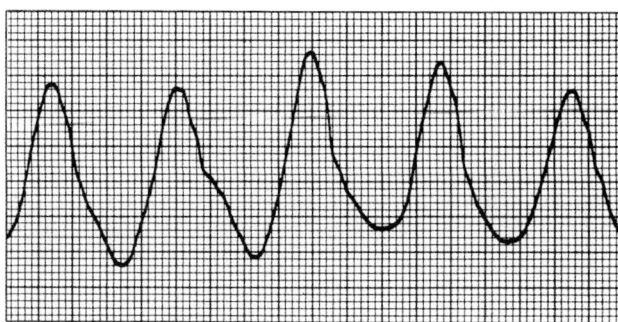

• **Fig. 8.36** Electrocardiographic pattern of marked hyperkalemia (K+ = 8.9) showing a "sine-wave" pattern.

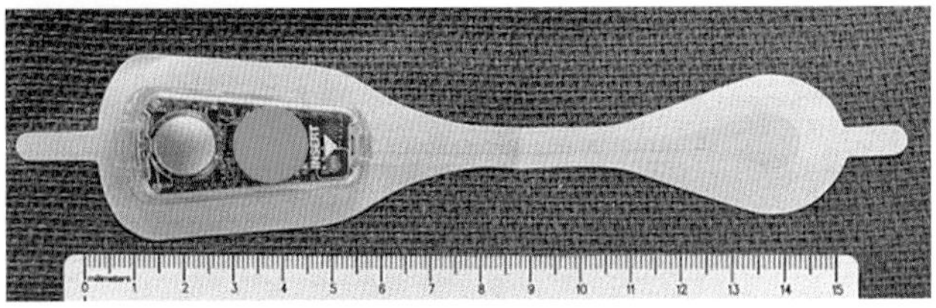

• **Fig. 8.37** Patch monitor for long-term ECG recording.

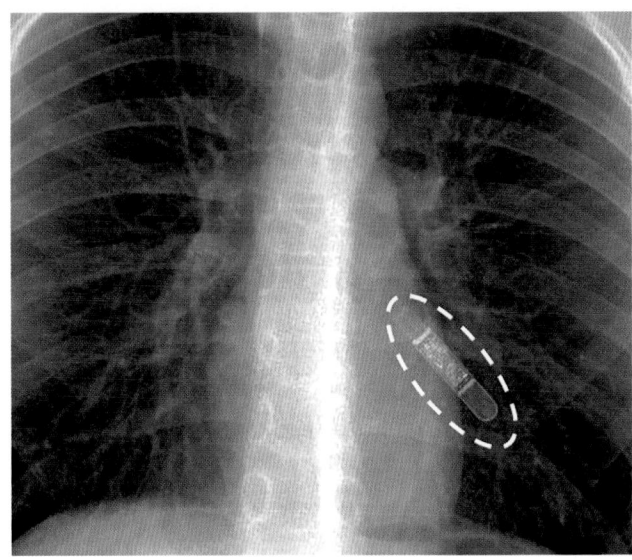

• **Fig. 8.38** Chest X-ray showing a subcutaneous implanted loop recorder *(dashed circle)*.

is the need to capture episodic events that may be caused by a cardiac arrhythmia or other notable ECG changes precisely when they occur. These include palpitations, chest pain, and unexplained syncope/near-syncope. Options for ambulatory monitors have expanded in recent years and differ in duration and in their ability to record continuously or intermittently. The most familiar choice is the traditional *Holter* monitor. This portable recording device is usually worn on a waist belt with wires running to multiple adhesive chest electrodes. The Holter monitor provides a continuous ECG recording for 24–48 hours. It is useful for routine surveillance of heart rate and rhythm, quantifying ectopy, and capturing symptoms that occur at least daily.

Patch monitors (Fig. 8.37) are a more modern variation of the Holter and provide continuous ECG recording for up to 2 weeks. A wireless patch adheres to the chest and records continuously, and contains a patient-triggered event button that can be used to flag portions of the recording that correlate with the occurrence of symptoms. Patch monitors offer increased comfort and convenience compared with wired monitors, as well as longer data collection and improved signal quality.

For infrequent symptoms unlikely to be captured by a Holter or patch monitor, an external event monitor may be used. This is a patient-activated monitor that may either be worn continuously until symptoms are captured (*loop monitor*) or carried and applied to the chest when symptoms occur (*event monitor*). A loop monitor records an ECG continuously but does not store data unless the symptom button is pressed. When this happens, the monitor records an ECG tracing just prior to, during, and for a brief period after the event. Some event monitors may be programmed to record without patient activation when preset heart rate parameters are met. Symptom monitors provide a brief ECG recording for a few seconds after the monitor is applied. Data from both types of monitor are transmitted wirelessly to be analyzed by a technician and forwarded to the provider. External event monitors are generally prescribed for 30 days.

While external event monitors have the advantages of being portable and noninvasive, they are of limited use in the documentation of very infrequent or debilitating symptoms. For these indications, an *implantable loop recorder* (ILR) may be required. An ILR is a small, leadless device implanted subcutaneously using local anesthesia (Fig. 8.38). This allows for ongoing data collection over a period of 3 or more years. Data collection is initiated either by the patient using a small activator, or when preset heart rate parameters

are met. Data may be obtained by interrogation with a programmer or transmitted wirelessly. ILRs are also useful for long-term monitoring of asymptomatic patients at known risk of arrhythmia in the setting of congenital heart disease or inherited arrhythmia substrates.

Recently developed smartphone-based apps also show promise in providing simple, easy-to-use, widely accessible ambulatory ECG monitoring.

References

1. Bartos DC, Grandi E, Ripplinger CM. Ion channels in the heart. *Compr Physiol.* 2015;5:1423-1464.
2. Bernstein SA, Morley GE. Gap junctions and propagation of the cardiac action potential. *Adv Cardiol.* 2006;42:71-85.
3. Davignon A, Rautaharju PM, Boisselle E, et al. Normal ECG standards for infants and children. *Pediatr Cardiol.* 1979;1: 123-131.
4. Saarel EV, Granger S, Kaltman JR, et al. Electrocardiograms in healthy North American children in the digital age. *Circ Arrhythm Electrophysiol.* 2018;11:e005808.
5. Miller MD, Porter C, Ackerman MJ. Diagnostic accuracy of screening electrocardiograms in long QT syndrome. *Pediatrics.* 2001;108:8-12.
6. Meziab O, Abrams DJ, Alexander ME, et al. Utility of incomplete right bundle branch block as an isolated ECG finding in children undergoing initial cardiac evaluation. *Congenit Heart Dis.* 2018; 13:419-427.
7. Tague L, Wiggs J, Li Q, et al. Comparison of left ventricular hypertrophy by electrocardiography and echocardiography in children using analytics tool. *Pediatr Cardiol.* 2018;39:1378-1388.
8. Arruda MS, McClelland JH, Wang X, et al. Development and validation of an ECG algorithm for identifying accessory pathway ablation site in Wolff-Parkinson-White syndrome. *J Cardiovasc Electrophysiol.* 1998;9:2-12.
9. Ariyarajah V, Spodick DH. Pericarditis: diagnostic cues and common electrocardiographic manifestations. *Cardiol Rev.* 2007;15: 24-30.

10. Finocchiaro G, Sheikh N, Biagini E, et al. The electrocardiogram in the diagnosis and management of patients with hypertrophic cardiomyopathy. *Heart Rhythm.* 2020;17:142-151.

11. Carlson AM, Turek JW, Law IH, Von Bergen NH. Pseudo-preexcitation is prevalent among patients with repaired complex congenital heart disease. *Pediatr Cardiol.* 2015;36:8-13.

12. Ozeke O, Cay S, Ozcan F, Karakurt M, Topaloglu S, Aras D. The fragmented QRS and epsilon wave in arrhythmogenic right ventricular dysplasia: does before-and-after the end of the QRS complex matter? *Pacing Clin Electrophysiol.* 2018;41:1269-1270.

13. Krahn AD, Laksman Z, Sy RW, et al. Congenital long QT syndrome. *JACC Clin Electrophysiol.* 2022;8:687-706.

14. Campuzano O, Sarquella-Brugada G, Cesar S, Arbelo E, Brugada J, Brugada R. Recent advances in short QT syndrome. *Front Cardiovasc Med.* 2018;5:149-154.

15. Marsman EMJ, Postema PG, Remme CA. Brugada syndrome: update and future perspectives. *Heart.* 2022;108:668-675.

16. Hoffman JI. Electrocardiogram of anomalous left coronary artery from the pulmonary artery in infants. *Pediatr Cardiol.* 2013;34:489-491.

9

Echocardiography

DAVID M. HARRILD AND ANDREW J. POWELL

KEY LEARNING POINTS

- Two-dimensional (2D) transthoracic echocardiography is the first-line tool for the diagnosis of congenital and acquired pediatric heart disease and should be performed in a systematic and rigorous fashion with the goal of producing images of the highest quality achievable.
- Doppler echocardiography can measure blood and myocardial velocity and thereby provide functional information about valve and ventricular function, and pressure differences in the heart and blood vessels.

- Three-dimensional echocardiography may be used to supplement 2D images particularly to elucidate valvar anatomy and dysfunction, and to qualify ventricular volumes.
- Transesophageal echocardiography provides a detailed pre- and postsurgical assessment in the operating room as well as procedural guidance in the cardiac catheterization laboratory.
- Fetal echocardiography enables the prenatal diagnosis of many forms of heart disease and can guide counseling and impact postnatal treatment plans.

Diagnostic imaging of the cardiovascular system has evolved dramatically over the past several decades. Until the advent of echocardiography in the 1970s, cardiac catheterization and angiography were the principal methods used to image the heart and thoracic vessels. During the second half of the 1970s, M-mode echocardiography—the first generation of cardiac ultrasound—provided limited anatomic information insufficient to replace angiography in most patients with congenital heart disease. During the 1980s, however, the rapid evolution of two-dimensional (2D) echocardiography transformed the field. Advances in transducer design and image processing along with the development of novel imaging planes led to accurate and complete diagnosis of complex congenital defects.[1-3] The introduction of Doppler ultrasound to investigate blood flow added the ability to perform more complete hemodynamic assessment. By the mid- to late 1980s, much of the necessary anatomic and hemodynamic information required for patient management could be obtained noninvasively, reducing the need for diagnostic catheterization in many patients. At present, an echocardiographic examination provides extensive anatomic and hemodynamic information noninvasively in real time and at relatively low cost. Current echocardiography systems can easily be deployed in the intensive care unit, operating room, or catheterization laboratory; newer handheld systems provide easy portability with good image quality.

This chapter reviews the general principles and applications of echocardiography in patients with pediatric and congenital heart disease. The role and findings of echocardiography for a specific condition are addressed in the chapters dedicated to each condition.

Technical Background

The imaging surface of an ultrasound transducer comprises multiple electronic elements containing piezoelectric crystals. When excited by an electrical impulse sent from a pulse generator, the molecules within the crystal vibrate, producing an ultrasound wave that travels through soft tissue at approximately 1540 m/s. When the ultrasound wave encounters an interface between tissues with different acoustic properties (e.g., blood and myocardium), a portion of the ultrasound energy is reflected back to the transducer, and the remainder continues onward until it encounters the next tissue interface. Returning ultrasound energy absorbed by the piezoelectric crystals is converted into electrical energy, which then goes through a series of electronic processes including amplification, filtering, postprocessing, and display. The distance of a reflecting surface from the transducer is calculated on the basis of the time it takes the sound wave to reach the structure and return to the transducer. This information then determines the location of the pixels representing that structure on a display screen.

The quality of echocardiographic images depends on multiple factors, some of which are controlled by the operator. For example, the frequency range of the selected transducer will impact tissue penetration (i.e., the brightness of

110

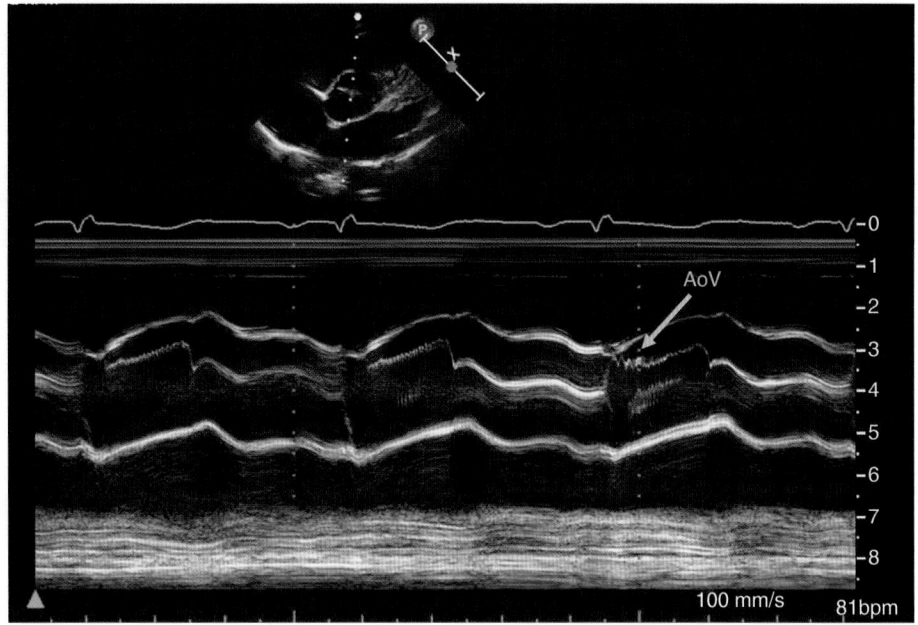

• **Fig. 9.1** M-mode view showing aortic valve fluttering motion in the setting of subvalvar aortic stenosis. *AoV,* Aortic valve leaflet.

more distant structures) and spatial resolution (i.e., the ability to distinguish two closely spaced structures). Temporal resolution (i.e., the time difference between two subsequent imaging frames) can be optimized by adjusting the sector width and depth, as well as the line density.

M-Mode Echocardiography

M-mode echocardiography demonstrates tissue interfaces at varying distances along a single narrow line or beam on the *y*-axis, with time on the *x*-axis (Fig. 9.1). This spatially one-dimensional image is characterized by excellent temporal resolution but provides limited anatomic information. Having been nearly completely replaced by 2D echocardiography imaging, M-mode is no longer practical for anatomic imaging of the heart, but is still used occasionally for evaluation of left ventricular (LV) dimensions and function. When superior temporal resolution is required, M-mode may also be useful for assessing motion of structures such as native and prosthetic valve leaflets.

Two-Dimensional Echocardiography

In current clinical practice, 2D echocardiography is the workhorse and primary tool for anatomic imaging. The ultrasound beam is swept rapidly and successively in an arc, creating multiple linear M-mode images, which are then aligned sequentially to create a cross-sectional image of the heart (Fig. 9.2). Individual lines within the 2D image are constructed at a rate termed the "pulse repetition frequency."[4] The speed of ultrasound in tissue and the depth of the image, in turn, govern the pulse repetition rate. Compared with adults, the shorter distance between the

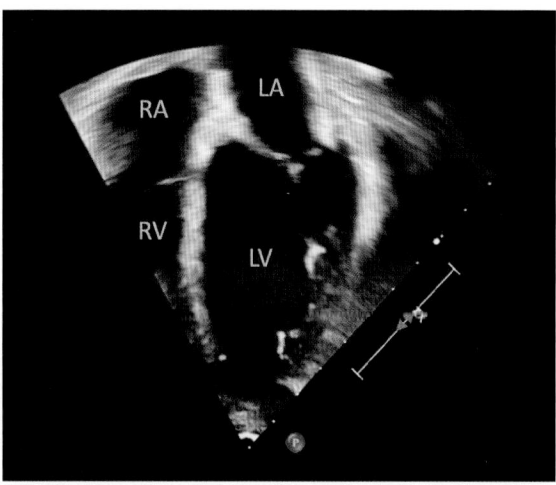

• **Fig. 9.2** Two-dimensional echocardiogram in the apical four-chamber view. *LA,* Left atrium; *LV,* left ventricle; *RA,* right atrium; *RV,* right ventricle.

transducer and the heart in infants and children allows higher pulse repetition frequency and may often result in higher image quality. Pulse repetition frequency influences frame rate, which is an important determinant of temporal resolution and is a vital contributor to good image quality in pediatric patients given their relatively rapid heart rates.

Three-Dimensional Echocardiography

An experienced examiner or observer can mentally construct a three-dimensional (3D) image of the heart from serial 2D echocardiographic images obtained by sweeping the transducer through anatomic structures. 3D echocardiography provides a more direct means of displaying information about cardiovascular structures and may give a clearer picture of the anatomical relationships. Early 3D echocardiography was based on computer reconstruction of contiguous 2D cross-sectional images, and was hampered by difficulties in accurately registering the ultrasound image data in time and space and by long image processing time. Development of 3D ultrasound transducers, gating techniques, improved computer technology and software, and refinement of the user interface have resulted in shorter acquisition and reconstruction times, and improved image quality.[5] 3D echocardiography sends and receives a pyramidal set of ultrasound data from several thousand piezoelectric transducer elements, and produces a 3D image using parallel image processing techniques (Fig. 9.3; Video 9.1). Its spatial and temporal resolution are inferior to 2D imaging, but this gap will likely narrow with continued technological developments, with expanding use in the areas of quantification of ventricular volumes and assessment of valvular anatomy and mechanism of dysfunction.

Doppler Echocardiography

Doppler ultrasound assessment of normal and abnormal hemodynamics is a fundamental part of the echocardiographic examination.[6] The 2D-guided Doppler interrogation has greatly enhanced the clinical utility of this technology, allowing comprehensive evaluation of flow characteristics within the heart and adjacent vessels. Spectral and color Doppler flow mapping are routinely used to measure velocity and direction of blood flow in healthy and diseased hearts (Fig. 9.4). Doppler-derived calculations provide quantitative

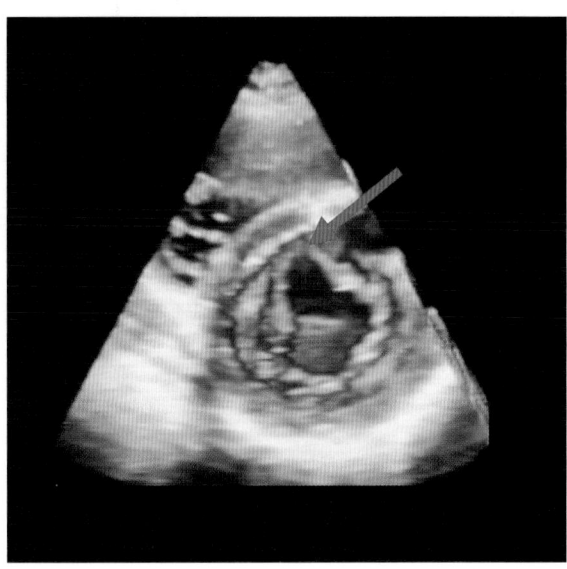

• **Fig. 9.3** Three-dimensional echocardiogram. Diastolic frame showing a cleft *(red arrow)* anterior mitral leaflet in a patient with primum atrial septal defect.

estimations of blood flow (such as stroke volume and cardiac output), pressure gradients, and cross-sectional area. Doppler echocardiography also allows qualitative and semiquantitative assessment of valve regurgitation, intra- and extracardiac shunts, and myocardial motion.

Doppler imaging is based on the physical principle that when a propagated sound wave encounters a moving target, the frequency of the reflected sound wave changes in a predictable fashion, shifting in proportion to the velocity of the target relative to the transducer. The frequency shift, known

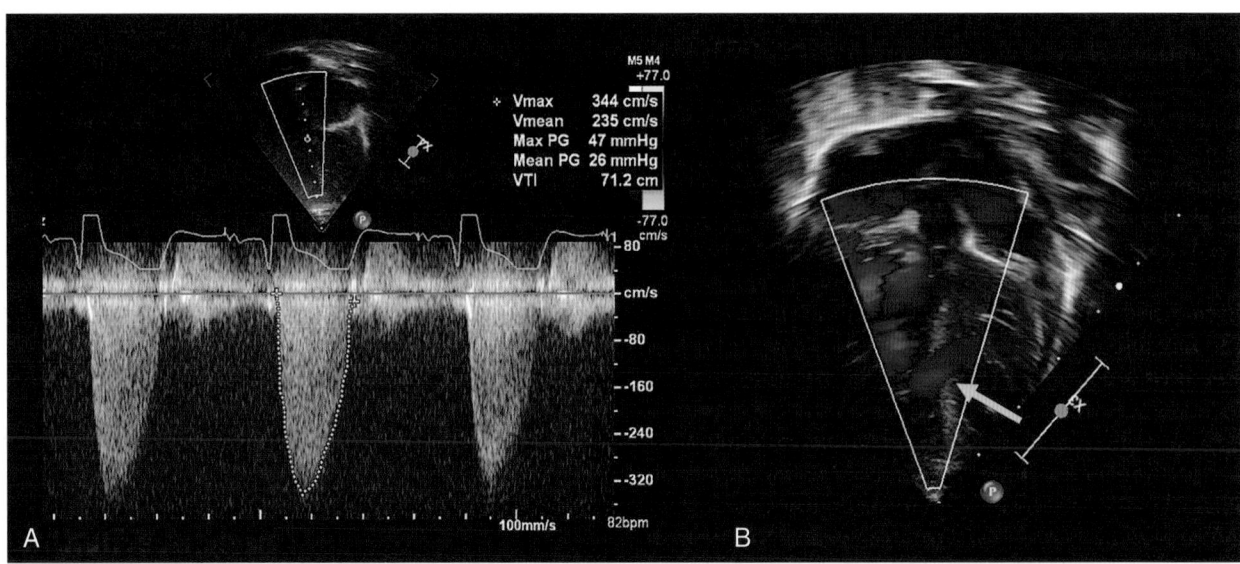

• **Fig. 9.4** Doppler echocardiography. (A) Interrogation of the left ventricular outflow tract from the apical window with continuous wave Doppler in a patient with subvalvar aortic stenosis. The peak velocity is ~3.4 m/seconds and the predicted maximum instantaneous gradient is ~47 mm Hg. Tracing the spectral Doppler signal yields a mean gradient of 26 mm Hg. (B) Color Doppler flow mapping from the apical window showing a moderate mid-muscular ventricular septal defect (location indicated by the *yellow arrow*).

as Doppler shift (Δf), is related to the transmitted frequency (Fo), the average velocity of sound (C) in tissue at 37°C (1540 m/seconds), the velocity (V) and the direction of the target relative to the ultrasound beam (ϕ), according to the formula

$$\Delta f = \frac{2Fo \cdot V \cdot \cos\phi}{C}$$

This equation can be rearranged to solve for the velocity of the moving target:

$$V = \frac{C \cdot \Delta f}{2Fo \cdot \cos\phi}$$

The cosine function in the Doppler equation predicts that when the ultrasound beam is parallel to the direction of the moving target (angle of incidence = 0), the Doppler frequency shift is maximal (cosine 0 degrees = 1), whereas when the target is moving perpendicular to the ultrasound beam (cosine 90 degrees = 0), no frequency shift will be detected regardless of the target's velocity. It is important to recognize that the angle of incidence has three dimensions, whereas image display is typically 2D and the third dimension is therefore not assessed. In 2D echocardiographic examination, the angle of incidence can be estimated but not confirmed, and the direction of flow may be unpredictable, particularly in high-velocity lesions such as aortic stenosis. As long as the angle of incidence relative to the actual direction of flow does not exceed 20 degrees, the true velocity will be underestimated by 6% or less (cosine 20 degrees = 0.94). When the angle of incidence exceeds 20 degrees, the degree of underestimation of velocity rapidly increases. Therefore, when performing a Doppler examination, every effort is made to align the ultrasound beam with the direction of motion so that the highest available spectral signals and corresponding velocities are recorded and the accompanying audio signals reach the highest pitch. Color Doppler imaging can show the direction of the target jet and may be used to help minimize the angle of incidence.

Continuous-Wave Doppler

This method uses two separate transducer elements, allowing continuous, simultaneous transmission and detection of the Doppler signal. As a result, all reflectors along the path of the ultrasound beam contribute to the recorded signal, and it is impossible to discern the location of the highest flow velocity, a phenomenon termed "range ambiguity." The advantage of this method is that any peak velocity within the physiologic range can be measured. Continuous-wave Doppler is most useful in assessing high-velocity flow jets and gradients at easily identifiable locations, such as semilunar valve stenosis and restrictive ventricular septal defects.

Pulsed-Wave Doppler

In this method, a brief burst of ultrasound energy is emitted by the transducer followed by a pause during which the transducer "listens" for the returning waves. By superimposing the range-gated Doppler beam on the 2D image, the operator can specify the region to be interrogated, limiting the timing and duration of reception to allow only the returning signals from a particular location to be processed. According to the sampling theorem, the maximum measurable frequency shift in one direction is half the sampling rate (or pulse repetition rate). In other words, the maximum velocity or Doppler shift that can be unambiguously recorded is limited by a finite sampling rate, and decreases with increasing distance from the transducer. The further the interrogated region is from the transducer, the longer it takes for the ultrasound wave to reach it and return. To avoid range ambiguity, the transducer must wait for the returning signal before emitting a new one. When the sampling rate is less than twice the frequency shift, aliasing results. The highest frequency shift (i.e., velocity) that can be unambiguously displayed is termed the "Nyquist limit." The lower the transducer frequency, the higher the Nyquist limit. From a practical perspective, this means that lower-frequency transducers should be used to resolve higher velocities and gradients by pulsed-wave Doppler.

High-Pulse Repetition Frequency (HPRF) Doppler

This method is an intermediate between continuous and pulsed-wave Doppler. Instead of waiting for the returning pulse before emitting the next one, the system sends a subsequent pulse during the "listening period" for the original one. By doing so, pulse repetition frequency is increased and the Nyquist limit is extended. The price is paid in range ambiguity; the examiner cannot be certain at which of several locations along the beam path the maximal recorded velocity was actually detected.

Color Doppler

In color Doppler imaging, the returning ultrasound signals from multiple locations along the scan line are assessed for frequency shift. For each gate assessed, the frequency shifts are averaged, and the mean velocity and direction of flow are color-coded and assigned to pixels within the display (Fig. 9.4B). By convention, flow toward the transducer is coded as red, and flow away from the transducer is coded as blue. The intensity of the color display is proportional to the averaged frequency shift and velocity. A second color, typically green or yellow, is assigned to pixels depending on the statistical variance of the frequency shifts within each gate. A color-coded Doppler image is constructed by combining adjacent lines of processed Doppler information, and superimposed on the gray-scale 2D image. Color Doppler imaging is particularly useful in pediatric echocardiography because it greatly enhances the ability to identify and investigate the sources of abnormal flow such as septal defects, stenotic and regurgitant valves, coronary artery fistulae, and patent ductus arteriosus.

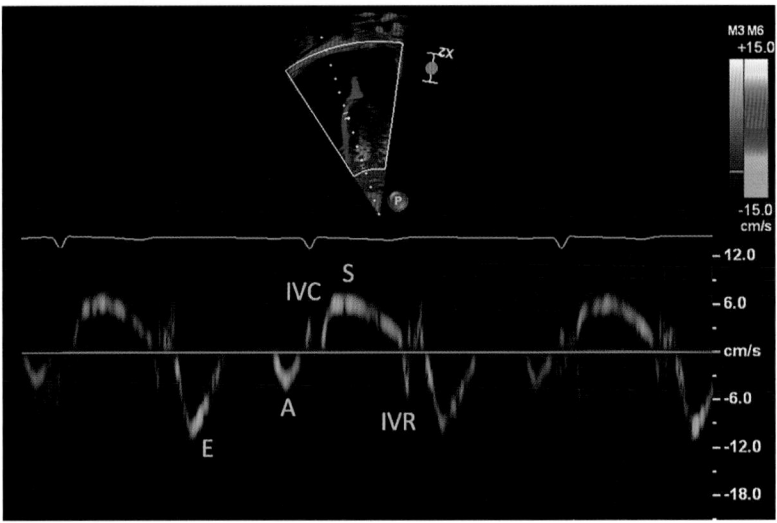

• **Fig. 9.5** Tissue Doppler interrogation of the basal septum from the apical window. *A,* Atrial (late) diastolic phase; *E,* early diastolic phase; *IVC,* isovolumic contraction; *IVR,* isovolumic relaxation; *S,* systolic phase.

Tissue Doppler

Tissue Doppler imaging is a technique used to assess myocardial velocity, strain, and function.[7] The technique is based on the differences in velocity and amplitude between the motion of blood and the myocardium. Whereas the velocity of moving blood is relatively high and the amplitude of the Doppler signal is low, the velocity of the contracting and relaxing myocardium is low and the amplitude of the Doppler signal is high. By filtering out the higher velocity, low-amplitude signals from the blood, myocardial velocities are readily measured. Tissue Doppler imaging is commonly used to assess longitudinal (base-to-apex) and radial (short-axis) myocardial velocities as well as time intervals such as isovolumic contraction and relaxation times, ejection time, and others (Fig. 9.5).

Contrast Echocardiography

As early as the late 1960s, Gramiak et al.[8] noted that intravascular injections of solution resulted in a contrast effect detectable by ultrasound. Initially, this technique was used to identify structures on M-mode images. More recently, contrast echocardiography has been used to detect systemic[9] and pulmonary venous[6] anomalies as well as shunt lesions. Agitating saline solution creates microbubbles and these microbubbles are highly reflective on ultrasound because they contain air. A bolus of agitated saline injected in a peripheral vein creates contrast that opacifies the right heart, but is essentially filtered (blocked) in a single pass through the capillaries of the pulmonary vascular bed. The appearance of contrast in the left heart identifies an intracardiac or intrapulmonary right-to-left shunt. In pediatric echocardiography, contrast studies are primarily used to investigate suspected intracardiac shunts not detectable by color Doppler, baffle leaks after cardiac surgery, and

TABLE 9.1	Common Indications for Echocardiography in Pediatric Patients
Congenital heart disease (known or suspected)	
Kawasaki disease	
Multisystem inflammatory syndrome in children	
Rheumatic heart disease	
Primary or secondary cardiomyopathy	
Cardiotoxic medications (such as anthracycline chemotherapy)	
Pericardial disease or effusion	
Suspected endocarditis or vegetation	
Persistent pulmonary hypertension of the newborn	
Primary pulmonary hypertension	
Cerebrovascular infarct (embolic)	
Chest pain	
Syncope	
Rhythm and conduction abnormalities	
Genetic syndromes and multiple congenital anomalies	
Cardiac and paracardiac tumors	
Arteriovenous malformations	

pulmonary arteriovenous malformations (Video 9.2). Newer non-saline ultrasound contrast agents are designed to cross the pulmonary capillaries and therefore opacify the left heart chambers. These agents are used to improve visualization of the LV cavity in patients with poor acoustic windows and to assess myocardial perfusion.

Objectives of the Echocardiographic Examination

Table 9.1 summarizes some of the common indications for echocardiography. In addition, appropriate use criteria for pediatric echocardiography have been defined.[10] The echocardiographic examination is tailored to the individual patient on the basis of physical examination and history, prior knowledge of the patient's cardiac and vascular anatomy, results of previous testing, clinical status, and expected level of cooperation. The first echocardiogram should strive to include a comprehensive survey of all components of the central cardiovascular system. Subsequent examinations may be targeted to answer specific clinical questions. It is often prudent, however, to perform a relatively complete study at follow-up, even in patients with previous comprehensive echocardiograms, because of the dynamic nature of congenital and acquired pediatric heart disease.

Examination Technique

A comprehensive anatomic examination includes determination of visceral situs, cardiac position, atrial situs, systemic and pulmonary venous connections, ventricular situs, atrioventricular and ventriculoarterial alignments and connections, and great arterial anatomy. Color and spectral Doppler examination of the valves, great vessels, atrial and ventricular septae, and proximal coronary arteries is an important component of the basic examination, as is an assessment of ventricular function. The examiner should proceed through the study in an orderly fashion, preferably obtaining views in a predetermined customary sequence to ensure local standardization of studies and facilitate subsequent review. It is helpful to go through a mental checklist of anatomic and functional information needed, both during and at the end of the exam, to ensure that a complete study has been obtained. In patients who are asleep or sedated and may awaken before the study is completed, and in those who are critically ill or unstable, it is advisable to prioritize the critical elements of the study. Mental 3D reconstruction of cardiac anatomy is facilitated by recordings of complete sweeps through the heart and vessels, from one side or end of the heart to the other, from each view. This method also increases the likelihood that subtle findings overlooked during image acquisition will be detected upon subsequent review.

After each imaging sweep is completed and recorded, focused color and spectral Doppler interrogation of the atrial and ventricular septa, valves, and vessels should be performed. To maximize color Doppler quality and frame rate, rather than trying to examine all structures in the field of view simultaneously, each relevant structure should be examined individually using as narrow a region of interest as possible. Color Doppler should be used to align the pulsed- or continuous-wave Doppler beam with the flow jet being examined. Images of important findings, and color and spectral Doppler of normal and abnormal flow jets, should be recorded in such a fashion that an interpreting physician who did not perform the examination nonetheless has enough information to confidently report the findings.

Sedation

To perform a complete echocardiographic examination in infants and uncooperative children, sedation is often necessary.

Adequate sedation for a complete echocardiographic examination can be accomplished with a variety of medications and techniques, often in collaboration with colleagues in pediatric cardiac anesthesia. Institutional guidelines for conscious and deep sedation, including nothing-by-mouth restrictions and availability of resuscitation equipment, should be adhered to, and qualified medical personnel not involved in performing the echocardiogram should be responsible for monitoring the patient's cardiorespiratory status.

Equipment

A variety of commercially available echocardiographic systems are suitable for examination of pediatric patients. For the degree of image resolution necessary for diagnosis of congenital anomalies, it is important that high-frequency transducers be available. For 2D imaging, one should use the highest-frequency transducer capable of obtaining high-quality images of the structures being examined; a lower-frequency probe may be needed for color and spectral Doppler examination of the same structures.

Echocardiographic Views

Standard Imaging Planes and Image Display

Standard echocardiographic imaging planes include long-axis planes parallel to the major (long) axis of the LV and short-axis planes perpendicular to the major axis of the LV. These views are obtained from subxiphoid (subcostal) and parasternal windows. A four-chamber view is obtained from the cardiac apex. Additional standard imaging planes include views that align with the long axis of the aortic arch and coronal views from the suprasternal notch. In addition, specialized views to optimally display the atrial septum, branch pulmonary arteries, ductus arteriosus, and coronary arteries are components of a complete anatomic survey. Unconventional imaging planes and windows may be necessary to obtain complete anatomic information, especially in the setting of complex congenital defects and distorted intrathoracic anatomy (e.g., diaphragmatic hernia). The examiner may need to improvise to obtain the necessary information.

By convention, the transducer is oriented so that images are displayed in an *anatomically correct* orientation, as if the patient were facing the viewer; right-sided structures are displayed on the left side of the screen and vice versa. To prevent confusion during interpretation and review, it is critical to follow this rule, regardless of the position of the cardiac apex (levo- or dextrocardia). The exception to this is the parasternal long-axis view, which, by convention, is displayed so that superior structures are on the right side of the displayed image and the cardiac apex is on the left side of the image, regardless of the position of the heart.

Subxiphoid (subcostal) (Fig. 9.6A)

Sweeps from the subxiphoid window provide a wide-angle view of the entire heart and great vessels. This view

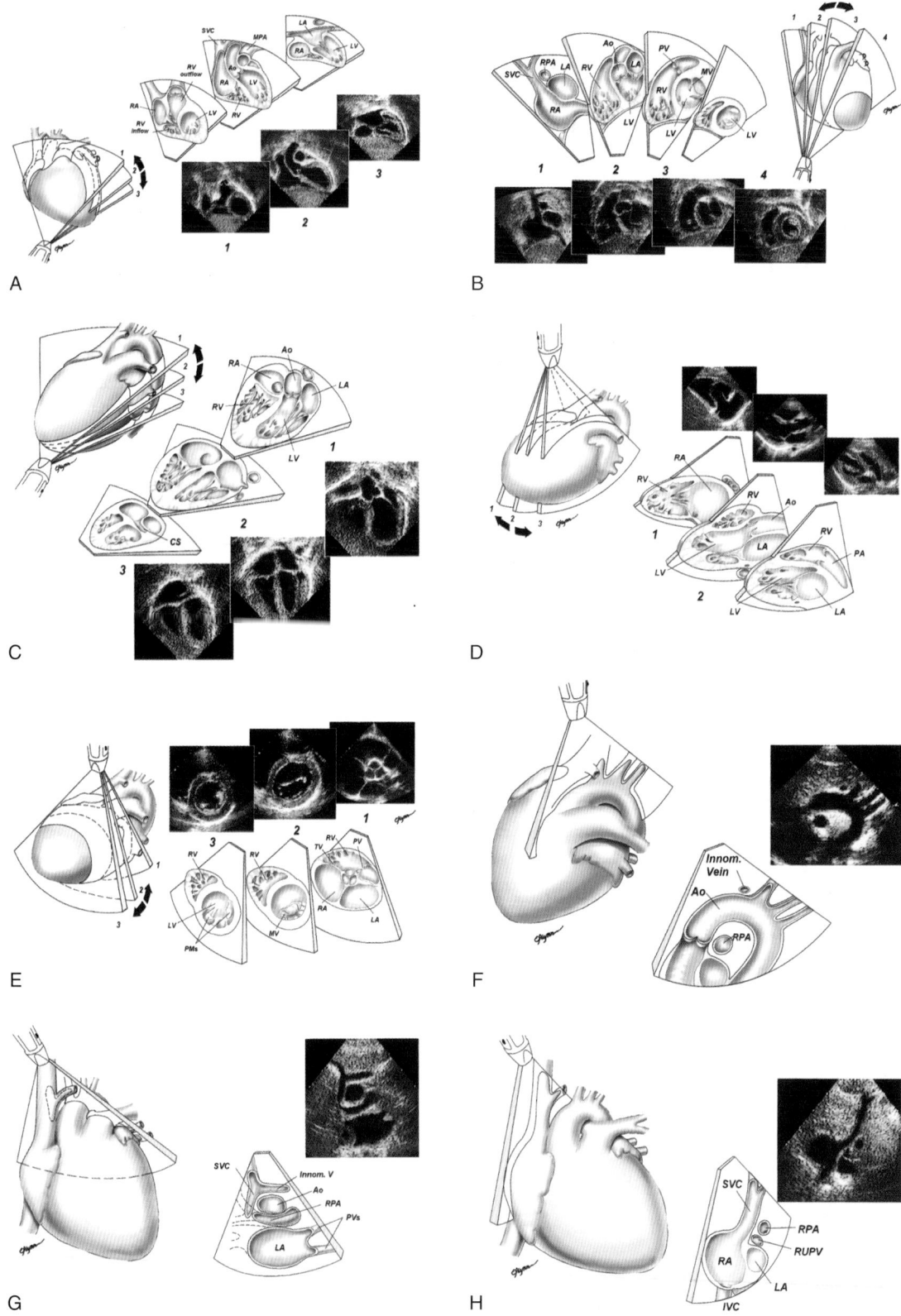

• **Fig. 9.6** Two-dimensional echocardiographic imaging planes (see text for details). (A) Subxiphoid long axis. (B) Subxiphoid short axis. (C) Apical four chamber. (D) Parasternal long axis. (E) Parasternal short-axis view. (F) Suprasternal notch view: long axis of aorta. (G) Suprasternal notch view: transverse view. (H) Right parasternal view. *Ao,* Aorta; *Innom,* innominate; *IVC,* inferior vena cava; *LA,* left atrium; *LV,* left ventricle; *MPA,* main pulmonary artery; *MV,* mitral valve; *PMs,* papillary muscles; *PV,* pulmonary valve; *PVs,* pulmonary veins; *RA,* right atrium; *RPA,* right pulmonary artery; *RUPV,* right upper pulmonary vein; *RV,* right ventricle; *SVC,* superior vena cava; *TV,* tricuspid valve. (From Geva T. Echocardiography and Doppler ultrasound. In: Garson, A, Bricker, JT, Fisher, DJ, Neish SR (eds). *The Science and Practice of Pediatric Cardiology.* Baltimore: Williams & Wilkins, 1997, pp. 789, with permission.)

is particularly useful in infants and small children because of the proximity of the transducer to the heart and lack of intervening bone or lung tissue. Beginning with subcostal sweeps is the most efficient way to assess cardiac position, and visceral and atrial situs; obtain an overview of the intracardiac and great vessel anatomy; and determine the relationships between structures.

Imaging from the subxiphoid window is performed with the patient supine, often with knees bent (to relax the abdominal muscles). Beginning with a cross-sectional view of the abdomen from just below and often slightly lateral to the xiphoid process, a cross-section of the abdominal aorta and inferior vena cava, and their relationship to each other and the spine, is displayed. The position of the stomach is usually evident due to highly reflective air within it. Angling slightly superiorly demonstrates the hemidiaphragms and their motion with respiration. The transducer plane is swept superiorly through the diaphragm, from the posterior inferior surface to the anterior surface of the heart, and ending with a coronal slice through the right ventricular (RV) outflow tract (Fig. 9.6A). Turning the transducer 90 degrees clockwise provides a subxiphoid short-axis view (Fig. 9.6B). Beginning with a plane demonstrating the superior and inferior vena cavae, the transducer plane is swept through the heart ending at the cardiac apex. In patients with high-quality images from the subxiphoid window, these two sweeps may serve to demonstrate much of the details regarding the systemic and pulmonary venous connections, atrial septum, atrioventricular valve morphology, ventricular septum, outflow tracts, proximal great arteries, and descending aorta. In patients with poor or inaccessible apical and parasternal windows, a nearly complete examination (with the exception of optimal images of the aortic arch and coronary artery origins) can be performed from the subxiphoid window.

If images are adequate in quality from this view, the atrial and ventricular septa, pulmonary veins, and outflow tracts should be examined with color Doppler. This window also provides a good angle for spectral Doppler interrogation of the outflow tracts, superior and inferior vena cavae, and abdominal aorta.

Apical (Fig. 9.6C)

Apical imaging is usually best performed with the patient lying approximately 45 degrees up on their left side (for levocardia), bringing the apex closer to the chest wall and displacing the lung. Positioning the transducer over the cardiac apex, one obtains a four-chamber view of the heart, displaying both atria, both atrioventricular valves at their maximum lateral dimensions, and both ventricles in long axis. Sweeping posteriorly, the coronary sinus and posterior ventricular septum are imaged. Sweeping anteriorly, the left and RV outflow tracts are imaged. The pulmonary veins are visible, but individual veins are usually better evaluated on other views. Rotating the transducer clockwise approximately 90 degrees displays a two-chamber view of the left ventricle.

Color Doppler interrogation of the atrioventricular valves, muscular ventricular septum, and LV outflow tract should be performed from the apical view, which also provides good angles for spectral Doppler interrogation of atrioventricular valves, LV outflow tract, aortic valve, and the right lower pulmonary vein. Moving the transducer slightly medially toward the left lower sternal border often allows imaging and Doppler evaluation of the RV outflow tract and pulmonary valve.

Parasternal Short and Long Axis (Fig. 9.6D and E)

Parasternal views are obtained just lateral to the sternum, usually in the third or fourth left intercostal space. Again, it is helpful to have the patient rolled up on his or her left side. The initial long-axis image is obtained with the transducer plane oriented from the patient's right shoulder to the left hip. With proper orientation, the left atrium, mitral valve, left ventricle, posterior LV free wall and septum, LV outflow tract, aortic valve, and ascending aorta are displayed (Fig. 9.6D). Sweeping inferiorly and rightward toward the right hip images the right atrium, tricuspid valve, and RV inflow, and sweeping superiorly and leftward displays the RV outflow tract, pulmonary valve, and main pulmonary artery. This view provides another opportunity for color Doppler interrogation of the atrioventricular valves, ventricular septum, outflow tracts, and semilunar valves.

The parasternal short-axis view is obtained from the same window, with the transducer rotated 90 degrees clockwise (Fig. 9.6E). Beginning with a cross-section of the LV at the level of the mitral valve, RV inflow and outflow tracts, sweeping apically provides images of the LV chamber and the muscular ventricular septum. Sweeping up toward the base of the heart, the aortic valve is viewed in cross-section, along with the coronary artery origins, the atrioventricular canal, the membranous and conoventricular septa, pulmonary valve and main pulmonary artery. Color Doppler and, if indicated, spectral Doppler interrogation of the ventricular septum and pulmonary veins is typically performed from this view, as is Doppler examination of the pulmonary valve.

The pulmonary artery bifurcation is usually best seen from one or two interspaces higher, with slightly more clockwise rotation. Rotating counterclockwise to a 1 o'clock view allows imaging of a ductus arteriosus in long axis. A right parasternal view is often helpful for imaging the atrial septum and superior vena cava, and provides a good angle for Doppler examination of the aortic valve and ascending aorta (Fig. 9.6H).

Suprasternal Notch (Fig. 9.6F and G)

For suprasternal notch imaging, it is usually helpful to have the patient lie flat on his or her back with a roll under the shoulders, hyperextending the neck and turning the head to the side to provide better exposure. This position may make younger children apprehensive, and repositioning sleeping infants and children may awaken them. Without repositioning the patient, it is sometimes possible to obtain satisfactory suprasternal notch views, or similar images from the top of the sternum or the right or left infraclavicular space.

Beginning with the transducer plane oriented from left to right and aimed inferiorly in a coronal plane, one sees a cross-section of the ascending aorta, the long axis of the right pulmonary artery, and a cross-section of the superior vena cava (Fig. 9.6G). In infants and many children, most or all of the pulmonary veins can also be imaged from this view, often referred to as a "crab view." Sweeping cranially through the ascending aorta and superior vena cava, one obtains a long axis of the left innominate vein and transverse aortic arch, and further cranial angulation demonstrates the brachiocephalic arteries. Color Doppler interrogation of the innominate vein (to assess for a persistent left superior vena cava) and pulmonary veins is typically performed from this view.

Counterclockwise rotation of the transducer images the entire aortic arch in long axis (Fig. 9.6F), allowing color and spectral Doppler examination of the ascending and descending aorta. To demonstrate a right aortic arch in long axis, some echocardiography laboratories recommend rotating the transducer 180 degrees to display the descending aorta on the left side of the screen.

Interpretation and Reporting

Interpretation of pediatric echocardiographic examinations requires a thorough knowledge of normal cardiac morphology and physiology, and the myriad of potential congenital and acquired anomalies. While reviewing the images, the interpreter builds a mental 3D image of the anatomy and systematically runs down a checklist to ensure that cardiac relationships and structures are clearly delineated, and any potential anomalies are either clearly demonstrated or excluded. The interested reader is referred to the earlier sections on morphologic anatomy and segmental approach to diagnosis (see Chapter 3), as well as subsequent chapters on acquired and congenital anomalies, for detailed descriptions.

Reports should be unambiguous in the description of the segmental anatomy and atrioventricular and ventriculoarterial relationships so that the reader has no doubt as to the sidedness of structures and ventricular looping. It is preferable to refer to the ventricles by their morphology rather than the side of the body on which they are located. For example, to eliminate ambiguity in a patient with L-looped ventricles (ventricular inversion), one might refer to the "right-sided morphologic left ventricle."

Quantitative Analysis

Cardiovascular structures can be measured on still-frame 2D echocardiographic images with a high degree of accuracy. Measurements of individual structures can be compared to published normal values to determine whether they fall within the expected range for the patient's

somatic size or age, and, if not, their extent of deviation from normal.

Description of Technique

Measurement of linear dimension (e.g., vessel or valve annulus diameter), cross-sectional area (e.g., valve area), or 3D volume (e.g., ventricular volume or mass) helps to determine the severity of disease and predict natural history and prognosis. Unlike in adult cardiology, because of the wide variation in size of pediatric patients and the considerable growth of cardiovascular structures between birth and adulthood, it is critical that normal ranges properly account for patient age or body size.

The growth of cardiac structures may not have a linear relationship to body surface area, height, weight, or age. In fact, most linear dimensions (such as valve and vessel diameters) are best indexed to the square root of body surface area.[11] This is expected, since the heart and great vessels grow much more rapidly during the first 2 to 4 years of life compared with later childhood and adolescence. For example, when the aortic valve annulus diameter is indexed to the square root of the body surface area, the mean annulus diameter in the normal population is 1.51 cm/$m^{0.5}$ in all children, from newborn to adult size. It follows that cross-sectional measurements are best indexed to body surface area.

Comparison of measurements between individuals is simplified by the use of Z scores.[12,13] The Z score indicates the deviation of a measurement relative to the regression line of a normal data set, and is expressed as the number of standard deviations from the expected mean. It is calculated as:

$$Z \text{ score} = \frac{\text{measured value} - \text{mean value of normal population}}{\text{standard deviation of normal population}}$$

Expression of measurements as Z scores allows comparison between patients and the normal population, regardless of the age or size of the patient.[12] Normal dimensions of cardiac structures with respect to size and age have been established (these are available online, for example, at: http://zscore.chboston.org).

Assessment of the volume of the LV chamber is an integral component of the echocardiographic evaluation of patients with suspected LV hypoplasia and those with lesions causing LV volume overload. Algorithms for calculating LV volume based on various geometric models have been developed and are reviewed in more detail elsewhere.[13] The biplane area–length method is a commonly used method. This technique uses the formula V = 5/6 × cross-sectional area of the LV in short axis × LV length in long axis (Fig. 9.7A). The biplane Simpson's rule is another frequently used technique. The left ventricle is imaged in two orthogonal views, which share a common long axis: for example, the apical four- and two-chamber views (Fig. 9.7B). LV volume is calculated using the formula:

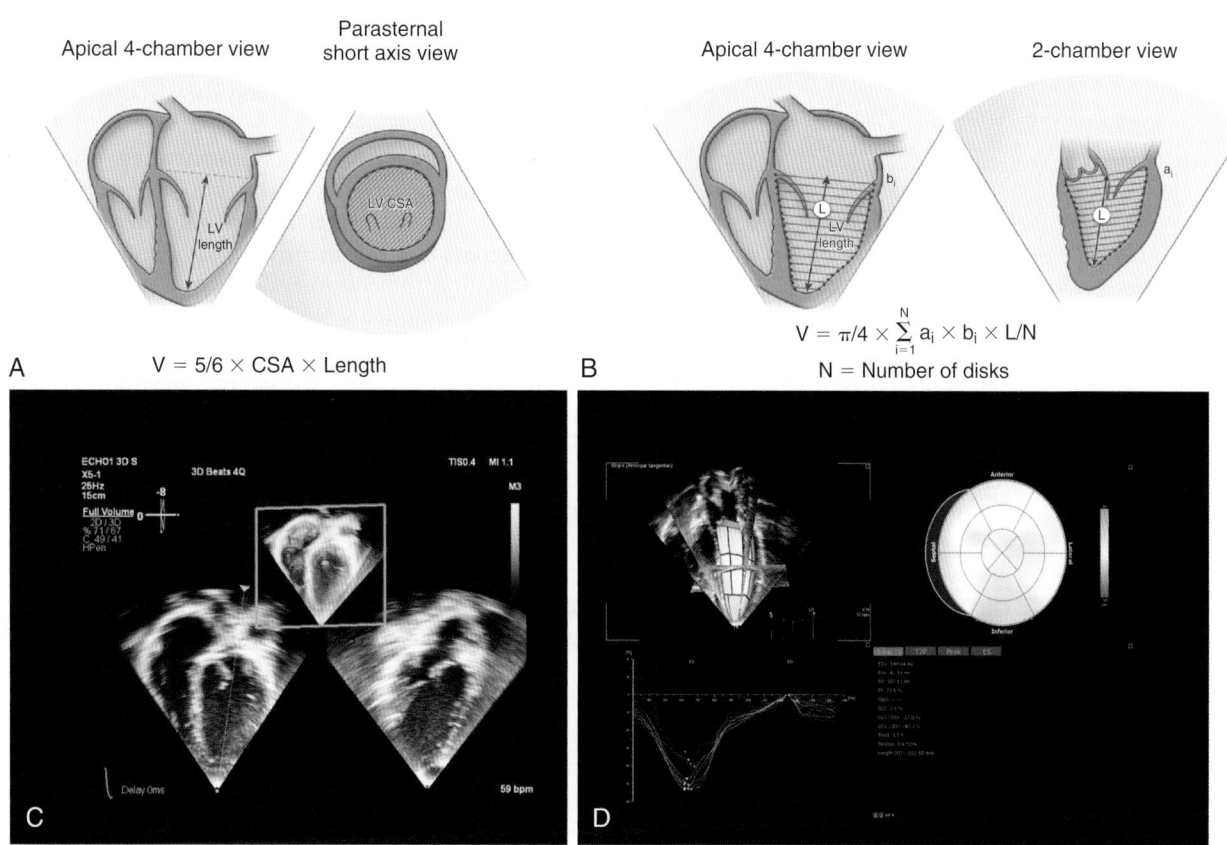

Apical 4-chamber view   Parasternal short axis view   Apical 4-chamber view   2-chamber view

$$V = \pi/4 \times \sum_{i=1}^{N} a_i \times b_i \times L/N$$
N = Number of disks

A $V = 5/6 \times CSA \times Length$ B

C   D

• **Fig. 9.7** Left ventricle volume calculation. (A) Simpson rule. (B) Area–length method. (C) 3D left ventricular volume, which may be used with analytical software (panel D) to calculate the ventricular volume directly. (Panels A and B from Geva T. Echocardiography and Doppler ultrasound. In: Garson, A, Bricker, JT, Fisher, DJ, Neish SR (eds). *The Science and Practice of Pediatric Cardiology*. Baltimore: Williams & Wilkins, 1997, pp. 789, with permission.)

$$V - \frac{\pi}{4} \times \sum_{i=1}^{N} ai \times bi \times \frac{L}{N}$$

Where a_i = slice radius in the apical two-chamber view, b_i = slice radius in the apical four-chamber view, L = LV length, N = number of slices, and V = volume. Measurement of LV and RV volumes using 3D echocardiography, based upon the method of summation of disks, indicates that it has the potential to be more accurate than 2D echocardiographic techniques (Fig. 9.7C and D; Video 9.3).[14] LV myocardial volume can be measured using 2D or 3D echocardiography by calculating the total volume of the LV including the myocardium and subtracting the LV chamber volume. LV mass is then calculated by multiplying the myocardial volume by the density of muscle (1.055 g/mL).

Ventricular Function

Commonly used indices of ventricular function include shortening fraction, fractional area change, ejection fraction, velocity of circumferential fiber shortening, peak dp/dt, and ventricular strain. All of these are measures reflective of global pump function. These indices are, however, unable to distinguish between the effects of altered loading conditions

and intrinsic abnormalities in myocardial contractility. Acutely decreasing preload or increasing afterload will depress the ejection fraction or strain which may be erroneously interpreted as being due to an intrinsic abnormality of myocardial contractility. Conversely, the ejection fraction or strain may be normal even in the setting of abnormal myocardial contractility if the loading conditions are abnormal. The advantage of most of these indices is their relative simplicity and ease of acquisition. Load-independent assessment of LV systolic function requires a more sophisticated analysis. The interested reader is referred to *Chapter 11: Assessment of Ventricular and Myocardial Performance.*

Doppler Evaluation of Pressure Gradients

Because congenital heart defects frequently result in elevated pressure in one or more cardiac chambers or vessels, it is valuable to have a noninvasive means of estimating pressure. Doppler measurement of blood velocity allows estimation of pressure across valves and between chambers. The Bernoulli equation, originally described by Daniel Bernoulli in the 1700s, allows prediction of the pressure difference (ΔP) between two points separated by a distance (s). It does so by using the velocity at the two points (V_1 and V_2), the fluid density (blood $\rho = 1060$ kg/m³), and the velocity-dependent viscous friction according to:

$$\Delta P = \overbrace{\frac{1}{2}\rho(V_2^2 - V_1^2)}^{\text{convective acceleration}} + \overbrace{\rho\int_1^2 \frac{d\vec{V}}{dt}\,d\vec{s}}^{\text{flow acceleration}} + \overbrace{R(\vec{V})}^{\text{viscous friction}}$$

For most clinical applications of the Bernoulli equation, the convective acceleration component of the formula is considered the most significant. The simplification of terms in that portion of the equation yields a coefficient value of 3.98, which for all physiologically relevant clinical situations can be rounded to 4. The second term of the equation representing flow acceleration is equal to zero when calculating mean and peak pressure differences and thus can be dropped for these common situations. The third term describes the force necessary to overcome viscous friction, which for pressure drops across a discrete orifice is negligible. Therefore, for most clinical applications, a simplified formula is used that relies upon the following assumptions: (a) the velocity proximal to the obstruction (V_1) is negligible compared with the velocity just distal to the obstruction (V_2); (b) flow acceleration occurs is negligible for mean and peak pressure gradients; (c) viscous friction is trivial; and (d) the flow is laminar. The Bernoulli equation can therefore be simplified to the following:

$$\Delta P = 4 \cdot V_2^2$$

This simplified formula has been proven valid in *in vitro* flow models and in a variety of clinical settings. However, it is important to note that the assumptions allowing for the simplification of the Bernoulli equation may not always be valid. For example, in long-segment narrowing such as a Blalock-Taussig-Thomas shunt, ignoring the viscous friction term of the Bernoulli equation will result in significant underestimation of the pressure drop.

A common application of the simplified Bernoulli equation is estimating the RV systolic pressure, which, in the absence of RV outflow tract obstruction, is equal to the pulmonary artery systolic pressure. This may be done by measuring the peak tricuspid regurgitation jet velocity and applying the simplified Bernoulli equation to calculate the RV to right atrium pressure difference in systole. One then adds an assumed right atrial pressure (e.g., 5 mm Hg) to the pressure difference to estimate the RV systolic pressure.

Special Echocardiographic Procedures

Transesophageal Echocardiography

Indications

Echocardiographic imaging from the esophagus using a specialized transducer typically provides high-quality images of the heart because of the absence of intervening structures such as lung and bone which interfere with the transmission of acoustic energy in transthoracic imaging.

Structures that are particularly well suited to transesophageal echocardiography (TEE) examination are those located closest to the esophagus including the atrial septum, pulmonary veins, superior vena cava, atrioventricular valves, LV outflow tract, aortic valve, coronary artery origins, and surgically created atrial baffles. More anterior structures, such as the RV outflow tract and pulmonary valve, and those obscured by adjacent airways (e.g., the left pulmonary artery) are more difficult to evaluate.

In combination with 3D imaging techniques, TEE images can be used to create very high-quality images of the cardiac structures, in particular the atrioventricular and semilunar valves (Video 9.4). One general indication for TEE is in patients who have poor transthoracic acoustic windows and image quality. TEE evaluation of prosthetic atrioventricular valve function, regurgitation, and perivalvar leaks is usually superior to that obtained by transthoracic imaging. Moreover, in older children and adults, TEE has greater sensitivity than transthoracic imaging for intracardiac thrombus and vegetations. Another general indication for TEE is when the chest is not accessible for transthoracic echocardiography such as during cardiac surgery or cardiac catheterization. Preoperative TEE can elucidate anatomic details that may have been incompletely evaluated on preoperative transthoracic studies and may thus serve to further inform the surgical plan. Postoperative TEE in the operating room plays a crucial role in evaluating surgical procedures. It is particularly helpful for assessing the efficacy of septal defect repair, relief of outflow tract obstruction, valvuloplasty, patency of intracardiac baffles, and ventricular function, and can identify residual lesions not otherwise suspected. If unsatisfactory results or significant residual lesions are found, the surgery can be revised before leaving the operating room and then reassessed by TEE. TEE is also useful for providing real-time guidance and assessment during interventional catheterization procedures such as device closure of atrial and ventricular septal defects, venous baffle obstruction relief and defect closure, and some valve implantations.

Equipment and Technique

TEE probes are available in different sizes including those small enough to be suitable in some newborns, and may have 3D imaging capability. Most TEEs are performed under general anesthesia. Experienced medical personnel should insert the probe to avoid injury to the patient's teeth, posterior pharynx, airway, or esophagus. Although the questions to be answered by TEE may be focused, once these have been addressed, a comprehensive examination for additional unsuspected findings is advisable if it is feasible to do so.

Fig. 9.8 shows representative TEE views. A comprehensive TEE examination often begins with the probe tip in the stomach, where anteflexion provides views of the left and right ventricles for assessment of myocardial function, atrioventricular valve morphology, and the muscular ventricular septum. The best angles for Doppler interrogation of RV

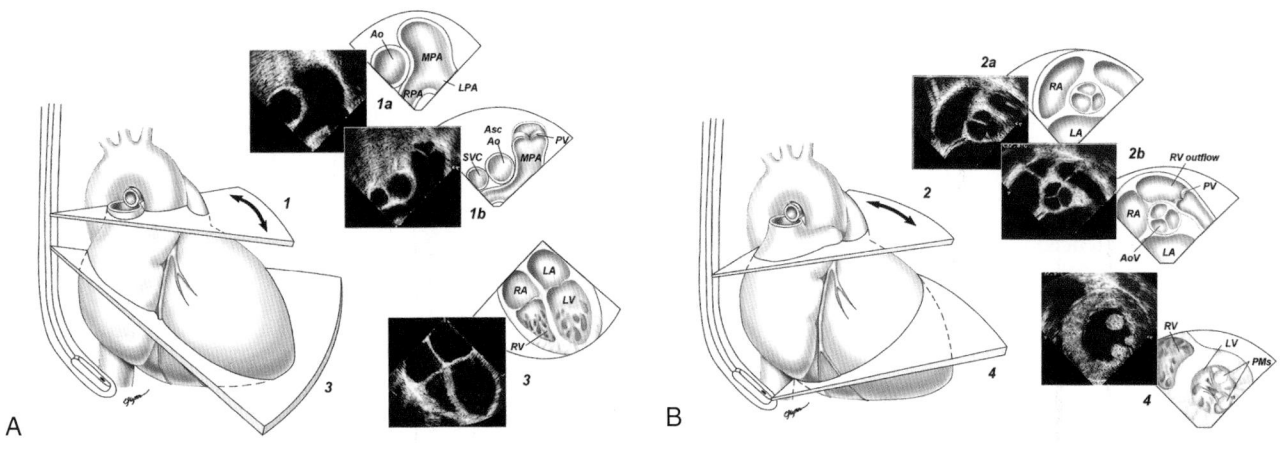

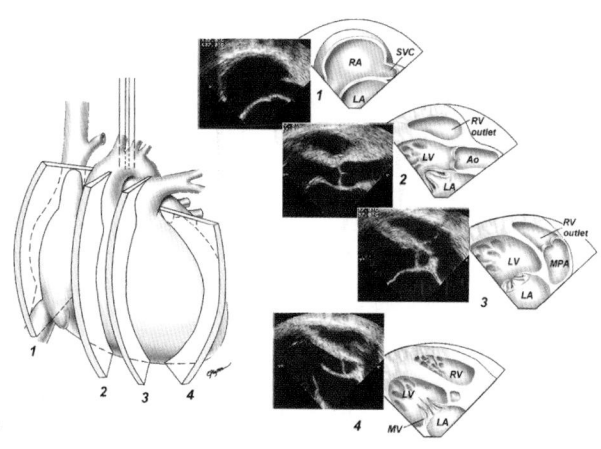

• **Fig. 9.8** Transesophageal imaging. (A) Transverse plane: cross-sectional view at level 1a depicts the proximal ascending aorta *(Ao)*, main pulmonary artery *(MPA)*, and left and right pulmonary arteries *(LPA and RPA*, respectively). A rightward tilt of the transducer shows the RPA as it passes behind the superior vena cava *(SVC)* and ascending aorta *(Asc Ao)*. To obtain a four-chamber view (level 3), the transducer is advanced in the esophagus with slight retroflexion of the scope. (B) Level 2 is parallel to the transthoracic parasternal short-axis view. In level 2a, the atrial septum is imaged by a slight rightward tilt of the transducer. In level 2B, the aortic valve *(AoV)* is seen in cross-section in the center of the image, the left atrium *(LA)*, right atrium *(RA)*, tricuspid valve, right ventricular outflow *(RV outflow)*, pulmonary valve *(PV)*, and the proximal main pulmonary artery are seen. By advancing the transducer into the lower esophagus and anteflexing the scope, a cross-sectional view of the left ventricle *(LV)*, mitral valve, and papillary muscles is obtained (level 4). Note that image orientation is the same as in transthoracic echocardiography. (C) Vertical (longitudinal) plane: the sweep begins at a plane that crosses the SVC, LA, RA, and atrial septum (level 1). Next, a leftward tilt of the transducer shows an image parallel to the transthoracic parasternal long-axis view of the LA, mitral valve, LV, left ventricular outflow tract, and proximal aorta (Ao) (level 2). Further leftward tilt of the transducer (level 3) shows the right ventricular outflow tract *(RV outlet)*, pulmonary valve, and main pulmonary artery *(MPA)*. The sweep continues leftward to show the leftward aspects of the left atrium, mitral valve, and LV (level 4). Further leftward tilt depicts the left atrial appendage and the left pulmonary veins (not shown). Note that image orientation is the same as in transthoracic echocardiography. (From Geva T. Echocardiography and Doppler ultrasound. In: Garson, A, Bricker, JT, Fisher, DJ, Neish SR (eds). *The Science and Practice of Pediatric Cardiology*. Baltimore: Williams & Wilkins, 1997, pp. 789, with permission.)

and LV outflow tract gradients are usually obtained from the stomach. This view, however, can be challenging to obtain in patients whose heart is not on the same side as the stomach. Withdrawal of the probe into the lower and mid-esophagus provides excellent images of the atrial septum, pulmonary veins, atrial appendages, atrioventricular valves, LV outflow tract, aortic and pulmonary valves, and coronary arteries. Straightening or retroflexion of the probe

results in a four-chamber view, and anteflexion visualizes the ventricles and aortic valve in cross-section. A higher esophageal view allows examination of the main and branch pulmonary arteries, ductus arteriosus, transverse aortic arch, and superior vena cava. Rotating the probe's imaging face posteriorly demonstrates the descending aorta. Standards for image display vary among institutions; displaying the TEE images with the same orientation as corresponding transthoracic images in the same plane, however, helps orient viewers more familiar with transthoracic images. The interested reader is referred to guidelines for TEE in children published by the American Society of Echocardiography in 2018.[15]

Patient Selection and Safety

Although in experienced hands TEE is very safe, complications such as oropharyngeal and esophageal injury and compression of airways and vascular structures can occur. Contraindications to TEE include unrepaired tracheoesophageal fistula, significant esophageal stricture, active upper gastrointestinal bleeding, and an uncontrolled airway in a patient with significant respiratory or cardiac compromise. Relative contraindications include previous esophageal surgery, esophageal varices or diverticulum, cervical spine instability, and severe coagulopathy.

Fetal Echocardiography

Early attempts to use M-mode echocardiography to diagnose abnormalities of fetal cardiac structure and rhythm were met with limited success.[16] With the advent of high-resolution 2D imaging in the 1980s, detailed examination of fetal cardiac anatomy and accurate diagnosis of even very complex congenital heart defects became possible (Fig. 9.9).[16,17] Today, congenital heart defects can be diagnosed by fetal echocardiography performed transabdominally as early as 14 weeks' gestation and transvaginally as early as 10 weeks' gestation.

Detection of Congenital Heart Disease on Routine Ultrasound

The detection rate of congenital heart disease on routine screening obstetrical ultrasound is variable and operator-dependent. Visualization of a four-chamber view alone has proven inadequate to rule out fetal heart disease; when accompanied by a view of the great arteries, the detection rate increases significantly. However, the defects most likely to be detected on routine ultrasound screening are those in which there is a significantly hypoplastic ventricle or great artery, large ventricular septal defect, obvious abnormality of the atrioventricular valves (e.g., absent or common atrioventricular valve), significant cardiomegaly, or non-immune hydrops. Particularly in fetuses thought to be at low risk for congenital heart disease, defects such as isolated semilunar valve stenosis, hypoplastic aortic arch with coarctation, transposition of the great arteries, and anomalies of the pulmonary and systemic veins are less likely to be detected. Whereas the initial scan in fetuses at risk for congenital heart defects may be performed as early as 14 to 18 weeks of gestation, image resolution later in gestation (20–28 weeks) is better in most instances. Indications for fetal echocardiography are summarized in Table 9.2.

Fetal Circulation

Accurate diagnosis of fetal congenital heart defects requires knowledge of the wide variety of possible lesions and their echocardiographic appearance as well as familiarity with the fetal circulation and the effects of structural and functional heart disease on this system. For example, in the setting of severe aortic or pulmonary valve stenosis with an intact ventricular septum, the ventricle on the affected side of the heart has diminished diastolic filling and poor systolic function; growth of this ventricle slows or even stops, which may render the ventricle severely hypoplastic by the third trimester.[18] For a detailed discussion of these issues, please see *Chapter 4: Fetal and transitional circulation.*

Technique

Fetal echocardiography should be performed by sonographers or physicians who are experienced in echocardiographic examination of congenital heart defects and understand how

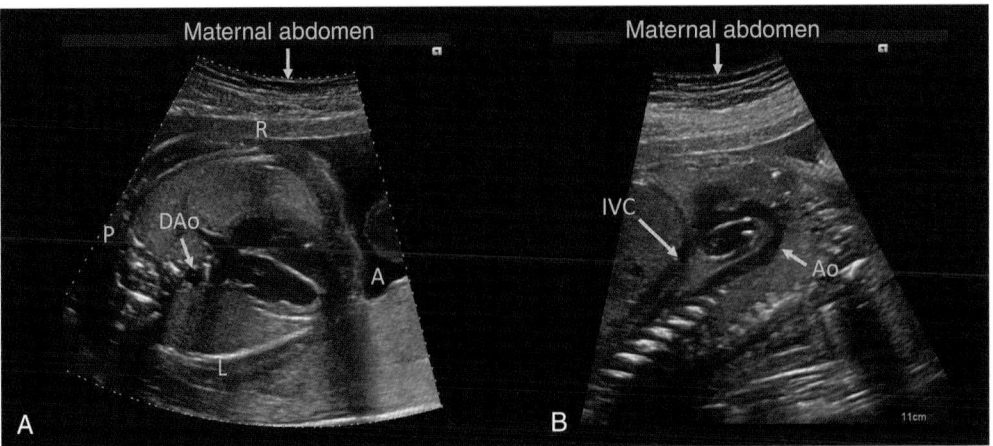

• **Fig. 9.9** Fetal echocardiogram. (A) Four-chamber view. (B) Oblique sagittal view of the thoracic and abdominal aorta. *A,* Anterior; *Ao,* aorta; *DAO,* descending aorta; *IVC,* inferior vena cava *L,* left; *P,* posterior; *R,* right.

TABLE 9.2   Indications for Fetal Echocardiography

Fetal Risk Factors

- Suspected cardiac anomaly on level I obstetrical ultrasound
- Abnormal visceral situs
- Abnormal cardiac position or axis
- Extracardiac structural anomalies associated with congenital heart disease including:
  - Single umbilical artery
  - Nuchal thickening/lucency
  - Diaphragmatic hernia
  - Duodenal atresia
  - Tracheoesophageal fistula
  - Cystic hygroma
- Chromosomal abnormalities including:
  - Trisomy 21
  - Chromosome 22q11 microdeletion (velocardiofacial syndrome)
  - Turner syndrome
- Fetal arrhythmias including tachy- and bradyarrhythmia
- Intrauterine growth retardation
- Nonimmune hydrops fetalis
- Structural anomaly affecting cardiovascular physiology, including:
  - Sacrococcygeal teratoma
  - Twin–twin transfusion
  - Acardiac twin
  - Vein of Galen malformation
  - Congenital pulmonary airway malformation

Maternal Risk Factors

- Exposure to teratogen
- Infection
- Autoantibodies (Anti-Ro/SSA antibodies)

Familial Risk Factors

- Congenital heart disease
- Syndromes such as Marfan, Noonan, trisomy 21, DiGeorge
- Tuberous sclerosis

these defects impact the fetal circulation. Familiarity with the examination of fetal structures outside the heart, including the ability to recognize significant lung hypoplasia, thoracic masses, hydrops fetalis, and fetal distress are essential.

Special attention should be paid to maternal comfort during the examination, with consideration given to a leftward laying position later in gestation, reducing compression of the maternal inferior vena cava by the uterus. The fetal position may change frequently during the examination and as such the examiner must reorient as the position of the fetus changes. If the fetus is in an unfavorable position for clear imaging, this may be altered by having the mother turn on her side or take a walk. After first assessing the position of the fetus in the uterus, one can identify the fetal right and left sides. The position of the fetal cardiac apex and stomach thus determined, these can then be used as markers of sidedness (i.e., right and left) if the fetus changes position.

Although a segmental approach to diagnosis is important, it is often difficult to obtain images of fetal cardiac structures in a predetermined sequence; it may be more time-efficient to image structures as they present themselves, eventually evaluating the entire heart. In some fortuitous circumstances, single sweeps may be adequate to image large portions of the fetal anatomy (Video 9.5). It is helpful to maintain a mental checklist of all of the components of a complete study, ensuring that all items are addressed before completing the examination. In addition to assessment of cardiac morphology, other features that are part of a comprehensive fetal echocardiographic examination include spectral and color Doppler assessment of valve and ventricular function, measurement of cardiac structures, and assessment of heart rate and rhythm. Normal dimensions of fetal cardiac structures with respect to gestational age have been established (these are available online, for example, at: http://zscore.chboston.org). An assessment of fetal size, using measurements of the head, femur, and abdomen, is useful for interpreting cardiac measurements, particularly if the fetus is large or small for gestational age.

Fetal Arrhythmia

Evaluation of fetal arrhythmias begins with an assessment of rate and regularity, followed by determination of the potential mechanism of arrhythmia. Simultaneous M-mode interrogation of contraction of the atrial wall (preferably the atrial appendage) and a ventricular wall or the aortic valve can demonstrate timing of contraction of the atria and ventricles and their relationship to each other. Simultaneous Doppler interrogation of the LV inflow and outflow can provide similar information and is usually easier to obtain; tissue Doppler techniques may be used as well. Finally, careful 2D imaging of the contraction of the appendages and ventricles can give clues as to the nature of the arrhythmia, distinguishing complete atrioventricular block from sinus bradycardia, for example. Determination of cardiac anatomy, ventricular and valve function, and signs of hydrops (pleural and pericardial effusion, ascites, skin thickening) are part of a comprehensive evaluation of any fetal arrhythmia.

Limitations of Fetal Echocardiography

Even in the setting of high-quality images of the fetal heart, there are some cardiac abnormalities that cannot reliably be excluded prenatally. These include small ventricular septal defects, mild valve abnormalities, coronary artery anomalies, some atrial septal defects, and persistent patency of the ductus arteriosus. Although predictors of postnatal coarctation of the aorta have been described,[19] potential coarctation remains challenging to exclude with certainty in any fetus. In addition, there are some cases in which a complete examination simply cannot be performed, usually due to poor acoustic windows or persistently suboptimal fetal position.

Counseling

Physicians or medical professionals who counsel parents about the results of fetal echocardiograms must be knowledgeable about the defect in question, including *in utero* and postnatal natural history, expected postnatal course, anticipated surgical or catheter interventions and their success rates, expected quality of life, and the range of possible outcomes from the best to worst case scenario. In addition, because many congenital heart defects are associated with syndromes or chromosomal anomalies, the counselor must have a thorough knowledge of these associations to provide the parents with a comprehensive picture of the disease and its implications for the child's life. The limitations of the echocardiogram and of fetal echocardiography in general should be explained.

A team approach is useful in preparing parents and families for perinatal and postnatal events. Early involvement of pediatric cardiologists, obstetricians, neonatologists, social workers, cardiothoracic surgeons, genetic counselors, and cardiac nurses may be beneficial in helping families obtain the information and resources they need. Meeting with various members of the medical team who will be caring for the infant after birth and a tour of the nursery or intensive care unit where the infant will be initially managed may help parents cope with the diagnosis of heart disease in their child and prepare them for postnatal events.

Clinical Implications

Prenatal diagnosis enables planning for a delivery in a tertiary care center where pediatric cardiologists, intensivists, cardiac surgeons, neonatologists, nurses, and other specialists are available to care for the infant. Postnatal management strategies can be developed and discussed with the parents in advance. Prostaglandin therapy can be instituted shortly after delivery for ductus-dependent lesions, thereby preventing harmful levels of hypoxia and acidosis in most instances. In addition, if urgent postnatal catheter or surgical therapy is anticipated, delivery timing can be coordinated to ensure that the necessary personnel are available. In rare instances, there may be a role for placing the newborn on an extracorporeal membrane oxygenator in the delivery room before separation from the placenta.

Although reports conflict as to whether prenatal diagnosis of congenital heart disease lowers mortality, evidence shows that morbidity is reduced.[20] Increased and earlier prenatal detection of the most severe types of congenital heart disease may result in decreased prevalence of these diseases in newborn populations in some countries due to elective terminations.

Prenatal diagnosis can affect management during pregnancy. Fetal tachyarrhythmias may be treated by administration of medication to the mother[21]; this, in turn, may prevent development of hydrops fetalis and the need for early delivery. Hydrops caused by structural or functional cardiac abnormalities may prompt early delivery if the fetus is deemed more likely to survive *ex utero*. Finally, there may be an increasing role for prenatal catheter and surgical interventions.

While early attempts at transcatheter balloon dilation of the aortic valve in fetuses with critical aortic stenosis were largely unsuccessful,[22] more recently efforts have demonstrated high rates of technical success, with indications including not only aortic valvuloplasty but also critical pulmonary stenosis, premature closure of the foramen ovale, and hypoplastic left heart syndrome with intact or nearly intact atrial septum.[23] The effect of transcatheter interventions on *in utero* natural history and long-term outcome have been reported, with selection criteria for this procedure becoming correspondingly increasingly refined.[24]

Safety and Complications

No pre- or postnatal adverse effects resulting from diagnostic ultrasound have been reported. Medical personnel using this technology must however be cognizant that ultrasound is a form of mechanical energy which under certain conditions can cause damage to the exposed tissue. This injury can result from conversion of mechanical energy to heat or from creation of gaseous microcavitations. Thus far, biologic damage has been observed only in nonclinical laboratory conditions. The American Institute of Ultrasound in Medicine has stated that "No confirmed biologic effects on patients or instrument operator caused by exposure at intensities typical of present diagnostic ultrasound instruments have ever been reported. Although the possibility that such biologic effects may be identified in the future, current data indicate that the benefits to patients of the prudent use of diagnostic ultrasound outweigh the risks, if any, that may be present."[25]

References

1. Sanders SP. Echocardiography and related techniques in the diagnosis of congenital heart defects: part i: veins, atria and interatrial septum. *Echocardiography*. 1984;1:185-217.
2. Snider AR, Serwer GA, Ritter SB. *Echocardiography in Pediatric Heart Disease*. St. Louis: Mosby; 1997.
3. Silverman NH. *Pediatric Echocardiography*. Baltimore: Williams & Wilkins; 1993.
4. Feigenbaum H. *Echocardiography*. Philadelphia: Lea & Febiger; 1994.
5. Simpson J, Lopez L, Acar P, et al. Three-dimensional echocardiography in congenital heart disease: an expert consensus document from the European Association of Cardiovascular Imaging and the American Society of Echocardiography. *J Am Soc Echocardiogr*. 2017;30:1-27.
6. Snider AR, Silverman NH, Turley K, Ebert PA. Evaluation of infradiaphragmatic total anomalous pulmonary venous connection with two-dimensional echocardiography. *Circulation*. 1982;66:1129-1132.
7. Edvardsen T, Gerber BL, Garot J, Bluemke DA, Lima JA, Smiseth OA. Quantitative assessment of intrinsic regional myocardial deformation by Doppler strain rate echocardiography in humans: validation against three-dimensional tagged magnetic resonance imaging. *Circulation*. 2002;106:50-56.

8. Gramiak R, Shah PM, Kramer DH. Ultrasound cardiography: contrast studies in anatomy and function. *Radiology*. 1969;92: 939-948.

9. Cohen BE, Winer HE, Kronzon I. Echocardiographic findings in patients with left superior vena cava and dilated coronary sinus. *Am J Cardiol*. 1979;44:158-161.

10. Campbell RM, Douglas PS, Eidem BW, Lai WW, Lopez L, Sachdeva R. ACC/AAP/AHA/ASE/HRS/SCAI/SCCT/SCMR/ SOPE 2014 appropriate use criteria for initial transthoracic echocardiography in outpatient pediatric cardiology: a report of the American College of Cardiology Appropriate Use Criteria Task Force, American Academy of Pediatrics, American Heart Association, American Society of Echocardiography, Heart Rhythm Society, Society for Cardiovascular Angiography and Interventions, Society of Cardiovascular Computed Tomography, Society for Cardiovascular Magnetic Resonance, and Society of Pediatric Echocardiography. *J Am Coll Cardiol*. 2014;64:2039-2060.

11. Tanner JM. Fallacy of per-weight and per-surface area standards, and their relation to spurious correlation. *J Appl Physiol*. 1949; 2:1-15.

12. Lopez L, Colan S, Stylianou M, et al. Relationship of echocardiographic Z scores adjusted for body surface area to age, sex, race, and ethnicity: The Pediatric Heart Network Normal Echocardiogram Database. *Circ Cardiovasc Imaging*. 2017;10:e006979.

13. Lopez L, Colan SD, Frommelt PC, et al. Recommendations for quantification methods during the performance of a pediatric echocardiogram: a report from the Pediatric Measurements Writing Group of the American Society of Echocardiography Pediatric and Congenital Heart Disease Council. *J Am Soc Echocardiogr*. 2010;23:465-495; quiz 576-577.

14. Arai K, Hozumi T, Matsumura Y, et al. Accuracy of measurement of left ventricular volume and ejection fraction by new real-time three-dimensional echocardiography in patients with wall motion abnormalities secondary to myocardial infarction. *Am J Cardiol*. 2004;94:552-558.

15. Puchalski MD, Lui GK, Miller-Hance WC, et al. Guidelines for performing a comprehensive transesophageal echocardiographic: examination in children and all patients with congenital heart disease: recommendations from the American Society of Echocardiography. *J Am Soc Echocardiogr*. 2019;32:173-215.

16. Kleinman CS, Hobbins JC, Jaffe CC, Lynch DC, Talner NS. Echocardiographic studies of the human fetus: prenatal diagnosis of congenital heart disease and cardiac dysrhythmias. *Pediatrics*. 1980;65:1059-1067.

17. Allan LD, Crawford DC, Anderson RH, Tynan MJ. Echocardiographic and anatomical correlations in fetal congenital heart disease. *Heart*. 1984;52:542-548.

18. Simpson JM, Sharland GK. Natural history and outcome of aortic stenosis diagnosed prenatally. *Heart*. 1997;77:205-210.

19. Hornberger LK, Sahn DJ, Kleinman CS, Copel J, Silverman NH. Antenatal diagnosis of coarctation of the aorta: a multicenter experience. *J Am Coll Cardiol*. 1994;23:417-423.

20. Copel JA, Tan AS, Kleinman CS. Does a prenatal diagnosis of congenital heart disease alter short-term outcome? *Ultrasound Obstet Gynecol*. 1997;10:237-241.

21. Copel JA, Friedman AH, Kleinman CS. Management of fetal cardiac arrhythmias. *Obstet Gynecol Clin North Am*. 1997;24: 201-211.

22. Kohl T, Sharland G, Allan LD, et al. World experience of percutaneous ultrasound-guided balloon valvuloplasty in human fetuses with severe aortic valve obstruction. *Am J Cardiol*. 2000; 85:1230-1233.

23. Tworetzky W, Wilkins-Haug L, Jennings RW, et al. Balloon dilation of severe aortic stenosis in the fetus: potential for prevention of hypoplastic left heart syndrome: candidate selection, technique, and results of successful intervention. *Circulation*. 2004;110:2125-2131.

24. Freud LR, McElhinney DB, Marshall AC, et al. Fetal aortic valvuloplasty for evolving hypoplastic left heart syndrome: postnatal outcomes of the first 100 patients. *Circulation*. 2014; 130:638-645.

25. Lizzi F, Mortimer A, Carstensen E, et al. Bioeffects considerations for the safety of diagnostic ultrasound. American Institute of Ultrasound in Medicine. Bioeffects Committee. *J Ultrasound Med*. 1988;7:S1-S38.

10

Advanced Cardiac Imaging

DANIEL A. CASTELLANOS AND ASHWIN PRAKASH

KEY LEARNING POINTS

- A cardiac MRI (CMR) examination uses cardiac and respiratory gating to perform an assessment of cardiovascular anatomy, ventricular function, blood flow quantification, and myocardial tissue characterization.
- While valvar regurgitant fractions and shunt volumes can be calculated by direct measurement, indirect calculation (e.g., quantifying flow before and after a shunt) is also utilized.
- Tissue characterization by CMR is performed by assessing how gadolinium-based contrast agents perfuse into and wash out of myocardium.

- There are three main types of cardiac CT (CCT) acquisitions that range from a relatively low radiation dose and highly accelerated scan to generate a still image of the heart to a retrospectively gated scan that acquires a full cardiac cycle and can be used for cine imaging.
- CCT is often used to assess the coronary arteries, to assess extracardiac vascular abnormalities, to plan catheter-based interventions, to assess ventricular function, and often in patients with pacemakers and implantable cardiac defibrillators.

Magnetic Resonance Imaging

Although MRI has been used for evaluation of the cardiovascular system since the early 1980s, its clinical implementation was initially slow due to long scan time and limited diagnostic information, which was predominantly confined to morphology. Rapid developments in hardware design, and imaging sequences during the 1990s led to an expansion in the clinical utility of cardiovascular magnetic resonance imaging (CMR) in patients with congenital and acquired heart disease. Anatomic and functional imaging by CMR complements echocardiography and x-ray angiography while avoiding many of the limitations of these modalities. For example, in contrast to echocardiography, acoustic windows and body size do not limit CMR, and, unlike cardiac catheterization, CMR does not use ionizing radiation. Currently, the diagnostic utility of CMR has extended beyond the assessment of cardiac anatomy and function to measures of blood flow, tissue characterization, the evaluation of myocardial perfusion and viability, lymphatic system assessment, and the assessment of myocardial iron overload. The following section reviews basic CMR techniques, clinical applications, indications, and contraindications.

Technical Aspects of CMR

Background

The primary source of signal used to construct MR images is derived from hydrogen protons (^1H). In MRI, the ^1H

protons are often referred to as spins because their angular momentum results in a precession (spinning) around the axis of the primary magnetic field. The highest concentrations of ^1H protons are in water and fat. Through the use of a strong static magnetic field, much weaker but rapidly varying magnetic field gradients, and short pulses of radiofrequency (RF) energy, the ^1H protons (spins) in selected regions of the body are stimulated to emit RF waves. These RF waves are then used to construct MR images. The strength of the static magnetic field in many clinical scanners used for CMR is 1.5 to 3 Tesla (T).

The building blocks of an MR examination are called pulse sequences. An MR pulse sequence describes the way the magnetic field gradients and RF pulses are applied to produce images with particular characteristics. During the course of a CMR examination, the examiner selects the pulse sequences and prescribes imaging locations and planes to acquire the image data in order to address specific clinical questions. Common pulse sequences used in clinical CMR practice are described briefly in the following paragraphs. A more detailed discussion of technical aspects of CMR is beyond the scope of this chapter and can be found in other sources.[1,2]

Cardiac and Respiratory Gating

Because most CMR techniques acquire data over multiple heartbeats, cardiac and respiratory motion during image acquisition can result in image blurring. In order to compensate for cardiac motion, image acquisition is synchronized with the cardiac cycle, using electrocardiographic (ECG) or vectorcardiographic gating. Blurring due to respiratory motion can be avoided either with breath-holding during image acquisition, synchronizing image data acquisition to the respiratory cycle, or using multiple signal averages. Respiratory motion can be tracked using a MR navigator pulse that concurrently tracks the position of the diaphragm or cardiac border, or by directly tracking heart motion during the respiratory cycle.[3]

Contrast Agents

Using modern CMR scanners, a larger proportion of CMR examinations can be performed without the use of a contrast agent. However, contrast agents can be useful in certain specific scenarios.

Gadolinium-Based Contrast Agents

Gadolinium is a small molecule that, while inherently toxic, is rendered safe by chelation with a larger molecule prior to administration. Several gadolinium-based contrast agents (GBCAs) using linear and cyclic chelates are available commercially. In CMR, GBCAs are used for contrast magnetic resonance angiography (MRA), assessment of myocardial perfusion, and assessment of fibrosis. In general, GBCAs are considered extremely safe with good patient tolerance. The most common reactions (~1% for each) are mild and include nausea and vomiting, headaches, and rash. GBCAs are not nephrotoxic; however, a serious systemic disorder called nephrogenic systemic fibrosis (NSF) can occur in a small proportion of patients with end-stage renal failure who receive GBCAs.[4] The risk and benefits of the administration of gadolinium should be assessed on a case-by-case basis for any patient with renal dysfunction.

Ferumoxytol

Ferumoxytol is commonly used in the intravenous treatment of iron deficiency anemia. However, it has unique properties that make is particularly suitable for MRA. Unlike GBCAs that rapidly diffuse out of the intravascular pool into the interstitium, ferumoxytol persists in the blood pool for days to weeks, allowing the time needed for high-resolution respiratory and ECG-gated MRA. This can be particularly useful in the evaluation of complex congenital cardiac defects in young children. Due to safety concerns related to hypersensitivity, this agent is administered using a slow intravenous infusion with cardiorespiratory monitoring.[5]

Clinical Applications

CMR is used to obtain diagnostic information in a wide range of congenital and acquired pediatric heart disease. It is usually performed in concert with other tests, including echocardiography, cardiac catheterization, and computed tomography (CT). The most common clinical scenarios in which CMR is requested involve one or more of the following: (a) when the existing diagnostic information is incomplete or inconsistent; (b) to avoid diagnostic catheterization

with its associated risks; and (c) for the unique capabilities of CMR (e.g., ventricular volumes and function, site-specific flow measurements, tissue characteristics, lymphatic assessment, or tumor characterization). In practice, CMR is increasingly used in patients with suboptimal echocardiographic windows, a relatively common problem in adolescents and adults with congenital heart disease (CHD), for assessment of ventricular dimensions and function, and for quantification of valve regurgitation. Detailed preexamination planning is crucial given the wide array of imaging sequences available and the often complex nature of the clinical, anatomic, and functional issues in patients with CHD.

Assessment of Cardiac and Extracardiac Anatomy

Several CMR pulse sequences can be used to assess intracardiac and extracardiac anatomy. CMR can be particularly useful in understanding complex spatial relationships in congenital defects and in the evaluation of abnormalities in extracardiac structures (such as the aortic arch, pulmonary arteries, and pulmonary veins), which can be difficult to assess using echocardiography (Video 10.1).

Cine Steady-State Free Precession Imaging

ECG-gated 2D cine steady-state free precession (SSFP) imaging has become the workhorse of CMR imaging. Typically performed during short breath holds, this pulse sequence yields high-quality cine images of the heart and extracardiac vasculature (Video 10.2). In these images, the blood appears bright while the myocardium and other tissues appear gray. In addition to assessment of anatomy, turbulent flow jets can also be visualized. While in-plane resolution is high, slice thickness (4–8 mm) limits resolution through the imaging plane. More recently, technical advances have made high-resolution 3D cine SSFP imaging possible, which allows interrogation of a cine 3D dataset post-acquisition to create unique imaging planes and 4D virtual models (Video 10.3). Of note, SSPF images are highly susceptible to artifacts caused by ferromagnetic implants or devices.

Black Blood (Fast Spin Echo) Imaging

This ECG-gated image sequence yields static images obtained during diastole that are characterized by black blood pool and gray appearance of myocardium and other tissues (Fig. 10.1). The main advantage of this pulse sequence is its high spatial resolution with thinner slices (0.8–6 mm) and lower susceptibility to artifact related to ferromagnetic implants. As it does not provide cine images, its use is limited to situations when high-resolution assessment of anatomy is necessary, especially in the presence of ferromagnetic implants. Recently, 3D versions of this image sequence have also become available.

Contrast-Enhanced 3D MRA

This technique uses the T1 reducing effects of GBCAs to markedly increase the contrast between vascular and nonvascular structures using a T1-weighted gradient echo pulse

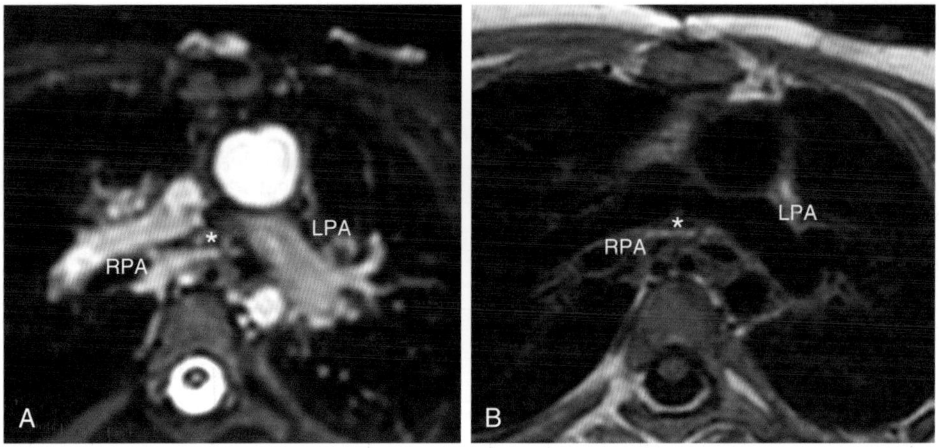

• **Fig. 10.1** Images from a 3-year-old male with hypoplastic left heart syndrome with mitral and aortic atresia, most recently S/P right bidirectional Glenn shunt to right pulmonary artery *(RPA)*, right modified Blalock-Taussig-Thomas shunt connected to left pulmonary artery *(LPA)*, and a fenestrated partition between right and left pulmonary arteries. **(A)** An image from a 3D balanced steady-state free precession angiogram at the level of the pulmonary arteries has flow-related artifact at the site of the intrapulmonary fenestration resulting in uneven blood pool image contrast. **(B)** A 3D black blood sequence at the same site demonstrates better visualization of the LPA lumen and the fenestrated partition. * is immediately adjacent to the intrapulmonary fenestrated partition.

sequence. A bolus of GBCA is injected intravenously and imaging is performed during passage of the bolus through the vessel of interest with a relatively short acquisition time (15–30 seconds). Imaging is typically performed during a breath hold to minimize blurring from breathing motion and is often repeated a few seconds later to obtain a delayed dataset to visualize venous anatomy. The 3D data set can be reconstructed to obtain multiplanar reconstruction and 3D volume rendering (Fig. 10.2). 3D MRA images provide excellent visualization of the extracardiac thoracic vasculature and is useful in the evaluation of abnormalities involving the systemic or pulmonary veins, pulmonary arteries, or the thoracic aorta and its branches. Because it does not utilize ECG gating, there is blurring of intracardiac structures related to cardiac motion, and therefore, it does not provide good visualization of intracardiac structures or coronary arteries.

Non-Contrast 3D MRA Using 3D SSFP

This is a newer technique that utilizes an ECG-gated 3D SSFP pulse sequence to perform 3D MRA without the need for contrast injection. It minimizes respiratory motion with the use of a respiratory navigator.[3] ECG gating is used to obtain a 3D dataset during a prespecified portion of the cardiac cycle while minimizing cardiac motion. Therefore, excellent imaging of both intracardiac and extracardiac structures is possible, including imaging of the origin and courses of the coronary arteries (Fig. 10.3). On most modern scanners, this image sequence has supplanted contrast-enhanced 3D MRA as the default MRA technique. Similar to other SSFP images, this pulse sequence is sensitive to artifacts caused by ferromagnetic implants.

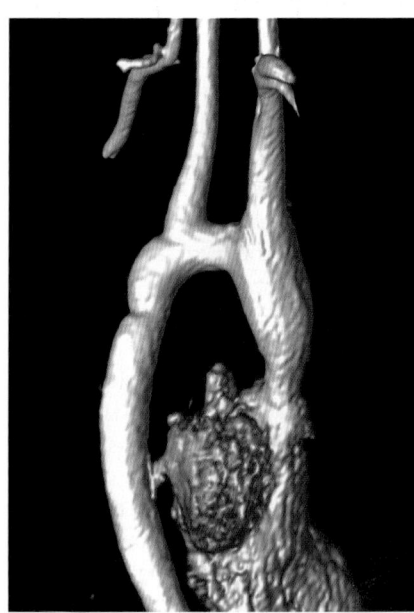

• **Fig. 10.2** A right lateral view of a 3D volume rendered magnetic resonance angiogram in an 18-year-old male with coarctation of the aorta and bicommissural aortic valve who underwent coarctation repair utilizing a left subclavian artery flap. A mildly small sino-tubular junction is also noted. Only two arch branches are visualized as the left subclavian artery is discontinuous from the arch (consistent with history of subclavian flap repair).

Quantification of Ventricular Volume, Mass, and Function

CMR is superior to echocardiography in quantifying ventricular size and function due to its lack of reliance on geometric assumptions regarding the shape of the left and

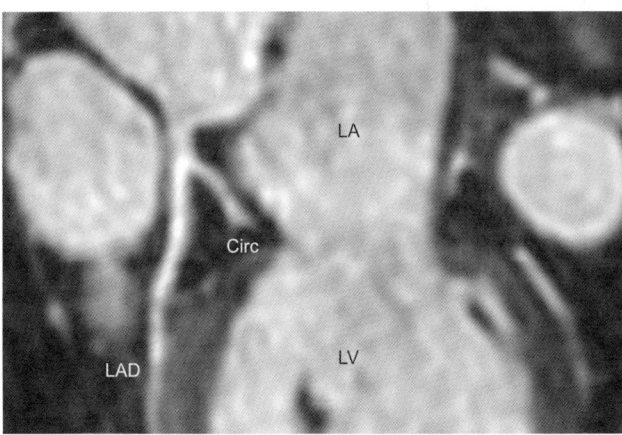

• **Fig. 10.3** Image from a 3D balanced steady-state free precession angiogram in a 35-year-old female with normal coronary artery anatomy. An oblique view demonstrates the left main coronary artery arising from the aortic root and bifurcating into the circumflex *(Circ)* and left anterior descending *(LAD)* coronary arteries. *LA,* Left atrium; *LV,* left ventricle.

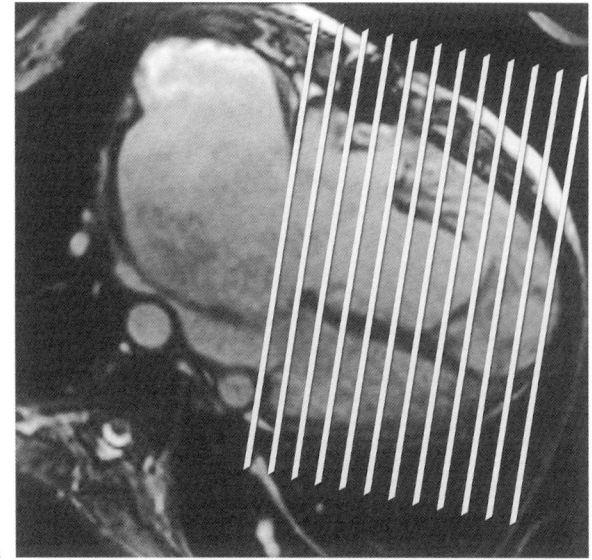

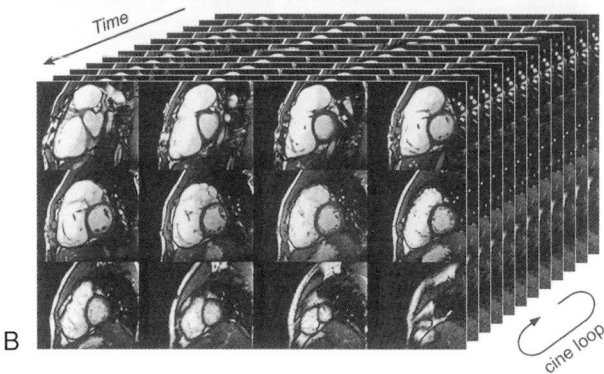

• **Fig. 10.4** Magnetic resonance imaging assessment of ventricular function in a patient with repaired tetralogy of Fallot and right ventricular dilatation. **(A)** A diastolic frame of an ECG-triggered steady-state free precession cine magnetic resonance imaging in the four-chamber plane is used to prescribe multiple contiguous slices perpendicular to the long axis from the base through the apex. **(B)** Multiple (usually 12) short-axis slices displayed in cine loop format.

right ventricles, and because image quality does not deteriorate with increasing body size. This is particularly true for the assessment of right ventricular size and function, which has a complex geometric shape, making quantification difficult by echocardiography. Multiple studies have demonstrated that measurements of left and right ventricular volume, mass, and function by CMR are highly accurate and reproducible.[6]

Ventricular dimensions and function are assessed on CMR by obtaining a series of 2D cine SSFP images that includes both left and right ventricles. This is typically performed using images in the short axis of the ventricles, but is also possible using a set of axial images.[7] The method for quantification of ventricular volume, mass, and function is shown in Fig. 10.4. The process involves tracing the endocardial border of each ventricle in each slice at end-systole and end-diastole. The volume of each slice is calculated as the product of its cross-sectional area and thickness, assuming an equal slice area throughout its thickness. Ventricular volume is then determined by summation of the volumes of all slices. From the end-systolic and end-diastolic volumes, one can calculate left and right ventricular stroke volume and ejection fraction. Ventricular mass is calculated by tracing the epicardial borders, subtracting the endocardial volumes, and multiplying the resultant muscle volume by the specific gravity of the myocardium (1.05 g/mm^3).

The quantification of ventricular volume, mass, and ejection fraction by CMR has been shown to be accurate and reproducible between readers and examinations. This can be useful in the follow-up of patients in whom management decisions are based on these data, for example, in patients with repaired tetralogy of Fallot and pulmonary regurgitation. Interpretation of ventricular volumes requires adjustment for body size. This is typically done with the use of z-scores. Although small normative CMR datasets are available for children, high-quality z-scores similar to those available for echocardiography are not available; therefore, interpretation usually relies on indexing values to body surface area.[7] It should be noted that ventricular volumes indexed to body surface area vary by age, and are smaller in younger children and infants, related to a faster heart rate.

Blood Flow Quantification

Blood flow can be measured with a pulse sequence known as cine phase contrast or velocity-encoded MRI. This gradient echo sequence is based on the principle that the signal from protons flowing through a magnetic field gradient accumulates a phase shift that is linearly proportional to its velocity. Multiple phase images are constructed during the cardiac cycle in which the signal amplitude of each voxel is proportional to the mean flow velocity within that voxel. Blood flow is measured by obtaining cross-sectional images of the vessel of interest, defining a region of interest around

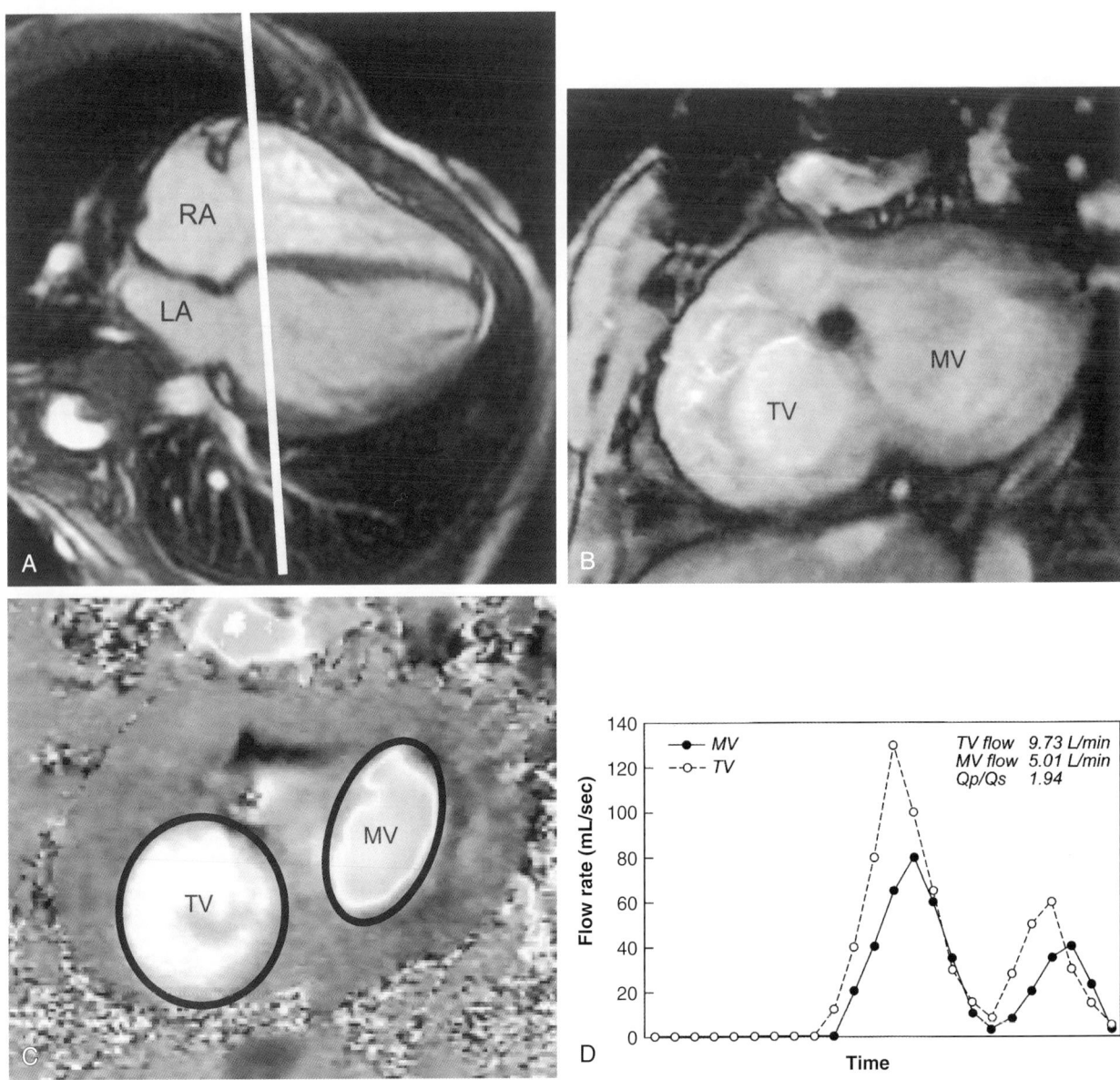

• **Fig. 10.5** Magnetic resonance imaging measurements of blood flow through the atrioventricular valves in a patient with left-to-right shunt from a secundum atrial septal defect. **(A)** An image in the four-chamber plane is used for placement of the ECG-triggered phase-contrast cine magnetic resonance imaging sequence perpendicular to plane of the atrioventricular valves. **(B)** Magnitude image reconstructed from the amplitude of the magnetic resonance radiofrequency signal provides anatomic depiction. **(C)** Phase image reconstructed from the phase difference of the magnetic resonance radiofrequency signal provides information on flow velocity and direction. A region of interest is drawn around the flow signals in the atrioventricular valves. **(D)** Instantaneous flow rates (mL/second) are calculated by integration of the velocities across the regions of interest. The areas under the flow curves represent stroke volumes *ECG*, electrocardiogram, *LA*, left atrium, *mL*, milliliters, *MV*, mitral valve, *RA*, right atrium, *RV*, right ventricle.

the vessel on the phase images, integrating the velocities of the enclosed voxels, and multiplying the product by the vessel's cross-sectional area (Fig. 10.5). *In vivo* and *in vitro* studies show that measurements of blood flow by velocity-encoded cine MRI are accurate and reproducible. Examples of clinical applications include measurements of valve regurgitation, pulmonary-to-systemic flow ratio (Qp/Qs) in patients with shunt lesions, measurement of differential pulmonary artery flow, and quantification of aortopulmonary collateral flow.[8-10]

Valve Regurgitation

Quantifying the severity of valve regurgitation is a particular strength of CMR and can help in management decisions. The use of phase-contrast flow data is integral in this calculation. The simplest method (typically used for the calculation of pulmonary regurgitation), involves obtaining phase-contrast images just above the valve of interest and tracing the outline of the vessel to obtain a flow rate curve over time. From this curve, forward and backward volume can be calculated and the regurgitation fraction is calculated as the

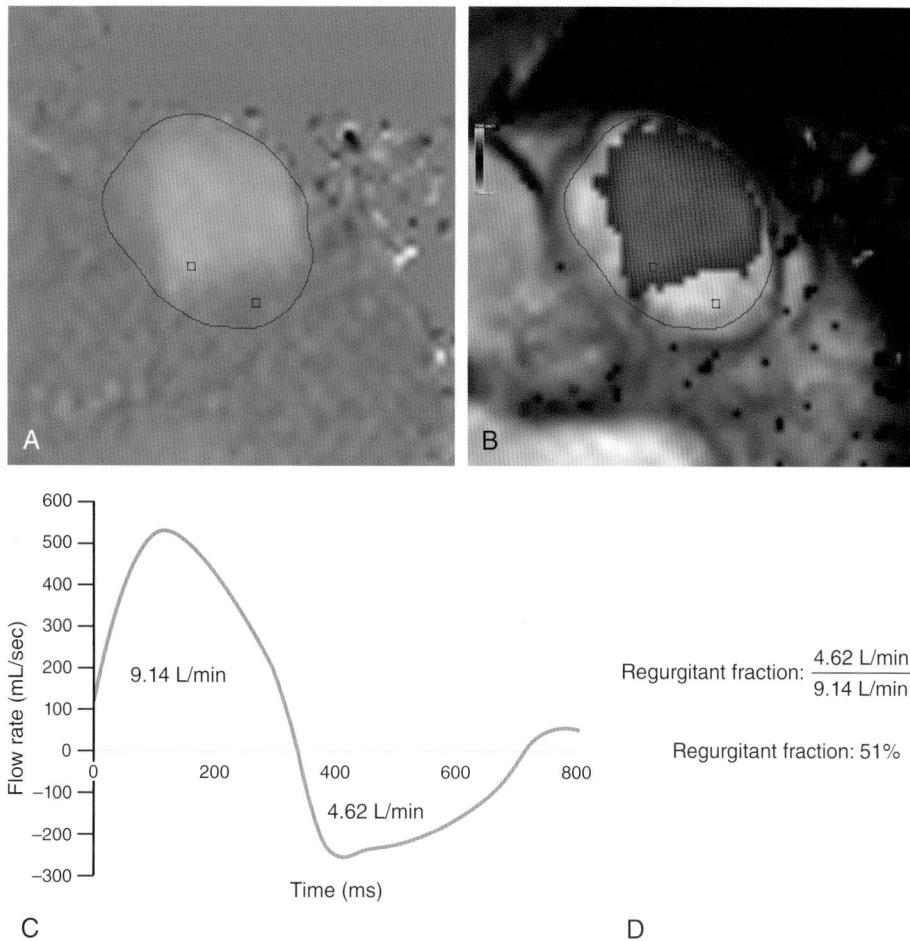

• **Fig. 10.6** Phase-contrast flow measurement at the proximal main pulmonary artery in a 33-year-old female with pulmonary atresia with intact ventricular septum, S/P repair with right ventricular outflow tract patch. Severe pulmonary regurgitation is noted with a regurgitation fraction of ~51%. **(A)** Phase image reconstructed from the phase difference of the magnetic resonance radiofrequency signal provides information on flow velocity and direction. A region of interest is drawn around the main pulmonary artery. **(B)** Magnitude image with color coding based on the phase image represents flow, with a region of interest drawn around the main pulmonary artery. **(C)** Flow-time curve demonstrating the change in flow rate over time (during one R-R interval). **(D)** The regurgitant fraction is calculated by dividing the regurgitant volume by the forward volume.

ratio of the regurgitant volume and the forward volume (Fig. 10.6). Other methods to calculate valvar regurgitant fractions involve using the difference in phase-contrast measurements from two different vessels, the difference in a phase-contrast flow measurement and a ventricular stroke volume, or the difference of ventricular stroke volumes. Each method has unique strengths and limitations. For instance, using the difference of ventricular stroke volumes to calculate atrioventricular valve regurgitation assumes the absence of intracardiac shunts and regurgitation of any of the other valves. For atrioventricular valves, since a vessel distal to the valve is not available for direct flow measurements and there is significant translation motion of the valve plane, regurgitation volume is calculated indirectly. One method to calculate atrioventricular valve regurgitation utilizes phase-contrast imaging to measure the volume of inflow into each atrioventricular valve. In cases where only one of the atrioventricular valves is regurgitant, the regurgitant volume can be calculated

as the difference between the inflow of the mitral and tricuspid valves, and the regurgitation fraction as the ratio of the regurgitant volume and the inflow into the regurgitant valve.

Shunts

Phase-contrast, velocity-encoded CMR can be used to quantitatively assess intracardiac and extracardiac shunts and to estimate the ratio Qp/Qs. Typically, shunt volume is calculated using a comparison of phase-contrast flow measurements on either end of the shunt. The site of Qp and Qs measurements is dictated by the location of the shunt (Fig. 10.7). For example, in the setting of a ventricular or atrial septal defect with left-to-right shunting, comparison of main pulmonary artery (Qp) and aortic (Qs) flow measurements can be used. On the other hand, in the setting of a patent ductus arteriosus with left-to-right flow, the aortic valve flow would have a higher amount of flow (Qp) than main pulmonary artery (Qs).

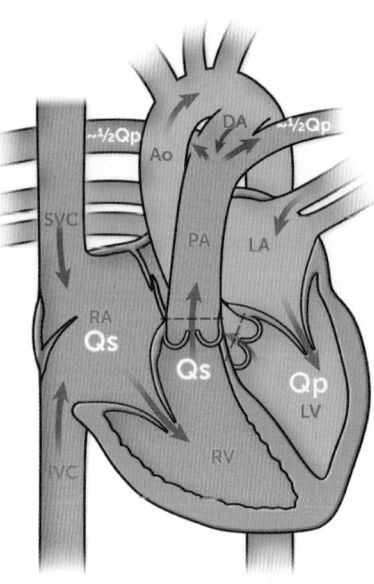

VSD

PDA

Qp:Qs = MPA:AoV

Qp:Qs = AoV:MPA

• **Fig. 10.7** Qp and Qs can be calculated using phase-contrast flow measurements. The site of Qp and Qs measurements is dictated by the location of the shunt. In the case of a ventricular septal defect *(VSD)*, Qp can be measured with a main pulmonary artery *(MPA)* flow measurement, while Qs can be measured with an aortic root flow measurement. In the case of a patent ductus arteriosus *(PDA)*, the shunt is distal to the MPA and aortic root. Therefore, Qp can be measured with an aortic root flow measurement, while Qs can be measured with MPA flow measurement. *Qp*, pulmonary flow; *Qs*, aortic flow.

Tissue Characterization

Myocardial Perfusion

CMR can assess myocardial perfusion by detecting the transit and distribution of GBCAs through the heart. Using an ultrafast multi-slice pulse sequence, the first pass of a bolus of a GBCA through the myocardium can be imaged. Myocardial regions with decreased perfusion exhibit delayed or lack of signal enhancement. This can be useful in detecting areas of reversible ischemia during stress, which can be achieved by administering a coronary vasodilator (e.g., adenosine or regadenoson) or an agent that increases myocardial oxygen demand, such as dobutamine. Stress perfusion imaging can be useful in evaluating the significance of coronary abnormalities in patients with Kawasaki disease and giant coronary aneurysms, and patients with congenital coronary anomalies.[11] It can also be useful in assessing the degree of vascularity of cardiac tumors.

Myocardial Viability

Myocardial viability can be assessed 10–20 minutes after administration of a GBCA using a technique known as late gadolinium enhancement (LGE). Normal viable myocardium consists of tightly packed myocytes, with little intercellular space for GBCA to seep into; while nonviable myocardium (due to infarction or fibrosis) allows GBCA to accumulate in expanded intercellular spaces (due to fibrosis). The signal from viable myocardium or blood pool is further suppressed using an inversion pulse, rendering normal myocardium dark, whereas nonviable myocardium exhibits high signal intensity (hyperenhancement) due to retention of the contrast agent. This technique is sensitive and specific in detecting irreversible myocardial injury.[12] LGE imaging can be useful in confirming the diagnosis of myocarditis and the extent of LGE is related to prognosis in a variety of acquired and congenital disorders such as hypertrophic cardiomyopathy, repaired tetralogy of Fallot, and single ventricular physiology. It can also be used to detect endocardial fibroelastosis (Fig. 10.8) and in identifying the type of cardiac tumors.[13]

Imaging of Diffuse Myocardial Fibrosis and Edema

This is performed using parametric mapping techniques. Every tissue has a unique T1 relaxation time in the presence of a strong magnetic field. An extracellular volume (ECV) fraction represents a physiologic parameter that is derived from the ratio of T1 signal values prior to and after the administration of GBCAs. An increased ECV fraction is usually indicative of fibrosis.[14] Unlike LGE imaging, which is most useful in separating areas of discrete scarring from normal myocardium, ECV fraction is useful in identifying diffuse fibrosis, for example in patients with myocarditis.[15] Each substance also has a unique T2 relaxation which can also be performed with the T2-weighting to obtain a T2 relaxation time. A parametric technique known as T2 mapping can be used to identify areas of myocardial edema, such as in acute myocarditis.[15]

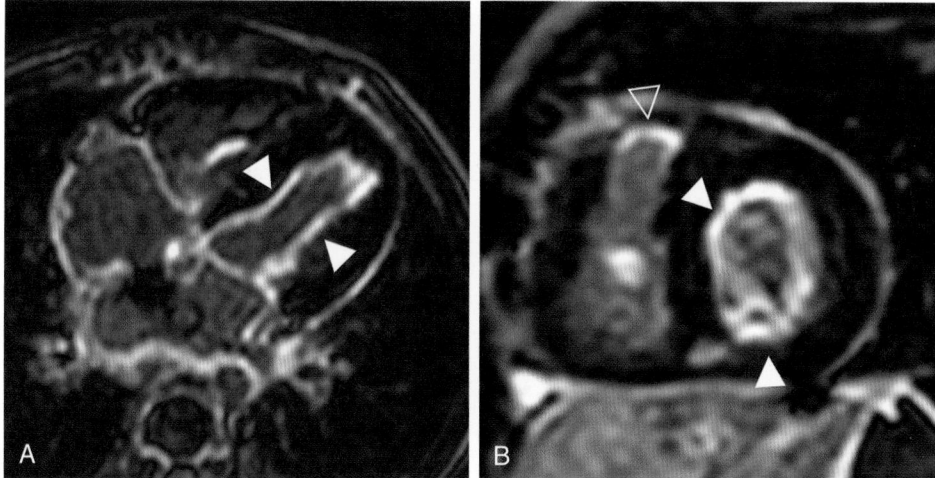

• **Fig. 10.8** Late gadolinium enhancement imaging is performed to assess for endocardial fibroelastosis in an 18-month-old female with a history of severe aortic stenosis who underwent fetal balloon valvuloplasty, then post-natal balloon valvuloplasty, followed by stage 1 operation with Sano modification, and most recently takedown of Sano conduit, bidirectional Glenn shunt, aortic valvotomy, endocardial fibroelastosis resection, and 7-mm fenestrated atrial septal defect closure. Late gadolinium enhancement of the entire left ventricular endocardial surface *(solid arrows)* is consistent with endocardial fibroelastosis. Late gadolinium enhancement is also present at former right ventricle to pulmonary artery conduit site *(hollow arrow)*. **(A)** Four-chamber view. **(B)** Short-axis view.

Characterization of Cardiac Tumors

CMR can be used to accurately predict the tissue type of common cardiac masses using a battery of pulse sequences that include cine SSFP imaging, T1- and T2-weighted black blood imaging, myocardial perfusion, and LGE imaging.[13] In addition to tissue characterization, CMR also provides a 3D assessment of the extent and size of the mass, and its relationship with surrounding structures, which is critical in surgical planning prior to resection.

Lymphatic Imaging

An emerging area of study in patients with CHD is the use of MRI to evaluate the lymphatic system. Patients with single ventricle physiology are known to have lymphatic complications. Non-invasive imaging techniques using T2-weighted pulse sequences can demonstrate areas of lymphatic leak and signal within the neck and thorax (Fig. 10.9). Such an evaluation has been shown to be related to clinical outcomes.[16] A more dynamic assessment of the lymphatic system can be performed using a dynamic contrast-enhanced magnetic resonance lymphangiogram (DCMRL), after direct injection of GBCA directly into an inguinal lymph node. DCMRL can help guide transcatheter treatment of serious lymphatic complications such as persistent chylous pleural and pericardial effusions, and protein-losing enteropathy in patients with single ventricular physiology.

Contraindications and Safety

There are no known deleterious biologic effects caused by the static magnetic fields used in clinical MRI scanners. Nevertheless, safety rules must be strictly observed in the MRI suite to prevent injury related to movement or heating

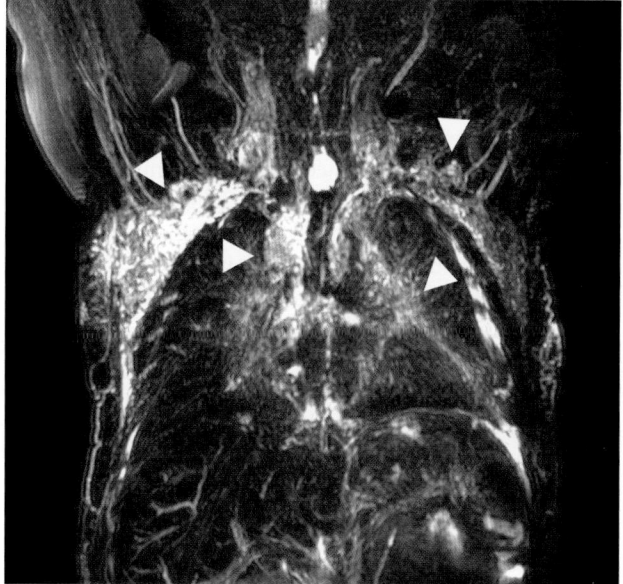

• **Fig. 10.9** T2-weighted lymphatic imaging in a 10-month-old male with hypoplastic left heart syndrome who underwent single ventricle palliation through Glenn circulation but developed functionally failing Glenn circulation with high pulmonary vascular resistance, minimal antegrade pulmonary blood flow, severe decompressing venovenous collateral burden, and significant aortopulmonary collateral burden. T2W signal (indicative of lymphatic leak, *solid arrows*) is noted in the bilateral supraclavicular region (extending laterally), in the mediastinum, and in the interstitium of the lungs.

of ferromagnetic objects. Patients and any accompanying individuals should be carefully screened for ferromagnetic objects or medical devices before entering the MRI suite.

Electronic devices such as pacemakers and implanted defibrillators can malfunction in the MRI environment, although several newer pacemakers are MR compatible under certain conditions. Fortunately, most implants used in patients with heart disease (e.g., sternal wires, heart valves, stents, and occluding devices and coils) are not considered a contraindication to MRI, although they may cause imaging artifacts in their vicinity. Information regarding the safety of individual devices can be determined either by consulting a published source on MRI safety or by contacting the manufacturer.

Sedation and Anesthesia

CMR examinations are inherently slow and acquisition of high-quality images requires the patient to lie still in the scanner for 60–90 minutes. In general, patients younger than 8 years are unable to cooperate with a typical CMR examination and require administration of general anesthesia. General anesthesia is safe when performed by experienced practitioners and has the added benefit of the ability to suspend respiration during image acquisition.

Cardiac Computed Tomography

Although CT technology has been available for several decades, its use in cardiac imaging, especially in children, was initially limited due to risk of exposure to high radiation doses and image blurring due to cardiac and respiratory motion. However, CT technology has witnessed a remarkably rapid evolution in recent years, with marked improvement in image quality related to higher temporal resolution, shorter scan times, and marked reduction in radiation doses. This has made cardiac CT (CCT) an attractive imaging modality in pediatric patients with CHD. It serves a complementary role to echocardiography and CMR. It is able to provide high spatial resolution angiography of cardiac and extracardiac structures along with additional diagnostic information regarding parenchymal lung disease. With modern scanners, scan duration is short and therefore sedation is not necessary in most cases.

Technical Aspects of CCT

CT uses rapidly rotating x-ray beams and detectors to create an image. The photons that are not absorbed by the tissue pass into multiple detectors in the scanner's gantry and are converted into digital signals, which are then combined by a computer program to form a cross-sectional image. Modern dual-source scanners have two sets of two x-ray tubes and detector arrays. This requires only a one-fourth rotation of the gantry to create an image, thereby reducing scan time.

Radiation Dose

Radiation exposure varies linearly with the x-ray tube current (mAs) and has a squared relationship with the voltage peak (KVp). Therefore, modern scanners minimize radiation exposure by scanning at lower KVp (70–80 KV) and

higher mAs, thereby maintaining image quality at markedly lower radiation doses. Many vendors provide automatic control of these parameters to create images of prespecified quality. Radiation doses delivered to the patient is expressed as the dose-length product (mGy-cm) which is used to calculate effective radiation doses (mSv) using standardized age- and organ-specific tables. Modern third-generation dual-source scanners are able to provide image quality equivalent to scanners from a decade ago using radiation doses that are 5–10 times lower. Although the acquired data has a high degree of noise due to lower radiation exposure, model-based iterative reconstruction techniques help improve the signal-to-noise ratio to create high-quality images.

CCT Scan Modes

Several types of CCT scans are available on modern scanners (Fig. 10.10). The type of scan is chosen based on the clinical question and the patient's age, heart rate, and breath-holding ability.

Highly Accelerated Scan

This scan type acquires images of the entire chest within 200–500 milliseconds and is the default scan mode on modern third-generation dual-source scanners, as it freezes most cardiac and respiratory motion and uses the lowest radiation dose. CT vendors use different techniques for this type of scan. The most common technique is a high-pitch spiral scan. Pitch is the distance the table travels during one 360-degree gantry rotation of the CT scanner divided by the total thickness of the slices acquired. As such, it allows for the acquisition of the entire heart within a single cardiac cycle, by using rapid table movement during a single gantry rotation. Other scanners utilize a larger detector that acquires images of the entire heart with a single gantry rotation without table movement. This scan provides a single set of static images of the chest, and cine imaging is not possible. As respiratory and cardiac motion is minimized by the speed of imaging, most children do not require sedation or anesthesia, except for coronary artery imaging. The scan can be performed with or without ECG triggering. ECG triggering is not necessary for most applications except coronary artery imaging. Scans can be triggered either in systole or diastole. For most applications, this scan is insensitive to heart rate, but for coronary artery imaging, heart rates below 70–75 beats/minute are essential.

Prospectively Gated Sequential Axial Scan

This scan acquires 2–5 sets of sequential axial images using a single gantry rotation at each station, with table movement between each axial set to move to the next station (also known as a step-and-shoot scan). The image sets are then fused seamlessly prior to image reconstruction to create a single CT dataset. This scan allows the acquisition of multiple prespecified cardiac phases within any portion of the cardiac cycle. Therefore, this scan is most useful for coronary artery imaging when the heart rate is too rapid for the highly accelerated scan. With faster heart rates, the ability to

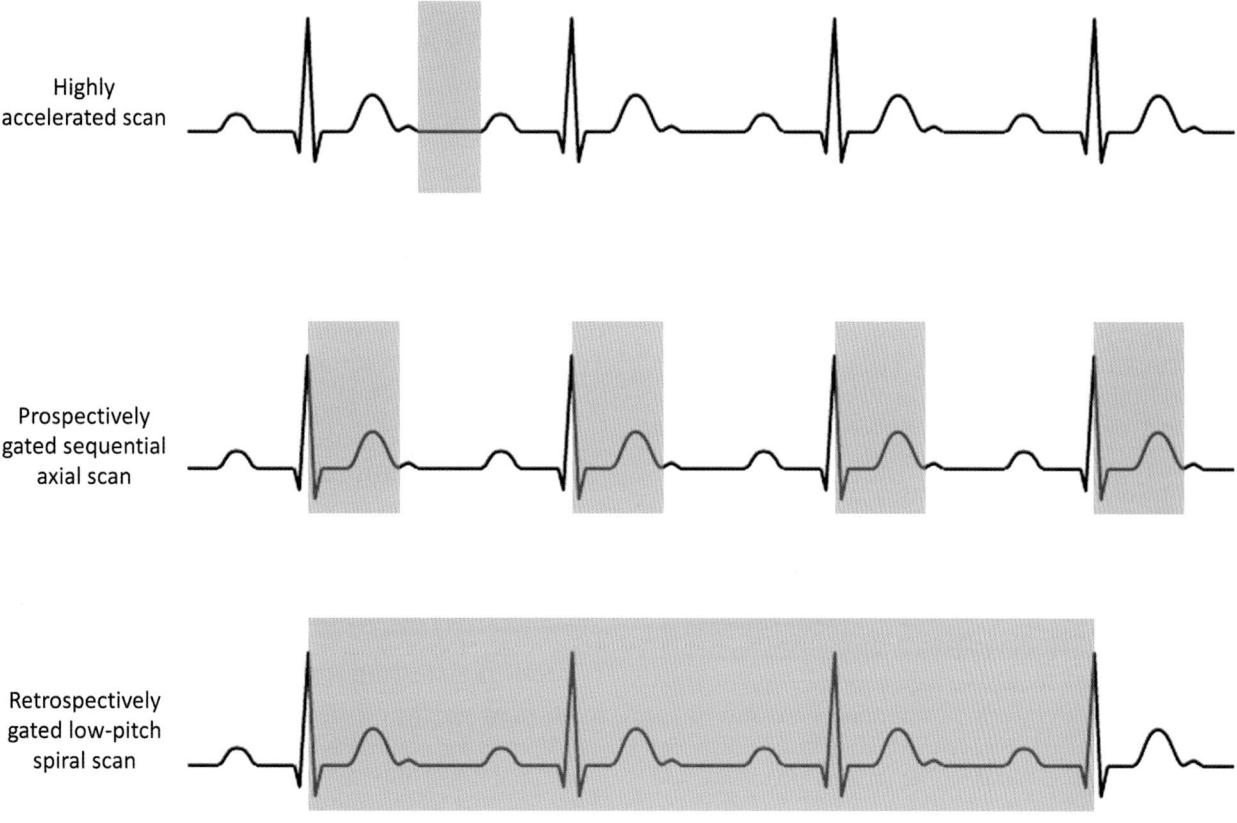

Highly
accelerated scan

Prospectively
gated sequential
axial scan

Retrospectively
gated low-pitch
spiral scan

• **Fig. 10.10** Three CCT scan modes are shown with blue-gray highlighting representing when imaging is being performed during the cardiac cycle. A highly accelerated mode captures a frozen image of the heart over a fraction of a second and is the lowest radiation dose of all the scan modes shown. In a prospectively gated sequential axial scan, sets of images are acquired with each heart beat at different anatomic locations and then fused to make the final image. A retrospectively gated low-pitch spiral scan captures data continuously over multiple cardiac cycles, then reconstructs the image retrospectively using ECG gating. A retrospectively gated scan can also utilize dose modulation in which lower radiation is used for most of the cardiac cycle and the full dose is reserved for a specific cardiac phase.

acquire multiple cardiac phases allows high-quality imaging of the coronary arteries. The radiation doses for this type of scan are higher than those for the highly accelerated scan, but lower than retrospectively gated scans. As this scan needs 3–8 seconds for image acquisition, breath holding is essential to avoid misregistration between the various axial stations. Therefore, younger children scanned using this mode require general anesthesia with breath holding. ECG gating is also essential for this scan type.

Retrospectively Gated Low-Pitch Spiral Scan

This is the oldest type of CCT scan and is available on all current CT scanners. The region of interest is scanned continuously during slow table movement and multiple cardiac phases are reconstructed retrospectively using ECG gating. On modern scanners, ECG dose modulation is available, such that highest radiation dose can be restricted to a certain portion of the cardiac cycle, typically diastole, with a lower radiation dose at all other time points within the cardiac cycle. This scan provides images throughout the cardiac cycle; therefore, cine images can be

created to quantify ventricular function. Multi-phase imaging is also useful in coronary artery imaging in patients with rapid heart rates. Due to the longer duration of this scan (3–6 seconds), breath holding is essential and therefore younger children require general anesthesia. ECG gating is also essential for this scan. This scan type delivers the highest radiation doses and should be used only when absolutely necessary.

Contrast Administration and Timing

Almost all CCT scans in patients with CHD require administration of iodinated contrast to visualize intravascular structures. Rapid contrast infusion using a large-bore intravenous line is essential to achieve high contrast concentration to achieve desired image quality. Iodinated contrast can be nephrotoxic and a clinical assessment of renal status is essential prior to administration. When renal status is questionable or impaired, serum blood urea nitrogen and creatinine levels should be obtained. In patients with impaired renal status, risk of kidney injury can be mitigated in select patients with prehydration.

Contrast Dose, Injection Protocol, and Injection Rate

Most CCT scans use 1 mL/kg of contrast. Higher doses (up to 2 mL/kg) are used for small infants and when a venous phase of imaging is needed (such as in patients with Fontan circulation). Contrast is usually injected using an automated power injector that allows for precise injection rates. Injection rate is typically adjusted to achieve a 7- to 10-second contrast injection. This allows for minor errors in contrast timing while providing high contrast concentrations in the region of interest. Typically, full-strength contrast injection is followed by injection of an equal volume of saline to flush the intravenous line and venous system of contrast (biphasic injection). In situations where both the left and right sides of the heart need to be opacified with contrast, such as for the assessment of ventricular function, a triphasic injection can be used. A triphasic injection uses full-strength contrast, followed by equal volume of half-strength contrast, followed by saline.

Contrast Timing

Since scan duration is short on most modern scanners, precise contrast timing to achieve high contrast concentration within the region of interest at the time of the scan is essential. Several available timing methods provide equivalent results and are chosen based on the imager's preference and institutional workflow.

Test Bolus. The passage of a small amount (0.3 ml/kg) of contrast is tracked through a single slice of the heart for 10–15 seconds after administration. Following this acquisition, image intensity (HU) at the region of interest is quantitatively analyzed to obtain the time to peak contrast concentration within the region. A further delay equal to 1/2 to 2/3 of the duration of contrast injection is added to this timing to correct the scan delay for the actual CCT acquisition. Although this method provides the most precise timing, results can be unsatisfactory if the heart rate changes significantly between the test bolus and final scan.

Bolus Tracking. The full dose of contrast is administered and image intensity at a prespecified location within the heart is monitored until a prespecified image intensity level (HU) triggers the CCT scan, followed by an additional delay equal to half the contrast duration (to a maximum of 6–7 seconds). This method minimizes contrast dose as a test bolus is eliminated. It is also resistant to changes in heart rate during acquisition and provides a more rapid workflow.

Manual Triggering. This method is similar to bolus tracking, but triggering is performed manually when contrast is visualized within the region of interest.

Special Considerations for Coronary CCT

Coronary CCT is particularly technically challenging as the coronary arteries are small and move rapidly during the cardiac cycle. Successful imaging relies on timing the acquisition during a phase of the cardiac cycle when the coronary arteries are "resting." Coronary CCT typically acquires images during of one of two rest periods within the cardiac cycle. The mid-diastolic rest period is longest at low heart rates, but the longest rest period shifts to end-systole when the heart rate is > 80 beats/minute. In addition, the highly accelerated scan mode can only be used for coronary CCT to acquire the mid-diastolic rest period when the heart rate is < 75 beats/minute. For these reasons, it is important to measure the heart rate upon arrival and administer a beta-blocker (oral metoprolol 1–2 mg/kg) if the heart rate is > 70 beats/minute. The scan is typically performed 1 hour after beta-blocker administration, when the effect of metoprolol peaks. In addition, administration of sublingual nitroglycerin 1–3 minutes prior to the scan facilitates visualization of the coronary arteries. In patients under general anesthesia, continuous intravenous infusions of esmolol and nitroglycerin can be used.

Clinical Applications of CCT

In recent years, several applications for CCT in children and adults with CHD have emerged and it has been demonstrated to be a reliable and accurate complement to other imaging techniques such as echocardiography and CMR.[17-19]

Coronary Artery Imaging

Due to its excellent spatial resolution, CCT is particularly well suited for noninvasive coronary angiography and has a well-established role in the assessment of atherosclerotic coronary artery disease in the adult population. Newer technical advances including a higher temporal resolution and lower radiation exposure have expanded applications to the pediatric population. Coronary CCT is rapidly becoming the standard of care for the evaluation of a wide variety of coronary abnormalities including congenital coronary artery anomalies, large coronary artery aneurysms after Kawasaki disease, coronary artery fistulae, and coronary artery origins and courses in the setting of complex CHD. In patients with anomalous aortic origin of a coronary artery, CCT imaging is useful in surgical planning and CCT features have been well validated against surgical findings (Fig. 10.11).[20,21] In patients with giant coronary artery aneurysms after Kawasaki disease, CCT can be used as a noninvasive alternate to conventional angiography for surveillance and to identify stenosis and thrombosis formation.[22] In complex CHDs where coronary anatomy is crucial to surgical or transcatheter treatment, CCT can be useful in delineating coronary artery anatomy when echocardiography is inconclusive. After surgical or transcatheter interventions, CCT can be useful for initial noninvasive evaluation when coronary artery injury or compression is suspected.

Extracardiac Vascular Abnormalities

CT is particularly well suited for the assessment of extracardiac vascular abnormalities involving the aortic arch and its branches, pulmonary and systemic veins, and the pulmonary arterial tree. This can be useful in patients in whom echocardiographic evaluation is insufficient or inconclusive. In addition, it can avoid the need for diagnostic catheterization. For example, CCT can be useful in initial evaluation

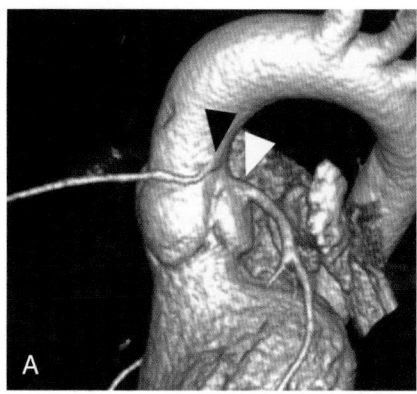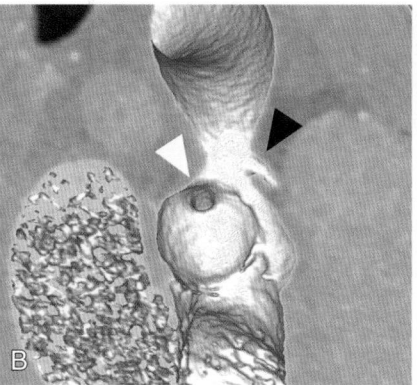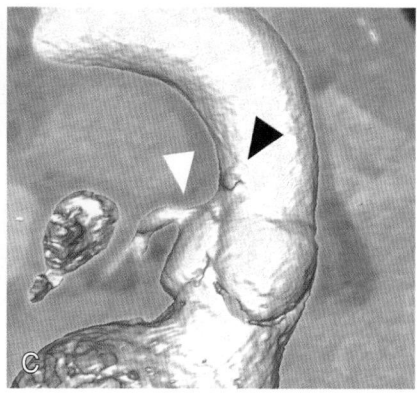

• **Fig. 10.11** Coronary computed tomography in a 6-year-old male with an anomalous aortic origin of the right coronary artery from the ascending aorta. **(A)** A 3D volume rendered image of the left main coronary artery *(white arrow)* and the right coronary artery *(black arrow)*. **(B)** Endoluminal view with the left main coronary artery origin *(white arrow)* shown *en face* and the right coronary artery origin *(black arrow)* shown in long axis. **(C)** Endoluminal view with the left main coronary artery origin *(white arrow)* shown in long axis and the right coronary artery origin *(black arrow)* shown *en face*.

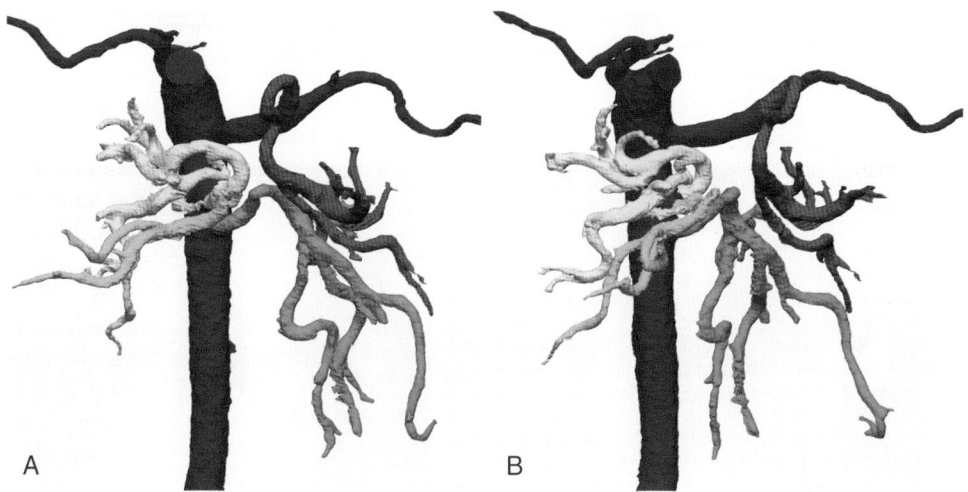

• **Fig. 10.12** Images of an 11-day-old male with tetralogy of Fallot with pulmonary atresia and a right aortic arch with aberrant left subclavian artery. Four major aortopulmonary collateral arteries (MAPCAs) were visualized. The image was segmented in Mimics (Materialize NV, Leuven, Belgium) and, to better demonstrate the anatomy, the vessels were color coded. The ascending aorta and anterior aspect of the aortic arch were removed to improve visualization of the MAPCAs. The superior-most MAPCA arises from the aberrant left subclavian artery, while all other MAPCAs arise from the thoracic descending aorta. Two MAPCAs course to the right lung and two course to the left lung. **(A)** A view facing from anterior to posterior. **(B)** A right oblique view.

of newborns with tetralogy of Fallot with pulmonary atresia and multiple aorticopulmonary collateral arteries (MAPCAs; Fig. 10.12). In addition, CCT can complement echocardiographic evaluation of newborns with complex CHD when aspects of the extracardiac anatomy are not fully delineated by echocardiography.[19]

Planning of Catheter-Based Interventions

CCT imaging is being increasingly used to plan catheter interventions. In newborns with ductal dependent pulmonary circulation, CCT can help plan ductal stenting by delineating the length and course of the ductus, especially in infants with a tortuous ductus (Fig. 10.13).[23] During interventional procedures in patients referred for complex CHD, CCT images can provide a 3D roadmap for the interventionalist, which can be superimposed on the fluoroscopic images. This can help reduce contrast and radiation doses (useful in cases where multiple dilations are necessary such as complex pulmonary artery or pulmonary vein disease). Prior to transcatheter pulmonary valve replacement, especially in the presence of a native outflow tract, CCT is crucial in assessing feasibility related to device fit and possible compression of adjacent coronary arteries. Similarly, CCT is an essential prerequisite to transcatheter aortic and mitral valve replacement in order to assess feasibility and risk of complications.[24] For electrophysiologic procedures,

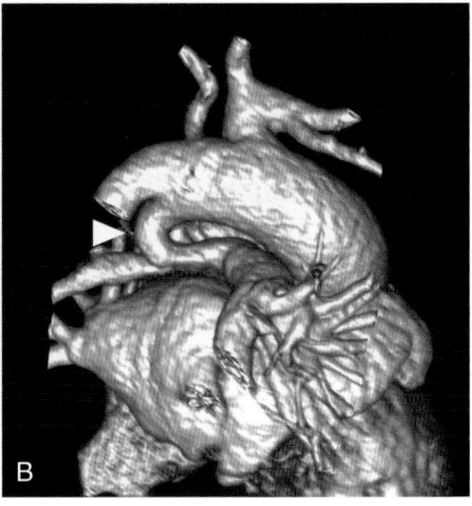

• **Fig. 10.13** Images from a 10-month-old female with dextrocardia, {I,D,D} transposition of the great arteries, pulmonary atresia, a large conoventricular septal defect, and a left aortic arch with a common origin of the right brachiocephalic and left common carotid arteries. Pulmonary blood flow was supplied solely by a patent ductus arteriosus (PDA, *white arrow*). **(A)** A lateral oblique image of the PDA as it arises from the aorta and inserts into the pulmonary arteries. The PDA origin in relation to the arch branches is appreciated. **(B)** A 3D volume rendered image of the PDA as it inserts into the pulmonary arteries. The descending aorta was removed from this image to improve visualization of the PDA.

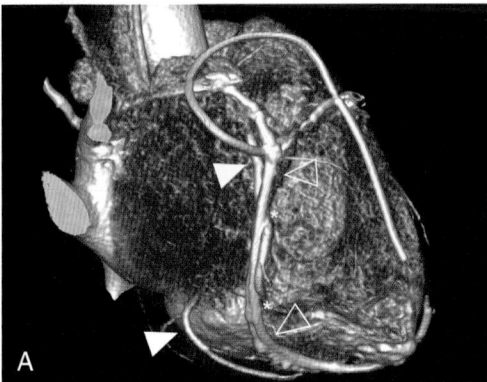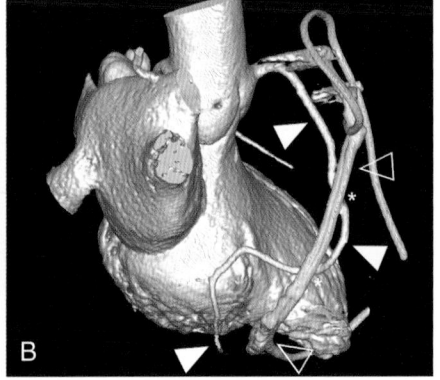

• **Fig. 10.14** Images from a 13-year-old male with complete heart block secondary to maternal lupus for which an epicardial pacemaker was placed. The patient has normal coronary artery origins and a right dominant coronary artery system. Epicardial leads *(hollow arrows)* course into the right atrioventricular grove and come into direct contact with the right coronary artery *(solid arrows)* in two locations *(*)*. These findings are concerning for coronary artery compression. **(A)** A 3D volume rendered image from the right lateral view. **(B)** A 3D volume rendered image from the right posterior view, after the right-sided cardiac structures have been removed.

CCT images can be beneficial by providing an anatomic overlay on the electrical map during ablation procedures.

Ventricular Function

CT can serve as an adjunct to other imaging modalities for the assessment of ventricular function. Patients who use CT for this indication typically have suboptimal visualization of the ventricles with other modalities or contraindication to cardiac MRI. Examples of such scenarios include patients with poor echocardiographic windows, significant device-related artifact on cardiac MRI, or patients with safety concerns for cardiac MRI (such as active epicardial pacemakers, Video 10.4).

CT in Patients with Pacemakers and Implantable Cardiac Defibrillators

CCT has an expanding role in the population of patients with pacemakers and implantable cardiac defibrillators. As these patients do not often undergo cardiac MRIs due to safety concerns, CCT provides a mechanism by which ventricular function can be assessed. Furthermore, CCT is particularly well suited for the identification of rare but serious adverse device-related complications, such as coronary artery compression by epicardial pacemaker leads (Fig. 10.14).[25]

References

1. Ridgway JP. Cardiovascular magnetic resonance physics for clinicians: part I. *J Cardiovasc Magn Reson*. 2010;12:71.

2. Biglands JD, Radjenovic A, Ridgway JP. Cardiovascular magnetic resonance physics for clinicians: part II. *J Cardiovasc Magn Reson*. 2012;14:66.

3. Moghari MH, Geva T, Powell AJ. Prospective heart tracking for whole-heart magnetic resonance angiography. *Magn Reson Med*. 2017;77:759-765.

4. Woolen SA, Shankar PR, Gagnier JJ, MacEachern MP, Singer L, Davenport MS. Risk of nephrogenic systemic fibrosis in patients with stage 4 or 5 chronic kidney disease receiving a group II gadolinium-based contrast agent: a systematic review and meta-analysis. *JAMA Intern Med*. 2020;180:223-230.

5. Nguyen KL, Yoshida T, Kathuria-Prakash N, et al. Multicenter safety and practice for off-label diagnostic use of ferumoxytol in MRI. *Radiology*. 2019;293(3):554-564.

6. Pattynama PM, Lamb HJ, Van der Velde EA, Van der Geest RJ, Van der Wall EE, De Roos A. Reproducibility of MRI-derived measurements of right ventricular volumes and myocardial mass. *Magn Reson Imaging*. 1995;13:53-63.

7. Fratz S, Chung T, Greil GF, et al. Guidelines and protocols for cardiovascular magnetic resonance in children and adults with congenital heart disease: SCMR expert consensus group on congenital heart disease. *J Cardiovasc Magn Reson*. 2013;15:51.

8. Iwamoto Y, Inage A, Tomlinson G, et al. Direct measurement of aortic regurgitation with phase-contrast magnetic resonance is inaccurate: proposal of an alternative method of quantification. *Pediatr Radiol*. 2014;44:1358-1369.

9. Powell AJ, Tsai-Goodman B, Prakash A, Greil GF, Geva T. Comparison between phase-velocity cine magnetic resonance imaging and invasive oximetry for quantification of atrial shunts. *Am J Cardiol*. 2003;91:1523-1525, A9.

10. Whitehead KK, Gillespie MJ, Harris MA, Fogel MA, Rome JJ. Noninvasive quantification of systemic-to-pulmonary collateral flow: a major source of inefficiency in patients with superior cavopulmonary connections. *Circ Cardiovasc Imaging*. 2009;2: 405-411.

11. Doan TT, Molossi S, Sachdeva S, et al. Dobutamine stress cardiac MRI is safe and feasible in pediatric patients with anomalous aortic origin of a coronary artery (AAOCA). *Int J Cardiol*. 2021;334:42-48.

12. Kellman P, Arai AE, McVeigh ER, Aletras AH. Phase-sensitive inversion recovery for detecting myocardial infarction using gadolinium-delayed hyperenhancement. *Magn Reson Med*. 2002;47:372-383.

13. Beroukhim RS, Prakash A, Buechel ERV, et al. Characterization of cardiac tumors in children by cardiovascular magnetic resonance imaging: a multicenter experience. *J Am Coll Cardiol*. 2011;58:1044-1054.

14. Flett AS, Hayward MP, Ashworth MT, et al. Equilibrium contrast cardiovascular magnetic resonance for the measurement of diffuse myocardial fibrosis: preliminary validation in humans. *Circulation*. 2010;122:138-144.

15. Ferreira VM, Schulz-Menger J, Holmvang G, et al. Cardiovascular magnetic resonance in nonischemic myocardial inflammation: expert recommendations. *J Am Coll Cardiol*. 2018;72:3158-3176.

16. Biko DM, DeWitt AG, Pinto EM, et al. MRI evaluation of lymphatic abnormalities in the neck and thorax after Fontan surgery: relationship with outcome. *Radiology*. 2019;291:774-780.

17. Han BK, Rigsby CK, Hlavacek A, et al. Computed tomography imaging in patients with congenital heart disease part I: rationale and utility. an expert consensus document of the Society of Cardiovascular Computed Tomography (SCCT): Endorsed by the Society of Pediatric Radiology (SPR) and the North American Society of Cardiac Imaging (NASCI). *J Cardiovasc Comput Tomogr*. 2015;9:475-492.

18. Han BK, Rigsby CK, Leipsic J, et al. Computed tomography imaging in patients with congenital heart disease, part 2: technical recommendations. an expert consensus document of the Society of Cardiovascular Computed Tomography (SCCT): Endorsed by the Society of Pediatric Radiology (SPR) and the North American Society of Cardiac Imaging (NASCI). *J Cardiovasc Comput Tomogr*. 2015;9:493-513.

19. Saengsin K, Pickard SS, Prakash A. Utility of cardiac CT in infants with congenital heart disease: diagnostic performance and impact on management. *J Cardiovasc Comput Tomogr*. 2022; 16:345-349.

20. Krishnamurthy R, Masand PM, Jadhav SP, et al. Accuracy of computed tomography angiography and structured reporting of high-risk morphology in anomalous aortic origin of coronary artery: comparison with surgery. *Pediatr Radiol*. 2021;51: 1299-1310.

21. Jegatheeswaran A, Devlin PJ, McCrindle BW, et al. Features associated with myocardial ischemia in anomalous aortic origin of a coronary artery: A Congenital Heart Surgeons' Society study. *J Thorac Cardiovasc Surg*. 2019;158:822-834.

22. Gellis L, Castellanos DA, Oduor R, et al. Comparison of coronary artery measurements between echocardiograms and cardiac CT in Kawasaki disease patients with aneurysms. *J Cardiovasc Comput Tomogr*. 2022;16:43-50.

23. Arar Y, Dimas VV, Nugent AW, et al. Pre-procedural CT imaging aids neonatal PDA stenting for ductal-dependent pulmonary blood flow with reduction in overall procedural morbidity. *Cardiol Young*. 2022;32:1401-1406.

24. Maschietto N, Prakash A, Del Nido P, Porras D. Acute and short-term outcomes of percutaneous transcatheter mitral valve replacement in children. *Circ Cardiovasc Interv*. 2021;14:e009996.

25. Mah DY, Prakash A, Porras D, Fynn-Thompson F, DeWitt ES, Banka P. Coronary artery compression from epicardial leads: more common than we think. *Heart Rhythm*. 2018;15:1439-1447.

11

Assessment of Myocardial Performance

STEVEN D. COLAN AND MING HUI CHEN

KEY LEARNING POINTS

- The primary myocardial properties of contractility, relaxation, and compliance are important determinates of myocardial and ventricular function, but are difficult to measure in the intact circulation. Consequently, current clinical management is primarily driven by measures of global ventricular function, which depend on afterload, preload, contractility, ventricular configuration and interaction, and synchrony of contraction.
- Diastolic ventricular function remains a major challenge for routine clinical management due to the need for measurement of diastolic ventricular pressure, often necessitating cardiac catheterization. Indirect measures of myocardial relaxation and compliance are in routine clinical use but have limited diagnostic accuracy.

- Ventricular torsion is an important mechanical determinant of ventricular performance that is underappreciated, at least in part because of challenges in measurement. Understanding torsion requires insight into myocardial fiber orientation and explains how a 65% ejection fraction can be generated by a mere 10% systolic reduction in the length of the individual sarcomeres.
- The cardiac response to exercise is poorly predicted by resting measurements of ventricular function but is a critical determinant of symptom status and quality of life. Exercise testing and exercise stress-echocardiography have developed into increasingly important tools for the assessment of cardiovascular health.

Introduction

Cardiac ventricular function represents the summation of pump function and muscle function. As a pump, the heart accepts blood at venous pressure and delivers that volume at arterial pressure, providing the force that distributes flow throughout the body. Extracardiac control of the pump function of the heart is mediated by reflex renal, vascular, and hormonal control systems that adjust pump function by influencing arterial and venous tone, heart rate, and contractility. The pump function also relies on the mechanical behavior of the cardiac musculature, which is influenced by preload, afterload, and contractility, and the health of the cardiac muscle can only be assessed through an evaluation of the complex interplay of these three determinants of myocyte fiber shortening. This dual perspective of the heart as a pump and the heart as a muscle is one of the most important aspects of cardiovascular physiology. For example, impaired myocardial function that results in inadequate blood pressure will activate a host of reflexes mediated by the neuroendocrine axis, resulting in systemic vasoconstriction that elevates systemic vascular resistance. The resulting increase in

afterload further impairs myocardial performance, leading to an adverse positive feedback loop. Pharmacologic manipulation of the pump function of the heart has proven to be one of the most fruitful therapeutic approaches to myocardial dysfunction, as reflected in the success of pharmacologic manipulation of the renin-angiotensin system and sympathetic nervous system for therapy of heart failure. Nevertheless, the function of the heart as a muscle is the primary determinant of ultimate outcomes, and the focus of this chapter is to discuss the physiology of the heart as a muscle, and the manner in which this muscular function interacts with the external forces imposed on the myocardium through filling pressure and impedance to ejection. The first section of this chapter discusses the physiology of myocardial fiber shortening and the relationship between fiber shortening and ventricular performance. The second section discusses several of the more important methods of evaluating myocardial systolic and diastolic properties and how these relate to ventricular function. This chapter represents an abbreviated and updated discussion of this topic that was previously presented in more detail as Chapter 15 of the second edition of this textbook.[1]

Preliminary Considerations

Terminology

The terminology used to describe ventricular and myocardial function relies in large part on terminology borrowed from disciplines such as mechanical engineering and is often used by cardiologists in a conceptual but inexact fashion. In general, physiologists attach a relatively restricted and specific meaning to terms that clinicians use in a broader, more inclusive sense. For example, the term "compliance" has a very specific definition in mechanical engineering terms referring to the change in volume per unit of applied force, but is frequently used in a more conceptual fashion in medicine, for example in reference to whether patients cooperate with a therapeutic regimen. To avoid confusion, the specific meanings of a number of these terms as used in this chapter in reference to **myocardial mechanics** are provided here. **Ventricular function or performance** refers to ejection (systolic ventricular ejection) and filling (diastolic ventricular filling). **Myocardial function or performance** is in turn used to refer to myocardial fiber shortening (systolic myocardial function) and lengthening (diastolic myocardial function). **Myocardial or ventricular mechanics** refers to the mechanical or physical properties and behavior of the myocardium or ventricle, and is used to distinguish this behavior from chemical, electrical, hormonal, and other properties. With reference to the myocardium, **strain** refers to the change in fiber length from the basal (relaxed) state. Because of this frame of reference, shortening is negative strain and elongation is positive strain. **Strain rate** is the amount of negative or positive strain per unit time. **Wall stress** is the force per unit area that causes myofibrillar lengthening (positive strain, diastolic strain) or myofibrillar shortening (negative strain, systolic strain). **Compliance** is displacement per unit of applied force. **Ventricular compliance** is calculated as change in volume per unit change in pressure. **Myocardial compliance** is the magnitude of strain induced by a specific stress, and **elastance** is the reciprocal of compliance.

Myocardial Versus Ventricular Mechanics

Myocardial mechanics are but one of the determinants of ventricular mechanics. Ventricular mechanics determine the amount of blood pumped during each cardiac cycle and the pressure at which the ventricle operates. Although common clinical practice is to equate myocardial and ventricular performance, the two are not equivalent because the mechanical behavior of the ventricle is highly dependent on myocardial synchrony, ventricular geometry, interventricular interaction, pericardial constraint, and other confounders. Determining the health of the myocardium is therefore dependent in large part on our ability to independently assess its properties, regardless of the behavior of the ventricle. Unfortunately, myocardial properties are generally not directly measurable but instead are derived from measurement of ventricular properties. This important issue accounts for much of the complexity associated with assessment of myocardial mechanics. The phases of the electrical and mechanical events during systole and diastole for the left ventricle are depicted in Fig. 11.1.

Systolic Myocardial and Ventricular Mechanics

Preload, afterload, and contractility are widely understood to be the determinants of the magnitude of fiber shortening. Although these terms are generally used in a conceptual fashion, the precise meaning of these terms reveals the potential shortcomings of the clinical methods of assessing loading conditions and contractility. Furthermore, under *in vivo* circumstances these variables are highly interdependent, creating the need to comprehend both the clinical indices of preload, afterload, and contractility, as well as the nature of their interrelationships.

Studies From Isolated Cardiac Muscle

Isolated muscle preparations have contributed substantially to our understanding of muscle physiology, and much of the terminology in common use has derived from this early work.[2] The experimental model consisted of an excised papillary muscle attached at one end to a tensiometer and at the other end to a lever. The lever transmitted the force of contraction to the opposing end of the lever, which was attached to a pan where weights could be added, thereby altering the force resisting myocardial shortening. This model has the advantage of having a parallel orientation of the myofibers, which contrasts with the normal transmural variation in myofibril orientation in the ventricular wall where the epicardial fibers are usually positioned at a 90-degree angle relative to the endocardial fibers. Weights are added to the other end of the lever until the desired resting muscle length is achieved, following which a "stop" is placed to prevent further muscle elongation. Because this is the force to which the muscle is exposed prior to the onset of contraction, it is referred to as the "preload." After placement of the stop, additional weight is added to the pan but the muscle is not exposed to this force until after it begins to contract, and hence it is referred to as the "afterload." Initial force generation after activation is isometric until force generation exceeds that required to lift the pan (equivalent to the isovolumic systolic phase of the ventricle), following which myocardial shortening against the isotonic force ensues, raising the weight. The isotonic nature of the systolic shortening phase in this model is an important difference from the phasic variation in pressure that characterizes the systolic phase in the ventricle. This type of isolated muscle preparation[2,3] was the primary investigative tool for the evaluation of cardiac muscle physiology for many years, as reviewed by Braunwald and Ross.[3]

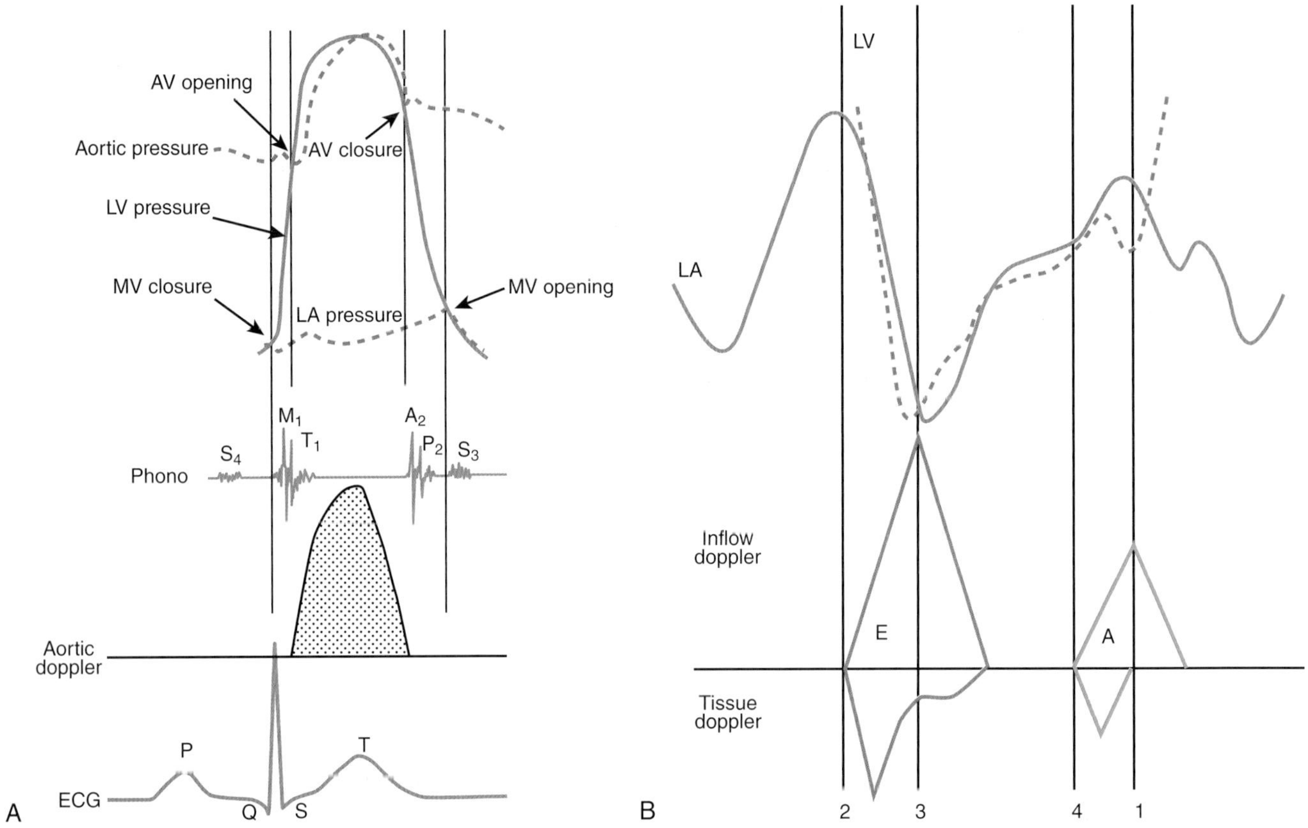

• **Fig. 11.1** Events in the systolic phase of the cardiac cycle. **(A)** The time interval between mitral closure and aortic valve opening constitutes the isovolumic contraction phase. The left ventricular ejection phase then begins and due to inertial forces continues to about 20 msec after ventricular pressure falls below aortic pressure, a time interval known as the left ventricular hang out interval. Progressive uptake of calcium into the sarcoplasmic reticulum leads to a fall in cytosolic calcium ion concentration and a higher percentage of myofibers enter the relaxation phase. After cessation of ejection, flow in the ascending aorta transiently reverses, closing the aortic valve. The abrupt cessation of retrograde flow in the aorta at the time of aortic valve closure creates a water-hammer effect in the aorta, accounting for the aortic component of the second heart sound. As force decay progresses, left ventricular pressure continues to fall until left atrial pressure exceeds ventricular pressure and the mitral valve opens. The time period from cessation of antegrade aortic flow until opening of the mitral valve is the isovolumic relaxation phase. *AV Closure,* time of aortic valve closure; *AV Opening,* time of aortic valve opening; *A2,* aortic component of second heart sound; *ECG,* electrocardiogram; *MV Closure,* time of mitral valve closure; *MV Opening,* time of mitral valve opening; *M1,* mitral component of first heart sound; *Phono,* phonocardiogram; *P2,* pulmonic component of second heart sound; *S3,* third heart sound; *S4,* fourth heart sound; *T1,* tricuspid component of first heart sound. **(B)** The interrelationships between the electrical and mechanical events during diastole for the left ventricle. Diastolic relaxation and elastic recoil of the compressed myocardium produce a period during which left ventricular pressure falls below atrial pressure, resulting in ventricular suction and augmenting the rate of early filling. Diastolic ventricular pressure rises until ventricular pressure exceeds atrial pressure (third VAPCP) which coincides with the peak velocity of the early diastolic inflow. During the deceleration phase of the early diastolic filling wave (E-wave), inflow continues due to blood inertia despite a negative pressure gradient between the left atrium and ventricle. A variable period of pressure equilibration and absence of flow during diastasis is followed by atrial activation and atrial pressure again exceeds ventricular pressure (fourth VAPCP) coincident with the atrial filling wave (A-wave). The cycle is completed when the peak velocity of the A-wave coincides with the first VAPCP when trans-mitral flow ceases, terminating the filling phase. *A,* Atrial component of mitral valve inflow Doppler; *E,* early component of mitral valve inflow Doppler; *Inflow Doppler,* Doppler tracing of mitral valve inflow; *LA,* left atrial pressure tracing; *LV,* left ventricular pressure tracing; *Tissue Doppler,* spectral Doppler recording of left ventricular lateral free wall tissue Doppler; *1, 2, 3, and 4,* the respective first, second, third, and fourth ventriculoatrial pressure crossover points.

Preload

This isolated muscle preparation defined many features of the mechanical behavior of cardiac muscle. For any fixed level of afterload, higher preload (stretching the muscle to a greater length) results in a greater magnitude and velocity of shortening, up to a sarcomere length of about 2.2 μ, after which further stretch leads to a fall in developed tension. The molecular explanation for this behavior is that stretching of the sarcomere increases the number of active sites between actin and myosin, leading to increased adenosine triphosphate (ATP) hydrolysis, increased rate of cross-bridge cycling, and increased tension development. The heart normally operates at sarcomere lengths of 1.8–2.0 μ; therefore, under normal circumstances there is some degree of "preload reserve" where an increase in sarcomere length results in an increase in tension development by the sarcomere. It is important to note that although the term "preload" implies a load or a force, at the molecular level the preload effect is actually mediated by sarcomeric length. Thus, at the myocardial level, preload is best defined as the *end-diastolic fiber length* (EDFL), a parameter that cannot be assessed in the intact heart.

The Frank–Starling Relationship

Observations by Otto Frank in isolated muscle preparations led him to conclude that the effects of "length and tension changes in skeletal muscle correspond to changes in volume and pressure in the heart." Subsequently, E.H. Starling observed that the mechanical energy generated by contracting muscle is a function of the length of the muscle fiber prior to onset of contraction, leading him to conclude that increased muscle length prior to the onset of contraction (within physiologic limits), leads to an increase in the number of interactions of actin and myosin that take place between the muscle filaments during contraction, augmenting the force of the contraction, a phenomenon known as the Frank–Starling mechanism. This property was confirmed when electron microscopy became available.

Clinical indices of Preload

At present, there is no clinically applicable method for measuring EDFL, leading to reliance on indirect indices of preload such as end-diastolic volume. End-diastolic volume has a relatively high predictive value for acute change in EDFL, but a poor predictive value when attempting to compare preload status between individuals or in the same individual over time. For example, an acute rise in end-diastolic volume usually, but not always, corresponds to an acute rise in EDFL, and therefore an acute rise in preload. However, the response is highly variable because the change in fiber length is dependent on the position on the nonlinear diastolic pressure-volume curve. The normal adaptation of the left ventricle to sustained changes in cardiac output is an increase or decrease in operant volume through the addition or removal of myofibers in series. This capacity for remodeling makes end-diastolic volume a poor index of preload between individuals and even in the same individual over time intervals of more than a few days. Reliance on end-diastolic volume as an index of preload has resulted in a number of clinically important misunderstandings. For example, because of the increased left ventricular size characteristic of lesions such as aortic regurgitation, it is often incorrectly assumed that preload is elevated. Although acute aortic regurgitation leads to a rise in EDFL, the chronic process of ventricular remodeling with the addition of myofibrils in series generally results in a return of preload (that is, EDFL) to normal.

The alternative preload indices in common use all rely on some measure of the force distending the ventricle rather than assessing the degree of distension. These include central venous pressure, left atrial pressure, left ventricular end-diastolic pressure, and end-diastolic wall stress. Of these, end-diastolic wall stress is the most direct measure of force exerted on the myofibers, but even this has a variable relationship to EDFL due to variation in ventricular compliance. Other potential confounders are pericardial constriction or tamponade physiology, or situations where diastolic interventricular interaction is increased, such as right ventricular volume overload.

The importance of abnormalities of preload in the evaluation of myocardial and ventricular performance primarily relates to the fashion in which it mimics contractility. Changes in preload or contractility have similar impacts on fiber shortening. Changes in preload are quite common and have been identified as the source of altered ventricular function in many clinical situations, including the acute fall in function after hemodialysis due to a fall in filling pressure and reduced systolic function due to reduced resting preload that is often seen in endurance athletes.[4] A particularly important clinical scenario is that of a patient who undergoes surgery for a volume overload lesion such as aortic regurgitation or ventricular septal defect and postoperatively the fall in preload results in an acute decrease in systolic ventricular function, potentially confounding detection of perioperative myocardial injury.

Afterload

As noted, in the isolated papillary muscle preparation, "afterload" refers to the load that is faced by the muscle after the onset of contraction, that is, it is the force resisting myofiber shortening. There is an inverse relationship between afterload and both the rate and extent of fiber shortening. Clinically, it is common practice to use hemodynamic variables such as arterial pressure and vascular resistance as indices of afterload. However, ultimately, when evaluating the heart as a muscle, we are interested in the behavior of individual myofibers. In the isolated muscle preparation described earlier, shortening is linear and afterload is represented by a weight on a lever. Because myocardium contains multiple muscle fibers, the afterload of the individual myofiber is represented by the proportion of the load it faces and is quantified as stress, the force per unit cross-sectional area. For the isolated muscle preparation, the stress is obtained as the afterload weight divided by the cross-sectional area of the papillary muscle and represents the force resisting shortening at the myofiber level. However, it is not possible to measure myocardial fiberstress *in situ* because of the impossibility of inserting a force gauge in series with the myofibers in the ventricular wall. Afterload, assessed as fiberstress, must therefore be calculated from secondary measures.

The individual myofibers are oriented circumferentially but at a variable angle with respect to the long axis of the left ventricle, depending on their position relative to the endocardium. Overall, myofiber contraction creates an inwardly, radially oriented force within the wall that elevates pressure within the cavity, a force that is at all points perpendicular to the cavity surface. The wall stress can be calculated based on the law of Laplace (tension = pressure $\times$ radius). For a thick-walled cylinder such as cardiac ventricle, the force is distributed across the wall thickness (h) and is therefore calculated as wall stress = (pressure $\times$ radius)/h. Since a cylindrical shape is a poor representation of the left ventricle, significant modifications to this basic relationship have been suggested to accommodate the complex geometry of the prolate ellipsoid shape that is characteristic of the left ventricle. Although there are differences in the absolute values obtained, the relative magnitude of the calculated stress is similar regardless of which formula is used.[5]

The cardiac cycle is a dynamic process that leads to cyclic variation in wall stress. Ventricular pressure, wall thickness, and radius of curvature are the determinants of stress and they undergo a predictable pattern of change, with ventricular radius falling and wall thickness rising while pressure rises and falls over the course of systole. The net result is that stress rises rapidly in early systole and peaks within the first 20% of ejection, followed by a nearly linear fall until aortic valve closure, following which there is an exponential fall during isovolumic diastole until mitral inflow begins (Fig. 11.2). There are several derived stress indices that have specific physiologic importance. Integrated systolic stress (the systolic force-time integral) is a primary determinant of myocardial oxygen consumption, reflecting the direct relationship between energy generation and oxygen consumption in the myocardium.[6] End-diastolic wall stress is a primary driver of eccentric hypertrophy (hypertrophy characterized by maintenance of a normal mass-volume ratio) that is characteristic of volume overload lesions and normal growth. A rise in diastolic wall stress stimulates the addition of new myofibers in series, increasing ventricular capacitance, thereby reducing end-diastolic stress in a servo mechanism feedback loop responding to both mechanical and hormonal components. Peak systolic stress is the primary determinant of concentric hypertrophy (an increase in the mass-to-volume and thickness-to-dimension ratios related

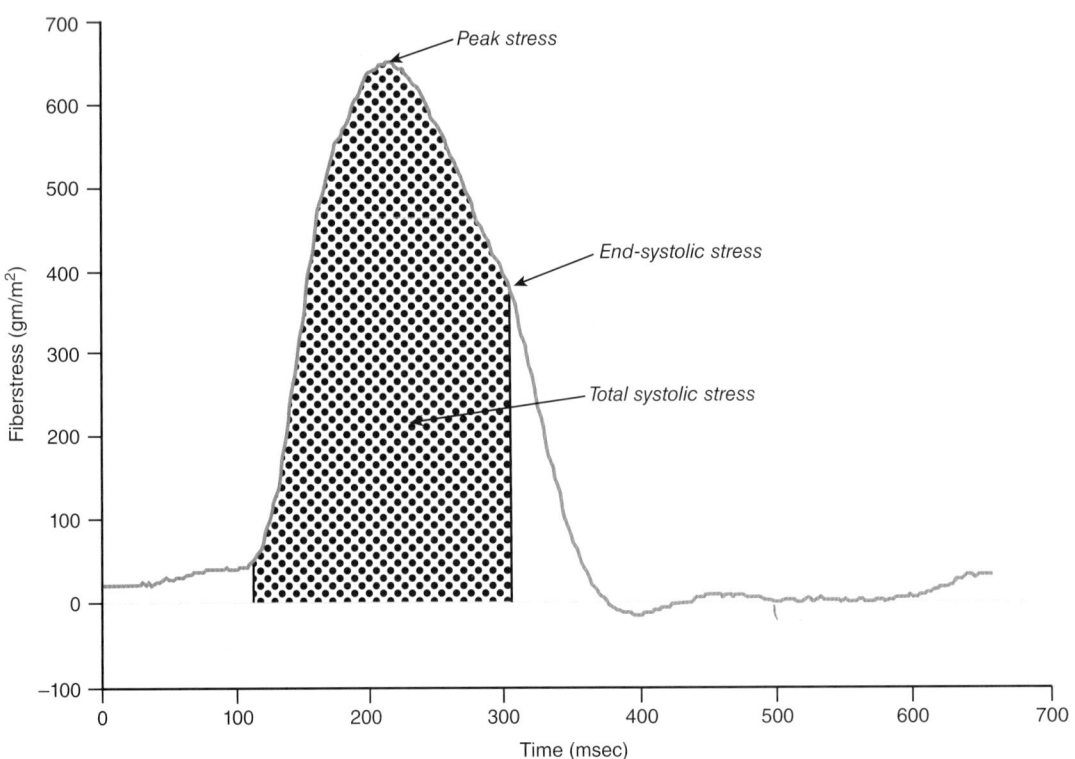

• **Fig. 11.2** Diagram of the time course of fiberstress over the course of the cardiac cycle. With onset of contraction (beginning of shaded area), stress rises rapidly and peaks early in the ejection phase. During the second two-thirds of ejection stress falls almost linearly until end-systole, when exponential force decay ensues. Depending on the magnitude of elastic recoil, stress may fall below zero in early diastole. During diastole, stress rises in a nonlinear fashion.

to addition of myofibers in parallel, as is characteristic of pressure overload lesions.

End-Systolic Fiberstress

End-systolic fiberstress is the primary determinant of the magnitude myocardial shortening, based on the end-systolic force-length relationship. This important property of myocardium has been the subject of extensive investigative work in isolated muscle and heart preparations, the results of which have wide implications with regard to myocardial mechanics. Perhaps the most important conclusion from this body of work is that for any constant contractile state, end-systolic pressure determines end-systolic volume regardless of events earlier in the cardiac cycle. An isolated heart experiment performed by Suga et al.[7] is particularly illustrative of this point. In isolated canine hearts, ventricular volume was controlled over the course of the cardiac cycle by a servo mechanism that permitted control over end-diastolic volume, end-systolic volume, and the time and rate of ventricular ejection, permitting the investigators control over the time course of ventricular pressure generation (Fig. 11.3). The experiment was conducted

with contractility held constant. The time course of the change in volume during systole was experimentally controlled to deviate substantially from beat-to-beat, although with the exception of Run III end-diastolic and end-systolic volume were constant. Because there were no acute changes in ventricular compliance, the constant end-diastolic volume resulted in a constant end-diastolic pressure, assuring that preload did not change over the course of the experiment. The net result was a preparation with constant preload, contractility, stroke volume, and ejection fraction, but variable wall stress over the course of ejection. Despite wide variation in wall stress at all points preceding end systole, as long as end-systolic volume was held constant, the end-systolic pressure also remained constant. The conclusion of this line of investigation was that when EDFL and myocardial contractility are held constant, end-systolic fiberstress is the sole determinant of the extent of systolic fiber shortening despite marked variation in peak, mean, and integrated fiberstress. Overall, the work done by this group of investigators demonstrated that: (1) integrated systolic fiberstress is an important determinant of myocardial oxygen consumption, (2) peak fiberstress is the most important

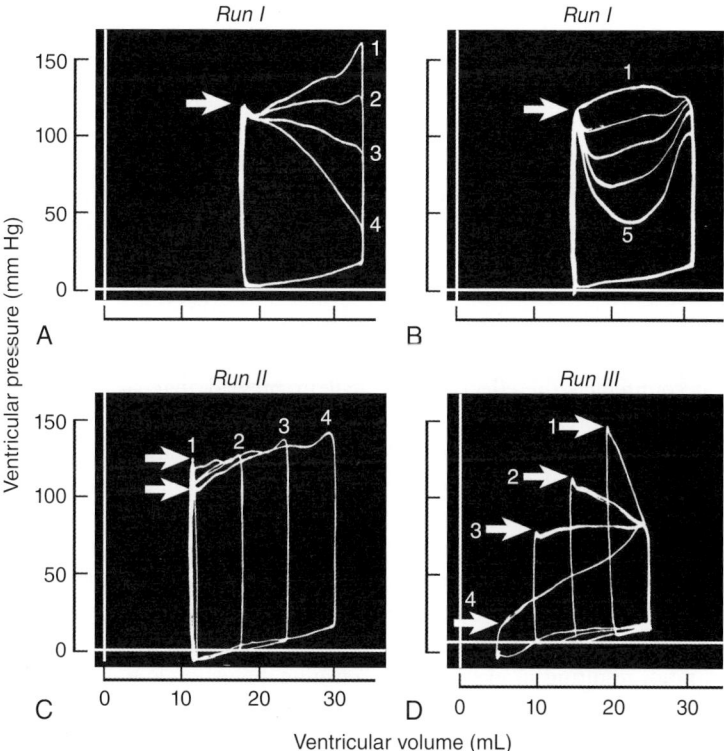

• **Fig. 11.3** Ventricular pressure-volume curves obtained in an isolated heart preparation at constant contractility with servo-controlled ventricular volume but highly variable outflow resistance. End sysole is marked by the arrows in each panel. Panels A and B indicate that when end-systolic volumes were clamped precisely at the specified volume, end-systolic volume was invariant despite of the marked changes in the pressure and volume courses during systole. Panel D illustrates the linear relation of the end-systolic pressure volume relations under variable outflow resistance within the normal physiologic range, and that this linear relation is not maintained at end-systolic pressures below the physiologic range. (From: Suga H, Kitabatake A, Sagawa K. End-systolic pressure determines stroke volume from fixed end-diastolic volume in the isolated canine left ventricle under a constant contractile state. *Circ Res.* 1979;44:238; with permission).

determinant of concentric myocardial hypertrophy, and (3) end-systolic fiberstress is the measure of afterload that is most determinant of end-systolic fiber length.

An alternative approach to the characterization of afterload in the intact cardiovascular system has been the investigation of the opposition to ejection imposed by the systemic or pulmonary circulation, quantified as arterial impedance.[8] Impedance is time-varying opposition to flow and is conceptually similar to resistance but is measured in a system that has oscillatory rather than continuous flow. The factors that determine impedance include the physical properties of blood (density and viscosity) and the vascular wall (compliance), the diameter of the vessel, the pulsatile nature of the flow, and the reflected pressure and flow waves generated in the distal parts of the vasculature. In fact, both arterial impedance and fiberstress are forms of afterload, but the determination of the appropriate measure of afterload depends on the frame of reference. With reference to the specific issue of myofiber shortening and hypertrophy, the importance of vascular impedance relates to the influence it exerts over end-systolic pressure. Arterial impedance is therefore an indirect determinant of myofiber shortening, whereas end-systolic fiberstress is the direct measure of afterload that is most predictive of systolic function.

In summary, afterload is a key determinant of myofiber shortening, ventricular function, and the quantity of blood ejected by the ventricle. In the intact heart, increasing or decreasing afterload while holding preload, contractility, and heart rate remain constant causes an immediate and reciprocal change in both the extent and velocity of fiber shortening. Net myocardial afterload is determined by factors both external (vascular impedance) and internal (ventricular size and shape and the mass-to-volume ratio) to the heart, and is best assessed as end-systolic fiberstress.

The importance of abnormalities of afterload in the evaluation of myocardial and ventricular performance primarily relates to the fashion in which it counteracts the effects of contractility. When contractile state and preload are constant, higher afterload leads to lower myofiber shortening. Chronic abnormalities of afterload are extremely common, both in normal cardiovascular physiology such as the physiologic hypertrophy associated with resistance exercise and in pathologic conditions such as aortic stenosis and dilated cardiomyopathy. The latter condition is particularly noteworthy because it is characterized by a dilated ventricle with reduced thickness-to-dimension ratio, resulting in elevated afterload (end-systolic fiberstress) based on altered ventricular structure that compounds the adverse impact of decreased contractility. In the normal heart, fiberstress falls progressively over the latter 70%–80% of systole (Fig. 11.3). This fall in instantaneous afterload is primarily related to fiber shortening and is consequently strikingly attenuated in dilated cardiomyopathy. Therefore, the cardiomyopathic heart labors under the combined adverse impact of reduced contractility and elevated afterload, even at low blood pressure and arterial impedance. Chronic elevation of fiberstress

plays a vital role in the "cardiomyopathy of overload," in which sustained elevation of afterload is recognized to eventually result in myocardial apoptosis and myocardial dysfunction.[9]

Contractility

Myocardial contractility specifically refers to the intrinsic force-generating capacity of myofibers, independent of preload and afterload. Assessment of contractility is therefore a definition of exclusion, based on measurement of net force generation after accounting for the effects of afterload and preload. It is common clinical practice for physicians to equate contractility with global ventricular function, assessed as ejection fraction or fractional shortening. Although contractility is a necessary contributor to fiber shortening, it is not the sole determinant, which also depends on initial fiber length and the load resisting muscle shortening. The usual clinical indices of cardiac function, including cardiac output, fractional shortening, ejection fraction, and stroke volume reflect only fiber shortening and fail to differentiate between the effects of contractility and loading conditions (preload and afterload).

Indices of Myocardial Contractility

There has been a large number of indices of cardiac contractility reported over the years. In many regards, this is not surprising because virtually any measurement that directly or indirectly reflects active myocardial force generation represents a measure of contractility. As discussed above, loading conditions (preload and afterload), which are subject to both cardiac and extra-cardiac factors, also affect most indices of cardiac function and can therefore lead to misinterpretation of the contractile state. For example, although a depressed ejection fraction is generally assumed to indicate depressed contractility, this is not a reliable interpretation. The acute fall in preload that accompanies elimination of a volume overload, for example after aortic valve repair or replacement for aortic regurgitation, will generally result in an acute fall in ejection fraction secondary to preload reduction, even if myocardial contractility remains normal. Since the therapeutic implications of abnormal ventricular function are quite different depending on whether it is due to abnormal load or abnormal contractility, there has been a great deal of interest in developing load-independent indices of contractility. The ensuing discussion is aimed at presenting the most important indices of contractility with their relative strengths and limitations, recognizing that there are many other contractility indices that have been reported that will not be discussed here. The focus of this discussion is on the left ventricle. Although the same myocardial physiology is applicable to the right ventricle, many of the functional indices are geometry dependent and therefore must be appropriately modified for use in the right ventricle.

Many indices of contractility have been proposed and used over time. A more comprehensive review of these can be found in Chapter 15 of the second edition of this textbook.[1] The current presentation will focus on those indices that are currently commonly employed in clinical practice.

Pre-Ejection Phase Indices of Contractility

First Derivative of Left Ventricular Pressure

The maximum value of the first derivative of left ventricular pressure ($LV\text{-}dP/dt_{max}$) is quite sensitive to changes in cardiac contractility, but although reasonably independent of afterload, $LV\text{-}dP/dt_{max}$ is affected by acute changes in preload. Although this shortcoming can be in large part overcome in controlled experimental situations, the preload dependence limits its clinical utility as an index of contractility. This index has number of advantages, including the ability to monitor contractility on a beat-by-beat basis and geometry independence. The technical aspects of the measurement are an impediment to its use, because the measurement of $LV\text{-}dP/dt_{max}$ requires use of high-fidelity, catheter tip micromanometers to achieve the higher-frequency response than is possible with standard transducers.

Ejection Phase Indices of Contractility

Systolic Time Intervals

Measurement of various time intervals in the cardiac cycle have at times been used to evaluate systolic function. The Tei index, also known as the **myocardial performance index**, is calculated as ([isovolumic contraction time + isovolumic relaxation time) ÷ systolic ejection time), measures that can be obtained from spectral Doppler and from mitral and aortic valve m-mode tracings. This index has been reported to be sensitive to changes in both systolic and diastolic ventricular function, but there are very few data concerning its relative load dependence and it is highly dependent on synchrony of activation and relaxation. The growth in popularity of this index can be in large part attributed to the ease of acquisition, its applicability in subjects with poor echocardiographic images, and absence of dependence on assumptions concerning ventricular geometry. However, despite common usage, at this juncture the relative diagnostic utility of this index as a measure of right ventricular contractility remains undefined.

Ejection and Shortening Fraction

These indices rely on measurements and calculations that provide an estimate of fiber shortening. For volume, area, diameter, surface area, and circumference of the left ventricle, it is possible to calculate the fractional systolic change for each as the difference between the diastolic and systolic value divided by the initial (diastolic) value. The fractional volume change is generally called the ejection fraction and is calculated from end-diastolic volume (V_{ED}) and end-systolic volume (V_{ES}) as ($V_{ED} - V_{ES})/V_{ED}$. Volume measurements can be performed by numerous imaging modalities, and although there are varying degrees of accuracy for each of the

methods, the limitations of ejection fraction as a measure of contractility are the same regardless of the method employed. Fractional diameter change is commonly known as **shortening fraction** or **fractional shortening**, and is calculated from short-axis left ventricular end-diastolic diameter (D_{ED}) and end-systolic diameter (D_{ES}) as ($D_{ED} - D_{ES})/D_{ED}$. If the cross-sectional configuration is circular, fractional shortening provides a direct measurement of endocardial circumferential fiber shortening. If the short-axis configuration of the left ventricle in not circular, as is the case with significant right ventricular volume or pressure overload and in other situations characterized by increased interventricular interaction (see discussion below), fractional shortening is not an accurate measure of ventricular function.

Evaluation of ejection fraction using 2D and 2D methods overcomes some of the issues related to abnormal ventricular geometry, and pediatric guideline recommendations have been published.[10] Nonetheless, although calculation of ventricular volumes can provide an accurate estimate of stroke volume and ejection fraction, their value as an index of contractility is limited by their load dependence. Ventricular shape change during contraction further confounds the accuracy. For example, patients with right ventricular volume overload secondary to an atrial septal defect are commonly noted to have depressed left ventricular ejection fraction due to abnormal left ventricular geometry at end diastole.[11] During early systole, about 20% of total fiber shortening is devoted to shape change (converting the ventricle to a circular configuration) before ejection ensues (Fig. 11.4). As a consequence, ejection fraction is generally depressed although myocardial fiber shortening is normal.

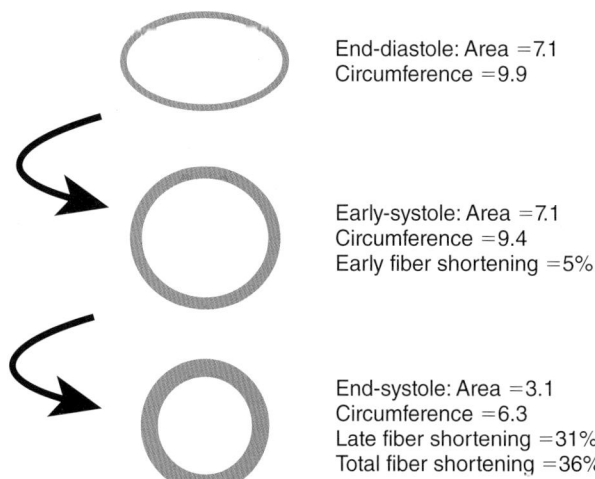

End-diastole: Area =7.1
Circumference =9.9

Early-systole: Area =7.1
Circumference =9.4
Early fiber shortening =5%

End-systole: Area =3.1
Circumference =6.3
Late fiber shortening =31%
Total fiber shortening =36%

• **Fig. 11.4** Time course of fiber shortening in the presence of right ventricular volume overload. During early systole, fiber shortening converts the ventricular configuration from elliptical to round without a change in volume. Ejection is due to the further fiber shortening over the course of systole. The net fiber shortening is normal although the fiber shortening during ejection and the ejection fraction may be depressed.

Load-Independent Indices of Contractility

Two different approaches have been followed in attempting to quantify myocardial contractility devoid of the effects of preload or afterload. Analysis of the end-systolic pressure-volume relation (time-varying systolic elastance, the E-max relationship) has been used to directly measure indices of contractility that are intrinsically load independent.[12] This method has identified important physiologic principles regarding ventricular function but has not been commonly implemented clinically due to the requirements for invasive pressure and volume measurements, manipulation of ventricular pressure during the evaluation, nonlinearity of the end-systolic pressure-volume relationship due to Frank–Starling relationship and shortening deactivation,[13] and uncertainty how to adjust for differences in body size.

Diastolic Myocardial and Ventricular Mechanics

The physiology of diastole and the impact of changes in diastole on systolic function are complex and are clinically challenging to evaluate. Diastolic heart failure (the clinical syndrome of congestive heart failure in the presence of normal systolic function) has been reported to account for 40%–50% of adults with congestive heart failure, and is seen in children,[14] although it is uncommon. Association of abnormal indices of diastolic dysfunction has been reported with a wide variety of etiologies in children including primary cardiomyopathies (restrictive and hypertrophic) but are far more commonly seen as a secondary manifestation in chronic hypertension, obesity. Although the primary restrictive cardiomyopathies are rare,[15] the clinical importance of secondary diastolic dysfunction has been increasingly recognized. Development of noninvasive methods for evaluating diastolic function has resulted in an explosion of relevant literature, despite the fact that the diagnostic accuracy of these methods remains largely unknown. There has been only limited evaluation of these noninvasive indices against the more physiologically meaningful invasive measures, limiting the ability to interpret their meaning.

Diastolic events must also be evaluated at both the myocardial and ventricular levels. Although in many regards the diastolic myocardial processes of relaxation and fiber lengthening represent the reciprocal of the systolic events of activation and fiber shortening, during diastole these two processes are largely temporally distinct, since at the ventricular cavity level, diastole is characterized by pressure decay followed by ventricular filling. It is important to recognize that similar to systolic ventricular properties, filling dynamics describe ventricular behavior and have only an indirect relationship to myocardial behavior. Although widely described as indices of diastolic function, the measures of filling dynamics reflect other factors in addition to the intrinsic diastolic chamber and myocardial properties.

Myocardial and Ventricular Relaxation

Myocardial relaxation ensues as a consequence of calcium sequestration by the sarcoplasmic reticulum, uncoupling the actin-myosin cross-bridge bonds. Calcium removal is an active, energy-consuming process that is impeded when cellular energy supplies are inadequate, and ischemia results in impaired myocardial relaxation prior to any impact on systolic function. Myocardial force decay begins early in systole but accelerates towards late systole and concludes as a rapid, exponential fall in wall stress that occurs primarily during isovolumic relaxation (Fig. 11.3) Relaxation continues into the early phase of diastolic filling, with the duration of overlap between these two phases of diastole primarily determined by the rate of relaxation. The decline in global fiberstress runs parallel to the fall in ventricular pressure during isovolumic relaxation because the other two determinants of fiberstress (ventricular mass and volume) are constant during this time period. The time (t) course of the fall in cavity pressure (P) can be fit to an exponential equation of the form:

$$P = \alpha \cdot e^{-t/\tau} + \beta$$

The exponent tau (τ) is known as the **time constant of ventricular relaxation** and mathematically is the length of time required for pressure to fall to 1/e of its end-systolic value. Measurement of tau has technical requirements similar to calculation of LV-dP/dt, necessitating the use of a high-fidelity pressure transducer.

The rates of myocardial and ventricular relaxation have other determinates beyond the intrinsic myocardial properties related to calcium handling. Both the myocardium and the ventricle are subject to the phenomenon of **elastic recoil** where some of the energy stored as myocardial compression is recovered in early diastole, as reflected in the fact that diastolic pressure can fall below atmospheric pressure.[16] The magnitude of elastic recoil is dependent on end-systolic volume and hence on afterload and contractility. Therefore, not surprisingly, the time constant of ventricular relaxation is dependent on heart rate, magnitude of hypertrophy, contractile state, and afterload.[17] Although myocardial relaxation is an intrinsic property of the myocardium, there is no currently available method for independently assessing relaxation properties.

Myocardial and Ventricular Compliance

Once maximum cross-bridge uncoupling is complete, the mechanical properties of the myocardium are determined by cytoskeletal and extracellular matrix properties. At short sarcomere lengths, the giant sarcomeric protein titin is the major determinant of passive tension,[18] but collagen is also important at longer sarcomere lengths. Shifts in titin isoforms and changes in collagen content and cross-linking are currently believed to explain most of the variation in passive myocardial properties.[19] Myocardial compliance is calculated from the myocardial stress-strain relationship, that is, the relative amount of lengthening (strain, σ) that results from a given force (stress, σ). Many biologic materials, including the myocardium, are viscous, which means that they are more resistant to rapid stretching than to gradual application of equivalent force. Because of this, the force resisting muscle lengthening depends on the rate of strain ($d\varepsilon/dt$), adding to the complexity of the model. The complexity of the data acquisition required to compute compliance has limited its use in routine clinical care. However, this is the property that quantifies the relaxed state of the myocardium and is an important determinant of ventricular compliance and filling.

Passive ventricular properties can be calculated from the diastolic pressure-volume curve and its derivative, the end-diastolic pressure-volume relationship (EDPVR). Cessation of filling at end diastole creates the only time point at which diastolic filling pressure is free of the effects of viscosity and is therefore below the dynamic diastolic pressure-volume curve, as illustrated in Fig. 11.5. Mitigating the impact of myocardial viscosity on the pressure-volume relationship requires measurement of diastolic pressure-volume curves at variable levels of preload (Fig. 11.6). Ventricular chamber stiffness is quantified as the instantaneous slope of the first derivative of the pressure-volume relationship (dP/dV) at any given volume (Fig. 11.7), and chamber compliance is the reciprocal of stiffness. The EDPVR is non-linear with higher volumes associated with lower compliance. In addition, the EDPVR is dependent on chamber geometry, right

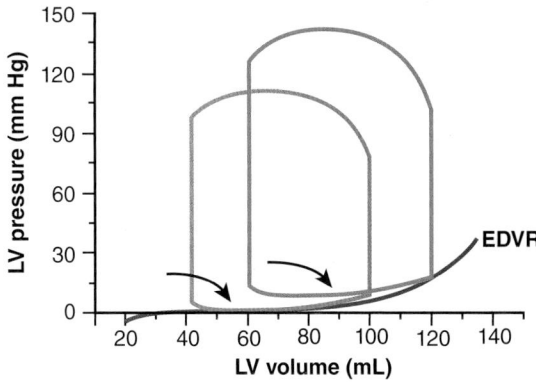

• **Fig. 11.5** Calculation of the end-diastolic pressure volume relationship requires acquisition of pressure-volume loops over multiple levels of end-diastolic pressure to exclude the impact of myocardial viscosity. *EDPVR,* End-diastolic pressure-volume relationship.

ventricular pressure, ventricular hypertrophy, and external pericardial and thoracic constraint in addition to myocardial compliance. Because filling is the end point of a complex set of interacting processes, it is not surprising that abnormal filling behavior is a sensitive indicator of disease. However, determining the relative importance of the many possible factors that contribute to abnormal filling behavior is generally quite difficult.

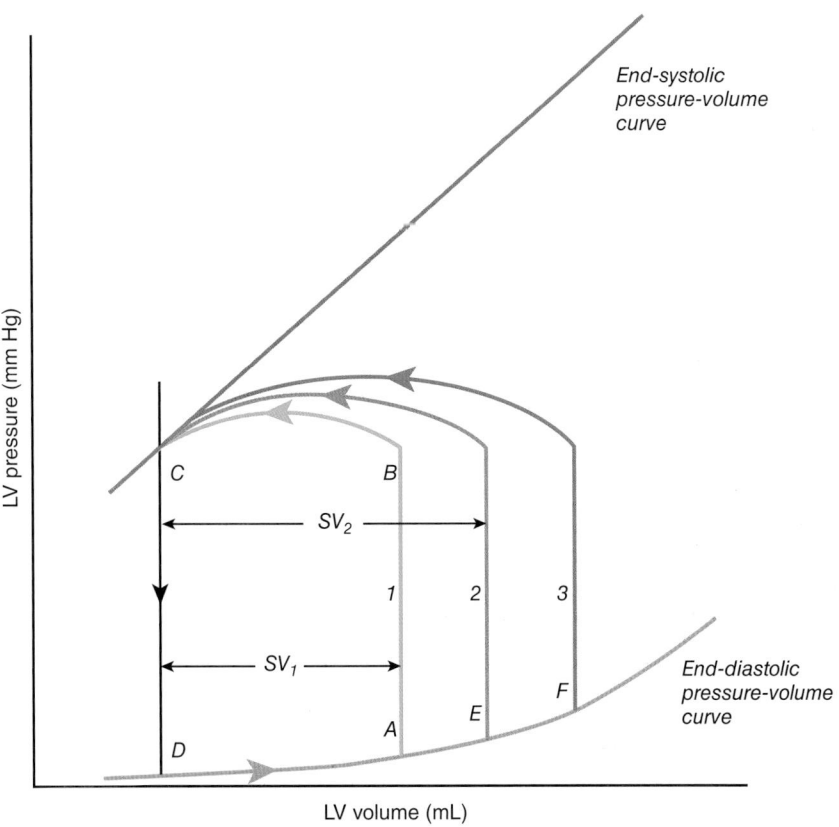

• **Fig. 11.6** Idealized pressure-volume loops at constant contractility (invariant end-systolic pressure-volume relationship) at multiple levels of end-diastolic pressure to calculate the end-diastolic pressure-volume relationship as a measure of ventricular compliance.

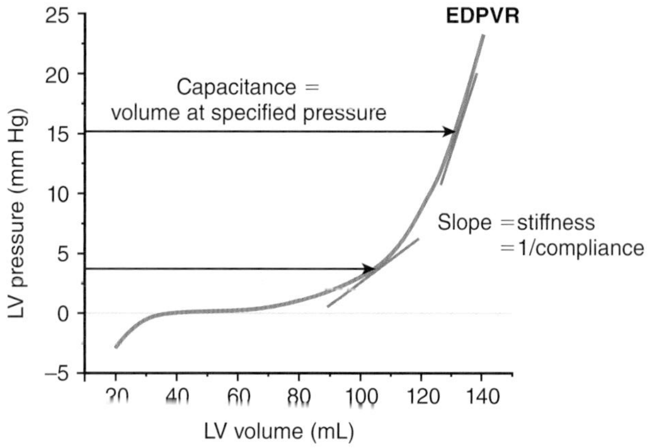

• **Fig. 11.7** The end-diastolic pressure volume curve allows measurement of pressure-specific ventricular capacitance and compliance, where the latter is measured as the slope of the end-diastolic pressure-volume curve. *EDPVR,* End-diastolic pressure-volume relationship.

Diastolic Function Indices

The complex and invasive methods that are required to evaluate the time constant of relaxation and the diastolic pressure-volume relationship have restricted their application to animal studies and occasional small research studies. The wide availability of Doppler echocardiography and the ease with which various indices of filling behavior can be obtained has resulted in the development of an extensive literature relating to these techniques. Much of this work is devoted to correlation between diastolic parameters and outcomes rather than investigation into the underlying physiology.

Normal diastolic filling proceeds in two phases (Fig. 11.1B), with a dominant passive E-wave followed by near cessation of flow followed by the A-wave in response to atrial contraction. At the ventricular level, the E-wave occurs during the period of overlap between relaxation and early filling and is therefore determined by both relaxation and compliance. The A-wave is the late diastolic flow augmentation secondary to atrial contraction, and at the ventricular level is determined primarily by ventricular compliance. Due to the beat-to-beat variation in maximum velocities secondary to respiratory effects, the E-wave/A-wave ratio (E/A) is generally relied upon, with elevated E/A interpreted as abnormal compliance, reduced E/A interpreted as abnormal relaxation, and normal E/A interpreted as either normal compliance and relaxation or as secondary to abnormalities in both ("pseudo-normalization"). Additional measurements have been added to the analysis in an effort to overcome the phenomenon of pseudo-normalization. The deceleration phase of the E-wave takes place after completion of relaxation and the rate of flow deceleration depends primarily on ventricular compliance with an abnormally rapid termination of antegrade flow indicating diminished compliance. Similarly, duration of the A-wave and the duration of flow reversal in the pulmonary veins depend on ventricular compliance.

Tissue-Doppler Diastolic Indices

Doppler samples obtained directly from myocardium can be used to assess the velocity of tissue motion. These indices do not directly assess inflow, relaxation, or compliance, but rather represent the directional tissue velocity resulting from the complex interplay of these factors. The diastolic tissue Doppler pattern is similar to the mitral inflow pattern, manifesting a rapid early diastolic phase followed by relatively little change in mid diastole and a late diastolic phase that corresponds to the A-wave (Fig. 11.1B). Although late diastolic tissue motion is passive, and therefore relates closely to filling in response to atrial contraction, early diastolic tissue velocity appears to be relatively independent of preload and has been reported to correlate with the time constant of relaxation. The ratio of the peak early transmitral flow velocity to the peak early myocardial tissue velocity correlates with filling pressure, although there are significant limits to the preload independence of this parameter. Left atrial strain has relatively recently been added to the available means of detecting elevated resistance to diastolic filling of the left ventricle. There are limited data on the performance of this method of detecting diminished compliance, but the early data are promising.[20]

Clinical Interpretation of Noninvasive Diastolic Indices

There has been considerable debate in the literature as to the meaning of Doppler-based diastolic indices. Verification of the physiologic significance of the Doppler indices has been in large measure based on correlation analysis. With regard to noninvasive indices of diastolic function, the primary limitation to correlation analysis is the potential failure to recognize the primary role played by covariates. The described abnormalities of Doppler indices of diastolic function are highly dependent on heart rate and filling pressure and are therefore accurate predictors of impaired compliance only insofar as the elevation in filling pressure relates to abnormal ventricular compliance. Because impaired compliance is commonly accompanied by elevated filling pressure, there is collinearity between filling pressure, ventricular compliance, and filling dynamics. However, abnormal filling pressure, although an important contributor to clinical status, is an extremely unreliable index of intrinsic myocardial properties because of its dependence on a myriad of confounding factors and the ease with which it is modified by therapeutic interventions.

One of the important areas of clinical application of the Doppler-derived indices of diastolic function has been in the adult population with diastolic heart failure, where the label "heart failure with normal ejection fraction" has been used. This clinical syndrome of congestive heart failure with preserved systolic function accounts for a significant percentage of heart failure in older adults, but is very uncommon in children and young adults.[21] The etiologies include myocardial diastolic dysfunction, valvular heart diseases such as mitral stenosis, pericardial diseases such as tamponade, and volume overload situations such as severe anemia. Diagnostically, the patients with intrinsic abnormalities of diastolic dysfunction secondary to cardiomyopathy (hypertrophic, restrictive, and infiltrative disorders) are of primary interest. The sensitivity and specificity of the noninvasive indices of diastolic function have not been extensively evaluated in the pediatric population, significantly limiting the confidence with which they can be employed.

Torsion

The normal configuration of the myocardial fibers in the left ventricular wall[22] is circumferential, but angulated relative to the long axis of the ventricle (Fig. 11.8). The myofibers run parallel to the endocardial surface at all layers, but there is a transmural change in the angle of the myofibers relative to the long axis of the left ventricle such that from an apical perspective, the subendocardial fibers exert a clockwise force and the subepicardial fibers exert a counterclockwise force. The larger radius for subepicardial fibers compared with subendocardial fibers results in a larger moment-arm for the subepicardial fibers and hence create a greater torsional force, resulting in net counterclockwise torsion. Detorsion (untwisting) occurs during isovolumic relaxation and the torsional recoil releases the potential energy (shear stress) stored during the systolic myocardial deformation. The untwisting rate correlates closely with the relaxation time constant.

Concentric hypertrophy secondary to factors such as hypertension, aortic stenosis, and hypertrophic cardiomyopathy augments torsion, resulting in diminished longitudinal shortening and increased circumferential shortening secondary to the change in systolic shape change and is not a sign of decreased contractility. Ultimately, torsion results in a more uniform transmural distribution of left ventricular fiberstress and hence fiber shortening. The mechanical advantage of torsion has been mathematically modeled and it has been estimated to result in a doubling of endocardial sarcomeric shortening at the expense of a 15% decrease in epicardial shortening compared to the absence of torsion, thereby increasing sarcomeric shortening efficiency.

The Effect of Heart Rate on Cardiac Performance

Changes in heart rate are associated with alterations in preload, myocardial oxygen consumption, and contractility. Ejection time diminishes as a function of the square root of cardiac cycle time, which means that there is a decrease in the percentage of the cardiac cycle available for filling. As a result, diastolic ventricular volume and stroke volume decrease unless there is an associated rise in filling pressure. Myocardial blood flow occurs primarily during diastole, and hence tachycardia potentially compromises blood flow during sustained tachycardia. The direct myocardial effect from an increase in contraction frequency has been labeled

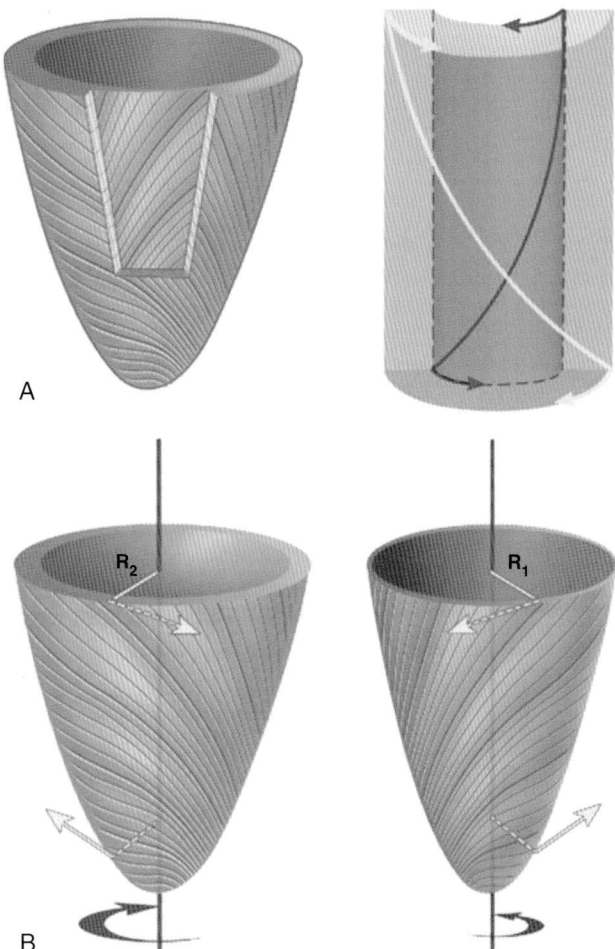

• **Fig. 11.8** (A) Illustration of the progressive 90-degree change in left ventricular myofiber orientation from a subepicardial left-handed helix to a subendocardial right-handed helix. The subepicardial fibers have a longer moment arm compared with the subendocardial (R2 > R1) and as a consequence exert a larger force. (B) The net result is a lesser endocardial rotation compared with the epicardial rotation in the opposite direction, and a net counterclockwise rotation of the heart when viewed from the apex. (From: Sengupta PP, Tajik AJ, Chandrasekaran K, Khandheria BK. Twist mechanics of the left ventricle. *JACC Cardiovasc Imag.* 2008;1:366; with permission).

the force-frequency relationship (FFR) and is associated with a positive inotropic effect independent of adrenergic augmentation of contractility.[23]

The FFR plays an essential role in adjusting myocardial performance of the heart to meet the changing hemodynamic needs of the body. The molecular mechanism responsible for the frequency-dependent modulation of the contractility of cardiac muscle has been shown to relate to an increase in the amount of Ca^{++} ions entering the myocardial cells with each beat. The essential role of Ca^{++} in excitation-contraction coupling means that greater amplitude intracellular Ca^{++} transients in response to higher contraction frequency results in augmented force generation over a broad range of frequencies. The FFR and the response of contractile force to arrhythmia such as post-extrasystolic potentiation reflect an essential mechanism for contractile regulation in the heart under physiologic and pathological conditions. Changes in sarcoplasmic reticulum Ca^{++} handling appears to account for the flattened FFR characteristic of failing human myocardium, although Na^+ influx and Na^+ homeostasis may also play a crucial role.

Understanding Stress Echocardiography Basics: Assessment of Ischemia

As previously discussed, multiple indices are used to define left ventricular contractility and function at baseline. By looking at LV global function and LV regional wall motion under conditions of increased need for cardiac output, such as during exercise, it is possible to evaluate ischemia in a patient. The basis for all noninvasive imaging with exercise or stress is grounded on the fundamentals of the ischemic cascade (Fig. 11.9). Ischemia begins when myocardial oxygen demand exceeds supply. Perfusion defects develop in the ischemic regions. As ischemia progresses, diastolic dysfunction (slowed/delayed ventricular relaxation) follows. Next, there is onset of regional wall motion abnormalities (WMAs) or systolic dysfunction, which can be detectable by stress echocardiography. It is only after the development of regional WMAs that ECG abnormalities become visible. Symptoms such as chest pain or shortness of breath occur late in the ischemic cascade, as do ECG changes. Therefore, patients may have evidence of ischemia and WMAs with stress, before they manifest definitive ECG changes or symptoms.

In pediatrics, exercise or dobutamine are typically used as the stressor to elicit potential ischemia. Exercise is preferred over pharmacologic stress (e.g., dobutamine), since exercise allows concurrent assessment of the patient's exercise capacity. In patients who cannot exercise, dobutamine stress echocardiography (DSE) can be used as an alternative to

exercise stress echocardiography (ESE). It is portable and may be particularly useful in patients in intensive care unit or patients too young to exercise on a bicycle or treadmill.

Although bicycle or treadmill can be used, treadmill achieves higher blood pressure and heart rate, indicating higher myocardial oxygen demands. For an ESE, ~5 minutes of imaging is acquired before exercise to assess all the 17 segments of the LV walls as defined by the American Society of Echocardiography guidelines (Fig. 11.10). The same imaging is acquired again immediately after exercise, with the goal of completing all ischemia imaging within 90 seconds after termination of exercise/stress. ESE is well tolerated in children, can be performed generally in children over 6 years of age without developmental delay, who can walk on a treadmill or bike, and requires no sedation, needle stick, or radiation exposure. At Boston Children's Hospital, ESE has almost completely replaced other stress imaging modalities, such as nuclear scintigraphy, which requires intravenous catheter placement and radiation exposure which can be equivalent to hundreds of chest X-rays per test. Please refer to stress echocardiography for pediatrics guidelines published by the *Journal of the American Society of Echocardiography* for protocols and further details.[24]

Children who may be at high risk for ischemia, including those with (1) history of coronary aneurysms with history of Kawasaki disease, (2) s/p cardiac transplantation, (3) anomalous aortic origin of a coronary artery, (4) s/p coronary manipulation or reimplantation following congenital heart surgery (i.e., s/p arterial switch operation in transposition of the great arteries), (5) s/p chest radiation, or (6) familial hyperlipidemia (Fig. 11.11). Kawasaki disease is the leading cause of acquired coronary artery disease (CAD) in children with inflammatory vasculitis, leading to coronary artery dilation, coronary aneurysms, and subsequent coronary thrombosis. ESE is useful for serial screening and prognosis, as is DSE.

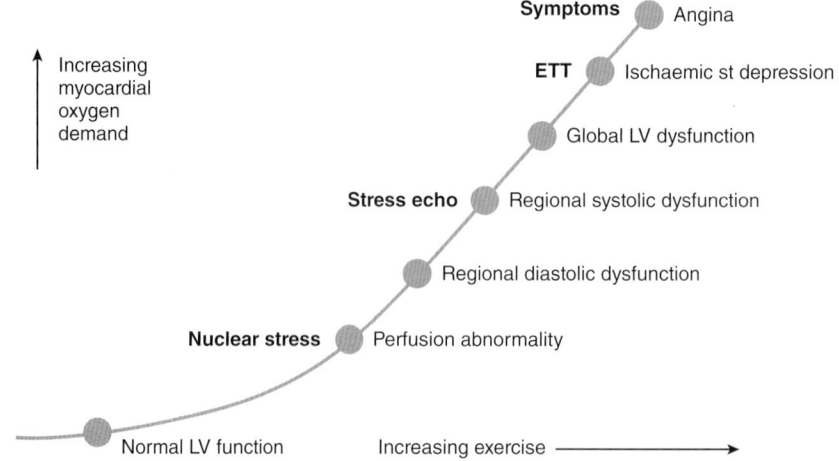

• **Fig. 11.9** Impact of ischemia on LV function with increasing myocardial oxygen demand outstripping myocardial oxygen supply. With increasing exercise, there is greater oxygen demand, and in patients with ischemia, a limited oxygen supply which results in ischemia. Stress echocardiography can detect regional systolic dysfunction in the initial stages of the ischemic cascade, and before the onset of ischemic EKGs changes or before patient symptoms such as chest pain or shortness of breath. *ETT,* Exercise tolerance test; *LV,* left ventricle.

| Pre-Exercise | Post-Exercise | | Pre-Exercise | Post-Exercise |

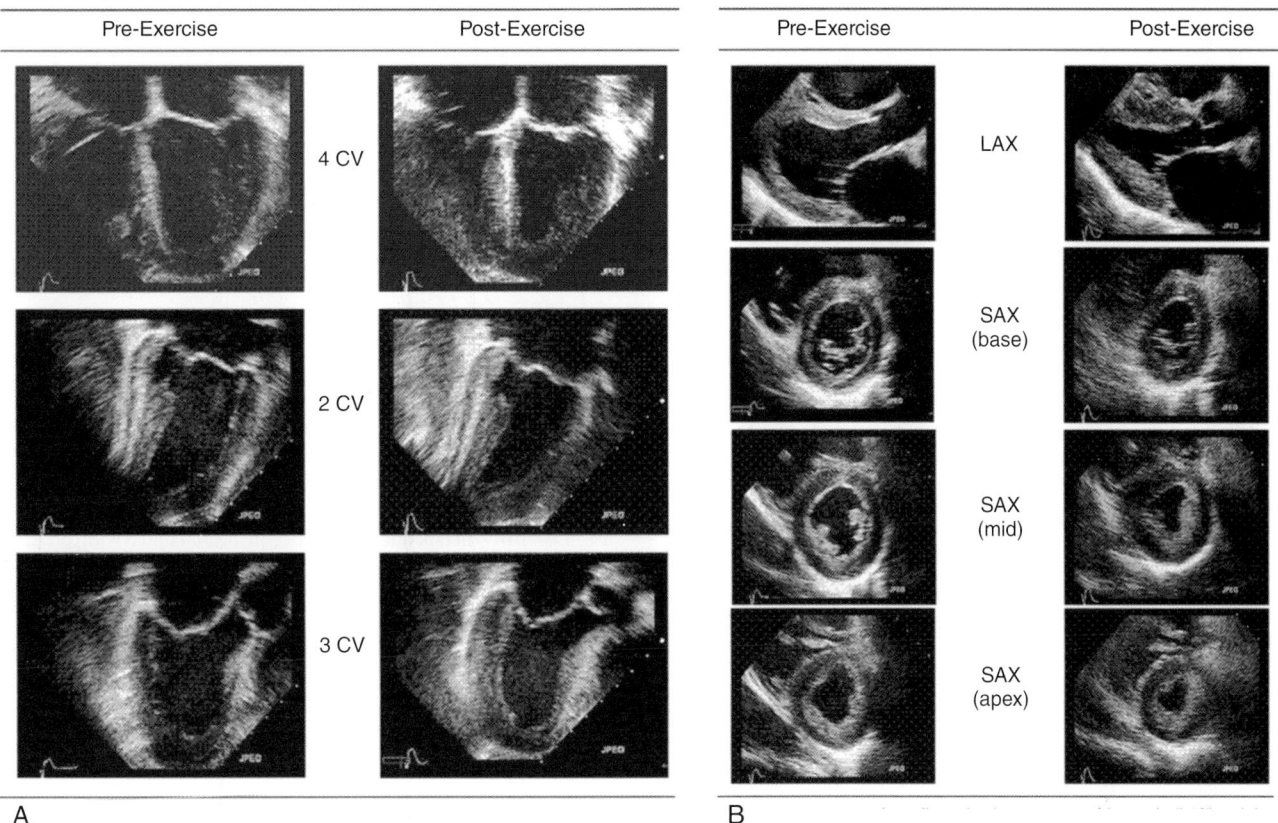

A   B

• **Fig. 11.10** Exercise stress echocardiography show **(A)** apical four-, three-, and two-chamber views and **(B)** parasternal long- and short-axis views of the left ventricle, pre- and post-exercise. Note the increase in myocardial wall thickening with stress as compared with rest, and also the decrease in LV chamber size as the heart becomes hyperdynamic. *CV,* chamber view; *LAX,* parasternal long-axis view; *SAX,* parasternal short-axis view. (Figures modified from Chen MH, Abernathey E, Lunze F, Colan SD, O'Neill S, Bergersen L, Geva T, Blume ED. Utility of exercise stress echocardiography in pediatric cardiac transplant recipients: a single-center experience. *J Heart Lung Transplant.* 2012;31:517–523.)

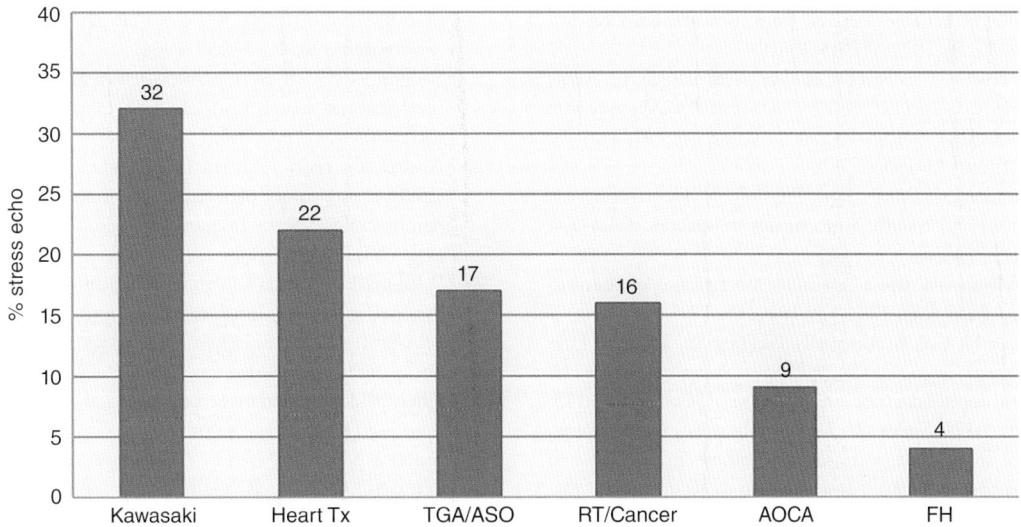

• **Fig. 11.11** Indications for stress echocardiography performed in children and young adults at Boston Children's Hospital for evaluation of ischemia from 2006 to 2021 (*n* > 2000). *AOCA,* Anomalous origin of a coronary artery; *FH,* familial homozygous hypercholesterolemia; *RT,* radiation therapy to the chest; *TGA/ASO,* transposition of the great arteries, status post-arterial switch operation; *Tx,* transplant.

Pediatric heart transplant recipients are at high risk for transplant-induced coronary vasculopathy. While annual coronary angiography has traditionally been used to screen for epicardial CAD, it is unable to visualize smaller coronary vessels and the microvasculature where transplant vasculopathy with diffuse intimal hyperplasia begins. Both DSE and ESE have been shown to be safe and feasible, with good sensitivity, specificity, and negative predictive value in excluding epicardial CAD.[25] At Boston Children's Hospital, routine use of ESE has decreased the annual interval of coronary angiography to now biannual in patients who have a normal stress echocardiography. An abnormal ESE has been associated with late cardiac outcomes and death in pediatric cardiac transplant recipients.[26] DSE can also help detect coronary vasculopathy and help risk-stratify patients, although ESE is preferred over DSE where feasible, given the lack of need for an IV and anesthesia in children.[24]

Overall, pediatric stress echocardiography has been shown to be feasible and aid in the diagnosis, risk stratification, and/or prognosis of acquired and congenital heart disease in children.[26,27] Beyond its use in the diagnosis of ischemia, it has been used to assess myocardial contractile reserve and identify patients at risk for future cardiac events. Patients identified as being at the highest risk of adverse events may be able to receive interventions earlier in the course of their cardiovascular disease, and better risk stratification may help improve the prognosis for conditions that affect a child's heart.

References

1. Colan SD. Assessment of ventricular and myocardial performance. In: Keane JF, Lock JE, Fyler DC, eds. *Nadas' Pediatric Cardiology.* 2nd ed. Philadelphia: Elsevier; 2006:251-274.
2. Elzinga G, Westerhof N. How to quantify pump function of the heart. The value of variables derived from measurements on isolated muscle. *Circ Res.*1979;44:303-308.
3. Braunwald E, Ross Jr. J. Control of cardiac performance. In: Berne RM, Sperclakis N, Geiger SR, eds. *Handbook of Physiology, Section 2: The Cardiovascular System, Volume 1.* Baltimore: Williams & Wilkins Co.; 1979:533-580.
4. Colan SD, Sanders SP, Borow KM. Physiologic hypertrophy: effects on left ventricular systolic mechanics in athletes. *J Am Coll Cardiol.* 1987;9:776-783.
5. Regen DM. Myocardial stress equations: fiberstresses of the prolate spheroid. *J Theor Biol.* 1984;109:191-215.
6. Dong H, Mosca H, Gao E, Akins RE, Gidding SS, Tsuda T. Integrated wall stress: a new methodological approach to assess ventricular workload and myocardial contractile reserve. *J Transl Med.* 2013;11:183.
7. Suga H, Kitabatake A, Sagawa K. End-systolic pressure determines stroke volume from fixed end-diastolic volume in the isolated canine left ventricle under a constant contractile state. *Circ Res.* 1979;44:238-249.
8. Bikia V, Rovas G, Pagoulatou S, Stergiopulos N. Determination of aortic characteristic impedance and total arterial compliance from regional pulse wave velocities using machine learning: an in-silico study. *Front Bioeng Biotechnol.* 2021;9:649866.
9. Wernig F, Xu QB. Mechanical stress-induced apoptosis in the cardiovascular system. *Prog Biophys Mol Biol.* 2002;78:105-137.
10. Lopez L, Colan SD, Frommelt PC, et al. Recommendations for quantification methods during the performance of a pediatric echocardiogram: a report from the Pediatric Measurements Writing Group of the American Society of Echocardiography Pediatric and Congenital Heart Disease Council. *J Am Soc Echocardiogr.* 2010;23:465-495.
11. Walker RE, Moran AM, Gauvreau K, Colan SD. Evidence of adverse ventricular interdependence in patients with atrial septal defects. *Am J Cardiol.* 2004;93:1374-1377.
12. Suga H. Cardiac energetics: from E(max) to pressure-volume area. *Clin Exp Pharmacol Physiol.* 2003;30:580-585.
13. Habigt MA, Michelle Krieger M, Gesenhues J, Ketelhut M, Mechelinck M, Hein M. Non-linearity of end-systolic pressure–volume relation in afterload increases is caused by an overlay of shortening deactivation and the Frank–Starling mechanism. *Sci Rep.* 2021;11:3353.
14. Das BB. Therapeutic approaches in heart failure with preserved ejection fraction (HFpEF) in children: present and future. *Paediatr Drugs.* 2022;24:235-246.
15. Ware SM, Bhatnagar S, Dexheimer PJ, et al. The genetic architecture of pediatric cardiomyopathy. *Am J Hum Genet.* 2022;109:282-298.
16. Udelson JE, Bacharach SL, Cannon RO III, et al. Minimum left ventricular pressure during β-adrenergic stimulation in human subjects: evidence for elastic recoil and diastolic "suction" in the normal heart. *Circulation.* 1990;82:1174-1182.
17. Mawad W, Friedberg MK. The continuing challenge of evaluating diastolic function by echocardiography in children: developing concepts and newer modalities. *Curr Opin Cardiol.* 2017;32:93-100.
18. Granzier HL, Labeit S. The giant protein titin - A major player in myocardial mechanics, signaling, and disease. *Circ Res.* 2004; 94:284-295.
19. Fukuda N, Takako Terui T, Ishiwata S, Kurihara S. Titin-based regulations of diastolic and systolic functions of mammalian cardiac muscle. *J Mol Cell Cardiol.* 2010;48:876-881.
20. Sabatino J, Di Salvo G, Prota C, et al. Left atrial strain to identify diastolic dysfunction in children with cardiomyopathies. *J Clin Med.* 2019;8:1243.
21. Beladan CC, Botezatu JS, Popescu BA. Reversible left ventricular diastolic dysfunction–Overview and clinical implications. *Echocardiography.* 2020;37:1957-1966.
22. Sengupta PP, Tajik AJ, Chandrasekaran K, Khandheria BK. Twist mechanics of the left ventricle: principles and application. *JACC Cardiovasc Imaging.* 2008;1:366-376.
23. Alvarez SV, Fortin-Pellerin E, Alhabdan M, et al. Strain rate in children and young piglets mirrors changes in contractility and demonstrates a force-frequency relationship. *J Am Soc Echocardiogr.* 2017;30:797-806.
24. Pellikka PA, Arruda-Olson A, Chaudhry FA, et al. Guidelines for performance, interpretation, and application of stress echocardiography in ischemic heart disease: from the American Society of Echocardiography. *J Am Soc Echocardiogr.* 2020;33:1-41.
25. Chen MH, Abernathey E, Lunze F, et al. Utility of exercise stress echocardiography in pediatric cardiac transplant recipients: a single-center experience. *J Heart Lung Transplant.* 2012;31:517-523.
26. Perez MT, Rizwan R, Gauvreau K, et al. Prognostic value of exercise stress echocardiography in pediatric cardiac transplant recipients. *J Am Soc Echocardiogr.* 2022;35:1133-1138.
27. Cifra B, Dragulescu A, Border WL, Mertens L. Stress echocardiography in paediatric cardiology. *Eur Heart J Cardiovasc Imaging.* 2015;16:1051-1059.

12

Exercise Testing

JONATHAN RHODES, SUELLEN YIN, AND NAOMI GAUTHIER

KEY LEARNING POINTS

- Interpretation of exercise data and appreciation of the capabilities of the technology require an understanding of the physiology and the mechanisms by which the cardiovascular system normally meets the metabolic demands of exercise.
- Cardiopulmonary metabolic stress testing can objectively measure a patient's exercise capacity and delineate contributing respiratory and cardiac factors.

- Exercise testing is a powerful tool for identifying the need for intervention, monitoring treatment efficacy, prognosticating, and determining safety of exercise for long-term cardiovascular health in patients with congenital and acquired heart disease.

The primary task of the cardiopulmonary system is to deliver oxygen (O_2) in quantities sufficient to support the metabolic needs of the body. This system is maximally stressed when the metabolic rate is increased, a condition that occurs most commonly during physical activity. Most clinical tests assess the cardiopulmonary system while the patient is at rest. Although valuable, these tests do not predict the manner in which the cardiopulmonary system will respond to the demands of exercise, nor do they reliably inform the clinician regarding a patient's capacity to perform physical activities. Moreover, subjective accounts of a patient's exercise function are often unreliable. Exercise testing, however, provides physicians with an opportunity to gain valuable, objective insights into these and other clinically important aspects of a patient's cardiopulmonary function.[1]

Physiology of Exercise

The energy required to perform exercise is derived from the hydrolysis of adenosine triphosphate (ATP). At rest, skeletal muscles possess limited quantities of ATP and other high-energy phosphate molecules. If exercise is to continue for more than a brief period, ATP must be continually replenished through the metabolism of fuels. Aerobic metabolism of fuels produces large quantities of ATP per molecule of substrate but requires an adequate supply of O_2. This O_2 must be delivered to the skeletal muscle by the cardiovascular system.[1] The factors responsible for this process are best understood through the Fick equation[a]:

$$\dot{V}_{O2} = [CO] \times [O_2 \text{ extraction}]$$
$$= [HR \times SV] \times [C_aO_2 - C_vO_2]$$
$$= [HR \times SV] \times [1.36\,(Hgb)(S_aO_2 - S_vO_2]$$

Normally, during exercise, each of these variables is altered to maximize O_2 delivery.

Heart Rate

During exercise, HR rises threefold from resting values of 60–80 bpm to ~200 bpm at peak exercise. This rise is mediated primarily by the autonomic nervous system via an increase in sympathetic activity and a reduction in parasympathetic activity.

Stroke Volume

During a progressive upright exercise test, SV rises rapidly and then plateaus at a level 1.5–2 times greater than baseline.

---

[a] $\dot{V}_{O2}$: O_2 consumption; CO: cardiac output; HR: heart rate; SV: stroke volume; C_aO_2: arterial O_2 content; C_vO_2: venous O_2 content; Hgb: hemoglobin concentration; S_aO_2: arterial O_2 saturation; S_vO_2: venous O_2 saturation. By convention, a "V" with a dot over it represents a flow (e.g., liters/minute), whereas a "V" without a dot over it represents a volume (e.g., liters).

Thereafter, increases in CO are due primarily to increases in HR. The increase in SV is mediated by: (1) increased cardiac contractility secondary to increased adrenergic stimulation; (2) decreased afterload secondary to a dramatic decline in systemic and pulmonary vascular resistance (PVR); (3) enhanced ventricular filling secondary to the pumping action of the skeletal muscles[2]; and (4) improved lusitropic function.[3] Hence, peak-exercise is typically associated with a fivefold increase in CO.

Oxygen Extraction

At rest, normal S_aO_2 approaches 100% and S_vO_2 is approximately 70%. Hence, the body extracts only 30% of its O_2 delivery. At peak-exercise, however, muscles extract a much greater percentage of the delivered O_2. S_vO_2 typically falls to less than 30% and total body O_2 extraction more than doubles at peak-exercise. The Fick equation elucidates the cardiovascular adaptations to exercise that permit $\dot{V}_{O_2}$ to increase more than 10-fold over resting values.

Exercise is also associated with a remarkable redistribution of CO (Fig. 12.1). At rest, the muscles receive only 20% of CO (~1 L/min; 0.025 mL/g of muscle tissue), whereas at peak-exercise they receive 80% of a much larger CO (~20 L/min; 0.5 mL/g of muscle tissue). The coronary blood flow also increases five-fold from ~0.25 L/min (0.7 mL/g cardiac tissue) to ~1.25 L/min (3.5 mL/g cardiac tissue). The redistribution of blood flow to the muscles

and heart is further enhanced by vasoconstriction within the renal and mesenteric vascular beds.[1]

In addition to consuming O_2, the aerobic metabolism of fuels produces carbon dioxide (CO_2). For each carbon atom of glucose that is metabolized, one molecule of O_2 is consumed and one of CO_2 is produced:

$$H\text{-}C\text{-}OH + O_2 \rightarrow H_2O + CO_2 \text{ (6 ATP/carbon atom)}$$

The respiratory quotient (RQ), the stoichiometrically determined ratio of the number of moles of CO_2 produced, divided by the number of moles of O_2 consumed, is 1.0.

The aerobic metabolism of each carbon atom from the hydrocarbon chain of a free fatty acid consumes 1.5 molecules of O_2 and produces 1 molecule of CO_2:

$$H\text{-}C\text{-}H + 1\tfrac{1}{2} O_2 \rightarrow H_2O + CO_2 \text{ (8 ATP/carbon atom)}$$

The RQ for this chemical reaction is 0.67.

Consequently, during aerobic metabolism, when a mixture of fats and carbohydrates are consumed, the respiratory exchange ratio (RER; ratio of the *measured* $\dot{V}_{CO_2}$/the *measured* $\dot{V}_{O_2}$) is typically approximately 0.80 (i.e., between 0.67 and 1.0).[1]

Although aerobic metabolism of fuels produces large quantities of ATP, the amount that may be derived from aerobic metabolism is limited by the amount of O_2 that is delivered. As the intensity of exercise increases, the energy requirements of muscle cells rise and ultimately exceed that which can be produced by aerobic metabolism. The muscle

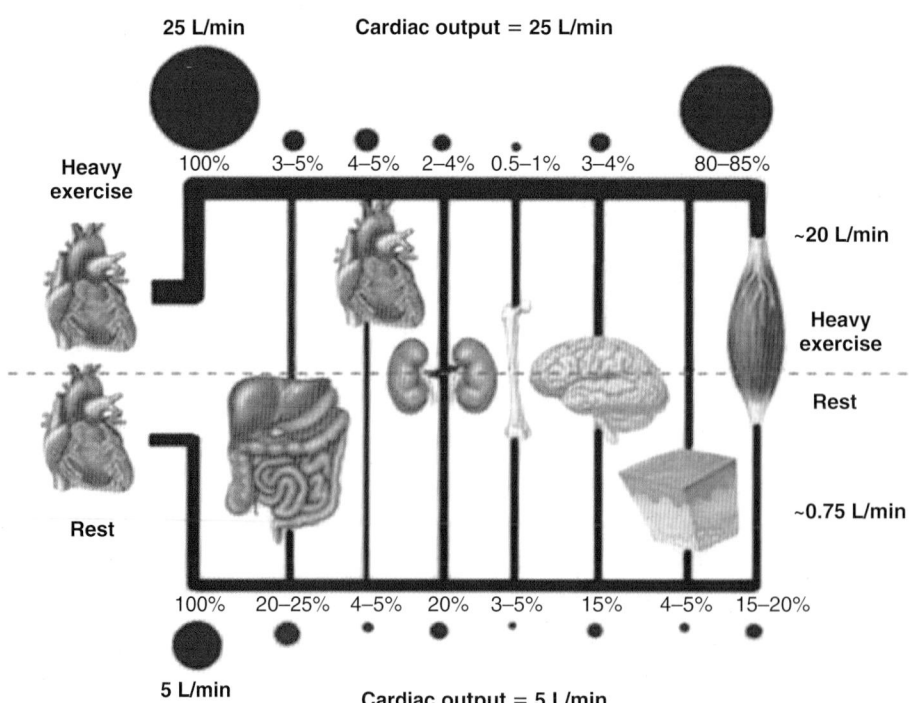

• **Fig. 12.1** Distribution of cardiac output at rest and with exercise. (Figure adapted from Astrand et al., *Textbook of work physiology: Physiological bases of exercise*, 4th ed., 2003.)

cell must then begin to rely on anaerobic metabolism of glucose to provide a portion of its energy needs:

$$C_6H_{12}O_6 \rightarrow 2(CH_3CHOHCOOH)(0.3\ ATP/carbon\ atom)$$
$$\text{Glucose} \qquad\qquad \text{Lactic acid}$$

Anaerobic metabolism does not produce as much ATP/carbon atom as aerobic metabolism, but it does not require O_2. It also produces lactic acid, which reacts with bicarbonate to produce CO_2:

$$CH_3CHOHCOOH\ +\ HCO_3^-\ \rightarrow\ CH_3CHOHCOO^-$$
$$\text{Lactic acid} \qquad \text{Bicarbonate} \qquad\qquad \text{Lactate}$$
$$+H_2O\ +\ CO_2$$
$$\text{Carbon dioxide}$$

When muscles begin to rely on anaerobic metabolism for ATP production, lactate levels abruptly rise and an increase in $\dot{V}_{CO2}$, out of proportion to the concomitant increase in $\dot{V}_{O2}$, is observed. During a progressive exercise test, the point at which these phenomena are detected is called "ventilatory anaerobic threshold (VAT)". Although some controversy exists concerning the mechanisms and physiology that underlie it, most exercise physiologists agree that VAT is a clinically useful and valid concept.[4]

The elimination of CO_2 is another function of the cardiopulmonary system that may be maximally stressed during exercise. The mechanisms employed by the lungs to excrete the large quantities of CO_2 produced during exercise are described by the alveolar ventilation equation[b]:

$$\dot{V}_{CO2} = RR \times V_T(1 - V_D/V_T) \times P_aCO_2/P_B$$

In a manner analogous to the delivery of O_2, the physiologic variables of this equation are altered to optimize CO_2 elimination during exercise.

Respiratory Rate

As exercise intensity increases, a normal subject's RR rises slowly initially. During later, more intense stages of exercise, the RR rises more rapidly; at peak-exercise it may increase to more than three times the resting values.[5]

Tidal Volume

V_T rises rapidly with exercise and then plateaus at a level approximately three times greater than resting values.[5]

Dead Space/Tidal Volume Ratio

Anatomic V_D, the volume of air in the trachea, bronchi and other airways that do not participate in gas exchange, does not change appreciably during exercise. Physiologic V_D actually declines secondary to improved matching of ventilation/perfusion. Hence, during exercise the V_D/V_T falls rapidly and then levels off at a level one-third to half of the resting value.[5]

---

[b]RR: respiratory rate; V_T: tidal volume; V_D: dead space; P_aCO_2: arterial pCO_2; P_B: barometric pressure.

Central Hemodynamics

In young adults, systemic arterial blood pressure (BP) rises as the intensity of exercise is increased. At peak-exercise, systolic BP typically exceeds resting values by 50%–75%. In contrast, diastolic pressure changes little during exercise. Consequently, mean arterial pressure (MAP) increases only 25%–30% above resting values. The relatively modest rise in MAP, despite the four- to fivefold increase in cardiac output that accompanies strenuous exercise, indicates that systemic vascular resistance (SVR) falls dramatically, typically to levels 30%–40% of resting values. Most of the decrease in SVR is due to dilation of blood vessels in the exercising muscles and cutaneous vascular beds.[6] Left ventricular (LV) filling pressures also rise during exercise, as the ventricle moves up its Starling curve to accommodate the hemodynamic demands of exercise.

Pulmonary artery (PA) systolic pressure rises progressively as the intensity of exercise is increased. Near peak-exercise, PA systolic pressures are typically 100% greater than resting values. PA diastolic pressures change little during exercise. Mean PA pressures rise to levels approximately 10 mm Hg (~70%) above resting values. Almost all the increase in mean PA pressure is due to the rise in left-sided filling pressures. The transpulmonary gradient changes little during exercise, indicating that the four- to fivefold increase in pulmonary blood flow (PBF) during exercise is accompanied by an almost reciprocal fall in PVR.[6] This fall is mediated by dilation of pulmonary resistance vessels and by recruitment of pulmonary vascular beds that are closed or only partially perfused at rest.

It can be seen from this analysis that the hemodynamic work performed by the LV at peak-exercise (pressure × flow) is more than six times greater than resting values. The hemodynamic work performed by the RV increases even more dramatically (more than eightfold) during exercise. This observation has important implications for patients in whom the RV may be absent or structurally abnormal.

The dramatic increase in ventricular work during exercise is supported by a concomitant increase in coronary blood flow during exercise. This increase in coronary blood flow results from a decline in coronary vascular resistance and other factors related to the structure of the coronary vascular bed and its unique relationship to the myocardium.[7] The myocardial blood supply during exercise may be compromised by congenital or acquired coronary artery lesions. It is also important to recall that coronary arterial blood flow occurs primarily during diastole. Consequently, aortic regurgitation and diastolic run-off lesions (e.g., aorto-pulmonary shunting lesions) can compromise coronary perfusion by lowering diastolic BP and, therefore, coronary perfusion pressure.

Conduct of an Exercise Test

The protocol chosen for an exercise test should be determined by the clinical questions to be addressed (Table 12.1). Most questions can be addressed with either a cycle or a

TABLE 12.1 Important Clinical Questions that May be Addressed in the Exercise Physiology Laboratory

- What causes a patient to stop exercising? Is the patient limited by cardiovascular, respiratory, musculoskeletal, hematologic, metabolic, neurologic, emotional, or other factors?
- If the patient's ability to exercise is limited by the function of his/her cardiovascular system, which specific cardiovascular factors are responsible for the limitation?
- If the patient's ability to exercise is limited by respiratory or other factors, can the pathophysiologic processes responsible of the poor exercise function be identified more clearly?
- How does the patient's condition compare to normal subjects?
- How does the patient's condition compare to his/her past status?
- What interventions might improve his/her status?
- How might the effectiveness of these interventions be assessed?
- Does exercise pose any risk for this patient?
- Can anything be done to minimize these risks?
- How can the effectiveness of these risk-lowering strategies be assessed?

TABLE 12.2 Relative Advantages of Bicycle and Treadmill Ergometers

Bicycle	Treadmill
Easy to measure external work	Can achieve slightly higher peak $\dot{V}_{O2}$ and peak HR and peak myocardial $\dot{V}_{O2}$
External work performed relatively independent of patient size	May more closely simulate a patient's usual physical activities
Ramp protocols → easier to determine VAT	Can easily accommodate very small patients
Can more easily accommodate extremely-fit individuals	
Less noisy → easier to determine BP	
Less motion artifact on EKG	
Less risk of injury	
Less expensive	
Requires less space	

TABLE 12.3 The Standard Bruce Protocol

Stage	Speed (mph)	Grade (%)	Duration (min)
1	1.7	10	3
2	2.5	12	3
3	3.4	14	3
4	4.2	16	3
5	5.0	18	3
6	5.5	20	3
7	6.0	22	3

TABLE 12.4 Physiologic and Clinical Parameters Determined During Exercise Tests

Measured Variables	Derived Variables	Clinical Parameters
RR	$\dot{V}_E$	$\dot{V}_{O2}$ max
V_T	$\dot{V}_{CO2}$	Peak work rate
P_ECO_2	$\dot{V}_{O2}$	VAT
P_EO_2	Heart rate	Peak RER
$P_{ET}CO_2$	Arrhythmias	Peak HR
$P_{ET}O_2$	ST changes	Peak O_2 pulse
Blood pressure		Peak $\dot{V}_E$
Work rate		Breathing reserve
Oxygen saturation		$\Delta\dot{V}_E/\Delta\dot{V}_{CO2}$
EKG		Peak V_T and RR

EKG, electrocardiogram; *HR*, heart rate; P_ECO_2, partial presure of carbon dioxide in expired gas; P_EO_2, partial pressure of oxygen in expired gas; $P_{ET}CO_2$; partial pressure of carbon dioxide in end-tidal gas; $P_{ET}O_2$, partial pressure of oxygen in end-tidal gas; *RER*, respiratory exchange ratio; *RR*, respiratory rate; V_T, tidal volume; *VAT*, ventilatory anaerobic threshold; V_E, minute ventilation; V_{CO2}, carbon dioxide output; V_{O2}, oxygen consumption

treadmill ergometer. The relative advantages of these modalities are listed in Table 12.2. The most popular cycle protocol is a "ramp" protocol in which the subject pedals at a rate of 60 rpm. After an initial 2- to 3-minute warm-up period against zero resistance, the resistance is increased progressively at a constant rate until the 60 rpm pedaling rate can no longer be maintained. The rate at which the resistance is increased is selected so that the subject will reach peak-exercise after about 10 minutes. The most popular treadmill protocol is the "Bruce protocol" (Table 12.3). In this protocol, the treadmill speed and elevation are increased by predetermined amounts every 3 minutes, until the subject can go no further or the desired information has been acquired.[8] The protocol has only seven stages and is therefore not ideal for extremely fit individuals whose exercise capacity exceeds that required to complete the seventh stage. Baseline, and sometimes post-exercise, spirometric measurements are commonly obtained at the time of exercise testing to aid in the interpretation of the exercise physiology data.

Interpretation of Exercise Physiology Tests

Table 12.4 lists the physiologic variables that are directly measured during a non-invasive exercise physiology test and

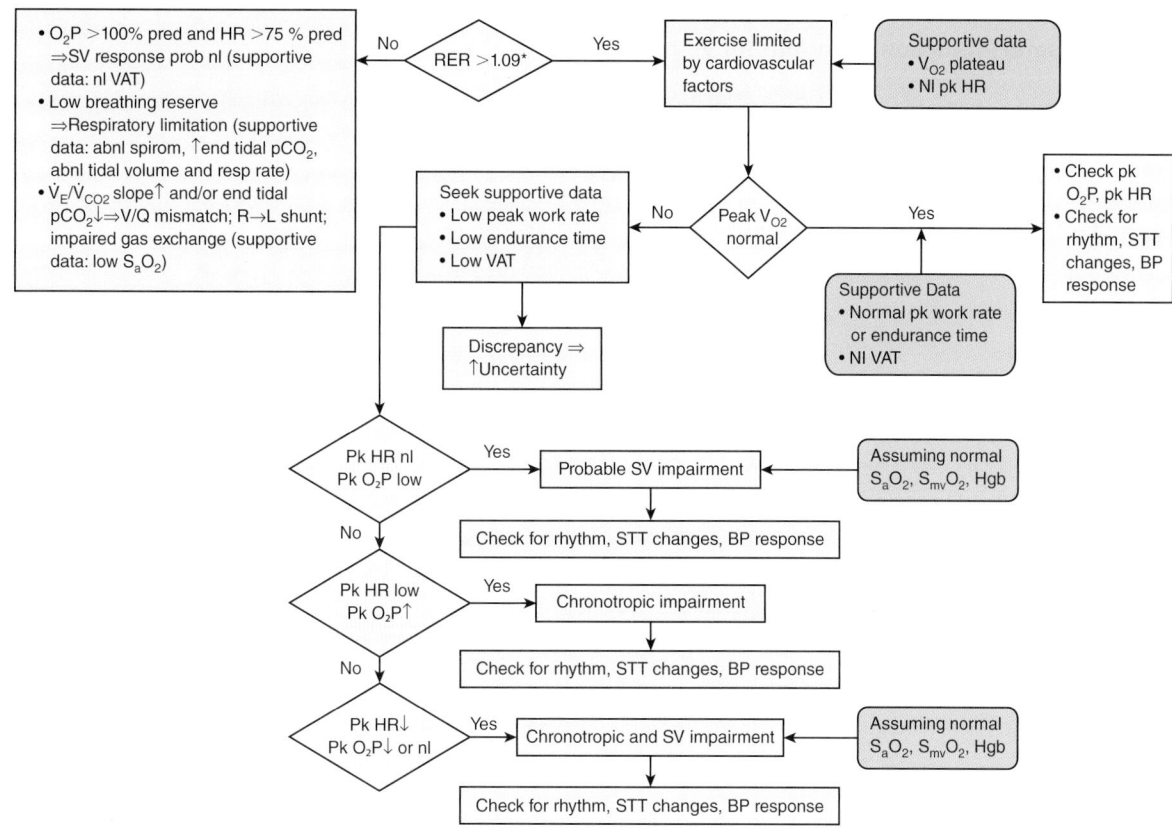

*$\dot{V}_E/\dot{V}_{CO2}$ slope, end tidal pCO$_2$, RR, tidal volume, breathing reserve and spirometry should also be assessed at the end of each branch point

• **Fig. 12.2** Algorithm for the assessment of cardiopulmonary exercise test data. *BP*, Blood pressure; *Hgb*, hemoglobin; *HR*, heart rate; *nl*, normal; *O$_2$P*, oxygen pulse; *pk*, peak; *RER*, respiratory exchange ratio; *S$_a$O$_2$*, arterial oxygen saturation; *S$_{mv}$O$_2$*, mixed venous oxygen saturation; *SV*, stroke volume; *VAT*, ventilatory anaerobic threshold; *V$_{O2}$*, oxygen consumption.

some of the clinically relevant derived physiologic parameters. An analytic approach to the interpretation of these data is presented in Fig. 12.2.

$\dot{V}_{O2}$ Max

During a progressive exercise test, $\dot{V}_{O_2}$ increases linearly in proportion to work rate (WR). However, near peak-exercise, $\dot{V}_{O_2}$ plateaus, and further increases in WR do not induce additional increases in $\dot{V}_{O_2}$. The level of $\dot{V}_{O_2}$ at this plateau is defined as $\dot{V}_{O_2}$max. The level of motivation and effort required to reach $\dot{V}_{O_2}$max is not always achieved during an exercise test, especially when the subject is a young child. Many will refer to the highest $\dot{V}_{O_2}$ achieved as the "peak $\dot{V}_{O_2}$" rather than the " $\dot{V}_{O_2}$max." When an exercise test is terminated due to motivational factors or factors other than the cardiopulmonary system's ability to deliver O$_2$ to the exercising muscles, peak $\dot{V}_{O_2}$ will be less than $\dot{V}_{O_2}$max.

$\dot{V}_{O_2}$ max is one of the best indicators of exercise capacity and cardiopulmonary fitness. However, defining a "normal" value for $\dot{V}_{O_2}$max is not straightforward. $\dot{V}_{O_2}$max, when expressed as milliliters O$_2$/min, increases as body mass increases.

$\dot{V}_{O_2}$max is therefore commonly normalized for weight. However, the relationship between $\dot{V}_{O_2}$max and body weight is nonlinear. Moreover, $\dot{V}_{O_2}$max is affected by other factors such as body habitus and composition; since adipose tissue consumes almost no O$_2$ during exercise, normalizing $\dot{V}_{O_2}$max for weight alone may be misleading and predispose to erroneous conclusions.

Some physiologists have suggested normalizing $\dot{V}_{O_2}$max using an exponent of body length or weight. There is no conformity of opinion concerning the optimal method and these approaches invariably result in rather unwieldy and unfamiliar units (e.g., mL O$_2$/kg$^{2/3}$/min). In addition, regression equations can produce unrealistic results when a subject's age and/or size are near or beyond the limits of the patient population from which the equation was derived.[1] Although each approach has its advantages and disadvantages, most pediatric exercise laboratories' estimates of $\dot{V}_{O_2}$max are generated using a regression equation that takes into account age, sex, height, and/or weight (Table 12.5).[9-12] It is important to use a regression equation generated from an appropriate protocol and study population.

Among patients with congenital heart disease (CHD), the most common factors responsible for a low $\dot{V}_{O_2}$max are:

TABLE 12.5	Some Useful Prediction Equations for $\dot{V}_{O_2}$max*	

Predicted $\dot{V}_{O_2}$ max (L/min) =	Comments
For males: $\quad 4.36 \times ht - 4.55$ For females: $\quad 2.25 \times ht - 1.84$	These equations, derived from normal subjects aged 6–17 years, are the ones used most frequently for pediatric patients.[11] They tend to generate unrealistically high estimates for extremely tall, thin subjects, and for extremely short subjects (<130 cm tall) paradoxically predict lower values for boys than for girls.
For males: $\quad 0.053 \times wt - 0.30$ For females: $\quad 0.029 \times wt - 0.29$	These equations, derived from normal subjects aged 6–17 years,[12] yield unrealistically high values for overweight subjects, but may provide superior estimates for tall, thin subjects.
For males: $\quad (3.45 \times ht) - (0.028 \times A) + (0.022 \times wt) - 3.76$ For females: $\quad (2.49 \times ht) - (0.018 \times A) + (0.010 \times wt) - 2.26$	These equations are for subjects > 17 years old.[10]
For males: $0.67 \times ht^{2.7}$ For females: $0.48 \times ht^{2.7}$	These equations are appropriate for subjects < 20 years old.[10] Because weight is not considered, they may produce unrealistically high values for tall, thin subjects.
For males: $\quad 5.14 \times ht^{1.88}/A^{0.49}$ For females: $\quad 3.55 \times ht^{1.88}/A^{0.49}$	These equations are appropriate for subjects > 20 years old.[10] Because weight is not considered, they may produce unrealistically high values for tall, thin subjects.

*Predicted values are for bicycle ergometry. Treadmill values are 5%–10% higher.
A, Age in years; *ht*, height in meters; *wt*, weight in kilograms.

(1) an inability to increase SV during exercise (e.g., patients with ventricular systolic or diastolic dysfunction, valvular disease, left-to-right shunts, elevated systemic afterload, preload limitation, or pulmonary vascular disease); (2) an inability to increase HR to appropriate levels at peak-exercise (e.g., patients with sinus or atrioventricular node dysfunction); and (3) systemic hypoxemia (e.g., patients with right-to-left shunts).[1]

Peak Work Rate

The peak WR achieved during a progressive exercise test is another useful index of exercise function. This parameter is not readily determined during treadmill exercise testing, because the work is a function not only of the speed and elevation of the treadmill but also of the weight borne by the subject's feet. This last variable is a function of the subject's body weight and the difficult-to-quantify degree to which he/she leans on the handrails. Due to these complexities, the endurance time on a standard protocol (e.g., the Bruce protocol) is used as a surrogate for the peak WR. Nomograms are available for the prediction of an individual's endurance time on the basis of age and sex (Table 12.6).[8] The normal ranges tend to be quite broad and it must be emphasized that endurance time on a treadmill does not provide quantitative information regarding the amount of work that an individual's cardiopulmonary system may support. It is therefore often inappropriate and misleading to compare the endurance times of different subjects. Endurance times from serial exercise tests on the same subject are frequently worthwhile, but the potential influence of changes in a subject's age, size, and exercise technique must be taken into account.[1]

The work performed on a cycle ergometer derives primarily from the work required to overcome the resistance in the pedals. WR is readily measured during these tests and generally expressed in the unit of Watts. Identifying a "normal value" for the peak WR is complicated by many of the same considerations that applied to peak $\dot{V}_{O_2}$. Consequently, regression equations are generally used to calculate predicted values for peak WR and results are expressed as a percentage of this predicted value.[9]

Because the amount of work performed during an exercise test is dependent upon the amount of O_2 that can be delivered to the exercising muscles, the peak WR is influenced by the same factors that influence peak $\dot{V}_{O_2}$. The peak WR may also be influenced by orthopedic, neurologic, and other mechanical issues that can affect the efficiency of exercise.

Ventilatory Anaerobic Threshold

During a progressive exercise test, the VAT occurs when aerobic metabolism, which is limited by the amount of O_2 delivered by the cardiovascular system, is insufficient to meet the energy requirements of the exercising muscles. The VAT is a physiologic phenomenon that is not affected

TABLE 12.6	Endurance Time on Bruce Protocol for Normal Children With Innocent Murmurs

Age group (yr)	Percentiles					Mean	SD
	10	25	50	75	90		
Boys							
4–5	8.1	9.0	10.0	12.0	13.3	10.4	1.9
6–7	9.7	10.0	12.0	12.3	13.5	11.8	1.6
8–9	9.6	10.5	12.4	13.7	16.2	12.6	2.3
10–12	9.9	12.0	12.5	14.0	15.4	12.7	1.9
13–15	11.2	13.0	14.3	16.0	16.1	14.1	1.7
16–18	11.3	12.1	13.8	14.5	15.8	13.5	1.4
Girls							
4–5	7.0	8.0	9.0	11.2	12.3	9.5	1.8
6–7	9.5	9.6	11.4	13.0	13.0	11.2	1.5
8–9	9.9	10.5	11.0	13.0	14.2	11.8	1.6
10–12	10.5	11.3	12.0	13.0	14.6	12.3	1.4
13–15	9.4	10.0	11.5	12.0	13.0	11.1	1.3
16–18	8.1	10.0	10.5	12.0	12.4	10.7	1.4

by patient effort or motivation and may be determined on a submaximal exercise test. Because anaerobic metabolism produces CO_2 but does not consume O_2, the VAT is marked by an increase in $\dot{V}_{CO2}$ out of proportion to the associated increase in $\dot{V}_{O2}$ during a progressive exercise test. This phenomenon is manifested by a change in the slope of the $\dot{V}_{CO2}$ versus $\dot{V}_{O2}$ curve or the $\dot{V}_E$ versus $\dot{V}_{O2}$ curve. The VAT may also be determined by detecting the point where the $\dot{V}_E/\dot{V}_{O2}$ reaches a minimum and begins to increase while the $\dot{V}_E/\dot{V}_{CO2}$ is flat or decreasing. End-tidal pO_2 also reaches a minimum at the VAT.[13] Computer algorithms are available for detecting the VAT. These algorithms are sometimes confounded by erratic breathing patterns which is a common problem among anxious young patients. It is therefore important to assure that the computer-determined VAT corresponds with the value determined by visual inspection of the appropriate graphs.

The VAT is usually expressed in the units "mL O_2/kg/min". Prediction equations exist for the calculation of normal values for the VAT based on age, size, and sex. VAT is also commonly expressed as a percentage of predicted $\dot{V}_{O2}$ max. In the absence of cardiovascular disease, VAT rarely falls below 40% of predicted $\dot{V}_{O2}$max. However, VAT is often depressed below this value in patients with conditions which impair the ability to increase CO or O_2 delivery appropriately during exercise.[5,14] VAT is also dramatically depressed in patients with coarctation of the aorta, peripheral vascular disease (e.g., patients with Takayasu's arteritis),

and other conditions which limit blood flow to the legs during exercise.[14]

The Respiratory Exchange Ratio

During a progressive exercise test, the RER rises progressively after the VAT has been passed and is therefore an objective physiologic index of effort.[13,14] For adults and older children, a peak RER < 1.09 implies that exercise was not terminated on account of a cardiovascular limitation. Young children tend to have less anaerobic capacity and their peak-exercise RER therefore tends to be slightly lower. Conversely, a peak-exercise RER > 1.09 suggests that a cardiovascular limitation (i.e., an inability to provide sufficient O_2 to the muscles to support ongoing exercise) was at least a major factor responsible for the termination of exercise. These considerations are of particular importance in patients with a compromised chronotropic response to exercise, a condition commonly encountered after surgery for CHD. In these cases, an elevated peak-exercise RER would indicate that the low peak HR is not due to a suboptimal effort. Determination of the peak-exercise RER is also very helpful in the interpretation of exercise tests of patients receiving beta-blockers or other antiarrhythmic agents which may depress the chronotropic response.

If a patient's peak-exercise RER is low, exercise was probably not terminated on account of a cardiovascular limitation. Under these circumstances, peak-exercise RER may not accurately reflect the patient's cardiovascular status and must be interpreted with caution. Data from submaximal exercise, however, may still be valid and useful.[1]

Heart Rate

The maximum HR achievable at peak-exercise tends to decline with age. For treadmill exercise, the normal peak HR is commonly estimated from the equation:

$$\text{Peak HR} = 220 - \text{age (in years)}$$

Peak HR on a cycle tends to be about 5%–10% less than on a treadmill.[15]

During a progressive exercise test, HR rises linearly in proportion to $\dot{V}_{O_2}$, from resting to peak values. In patients with isolated chronotropic defects, the slope of the HR versus $\dot{V}_{O_2}$ curve is depressed and a normal peak HR is not achieved. Patients with a depressed SV response to exercise rely excessively on a rise in HR to increase their CO, and the slope of the HR vs. $\dot{V}_{O_2}$ curve is abnormally steep. This abnormal HR response may be seen even in patients with co-existing chronotropic defects. In these individuals, the stimulus to increase HR in compensation for the depressed SV response partially overwhelms the chronotropic defect and causes the HR rise to be abnormally steep relative to the rise in $\dot{V}_{O_2}$, even though the peak-exercise HR remains abnormally low. In contrast, athletes tend to have larger-than-normal SVs and therefore at submaximal levels of exercise tend to have a low HR for any given $\dot{V}_{O_2}$. The athlete's peak-exercise HR, however, is normal (Fig. 12.3).[1]

The Oxygen Pulse

The oxygen pulse (O_2P) at peak-exercise is related to the SV at peak-exercise and is, therefore, one of the most useful indices available from the exercise physiology laboratory. The relationship between the O_2P and SV is best understood by dividing both sides of the Fick equation by HR:

$$\dot{V}_{O_2}/HR = O_2P = CO/HR \times O_2 \text{ extraction}$$
$$= SV \times O_2 \text{ extraction})$$

At peak-exercise, O_2 extraction is maximized and may be assumed to be the same value in most patients. Therefore, at peak-exercise, O_2P is proportional to SV provided the assumption regarding the O_2 extraction at peak-exercise and the blood's O_2 content is valid. Normal values for O_2P at peak-exercise may be calculated by dividing the predicted peak $\dot{V}_{O_2}$ by the predicted peak HR. Peak-exercise O_2P is best expressed as an absolute value (mL O_2/beat) and as a percentage of the predicted peak-exercise O_2P.

When using the O_2P to draw conclusions concerning a subject's SV at peak-exercise, it is important to recall that O_2 extraction is equal to the C_aO_2 minus the C_vO_2. Consequently, in patients with depressed C_aO_2 at peak-exercise (e.g., patients with anemia or patients with significant arterial desaturation at peak-exercise), O_2 extraction at peak-exercise would be less than normal and the O_2P would

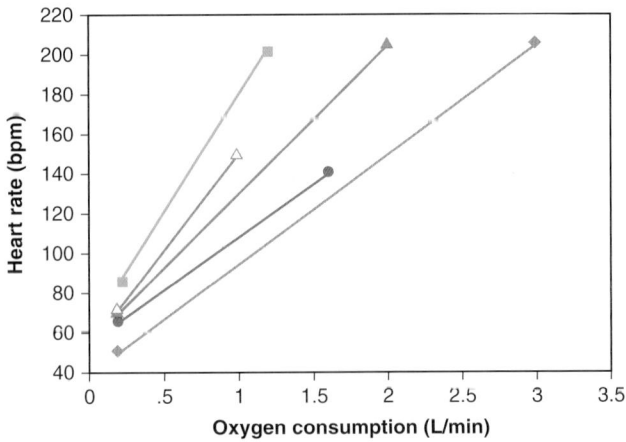

• **Fig. 12.3** Influence of various clinical conditions upon the relationship between heart rate and oxygen consumption during exercise. Variation of heart rate with respect to oxygen consumption during a progressive exercise test for a hypothetical 50-kg 15-year-old normal subject (*solid triangle*), athlete (*diamond*), patient with a depressed chronotropic response (*circle*), patient with a depressed stroke volume response (*square*), and a patient with both a depressed chronotropic and stroke volume response (*open triangles*). Note that the athlete's peak oxygen pulse (peak oxygen consumption divided by peak heart rate) is above normal. The patient with a depressed stroke volume response has a below-normal peak oxygen pulse and partially compensates for this condition by increasing heart rate more rapidly than normal, causing the slope of the heart rate-oxygen consumption curve to be abnormally steep. In contrast, the patient with a depressed chronotropic response has an abnormally flattened curve and cannot achieve a normal peak heart rate, although a partial compensation for the chronotropic deficiency is achieved by increasing the peak oxygen pulse (i.e., stroke volume) to above-normal levels. The patient with the depressed chronotropic and stroke volume response still has a steeper-than-normal slope but cannot achieve a normal peak heart rate and cannot compensate for this chronotropic deficiency by increasing stroke volume. This individual's peak oxygen consumption is therefore more depressed than any of the other subjects'.

therefore underestimate SV. In contrast, polycythemia increases C_aO_2 and would therefore cause the O_2P to overestimate SV. Similarly, among athletes, the peak O_2P tends to overestimate SV because their O_2 extraction at peak-exercise is slightly higher than that of normal subjects. If these potential confounding factors are borne in mind, calculation of the O_2P can permit clinicians to make valid and valuable inferences regarding a subject's cardiovascular response to exercise.[c]

The O_2P tends to be depressed in patients with conditions that impair their ability to increase SV to appropriate levels at peak-exercise. Patients with depressed ventricular function, severe valvular disease, systemic hypertension, coronary artery disease, and pulmonary vascular obstructive disease often have a low peak-exercise O_2P.[1] The O_2P is often depressed in patients who have undergone a Fontan

---

[c]For the purposes of this discussion, the term SV refers to the forward, or physiologic SV (i.e., the amount of blood that goes to the body with each heartbeat). It is therefore not equivalent to the anatomic SV (i.e., end-diastolic volume minus end-systolic volume) when valvular regurgitation or shunt lesions are present.

procedure, even in the absence of ventricular or valvular dysfunction.[16] In these patients, the low O_2P probably reflects the absence of a subpulmonary ventricle, the inability of the passively perfused pulmonary vascular bed to accommodate the high rate of blood flow normally present at peak-exercise, and the consequent underfilling (i.e., preload limitation) of the systemic ventricle.[1]

Young patients with chronic aortic regurgitation usually have well-preserved exercise function and peak-exercise O_2P.[17] In these patients, the fall in SVR that normally accompanies exercise tends to lessen the severity of the regurgitation during exercise. In addition, the LV dilation typically present in chronic aortic regurgitation helps to maintain SV and usually compensates effectively for the hemodynamic burden imposed by the leaky valve. Similar factors may also help to preserve the exercise function of patients with other valvular insufficiency lesions.

Minute Ventilation and Breathing Reserve

At peak-exercise, minute ventilation ($\dot{V}_E$) is usually less than the maximum voluntary ventilation (MVV, the maximum amount of air that a subject can breathe in and out in 1 minute). MVV is usually estimated by measuring the maximum amount of air a subject can breathe out during 12 seconds of maximal hyperventilation and multiplying this quantity by 5. This maneuver requires a degree of patient cooperation that is often beyond the capacity of most young subjects and many older participants as well. Alternatively, MVV may be estimated by multiplying FEV_1 from baseline spirometry by 40.[18] Breathing reserve (BR) is the percentage of a subject's MVV that is not used at peak-exercise.

The normal BR at peak-exercise is 20–45%.[5] Patients with isolated cardiovascular disease tend to have normal MVVs, but their peak $\dot{V}_E$ tends to be low because their exercise capacity is depressed due to their cardiovascular disease. Consequently, these patients have higher-than-normal BRs. In contrast, patients with severe lung disease are often "respiratorily limited." They will typically have a lower-than-normal MVV and will have little or no BR at peak-exercise.

$$\Delta\dot{V}_E/\Delta\dot{V}_{CO2}$$

Normally, during a progressive exercise test, $\dot{V}_E$ rises linearly in proportion to $\dot{V}_{CO2}$ until the respiratory compensation point, a point above the anaerobic threshold when the accumulating lactic acidosis causes a compensatory increase in $\dot{V}_E$ out of proportion to the increase in $\dot{V}_{CO2}$. The slope of the linear portion (i.e., the portion of the curve below the respiratory compensation point) of the $\dot{V}_E$ versus $\dot{V}_{CO2}$ curve ($\Delta\dot{V}_E/\Delta\dot{V}_{CO2}$, i.e., the number of liters of air that must be breathed out in order to eliminate 1 L of CO_2) is a useful index of pulmonary function that reflects the efficiency of gas exchange during exercise. For adolescents and young adults, the normal value for $\Delta\dot{V}_E/\Delta\dot{V}_{CO2}$ is less than 28. It tends to be higher in children because their anatomic

V_D is higher relative to their lung volumes and their V_D/V_T ratio is therefore higher than that of older individuals,[19] as well as in older adults when gas exchange efficiency declines with age.

For gas exchange to proceed optimally, ventilation and perfusion must be optimally matched. Consequently, conditions which cause maldistribution of PBF are associated with an elevated $\Delta\dot{V}_E/\Delta\dot{V}_{CO2}$. This phenomenon is commonly encountered among patients with residual PA stenoses following repair of tetralogy of Fallot (TOF). In these subjects there is a positive correlation between $\Delta\dot{V}_E/\Delta\dot{V}_{CO2}$ and the degree of PBF maldistribution present on radionuclide lung perfusion scans. A pulmonary balloon angioplasty that effectively improves PBF distribution also improves (lowers) the $\Delta\dot{V}_E/\Delta\dot{V}_{CO2}$.[20]

The $\Delta\dot{V}_E/\Delta\dot{V}_{CO2}$ has also been found to be one of the best predictors of peak $\dot{V}_{O2}$ in postoperative TOF patients.[21] This observation probably reflects the critical, deleterious impact that PA stenoses combined with the pulmonary regurgitation may have upon the RV's ability to increase cardiac output during exercise.[22] Over time, this pernicious physiology has an adverse effect upon a patient's cardiovascular health; consequently, the $\Delta\dot{V}_E/\Delta\dot{V}_{CO2}$ is an excellent predictor of survival in patients with repaired TOF.

Patients with congestive heart failure (CHF) have PBF maldistribution as a consequence of the elevated pulmonary capillary wedge pressure (PCWP) that accompanies CHF. As ventricular function deteriorates and PCWP rises, the PBF maldistribution, and consequent ventilation/perfusion mismatch, worsens and the $\Delta\dot{V}_E/\Delta\dot{V}_{CO2}$ progressively rises. This strong link between PCWP and the $\Delta\dot{V}_E/\Delta\dot{V}_{CO2}$ probably accounts for the prognostic power of the $\Delta\dot{V}_E/\Delta\dot{V}_{CO2}$ in this patient population.[23] In a similar manner, for patients with an atrial switch procedure (Mustard or Senning) for transposition of the great arteries, elevation of the $\Delta\dot{V}_E/\Delta\dot{V}_{CO2}$ probably reflects the progressive systemic ventricular dysfunction that often develops in these patients and has been found to be a good predictor of prognosis in this population.[24]

In patients with pulmonary hypertension, PBF maldistribution results from pulmonary vascular disease. As the disease progresses, the PBF maldistribution worsens, gas exchange within the lungs becomes more and more inefficient, and $\Delta\dot{V}_E/\Delta\dot{V}_{CO2}$ rises. Hence, for patients with this condition, $\Delta\dot{V}_E/\Delta\dot{V}_{CO2}$ reflects the extent of disease within the pulmonary vasculature and has been found to be an excellent prognostic indicator.[25]

The $\Delta\dot{V}_E/\Delta\dot{V}_{CO2}$ is often elevated in Fontan patients.[26] This observation is probably due to the absence of a subpulmonary ventricle. The consequent loss of the normal PA pulsatility results in ventilation/perfusion mismatch secondary to a suboptimal PBF distribution. However, $\Delta\dot{V}_E/\Delta\dot{V}_{CO2}$ has not been found to be a good prognostic indicator in these patients, as the PBF maldistribution is related to their single ventricle physiology and unlike the conditions mentioned above, is not strongly related to the severity or progression of their disease. Elevations of $\Delta\dot{V}_E/\Delta\dot{V}_{CO_2}$ may also be seen in patients in whom the transport of gases across the alveolar-capillary membrane is impaired (e.g., patients with PCWP and/or alveolar disease).

Right-to-left shunting will also cause elevation of $\Delta\dot{V}_E/\Delta\dot{V}_{CO_2}$. This phenomenon results from the fact that the right-to-left shunting blood contains high levels of carbon dioxide during exercise. Chemoreceptors in the aorta will sense this elevated pCO_2 and stimulate hyperventilation so that the blood returning from the lungs will have a lower-than-normal pCO_2. When this blood mixes with the right-to-left shunting blood, the pCO_2 of the resulting admixture will be normal.[27]

Tidal Volume and Respiratory Rate

The V_T at peak-exercise typically increases to about 60% of the baseline forced vital capacity (FVC).[5] The FVC of patients who have undergone multiple cardiothoracic surgical procedures is often reduced, however, and their V_T at peak-exercise may comprise an abnormally large percentage of their baseline FVC. Patients with reactive airway disease may develop bronchoconstriction and air trapping during exercise and have abnormally small tidal volumes at peak-exercise. In these patients, post-exercise spirometric measurements would typically demonstrate an obstructive pattern more severe than that present on baseline spirometry. In contrast, upper airway obstruction (e.g., tracheal compression secondary to a vascular ring) tends to result in unusually large, slow breaths during exercise. The peak RR usually does not exceed 60 breaths/min (70 breaths/min in young children).[5] More rapid RRs are often seen in patients with restrictive or interstitial lung disease.

End-Tidal pCO$_2$

Normally, end-tidal pCO_2 ($P_{ET}CO_2$) approximates P_aCO_2. In fact, at rest $P_{ET}CO_2$ slightly underestimates P_aCO_2, and during heavy exercise it slightly overestimates P_aCO_2. However, in the presence of ventilation/perfusion mismatch, the close relationship between $P_{ET}CO_2$ and P_aCO_2 is disrupted. Under these circumstances, end tidal air is disproportionately derived from alveoli with high ventilation/perfusion ratios and consequently low pCO_2; $P_{ET}CO_2$ would therefore be less than P_aCO_2. Hence, a persistently low $P_{ET}CO_2$ throughout an exercise test is most often encountered in patients with ventilation/perfusion mismatch. Low $P_{ET}CO_2$ is also seen in patients with chronic metabolic acidosis due to an associated compensatory respiratory alkalosis and in patients with right-to-left intracardiac shunts. In these latter individuals, the pCO_2 of the blood returning from the lungs in the pulmonary veins (equal to the $P_{ET}CO_2$) must be reduced to below normal values. This adaptation allows the blood entering the systemic circulation, a mixture of pulmonary venous and right-to-left shunting blood, to have a normal pCO_2. In patients with right-to-left intracardiac shunts following a fenestrated Fontan procedure, the $P_{ET}CO_2$ (and the $\Delta\dot{V}_E/\Delta\dot{V}_{CO_2}$) during exercise trend

toward normal values following transcatheter closure of the Fontan fenestration.[27]

Rarely, a persistently low $P_{ET}CO_{22}$ may be due to hyperventilation secondary to emotional or psychological factors. In these situations, however, it is unusual for one to continue to hyperventilate throughout an exercise test. Arterial blood sampling is helpful in circumstances where doubt exists concerning the factors responsible for a $P_{ET}CO_2$. An elevated $P_{ET}CO_2$ almost invariably reflects CO_2 retention, usually secondary to respiratory disease. An exception to this generalization is encountered in athletic individuals at high exercise intensities.

Blood Pressure

Peak systolic BP rarely exceeds 200 mm Hg in normal adolescents.[15] In pediatric patients, an excessive rise in right upper extremity BP during exercise is most commonly encountered in patients with coarctation of the aorta; this may persist even after a successful repair. An excessive rise in BP may also be seen in patients with renal vascular disease, essential hypertension, and in patients with diffuse arteriopathies. At peak-exercise, systolic BP should exceed resting values by at least 25%. A depressed BP response may be seen in patients with cardiomyopathies, ventricular outflow tract obstruction, severe atrioventricular valve insufficiency, severe pulmonary insufficiency, pulmonary vascular obstructive disease, and coronary artery disease. Systolic BP should never fall during exercise and a fall in systolic BP is an indication for termination of an exercise test. Abrupt, dramatic declines in BP following exercise are sometimes seen in patients with vasodepressor syncope.

The Exercise EKG

Analysis of exercise EKG data is an integral component of an exercise test. The influence of exercise on the incidence and nature of rhythm disturbances should be assessed. In normal hearts, ectopy that is suppressed by exercise is thought to be benign. In contrast, myocardial ischemia, cardiomyopathies, and conditions such as the prolonged QT syndrome and catecholaminergic polymorphic ventricular tachycardia are often characterized by an increase in the frequency and complexity of ectopy during exercise. Rhythm disturbances are also commonly encountered in patients who have had surgery for CHD. In these patients, the absence or suppression of an arrhythmia during an exercise test may have little predictive value. Patients whose arrhythmias develop or worsen with exercise, however, appear to be at greater risk for future serious arrhythmic events. Exercise testing therefore plays an important role in the assessment and management of this difficult clinical issue.[1]

The influence of exercise on conduction abnormalities should also be assessed. Patients with significant AV nodal disease may develop progressively higher-grade AV block during exercise. In contrast, patients with AV block secondary to elevated resting vagal tone (e.g., many athletes) typically develop normal AV conduction during exercise.

In patients with Wolff-Parkinson-White syndrome, an abrupt loss of pre-excitation during exercise, a phenomenon encountered in ~15% of cases, may indicate that the bypass tract has a relatively long anterograde effective refractory period and that the subject is therefore at low risk for sudden cardiac death. However, there is not universal agreement on this point. A gradual loss of pre-excitation merely reflects enhancement of AV node conduction secondary to the changes in autonomic tone associated with exercise and indicates nothing about the electrophysiologic properties of the bypass tract. Borderline cases, in which categorization is somewhat subjective, are often encountered.[1]

Patients with the prolonged QT syndrome may have normal QT intervals at rest but may be unable to shorten their QT interval appropriately during exercise and/or in early recovery.[1] In patients with pacemakers, analysis of the exercise EKG may help assess whether the pacemaker is functioning properly and whether the pacemaker settings are optimal.[1]

The influence of exercise on the ST segment and T wave morphology should also be analyzed. It must be emphasized, however, that the incidence of coronary artery disease in the pediatric population is quite low, and the sensitivity and specificity of ST-T wave changes for the detection of coronary artery anomalies in pediatric subjects is unknown. Exercise-induced ST-T wave changes are more commonly encountered in pediatric patients with cardiomyopathies and/or myocardial ischemia secondary to excessively high myocardial O_2 demand during exercise (e.g., patients with aortic stenosis). More severe ST changes are certainly more suggestive of myocardial ischemia, especially when associated with chest pain and other abnormalities. However, the correlation between ST changes and myocardial ischemia in pediatric patients, although not precisely known, is probably no more than moderate. Radionuclide-based myocardial perfusion imaging is often employed to help in the assessment of at-risk patients and has been helpful in patients with Kawasaki disease and hypertrophic cardiomyopathy. Of note, perfusion abnormalities unassociated with significant detectable coronary artery pathology, are commonly found in patients following the arterial switch operation and are of questionable significance.[28] The value of myocardial perfusion studies in patients with congenital coronary artery malformations has not been established. Stress echocardiography has emerged as a radiation-free alternative to myocardial perfusion imaging. However, it too is encumbered by issues of low sensitivity and specificity.

It is with great sadness that we note the passing of Dr. Rhodes between his revising of this chapter and the publication of this edition of the textbook. For all of us who were lucky enough to work with Dr. Rhodes, we know that in addition to exceptional clinical care, teaching was his greatest passion. Every trainee and colleague who worked with Dr. Rhodes can recall the many lessons he passed on during our time with him. Each of us know of some element of cardiology "from the world according to Jonathan Rhodes". His legacy is one-of-a-kind, compassionate and dedicated person, clinician, teacher, and exercise physiologist with an unmatched love for his family, patients, and colleagues.

- Fellows of the Department of Cardiology, Boston Children's Hospital

References

1. Rhodes J, Alexander ME, Optowsky AR. *Exercuse Physiology for the Pediatric and Congenital Cardiologist.* Cham, Switzerland: Springer; 2019.
2. Braunwald E, Sonnenblick EH, Ross Jr J, Glick G, Epstein SE. An analysis of the cardiac response to exercise. *Circ Res.* 1967; XXII(suppl 1) I-44-I-58.
3. Udelson JE, Bacharach SL, Cannon RO III, Bonow RO. Minimum left ventricular pressure during beta-adrenergic stimulation in human subjects: evidence for elastic recoil and diastolic "suction" in the normal heart. *Circulation.* 1990;82:1174-1182.
4. Wasserman K. The Dickinson W. Richards lecture. New concepts in assessing cardiovascular function. *Circulation.* 1988;78: 1060-1071.
5. Hansen JE, Sue DY, Wasserman K. Predicted values for clinical exercise testing. *Am Rev Respir Dis.* 1984;129(2 Pt 2):S49-S55.
6. Ekelund LG, Holmgren A. Central hemodynamics during exercise. *Circ Res.* 1967;20-21(suppl I):I-33-I-43.
7. Goodwill AG, Dick GM, Kiel AM, Tune JD. Regulation of coronary blood flow. *Compr Physiol.* 2017;7:321-382.
8. Cumming GR, Everatt D, Hastman L. Bruce treadmill test in children: normal values in a clinic population. *Am J Cardiol.* 1978; 41:69-75.
9. Jones NL. *Clinical Exercise Testing.* 4th ed. Philadelphia: W.B. Saunders; 1997:131-134.
10. Jones NL. *Clinical Exercise Testing.* Philadelphia: W.B. Saunders; 1997:243, 4th ed.
11. Cooper DM, Weiler-Ravell D. Gas exchange response to exercise in children. *Am Rev Respir Dis.* 1984;129:S47-S48.
12. Cooper DM, Weiler-Ravell D, Whipp BJ, Wasserman K. Aerobic parameters of exercise as a function of body size during growth in children. *J Appl Physiol.* 1984;56:628-634.
13. Wasserman K. Determinants and detection of anaerobic threshold and consequences of exercise above it. *Circulation.* 1987; 76(suppl VI):VI-29-VI-39.
14. Wasserman K. The anaerobic threshold measurement to evaluate exercise performance. *Am Rev Respir Dis.* 1984;129(2 Pt 2):S35-S40.
15. Braden DS, Carroll JF. Normative cardiovascular responses to exercise in children. *Pediatr Cardiol.* 1999;20:4-10.
16. Paridon SM, Mitchell PD, Colan SD, et al. A cross-sectional study of exercise performance during the first two decades of life following the Fontan operation. *J Am Coll Cardiol.* 2008;52:99-107.
17. Rhodes J, Fischbach PS, Patel H, Hijazi ZM. Factors affecting the exercise capacity of pediatric patients with aortic regurgitation. *Pediatr Cardiol.* 2000;21:328-333.
18. Campbell SC. A comparison of the maximum voluntary ventilation with the forced expiratory volume in one second: an assessment of subject cooperation. *J Occup Med.* 1982;24:531-533.
19. Giardini A, Odendaal D, Khambadkone S, Derrick G. Physiologic decrease of ventilatory response to exercise in the second decade of life in healthy children. *Am Heart J.* 2011;161:1214-1219.

20. Rhodes J, Dave A, Pulling MC, et al. Effect of pulmonary artery stenoses on the cardiopulmonary response to exercise following repair of tetralogy of Fallot. *Am J Cardiol.* 1998;81:1217-1219.

21. Anderson PA, Sleeper LA, Mahony L, et al. Contemporary outcomes after the Fontan procedure: a Pediatric Heart Network multicenter study. *J Am Coll Cardiol.* 2008;52:85-98.

22. Sutton NJ, Peng L, Lock JE, et al. Effect of pulmonary artery angioplasty on exercise function after repair of tetralogy of Fallot. *Am Heart J.* 2008;155:182-186.

23. Uren NG, Davies SW, Agnew JE, et al. Reduction of mismatch of global ventilation and perfusion on exercise is related to exercise capacity in chronic heart failure. *Br Heart J.* 1993;70:241-246.

24. Giardini A, Hager A, Lammers AE, et al. Ventilatory efficiency and aerobic capacity predict event-free survival in adults with atrial repair for complete transposition of the great arteries. *J Am Coll Cardiol.* 2009;53:1548-1555.

25. Wensel R, Opitz CF, Anker SD, et al. Assessment of survival in patients with primary pulmonary hypertension: importance of cardiopulmonary exercise testing. *Circulation.* 2002;106:319-324.

26. Fernandes SM, McElhinney DB, Khairy P, et al. Serial cardiopulmonary exercise testing in patients with previous Fontan surgery. *Pediatr Cardiol.* 2010;31:175-180.

27. Meadows J, Lang P, Marx G, Rhodes J. Fontan fenestration closure has no acute effect on exercise capacity but improves ventilatory response to exercise. *J Am Coll Cardiol.* 2008;52:108-113.

28. Mahle WT, McBride MG, Paridon SM. Exercise performance after the arterial switch operation for D-transposition of the great arteries. *Am J Cardiol.* 2001;87:753-758.

Cardiac Catheterization

13

Fundamentals of Cardiac Catheterization

BRIAN QUINN AND DIEGO PORRAS

KEY LEARNING POINTS

- Pediatric interventional catheterization can aid in the diagnosis and management of patients with congenital heart disease.
- This field has evolved from a primarily diagnostic procedure into a field that provides various therapeutic and palliative interventional techniques for this complex and heterogenous patient population.
- Safety has improved over time with the advent of newer technologies and techniques, along with a better understanding of patient and procedural risk.

- Hemodynamic information obtained during the catheterization procedure can allow for the measurement of cardiac output, shunt calculations, assessment of vascular resistance, and valve area measurements through precise data collection acquired during the procedure.
- Modern technology and novel invasive imaging techniques have expanded the capability of cardiac catheterization to provide diagnostic information outside of standard fluoroscopy and angiography.

Introduction

Stephen Hales' measurement of equine arterial pressure,[1] Werner Forssman's celebrated auto-cannulation,[2] and Andre Cournand's assessment of pulmonary arterial pressures in human disease[3] mark the known beginnings of cardiac catheterization. The first cardiac catheterization in a case of congenital heart disease was reported in 1946, and the first interventional catheterization was described in the remarkable reports from the Institute for Cardiology from Mexico City where Rubio-Alvarez and his colleagues used their own blade-equipped catheter to successfully open a stenotic pulmonary valve.[4] Despite such successes, transcatheter therapy remained dormant until the lifesaving balloon septostomy technique for transposition of the great arteries by Rashkind and Miller.[5]

Since these pioneering studies, the capabilities of cardiac catheterization in children have increased enormously. Over time, this field of medicine has evolved from a historically diagnostic procedure into a field that provides various therapeutic and palliative interventional techniques, due inpart to expanding noninvasive diagnostic modalities and rapid advancements in congenital cardiac catheterization. Similarly, patient populations undergoing congenital catheterization have expanded with increasing numbers of adults living with congenital heart disease requiring invasive diagnostic and interventional therapies, along with small and low-birth-weight infants requiring treatment in the catheterization laboratory with novel techniques and tools that improve the safety profile in this population.

Indications for Cardiac Catheterization

Prior to the consideration of performing a cardiac catheterization, a complete anatomic assessment using noninvasive imaging modalities such as echocardiography, computed tomography, and magnetic resonance imaging should be considered in all patients. Because of the advancements in noninvasive imaging, diagnostic catheterization is not considered standard of care for the routine diagnosis of congenital heart defects, as it unnecessarily exposes a patient to additional radiation along with procedural and anesthetic risks. These noninvasive techniques have the ability to show excellent anatomic detail and physiologic estimates (e.g., pressure gradients, myocardial function, and systemic and pulmonary flow calculations), and can be performed repeatedly. Furthermore, these technologies have become complementary for both diagnostic and interventional catheterization, providing detailed anatomic assessment resulting in reduced radiation exposure during the catheterization along with improved preoperative planning for the intended intervention.

In general, diagnostic cardiac catheterization should be performed (1) when precise physiologic measurements are needed (e.g., studying the feasibility of a Fontan procedure, measuring the degree of pulmonary arterial hypertension); (2) when the anatomic features are poorly visualized by other noninvasive modalities (e.g., coronary anatomy, peripheral pulmonary arterial or venous structures); (3) when there is conflicting noninvasive data where cardiac catheterization remains the gold standard for determining need for surgical intervention on lesions such as mitral and aortic stenosis; or (4) postsurgical evaluation of the patient who may be too unstable for advanced imaging techniques or there is the possibility of residual lesions where the diagnostic catheterization may become an interventional procedure.[6]

Given the enormous variabilities in congenital heart disease in a heterogenous patient population, along with institutional variations in surgical versus transcatheter palliation, listing the indications for cardiac catheterization that would apply to each cardiac institution simply is not possible. Further discussion of indications will be presented in the chapters on individual lesions.

Risks of Catheterization

There is inherent risk of unanticipated adverse events (AEs) in pediatric cardiac catheterization due to procedural complexity combined with a complex patient population with intrinsic hemodynamic vulnerabilities, which have the potential to result in patient harm and, at times, mortality. Due to these patient complexities and increasing number of heterogenous procedures performed in infants, children, and adults with congenital heart disease, there is an ever-expanding roll of multicenter collaboration to study outcomes in this population.

In a review of the 2014–2017 Congenital Cardiac Catheterization Project on Outcomes (C3PO) multicenter registry, clinically significant high-severity adverse events (HSAEs) occurred in 5.2% of all cases performed in the registry.[7] Major events resulting in emergent surgical intervention or need for extracorporeal membrane oxygenation (ECMO) occurred in 1.3% of procedures, whereas death as a result of the catheterization was low 0.07% (17 of 23,119 patients). Interventional procedures (8.1%) tend to have higher rates of HSAEs than diagnostic-only procedures (3.9%). Biopsy procedures have a good safety profile with only 1.1% of cases resulting in an AE. Risk during a diagnostic catheterization procedure should be stratified further by age. Infants < 30 days of age have complications rates of 9.0%, whereas older children ≥ 1 year have AE rates of only 2.8%.

Risk occurred during interventional procedures varies greatly based on the procedural complexity. For instance, pulmonary valvuloplasty, atrial septal defect closure, and patent ductus arteriosus closure are both safe and efficacious procedures with HSAE rates similar to diagnostic-only procedures at 2.2%–3.9%. Higher-risk procedures such as aortic valvuloplasty, multiple pulmonary artery dilations, ventricular septal defect closure, and pulmonary vein interventions can have AE rates between 10.6% and 13.3%. To create a broad understanding of risk for both preprocedural planning and patient/family consultation, common congenital cardiac catheterization procedures have been stratified into six categories (0–5) of risk with clinically significant AE rates of 1.1%, 2.7%, 4.2%, 7.7%, 10.8%, and 13.9%, respectively (Table 13.1).

Common HSAEs include vascular access–related complications including vessel thrombosis, vessel injury, and, less likely, surgical management in 15% of all clinically

---

TABLE 13.1 Case Types by Frequency of High-Severity Adverse Event (HSAE)

	Percent Occurrence of HSAE (%)
Risk Category 0	1.1
Endomyocardial biopsy	<1
Endomyocardial biopsy with coronary angiography	1.9
Risk Category 1	2.7
Fontan fenestration or baffle leak device closure	<1
Pulmonary valvuloplasty, age > 30 days	2.2
Diagnostic only, age ≥ 1 year	2.8
Risk Category 2	4.2
Pulmonary valvuloplasty + procedure, age > 30 days	3.2
ASD or PFO device closure	3.3

Continued

<table>
<tr><td>**TABLE 13.1**</td><td>**Case Types by Frequency of High-Severity Adverse Event (HSAE)—cont'd**</td></tr>
</table>

	Percent Occurrence of HSAE (%)
Venous collateral device or coil occlusion	3.6
PDA device or coil closure	3.9
Diagnostic only, age >30 days to < 1 year	5.1
Risk Category 3	**7.7**
Pulmonary artery dilation and/or stent (only 1 vessel)	6.9
Fontan fenestration or baffle leak device closure + procedure	7.1
Aorta (coarctation) dilation and/or stent	7.5
Systemic pulmonary collateral device or coil closure +/− procedure	7.5
Pulmonary valvuloplasty +/− procedure age, age ≤ 30 days	8.5
Pulmonary artery dilation and/or stent (only 1 vessel) + RVOT conduit dilation and/or stent	8.5
Atrial septostomy	8.7
Diagnostic only, age ≤ 30 days	9.0
Risk Category 4	**10.8**
Pulmonary artery dilation and/or stent (only 1 vessel) + procedure	10.2
ASD or PFO device closure + procedure	10.3
Pulmonary vein dilation and/or stent	10.6
Pulmonary artery dilation and/or stent (≥2 vessels)	10.9
RVOT conduit dilation and/or stent	11.3
PDA dilation and/or stent	11.3
Risk Category 5	**13.9**
Aorta (coarctation) dilation and/or stent + procedure	12.2
Aortic valvuloplasty +/− procedure, age > 30 days	12.8
Aortic valvuloplasty +/− procedure age ≤ 30 days	13.0
Pulmonary artery dilation and/or stent (≥2 vessels) + RVOT and/or other procedure	13.2
VSD device closure	13.3
Mitral valvuloplasty	13.3
Atrial septostomy + procedure	13.9
TPV implantation +/− procedure	14.4
Atrial septum static dilation and/or stent placement	16.4
Atretic valve perforation +/− valvuloplasty	20.3

ASD, Atrial septal defect; *PDA,* patent ductus arteriosus; *PFO,* patent foramen ovale; *RVOT,* right ventricular outflow tract; *TPV,* transcatheter pulmonary valve; *VSD,* ventricular septal defect.

significant events. The majority of these complications (88%) can be treated conservatively or with minor medical or interventional therapy. Similarly, atrial arrythmias induced during the procedure are relatively common complications (12% of all events) and may be self-resolved or require medical or electrical cardioversion. Other common HSAEs that typically can be treated with minor medical or

transcatheter therapy include angioplasty-related complications, respiratory or anesthesia-related events, and hemodynamic instability necessitating medical therapy (e.g., hypotension and metabolic acidosis).

Furthermore, there has been major developments in the understanding of patient-specific determinants of risk, such as hemodynamic vulnerability, in this complex

TABLE 13.2	Hemodynamic Indicator Variables by Presence of High-Severity Adverse Event (HSAE)		
Hemodynamic Indicator Variables	**Presence of HSAE***	**Weighted Score Value (0–2)**	
Low systemic arterial saturation			
BiV (<95%)	5.0%	1	
SV (<78%)	9.0%	2	
Low mixed venous saturation			
BiV (<60%)	5.9%	1	
SV (<50%)	5.6%	1	
High pulmonary artery pressure			
BiV (≥45 mm Hg)	11.1%	2	
SV (mean ≥17 mm Hg)	12.7%	2	
High systemic ventricle EDp (≥18 mm Hg)	4.6%	1	
High Qp:Qs (>1.5)	4.2%	1	
High PVR (>3 iWU)	3.1%	0	

*The percent HSAE listed for each hemodynamic indicator variable in this table includes only cases with a single independent abnormal indicator variable.

BiV, Biventricular; *EDp,* end-diastolic pressure; *PVR,* pulmonary vascular resistance; *SV,* single ventricle; *iWU,* indexed Wood units.

patient population. Not uncommonly, patients undergoing congenital cardiac catheterization may have unique derangements in their hemodynamics, which may impact risk during the procedure. The most predictive hemodynamic variables, stratified by single or biventricular circulation, have been used to calculate procedural risk independent of the procedure type being performed (Table 13.2).[7] Each positive value is given a weighted score, which, when added together, correlates with higher risk of HSAE.[7] These include systemic arterial saturation, mixed venous saturation, pulmonary artery pressure, systemic ventricle end-diastolic pressure, Qp:Qs, and indexed pulmonary vascular resistance. Cumulative hemodynamic scores of 0, 1, 2, and ≥3 are associated with HSAE rates of 3.4%, 5%, 8.7%, and 9.5%, respectively.

Hemodynamic Evaluation

A complete description of the methods used to evaluate physiologic variables in congenital heart disease is beyond the scope of this book and has been discussed elsewhere.[8-10] What follows is an overview designed to help the reader gain understanding of the techniques being used.

Pressure Measurements

Recording systems consist of a fluid-filled catheter, a pressure transducer, an amplifier, and a computer. The fluid-filled catheter transmits the pressure wave from the heart to a transducer, which converts the energy of pressure to an electrical impulse proportional to the displacement of the diaphragm and, therefore, to the pressure. By convention, the pressure at the level of the heart is set at 0 mm Hg by opening the transducer to air at the level of the heart and adjusting the recorder to read zero. It is also

important to note that the stability of the system may change over time, making it prudent to check the calibration throughout the catheterization for periods where the system may "drift."

The response of the system depends, in part, on damping (i.e., anything that dissipates energy and changes the amplitude of oscillations in the diaphragm). Underdamping (which causes an artificial increase in pressure fluctuation) can occur when the catheter tip or shaft is moved during recording. Overdamping (artificial reduction in pressure fluctuation) is more common. Overdamping increases as the catheter diameter decreases and its length and compliance increase. Similarly, the presence of air, blood, and clots in the system or loose connections may contribute to overdamping.

Pressure recorders allow pressures to be displayed or recorded at different attenuations; that is, the scale of the pressure tracing can be changed. Pressures are also displayed or recorded as phasic or mean pressures. A phasic recording shows the instantaneous fluctuations in a pressure and is important for determining systolic and diastolic pressures and the presence of normal and abnormal waves. Modern pressure recorders automatically determine and display the mean pressure using electronic damping. The mean pressures of atria and arteries are routinely recorded and used, for example, to calculate vascular resistance.

Catheter selection is determined by the size of the patient and the vessel to be entered. The number and position of holes are also important. Endhole catheters are required to record pulmonary capillary or venous wedge pressures and are optimal for localizing gradients. Endhole catheters, especially balloon-tipped catheters, can become entrapped (for example, in the atrial appendage, ventricular apex, or trabeculae), leading to falsely elevated pressure. Because such tracings often have a normal contour, entrapment can be difficult to recognize. The use of catheters with multiple side holes reduces the problem of entrapment. However, they cannot be used for wedge pressures and are not optimal for localizing gradients.

Right Atrial Pressure

The normal right atrial pressure consists of the a, c, and v waves and x and y descents (Figs. 13.1 and 13.2) and the normal mean right atrial pressure is 2–6 mm Hg. The a wave is associated with atrial contraction at the end of diastole.

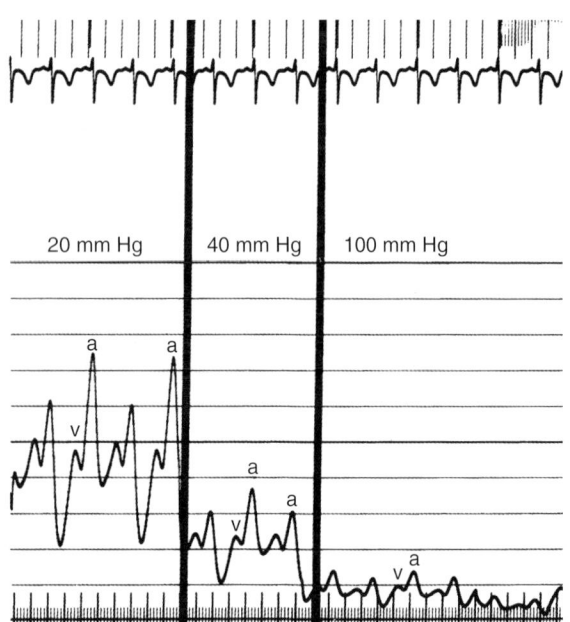

• **Fig. 13.1** Right atrial tracing at three different attenuations. In addition to phasic intracardiac changes, the pressure falls during inspiration. (From Fyler DC (ed). *Nadas' Pediatric Cardiology*, Philadelphia: Hanley & Belfus, 1992.)

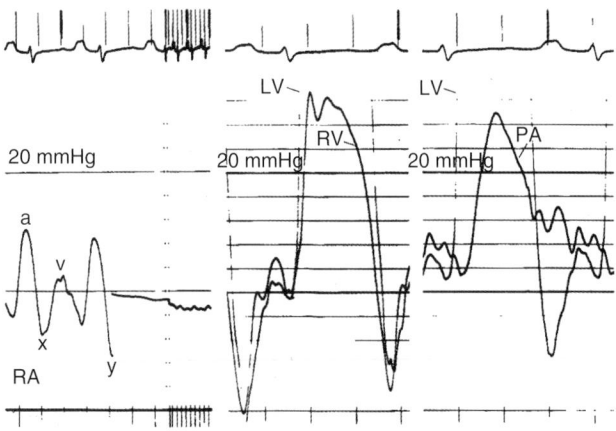

• **Fig. 13.2** Normal pressure tracings. Note the similarity of the right ventricular and pulmonary artery systolic trace and the similarity of the right and left ventricular diastolic pressure tracings. *LV*, Left ventricular tracing, which is only partially seen; *PA*, pulmonary artery tracing; *RA*, right atrial pressure tracing; *RV*, right ventricular pressure tracing. (From Fyler DC (ed). *Nadas' Pediatric Cardiology*, Philadelphia: Hanley & Belfus, 1992.)

It is usually the dominant wave in the right atrium. The c wave, a small notch on the descending side of the a wave, is clinically unimportant, and is associated with displacement of the tricuspid valve toward the right atrium in early systole. The v wave peaks during late systole and is related to continued atrial filling against the closed tricuspid valve. The x descent is the fall in pressure following the a and c waves due to a decrease in pericardial pressure and movement of the tricuspid valve away from the right atrium during ventricular ejection. The y descent is the decrease in pressure following the v wave and is due to opening of the tricuspid valve at the beginning of diastole.

Flow in the venae cavae is greatest during the x and y descents and ventricular filling is greatest during early diastole, with only about 30% of filling associated with atrial contraction. Pressure and flow also vary with respiration. Right atrial pressure is highest at the end of expiration and drops during inspiration, because of variation in intrathoracic pressure. This normal variation becomes exaggerated during periods of airway obstruction. Because of the low pressure, right atrial and ventricular filling are increased during inspiration. By convention, right atrial pressure is measured at the end of expiration.

Abnormalities of right atrial pressure include changes in mean pressure and changes in the normal pattern and relationships among the waves and troughs. Increases in right atrial mean pressure are associated with right ventricular dysfunction (decreased compliance) and outflow obstruction (tricuspid stenosis or atresia associated with a restrictive interatrial communication). In tricuspid regurgitation, the v wave may be dominant.

Superior and Inferior Vena Caval Pressure

Pressures in the superior and inferior venae cavae have contours similar to the right atrial pressure, and are not recorded routinely, except in any patient suspected of having caval obstruction.

Left Atrial Pressure

The a, c, and v waves and x and y descents are also seen in the left atrial pressure tracing. In contrast to right atrial pressure, the v wave is dominant in the normal left atrium. The mean left atrial pressure is normally 8 mm Hg. Elevations in left atrial pressure occur in patients with left ventricular dysfunction and in those with outflow obstruction (mitral stenosis or atresia with a restrictive interatrial communication). The v wave is increased in mitral regurgitation and decreased in total anomalous pulmonary venous return.

Pulmonary Artery "Wedge" Pressure

The pulmonary artery wedge pressure is measured by advancing an endhole catheter, with or without a balloon, into a branch of the pulmonary artery until the vessel is occluded by the catheter or, more commonly, by inflating the balloon. The pressure recorded through the endhole reflects distal pressure, that is, the left atrial pressure. The wedge pressure is routinely recorded simultaneously with the left ventricular end-diastolic pressure; normally there is no gradient. Differences in pressure suggest disease, improperly calibrated transducers, or a defective wedge pressure. The latter occurs when the catheter is overwedged or only partially wedged. The wedge pressure should look like a left atrial tracing, demonstrate respiratory variation, and be lower than the pulmonary artery pressure. However, because of the intervening capillaries and pulmonary veins, the wedge pressure is delayed and damped compared with direct measurement of the left atrial pressure. When important left atrial gradients are suspected, they should be measured directly.

Pulmonary Vein Pressure

Normal pressure tracings of pulmonary veins are similar to left atrial tracings. Abnormal elevation of pulmonary vein pressure in the presence of a normal left atrial valve suggests stenosis of the pulmonary veins. However, if only one or two of the veins are stenotic, flow within the lungs is redistributed and a minimal gradient may be measured across the stenotic veins.

Pulmonary Vein "Wedge" Pressure

If a catheter is wedged in a pulmonary vein, with or without a balloon, the pressure measured may reflect pulmonary artery pressure. This technique is conceptually similar to that used to measure pulmonary arterial wedge pressure. Achieving proper wedge position involves similar attention to detail. Although not employed routinely, obtaining pulmonary vein wedge pressure is the only way to estimate pulmonary artery pressure when the pulmonary arteries cannot be measured directly (e.g., patients with pulmonary atresia without shunts or with shunts that cannot be crossed). Although the wedge pressure estimate tends to be lower than actual pulmonary artery pressure, it is relatively accurate in patients with low or normal pulmonary artery pressure.

Right Ventricular Pressure

Normal ventricular pressures are easily distinguishable from atrial and arterial pressures. The right ventricular pressure wave consists of a rapid upstroke during isovolumic contraction, a systolic plateau, and a fall to near zero during isovolumic relaxation. There is, then, a gradual increase in pressure during diastole with a late diastolic increase associated with the a wave of atrial contraction (Fig. 13.2). The peak systolic and end-diastolic pressures, which vary with respiration, are measured routinely. End-diastole is identified as the point where the right atrial and ventricular tracings cross at the end of diastole or at the junction of the a wave and the rapid upstroke in the ventricular tracing. The former is the most accurate, but because simultaneous right atrial and right ventricular pressures are not routinely recorded, the latter is often utilized. The normal right ventricular systolic pressure is less than 30 mm Hg and the end-diastolic pressure is about 5 mm Hg.

Abnormal elevation of right ventricular systolic pressure occurs in outflow obstruction (e.g., pulmonary valve stenosis, pulmonary artery bands, or stenosis of the pulmonary artery branches), pulmonary artery hypertension, or lesions such as ventricular septal defects. In double-chambered right ventricle, anomalous muscle bundles obstruct the outflow portion of the right ventricle and create a proximal high-pressure chamber and a distal low-pressure chamber (Fig. 13.3).

Left Ventricular Pressure

The left ventricular pressure contour is similar to that of the right ventricle except the upstroke is more rapid, the systolic plateau flatter, and the a wave more prominent

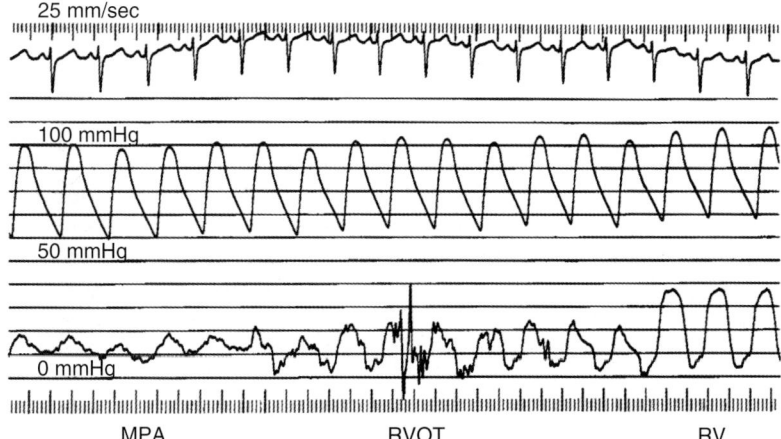

• **Fig. 13.3** Pressure pullback in a patient with double-chambered right ventricle *(RV)*. Upper tracing, electrocardiogram; middle tracing, arterial pressure; and lower tracing, obtained from the catheter as it was withdrawn from the pulmonary artery to the RV. Note that the pressure gradient occurs within the ventricle. Stenosis below the pulmonary valve will produce a characteristic pressure tracing in the right ventricular outflow tract *(RVOT)*, with a further gradient into the body of the RV. *MPA,* Main pulmonary artery. (From Fyler DC (ed). *Nadas' Pediatric Cardiology,* Philadelphia: Hanley & Belfus, 1992.)

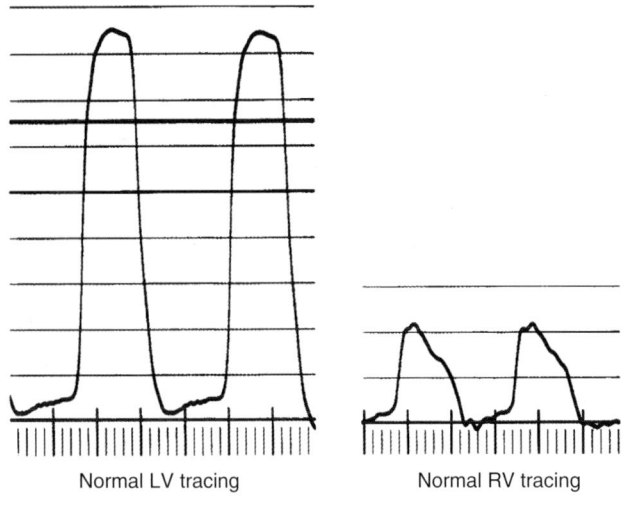

Normal LV tracing   Normal RV tracing

• **Fig. 13.4** Normal right *(RV)* and left ventricular *(LV)* pressure tracing. A normal LV pressure tracing has a flattened systolic pressure phase and very rapid upslopes and downslopes. (From Fyler DC (ed). *Nadas' Pediatric Cardiology*, Philadelphia: Hanley & Belfus, 1992.)

(Fig. 13.4). End-diastolic pressure varies with respiration and is measured as described for the right ventricle. Normally, left ventricular systolic pressure equals the aortic systolic pressure; both increase with age. The end-diastolic pressure is normally less than 12 mm Hg and is slightly higher than the left atrial mean pressure.

Pulmonary Artery Pressure

The normal systolic pressure in the pulmonary artery equals the right ventricle, but the diastolic pressure is higher because of closure of the pulmonary valve. Respiratory variation is common and, by convention, pressures are measured at the end of expiration. Normal mean pulmonary artery pressure is less than 20 mm Hg.

Aortic Pressure

The normal central aortic pressure wave consists of a systolic rise and a plateau, with a dicrotic notch on the downstroke. Closure of the aortic valve causes the diastolic pressure to remain well above the ventricular diastolic pressure. The aortic pressure and contours of the tracing vary, depending on where the pressure is measured. As the catheter is moved more peripherally (e.g., in the brachial or iliac arteries), the systolic pressure increases and the diastolic pressure decreases owing to "standing wave" amplification of the pulse. Thus, for example, when measuring gradients across the aortic valve, it is improper to compare left ventricular systolic pressure directly with femoral artery systolic pressure.

Aside from systemic hypertension or hypotension, abnormalities in aortic pressure usually are related to the presence of gradients (e.g., supravalvar aortic stenosis or coarctation of the aorta), a wide pulse pressure (e.g., aortic regurgitation, shunts such as a patent ductus arteriosus, systemic arteriovenous malformations, and decreased systemic resistance), or a narrow pulse pressure due to low output.

Gradients

A pressure gradient is the difference in pressure between two sites in the cardiovascular system and can be measured as a mean gradient, a peak gradient, or an instantaneous gradient. The severity of stenotic lesions commonly is described in terms of pressure gradients, although, in fact, the gradient depends on both the cross-sectional area of the obstruction and the flow across it. Thus, a severe narrowing may be associated with only a minimal gradient if the flow across the lesion is low.

Most commonly, a catheter is withdrawn across the obstruction while the pressure is being continuously recorded. Although this provides nearly simultaneous pressure recordings and allows easy measurement of peak and mean gradients, determination of instantaneous gradients requires that the two tracings be superimposed.

When assessing gradients, it is vital to assess flow across the lesion. In aortic or mitral valve stenosis, one should always estimate cardiac output. However, some lesions are so complex that accurate assessment of severity, using gradients and flows, becomes nearly impossible. For example, in stenosis of multiple branches of the pulmonary artery, it is not possible to measure flow across each lesion. In such situations, assessment of obstruction must rely on imaging techniques, lung scan data, or both.

Oxygen Content and Saturation

The oxygen content, or the saturation of the blood from the various chambers of the heart and great vessels, detects and quantifies shunts and, when combined with oxygen consumption, determines cardiac output. Oxygen saturation is the percentage of hemoglobin that is present as oxyhemoglobin, and it can be measured using reflectance oximetry. Oxygen content is defined as the total amount of oxygen present in the blood, both as oxyhemoglobin and that dissolved in the plasma. Formerly, it was measured directly, using the method of Van Slyke, but now oxygen sensing cells are used. Oxygen content per liter of blood may be calculated from oxygen saturation:

$$O_2 \text{ content} = (O_2 \text{ sat} \times 1.36 \times 10 \times \text{Hgb concentration})$$

The O_2 Sat is the percentage of oxygenated hemoglobin. The value of 1.36 is the amount of O_2 a gram of hemoglobin will carry when fully saturated. The number 10 is used to convert 100 mL to liters. The contribution of dissolved O_2 is small and commonly ignored except when the pO_2 is very high, such as when 100% oxygen is being administered.

Oxygen contents (O_2 con) and oxygen consumption (VO_2) are used to calculate blood flow using the equations:

$$\text{Pulmonary blood flow} = \frac{VO_2 (\text{mL/min})}{PV\,O_2\text{con} - PA\,O_2\text{ con}}$$

$$\text{Systemic blood flow} = \frac{VO_2 (\text{mL/min})}{SA\,O_2\text{con} - MV\,O_2\text{ con}}$$

where PV is pulmonary vein, PA is pulmonary artery, SA is systemic artery, and MV is mixed (systemic) venous.

If complete mixing of inferior vena caval, superior vena caval (SVC), and coronary sinus blood occurred, the right atrial, right ventricular, and pulmonary arterial oxygen saturations would equal the mixed venous content. In fact, studies have shown that variability in oxygen content is greatest in the right atrium[11] and least in the pulmonary artery, owing to incomplete mixing in the right atrium. Thus, in the absence of shunts, the pulmonary arterial saturation is used as the mixed venous oxygen saturation. In the presence of left-to-right shunts (see below), mixed venous oxygen contents must be obtained proximal to the site of the shunt.

In the absence of right-to-left shunts, mixing in the left side of the heart is insignificant because there is little variation in the oxygen content in the various pulmonary veins. In the presence of right-to-left shunts, the oxygen content must be measured proximal to the site of the shunt to calculate pulmonary blood flow.

Shunts

Both extracardiac and intracardiac defects allow shunting of blood between the pulmonary (right-sided) and systemic (left-sided) circulations. Shunts may be left-to-right, right-to-left, or bidirectional. Shunts can be localized using angiography, Doppler echocardiography, or a variety of indicators, including oxygen saturation, radionucleotides, and indocyanine green dye. This section will focus on detection and quantification of shunts using oxygen content or saturations.

Left-to-Right Shunts

In a left-to-right shunt, the flow of blood from the left side of the heart to the right leads to an increase in oxygen saturation in the right side of the heart. To detect this increase, samples are drawn from each right heart chamber. Significant increases in saturation between chambers must exceed the normal variation for that chamber.[12] Thus, the saturation in the right atrium varies 5% even without a shunt; a rise would be diagnostic only if the right atrial saturation exceeded SVC saturation by at least 6%.

Right-to-Left Shunt

With a right-to-left shunt, oxygen saturation decreases in the left heart. Unlike evidence for a left-to-right shunt, virtually any consistent decrease in oxygen saturation is diagnostic. For practical purposes, any decrease from normal arterial saturation (i.e., 95%) is considered as evidence of a right-to-left shunt in a child with heart disease until proven otherwise.

Shunt Calculations

A left-to-right shunt (Q_{L-R}) increases pulmonary blood flow (Q_p) compared with systemic blood flow (Q_s), and the shunt can be quantified by the equation:

$$Q_{L-R} = Q_p - Q_s$$

Usually, in children, the SVC oxygen content is taken as the mixed venous oxygen content. In discussing shunts, it is common to refer to the pulmonary-to-systemic flow ratio (Q_p/Q_s).

$$\frac{PV\,O_2\% - PA\,O_2\%}{SA\,O_2\% - MV\,O_2\%} = \frac{Q_p}{Q_s} = \frac{SA\,O_2 - MV\,O_2}{PV\,O_2 - PA\,O_2}$$

(Oxygen Consumption / Oxygen Consumption)

Thus, Q_p/Q_s can be determined without measuring or assuming an oxygen consumption, using only oxygen saturations.

In addition to pulmonary and systemic flows, the concept of effective flow (Q_{EFF}) is useful in calculating shunts. The effective pulmonary blood flow is the volume of unoxygenated blood flowing to the lungs (i.e., the amount of blood that picks up oxygen on passing through the lungs). For example, with a pure left-to-right shunt, effective pulmonary blood flow (Q_{EFF}) would equal the total pulmonary blood flow (Q_p) minus the shunt flow (Q_{L-R}), which equals systemic blood flow (Q_s). In bidirectional shunts, the left-to-right shunt is calculated as $Q_p - Q_{EFF}$, and the right-to-left shunt is calculated as $Q_s - Q_{EFF}$.

When quantifying shunts, saturations should be obtained as nearly simultaneously as possible to reduce hemodynamic variation. If the values of two series are different or if they suggest a shunt of borderline significance, more series are performed or another indicator is used. In general, shunt size measurements are estimates. To suppose that one can distinguish Q_p/Q_s ratios of 2 versus 2.2 or 1.8 is to ignore the variations inherent in the measurements. Thus, if the SVC saturation is 80, the pulmonary artery saturation 95, and the systemic artery saturation 100, the Q_p/Q_s is $(100 - 80)/(100 - 95)$. If the oximetry run is repeated and the SVC saturation is 78, the pulmonary artery saturation 96, and systemic artery saturation 99, the Q_p/Q_s ratio is $(100 - 80)/(100 - 95)$ or 7.

In certain lesions, it may be impossible to obtain adequately mixed samples to calculate shunt size. With a patent ductus arteriosus, the left pulmonary artery saturation is commonly higher than the right, and it is not possible to obtain truly mixed pulmonary arterial saturations. Averaging the values assumes that flow to both lungs is equal. With total anomalous pulmonary venous connections, it may be impossible to obtain mixed venous saturations.

Finally, some patients have more than one defect associated with left-to-right shunts. Thus, a patient may have an atrial septal defect, a ventricular septal defect, and a patent ductus arteriosus. Analyzing saturations from oximetry runs in a stepwise fashion, one might attempt to calculate the magnitude of the left-to-right shunt associated with each lesion. This assumes, incorrectly, complete mixing at each level. It also assumes that the increase at each level is due to only the lesion at that level. This may not be the case if, for example, the ventricular septal defect is associated with a left ventricular–right atrial shunt or there is tricuspid regurgitation.

Calculations for right-to-left shunts are fundamentally similar to calculations for left-to-right shunts. A right-to-left shunt (Q_{R-L}) leads to a decrease in left-sided saturations at or distal to the site of the shunt, and systemic blood flow (Q_s) is higher than pulmonary blood flow. It can be calculated as:

$$Q_{R-L} = Q_p - Q_s$$

and:

$$Q_p/Q_s = \frac{SA\ Q_2 - MV\ O_2}{PV\ O_2 - PA\ O_2}$$

In addition to right-to-left shunts, left-sided desaturation can be caused by pulmonary venous hypoxemia in a patient with lung disease. If the left atrium and pulmonary veins can be entered, the pulmonary venous saturation should be measured in as many pulmonary veins as possible. If the measurements are low, lung disease is suggested and 100% oxygen administered to the patient will significantly increase the pulmonary venous saturation. If the intrapulmonary shunt is due to a pulmonary arteriovenous malformation, the low saturation will increase modestly. Alternatively, if there is an atrial septal defect, an attempt should be made to occlude the defect with a balloon and measure the left atrial or systemic arterial saturation, which will normalize if the desaturation is due to a right-to-left shunt through the defect.

Cardiac Output

Cardiac output is the volume of blood pumped into the systemic circulation by the heart, expressed as liters per minute. When corrected for body surface area (BSA; liters/minute/m^2), cardiac output is referred to as the cardiac index. In patients with no shunts, pulmonary, systemic, and effective blood flows are equal (ignoring the minimal contribution of the bronchial circulation), and under stable conditions the term *cardiac output* can be used without confusion. However, in the presence of shunts, pulmonary, systemic, and effective blood flows may be unequal. In these patients, the more specific terms *pulmonary*, *systemic*, and *effective* blood flows are used.

Measurements or estimates of cardiac output, resistances, and valve areas are a routine part of most cardiac catheterizations. Indicator-dilution measurements are most commonly used to measure cardiac output. In general, if one knows the amount of indicator (I) added to (or subtracted from) a flowing fluid and the concentration of the indicator before (upstream) (C_b) and after (downstream) (C_a),

$$V = \frac{I}{C_a - C_b}$$

Assuming constant flow during the period of measurement, flow (Q) can be calculated by the introduction of a time term (t) into the equation

$$Q = \frac{I}{(C_a - C_b)t}$$

Numerous indicators have been used to measure cardiac output. The most common methods currently used are thermodilution and the Fick methods.

Thermodilution Cardiac Output

For thermodilution cardiac output determination, the indicator is rapidly injected cold saline. The cardiac output is calculated as

$$CO = \frac{V \times D_i \times S_i \times (T_b - T_i)}{dT \times t \times D_b \times S_b \times 1000/60}$$

where CO = cardiac output, V = volume injected minus dead space, D_i = density of injectate, S_i = specific heat of injectate, T_b = temperature of blood, T_i = temperature of injectate, dT = average temperature change, t = duration of temperature change (sec), D_b = density of blood, S_b = specific heat of blood, and 1000/60 = 1000 mL per 60 seconds.

The chilled saline solution is commonly injected in the right atrium, and a thermistor in the pulmonary artery measures blood temperature. The measured flow is equal to pulmonary blood flow and, in the absence of shunts, to the systemic blood flow. Thermodilution catheters have two lumens with a thermistor at the distal end. Various sizes are available so that when the thermistor is in the pulmonary artery, the proximal port, which is in the right atrium, can be used for injection. A curve shows the change in temperature with time at the thermistor, and calculations of output are made by dedicated computers.

The term dT $\times$ t in the denominator is the area under the curve, and cardiac output is inversely proportional to this area. The temperature at the thermistor is determined by the temperature of the blood, the temperature of the injectate, and the flow. The higher the flow, the more the injectate will be warmed, reducing the cold signal. However, the injectate is also warmed by contact with the catheter and the vessel walls. If the thermistor is in direct contact with a vessel wall, warming is increased, and cardiac output will be overestimated. Previously, thermodilution techniques were used to measure flows in specific vessels or organs by positioning the thermistor and injection port at appropriate sites. This technique, which assumes complete mixing of the thermal bolus, has now been largely supplanted by newer MRI techniques for output determinations.

Fick Method

Using the Fick method, the indicator is oxygen and cardiac output or flow (Q) is calculated from oxygen consumption/

minute (VO_2) divided by the difference in oxygen content between arterial (C_a) and venous (C_v) blood:

$$Q = \frac{VO_2\,(L/min)}{(C_a - C_v)}$$

As above, in the absence of shunts, pulmonary blood flow equals systemic blood flow. Pulmonary blood flow (Q_p) is:

$$Q_P\,(L/min) = \frac{VO_2\,(L/min)}{PV\,O_2\,con - PA\,O_2\,con}$$

where $PV\,O_2$ con and $PA\,O_2$ con are the pulmonary venous and the pulmonary arterial oxygen contents. Similarly, the systemic blood flow (Q_s) is:

$$Q_s\,(L/min) = \frac{VO_2\,(L/min)}{SA\,O_2\,con - MV\,O_2\,con}$$

where $SA\,O_2$ con and $MV\,O_2$ con are the systemic arterial and mixed venous oxygen contents.

Several devices are available for measuring oxygen consumption. Often, the entire volume of air expired gas is determined, as well as the relative volumes of oxygen, nitrogen, and/or carbon dioxide. Comparing the concentrations of gases in inspired (room air) and expired air allows calculation of the oxygen consumption. A second method does not involve collecting all the expired air, but uses a hood and a pump to withdraw air from the hood to an oxygen sensing device. If air is withdrawn from the hood at a rate (V_m) so that the fractional content of O_2 at the oxygen sensor remains constant at 0.122, O_2 consumption can be estimated.

Vascular Resistance

Calculations of vascular resistance (R) are made by relating the mean pressure change (delta P) across a circuit to the flow (Q) across the circuit, using the equation:

$$R = \frac{delta\ P}{Q}$$

Thus, systemic vascular (SVR) and pulmonary vascular (PVR) resistances are calculated as follows:

$$SVR = \frac{Ao - RA}{Q_s} - and - PVR = \frac{PA - LA}{Q_p}$$

where Ao is the mean aortic pressure, RA is the mean right atrial pressure, PA is the mean pulmonary artery pressure, and LA (or pulmonary capillary wedge) is the mean left atrial pressure. The pressures are in mm Hg and the flows in L/minute, and thus resistance is expressed as mm Hg/L/min (or Wood units). Resistance is commonly normalized for BSA by multiplying the calculated resistance by BSA.

Valve Areas

The most commonly used formulas for calculating valve areas are based on the work of Gorlin and Gorlin[11] in 1951. The first is $A = V/VC_c$, where A is the valve area, F is the flow rate, V is the velocity of flow, and C_c is the coefficient of orifice contraction. The second, which relates velocity to pressure gradient, is $V = C_v\,2gh$, where C_v is the coefficient of velocity, g is acceleration due to gravity (980 cm/sec/sec), and h is the pressure gradient. Combining these equations yields:

$$Valve\ area = \frac{F}{(C)(44.3)\,h}$$

where C is a constant. Flow across a valve occurs during diastole at the mitral and tricuspid valves, and during systole at the aortic and pulmonary valves. The final formula takes this into account by including the diastolic filling period (DFP, seconds per beat) or the systolic ejection period (SEP, seconds per beat) and the heart rate (HR beats sec):

$$A = \frac{CO/(DFP\ or\ SEP)\,HR}{44.3\,(C)}$$

where A is the area in cm^3, CO is the cardiac output in cm^3/min, and delta is the mean pressure gradient. The beginning and end of the DSP are the points where the atrial and ventricular pressure tracings intersect; the intersections of ventricular and arterial tracings at the beginning and end of systole define the SEP. When determined in this way, the constant, C, is 0.85 for the mitral valve and 1 for the aortic, pulmonary, and tricuspid valves.

The equations predict that, for any given valve area, decreasing the flow across the valve decreases the gradient and increasing the flow increases the gradient. Therefore, it is logical to classify severity of valvar stenoses in terms of valve area. Because most children with stenosis of pulmonary or aortic valves have normal cardiac outputs, the flow term in the equation tends to be a constant and severity varies directly with the gradient.

Angiographic Evaluation

Image Production

Basic equipment for image production includes the generator, the x-ray tube, and the image chain mounted opposite each other on a fixed stand or C-arm. The image chain consists of an image intensifier and a flat plane detector (Fig. 13.5). For pediatric studies, simultaneous biplane cineangiography is often necessary to provide sufficient anatomic information with minimal contrast material. Biplane systems are set up with the image intensifier positioned anterior to the patient and the x-ray tube located posteriorly so that x-rays enter through the back of the patient and exit the chest

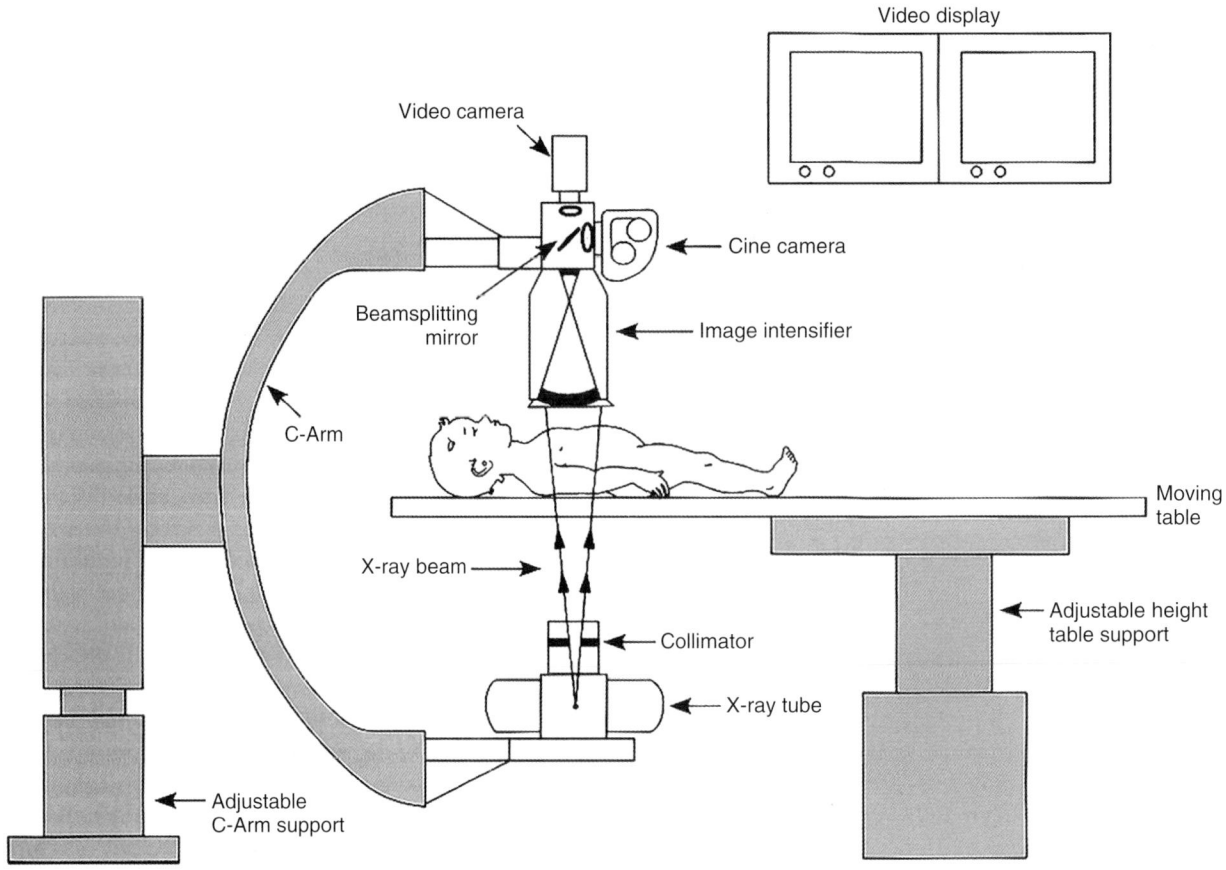

• **Fig. 13.5** Schematic representation of a single C-arm with x-ray tube, image intensifier, and cine camera over moving table top. (From Fyler DC (ed). *Nadas' Pediatric Cardiology*, Philadelphia: Hanley & Belfus, 1992.)

anteriorly to be captured by the image intensifier. Similarly, the lateral camera is positioned so that the image intensifier is located to the patient's left and the x-ray tube on the patient's right.

To produce an image, a current is passed through a filament in the cathode within the x-ray tube causing it to emit electrons.[13] The x-ray tube controls three variables: kilovoltage (kV) (which determines the energy spectrum of the x-rays), milliamperes (mA, the tube current that determines the number of x-ray photons produced), and milliseconds (msec, the length of exposure or pulse width in cineangiography). The image intensifier produces visible light when struck by x-ray photons through an interaction with input phosphor and the photocathode. The distribution of light produced corresponds to the spatial information formed by the attenuation of the x-rays by the patient's heart or by contrast agents used in angiocardiography.

During standard fluoroscopy and cineangiography, x-rays are delivered in short pulses instead of continuously. Radiation is delivered at a much higher level during angiography. The length of each pulse, or pulse width, determines the exposure for each individual frame. Pulse widths should be kept short to prevent blurring, but need to be long enough to provide a sufficient number of photons so that the image will not be too grainy. The pulse width in cineangiography

should not exceed 5 msec in pediatrics and 10 msec in adults.

Pulsed fluoroscopy is used throughout the case for live viewing of catheters, wires, and other equipment while traversing vascular and cardiac structures, providing sufficient image quality. Fluoroscopy images can be stored permanently for review to help reduce unnecessary radiation and contrast exposure. For digital acquisitions and permanent storage using cine angiography, the current is boosted by about 10- to 15-fold to produce a higher-quality image with typical pulsed rates of 10, 15, or 30 frames/sec. In addition, some modern catheterization laboratories come equipped with the ability to perform three-dimensional rotational angiography using the standard c-arm. This newer technology allows the interventionalist to obtain a full three-dimensional dataset used to evaluate complex vascular anatomy (e.g., the pulmonary arterial tree, coronary anatomy) with limitless potential. For instance, coronary artery location in relationship to a right ventricle to pulmonary artery conduit can be obtained during the case to understand the risk of potential coronary artery compression during stenting of the right ventricle to pulmonary artery conduit. Additionally, relationship of nonvascular structures, such as the airway, can be viewed prior to performing stent implantation on a nearby cardiac structure (e.g., left pulmonary artery). These images can also be used to provide an "overlay" with live fluoroscopy used during the procedure to assist with various interventions. Similarly, preoperative cardiac computed tomography and magnetic resonance imaging can be overlayed during the case using similar modern technology.

Other modern technology and invasive imaging techniques, outside of standard fluoroscopy and angiography, are currently being used in both adult and pediatric centers. These modalities include:

- Intravascular ultrasound (IVUS): Currently used extensively in the adult population to aid in diagnostic coronary angiography and pivotal in the detection of coronary artery abnormalities to guide possible need for transcatheter intervention. In the pediatric setting, IVUS is also routinely used to assess vascular information including vessel wall abnormalities, arteriopathy disorders, understand mechanisms of obstruction of particular lesions, and obtain measurements of vessel and vessel wall diameters.[14,15]
- Intracardiac echocardiogram (ICE): ICE has the ability to provide high-resolution imaging and real-time visualization of cardiac structures and can aid in device closure of cardiac defects such as atrial septal defect closure and closure of paravalvar leaks.[16]
- Optical coherence tomography (OCT): OCT use in coronary evaluation has emerged as an important tool to evaluation of vascular structure with high-resolution *in vivo* imaging.

Radiation Exposure and Protection

Numerous metrics exist to quantify radiation exposure used during fluoroscopy procedures. Absorbed dose is expressed as units of *gray* (Gy) compared with other metrics such as units of rads where 1 mGy = 100 mrad.[17] Fluoroscopic equipment used in pediatric interventional laboratories typically display cumulative air kerma ($K_{a,r}$) in units of mGy during the procedure to approximate the entrance skin plane of the patient.[17] Currently there is a movement to standardize the quantification of radiation dose used during pediatric interventional catheterization as dose area product (DAP) where DAP is the product of air kerma dose and the cross-sectional area exposed to the x-ray beam (μGy $\times$ m2). DAP provides a better reflection of stochastic risk acquired during the procedure compared with cumulative air kerma alone.[18]

It is important to consider the use of ionizing radiation in pediatric patients undergoing congenital cardiac catheterization, whereby pediatric patients are vulnerable to the effects of ionizing radiation as this may contribute to long-term health consequences and lifetime attributable cancer risk. This is particularly important for patients with complex congenital heart disease who may undergo repeated catheterization, and thus cumulative exposure over their lifetime.

Numerous methods exist in the modern laboratory to reduce radiation exposure for both the patient and operator(s)

to doses *As Low as Reasonably Achievable* (ALARA).[13,17] These methods are characterized in great detail within the literature.[13,17,18] Important methods to optimize equipment and technique reduce radiation exposure are as follows:

- Limit live fluoroscopy use for catheter manipulations and test injections
- Reduce frame rate and dose for acquisitions
- Utilize store fluoroscopy when lower image resolution is acceptable
- Single-plane acquisitions when bi-plane imaging is not necessary for anatomic assessment
- Use of filtration and low-dose imaging settings
- Collimation of image to enhance image quality and reduce effective dose
- Lowering of the image intensifier
- Use of digital subtraction angiography

Contrast Agents

Contrast agents can be either high-osmolality, low-osmolality, or iso-osmolality agents. Low- and iso-osmolality agents cause less patient discomfort, are safer, and are now routinely used. Complications and toxicity related to contrast use decrease as the osmolality approaches that of serum.[8-10]

Chemistry

High-osmolality ionic agents are salts of tri-iodinated benzene derivatives of diatrizoic or iothalamic acid (the anions), which are bound to sodium or methylglucamine (the cations). When in solution, the number of particles is immediately doubled; this results in a solution that is extremely hypertonic, with osmolality six to seven times that of blood. The hypertonicity of these agents not only causes the pain and warmth that the patient feels but is responsible in part for a number of other adverse physiologic responses.

Non-ionic contrast is formulated by replacing the carboxyl group of the benzene ring with a nonionizing side chain so that the compound does not dissociate in solution; thus, its osmolality is half as great as an ionic compound. Nonionic agents include iohexol and iopamidol.

Osmolality may also be reduced by linking two tri-iodinated benzoic acids together to form a dimer. This is prepared as a salt of sodium or meglumine, which then dissociates in solution into two particles as conventional ionic agents do. Because each anionic particle contains six rather than three iodine atoms (as in conventional contrast), fewer particles are needed for a given iodine concentration, and the osmolality is reduced by half.[19]

Physiology

When contrast agents are injected, there is a shift of fluid from interstitial and intracellular spaces into the intravascular space, causing volume expansion, a slight drop in hematocrit, and a change in electrolyte concentration.[20] Thus, important pressure and flow measurements should always be made prior to contrast injections. With normal renal excretion, values can be expected to return to baseline within a few minutes, but newborns, fragile infants, and any patient with severely compromised cardiac function will be adversely affected.[21,22]

Injection of contrast into the pulmonary vascular bed causes a rise in pulmonary artery pressure owing to a combination of vasospasm[22] and elevation of left atrial pressure. The release of histamine from mast cells and basophils, platelet dysfunction, and sludging of distorted red cells may play a role also.

Reflex tachycardia occurs in response to contrast-induced hypotension, and with increased intravascular volume, there is transient increase in cardiac output, along with a rise in ventricular diastolic pressure.[23] In the already compromised patient, this depressant effect, combined with volume expansion secondary to injection of the contrast, may precipitate pulmonary edema. These effects are all reduced through the use of low- and iso-osmolality agents.

Other toxic effects of high-osmolar contrast agents include decreased red cell pliability and increased viscosity, osmotic diuresis, proteinuria, hematuria, and, occasionally, renal failure.

Adverse Reactions

Arterial injection of contrast agent produces warmth; injection into pulmonary vessels produces coughing. Life-threatening reactions, including bronchospasm, laryngeal edema, and vascular collapse, are rare but documented complications. For patients who are at risk of having an anaphylactoid reaction or have had a prior reaction to contrast, premedication with methylprednisolone and diphenhydramine may be used.

Nephrotoxicity related to the contrast agent may result in episodes of acute renal failure, particularly in patients with underlying renal insufficiency, end-stage liver disease, or congestive heart failure. Clinical manifestations are variable, but most cases are temporary and reversable.[8-10]

Neurotoxicity is a rare complication, minimized through the use of low- and iso-osmolar agents, and may result in reactions such as headache, confusion, seizures, altered consciousness, visual disturbances, and dizziness.[8-10]

Angiocardiography

The first step in any selective angiography is vascular access to the necessary chamber with an appropriate catheter. Usually, femoral vessels are used for percutaneous vascular access in nearly all forms of CHD, with the umbilical, subclavian, jugular, and upper limb vessels available for special circumstances. In general, angiograms are performed with sidehole catheters adequate to deliver a large volume of contrast rapidly (e.g., up to 1.5 mL/kg in a second or less); the volume and speed are determined by multiple factors, including chamber size and flow. A more complete discussion of angiographic techniques in general, and special procedures such as balloon occlusion angiography, wedge

angiography, and coronary angiography in children, is available elsewhere.[8]

Modern biplane C-arm equipment has facilitated the acquisition of the axial views, introduced in the late 1970s, which accurately delineate various parts of the cardiac anatomy. Because in most cases today the basic diagnosis has been established by echocardiography before arrival in the catheterization laboratory, each angiographic view can be chosen to answer a specific anatomic question.

Axial angiography was developed to profile specific parts of the heart along the x-ray beam. For example, the ventricular septum runs neither in the sagittal nor the coronal plane, but obliquely such that a left anterior oblique view shows the midportion of the curved ventricular septum better than a simple lateral view does. Thus, the long axis of the heart is between horizontal and vertical, the bifurcation of the pulmonary artery is horizontal, and the aortic arch runs obliquely from front to back. Axial views were developed to take these anatomic facts into account and provide specific information about each chamber or vessel. However, simple frontal and lateral views are still useful, or even preferred, for demonstration of certain anatomic areas or when the abnormalities are so deranged that a preliminary view is desired.

The most common and useful views are posterior-anterior, lateral, long axial oblique, and hepatoclavicular. A long axial oblique view is obtained by placing the intensifier at 70-degree left anterior oblique with a 20-degree cranial angulation. Usually this is combined with the orthogonal right anterior oblique view (Fig. 13.6A). In left ventriculography, the long axial oblique projection provides good visualization of the mid and apical muscular septum, the membranous septum, and the subaortic area (Fig. 13.6B). This enables the viewer to see the motion of the anterior leaflet of the mitral valve, and the ventricular wall motion in the septal, apical, and posterior aspects, as well as mitral regurgitation and left ventricular–right atrial shunts. The aortic valve, the coronary arteries, and the arch and great vessels are well displayed. The right anterior oblique, orthogonal view provides information about anterior muscular septal and subpulmonary defects, both of which are difficult to pinpoint on other views. In tetralogy of Fallot, the infundibulum, pulmonary valve, and right pulmonary artery are nicely demonstrated.

The hepatoclavicular view was so named to describe the direction of the x-ray beam from the liver below to the left clavicle above. Technically, it is a shallower (40 degree) long axial oblique view with steeper (40 degree) cranial angulation than the long axial oblique (Fig. 13.7). This view focuses on the posterior aspect of the ventricular septum, in the region of the atrioventricular canal. In this projection, one can actually visualize a common atrioventricular valve, rather than infer its presence by an angiographic sign such as the gooseneck. This view is also called the four-chambered view because both atria and both ventricles can be seen in each of four quadrants of the image, so that valvular

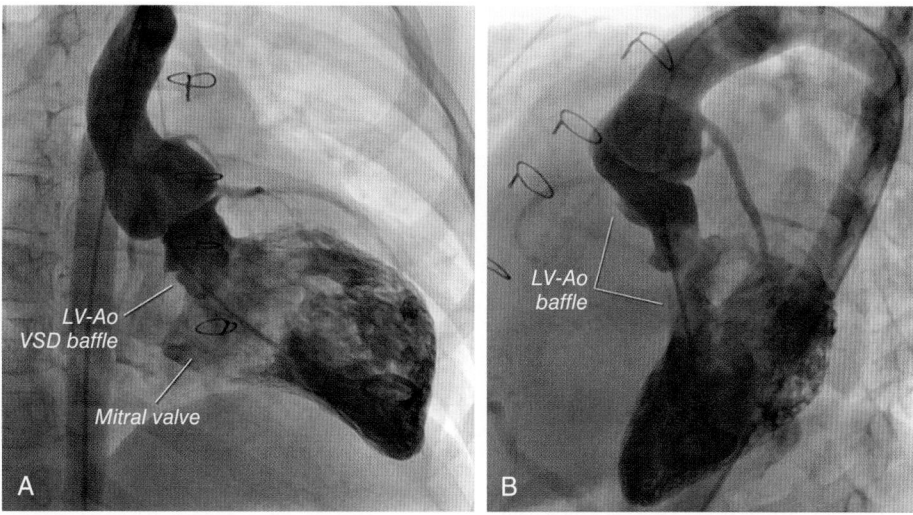

• **Fig. 13.6** **(A)** Left ventriculogram taken in the right anterior oblique view illustrating a patient who had a left ventricle to aorta baffle *(LV-Ao)*. **(B)** Left ventriculogram taken in the long axial oblique view again noting the LV-Ao baffle. *VSD,* Ventricular septal defect. (From Verma A. Congenital Heart Disease: The Catheterization Manual. *Congenit Heart Dis.* 2009;4. doi:10.1111/j.1747-0803.2009.00315.x (36-37))

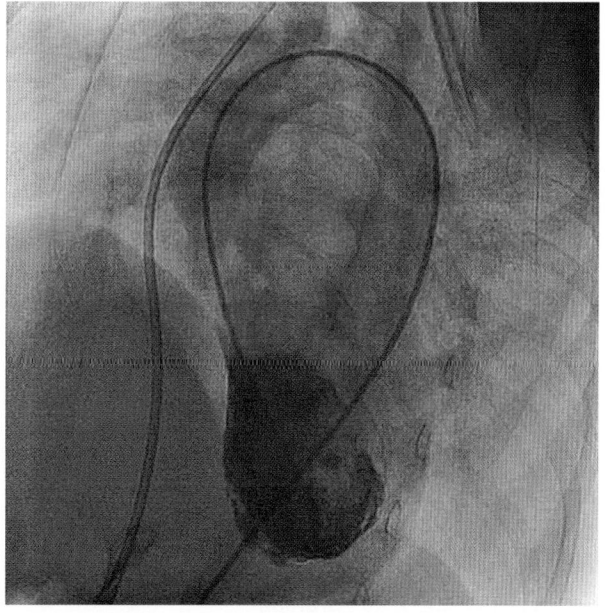

• **Fig. 13.7** Left ventriculogram taken in the hepatoclavicular view illustrating a view similar to an apical four-chamber echo view. (From Verma A. Congenital Heart Disease: The Catheterization Manual. *Congenit Heart Dis.* 2009;4.)

regurgitation, defects from the left ventricle to the right atrium and left or right overriding or atresia of the atrioventricular valves can be recognized.

The frontal view with 40-degree cranial angulation (Fig. 13.8A) is particularly useful for displaying the pulmonary artery bifurcation. The complementary orthogonal lateral view of the right ventricle (Fig. 13.8B) displays the pulmonary infundibulum and valve as well as the main and left pulmonary artery in profile. In tetralogy, septal alignment is particularly well illustrated, as the conal septum is profiled in its excessively anterior position. The most common angiographic views and the diagnoses and injected chambers in which they are most helpful are displayed in Table 13.3.

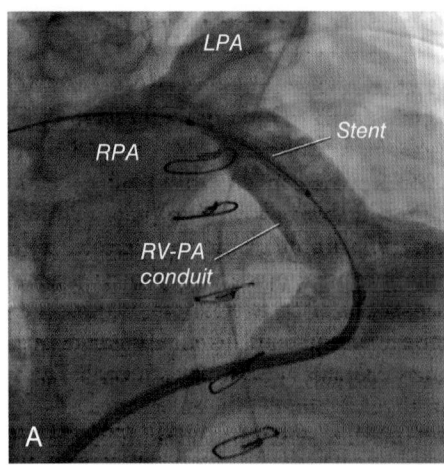
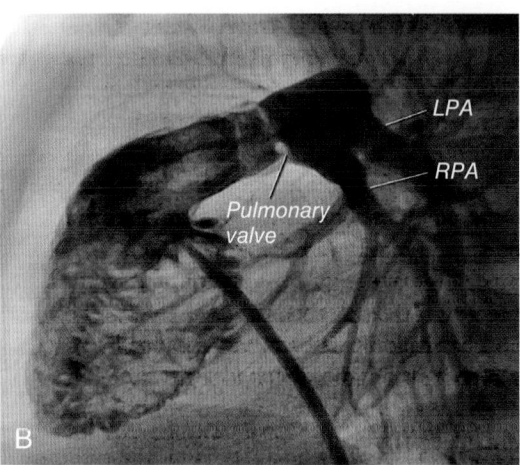

• **Fig. 13.8** **(A)** Right ventriculogram in a frontal projection with cranial angulation demonstrating the pulmonary artery bifurcation in a patient with a right ventricle to pulmonary artery conduit. **(B)** Right ventriculogram in the lateral projection demonstrating an unobstructed right ventricular outflow tract and the pulmonary artery bifurcation. *LPA,* Left pulmonary artery; *RPA,* right pulmonary artery; *RV,* right ventricle. (From Verma A. Congenital Heart Disease: The Catheterization Manual. *Congenit Heart Dis.* 2009;4.)

TABLE 13.3	Projections, Contrast Injection Site, and Highlighted Anatomic Details in Various Congenital Heart Defects	
Long Axial Oblique View: (70° LAO, 20° Cranial)		
Left Ventriculovgram		
VSD	Membranous, apical, and midmuscular VSDs	
Tetralogy of Fallot	Malalignment VSD, multiple VSDs	
D-TGA	Subpulmonary area and VSDs	
DORV	VSD location and size	
Sub AS	LV outflow and mitral valve	
Aortogram		
PDA	Size and location of ductus	
Tetralogy of Fallot	Coronary arteries	
AS	Aortic valve morphology and aortic insufficiency	
Aortic arch	Arch hypoplasia and coarctation	
Hepatoclavicular Four-Chamber View: (40° LAO, 40° Cranial)		
Left Ventriculogram		
VSD	AV canal type, posterior muscular VSDs	
Tricuspid atresia	VSD size, RV outflow chamber size	
Straddling TV	Valve attachments and flow pattern	
Single ventricle	Type, size, orientation	
Right Ventriculogram		
Tetralogy of Fallot	PA bifurcation and proximal LPA	
Frontal View With 30°–40° Caudal Angulation		
Aortogram (performed using temporary balloon occlusion)		
D-TGA	Coronary artery pattern	

TABLE 13.3   Projections, Contrast Injection Site, and Highlighted Anatomic Details in Various Congenital Heart Defects—cont'd

Standard RAO (Performed Along With Either Long Axial Oblique or Hepatoclavicular Views)

Left Ventriculogram

VSD	Subpulmonary and anterior muscular
Tetralogy of Fallot	Pulmonary infundibulum
Mitral valve	Prolapse and insufficiency

Aortogram

	Coronary artery pattern

Pulmonary Arteriogram

	Proximal right pulmonary artery

Right Ventriculogram

Tetralogy of Fallot	PA bifurcation, outflow obstruction

Frontal View with Cranial Angulation

Right Ventriculogram

Tetralogy	PA Bifurcation

Pulmonary Arteriogram

Tetralogy	Postop. bifurcation

Innominate Vein

LSVC	Drainage pattern

Right Ventriculogram

Pulmonary stenosis	Valve anatomy, level of stenosis
Pulmonary atresia	Level of atresia
DORV	Relationship of great vessels

Vena Cavae

Heterotaxy	Systemic venous drainage pattern

Pulmonary Veins

PV stenosis	Severity, type of stenosis
Pulmonary atresia	Find true pulmonary arteries (wedge injection)

Aortopulmonary Collateral

Pulmonary atresia	Identify collateral number, size, distribution

Standard Frontal and Lateral Views

Pulmonary Arteriogram

TAPVR	Branch PA anatomy and venous return pattern

Innominate Vein

LSVC	Drainage pattern

Right Ventriculogram

Pulmonary stenosis	Valve anatomy, level of stenosis
Pulmonary atresia	Level of atresia
DORV	Relationship of great vessels

Vena Cavae

Heterotaxy	Systemic venous drainage pattern

Continued

TABLE 13.3	Projections, Contrast Injection Site, and Highlighted Anatomic Details in Various Congenital Heart Defects—cont'd
Pulmonary Veins	
PV stenosis	Severity, type of stenosis
Pulmonary Atresia	Find true pulmonary arteries (wedge injection)
Aortopulmonary collateral	
Pulmonary Atresia	Identify collateral number, size, distribution

AS, Aortic stenosis; *DORV*, double outlet right ventricle; *D-TGA*, D-transposition of the great arteries; *LAO*, left arterior oblique; *LPA*, left pulmonary artery; *LSVC*, left superior vena cava; *LV*, left ventricle; *PA*, pulmonary artery; *PDA*, patent ductus arteriosus; *PV*, pulmonary vein; *RAO*, right anterior oblique; *RV*, right ventricle; *TAPVR*, total anomalous pulmonary venous return; *VSD*, ventricular septal defect

References

1. Hales S. *Statical Essays Containing Haemastaticks West End of St. Paul's.* London: W. Innys and R. Manby; 1733.
2. Forssman W. Die Sondierung des rechten Herzens. *Klin Wochenschr.* 1929;8:2085.
3. Cournand AF, Ranges HS. Catheterization of the right auricle in man. *Proc Soc Ex Biol Med.* 1941;46:462-466.
4. Rubio-Alvarez V, Limon RL, Soni J. Valvulotomias intracardias pormedico de un cateter. *Arch Inst Cardiol Mexico.* 1953;23:183-192.
5. Rashkind WJ, Miller WW. Creation of an atrial septal defect without thoracotomy: a palliative approach to complete transposition of the great vessels. *J Am Med Assoc.* 1966;196:991-992.
6. Feltes TF, Bacha E, Beekman RH, et al. Indications for cardiac catheterization and intervention in pediatric cardiac disease: a scientific statement from the American Heart Association. *Circulation.* 2011;123:2607-2652.
7. Quinn BP, Yeh M, Gauvreau K, et al. Procedural risk in congenital cardiac catheterization (PREDIC3T). *J Am Heart Assoc.* 2022;11:e022832.
8. Lock JE, Keane JF, Perry SB, eds. *Diagnostic and Interventional Catheterization in Congenital Heart Disease.* Norwell, MA: Kluwer Academic Publishers; 2000.
9. Bergersen L, Foerster S, Marshall A, Meadows J. *Congenital Heart Disease: The Catheterization Manual.* New York: Springer; 2009.
10. Butera G, Chessa M, Eicken A, Thomson J. *Cardiac Catheterization for Congenital Heart Disease: From Fetal Life to Adulthood.* 2nd ed. Cham: Springer; 2021.
11. Gorlin R, Gorlin G. Hydraulic formula for calculation of stenotic mitral valves, and central circulatory shunts. *Am Heart J.* 1951;41:1-29.
12. Freed MD, Miettinen OS, Nadas AS. Oxymetric detection of intracardiac left-to-right shunts. *Br Heart J.* 1979;42:690.
13. Justino H. The ALARA concept in pediatric cardiac catheterization: techniques and tactics for managing radiation dose. *Pediatr Radiol.* 2006;36:146-153.
14. Callahan R, Gauthier Z, Toba S, Sanders SP, Porras D, Vargas SO. Correlation of intravascular ultrasound with histology in pediatric pulmonary vein stenosis. *Children.* 2021;8:193.
15. Callahan R, Jenkins KJ, Gauthier Z, Gauvreau K, Porras D. Preliminary findings on the use of intravascular ultrasound in the assessment of pediatric pulmonary vein stenosis. *Catheter Cardiovasc Interv.* 2021;97:E362-E370.
16. Enriquez A, Saenz LC, Rosso R, et al. Use of intracardiac echocardiography in interventional cardiology. *Circulation.* 2018;137:2278-2294.
17. Hill KD, Frush DP, Han BK, et al. Radiation safety in children with congenital and acquired heart disease: a scientific position statement on multimodality dose optimization from the image gently alliance. *JACC Cardiovasc Imaging.* 2017;10:797-818.
18. Quinn BP, Armstrong AK, Bauser-Heaton HD, et al. Radiation risk categories in cardiac catheterization for congenital heart disease: a tool to aid in the evaluation of radiation outcomes. *Pediatr Cardiol.* 2019;40:445-453.
19. Swanson DP, Thrall JH, Shetty PC. Evaluation of intravascular low-osmolality contrast agents. *Clin Pharm.* 1986;5:877-891.
20. Friesinger G, Schaffer J, Cooley JM, et al. Hemodynamic consequences of the injection of radiopaque material. *Circulation.* 1965;31:730-740.
21. Sagy M, Aladjem M, Shem-Tov A, et al. The renal effect of radiocontrast administration during cardioangiography in two different groups with congenital heart disease. *Eur J Pediatr.* 1984;141:236-239.
22. Dawson P. Chemotoxicity of contrast media and clinical adverse effects: a review. *Invest Radiol.* 1985;20:84-91.
23. Hayward R, Dawson P. Contrast agents in angiocardiography. *Br Heart J.* 1984;52:361.

14

Interventional Cardiac Catheterization

DIEGO PORRAS AND NICOLA MASCHIETTO

KEY LEARNING POINTS

- A well-developed interventional program is one of the essential pillars of any center treating complex congenital heart disease.
- It is of paramount importance for pediatric and congenital cardiologists to be familiar with the indications and outcomes of both surgical and transcatheter strategies for specific lesions.

- The field of pediatric and congenital interventional cardiology is constantly evolving. Therefore, having a strong knowledge base and understanding the principles behind the current interventions represent only a starting point and will help the reader adapt, and hopefully contribute, to the evolution of the field.

Transcatheter Valve Dilation

Valvar Pulmonary Stenosis

Since Kan and colleagues reported the first static balloon dilation of the pulmonary valve in 1982, this procedure has become the first-line therapy for isolated valvar pulmonary stenosis.[1] Indications, technical aspects, goals, and acute outcomes are summarized in Table 14.1. A typical procedure can be seen in Video 14.1. The balloon size to be used is based on the measurement of the pulmonary valve annulus. A balloon-to-annulus ratio (BAR) of 1.2 to 1.25 has been demonstrated to be as effective as larger BARs, while resulting in less pulmonary regurgitation (PR).[1] The peak-to-peak gradient across the pulmonary valve is assessed before and after each balloon dilation. Significant residual gradients should be carefully characterized to differentiate between the supravalvar, valvar, and subvalvar (infundibular) components of the residual gradient, since repeat balloon dilation can only address the valvar component and any infundibular gradient (due to hyperdynamic and hypertrophied right ventricular outflow tract [RVOT] muscle) tends to decrease or resolve over time as the muscle remodels once the valvar stenosis is relieved. A right ventricular cineangiogram can help confirm the hyperdynamic infundibulum and muscle bundles (Video 14.1), when present,

and is also obtained after interventions to ensure there is no extravasation of contrast or tears.

The procedure has been shown to be safe and effective in multiple reports since the 1980s.[1] Restenosis is quite rare outside of the newborn period, and thus a single valvotomy is likely to last decades, if not a lifetime. There are two subpopulations that may have less-than-ideal outcomes: (1) neonates with critical pulmonary valve stenosis, in whom restenosis is quite common and reintervention often required; and (2) patients with a dysplastic pulmonary valve, such as that seen in patients with Noonan syndrome.

PR after pulmonary balloon valvuloplasty is common, with nearly 50% of patients having at least mild PR immediately after the procedure. In long-term follow-up, at least moderate PR has been reported in up to 60% of the patients.[1] However, it is important to note that the incidence and severity of regurgitation have been shown to be lower after pulmonary balloon valvuloplasty than after surgical valvotomy. While PR had traditionally been seen as benign and thought to be well tolerated, its long-term deleterious effects are increasingly being recognized in this population and many of these patients may require further interventions to re-establish pulmonary valve competence later in life.

TABLE 14.1 Indications, Technical Aspects and Goals of Transcatheter Balloon Valvuloplasty

Intervention	Class I Indications[2]	Technical Aspects	Goals	Success Rates
Pulmonary valve balloon dilation for congenital pulmonary stenosis	1. Critical valvar pulmonary stenosis (defined as pulmonary stenosis present at birth with cyanosis and evidence of patent ductus arteriosus dependency) 2. Moderate or worse valvar pulmonary stenosis, defined by a cath gradient ≥ 40 mm Hg across the pulmonary valve 3. Clinically significant pulmonary valve stenosis in the presence of RV dysfunction	• Balloon-to-annulus ratio 1.2 +/− 0.1	• Procedural success defined as one or more of the following: • Post-BPV peak systolic valvar gradient < 25 mm Hg • Decrease in gradient by 50% • Reduction of RV/systemic pressure ratio by 50%	• Reported acute success rates > 90%
Pulmonary valve perforation and balloon dilation for PA/IVS	No class I indication, but reasonable to perform pulmonary valvuloplasty in newborns with PA/IVS who have favorable anatomy that includes the exclusion of RV-dependent coronary circulation	• After successful perforation of the valve, serial balloon dilations starting with small balloons (~2.5–4 mm) to allow passage of larger balloons • Final balloon-to-annulus ratio 1.2 +/− 0.1	• Perforate and balloon dilate the atretic pulmonary valve, establishing antegrade pulmonary flow across the RVOT and reducing the RV pressure	• >90% acute success rates
Aortic valve balloon dilation	1. Isolated critical aortic stenosis in the newborn, regardless of gradient 2. Asymptomatic patients with resting peak systolic gradient by cath ≥ 50 mm Hg 3. Symptomatic patients (angina or syncope or ischemic ST-T-wave changes on electrocardiography at rest or with exercise) with gradient by cath ≥ 40 mm Hg	Balloon-to-annulus ratio of ~0.8 to start; increase by 5%–10%, serially dilating the valve until a ratio of ~1 is reached	1. Peak-to-peak gradients < 35 mm Hg or at least 50% reduction in peak-to-peak gradient compared to the start of the case) 2. Mild or less AR (or an increase in the degree of AR of no more than 1 grade for patients with pre-existing AR)	• >85% with residual peak-to-peak gradient at the end of the procedure of ≤ 35 mm Hg) with no or only mild increase in AR (nearly half with no AR and over 80% with mild or less AR at the end of the procedure). • ≥ Moderate AR reported in 7%–22% of patients • Severe AR between 1% and 2%.[3,4-9]
Mitral balloon valvuloplasty for congenital MS	None (see text)	• BSA-based method for initial balloon size: 8 mm for BSA 0.4–0.8 m[10], 10 for BSA 0.8–1.2 m[10], and 12 mm for BSA 1.2 m[10] • Height-based method: Balloon diameter (mm) = (height (cm)/10) + 10	• Reduce LV inflow obstruction and LA pressure enough to improve symptoms and delay MVR until the patient is older and larger • Avoid a significant increase in mitral regurgitation	• Results reported by McElhinney et al.[11] • MS gradient reduced by a median of ~40% • Calculated effective MV orifice area nearly doubled • Symptomatic improvement sufficient to avoid further MV intervention for at least 1 year in > 50% • 40% survival free from MV reintervention at 5 years • MVR-free survival 55% at 5 years • Moderate or severe mitral regurgitation in nearly 30% of patients

AR, Aortic regurgitation; BPV, balloon pulmonary valvuloplasty; BSA, body surface area; LA, left atrial; LV, left ventricular; MS, mitral stenosis; MVR, mitral valve replacement; PA/IVS, pulmonary atresia and intact ventricular septum; RV, right ventricular; RVOT, right ventricular outflow tract.

Pulmonary Atresia With Intact Ventricular Septum

In some neonates with membranous pulmonary atresia and intact ventricular septum (PA/IVS) who have non-RV-dependent coronary circulation, neonatal RV decompression can be accomplished percutaneously as a first step in management. The atretic valve is preferably perforated in antegrade fashion (from RV to MPA). The most commonly used techniques for valve perforation in PA/IVS include use of a radiofrequency ablation wire or use of a specialized chronic total occlusion wire (Video 14.2). After the valve is crossed, serial balloon dilations can eliminate the valvar contribution to RV outflow obstruction. Establishment of sufficient pulmonary blood flow through stenting of the patent ductus arteriosus (PDA) or through a surgical aorto-pulmonary shunt may be necessary if the patient is unable to maintain sufficient pulmonary blood flow in the absence of a PDA. It can take several weeks for the RV to remodel enough to be able to accommodate sufficient inflow. Once this occurs, the additional source of pulmonary blood flow can be occluded using transcatheter techniques or, in the case of ductal stents, allowed to close over time.

The initial part of the procedure focuses on delineation of the coronary supply, to ensure that it is not dependent on RV-coronary fistulae (see Chapter 37 on PA/IVS for further details). Once the decision has been made to perforate the valve, the best approach (surgical vs. transcatheter) depends on multiple factors, including the right ventricular inflow and outflow anatomy and the size of the pulmonary valve annulus. For those patients with adequately sized tricuspid valve, right ventricle, and a pulmonary valve annulus of at least 4 mm in diameter, transcatheter perforation is an excellent alternative to surgery. In general, we reserve surgery for patients in whom transcatheter valve perforation and balloon valvuloplasty fail to reduce the RV pressure significantly or in those in whom surgical remodeling of the RV cavity/RVOT is necessary.

The results of this procedure are less satisfactory than those for critical pulmonary stenosis. Complication rates are higher and cyanosis frequently persists for days or longer, necessitating prolonged management in the intensive care unit with prostaglandin infusion and/or placement of a ductal stent or surgical aorto-pulmonary shunt to ensure adequate pulmonary blood flow while the RV remodels.[10] PA/IVS includes a wide spectrum of anatomic severity, and certainly patients on the milder end of the spectrum tend to have better outcomes after transcatheter therapy and are often able to avoid surgery altogether.

Valvar Aortic Stenosis

Randomized studies have never been performed to compare the outcomes of balloon aortic valvuloplasty (BAVP) with those of surgical aortic valvotomy. The steady adoption of the procedure has been mainly supported by several retrospective studies comparing historical and contemporaneous outcomes, and showing that the two procedures are comparable with respect to survival, relief of stenosis, and incidence of aortic regurgitation (AR).

Class I indications for intervention are shown in Table 14.1. It is also important to know that using the gradient as the sole determinant for intervention has several limitations. The gradients specified in Table 14.1 assume normal cardiac output through the valve. Those thresholds have to be adjusted in patients with ventricular dysfunction and/or low cardiac output. There are also clinical circumstances that may warrant balloon dilation even if the gradient is 35–50 mm Hg, like patients planning pregnancy, athletes, and patients with consistently high echo-derived gradients (mean gradients > 50 mm Hg) who are under deep sedation or general anesthesia at the time of the procedure.

The most commonly used approach for BAVP is retrograde from a femoral artery. However, there are several other options in terms of approach (antegrade from a femoral or umbilical vein) and access site (carotid artery, axillary artery, umbilical artery, perventricular), which can be chosen in specific situations. Following routine right and left heart catheterization, including angiograms in the aortic root and the LV, the valve annulus is measured from a left ventricular angiogram taken in the long axial oblique view (Fig. 14.1). A balloon of appropriate size (see Table 14.1) is advanced over a guidewire, the distal end of the wire having been looped in the ventricle. As shown in Table 14.1, serial balloon dilations are performed, starting with a BAR between 0.8 and 0.9 and increasing the balloon diameter progressively by 10% or less with each subsequent dilation. Depending on the diameter, this can be achieved by using a larger balloon or by inflating the same balloon at a higher inflation pressure using a pressure gauge and the manufacturer guidelines to achieve the desired effective diameter. This process of balloon dilation followed by repeat assessment of the gradient and the degree of AR is repeated until the desired result is achieved (see Table 14.1). Balloon stabilization during the inflation and deflation is an important part of the procedure, as each ventricular contraction forcefully pushes the balloon out of the left ventricular outflow tract (LVOT). Some commonly used techniques that help stabilize the balloon include: (1) stiffer guidewire with a short or looped floppy tip to ensure that the part of the wire that provides the most support is across the aortic valve; (2) longer balloons (depending on the patient's age/size, a 4- or 6-cm long balloon may be appropriate; (3) rapid pacing to reduce stroke volume (often rates of > 200 bpm are necessary); and (4) double balloons (which allows for some blood to exit the ventricle between the balloons and, therefore, makes the system more stable). Other techniques that have been described but are rarely used include special balloons that are designed to allow some output while the balloon is inflated, adenosine bolus to cause a pause in ventricular contraction, and even induction of ventricular fibrillation by delivering a defibrillation shock on the T wave.

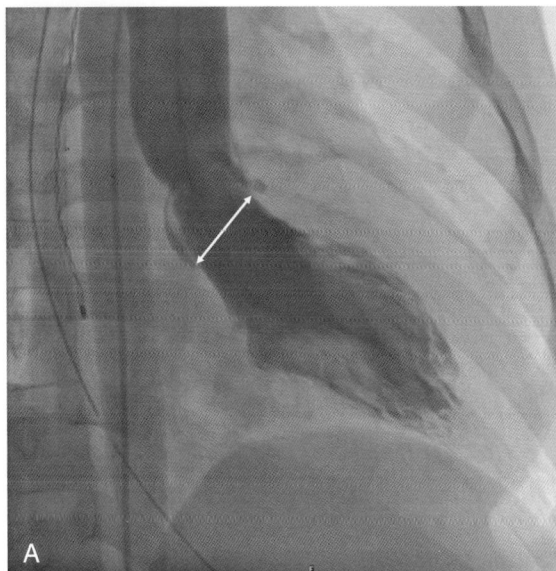

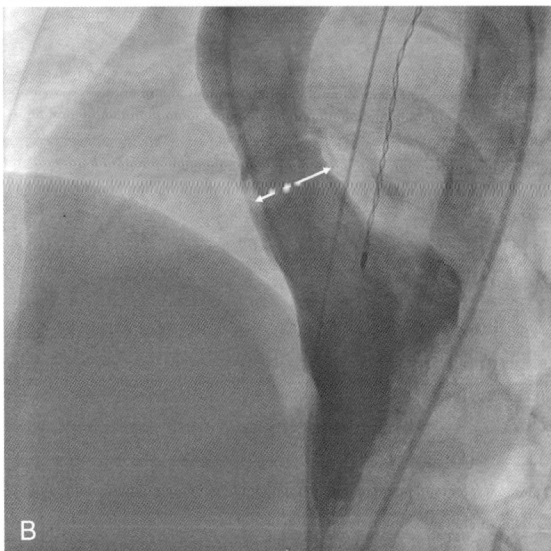

• **Fig. 14.1** Still-frames during systole from a left ventriculogram in 30-degree right anterior oblique **(A)** and long-axial oblique **(B)** views showing measurements of the aortic valve annulus in a patient with aortic valve stenosis and a bicuspid aortic valve. Note that the aortic valve leaflets are thickened and dome in systole. The measurement is performed from hinge-point to hinge-point *(double-headed arrows)*.

Neonates with critical aortic stenosis (AS; defined as ductal dependent systemic output) are particularly fragile and often have low gradients across the valve because of diminished cardiac output. In patients with low gradients, it is difficult to assess the results of each balloon dilation in the acute setting, and therefore it is difficult to know whether further inflations (with the associated risk of increasing AR) are necessary. In these cases, we generally perform serial dilations as for older patients until we see an improvement in left ventricular output and/or function as assessed angiographically, until we reach 100% of the valve annulus or until there is some AR. The goal in these patients is to palliate them enough to allow improvement in LV function and so that they are no longer dependent on PDA flow to maintain systemic output. It is imperative to avoid a significant increase in AR in these patients, and therefore we often accept a partial result, even if that makes reintervention more likely in the next few weeks to months.

The efficacy of BAVP as a palliative procedure for congenital aortic valve stenosis has been well established. Acute results are summarized in Table 14.1. Long-term outcomes of BAVP in over 500 patients at our institution were reported by Brown et al.[3] and underscore the procedure's palliative nature, with survival free from surgical aortic valve reintervention of 82% at 5 years and only 45% at 20 years. Not surprisingly, patients with better acute outcomes (residual AS gradient ≤ 35 mm Hg and trivial or no AR) had the longest freedom from aortic valve replacement (AVR; 95% at 10 years), while those with AS gradient > 35 mm Hg and moderate or severe AR immediately after the intervention had the shortest freedom from AVR (35% at 10 years).[3]

In summary, while BAVP is highly effective for acute relief of congenital AS, there are steady long-term hazards for surgical aortic valve reintervention and for AVR that are independent of age at balloon dilation and severity of presenting AS. While the majority of patients with a favorable acute outcome from BAVP can be expected to be free from AVR even 20 years after BAVP, patients with a less favorable acute outcome need particularly close follow-up and can be expected to require surgery in the first decade after the procedure.

Mitral Valvar Stenosis

The technique of percutaneous transcatheter balloon mitral valvuloplasty was first reported by Lock et al.[12] They performed the procedure in eight patients with rheumatic mitral stenosis (MS) between the ages of 9 and 23 years in India and showed that this approach resulted in good acute and short-term outcomes. In patients with rheumatic mitral valve stenosis, balloon dilation has become the first-line therapy. The mechanism of a successful balloon mitral valvuloplasty in rheumatic heart disease has been shown by pathological studies to be a fracture or tear of the commissures. On the other hand, the mechanism of MS in patients with congenital MS is much more complex than that of rheumatic MS. The morphology in congenital MS is quite heterogenous and the abnormalities can involve not only the leaflets but also the annulus and the subvalvar tensor apparatus. It often occurs in conjunction with other left heart obstructive lesions and intrinsic left ventricular myocardial abnormalities, which can significantly complicate its management. While this disease is heterogenous and includes different levels of severity, in the more severe end of the spectrum it is associated with significant morbidity and mortality and the current therapeutic options, both medical and surgical, have had limited success. This is especially true in neonates and infants, and often mitral valve replacement (MVR) becomes unavoidable. Although MVR can successfully relieve MS and MR, it is not an ideal solution in a growing child, since they will tend to quickly "outgrow" the prosthesis and are likely to require early replacement. In the setting of limited alternatives in young patients, balloon mitral valvuloplasty offers a less invasive palliative alternative for patients with medically refractory congenital MS. While the mechanism by which balloon mitral valvuloplasty works is less clear for these patients than for those with rheumatic MS, clinical experience has shown that it can relieve obstruction to more manageable levels and it can often delay surgery.[11] While these results are limited, delaying surgery in infants and young children can help tremendously in their management, since surgical options are better as the child becomes older and larger.

Indications for the procedure, technical aspects, goals, and acute outcomes are summarized in Table 14.1. It is important to note that the only class I indication for this procedure is for patients with rheumatic mitral valve stenosis and there are no class I indications for balloon dilation of the mitral valve in patients with congenital MS.[2] In general, we consider balloon mitral valvuloplasty in patients with severe congenital MS (defined as mean mitral valve inflow gradient > 10 mm Hg) if they have (1) systemic or higher pulmonary artery pressures, (2) failure to thrive or frequent respiratory infections requiring intensive medical management, or (3) in asymptomatic patients with mean mitral gradients greater than 15 mm Hg. After obtaining hemodynamics, including simultaneous LA and LV pressure tracings to determine the mitral valve inflow gradient, a balloon-tipped catheter is advanced from the LA to the LV. Care is taken to ensure that the balloon is at least partially inflated when it crosses the left ventricular inflow in order to avoid passing through mitral valve chordae. A guidewire is advanced into the apex of the LV using preformed curves to ensure a stable position, and a balloon is inflated across the mitral leaflet tips. Serial dilations are performed, starting with smaller balloon sizes and gradually increasing the balloon size with the goal of producing reasonable gradient reduction without causing significant mitral regurgitation (MR). Since the anatomic substrate of obstruction is unpredictable, we generally start with balloons that are related to either the patient's body surface area or the patient's height, rather than annulus size (see Table 14.1). Gradients are measured before and after every dilation, hoping to reduce the gradient by at least 50%, although reducing the mean gradient by 25% to 30% is frequently clinically significant (see Table 14.1). Angiography can be used to assess for the presence of MR after dilations, although we currently tend to use intraprocedural echocardiography for this purpose. This approach gives a more accurate assessment of the degree of MR, since left ventricular angiograms often give an overestimate of MR by inducing ectopic ventricular beats. It not only helps reduce radiation dose but also significantly reduces the contrast load (even eliminating the need for contrast in select patients), which is especially important in this patient population with elevated left atrial pressures and left ventricles with steep compliance curves. As noted in Table 14.1, the incidence of moderate or severe MR after

balloon dilation in congenital MS is not trivial, and this limits the appeal of the procedure.

Transcatheter Valve Replacement

Transcatheter Pulmonary Valve Replacement

The implant of the first transcatheter pulmonary valve into a human by Bonhoeffer et al.[13] in 2000 and the subsequent development of the Melody transcatheter pulmonary valve (Medtronic Inc, Minneapolis, MN) changed the field of interventional cardiology. It created, for the first time, the opportunity not only to treat stenotic valvar lesions in the catheterization laboratory but to relieve regurgitation at the same time. Published guidelines are largely derived from data from patients with tetralogy of Fallot and advocate for pulmonary valve replacement (PVR) in patients with severe PR, RV dilation, and symptoms of right heart failure.[1] Indications for PVR in the asymptomatic patient, those with other types of CHD (e.g., isolated pulmonary valve stenosis/regurgitation), and the question of whether those indications should differ depending on how invasive the PVR will be for a particular patient (surgical vs. transcatheter) remain controversial and are reviewed in other chapters. Both the Melody valve and the Sapien valve (Edwards Life Sciences, Irvine, CA) are FDA approved for use in dysfunctional RV to pulmonary artery conduits. Their use has quickly expanded to placement into existing surgical bioprostheses (valve-in-valve), amenable native RVOTs, and other off-label uses, with excellent results. Intentional fracture of existing bioprosthetic valve rings also allows for increased inner diameter of the new transcatheter valve despite the presence of a relatively small surgical bioprosthesis (Video 14.3). These uses and indications allow for transcatheter PVR in approximately one-third of the patients meeting indications for PVR. However, until recently, the majority of patients with large, postoperative native RVOTs and significant PR required open-heart surgery in order to restore pulmonary valve competence. With the development of "native outflow devices," the options for transcatheter PVR are quickly expanding to these patients as well. The Medtronic Harmony valve consists of a large, hourglass-shaped, covered self-expanding stent with a porcine pericardial valve mounted inside of it. The Alterra Adaptive Prestent (Edwards Lifesciences, Irvine, CA) has a similar design but no valve inside of it. Instead, the self-expanding frame serves as a "lumen reducer" and is designed for a 29-mm Sapien valve to be implanted inside of it. Both devices are designed with future valve-in-valve transcatheter PVR in mind, allowing for the possibility of avoiding open-heart surgery for PVR altogether in these patients as the bioprostheses start to fail over time.

Before placing a transcatheter pulmonary valve, it is very important to ensure that expansion of stents or the transcatheter valve at the desired diameter will not cause compression of the aortic root and/or the coronary arteries.

This requires balloon compression testing, using a balloon of the final desired stent diameter and performing simultaneous aortic root and/or selective coronary angiography while the balloon is fully inflated. If there is enough compression of the aortic root to cause any AR or if there is any coronary compression (Video 14.4), transcatheter PVR is contraindicated.

It is important to keep in mind that there has never been a randomized trial comparing surgical and transcatheter PVR; therefore, there is currently no available data to guide clinical decision-making or to elucidate how the long-term outcomes compare. Despite this limitation, all of these developments in combination have allowed for a paradigm shift in the treatment of right-sided congenital heart lesions involving the RVOT.

Transcatheter Aortic Valve Replacement in Congenital Heart Disease

While the experience with transcatheter aortic valve replacement (TAVR) in adults with calcific AS has grown exponentially over the last 10 years, the use of TAVR in congenital heart disease (CHD; Video 14.5) is significantly more limited.[14] In most centers, the use of TAVR for this indication is reserved for patients with bioprosthetic aortic valves and/or patients with high surgical risk. A cardiac CT is obtained for procedural planning and is essential to determine candidacy for TAVR, to ensure the size of the annulus is appropriate and that the coronary arteries are not at risk for obstruction once the existing leaflets of the aortic valve are trapped in an open position by the new transcatheter valve stent. The experience with this procedure in children and young adults with CHD has been encouraging. Although the number of patients is limited and long-term outcomes unknown, short-term outcomes compare favorably with surgical replacement using a bioprosthesis.[14] It is possible that as technology develops further, more patients in the congenital population will be eligible for this procedure.

Transcatheter Mitral Valve Replacement

In recent years, surgical implantation of the Melody transcatheter valve in the mitral position has gained popularity, especially for small infants and children, in whom the options for MVR are limited. This option allows for serial balloon expansion of the valve to adjust for the child's somatic growth. Once the valve leaflets degenerate and MR becomes significant, transcatheter mitral valve replacement (TMVR; valve-in-valve) is a possibility and has been shown to feasible and associated with good acute outcomes even in small children weighing less than 20 kg (Video 14.6).[15] TMVR in children has also been successfully performed with excellent acute and short-term outcomes in patients with other types of bioprosthetic valves (valve-in-valve), mitral annuloplasty rings (valve-in-ring), and even in the native, non-calcified, mitral valve annulus in a postsurgical patient.[15] A cardiac CT is used to evaluate candidacy for TMVR and helps predict whether the new valve would be at risk of producing LVOT obstruction (Fig. 14.2). While this type of experience is currently limited and its long-term results are unknown, it represents an important step forward in the management of congenital MS.

Transcatheter Tricuspid Valve Replacement

There are multiple emerging technologies for transcatheter tricuspid valve therapies that are being used in adults with acquired TR and are reviewed elsewhere.[16] These strategies are likely to mature over the coming years and some of them may be applicable to patients with CHD. Similar to TMVR, currently, transcatheter tricuspid valve replacement (TTVR) in patients with CHD is usually performed as a valve-in-valve procedure, although there are some reports of valve-in-ring TTVR. Heterotopic TMVR has also been reported.[16] While the acute results for TMVR are typically quite encouraging, there is a tendency for the valve to fail earlier than in other positions, similar to the experience reported for surgical TVR.

Vascular Interventions

Stenting of the Patent Ductus Arteriosus in Newborns

The Blalock-Taussig-Thomas (BTT) shunt was the first operation to palliate cyanotic CHD. Despite the fact that the operation has been performed since the 1940s, it continues to be associated with significant mortality, varying between 7% and 14%.[17,18] Gibbs et al.[19] first reported ductal stenting as an alternative to a BTT shunt in 1992. As technology has evolved and experience has accrued, ductal stenting for newborns with ductal dependent pulmonary blood flow has emerged as an acceptable alternative to surgical BTT shunts. Case planning and preprocedural imaging are an important consideration in these cases (Fig. 14.3). A detailed echocardiogram to show the ductal, aortic, and pulmonary artery anatomy in detail is usually the first step. If the PDA is tortuous, the duct inserts into a branch pulmonary artery (which can be a risk factor for branch pulmonary artery coarctation or isolation) or the anatomy is not sufficiently understood by echocardiography, a computed tomography angiography (CTA) is obtained to plan the procedure. The ideal site of vascular access is chosen based on this preprocedural imaging and which site would give the most coaxial alignment. Vertical ducts (arising from the lesser curvature of the aortic arch and having a general trajectory that is cephalad to caudad) are best approached from a carotid or axillary artery. Horizontal ducts are best approached from femoral arterial access. In neonates, carotid and axillary artery access have the added advantage that these vessels are two to three times larger than the femoral/iliac arteries, making vascular complications less likely. The ultimate size of the stent needs to be between 3 and 4 mm

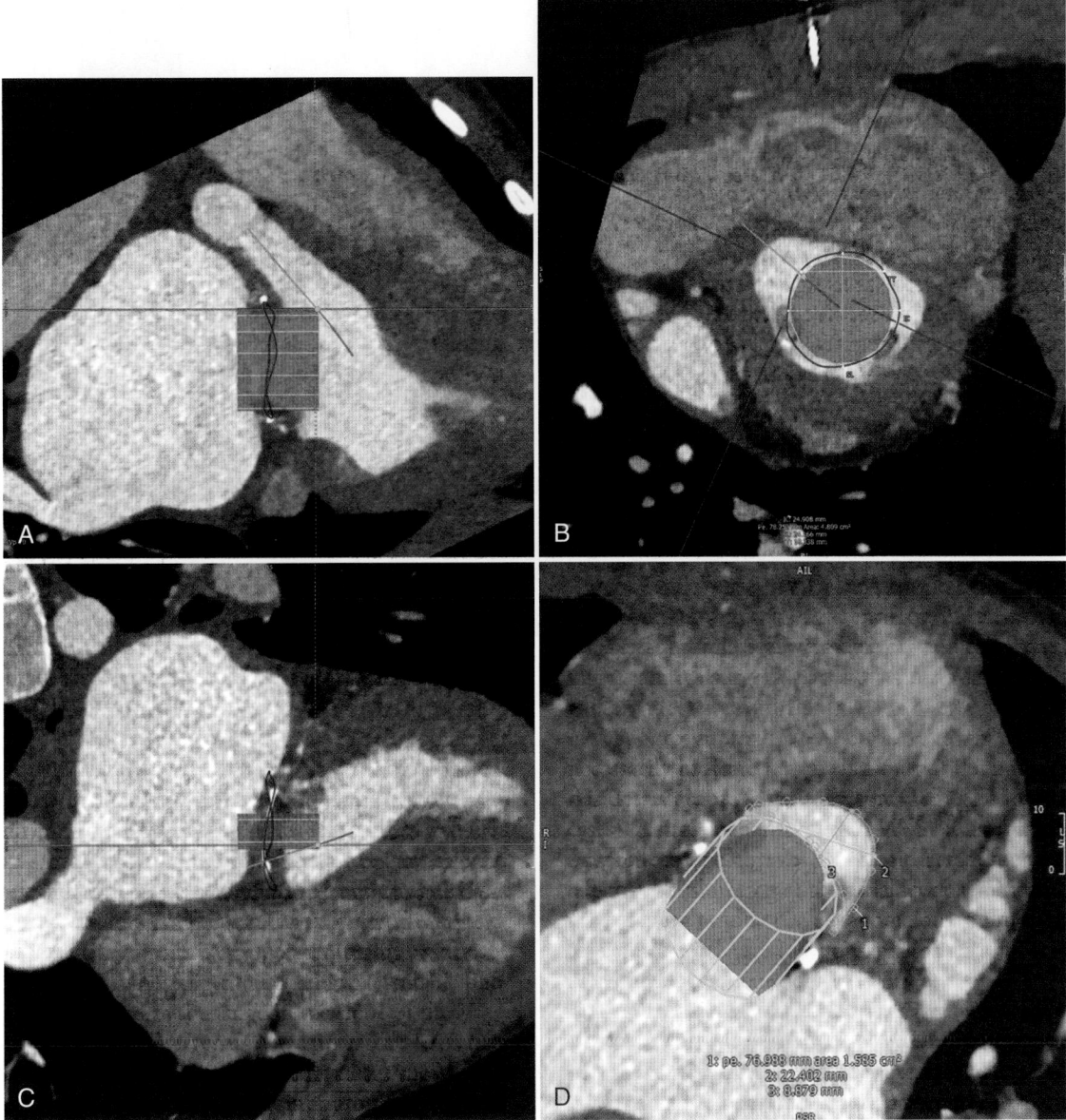

• **Fig. 14.2** Use of cardiac computed tomography for planning of transcatheter mitral valve-in-valve replacement procedure. **(A)–(D)** Segmentation of the mitral annulus and embedding virtual valve to assess the risk of left ventricular outflow tract (LVOT) obstruction. A simulated neo-LVOT area *(orange dotted line panel* **D)** is obtained in the narrowest portion of the LVOT in a mid-systolic phase with a virtual valve in place *(green line* indicates outer edges of virtual valve at the level of cross section).

in diameter, depending on patient size and length of the PDA. Therefore, the prostaglandin infusion needs to be stopped in advance of the procedure so that the patient arrives in the catheterization laboratory with a sufficiently constricted PDA, but not so constricted that it results in profound systemic hypoxemia. Coronary stents, bare-metal or drug-eluting, are used for this procedure and can be inserted through a 3.3 French sheath. Drug-eluting stents are used most commonly because of data from animal models of ductal stenting showing less in-stent stenosis over time,[20] although this remains to be confirmed in humans. While clinically evident toxicity from the medication on these stents has not been reported in neonates, one study found

that sirolimus levels were up to 20 times higher in neonates than in older children and adults.[21] Once the stent is deployed to the desired diameter, repeat angiography can confirm appropriate placement and assess for the necessity of a second, telescoping stent if any portion of the duct is not covered by stent material, since any portion that remains uncovered will tend to close over time and produce restriction to pulmonary blood flow (Fig. 14.4). Complications include vascular access site complications, ductal spasm or dissection, hyperacute stent thrombosis, and stent migration, embolization, or malposition. Most of these complications are temporary or can be resolved in the catheterization laboratory, but having surgical and extracorporeal membrane

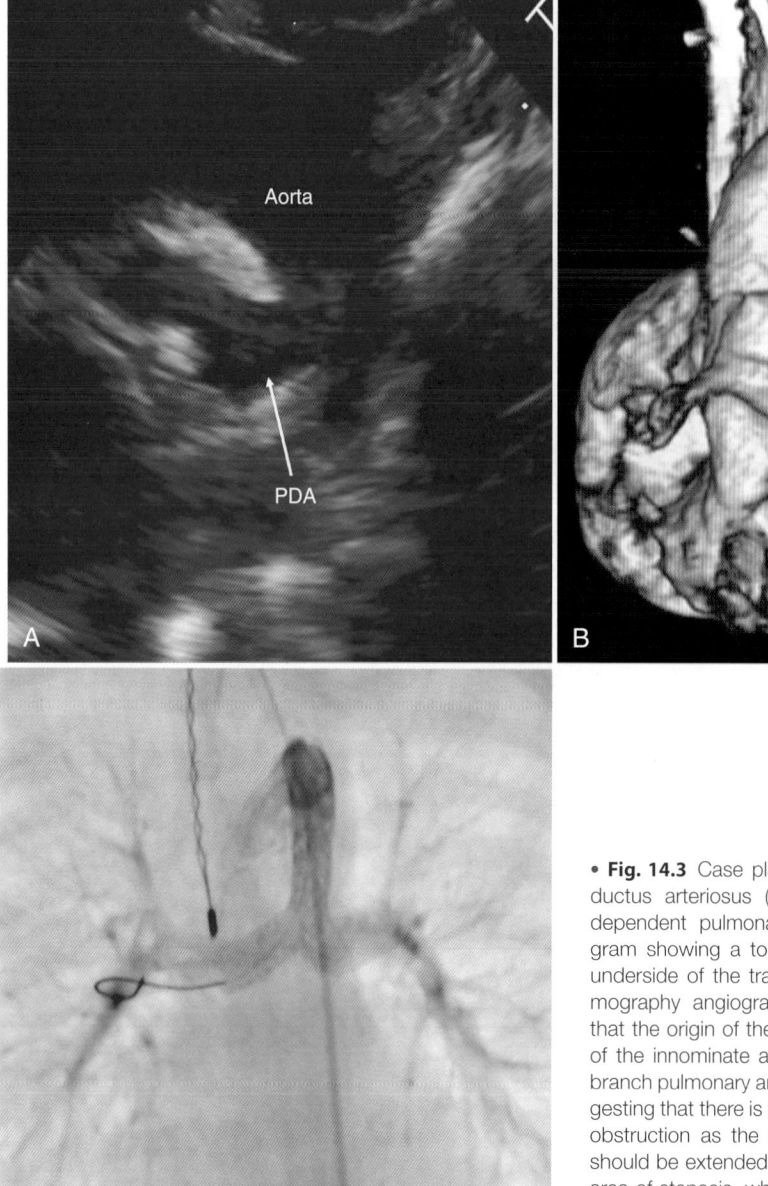

• **Fig. 14.3** Case planning for stenting of the patent ductus arteriosus (PDA) in a patient with ductal-dependent pulmonary blood flow. **(A)** Echocardiogram showing a tortuous PDA that arises from the underside of the transverse arch. **(B)** Computed tomography angiography 3D reconstruction showing that the origin of the PDA is aligned with the take-off of the innominate artery. There is narrowing of both branch pulmonary arteries at the ductal insertion, suggesting that there is potential for worsening branch PA obstruction as the PDA closes and that the stents should be extended into the branch Pas to cover the area of stenosis, which is likely surrounded by ductal tissue. **(C)** Angiography following Y-stents from the PDA into the branch Pas, resolving the narrowing of the branches.

oxygenation (ECMO) backup is important for these procedures. Over time, ductal stents tend to develop progressive narrowing due to in-stent stenosis, so it is important to follow these patients closely. Depending on how long the patient needs to wait for the next surgery, reintervention is often required at around 2–3 months to improve systemic hypoxemia that develops as the stent gets narrow and the patient grows (Fig. 14.5). While ductal tortuosity (Fig. 14.6), potential for branch pulmonary artery stenosis/coarctation and complex anatomy were considered contraindications for ductal stenting in the past, as experience has grown and equipment has improved, these kind of situations are routinely encountered and overcome in centers experienced in this procedure. As in other forms of CHD therapy with

transcatheter and surgical options, there has never been a randomized trial comparing BTT shunt with ductal stenting. Until that is available, it will be difficult to know for certain which approach is better and the field will have to continue to rely on expert opinion and nonrandomized, retrospective data to make these decisions.

Transcatheter Therapies for Vascular Stenoses

Venous and arterial stenotic lesions can be treated with transcatheter balloon and/or stent angioplasty. Although the approach to each type of lesion varies slightly, the principles of balloon angioplasty are the same for all vessels. The goal of balloon angioplasty is to produce a so-called

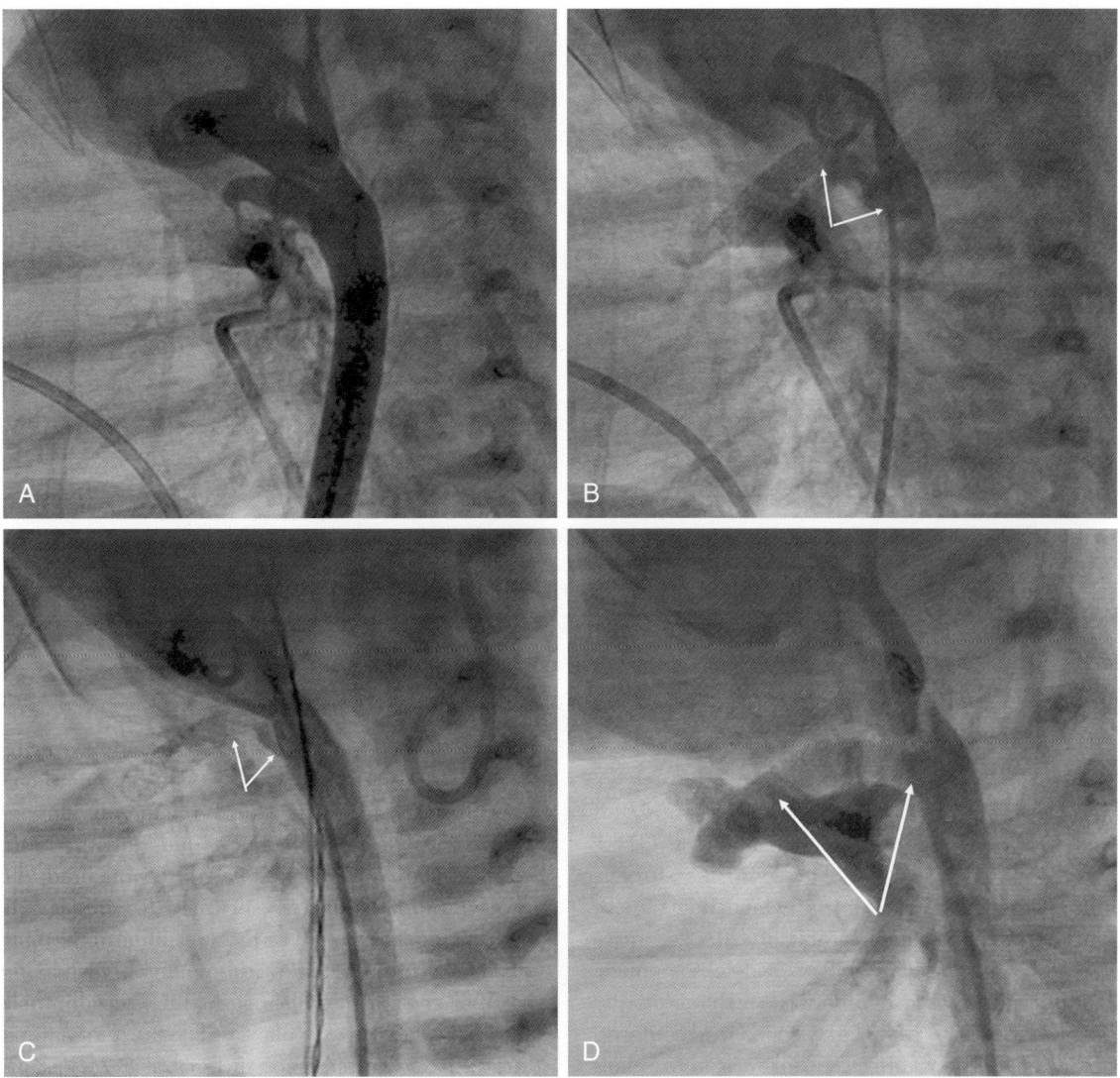

• **Fig. 14.4** Ductal stenting complicated by narrowing of the uncovered aortic portion of the patent ductus arteriosus (PDA). **(A)** Initial angiogram shows a PDA with significant constriction on the pulmonary artery end. **(B)** Follow-up angiogram shows that the stent extends into the main pulmonary artery but appears to leave the aortic end of the PDA uncovered. **(C)** Angiogram the following day, after prostaglandins were stopped the aortic end of the PDA, which was uncovered by the stent has constricted significantly and there is minimal flow through the PDA. **(D)** Follow-up angiography after restenting the PDA, now with good flow and a telescoping stents that covers the aortic end of the PDA.

"therapeutic tear," which consists of a partial-thickness tear (involving the intima and part of the media) of the target vessel at the level of stenosis. Techniques to achieve this type of tear vary according to the type of vessel and location and have been developed empirically. If the stenosis persists despite causing a satisfactory therapeutic tear, stenting may be indicated. Highly compliant lesions, like kinks or folds in the vessel, are typically resistant to balloon angioplasty and tend to respond well to stenting.

Recurrent Coarctation of the Aorta

The acute results of balloon angioplasty for re-coarctation (defined as recurrent obstruction after surgical repair of native coarctation of the aorta) in 200 patients were reported in 1990, showing that the pressure gradient could be reduced to less than 20 mm Hg in almost 80% of patients with a safety profile that compared favorably to reoperation.[22] Further experience, characterization of the mid- and long-term results of the procedure, and improvements in technique and technology quickly made balloon angioplasty the generally accepted first-line therapy for re-coarctation.[23]

Native Coarctation of the Aorta

Balloon angioplasty as primary therapy for native coarctation of the aorta can also be used as an alternative to

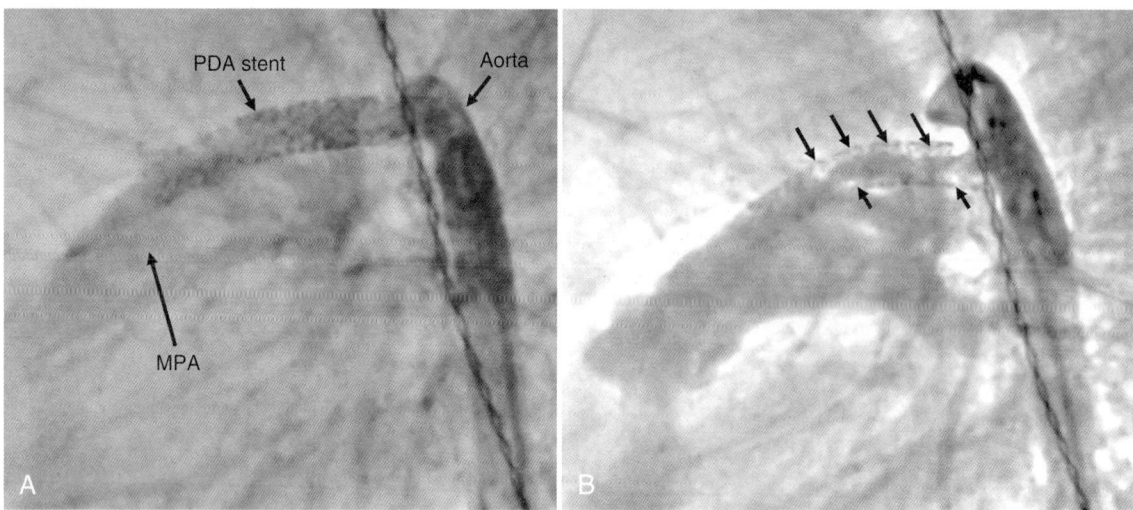

• **Fig. 14.5** Development of in-stent stenosis over time in a patient with ductal-dependent pulmonary blood flow. **(A)** Angiogram after stent placement shows good flow through the patent ductus arteriosus *(PDA)* with no in-stent stenosis. **(B)** Five months later, repeat angiogram shows significant in-stent stenosis. *MPA,* Main pulmonary artery.

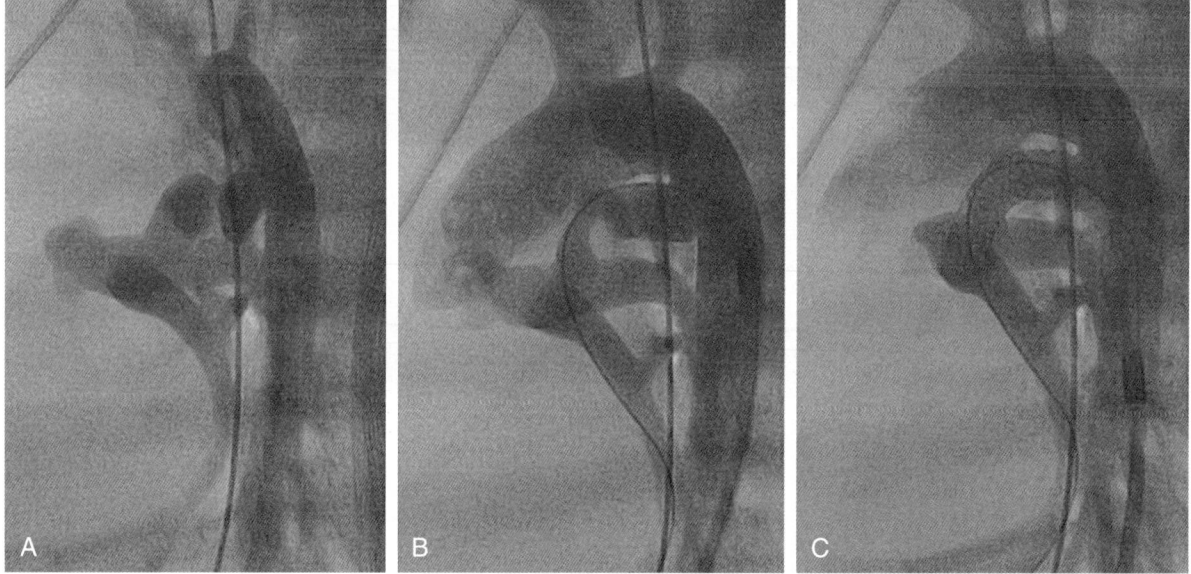

• **Fig. 14.6** Tortuous patent ductus arteriosus (PDA) in a patient with ductal-dependent pulmonary blood flow. **(A)** Initial angiogram shows tortuous PDA. **(B)** Once the PDA is crossed with a guidewire, it is significantly straightened by the wire. **(C)** Angiogram after PDA stent showing good flow through the PDA and stents covering the entire length of the PDA.

surgery. However, high recurrence and reintervention rates, and the incidence of aneurysm formation and vascular complications have tempered the enthusiasm for the procedure.[23]

Stent angioplasty (Fig. 14.7) has become the standard of care for native coarctation in adolescents and adults in most centers. While there are no randomized trials comparing surgery with stent placement, current data supports the noninferiority of stents in the short- and mid-term follow-up for patients in this age range.[23] For infants and growing children, implanting a stent guarantees the need for repeat

interventions to increase the size of the stent to account for the patient's somatic growth. Also, in small patients, the size of the sheath required to place a stent that can eventually reach adult size (18 mm or more) can be prohibitive. All of this, coupled with very good results of surgery for native coarctation, has kept surgery as the treatment of choice for native coarctation in infants and young children. Where the line is drawn, in terms of patient age and size, varies greatly from one institution to another and is likely to continue to change as improved technology becomes available. Overall, head-to-head comparisons of surgery versus transcatheter

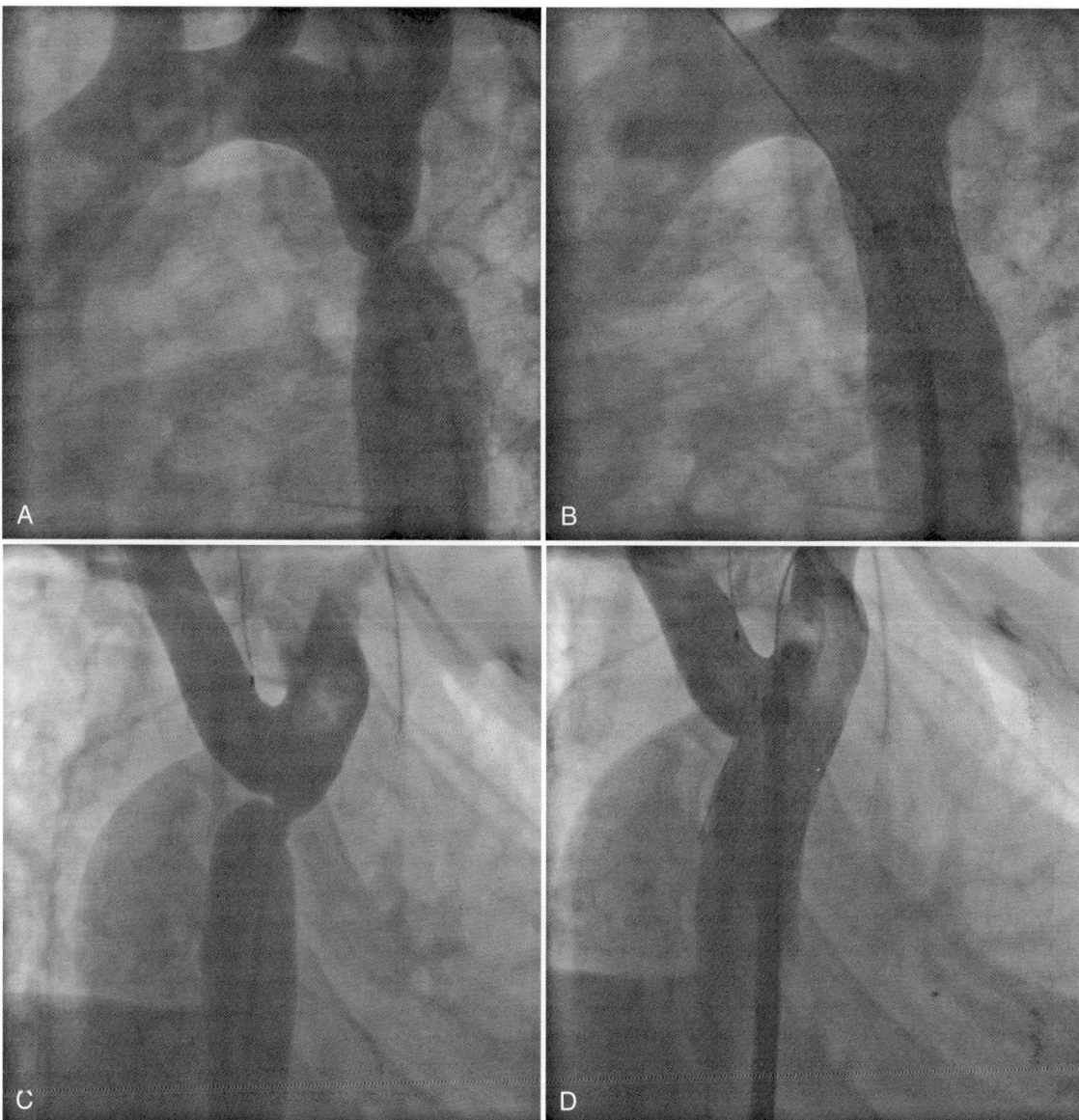

• **Fig. 14.7** Stent angioplasty for coarctation of the aorta. **(A)** and **(B)** Angiograms before and after stent angioplasty in a patient with native coarctation of the aorta. **(C)** and **(D)** Angiograms before and after stent angioplasty in a patient with native coarctation of the aorta and an aberrant right subclavian artery.

interventions for native coarctation of the aorta have shown that clinical outcomes are similar in both groups and the transcatheter procedures are associated with less procedural complications, a shorter length of hospital stay, and lower cost.[24] The transcatheter group tends to have more long-term complications (aneurysms, pseudoaneurysms, and/or reintervention), although the incidence has decreased significantly as the techniques have been refined empirically over the years and technology has improved. The advent of covered stents expanded the population of patients that can be treated with stenting to those with aneurysms and other vessel-wall abnormalities. It also allows for the possibility of transcatheter therapy for iatrogenic wall injury resulting from surgery (Fig. 14.8), or as a complication of balloon or stent angioplasty (Video 14.7). Primary therapy with

covered stents for native or recurrent coarctation of the aorta has not, however, been shown to decrease the incidence of aortic wall injury (aneurysms or pseudoaneurysms) in long-term follow-up, although this is a relatively new technology and data are limited. It is also important to note that the long-term implications of a stent in the aorta remain unknown and close follow-up of both surgical and transcatheter therapy patients is essential, since aortic wall complications (aneurysms, dissections, pseudoaneurysms, etc.) have been reported in both groups even over a decade after the index procedure. These patients also have abnormal peripheral vasculature and have a high risk of systemic hypertension and hypertensive response to exercise in long-term follow-up. While the risks of these findings are lower for patients that underwent repair before 2 years of age,

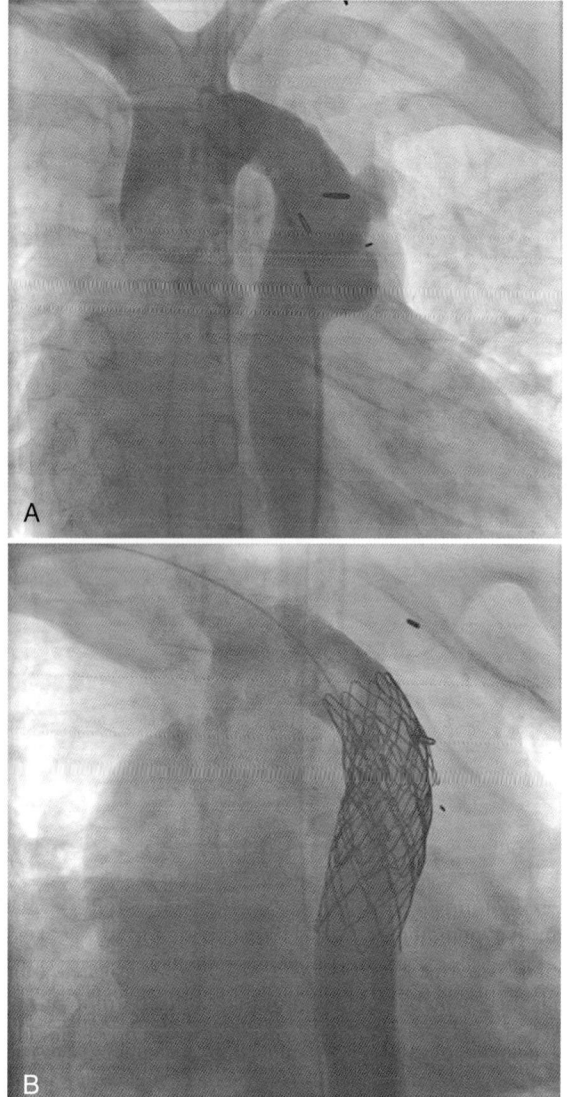

• **Fig. 14.8** Use of covered stents to exclude aortic aneurysms in a patient with a history of coarctation of the aorta treated surgically. Angiograms before **(A)** and after **(B)** covered stent placement, excluding the aneurysms effectively.

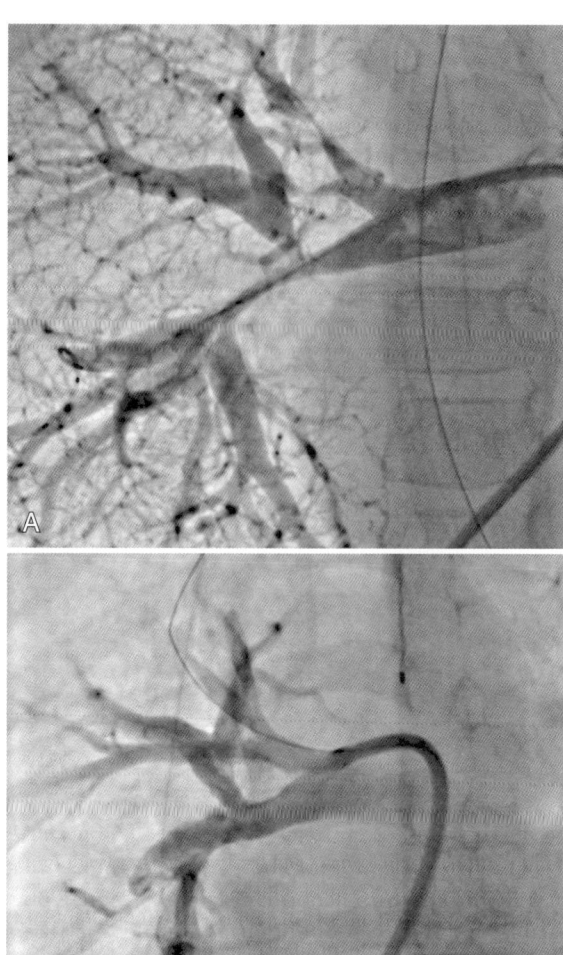

• **Fig. 14.9** Right pulmonary angiograms in a patient with Williams syndrome and severe peripheral pulmonary artery stenosis, before **(A)** and after **(B)** serial transcatheter interventions.

early repair does not guarantee freedom from these long-term issues, which may require medical therapy and close follow-up.[25]

Balloon and Stent Angioplasty of Branch Pulmonary Arteries

Pulmonary artery stenosis can be congenital or acquired. Some examples of acquired branch pulmonary artery stenosis include postoperative changes in patients with repaired or palliated conotruncal anomalies and chronic pulmonary thromboembolic disease. It may also be associated with genetic conditions such as Williams (Fig. 14.9), Alagille, and Noonan syndromes and has been reported as part of congenital rubella syndrome. It may affect the pulmonary arteries within the mediastinum (central

pulmonary artery stenosis) and/or peripheral branches beyond the hilum (peripheral pulmonary artery stenosis or PPS). Transcatheter interventions have become the standard of care for pulmonary artery stenosis, with surgical intervention reserved for specific scenarios, like concomitant surgery for other lesions, complex or resistant lesions that have not responded to transcatheter therapies or specific vasculopathies. Most commonly, however, the management of patients with CHD and pulmonary artery stenosis requires a team approach, with both surgical and transcatheter interventions used when appropriate throughout the lifetime of the patient.

Transcatheter therapies for branch pulmonary artery stenosis should be considered in patients who have one or more of the following abnormalities attributable, at least in part, to the stenotic lesions: (1) cyanosis, (2) signs or symptoms of right heart failure, (3) more than half systemic right ventricular pressures, (4) <25% of the pulmonary blood flow directed to one lung, (5) reduced or absent flow to the lung supplied by the stenotic vessel, (6) pulmonary hypertension in unobstructed lobes, or (7) moderate distal obstruction in the setting of severe PR.

Pulmonary arterial anatomy is determined from selective biplane right and left pulmonary arteriograms; care is taken to outline distal as well as proximal arterial anatomy. Cardiac CTA can be used for preoperative planning and intraprocedural guidance. Three-dimensional rotational angiography can also be performed during the procedure and provides detailed delineation of the anatomy of the entire pulmonary vascular tree in one single angiogram. The most severely affected vessels and the most distal lesions are typically dilated first. The choice of balloon depends on the desired diameter and how resistant the lesion is expected to be. An initial balloon about 2.5 to 3.5 times the size of the minimal luminal diameter (and no more than 2 times the diameter of the distal "normal" vessel) is selected. If a modest (about 75% to 90% of the balloon diameter) waist is seen, the balloon is inflated using a pressure gauge until the waist disappears. For vessels that require a balloon of 8 mm of diameter or smaller, we generally will not exceed 10–12 atm if the waist is persistent. In these cases, it is generally preferable to remove the balloon and replace it for an appropriately sized cutting balloon. The size of the required cutting balloon is typically smaller, no more than 0.5–1.0 mm larger than the diameter of the persistent waist on the prior balloon.[26] If the cutting balloon does not resolve the waist either, or if the vessel requires a balloon larger than 8 mm, we tend to use ultra-high-pressure balloons, which can be inflated to 30–40 atm if necessary, until the waist is resolved. If a tighter waist is seen (<75% of the balloon diameter), the balloon is deflated and the process is repeated using a smaller diameter balloon. If no waist is seen, larger balloons or better balloon positions are needed. Care is taken when crossing recently dilated vessels; angiograms and pressure measurements are repeated after each angioplasty. Post-dilation angiograms delineate success or failure, identify iatrogenic vascular trauma, and outline any residual lesions.

While stent implantation is feasible, safe, and is associated with excellent acute outcomes, our general approach to stenotic pulmonary artery lesions is to attempt balloon angioplasty first, and limit stent use to resistant lesions that recoil despite appropriate balloon-waist resolution and creation of a therapeutic tear, to treat obstructive intimal flaps produced by balloon angioplasty or for lesions that are highly compliant or caused by kinking or compression from other structures. It is especially important to avoid stents in growing patients, in whom stent implantation guarantees the need for further procedures as the child grows. Covered stents are rarely used in pulmonary arteries, with the exception of proximal branch pulmonary arteries, to treat uncontained tears, ruptures or aorto-pulmonary windows produced by balloon or stent angioplasty (Fig. 14.10). For lesions that are highly resistant, like those seen in patients with unifocalized aorto-pulmonary collaterals, it is also important to avoid stenting until the waist on the balloons has been resolved completely, since a narrowing that is resistant to ultra-high-pressure balloons and cutting balloons is unlikely to be resolved by a stent, and adding a stent will only result in further loss of luminal diameter at the site of the lesion.

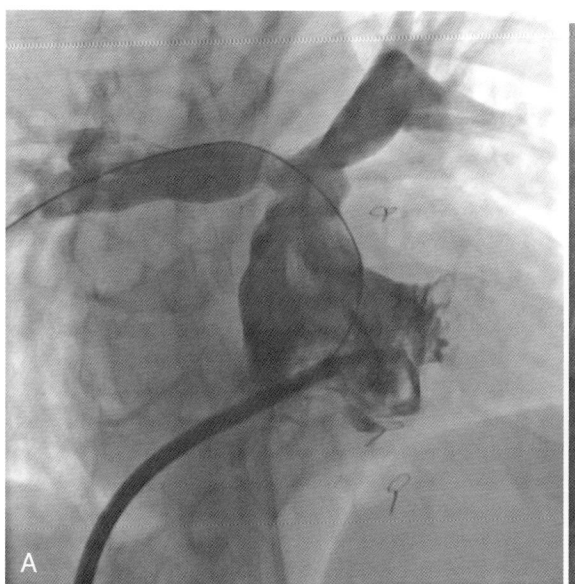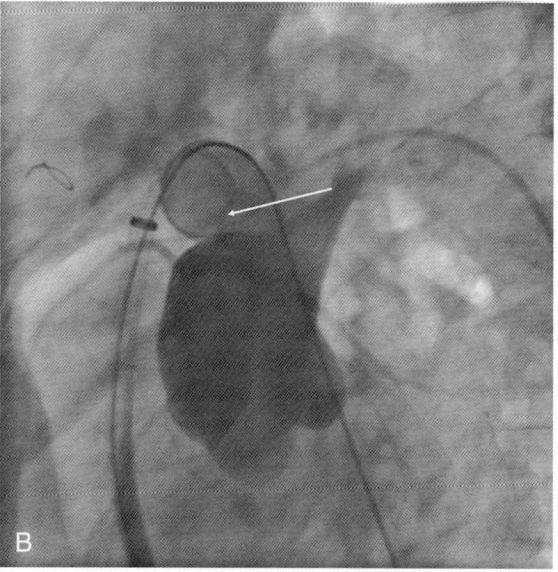

• **Fig. 14.10** Transcatheter management of a traumatic aortopulmonary (AP) window using a covered stent. **(A)** Initial angiogram in a patient who had previously undergone an arterial switch operation with LeCompte maneuver, presenting with obstruction of the right pulmonary artery (RPA). **(B)** After balloon and stent angioplasty of the RPA, an aortic angiogram in the lateral projection shows contrast entering the RPA from the aorta.   *Continued*

• **Fig. 14.10, cont'd** **(C)** After deployment of a covered stent, repeat aortogram in the same projection shows resolution of the AP window. **(D)** Pulmonary artery angiogram with similar angulation to panel A shows final result with improved caliber of the RPA.

The combination of standard balloons, high-pressure balloons, ultra-high-pressure balloons, cutting balloons, and stents leads to a high rate of success overall for transcatheter therapies for pulmonary artery stenosis, upward of 90%.[23] Reintervention is common, however, with about one-fourth of patients requiring reintervention in mid-term follow-up and with reinterventions being more common in smaller patients, patients with elastinopathies or Alagille syndrome, and in those with peripheral lesions.[23]

Mortality for this procedure has fallen steadily since it was introduced almost four decades ago, and is currently quite rare, with reported rates < 0.2%.[23] Morbidity includes vessel trauma (aneurysms, pseudoaneurysms, intimal flaps) and pulmonary hemorrhage that can occur from wire injury, vessel trauma, and/or reperfusion pulmonary edema. Aneurysms in the pulmonary artery tree following angioplasty have been generally benign (as long as the perfusion pressure is low) and can be managed conservatively. Patients with pulmonary artery obstructions in the early postoperative period are particularly vulnerable to vessel rupture if the site of the lesion was part of the anatomical dissection during surgery (since this removes some of the surrounding tissues that can help contain a tear) or if the lesion is at or near suture lines. In such patients, the use of primary stenting has largely replaced standard balloon angioplasty and has been proven to be acutely safe and effective.

Right Ventricle to Pulmonary Artery Conduits

The cause of stenosis of these conduits can be variable, including neointimal growth, kinking of the conduit, thrombus formation, deterioration/calcification of the conduit valve or the conduit wall itself, or a combination of these causes. Balloon angioplasty may give a satisfactory acute result, but the obstruction tends to recur within weeks unless a stent is placed. Before a stent can be placed, it is important to carefully characterize the location of the coronary arteries in relation to the conduit and ensure that a stent would not compress a coronary artery. This may require balloon compression testing, which involves inflation of a balloon of the diameter of the planned stent with simultaneous aortography or selective coronary angiography (Video 14.4). In growing patients with conotruncal malformations and an RV-PA conduit, stenting of an obstructed conduit can delay reoperation for several years. These stented conduits can also be further expanded by balloon angioplasty and/or re-stenting if the obstruction recurs or the patient outgrows the stented conduit. Covered stents can also be used to exclude pseudoaneurysms that may occur after surgery (Fig. 14.11) or to treat conduit ruptures or tears caused by balloon and/or stent angioplasty. In the era of transcatheter PVR, it is certainly possible to not only delay surgery for a longer period but also in some cases avoid surgery altogether, depending on the specific anatomy, patient size, and details of the specific conduit used.

Systemic Venous Obstruction

Systemic venous obstruction occurs in a number of postoperative congenital cardiac settings, most notably in patients who have undergone an atrial switch operation (Video 14.8). In both cardiac and noncardiac patient populations, systemic venous obstruction occurs with increasing frequency as a result of chronic indwelling catheters and, in some cases, cannulation for ECMO. Both angioplasty and stent placement have been applied successfully in the setting of superior vena cava obstruction. It is also important to remember that chronic elevation of systemic venous pressures can result

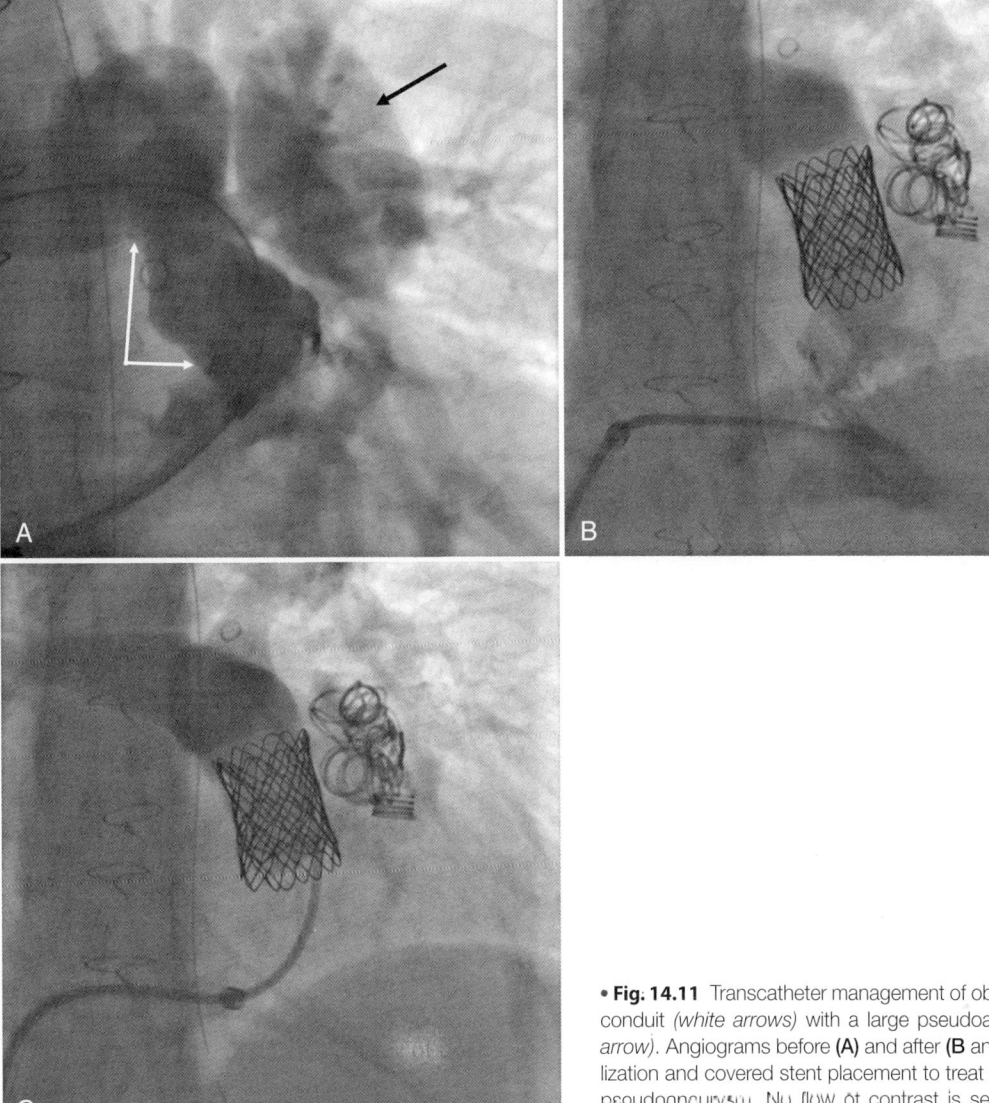

• **Fig. 14.11** Transcatheter management of obstructed RV-PA conduit *(white arrows)* with a large pseudoaneurysm *(black arrow)*. Angiograms before **(A)** and after **(B** and **C)** coil embolization and covered stent placement to treat obstruction and pseudoaneurysm. No flow of contrast is seen entering the large pseudoaneurysm after interventions.

in lymphatic dysfunction, leading to chylothorax, chronic pulmonary edema, and chronic pulmonary dysfunction. Treating the venous obstruction can help improve lymphatic drainage in this setting and should be a mainstay of therapy when patients have clinical evidence of lymphatic dysfunction associated with systemic venous obstruction.

Occlusion of Shunts

Patent Ductus Arteriosus

Several devices have been developed specifically for this indication, and the procedure has become the standard of care for patients of all ages with some exceptions related to specific anatomical types and patient factors.

The PDA occlusion procedure is relatively straightforward. Rare complications have been reported, including temporary left ventricular dysfunction from the acute change in preload and afterload associated with sudden closure of a large left-to-right shunt, inadvertent device embolization, and obstruction of the left pulmonary artery or the aorta by the device protruding into these structures, especially in small patients. Hemolysis has also been reported and is usually self-limited and, in persistent or severe cases, responds well to elimination of the residual flow.

One group of patients that remained a challenge until recently was premature infants with extreme low birth weight (ELBW). However, in recent years miniaturized versions of vascular occlusion devices have been used successfully. Early experience with these devices has been quite encouraging. In a multicenter trial which included 200 ELBW infants,[27] the implant success rate was 99% and the effective closure rate at the 6-month follow-up echocardiogram was 100% in patients weighing between 0.7 and 2 kg. Four patients experienced a primary safety endpoint event (two transfusions, one temporary hemolysis, and one aortic arch obstruction). Additionally, five patients < 2 kg (5%) developed new-onset moderate tricuspid regurgitation post procedure, likely related to tricuspid valve trauma during the procedure. Although fluoroscopy is necessary, device position and effect on adjacent structures are primarily assessed using intraprocedural transthoracic echocardiography, reducing exposure to iodinated contrast and radiation, and allowing the procedure to be performed without arterial access. The procedure can be performed in the catheterization laboratory or at the bedside. While there has not been a randomized controlled trial comparing device closure with surgical ligation, early experience suggests that post-ligation cardiac syndrome may be less

common and that improvement in respiratory status may be faster after device closure. Although these types of transcatheter devices provide the healthcare community with a nonsurgical alternative to achieve definitive ductal closure in ELBW infants, important questions on the optimal use of the device and long-term outcomes remain to be answered.

Secundum Atrial Septal Defect Closure

Device closure is currently the preferred treatment for hemodynamically significant secundum atrial septal defects (ASDs; Fig. 14.12), and it has also gained widespread application in

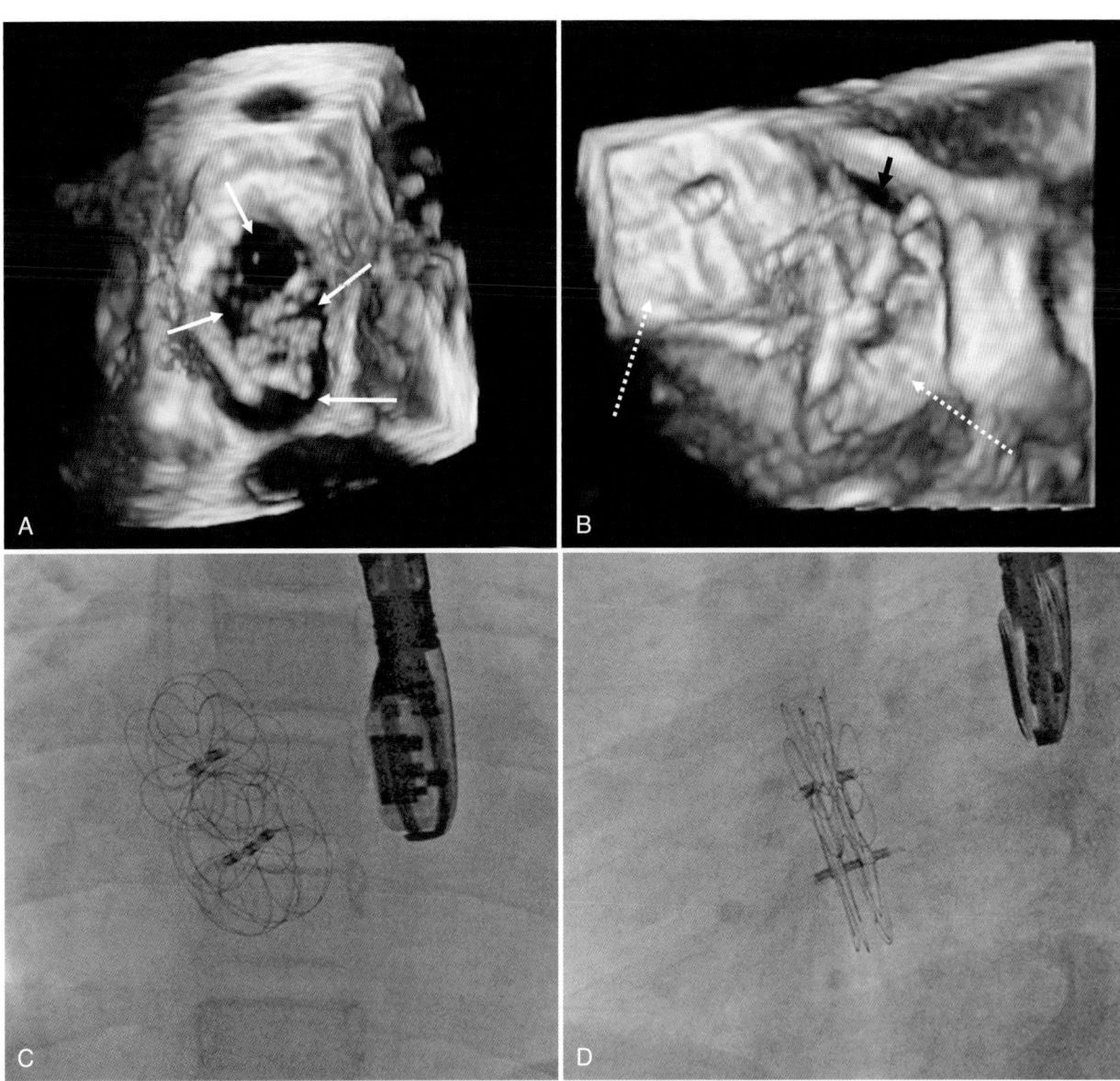

• **Fig. 14.12** Device closure of multifenestrated secundum atrial septal defect (ASD). **(A)** and **(B)**. Three-dimensional transesophageal echocardiogram showing a large multifenestrated secundum ASD *(white arrows)* before **(A)** and after device closure with two devices *(dotted white arrows)* **(B)**. Note there is a small residual defect between the two devices and the atrial wall *(black arrow)*. This residual shunt was present on the transthoracic echocardiogram the day after the procedure, but had resolved by the 1-year follow-up echocardiogram (not shown). **(C)** and **(D)** Fluoroscopic oblique AP and lateral projections showing the two ASD devices at the end of the procedure.

closure of the patent foramen ovale in patients with presumed paradoxical embolism after cryptogenic stroke.

There are specific anatomic requirements for a device to be placed safely, including the presence of sufficient rims around the defect and a defect size that allows for placement of an appropriately sized device relative to the patient's heart size so that it will not impinge on other structures (pulmonary veins, atrioventricular valves, conduction system). Echocardiography, either intracardiac or transesophageal (Fig. 14.12), plays a significant role in the guidance of these procedures and in the assessment of the final result. This also allows for reduction in the amount of radiation necessary for the procedure. There are currently many commercially available devices for transcatheter secundum ASD device closure. These can be generally divided into two groups: (1) self-centering devices (thick central portion between the two discs is meant to close the ASD completely with the discs providing additional stability), and (2) non-self-centering devices (central portion is thin and the defect is closed only by the discs). Self-centering devices can be used for small, moderate, or large defects (≤ 38 mm), while non-self-centering devices are intended for use only in small to moderate ASDs (≤ 18 mm). These devices have been successfully implanted in children aged < 2 years, although if a case is elective, common practice is to wait until the patient is > 15 kg, since this may offer some technical advantages. Complications are rare but include device embolism (which can usually be removed in the cath lab but sometimes requires surgical removal), cardiac arrhythmia requiring treatment, left atrial thrombus related to the device, and cerebral embolism. Early and late erosion of the device through the atrial wall into the pericardial space and/or the aorta has been reported in rare cases after device closure, primarily with the Amplatzer Septal Occluder. This is a major concern since it can happen even years after the procedure and can result in acute tamponade and even death. The incidence of this complication is difficult to establish, but most estimates vary between 1 and 3 cases of erosion for every 1000 implants.[28]

Ventricular Septal Defect Closure

Surgical closure continues to be the treatment of choice for patients with a hemodynamically significant ventricular septal defect (VSD), especially for perimembranous VSDs, which are the most common type of VSD. Patients with hemodynamically significant muscular VSDs may be offered percutaneous or hybrid-approach device closure. Exclusion criteria include weight < 3.0 kg (unless the hybrid perventricular approach is used); distance of < 4 mm between the VSD and any cardiac valve and pulmonary vascular resistance > 7 indexed Wood units.[2] Risks include device embolization, damage to atrioventricular valves, cardiac perforation and hemopericardium, embolic phenomena, ventricular tachycardia, and hemolysis. Complete heart block (CHB) is quite rare when closing muscular VSDs. However, the incidence of CHB in patients undergoing device closure of perimembranous VSDs has historically been reported to occur at a significantly higher incidence compared to surgical repair. This difference in CHB incidence has been a major hurdle in the wide adoption of this procedure for closure of perimembranous VSDs. While recent device design changes have shown promise, long-term follow-up data is currently limited.

Collateral Vessels and Surgically Created Aortopulmonary Shunts

Aortopulmonary collaterals can be found in association with various types of CHD, including Scimitar syndrome, tetralogy of Fallot with pulmonary atresia, and in patients with single ventricle physiology. Occlusion should be considered in patients with hemoptysis, patients in whom the left-to-right shunt is having or may have deleterious effects on their pulmonary vasculature and/or ventricular function or could result in worsening atrioventricular valve function over time. There are a variety of materials and devices used for this purpose, but the most commonly used in the current era include particulate agents, vascular plugs, and embolization coils. It is important to recognize that aortopulmonary collaterals may have multiple sources of arterial supply, and therefore materials or devices should be delivered as selectively and as distally in the vessel as possible to avoid persistent shunt from other sources.

Veno-venous collaterals can be seen in various forms of CHD. Systemic to pulmonary venous collaterals, or in the case of a Glenn circulation, even systemic to systemic venovenous collaterals, can result in right-to-left shunting and cyanosis. After a bidirectional Glenn procedure, the ligament of Marshall can recanalize and become a patent left superior vena cava draining to the coronary sinus, acting as a right-to-left shunt (Fig. 14.13). Devices and embolization coils can be used for transcatheter closure of these collaterals and vessels. However, these veno-venous collaterals form in response to elevated systemic venous pressures, so it is important to treat the underlying cause whenever possible in order to avoid recurrence and formation of new collaterals over time.

Surgical shunts that become unnecessary can also be closed definitively using coils or devices via a transcatheter approach. The techniques are similar to those used to close collaterals and the efficacy and safety profile of these procedures are similar. Closure devices have also been used to close a variety of clinically significant vascular communications including coronary arteriovenous fistulae, paravalvar leaks, pulmonary and systemic arteriovenous malformations, and other lesions.

Diagnostic and Interventional Catheterization in Postoperative Management

If a patient struggles in the postoperative period, requires mechanical support, or is unable to progress along the expected recovery pathway for their particular type of repair, it is important to have a programmatic approach that involves

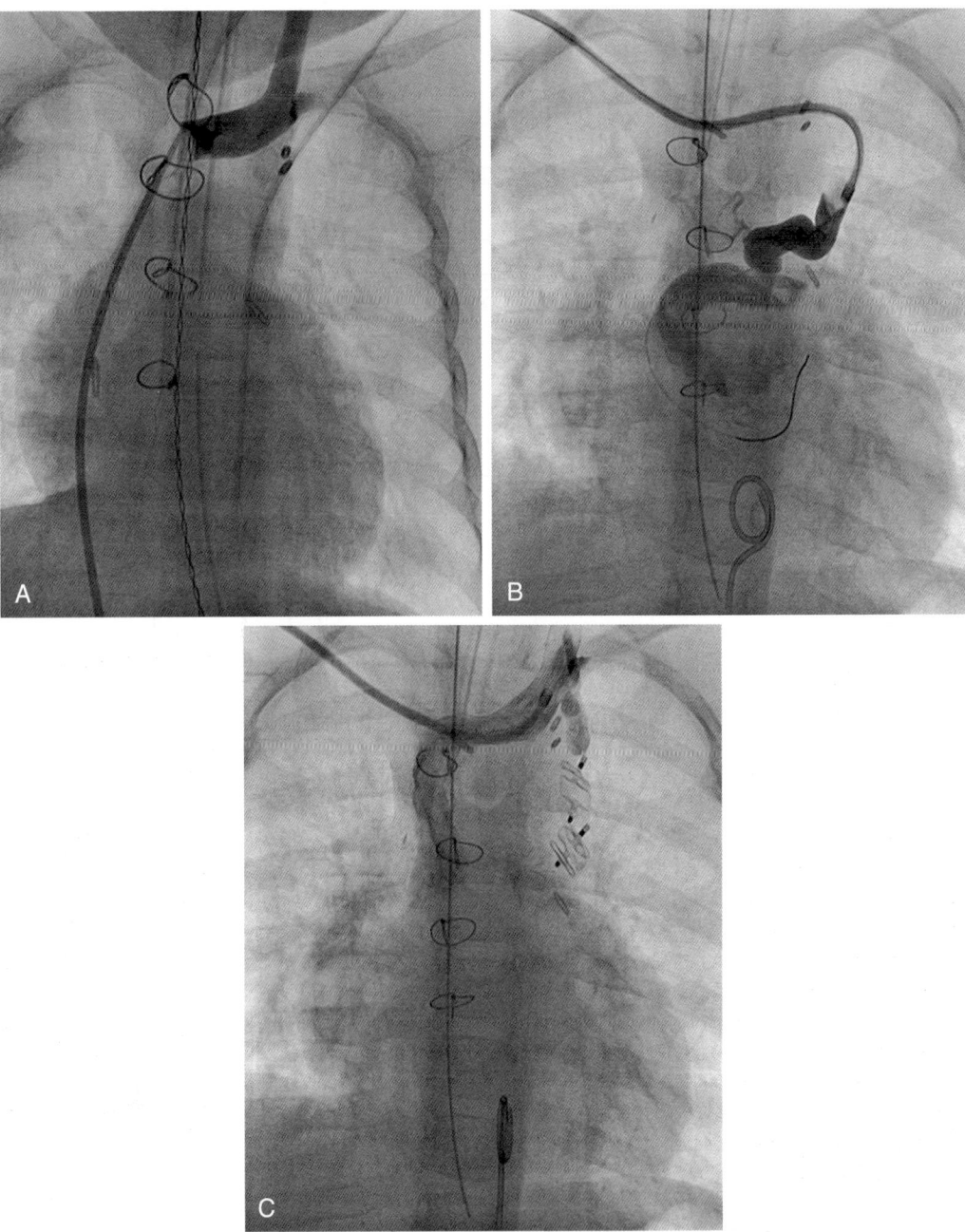

• **Fig. 14.13** Spontaneous recanalization of the left superior vena cava (LSVC) after a bidirectional Glenn (BDG) operation. **(A)** Balloon occlusion angiogram in the left innominate vein at the pre-Glenn catheterization shows no evidence of an LSVC. **(B)** Several months after the BDG, the LSVC has become patent and enlarged, decompressing the Glenn circulation by shunting blood away from the lungs, from the left innominate vein into an unroofed coronary sinus and left atrium. **(C)** Left innominate vein angiogram after device occlusion of the LSVC showing no residual flow.

early cardiac catheterization to rule out residual lesions and/or coronary obstruction. Postoperative cardiac catheterization in this scenario has been reported to yield information that leads to a change in clinical management in approximately 70% of the cases.[29] Early intervention on residual postoperative lesions has been shown to be safe and may shorten hospital length of stay by reducing residual hemodynamic burden.[29,30] Coronary lesions after congenital cardiac surgery are an important example (Fig. 14.14). While this is

a relatively rare lesion, it can be particularly difficult to diagnose by other modalities and requires a high index of suspicion. They usually present with significant sentinel events like inability to separate from cardiopulmonary bypass, cardiac arrest in the early postoperative period, malignant arrhythmias (ventricular fibrillation or ventricular tachycardia), or CHB. Timely diagnosis and intervention on coronary lesions are essential and has been shown to directly impact survival.[31]

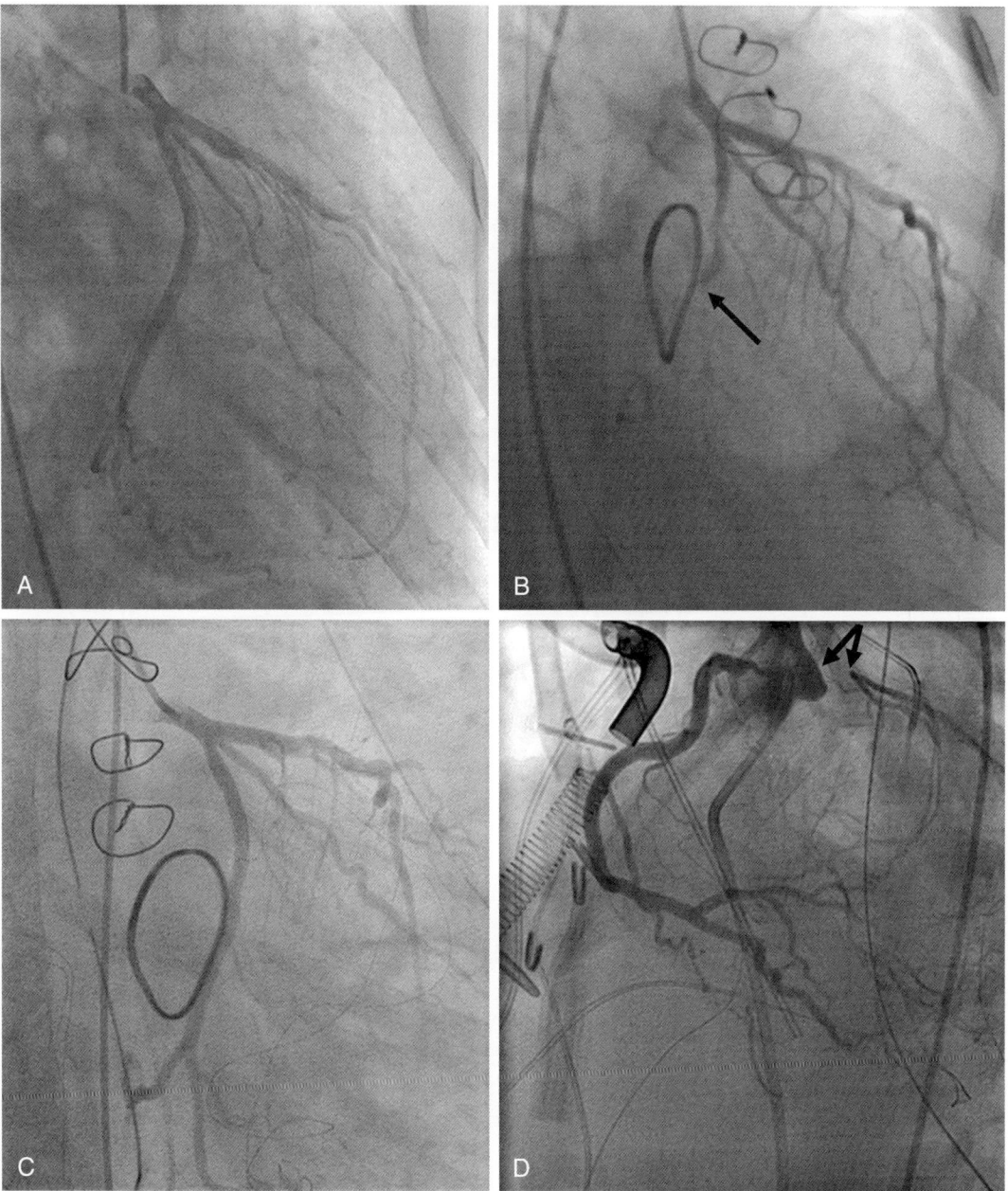

• **Fig. 14.14** Coronary artery lesions diagnosed in the immediate postoperative period. **(A)** to **(C)** Left coronary angiograms in a patient who underwent mitral valvuloplasty and placement of a mitral annuloplasty ring. Preoperatively, the circumflex coronary artery is widely patent **(A)**. However, in the immediate postoperative period, the circumflex is interrupted at the level of the annuloplasty ring (B) *(black arrow)*. Angiogram after surgical revision shows a patent circumflex coronary artery again **(C)**. **(D)** Aortogram in a patient on ECMO in the immediate postoperative period shows a large right coronary artery with small networks of collaterals filling the left coronary artery in retrograde fashion. The left main coronary artery is no longer in continuity with the aortic root *(black arrows)*. *Continued*

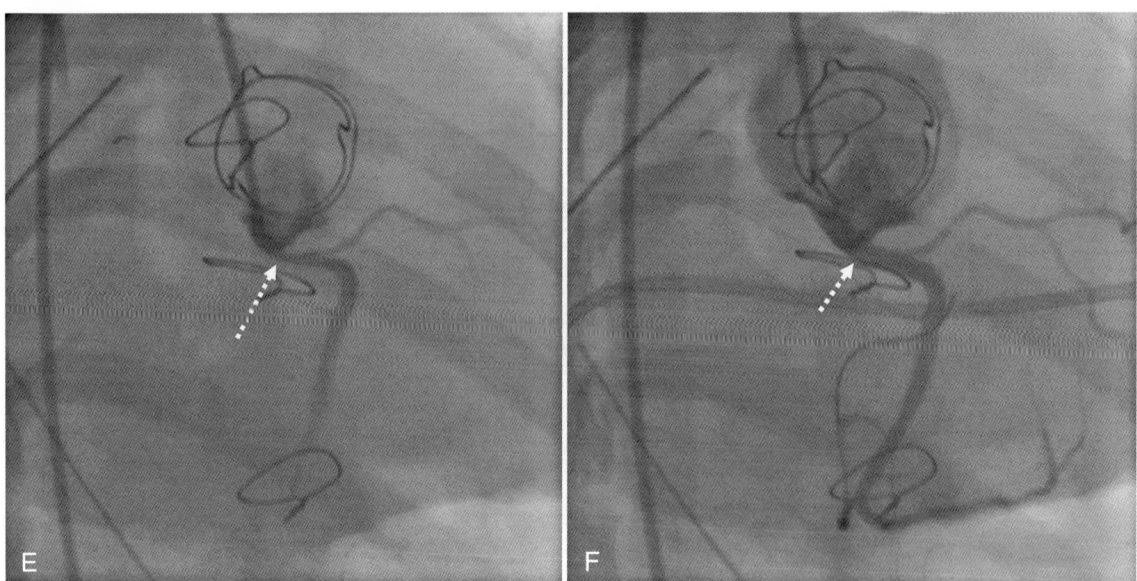

• **Fig. 14.14, cont'd** **(E)** and **(F)** Right coronary angiogram in a patient who underwent replacement of the aortic valve with a bioprosthesis. Initial angiogram shows severe obstruction of the proximal right coronary artery (*dotted white arrow*) **(E)**. After stent angioplasty, the right coronary artery is widely patent (*dotted white arrow*) **(F)**.

References

1. Morray BH, McElhinney DB. Semilunar valve interventions for congenital heart disease: JACC state-of-the-art review. *J Am Coll Cardiol.* 2021;77:71-79.

2. Feltes TF, Bacha E, Beekman RH III, et al. Indications for cardiac catheterization and intervention in pediatric cardiac disease: a scientific statement from the American Heart Association. *Circulation.* 2011;123:2607-2652.

3. Brown DW, Dipilato AE, Chong EC, Lock JE, McElhinney DB. Aortic valve reinterventions after balloon aortic valvuloplasty for congenital aortic stenosis intermediate and late follow-up. *J Am Coll Cardiol.* 2010;56:1740-1749.

4. Maskatia SA, Ing FF, Justino H, et al. Twenty-five year experience with balloon aortic valvuloplasty for congenital aortic stenosis. *Am J Cardiol.* 2011;108:1024-1028.

5. McCrindle BW, Blackstone EH, Williams WG, et al. Are outcomes of surgical versus transcatheter balloon valvotomy equivalent in neonatal critical aortic stenosis? *Circulation.* 2001;104:I152-I158.

6. McElhinney DB, Lock JE, Keane JF, Moran AM, Colan SD. Left heart growth, function, and reintervention after balloon aortic valvuloplasty for neonatal aortic stenosis. *Circulation.* 2005;111:451-458.

7. Moore P, Egito E, Mowrey H, Perry SB, Lock JE, Keane JF. Midterm results of balloon dilation of congenital aortic stenosis: predictors of success. *J Am Coll Cardiol.* 1996;27:1257-1263.

8. Porras D, Brown DW, Rathod R, et al. Acute outcomes after introduction of a standardized clinical assessment and management plan (SCAMP) for balloon aortic valvuloplasty in congenital aortic stenosis. *Congenit Heart Dis.* 2014;9:316-325.

9. Torres A, Vincent JA, Everett A, et al. Balloon valvuloplasty for congenital aortic stenosis: Multi-center safety and efficacy outcome assessment. *Catheter Cardiovasc Interv.* 2015;86:808-820.

10. Hasan BS, Bautista-Hernandez V, McElhinney DB, et al. Outcomes of transcatheter approach for initial treatment of pulmonary atresia with intact ventricular septum. *Catheter Cardiovasc Interv.* 2013;81:111-118.

11. McElhinney DB, Sherwood MC, Keane JF, del Nido PJ, Almond CS, Lock JE. Current management of severe congenital mitral stenosis: outcomes of transcatheter and surgical therapy in 108 infants and children. *Circulation.* 2005;112:707-714.

12. Lock JE, Khalilullah M, Shrivastava S, Bahl V, Keane JF. Percutaneous catheter commissurotomy in rheumatic mitral stenosis. *N Engl J Med.* 1985;313:1515-1518.

13. Bonhoeffer P, Boudjemline Y, Saliba Z, et al. Percutaneous replacement of pulmonary valve in a right-ventricle to pulmonary-artery prosthetic conduit with valve dysfunction. *Lancet.* 2000;356:1403-1405.

14. Robertson DM, Boucek DM, Martin MH, et al. Transcatheter and surgical aortic valve implantation in children, adolescents, and young adults with congenital heart disease. *Am J Cardiol.* 2022;177:128-136.

15. Maschietto N, Prakash A, Del Nido P, Porras D. Acute and short-term outcomes of percutaneous transcatheter mitral valve replacement in children. *Circ Cardiovasc Interv.* 2021;14:e009996.

16. Bhardwaj B, Cigarroa JE, Zahr F. Tricuspid valve percutaneous therapies. *Curr Cardiol Rep.* 2022;24:1209-1226.

17. Dorobantu DM, Pandey R, Sharabiani MT, et al. Indications and results of systemic to pulmonary shunts: results from a national database. *Eur J Cardiothorac Surg.* 2016;49:1553-1563.

18. Petrucci O, O'Brien SM, Jacobs ML, Jacobs JP, Manning PB, Eghtesady P. Risk factors for mortality and morbidity after the neonatal Blalock-Taussig shunt procedure. *Ann Thorac Surg.* 2011;92:642-651; discussion 651-652.

19. Gibbs JL, Rothman MT, Rees MR, Parsons JM, Blackburn ME, Ruiz CE. Stenting of the arterial duct: a new approach to palliation for pulmonary atresia. *Br Heart J.* 1992;67:240-245.

20. Lee KJ, Hinek A, Chaturvedi RR, et al. Rapamycin-eluting stents in the arterial duct: experimental observations in the pig model. *Circulation.* 2009;119:2078-2085.

21. Lee KJ, Seto W, Benson L, Chaturvedi RR. Pharmacokinetics of sirolimus-eluting stents implanted in the neonatal arterial duct. *Circ Cardiovasc Interv.* 2015;8:e002233.

22. Hellenbrand WE, Allen HD, Golinko RJ, Hagler DJ, Lutin W, Kan J. Balloon angioplasty for aortic recoarctation: results of Valvuloplasty and Angioplasty of Congenital Anomalies Registry. *Am J Cardiol.* 1990;65:793-797.

23. Goldstein BH, Kreutzer J. Transcatheter intervention for congenital defects involving the great vessels: JACC review topic of the week. *J Am Coll Cardiol.* 2021;77:80-96.

24. Forbes TJ, Kim DW, Du W, et al. Comparison of surgical, stent, and balloon angioplasty treatment of native coarctation of the aorta: an observational study by the CCISC (Congenital Cardiovascular Interventional Study Consortium). *J Am Coll Cardiol.* 2011;58:2664-2674.

25. Bocelli A, Favilli S, Pollini I, et al. Prevalence and long-term predictors of left ventricular hypertrophy, late hypertension, and hypertensive response to exercise after successful aortic coarctation repair. *Pediatr Cardiol.* 2013;34:620-629.

26. Bergersen LJ, Perry SB, Lock JE. Effect of cutting balloon angioplasty on resistant pulmonary artery stenosis. *Am J Cardiol.* 2003;91:185-189.

27. Sathanandam SK, Gutfinger D, O'Brien L, et al. Amplatzer Piccolo Occluder clinical trial for percutaneous closure of the patent ductus arteriosus in patients ≥700 grams. *Catheter Cardiovasc Interv.* 2020;96:1266-1276.

28. Thomson JD, Qureshi SA. Device closure of secundum atrial septal defect's and the risk of cardiac erosion. *Echo Res Pract.* 2015;2:R73-R78.

29. Siehr SL, Martin MH, Axelrod D, et al. Outcomes following cardiac catheterization after congenital heart surgery. *Catheter Cardiovasc Interv.* 2014;84:622-628.

30. Nicholson GT, Kim DW, Vincent RN, Kogon BE, Miller BE, Petit CJ. Cardiac catheterization in the early post-operative period after congenital cardiac surgery. *JACC Cardiovasc Interv.* 2014;7:1437-1443.

31. Goldsmith MP, Allan CK, Callahan R, et al. Acute coronary artery obstruction following surgical repair of congenital heart disease. *J Thorac Cardiovasc Surg.* 2020;159:1957-1965.e1.

15

Lymphatic Anomalies and Interventions

JESSE J. ESCH

KEY LEARNING POINTS

- The lymphatic system clears interstitial fluid, which is produced in response to hydrostatic and oncotic forces that vary between organs and patients.
- The thoracic duct forms the most important lymphovenous connection in the body. It demonstrates significant anatomic variation.
- Genetic syndromes may be associated with both congenital heart disease and lymphatic abnormalities. Turner syndrome should be suspected in any female neonate with edematous hands/feet.

- Any child undergoing cardiac surgery may suffer lymphatic complications such as chylothorax. Patients with palliated single ventricle face longer-term risk given the effects of venous hypertension on the thoracic duct and liver.
- With advances in conventional and magnetic resonance lymphangiography, targeted interventions can now be offered for many clinical lymphatic derangements.

Introduction

The lymphatic system is intricate, complex, and incompletely understood. Its key function is the collection of interstitial fluid—called *lymph* once it enters the lymphatic system—and transport of this fluid back into the circulation via lymphovenous connections. It also plays an important role in immune cell trafficking and activation, and is the major route of dietary fat absorption from the small intestine (with chylomicron-rich lymph called *chyle*). A thorough review of the lymphatic system in health and disease is well beyond the scope of this chapter. Nevertheless, some understanding of the lymphatic abnormalities most commonly seen in children with heart disease is essential to the practice of pediatric cardiology.

Basic Lymphatic Physiology and Anatomy

In most tissues, interstitial fluid is produced by filtration of plasma through a complex "filter" comprising intercellular clefts, endothelial glycocalyx, and pore/leak pathways.[1] The permeability of this filter varies by organ, with the hepatic sinusoids being particularly permeable. In general, there is net fluid production throughout the capillary bed, with all clearance occurring via lymphatics.

Inadequate lymph clearance results in edema. In health, the amount of interstitial fluid produced by an adult is approximately 4–7 L/day.

Human lymphatics form a non-circulatory vascular network: the direction of flow is one way, from interstitial space toward the systemic veins. Initial lymphatic vessels (blind ending and thin-walled) absorb lymph and coalesce to form collecting lymphatics. In the presence of one-way valves, lymph is driven centrally by intrinsic contraction of the muscular wall of collecting lymphatics, as well as by extrinsic contraction by surrounding skeletal muscle. Lymph passes through lymph nodes, which play an important immune function but also allow for absorption of up to half of lymph volume into the systemic venous system.[2]

Specialized lymphatics (*lacteals*) in intestinal villi receive chylomicrons from enterocytes, forming chyle. Intestinal lymphatics pass through mesenteric lymph nodes before coalescing to form the intestinal trunk. The intestinal trunk joins with at least one lumbar trunk to form the cisterna chyli, typically at the level of L1-L2, which is the caudal end of the thoracic duct (TD).

Lacking a basement membrane, hepatic sinusoids are very permeable, such that liver lymph is very protein-rich. This reduces the oncotic pressure gradient, which in most tissues moderates lymph production. As a result, liver lymph production is (1) high in volume at baseline and (2) sensitive to changes in hepatic/portal venous pressures and sinusoid transit time. It is estimated that mesenteric and hepatic lymph together constitute 80% of total body lymphatic flow, with the percentage rising even higher in the setting of congestive heart failure, hepatic cirrhosis, or hepatic venous hypertension. The lymphatic drainage of the liver is complex and includes connections with mesenteric lymphatic channels/nodes.[3]

The TD is the largest central collecting lymphatic channel and is estimated to handle ~75% of post-nodal lymphatic flow. In the most typical anatomical pattern, the TD ascends to the right of the midline, crosses leftward at approximately T5, arcs above the thoracic inlet, and then curves down to form the body's main lymphovenous connection at the junction of the subclavian and internal jugular veins (left venous angle). In this arrangement, lymph from the right chest/arm/head/neck drain via a right lymphatic duct, typically into the right venous angle. It is important to note that there are numerous anatomic variations in the tributaries forming the cisterna chyli, whether the TD is single or paired, whether a single TD ascends to the left or right of the midline, and whether the TD(s) drain to the left or right venous angle (Fig. 15.1).[4]

There are additional sites of lymphovenous connection beyond the insertions into the right and left venous angles. Such connections may exist, in particular, with the lumbar veins, portal vein, and renal veins.[5] These connections may have increased importance in disease states, and help explain why, for example, TD ligation is possible.

Lymphatic Abnormalities in Congenital Heart Disease

Many of the signs and symptoms of congestive heart failure (pulmonary edema, dyspnea, hepatomegaly, pedal edema) may be viewed as an imbalance between interstitial fluid production and lymphatic clearance. Beyond that, patients with congenital heart disease typically develop lymphatic abnormalities through one of three mechanisms: (1) underlying genetic syndrome, (2) traumatic injury to the TD (or another collecting lymphatic) during cardiac surgery, or (3) abnormal lymphatic flow patterns in the setting of abnormal anatomy/hemodynamics.

Underlying Genetic Syndrome

Turner syndrome is strongly associated with lymphatic abnormalities, likely due to hypoplasia of initial lymphatic vessels. Approximately 60% of affected infants display swollen hands and feet, and any newborn female with these findings should be suspected of having Turner syndrome.

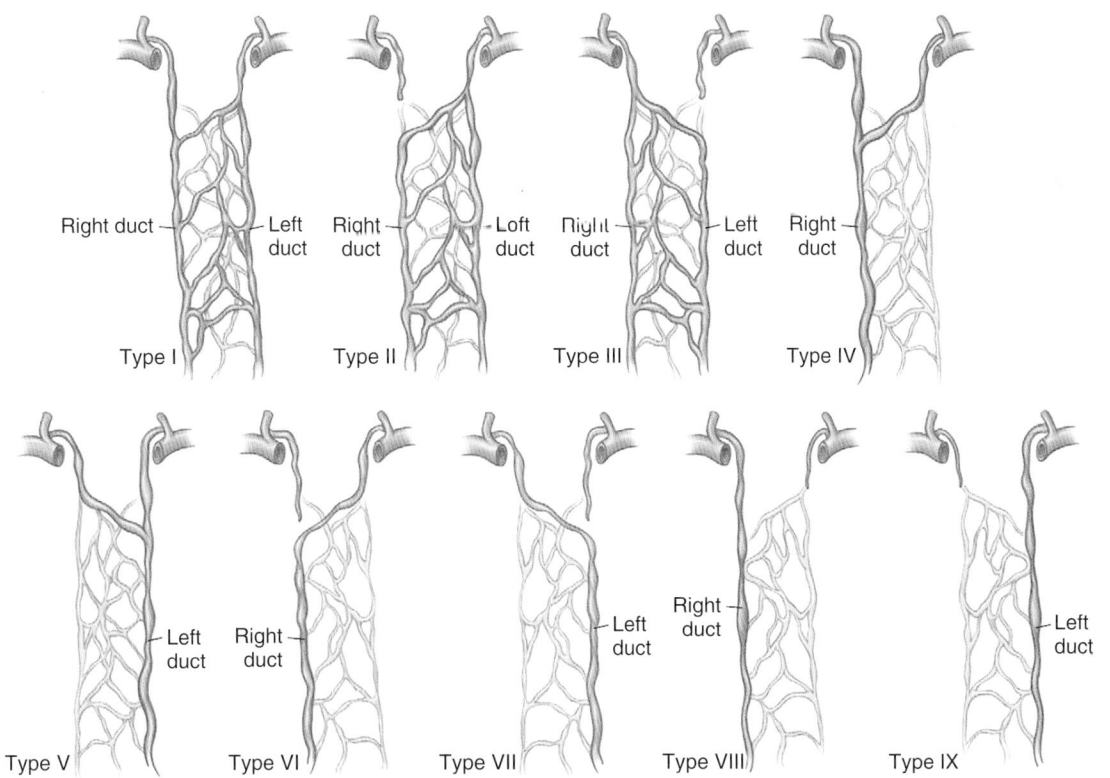

• **Fig. 15.1** Variations in thoracic duct anatomy described from cadaveric studies. The configuration most typically depicted in anatomical diagrams (type VI) is accurate in approximately 65% of individuals. (From Hematti H, Mehran RJ. Anatomy of the thoracic duct. *Thorac Surg Clin.* 2011;21:229-ix, used with permission.)

Characteristic features such as webbed neck and low posterior hairline are thought to follow from impaired cervical lymphatic drainage.[6]

Patients with Noonan syndrome display a wide range of lymphatic abnormalities, including lymphedema (which may be congenital), pulmonary/intestinal lymphangiectasia, lymphatic malformations, chylothorax, and protein-losing enteropathy (PLE).[7]

Injury to the Thoracic Duct and Its Tributaries

The TD and its branches travel in close proximity to the aorta, esophagus, and major systemic veins, and may be difficult to visualize. Traumatic injury to these lymphatic vessels can result in postoperative chyle leak syndromes, most typically chylothorax.

Chylothorax is often suspected by the milky appearance of pleural fluid, although in an *NPO* patient the appearance may be deceiving. Laboratory analysis is required to confirm the diagnosis, with the most definitive finding being presence of chylomicrons on lipoprotein electrophoresis. Total triglyceride level > 110 mg/dL is strongly suggestive of chylothorax, whereas triglyceride level < 50 mg/dL typically rules it out. Lipoprotein electrophoresis is often reserved for clarification of borderline triglyceride levels. In some situations, an enteral fat challenge can clarify the diagnosis. Chylous effusions usually demonstrate a predominance of lymphocytes on cell count (>70%).

Postoperative chylothorax complicates approximately 3%–5% of cases of pediatric cardiac surgery, although there is variation based on center/surgical technique.[8,9] Neonates and infants are at higher risk than older patients. With lymphatic imaging, it is often possible to visualize the level of TD injury and see the site of leakage of lymphatic fluid into the pleural space.

Abnormal Lymphatic Flow Patterns

Thrombotic occlusion of systemic veins affecting the site of lymphatic duct insertion (in particular involving the left/right venous angles at the thoracic inlet) can lead to non-traumatic chylothorax. Perhaps one of the most satisfying "lymphatic interventions" is percutaneous recanalization of such a thrombosis, with resolution of the chyle leak.

The surgically palliated single-ventricle patient presents a more complex example. Following superior cavopulmonary anastomosis, the cranial veins receiving the TD (and right lymphatic duct) often sustain supranormal pressures. A subset of patients go on to develop pulmonary lymphatic perfusion syndrome (PLPS), with lymph proceeding from the TD into the pleural spaces and/or peribronchial/parenchymal lymphatics.[10] Clinically, this results in chylothorax (which may present late after cardiac surgery) when the lymph flows into the pleural space, and plastic bronchitis when the lymph flows into the peribronchial/parenchymal lymphatics. Even in the absence of a clinical leak syndrome, many Glenn patients demonstrate increased number and

prominence of supraclavicular and mediastinal lymphatics on MRI imaging.[11]

The biology resulting in PLPS remains incompletely defined. Some have observed that the absolute cranial venous pressure measured at cardiac catheterization does not tightly correlate with the development of PLPS following bidirectional Glenn (patients with plastic bronchitis/chylothorax may have relatively "typical" pressures in the Glenn pathway, and some patients with severely elevated cranial venous pressures never display clinical signs of PLPS). One hypothesis is that elevation of venous pressure must be coupled with an additional lymphatic vulnerability to result in clinical lymphatic derangement. Pulmonary lymphangiectasia has been reported in a subgroup of fetuses with hypoplastic left heart syndrome, but whether similar preexisting abnormalities are indeed present in other single-ventricle patients who develop PLPS remains an open question.[12]

Fontan completion stresses the lymphatic system further by raising the venous pressure of the liver and intestines. As described above, the liver sinusoids are highly permeable, such that this rise in hepatic (and therefore portal) venous pressure significantly increases hepatic lymph production, with TD flow potentially increasing several-fold. This increased burden of lymphatic flow may unmask clinical chylothorax or plastic bronchitis. It may also result in PLE.

PLE is characterized by loss of proteins into the gut, and may result in diarrhea/abdominal pain, symptomatic hypo-albuminemia (edema, ascites), nutritional insufficiency, immunodeficiency due to both hypogammaglobulinemia and lymphopenia (with markedly low CD4+ T cells), and hypercoagulability (due to losses of proteins C and S).[13,14] Diagnosis is by detection of elevated fecal alpha 1-antitrypsin. Fontan-associated PLE appears to be due at least in part to disordered flow of hepatic lymph towards the small intestine (especially duodenum) and then spillage of this lymph into the intestinal lumen. PLE may affect up to 5%–15% of patients with Fontan physiology. Mortality from PLE has improved in the current era, but for some patients the symptoms remain chronic, intractable, and life limiting.

Lymphatic Imaging and Interventions

Surgical manipulation of the TD (including ligation) has been possible for many decades. As techniques for imaging lymphatic vessels have improved, so too have the range of potential interventions. Key advances include the evolution of magnetic resonance lymphangiography (MRL) and the development of transabdominal lymphatic interventions, both of which will be briefly discussed below.

Magnetic Resonance Lymphangiography

Thoughtful application of existing technology has allowed the cisterna chyli, TD, and other lymphatic vessels to be imaged using MRI techniques.

Lymphatic fluid has MRI characteristics similar to water and distinct from blood. Thus, T2-weighted non-contrast sequences can demonstrate the central lymphatics, as well as areas of ectatic or abundant lymphatic vessels. Pleural fluid has similar MRI characteristics, so the presence of effusions may obscure the lymphatic vasculature. Such MRL may be able to demonstrate the presence, size, and location/course of the TD.[15] Recent data suggests that in single-ventricle patients following bidirectional Glenn palliation, extensive lymphatic signal in the supraclavicular, mediastinal, and intrapulmonary regions on MRL may portend worse outcomes following Fontan completion[11] (Fig. 15.2).

The addition of MRI contrast—administered directly into the lymphatic system, most commonly through a femoral/inguinal node—allows for better spatial resolution of lymphatic vessels and adds a temporal component to elucidate flow patterns. This technique results in a dynamic contrast-enhanced magnetic resonance lymphangiogram (DCMRL).

Being somewhat invasive, DCMRL is typically reserved for patients with clinically significant lymphatic abnormalities (chylothorax or chylopericardium, plastic bronchitis, PLE). High-quality DCMRL imaging may identify therapeutic targets for intervention, such as TD interruption or lymphatic vessels coursing towards the lung/pleural space/pericardium (Fig. 15.3). In other cases, imaging may demonstrate disordered intrathoracic lymphatics and retrograde drainage to the abdomen/periphery; in these instances, no intervention may be possible.

Although DCMRL with lower extremity lymph node access can be incredibly useful, it does have limitations. As described above, much of the body's lymph is produced by the liver and small intestine, and this imaging strategy may miss important features of hepatic/mesenteric lymphatic physiology. Indeed, DCMRL studies with contrast administered through liver lymphatics (periportal thickening) were crucial in demonstrating that in Fontan-related PLE there is abnormal drainage of hepatic lymph to the duodenum.[16] More recently, DCMRL with intramesenteric contrast injection has been shown to be feasible, and could shed further light on the pathophysiology of PLE and chylous ascites.[17]

Conventional Lymphangiography and Percutaneous Interventions

Conventional lymphangiography is performed in the fluoroscopy suite by instillation of radiopaque contrast into peripheral or central lymphatics. Ideally this is performed using ethiodized oil as the contrast agent, as less viscous water-soluble contrast typically seeps out of the lymphatics before detailing the central lymphatic anatomy. Care must be taken to rule out right-to-left shunt prior to performing ethiodized oil lymphangiography, as this viscous agent can cause arterial occlusion (including stroke).[18] Historically, conventional lymphangiography was performed by dissection and cannulation of peripheral lymphatics. In the current era, direct nodal (or periportal) contrast administration is preferred.[19]

In patients with right-to-left shunt (e.g., status post Glenn or fenestrated Fontan), conventional lymphangiography may be performed using water-soluble contrast. Such imaging is unlikely to fully define the central lymphatic

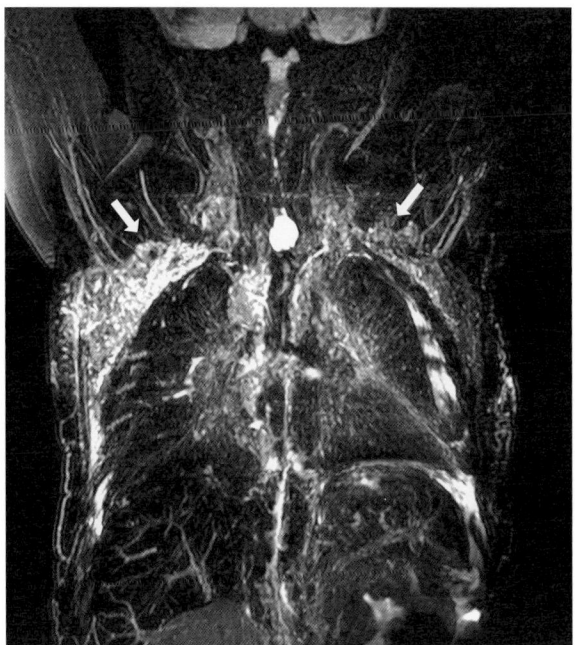

• **Fig. 15.2** T-2 weighted (non-contrast) magnetic resonance lymphangiogram in single-ventricle patient, status post-bidirectional Glenn. Note extensive dilated lymphatics in the supraclavicular regions *(white arrows)*, with extension into the mediastinum. There is also significant signal extending into the pulmonary parenchyma bilaterally.

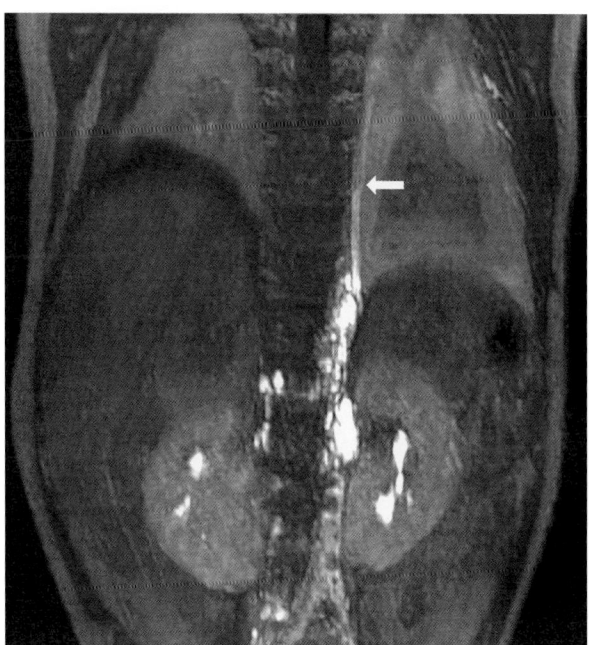

• **Fig. 15.3** Image from dynamic contrast-enhanced magnetic resonance lymphangiogram (DCMRL) in a single-ventricle patient with chylothorax following bidirectional Glenn. Contrast is seen to extend through dilated lymphatics along the leftward aspect of the spine, and then to leak into the left pleural space *(white arrow)*. No contrast is seen in the expected location of the thoracic duct.

anatomy, but may opacify the cisterna chyli or caudal TD. It is then possible to access these central lymphatic structures with a small-gauge needle via a transabdominal approach to allow more robust angiography of the more cranial lymphatics (Fig. 15.4).

Around the beginning of this century, interventional radiologists expanded these imaging techniques to develop percutaneous lymphatic interventions to treat chylothorax.[20] Initially the strategy involved either disruption of the TD below the level of the diaphragm or embolization of the TD along its length (most commonly with cyanoacrylate glue). In the current era, the goal is often selective occlusion of tributaries of the TD, which travel toward the pleural space (chylothorax), lung parenchyma/bronchial tree (plastic bronchitis), or pericardial space (chylopericardium).[10,21] In patients with amenable lymphatic anatomy, such interventions can be strikingly successful in resolving the clinical lymphatic disorder. Although complete TD occlusion is sometimes performed, concerns remain in single-ventricle patients about possible increased risks of PLE.

Ethiodized oil itself can have therapeutic effects, essentially occluding and sealing off culprit lymphatics.[22] This may be effective in congenital chylothorax as may be seen in Noonan syndrome, for example.

The percutaneous treatment of PLE and chylous ascites remain at the frontier of lymphatic intervention. Embolization of liver lymphatics draining toward the duodenum can

have at least short-term benefit in some patients with PLE; however, this is primarily a debulking-type procedure, and symptoms may recur.[23] Intervention directly on intestinal lymphatics remains challenging, although newer techniques such as retrograde access to the TD at the venous angle followed by navigation caudally to the mesenteric lymphatics may hold promise.

Surgical Lymphatic Interventions

Surgical TD ligation and pleurodesis remain options in the management of chylothorax. However, given the small size of pediatric lymphatic vessels, the anatomic variability of the TD, and the potential for accessory lymphatic channels arising caudal to the site of ligation, it is perhaps not surprising that TD ligation is not always curative.[24] Pleurodesis can carry significant morbidity. In the current era, many cardiologists prefer to reserve these surgical treatments for refractory cases or for when the patient is too unstable to undergo targeted lymphatic imaging/intervention.

Surgery to establish lymphovenous connections in the setting of interruption/occlusion of the TD is possible. Its role in the congenital heart population remains unclear.

In the setting of persistent lymphatic dysfunction in Fontan patients (PLE, plastic bronchitis, chylothorax), some have advocated for an "innominate vein turn-down" as a modification of the typical Fontan technique (Fig. 15.5).[25]

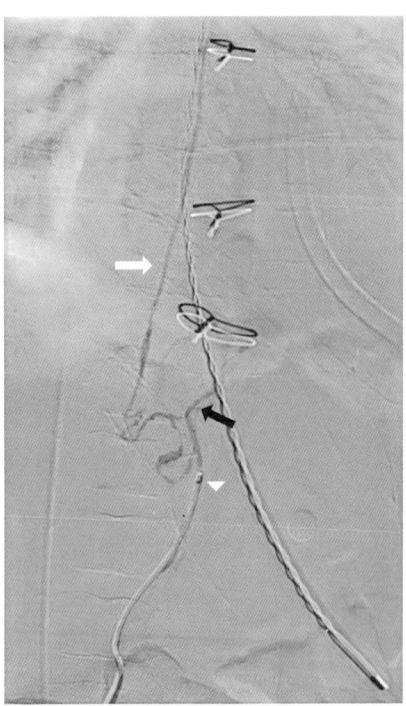

• **Fig. 15.4** Conventional lymphangiogram (with digital subtraction angiography image processing) in a single-ventricle patient status post bidirectional Glenn complicated by persistent left-sided chylothorax. A microcatheter has been inserted into an intra-abdominal lymphatic vessel (tip, *white arrowhead*). Contrast is seen filling a network of lymphatics which courses towards the base of the left lung (*black arrow*), and opacifies the thoracic duct (*white arrow*). The lymphatic network was selectively occluded, with subsequent resolution of chylothorax.

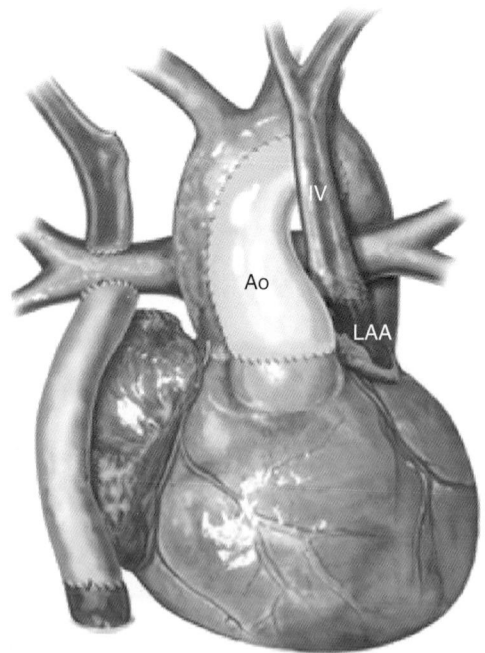

• **Fig. 15.5** Illustration of innominate vein "turn down" modification of Fontan. This procedure is intended to allow the thoracic duct to drain into the lower-pressure pulmonary venous atrium rather than the higher-pressure Fontan circuit. (Adapted from Hraska V Mitchell ME, Woods RK, Hoffman GM, Kindel SJ, Ginde S. Innominate vein turn-down procedure for failing Fontan circulation. *Semin Thorac Cardiovasc Surg Pediatr Card Surg Annu.* 2020;23:34-40, used with permission.)

At the cost of worsened cyanosis, this may allow the TD to drain directly into the lower-pressure pulmonary venous atrium (as opposed to the higher-pressure Fontan circuit). The indications for—and longer-term results of—this procedure have yet to be defined.

References

1. Michel CC, Woodcock TE, Curry FE. Understanding and extending the Starling principle. *Acta Anaesthesiol Scand*. 2020;64: 1032-1037.
2. Moore Jr JE, Betram CD. Lymphatic system flows. *Annu Rev Fluid Mech*. 2018;50:459-482.
3. Tanaka M, Iwakiri Y. The hepatic lymphatic vascular system: structure, function, markers, and lymphangiogenesis. *Cell Mol Gastroenterol Hepatol*. 2016;2:733-749.
4. Hematti H, Mehran RJ. Anatomy of the thoracic duct. *Thorac Surg Clin*. 2011;21:229-238.
5. Hsu MC, Itkin M. Lymphatic anatomy. *Tech Vasc Interv Radiol*. 2016;19:247-254.
6. Atton G, Gordon K, Brice G, et al. The lymphatic phenotype in Turner syndrome: an evaluation of nineteen patients and literature review. *Eur J Hum Genet*. 2015;23:1634-1639.
7. Cox TP, Vance CJ, Daley SK, et al. Systematic literature review of lymphatic imaging-guided procedural management of Noonan syndrome. *J Vasc Surg Venous Lymphat Disord*. 2022;10:1192-1196.
8. Buckley JR, Graham EM, Gaies M, et al. Clinical epidemiology and centre variation in chylothorax rates after cardiac surgery in children: a report from the Pediatric Cardiac Critical Care Consortium. *Cardiol Young*. 2017;27:1678-1685.
9. Mery CM, Moffett BS, Khan MS, et al. Incidence and treatment of chylothorax after cardiac surgery in children: analysis of a large multi-institutional database. *J Thorac Cardiovasc Surg*. 2014;147: 678-686.
10. Salva JJ, Itkin M, Rossano JW, et al. Post-operative chylothorax in patients with congenital heart disease. *J Am Coll Cardiol*. 2017;69:2410-2422.
11. Biko DM, DeWitt AG, Pinto, EM, et al. MRI evaluation of lymphatic abnormalities in the neck and thorax after Fontan surgery: relationship with outcome. *Radiology*. 2019;291:774-780.
12. Saul D, Degenhardt K, Iyoob SD, et al. Hypoplastic left heart syndrome and the nutmeg lung pattern in utero: a cause and

effect relationship or prognostic indicator? *Pediatr Radiol*. 2016; 46:483-489.
13. John AJ, Johnson JA, Khan M, et al. Clinical outcomes and improved survival in patients with protein-losing enteropathy after the Fontan operation. *J Am Coll Cardiol*. 2014;64:54-62.
14. Magdo HS, Stillwell TL, Greenhawt MJ, et al. Immune abnormalities in Fontan protein-losing enteropathy: a case control study. *J Pediatr*. 2015;167:331-337.
15. Dori Y. Novel lymphatic imaging techniques. *Tech Vasc Interv Radiol*. 2016;19:255-261.
16. Lemley BA, Biko DM, DeWitt AG, et al. Intrahepatic dynamic contrast-enhanced magnetic resonance lymphangiography: potential imaging signature for protein-losing enteropathy in congenital heart disease. *J Am Heart Assoc*. 2021;10(19):e021542.
17. Dori Y, Smith CL, DeWitt A, et al. Intramesenteric dynamic contrast pediatric MR lymphangiography: initial experience and comparison with intranodal and intrahepatic MR lymphangiography. *Eur Radiol*. 2020;30:5777-5784.
18. Kirschen MP, Dori Y, Itkin M, et al. Cerebral Lipiodol embolism after lymphatic embolization for plastic bronchitis. *J Pediatr*. 2016;176:200-203.
19. Rajebi MR, Chaudry G, Padua HM, et al. Intranodal lymphangiography: feasibility and preliminary experience in children. *J Vasc Interv Radiol*. 2011;22:1300-1305.
20. Itkin M, Kucharczuk JC, Kwak A, et al. Nonoperative thoracic duct embolization for traumatic thoracic duct leak: experience in 109 patients. *J Thorac Cardiovasc Surg*. 2010;139:584-590.
21. Dori Y, Keller MS, Rome JJ, et al. Percutaneous lymphatic embolization of abnormal pulmonary lymphatic flow as treatment of plastic bronchitis in patients with congenital heart disease. *Circulation*. 2016;133:1160-1170.
22. Gray M, Kovatis KZ, Stuart T, et al. Treatment of congenital pulmonary lymphangiectasia using ethiodized oil lymphangiography. *J Perinatol*. 2014;34:720-722.
23. Itkin M, Piccoli DA, Nadolski G, et al. Protein-losing enteropathy in patients with congenital heart disease. *J Am Coll Cardiol*. 2017;69:2929-2937.
24. Nadolski GJ, Itkin M. Lymphangiography and thoracic duct embolization following unsuccessful thoracic duct ligation: imaging findings and outcomes. *J Thorac Cardiovasc Surg*. 2018; 156:838-843.
25. Hraska V, Mitchell ME, Woods RK, et al. Innominate vein turndown procedure for failing Fontan circulation. *Semin Thorac Cardiovasc Surg Pediatr Card Surg Annu*. 2020;23:34-40.

16

Fetal Cardiac Interventions

WAYNE TWORETZKY AND RYAN CALLAHAN

KEY LEARNING POINTS

- The goal of fetal cardiac intervention (FCI) is to promote a biventricular circulation in a heart defect that would otherwise require univentricular palliation after birth. Examples of this are severe aortic valve stenosis with evolving hypoplastic left heart syndrome (HLHS) and pulmonary atresia with intact ventricular septum (PAIVS) with evolving hypoplastic right heart syndrome. Another goal is to improve perinatal survival in a heart defect that is otherwise highly lethal, such as HLHS with intact or severely restrictive atrial septum.
- In all fetal procedures, the most important patient is the healthy mother undergoing a procedure in an attempt to improve or treat a fetus with a serious anomaly; maternal safety is the priority.

- When evaluating fetuses with aortic stenosis for FCI, two important questions are considered. First, if left alone, will this fetus develop HLHS? Second, if the FCI is technically successful, will the left heart respond and be salvageable for a biventricular outcome after birth, thereby avoiding HLHS?
- The procedure itself is not without risk to the fetus, with ~5% to 10% rate of pregnancy loss. This risk assessment has to take into account the even higher risk of palliative surgery for HLHS as well as the potential benefit of preventing HLHS altogether.
- There is much research to be done on the natural history of these heart defects, patient selection for FCI, the sometimes novel surgeries performed after birth, and longer-term outcomes after FCI.

This chapter will focus predominantly on ultrasound (US)-guided catheter-based fetal cardiac interventions (FCIs). It will not cover fetal therapy such as transplacental antiarrhythmic drugs for fetal arrhythmias; that topic has been covered in Chapter 17.

Introduction

The goal of FCI is:

1. To promote a biventricular circulation in a heart defect that would otherwise require univentricular palliation after birth. Examples of this are severe aortic valve stenosis (AS) with evolving hypoplastic left heart syndrome (HLHS) and pulmonary atresia with intact ventricular septum (PA/IVS) with evolving hypoplastic right heart syndrome. Procedures are not performed for this indication if there is already clearly established HLHS.

2. To improve perinatal survival in a heart defect that is otherwise highly lethal, such as HLHS with intact or severely restrictive atrial septum (IAS).

Aortic Stenosis With Evolving Hypoplastic Left Heart Syndrome

The first reported FCIs were performed in the United Kingdom in the late 1980s, and this was followed by a few additional procedures at centers around the world.[1-4] Although in some cases there was reported procedural success, overall outcomes were poor and the concept was discontinued until a decade later. In the year 2000, the FCI program was initiated at Boston Children's and Brigham and Women's Hospitals. The team consisted of specialists from maternal-fetal medicine, obstetric U/S as well as pediatric interventional and fetal cardiologists, nurses, and fetal anesthesiologists. There has been a significant learning curve in refining FCI procedural techniques as well as patient selection and postnatal management.[5-7]

AS in the fetus has a range of outcome, depending on the timing in gestation and severity. At one end, AS can be mild, progress slowly, and result in neonatal AS with a biventricular heart requiring balloon dilation and/or surgery at some point in infancy. At the more severe end, in particular if the AS is more severe in early or mid-gestation, left heart growth arrest ensues resulting in HLHS at birth. In between these ends of the spectrum are patients born with so-called borderline left heart in whom neonatal decision-making regarding the appropriate therapy can be challenging. Patient selection for FCI requires an understanding of the natural history. This has been delineated in several publications, but more research needs to be done to understand the complete spectrum.[1,3,6,8,9] When evaluating fetuses with AS for FCI, two important questions are considered. First, if left alone, will this fetus develop HLHS? Second, if the FCI is technically successful, will the left heart respond and be salvageable for a biventricular outcome after birth, thereby avoiding HLHS?

Fetuses considered for FCI usually have anatomic abnormalities such as severe AS with thickened, doming aortic valve (AOV) leaflets, (Fig. 16.1) a normal-sized or dilated left ventricle (LV), and varying severity of endocardial fibroelastosis (EFE, Fig. 16.2). In addition are physiologic or Doppler aberrations that would predict evolution to HLHS. These include fused mitral valve inflow pattern, left-to-right or reversed flow at the patent foramen ovale (PFO) and retrograde flow in the transverse aortic arch supplied via the ductus arteriosus (Figs. 16.3 and 16.4). The retrograde arch flow occurs because the LV is unable to provide adequate antegrade flow due to severe AS and secondary LV dysfunction. Important predictors, amongst others, of LV salvageability are higher estimates of LV pressure as measured by mitral regurgitation or AS jet, minimal EFE, and at least normal length LV.[6,7,10,11]

Preoperative workup for FCI includes fetal echo, high-level obstetric US to rule out additional non-cardiac anomalies, consultations by fetal and interventional cardiology, maternal-fetal medicine, maternal anesthesia, as well as nursing and social work teams.

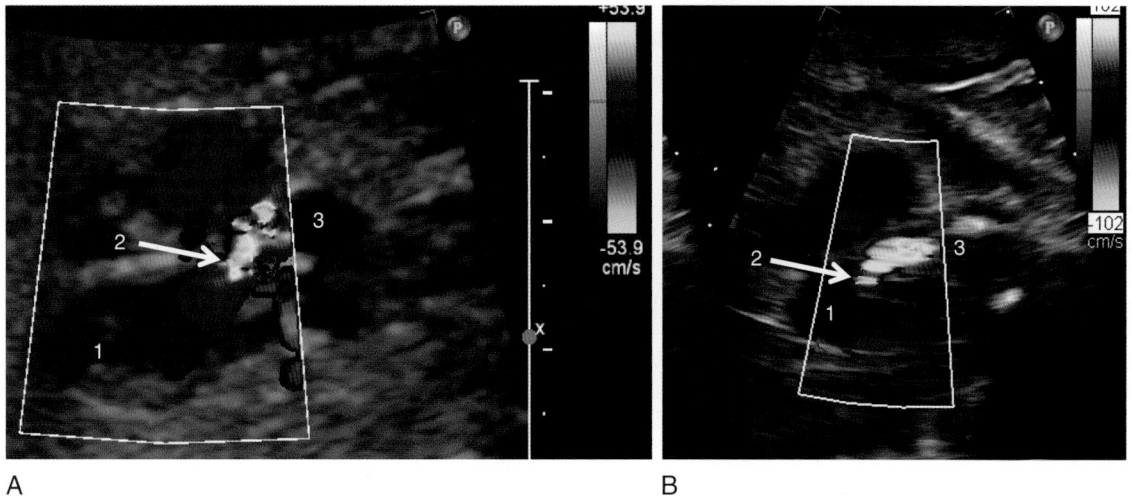

A   B

• **Fig. 16.1** Fetal echo image depicting the natural history and effect of aortic stenosis on the left ventricle. **(A)** 22 weeks' gestational age (GA). Normal-shaped LV. **(B)** 25 weeks' GA. Dilated, globular-shaped LV with patches of echogenicity (endocardial fibroelastosis). *1*, Left ventricle; *2*, right ventricle; *3*, left atrium; *4*, right atrium.

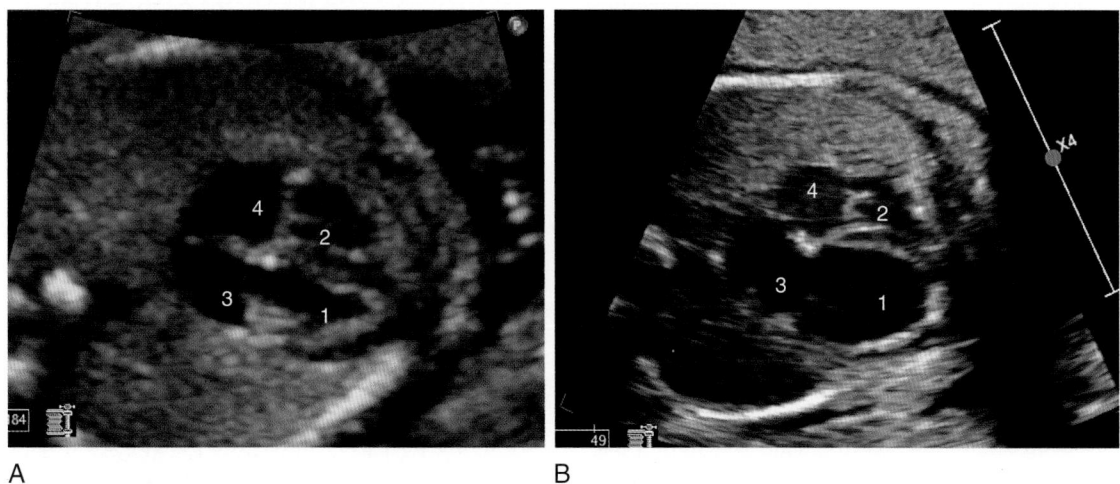

A   B

• **Fig. 16.2** **(A)** 22 weeks' gestation age (GA). Mild aortic stenosis. **(B)** 25 weeks' GA. Worsening aortic stenosis. *1*, Left ventricle; *2*, stenotic jet; *3*, aorta.

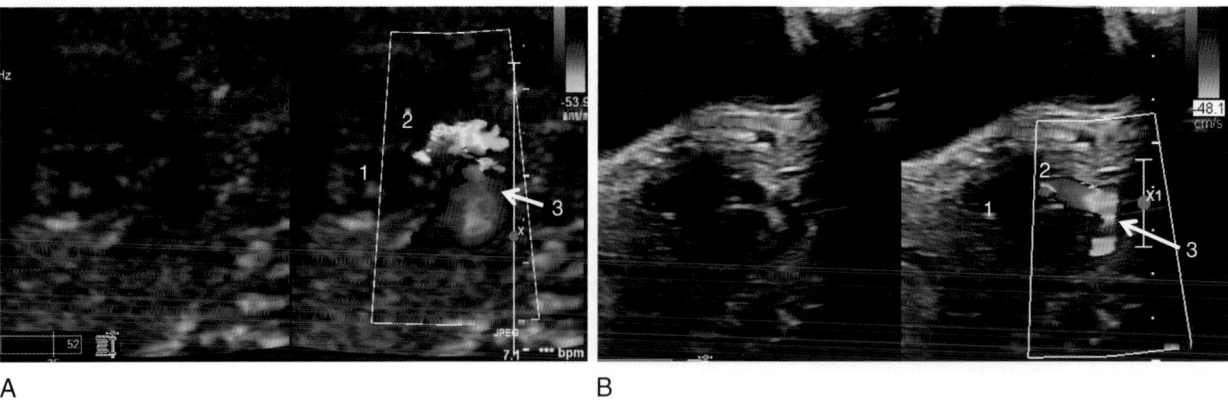

• **Fig. 16.3 (A)** Antegrade arch flow. Aortic arch flow changing from antegrade (22 weeks) to retrograde **(B)** retrograde arch flow (25 weeks) with worsening aortic stenosis and LV function. *1*, Left ventricle; *2*, Aortic stenosis color Doppler jet; *3*, aortic arch flow.

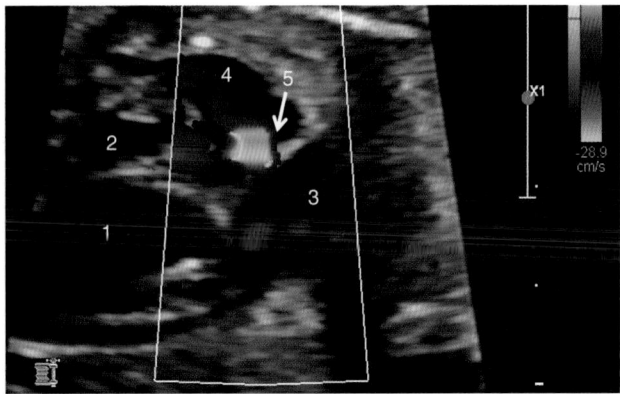

• **Fig. 16.4** Fetal aortic stenosis and LV dysfunction at 25 weeks' gestational age. Patent foramen ovale (PFO) with left-to-right flow. Reversal of the normal fetal flow pattern. *1*, Left ventricle; *2*, right ventricle; *3*, left atrium; *4*, right atrium; *5*, PFO with left-to-right flow.

In all fetal procedures, the most important patient is the healthy mother undergoing a procedure in an attempt to improve or treat a fetus with a serious anomaly. Maternal safety is the priority and mothers are screened for conditions that would preclude undergoing the procedure. Maternal contraindications for FCI include a bleeding or thrombotic disorder, rupture of membranes or premature labor, other significant medical conditions, and serious maternal congenital heart disease (CHD).

Fetal Cardiac Intervention for Aortic Stenosis: Procedure Technique

The FCI procedures are performed in the obstetric operating room. Maternal epidural is placed to relax the uterus and ensure minimal movement during the procedure. Although general anesthesia was used in the past, it is rarely used currently. If needed, the mother receives light sedation. Fetal position is assessed with US and if deemed suboptimal up to 1 hour can be spent repositioning the fetus. Once in optimal position with the LV apex pointing superior, fetal anesthesia

and paralysis are administered intramuscularly. Medications include fentanyl and pancuronium as well as atropine to counteract the vagal stimulus. For AS procedures, a 19-gauge 11.5–13.5-cm cannula with stylet is advanced under US guidance through the maternal abdominal wall, uterine wall, an intercostal space, and into the LV. The tip of the cannula is positioned in the LV outflow tract and the stylet removed. Blood return should be noted to confirm intracardiac position. A 0.014-inch guidewire with preloaded coronary artery balloon dilation catheter is inserted into the cannula and advanced out the tip. The wire is manipulated across the stenotic AOV and once position is confirmed in the ascending aorta the balloon dilation catheter is advanced over the wire and positioned across the AOV annulus (Fig. 16.5). Usually, two to three inflations are performed up to 120–130% of the measured AOV annulus size. After the last balloon deflation, all equipment is removed from the mother and color Doppler used to evaluate flow across the AOV. Technical success is considered when there is unequivocally improved color Doppler flow across the AOV.

Complications During Fetal Cardiac Intervention Procedure

The most frequent complications are bradycardia, commonly along with biventricular dysfunction and hemopericardium. Rarely, stasis or early thrombus formation is noted. Bradycardia and dysfunction are treated immediately with intracardiac epinephrine, usually with favorable and rapid response. Hemopericardium, if small, is well tolerated and usually resolves, but if moderate to large, is drained, usually with favorable response.

The procedure itself is not without risk to the fetus, with ~5% to 10% rate of pregnancy loss. The mother recovers overnight in the hospital with US and fetal echo repeated 24 hours post procedure. The patient is subsequently followed up at the referring institution and undergoes repeat fetal echoes 1 week post and approximately every month until delivery.

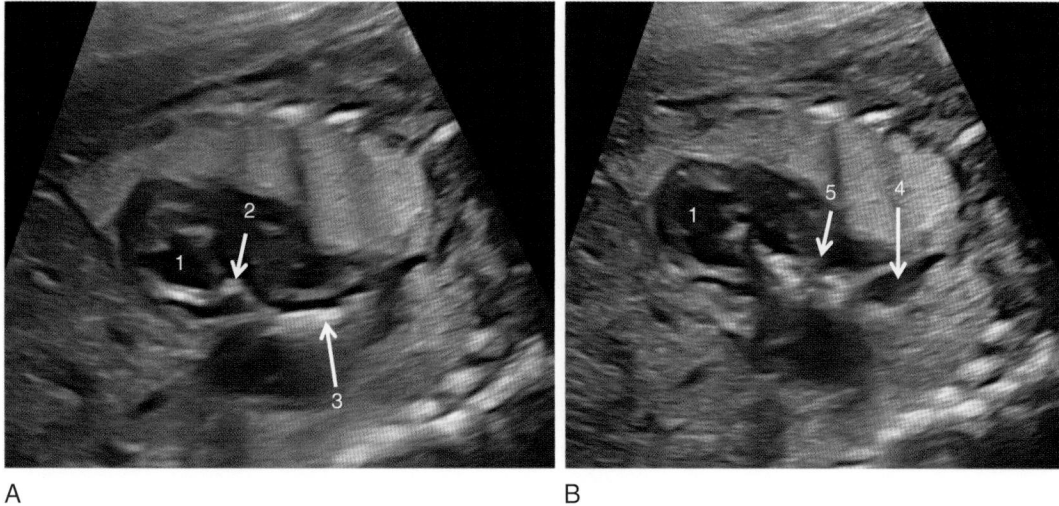

• **Fig. 16.5** **(A)** Guidewire across the aortic valve into the ascending aorta. **(B)** Balloon inflation across the aortic valve. Percutaneous, ultrasound-guided fetal aortic valvuloplasty. 25 weeks' gestational age. *1,* Left ventricle; *2,* tip of the cannula; *3,* guidewire in ascending aorta; *4,* ascending aorta; *5,* inflated balloon across the aortic valve.

The goal of FCI for AS is to prevent progression to HLHS. The most desired outcome is an unequivocal biventricular circulation after birth. Even with a biventricular circulation, most patients will require repeat balloon dilation of the AOV after birth. Some require a Ross procedure if there is significant post-neonatal valvuloplasty aortic regurgitation or a hypoplastic AOV annulus. The neonatal management and decision-making in this cohort can be complex, and there remain controversies in the management of borderline ventricles. At one end of the spectrum, the heart will unequivocally undergo a biventricular repair and at the other end HLHS. In the middle spectrum, the so-called borderline left heart, patients may undergo modified palliative surgery to promote growth of the left heart structures with a goal of an eventual biventricular repair if deemed appropriate. The postnatal management is the subject of ongoing innovation and research.[11-13]

Hypoplastic Left Heart Syndrome With Intact or Highly Restrictive Atrial Septum

This section will focus on HLHS with IAS, our experience, and the potential for FCI. The anatomic details, treatment, and outcomes of HLHS in general are discussed elsewhere in this book. HLHS with IAS is amongst the most severe form of CHD that we manage. Without treatment, patients usually die within minutes of birth. Standard neonatal management is emergent transfer from the delivery room to the cath lab for stenting of the atrial septum. Given the need for emergent postnatal treatment, fetal therapy has validity, and if successful can preclude the need for an emergent neonatal procedure. Moreover, at least in theory, decompressing the left atrium (LA)

in utero has the potential to improve lung and pulmonary vascular function. In standard risk fetal HLHS, the direction of flow at the PFO is left to right, reversed compared with the normal fetal circulation. The left heart is hypoplastic, cannot accommodate the pulmonary venous return, and consequently the pulmonary venous and left atrial flow decompresses from LA to right atrium (RA). When the atrial septum is intact, LA pressure is elevated, pulmonary veins dilated with bidirectional flow, and the lung parenchyma, lymphatics, and pulmonary arteries affected (Fig. 16.6). Damage to the lungs and pulmonary vasculature can have adverse consequences for short- and longer-term survival. Patients with HLHS with IAS have at least twice the early mortality compared to standard risk HLHS with an unrestrictive atrial septum. Fetal MRI can be used to assess the lungs with so-called "nutmeg lung"—a sign of dilated lymphatics and lung damage. Given the serious nature of CHD, the parents are given a very guarded prognosis.[14-16]

The general principles and techniques of FCI are similar for most cardiac lesions. For HLHS with IAS, the goal is to create a defect in the atrial septum to decompress blood flow from LA to RA. The initial procedures consisted of balloon dilation of the thick and fibrotic atrial septum. However, the defects tended to get smaller close to or over the rest of gestation. We subsequently changed the strategy by placing a coronary stent across the atrial septum (Fig. 16.7). If correctly positioned, the stent has potential to stay open and provide stability at birth. Access to the atrial septum can be achieved via either the RA or LA. From the RA, the cannula punctures the atrial septum and guidewire placed in a pulmonary vein. The balloon with preloaded stent is placed across the atrial septum and inflated to between 2.5 and 3 mm. Access can also be achieved via the LA with placement of the guidewire in the

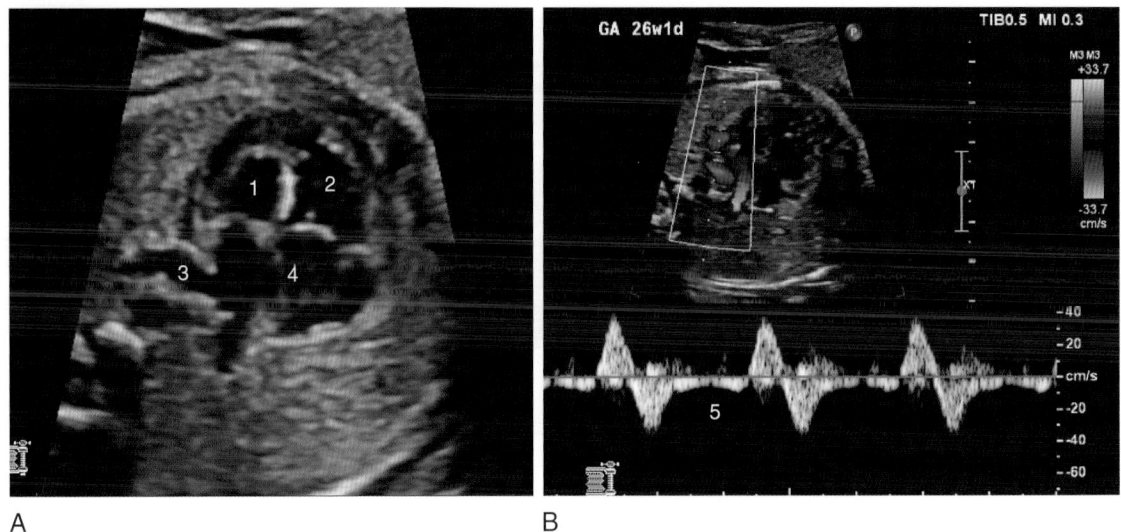

• **Fig. 16.6 (A)** Hypoplastic left heart syndrome (HLHS) with intact atrial septum (IAS). Four-chamber view demonstrating the hypoplastic left ventricle and dilated pulmonary veins. **(B)** HLHS with IAS with abnormal pulmonary venous Doppler. Pulmonary vein Doppler demonstrating bidirectional flow. *1,* Hypoplastic left ventricle; *2,* right ventricle; *3,* dilated pulmonary veins; *4,* intact atrial septum; *5,* pulmonary vein Doppler.

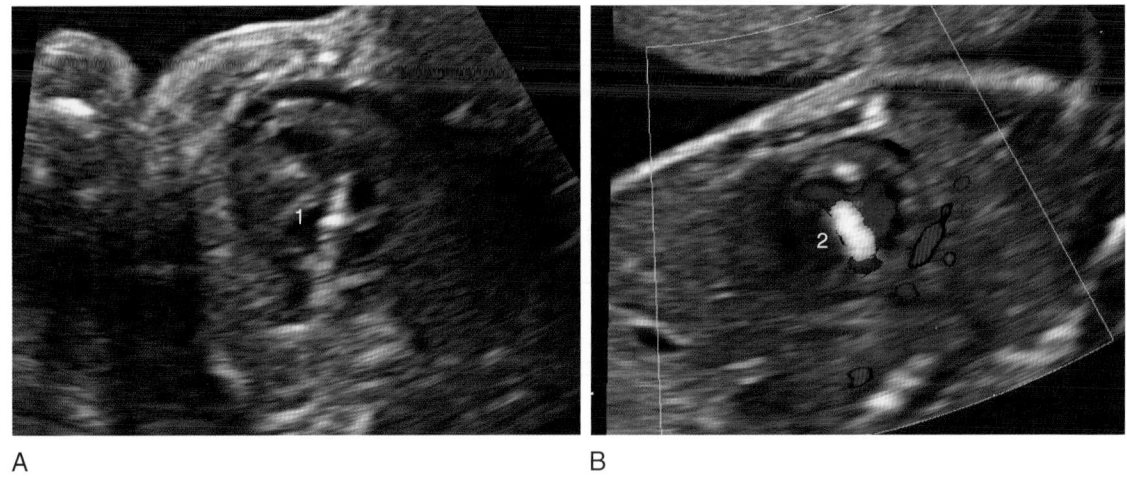

• **Fig. 16.7** Hypoplastic left heart syndrome with intact atrial septum. **(A)** Cannula across the atrial septum. **(B)** Stent across the atrial septum with color Doppler flow. *1,* Cannula across atrial septum; *2,* stent across atrial septum.

right ventricle (RV). The risk of puncturing the thin-walled RA is hemopericardium, which can be drained as described above. The left atrial wall in HLHS with IAS is usually thick and fibrotic and self-tamponaded by the surrounding lung. Once the stent is in place, all equipment is removed and patency confirmed by color Doppler. Creating a defect in the atrial septum might make the baby more stable at birth but is unlikely to remodel the pulmonary vasculature and lung parenchyma. In theory, for meaningful remodeling to occur, we would have to create a large defect early in gestation. At present, there are technical limitations to achieving this.[17-20]

The risks of FCI for HLHS with IAS are similar to other FCIs. Bradycardia is unusual when puncturing the atrium, but the risk of hemopericardium may be greater given the thin-walled RA. Much research and innovation needs to be

done to miniaturize equipment in order to improve success in younger fetuses.

Pulmonary Atresia With Intact Ventricular Septum

This section will discuss indications and contraindications for FCI for PA/IVS. The details of this cardiac defect are described elsewhere in this book.

The goal of FCI for PA/IVS is to promote sufficient RV growth to prevent the need for a palliative Fontan circulation and its long-term consequences. On fetal echo, anatomic and physiologic characteristics can predict the natural history and eventual postnatal circulation in most patients (Fig. 16.8). However, predictions in the middle range of

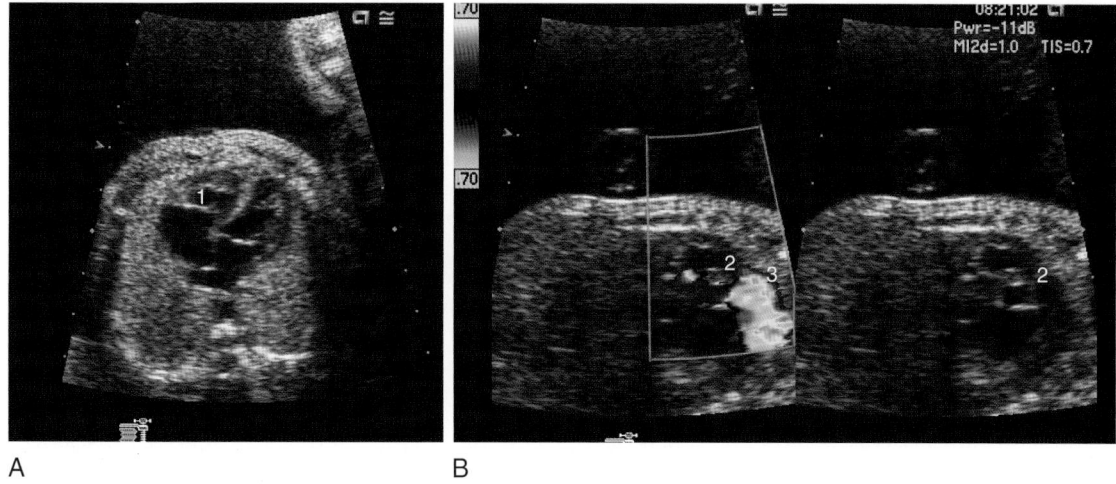

A

B

• **Fig. 16.8** Pulmonary atresia with intact ventricular septum. **(A)** Four-chamber view demonstrating a hypoplastic right ventricle. **(B)** Atretic pulmonary valve with retrograde flow in the main pulmonary artery. *1*, Right ventricle; *2*, atretic pulmonary valve; *3*, retrograde flow in the main pulmonary artery.

severity are imperfect. Moreover, the postnatal management strategy varies between institutions, a major determinant of outcome and the eventual circulation.[21,22]

All FCIs carry the risk of pregnancy loss. Therefore, FCI is not indicated in patients with good options for postnatal therapy. In PA/IVS, at the better end of the spectrum with mild to moderately hypoplastic right heart structures, postnatal therapy is usually sufficient for a good outcome. Favorable features include an identifiable plate-like pulmonary valve (PV), at most a mildly hypoplastic tricuspid valve (TV) annulus, and tricuspid regurgitation to decompress the RV. Although such patients may be the most enticing and easiest in whom to perform a FCI, they will do well with postnatal treatment, possibly staged therapy to achieve a biventricular circulation. An important predictor of eventual postnatal circulation is the TV annulus z-score. Several papers have shown that either prenatal or postnatal z-score of better than −3 can predict an eventual biventricular circulation. At the worst end of the spectrum are fetuses with PA/IVS with fibromuscular infundibular atresia and no identifiable PV. This is commonly associated with a small TV and RV. With no identifiable PV, FCI is contraindicated. In addition, such patients commonly have RV-dependent coronary circulation, precluding postnatal attempts at rehabilitating the RV. The absence of TV regurgitation and prominent color Doppler flow in the myocardium might be signs of coronary anomalies. If there is TV inflow, the blood has to decompress somewhere; in this case most likely retrograde through the myocardium to the coronary circulation. The middle group in the spectrum of severity is the target group for FCI. The hypoplastic right heart structures would predict the natural history resulting in a postnatal univentricular circulation. In order for such patients to be candidates for FCI, there needs to be an identifiable PV and unlikely to have RV-dependent coronary circulation. For above-described reasons, most patients with PA/IVS are not candidates for FCI.

Technique: Fetal Cardiac Intervention for Pulmonary Atresia With Intact Ventricular Septum

FCI for PA/IVS is technically more challenging than FCI for AS or HLHS with IAS. The RV is hypertrophied with a small cavity and complex geometry with the RV outflow tract and PV located behind the sternum. Procedures are usually performed between 22 and 30 weeks of gestational age. Maternal epidural and fetal intramuscular anesthesia are utilized as described above. Fetal positioning and optimal image quality are paramount. Access to the RV outflow tract is achieved through the RV apex or anterior RV to the left or right of the sternum. The atretic PV is perforated with the sharp tip of the cannula stylet. Once in the main pulmonary artery, the stylet is removed and the guidewire with preloaded balloon dilation catheter inserted and advanced into the pulmonary artery. The balloon is positioned across the PV annulus and inflated several times up to 150% of the annulus, after which all equipment is removed from the patient. Imaging with color Doppler will show antegrade flow as well as pulmonary regurgitation. Bradycardia and hemopericardium of the most frequently encountered complications and can be treated similar to other FCIs. Some institutions perform FCI for valvar pulmonary stenosis as well as PA/IVS with favorable anatomic features for biventricular circulation with standard postnatal therapy. Our institutional approach is to not perform FCI on this group as they have good options for postnatal therapy. Even when performing FCI for PA/IVS, it is unlikely to be the only therapeutic procedure. These patients will almost certainly require repeat balloon dilation postnatally as well as surgical enlargement of the outflow tract and RV muscle resection. The postnatal management will follow the standard algorithm for this cardiac defect regardless of whether FCI was performed. Further research is underway, including a multicenter retrospective study, to improve prenatal predictors of postnatal outcome in this cardiac defect.[23-25]

References

1. Allan LD, Sharland G, Tynan MJ. The natural history of the hypoplastic left heart syndrome. *Int J Cardiol.* 1989;25:341-343.

2. Allan LD, Maxwell DJ, Carminati M, Tynan MJ. Survival after fetal aortic balloon valvoplasty. *Ultrasound Obstet Gynecol.* 1995;5:90-91.

3. McCaffrey FM, Sherman FS. Prenatal diagnosis of severe aortic stenosis. *Pediatr Cardiol.* 1997;18:276-281.

4. Kohl T, Sharland G, Allan LD, et al. World experience of percutaneous ultrasound-guided balloon valvuloplasty in human fetuses with severe aortic valve obstruction. *Am J Cardiol.* 2000; 85:1230-1233.

5. Tworetzky W, Wilkins-Haug L, Jennings RW, et al. Balloon dilation of severe aortic stenosis in the fetus: potential for prevention of hypoplastic left heart syndrome: candidate selection, technique, and results of successful intervention. *Circulation.* 2004; 110:2125-2131.

6. Mäkikallio K, McElhinney DB, Levine JC, et al. Fetal aortic valve stenosis and the evolution of hypoplastic left heart syndrome: patient selection for fetal intervention. *Circulation.* 2006;113:1401-1405.

7. McElhinney DB, Marshall AC, Wilkins-Haug LE, et al. Predictors of technical success and postnatal biventricular outcome after in utero aortic valvuloplasty for aortic stenosis with evolving hypoplastic left heart syndrome. *Circulation.* 2009;120:1482-1490.

8. Friedman KG, Schidlow D, Freud L, Escobar-Diaz M, Tworetzky W. Left ventricular diastolic function and characteristics in fetal aortic stenosis. *Am J Cardiol.* 2014;114:122-127.

9. Freud LR, Moon-Grady A, Escobar-Diaz MC, et al. Low rate of prenatal diagnosis among neonates with critical aortic stenosis: insight into the natural history in utero. *Ultrasound Obstet Gynecol.* 2015;45:326-332.

10. McElhinney DB, Vogel M, Benson CB, et al. Assessment of left ventricular endocardial fibroelastosis in fetuses with aortic stenosis and evolving hypoplastic left heart syndrome. *Am J Cardiol.* 2010;106:1792-1797.

11. Friedman KG, Sleeper LA, Freud LR, et al. Improved technical success, postnatal outcome and refined predictors of outcome for fetal aortic valvuloplasty. *Ultrasound Obstet Gynecol.* 2018;52: 212-220.

12. Freud LR, McElhinney DB, Marshall AC, et al. Fetal aortic valvuloplasty for evolving hypoplastic left heart syndrome: postnatal outcomes of the first 100 patients. *Circulation.* 2014;130: 638-645.

13. Beattie MJ, Friedman KG, Sleeper LA, et al. Late gestation predictors of a postnatal biventricular circulation after fetal aortic valvuloplasty. *Prenat Diagn.* 2021;41:479-485.

14. Rychik J, Rome JJ, Collins MH, DeCampli WM, Spray TL. The hypoplastic left heart syndrome with intact atrial septum: atrial morphology, pulmonary vascular histopathology and outcome. *J Am Coll Cardiol.* 1999;34:554-560.

15. Vlahos AP, Lock JE, McElhinney DB, van der Velde ME. Hypoplastic left heart syndrome with intact or highly restrictive atrial septum: outcome after neonatal transcatheter atrial septostomy. *Circulation.* 2004;109:2326-2330.

16. Chintala K, Tian Z, Du W, Donaghue D, Rychik J. Fetal pulmonary venous Doppler patterns in hypoplastic left heart syndrome: relationship to atrial septal restriction. *Heart.* 2008;94:1446-1449.

17. Marshall AC, Levine J, Morash D, et al. Results of in utero atrial septoplasty in fetuses with hypoplastic left heart syndrome. *Prenat Diagn.* 2008;28:1023-1028.

18. Chaturvedi RR, Ryan G, Seed M, van Arsdell G, Jaeggi ET. Fetal stenting of the atrial septum: technique and initial results in cardiac lesions with left atrial hypertension. *Int J Cardiol.* 2013;168:2029-2036.

19. Kalish BT, Tworetzky W, Benson CB, et al. Technical challenges of atrial septal stent placement in fetuses with hypoplastic left heart syndrome and intact atrial septum. *Catheter Cardiovasc Interv.* 2014;84:77-85.

20. Mackesy MM, Kalish BT, Tworetzky W, et al. Sonographic pulmonary abnormalities in fetuses with hypoplastic left heart syndrome and intact atrial septum undergoing attempted atrial septostomy in utero. *Ultrasound Q.* 2017;33:82-85.

21. Salvin JW, McElhinney DB, Colan SD, et al. Fetal tricuspid valve size and growth as predictors of outcome in pulmonary atresia with intact ventricular septum. *Pediatrics.* 2006;118:e415-e420.

22. Gardiner HM, Belmar C, Tulzer G, et al. Morphologic and functional predictors of eventual circulation in the fetus with pulmonary atresia or critical pulmonary stenosis with intact septum. *J Am Coll Cardiol.* 2008;51:1299-1308.

23. Tworetzky W, McElhinney DB, Marx GR, et al. In utero valvuloplasty for pulmonary atresia with hypoplastic right ventricle: techniques and outcomes. *Pediatrics.* 2009;124:e510-e518.

24. Tulzer A, Arzt W, Gitter R, et al. Immediate effects and outcome of in-utero pulmonary valvuloplasty in fetuses with pulmonary atresia with intact ventricular septum or critical pulmonary stenosis. *Ultrasound Obstet Gynecol.* 2018;52:230-237.

25. Hogan WJ, Grinenco S, Armstrong A, et al. Fetal cardiac intervention for pulmonary atresia with intact ventricular septum: International Fetal Cardiac Intervention Registry. *Fetal Diagn Ther.* 2020;7:1-9.

Electrophysiology

17

Cardiac Arrhythmias and Antiarrhythmic Drugs

EDWARD P. WALSH AND MARK E. ALEXANDER

KEY LEARNING POINTS

- There are three potential mechanisms for tachycardia: (1) reentry, (2) abnormal focal automaticity, and (3) triggered activity.
- Proper treatment of tachycardia requires an understanding of the underlying mechanism and site of origin. This information can be determined with reasonable accuracy by systematic analysis of the standard electrocardiogram.

- Tachycardia with a wide QRS in the acute setting should be managed as ventricular tachycardia unless proven otherwise.
- Chronic treatment options (medications, catheter ablation, pacemakers, implantable defibrillators) need to be chosen carefully after consultation with an electrophysiologist.
- Safe use of antiarrhythmic drugs requires clear knowledge of their potential side effects, including negative inotropy and proarrhythmia.

This chapter is intended as a practical overview of the diagnosis and treatment of cardiac arrhythmias in young patients. Although the subject has occupied entire textbooks,[1] the purpose here is to focus on select material that would be most beneficial to trainees and clinicians working in an acute care setting. Accordingly, emphasis has been placed on the electrocardiogram (ECG) as the principle tool for diagnosis, with pharmacology as the mainstay of acute therapy. More advanced therapies, such as catheter ablation and pacemakers, will be covered as separate topics in subsequent chapters. Readers who are inexperienced or tentative with ECG interpretation and basic cellular electrophysiology may wish to review Chapter 8 before proceeding with discussion of rhythm disorders.

Pathophysiology of Arrhythmias

Arrhythmias may result from disorders of impulse generation (too fast or too slow), disorders of impulse conduction (reentry or block), or any combination thereof. These abnormalities are best understood by first examining their underlying mechanisms.

Mechanisms for Premature Beats and Tachycardias

Normally, by virtue of its rapid spontaneous depolarization, the sinoatrial (SA) node can claim priority as the natural pacemaker of the heart. Premature beats and tachycardias may preempt SA node activity due to either reentry, abnormal automaticity, or triggered activity.[2]

Reentry

By far the most common mechanism for tachycardia is the phenomenon of reentry. Reentry implies that a single impulse can propagate through cardiac tissue and return to reactivate the same tissue from whence it came (Fig. 17.1). Because cardiac cells require a refractory period after initial depolarization, the returning wavefront cannot simply walk backwards in its old footsteps. There must be a second pathway in the circuit, and the excitation wavefront must be sufficiently delayed at some point in the circuit to allow recovery of the original tissue (limb A). An additional requirement is that the return limb (limb B) be protected against the initial depolarization, which is to say there must be unidirectional antegrade block of the original impulse in limb B so that it will not be refractory to retrograde conduction. When all three conditions (dual pathways, conduction delay, and unidirectional block) are satisfied, single echo beats or a sustained reentrant arrhythmia can follow. Reentry will terminate promptly whenever conduction in one limb is sufficiently modified or interrupted, using techniques such as vagal stimulation, medications, overdrive pacing, electrical cardioversion, or catheter ablation.

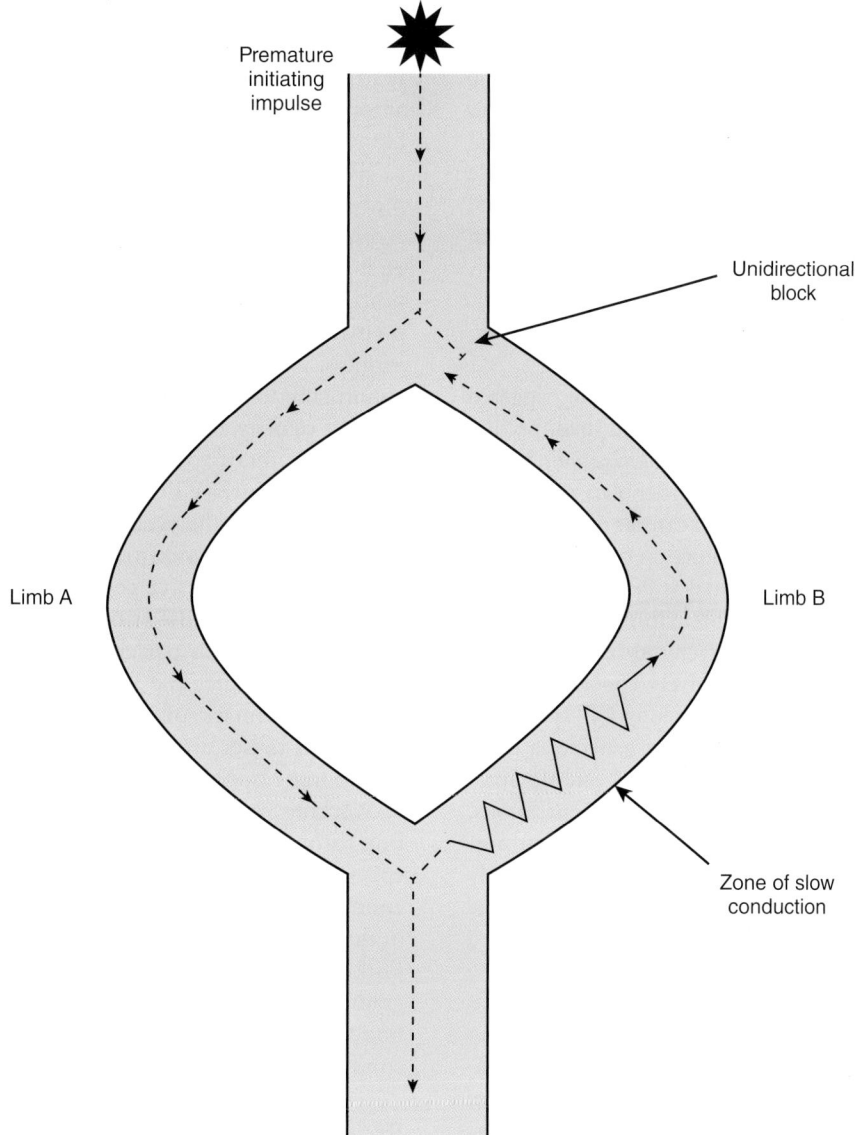

Premature
initiating
impulse

Unidirectional
block

Limb A

Limb B

Zone of slow
conduction

• **Fig. 17.1** The three classic requirements for reentry: (1) dual pathways, (2) unidirectional antegrade block in limb B, and (3) an area of slow conduction (wavy line in limb B) that allows time for limb A to recover from initial depolarization. The zone of slow conduction can be located anywhere along the circuit.

A classic example of reentry occurs in the *Wolff-Parkinson-White (WPW) syndrome*, which utilizes the atrioventricular (AV) node and an accessory pathway (AP) as the two limbs of the circuit. Reentry also appears to be the operative mechanism for atrial flutter (reentry within atrial muscle), atrial fibrillation (multiple shifting atrial reentry circuits), AV node reentry (via dual pathways within the AV node), and certain forms of ventricular tachycardia (VT; reentry within the ventricular muscle).

The general clinical features of reentry include: (1) ability to initiate and terminate tachycardia with appropriately timed premature beats, (2) abrupt *paroxysmal* onset and termination, (3) minimal rate variation during an episode, (4) fairly predictable pharmacologic response, (5) successful conversion with direct current (DC) shock, and (6) elimina-

tion with strategic ablation of one limb of the circuit. Such characteristics can be used to assign a mechanism of reentry to a clinical arrhythmia with a high degree of certainty.

Abnormal Focal Automaticity

Enhanced automaticity of a focus outside the SA node can result from any change in cell membrane conditions that promotes early achievement of threshold potential (Fig. 17.2 online). A single abnormal discharge can generate an isolated ectopic beat, while repetitive discharge can create salvos of automatic tachycardia. Abnormal focal automaticity has been implicated as the mechanism for several arrhythmias in children, including ectopic atrial tachycardia (EAT), junctional ectopic tachycardia (JET), and some VTs. Clinical characteristics that suggest such a mechanism include: (1) inability to initiate or terminate the arrhythmia with pacing maneuvers, (2) resistance to DC cardioversion, (3) wide variation in rate proportional to sympathetic tone with *warm-up* at initiation and *cool-down* at termination, (4) unpredictable pharmacologic response, and (5) a focal disorder that can be mapped and eliminated with a single well-positioned ablation lesion at the epicenter of electrical activation. These characteristics stand in sharp contrast with the behavior of reentrant tachycardia, and are easily distinguished in the clinical setting.

Triggered Activity

A third possible mechanism is the phenomenon of triggered activity. The electrical triggers in this case are small oscillations in cellular voltage known as *afterdepolarizations*, which can occur during phase 3 (*early* afterdepolarizations) or phase 4 (*late* afterdepolarizations) of a cardiac action potential (Fig. 17.3 online). If the oscillations are sufficiently high in amplitude, the threshold potential is exceeded and the cell will be triggered to generate a premature beat or, if the oscillations are repetitive, salvos of tachycardia. Early afterdepolarizations serve to initiate relatively chaotic types of tachycardia (e.g., torsades de pointes in long QT syndrome [LQTS]), while the delayed type typically generate a more organized focal disorder (e.g., some cases of ectopic atrial tachycardia [EAT] or VT). In experimental preparations, hypokalemia, high levels of catecholamines, drugs that prolong the QT interval, and hypoxic injury can produce early afterdepolarizations. Toxic levels of cardiac glycosides, acute hyponatremia, and catecholamines can produce the delayed type.

Efforts to define clinical features of triggered tachycardias in the intact heart can be frustrating because there is overlap with characteristics of both reentry and abnormal automaticity. Features in common with reentry include the ability to initiate and terminate tachycardia with pacing maneuvers and termination with DC shock. Features in common with abnormal automaticity include variation in rate (with warm-up and cool-down) and focal origin. Microelectrode studies of human atrial and ventricular tissue have convincingly demonstrated early and late afterdepolarizations *in vitro*, and it is quite certain that triggered activity is operative in clinical rhythm disorders such as LQTS and some focal tachycardias. However, at present, there is no clinical recording tool that can positively confirm afterdepolarizations in the intact heart, and one can only infer the mechanism based upon gross clinical behavior.

Mechanisms for Bradycardia and Block

Slow heart rates result from depressed depolarization in natural pacemaker cells and/or block of electrical activation. When SA node automaticity is impaired, one of several latent pacemaker sites in the atrium or AV conducting tissue normally assumes responsibility for generating cardiac rhythm. The escape rate depends on the level of the new pacemaker; foci located in more distal portions of the

conducting system have very slow spontaneous depolarization and, hence, generate slower rates. Latent pacemakers (particularly those below the AV node) also lack the rich autonomic influence found at the SA node and exhibit a blunted chronotropic response to exertion and stress.

Block may occur at any stage of the cardiac excitation process. This includes *exit block* (Fig. 17.4 online) and *entrance block* at a pacemaker focus, or *conduction block* of an established depolarization wavefront at various levels of the heart. Block is a physiologic event if an initiating impulse is premature and arrives at a cardiac site during normal refractoriness, whereas pathologic block occurs in the setting of abnormally long refractory periods, abnormally slow conduction velocity, or complete electrical discontinuity.

There is merit to a scheme that correlates patterns of block on the surface ECG with the specific type of cardiac cells involved in the event. Generally, slow-response cells of the AV node demonstrate a characteristic sequence of gradual and progressive conduction delay in response to increasingly premature stimuli, culminating in block of a single impulse. This pattern is known as *decremental conduction* and creates the familiar Wenckebach periodicity that is a hallmark of conduction delay within the AV node. It is rather unusual to observe this same phenomenon in fast-response cells of the His Purkinje system, APs, or working myocardium. With few exceptions, conduction through these areas tends to be all-or-none, such that episodic block is an unheralded event. This creates the contrast between conduction disturbances due to disease in the AV node (Mobitz I block) versus disease in the His-Purkinje system (Mobitz II block). The former shows gradual lengthening of the PR interval before a blocked impulse, whereas the latter shows only an abrupt nonconducted beat (Fig. 17.5).

Premature Beats

Premature beats are common in the pediatric age group, with atrial ectopy predominating in infants or young children, and ventricular ectopy during adolescence. Although isolated premature beats are generally benign, they may serve as markers of more serious underlying pathology, or as the initiating impulses for reentry tachycardias in susceptible individuals.

Atrial Premature Beats

Atrial ectopy appears on the ECG as an early P wave with an axis and morphology differing from the normal sinus P wave. Atrial premature beats (APBs) are usually followed by a normal QRS (Fig. 17.6A), but when sufficiently early, can conduct with QRS aberration (Fig. 17.6B) or block at the AV node (Fig. 17.6C). If the patient is completely asymptomatic and the physical examination is otherwise normal, occasional APBs are most always benign and do not necessarily warrant further investigation. However, in any child with symptoms of dizziness or sustained palpitations, APBs

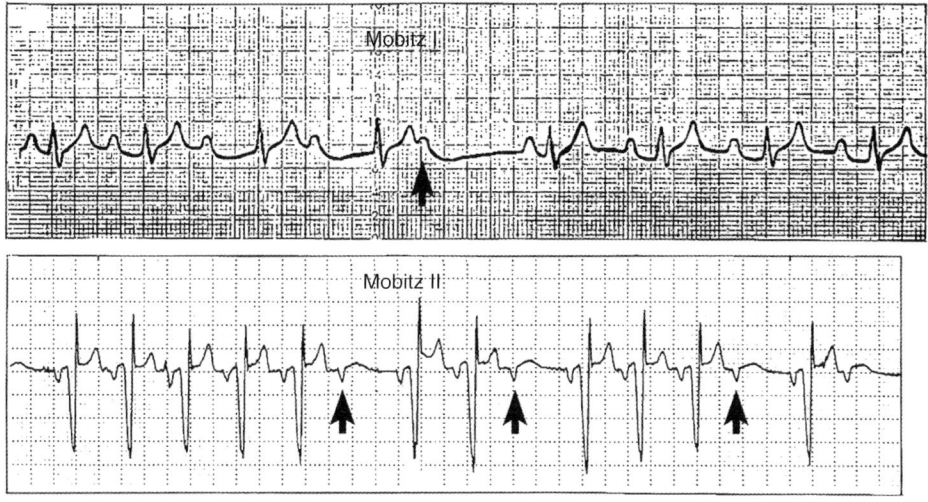

• **Fig. 17.5** Comparison of second-degree atrioventricular (AV) block in the slow-response cells of the AV node (Mobitz I) and the fast-response cells of the His Purkinje system (Mobitz II).

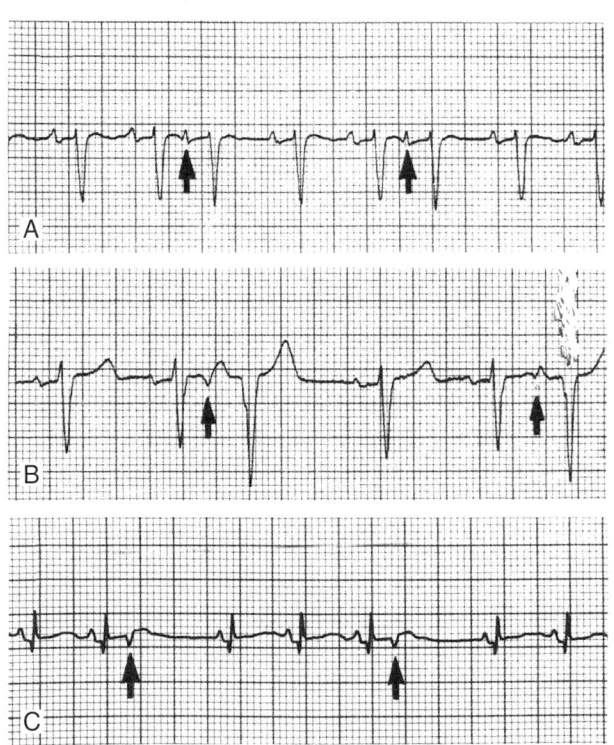

• **Fig. 17.6** Atrial premature beats *(arrows)* causing: **(A)** normal QRS, **(B)** conduction with aberration, and **(C)** block.

could be a manifestation of an underlying reentry circuit or automatic focus with the potential for supraventricular tachycardia (SVT). Surveillance testing with ambulatory monitoring may be indicated for such patients. In asymptomatic individuals, the diagnostic evaluation is expanded only if the beats are very frequent and/or seem to arise from multiple foci (i.e., variable morphologies for the P wave), in which case hyperthyroidism, structural heart disease, and cardiomyopathy may need to be considered as possible causes.

Junctional Premature Beats (JPBs)

Single ectopic beats arising from the AV node or proximal His-Purkinje system are rather rare. The ECG reveals an early normal QRS but no preceding P wave (Fig. 17.7 online). Prognostic and diagnostic considerations are generally similar to those for APBs. Occasionally, junctional premature beats (JPBs) can affect AV conduction if their timing coincides with a normal atrial depolarization. Collision of the premature beat with a normal atrial impulse can mimic abrupt AV block by the mechanism of *concealed conduction* and, thus, JPBs may be considered in the differential diagnosis of some atypical AV conduction abnormalities.

Ventricular Premature Beats

Ventricular ectopy is characterized by an early beat with a wide and abnormal QRS complex without a preceding P wave (Fig. 17.8 online). The T-wave axis is typically directed opposite to the QRS. Ventricular ectopy can usually be distinguished from aberrant APBs by the absence of a premature P wave and the presence of a fully *compensatory pause* (Fig. 17.9).

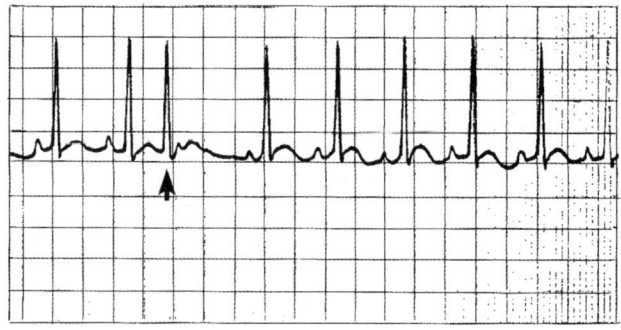

• **Fig. 17.7** Junctional premature beat. Note that the early QRS is identical to a sinus beat but is not preceded by a P wave.

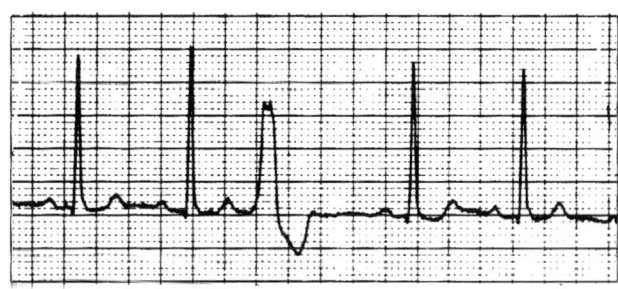

• **Fig. 17.8** Ventricular premature beat showing distortion of the QRS and inverted T wave.

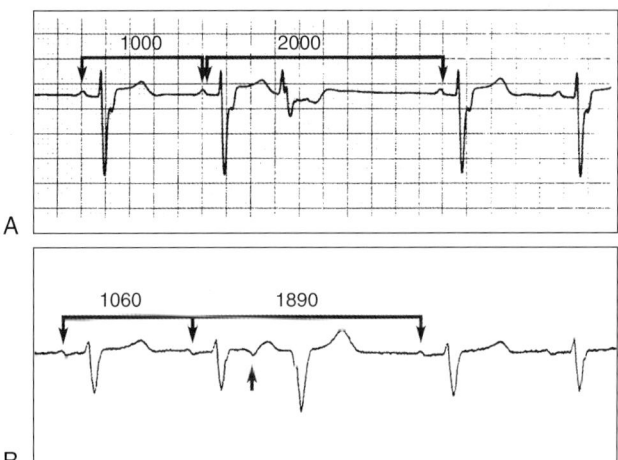

• **Fig. 17.9** Comparison of a ventricular premature beat **(A)** and an atrial premature beat with aberration **(B)**. Note that the pause following ventricular ectopy is typically "compensatory" (i.e., the interval between P waves for the sinus beats flanking the ectopic beat is exactly twice that for sinus rhythm). The pause following atrial ectopy is "noncompensatory," and the premature P wave *(arrow)* can be seen.

Ventricular premature beats (VPBs) are rather common in pediatric patients with ostensibly normal hearts, especially after puberty, and clinical follow-up of such patients has revealed a generally benign prognosis. Unfortunately, ventricular ectopy on a routine ECG cannot always be dismissed out of hand since it may be a manifestation of more serious underlying arrhythmias. For this reason, most patients with VPBs should undergo ambulatory monitoring. The appearance of very frequent and/or higher-grade ectopy may indicate the need for an expanded diagnostic evaluation, including an echocardiogram to rule out myopathy. Some reports suggest that suppression of VPBs with exercise testing indicates a benign condition, although this is not universally true and cannot be relied upon for risk stratification.

Asymptomatic patients with occasional isolated VPBs and normal hearts do not require treatment. The management of patients with frequent and/or high-grade ventricular ectopy will be discussed later in this chapter.

Tachycardias

The key to effective management of a tachycardia is accurate identification of the underlying mechanism. This must be understood in terms of both site of origin as well as the electrophysiologic generator (reentry vs. automaticity vs. triggered activity).

Terminology

The terms *SVT* and *VT* are practical starting points for describing a tachycardia, but they are sorely lacking in specificity. The label SVT is a broad category that includes any rapid rhythm arising from the atrium, the AV junction, or involving an AP, whereas VT refers to any disorder confined to cardiac sites below the bifurcation of the His bundle. Because SVT and VT convey so little mechanistic information, they are too imprecise for directing complex therapeutic decisions. A more meaningful nomenclature involves a classification as depicted in Table 17.1. The list is long, but it underscores the diverse nature of clinical tachycardias, each of which requires a fairly unique approach to therapy. From among these diverse mechanisms, it is necessary to narrow the differential diagnosis to only one or two choices at the bedside in order to plan therapy and organize further diagnostic testing. Systematic review of the standard ECG is usually sufficient to accomplish this task.

The first step is to examine a full 12- or 15-lead ECG obtained during tachycardia. A single-lead rhythm strip is hopelessly inadequate for this purpose because it lacks definition of the P wave axis and details of QRS morphology. The ECG is initially scrutinized for duration and morphology of the QRS complex. If the QRS is narrow and normal appearing (i.e., identical to a conducted sinus beat in all leads), it can be assumed that the ventricles were activated over the AV node and the His-Purkinje system, a finding that effectively eliminates VT from the differential diagnosis. Similarly, if the patient is known to have preexistent bundle branch block (e.g., following surgical repair of tetralogy of Fallot) and the QRS in tachycardia is identical to baseline sinus rhythm, it is reasonably safe to dismiss VT as a concern. However, if a wide or different QRS is observed, VT must be the primary initial consideration. Although the differential diagnosis may still include SVT that is distorted by rate-related bundle branch aberration or antegrade conduction over a preexcitation pathway, bear in mind that no harm will be done treating an SVT with wide-QRS according to VT recommendations, whereas treating VT under the incorrect assumption that it is SVT with aberration can be hazardous.

Differential Diagnosis of Narrow QRS Tachycardia

The possible mechanisms for narrow QRS tachycardias are shown in Fig. 17.10. Each diagram is accompanied by a hypothetical lead II ECG that emphasizes the diagnostic clues to be found in the timing and axis of the P wave.

The first item is *sinus tachycardia*, which is the prototype automatic arrhythmia. Although not strictly pathologic, it exemplifies the behavior for an automatic focus in that it accelerates and decelerates in a gradual manner, and varies

TABLE 17.1 Clinical Tachycardias

	Reentry	Automatic Focus	Triggered Activity
SA node	—————-	Sinus tachycardia	————————
Atrium	Atrial flutter/IART Atrial fibrillation	Ectopic atrial tachycardia Multifocal/chaotic atrial tachycardia	Ectopic atrial tachycardia (some cases)
av node/junction	AV nodal reentry Twin AV node reentry (heterotaxy)	Junctional ectopic tachycardia	————————
Accessory pathway	Orthodromic reciprocating tachycardia Antidromic reciprocating tachycardia Preexcited atrial fibrillation Permanent junctional reciprocating tachycardia	————————	————————
Ventricle	Monomorphic VT LV septal/Belhassen's VT Polymorphic VT	Focal VT	Torsades de pointes Bidirectional VT Focal VT (some cases)

AV, Atrioventricular; *IART,* intra-atrial reentrant tachycardia; *SA,* sinoatrial; *VT,* ventricular tachycardia.

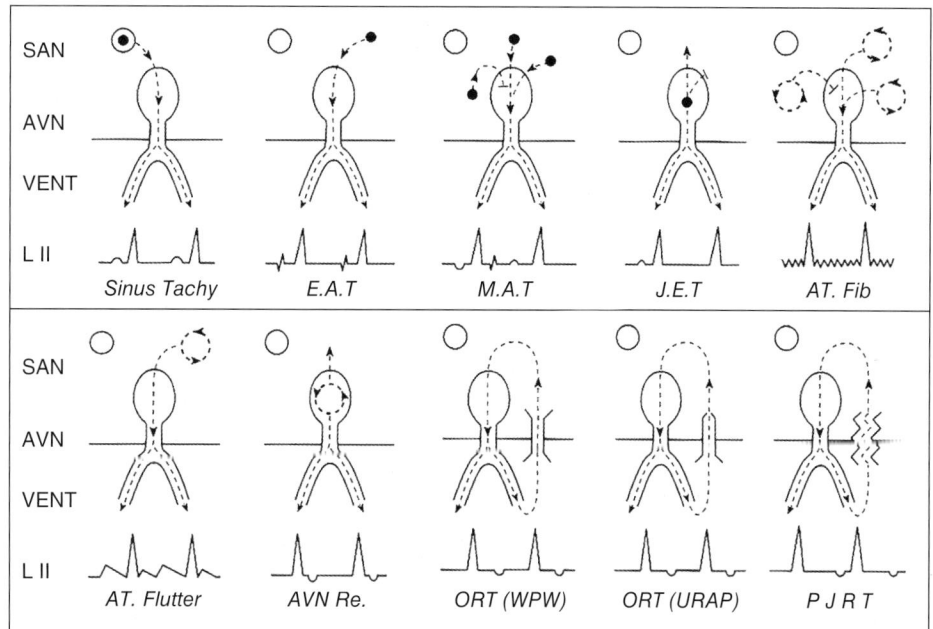

• **Fig. 17.10** Mechanisms for "narrow" QRS tachycardia. Diagrams show the sinoatrial node *(SAN)* upper left, with the atrioventricular node *(AVN)* and bundle branches crossing to the ventricle *(VENT)*. ECG lead II emphasizes the P wave timing and morphology. *AT,* Atrial; *EAT,* ectopic atrial tachycardia; *Fib,* fibrillation; *JET,* junctional ectopic tachycardia; *ORT,* orthodromic reciprocating tachycardia; *PJRT,* permanent form of junctional reciprocating tachycardia; *Tachy,* tachycardia; *URAP,* unidirectional retrograde accessory pathway; *WPW,* Wolff Parkinson White.

in rate with changes in autonomic tone. Note that P waves arising from the SA node register a normal axis of about +60 degrees (i.e., upright in lead II). Because sinus tachycardia usually occurs under conditions of high circulating catecholamines, conduction through the AV node is robust, so the A:V ratio is 1:1 and the PR interval is normal.

In *EAT,* an abnormal focus generates rapid depolarization from an atrial site outside the SA node. Several features distinguish it from sinus tachycardia. First, the P-wave axis is abnormal because of eccentric atrial depolarization.

Second, because catecholamine levels are not necessarily elevated and the mechanism does not directly involve the AV node or ventricles, episodic first- and second-degree block of AV conduction can often be observed without interruption of the atrial arrhythmia, especially during vagal stimulation or sleep. *Multifocal atrial tachycardia (MAT)* presents a similar picture, although in this instance multiple rapid P-wave morphologies are observed.

JET is a rare condition that can develop as a transient condition in young children following congenital heart surgery, but occasionally occurs as a congenital disorder. Note in Fig. 17.10 that the focus of rapid discharge is centered in the AV node or the proximal bundle of His. As with other automatic tachycardias, the rate accelerates gradually and exhibits perceptible variation over time. However, the key feature here is potential dissociation between the P and QRS, a consequence of the fact that atrial tissue is not directly linked to the arrhythmia mechanism. In some patients, there may be passive 1:1 retrograde atrial activation with a P axis of −120 degrees, while in others retrograde conduction may be variable or absent altogether. JET is the only narrow QRS tachycardia during which the ventricular rate can be faster than the atrial rate.

The automatic SVTs mentioned above are sometimes difficult to identify from a surface ECG alone, particularly when the P wave is not clearly discernable. Perhaps their most notable characteristic is refractoriness to electrical cardioversion, overdrive pacing, and conventional medications. Sometimes the diagnosis is only considered in retrospect after these remedies have been attempted unsuccessfully.

Reentry mechanisms are the more common cause of a narrow QRS tachycardia. Reentry within atrial muscle produces two familiar clinical arrhythmias: a single atrial reentry circuit referred to as *atrial flutter or IART*, and multiple small reentry circuits referred to as *atrial fibrillation*. Atrial fibrillation is readily recognized on the ECG, but flutter/IART is sometimes more difficult. The atrial rate during flutter/IART (classically 300 beats/min) may vary widely from patient to patient. Atrial rates as fast as 400/min may be seen in infants, and rates as slow as 120/min may occur in older patients after surgery for congenital heart defects. The hallmark sawtooth pattern in leads II, III, and aVF may also be difficult to demonstrate at times, particularly during 1:1 AV conduction of slower IART rates, or during 2:1 conduction when every other P wave is buried under a QRS. Careful ECG monitoring during vagal maneuvers or adenosine administration to transiently slow AV conduction can uncover hidden P waves.

The remaining reentrant circuits for narrow QRS tachycardia include reentry within the AV node, and those tachycardias that reciprocate between the atrium and ventricle via an AP. In these conditions, a 1:1 ratio is maintained between the atrium and ventricle, and SVT will terminate immediately when this ratio is disturbed. The atria are depolarized in the retrograde direction to produce a P wave axis of approximately −80 to −120 degrees. These tachycardias start abruptly, operate at fixed and regular rates, and react to vagal stimulation with either minimal change or abrupt termination. The timing of the retrograde P wave can be used as a marker to differentiate the disorders. In classic *AV node reentry*, retrograde atrial activation occurs nearly simultaneously with ventricular activation, so the P wave and QRS tend to be superimposed or at least very close in timing. This is reflected in a *ventriculoatrial (VA) interval* less than 70 msec on ECG. By comparison, the circuit in reciprocating tachycardias involving an AP must traverse a physically longer path so that the P wave occurs 70 msec or more after the QRS complex.

Further differentiation among these AV reciprocating circuits is possible by examining the ECG after tachycardia has been terminated. For AV node reentry, the ECG is normal between episodes. For a bidirectional accessory connection (i.e., *WPW syndrome*), the diagnosis is made by observing the delta wave and short PR interval after sinus rhythm is restored. *Concealed APs*, which only operate as unidirectional retrograde connections, are harder to diagnose because the ECG in sinus rhythm is completely normal. Differentiation between AV node and concealed pathway reentry may require electrophysiologic study for final resolution. However, one variety of concealed pathway (the *permanent form of junctional reciprocating tachycardia [PJRT]*) can usually be diagnosed with certainty. As the name implies, this form of SVT is very difficult to terminate for more than a few beats and exhibits a dramatically long VA interval during the tachycardia.

Differential Diagnosis of Wide QRS Tachycardias

A wide QRS tachycardia should be managed as VT until proven otherwise. Often, the surface ECG offers no reliable features to eliminate VT from consideration, and proof may come only from invasive electrophysiologic testing. Likewise, patient age and prior medical status should never persuade one to assume that a wide QRS rhythm is a relatively benign SVT. Although rare in the pediatric population, VT may occur at any age, even in previously healthy children.

The possible mechanisms and ECG features of wide QRS tachycardias in pediatric patients are diagrammed in Fig. 17.11. One of the most valuable diagnostic observations on ECG is the presence of *VA dissociation* between the rapid QRS and a slower P wave. If the ventricles are seen to beat independently of the atrium, the differential diagnosis is effectively limited to VT. One of the potential consequences of VA dissociation is the finding of *fusion beats*, caused by intermittent penetration of the slower atrial impulses. Always remember that the absence of VA dissociation does not rule out VT, since there can be passive retrograde 1:1 atrial depolarization over the normal AV node.

After restoration of sinus rhythm, the ECG provides additional diagnostic clues. If the patient is noted to have permanent bundle branch block at rest that is identical to the QRS in tachycardia, it is a safe assumption that the primary arrhythmia was SVT. Similarly, if a WPW pattern is seen, the pathway was likely to have participated in the tachycardia. The most difficult differential diagnosis involves the choice between VT and SVT with rate-related QRS aberration. In children with SVT, aberration may involve either the right or left bundle branch, often making the ECG indistinguishable at first glance from that of VT.

A flow chart highlighting the diagnostic ECG features for the various tachycardias is provided in Fig. 17.12. Note that the degree of diagnostic resolution from the ECG is much less exact for wide QRS compared with narrow QRS

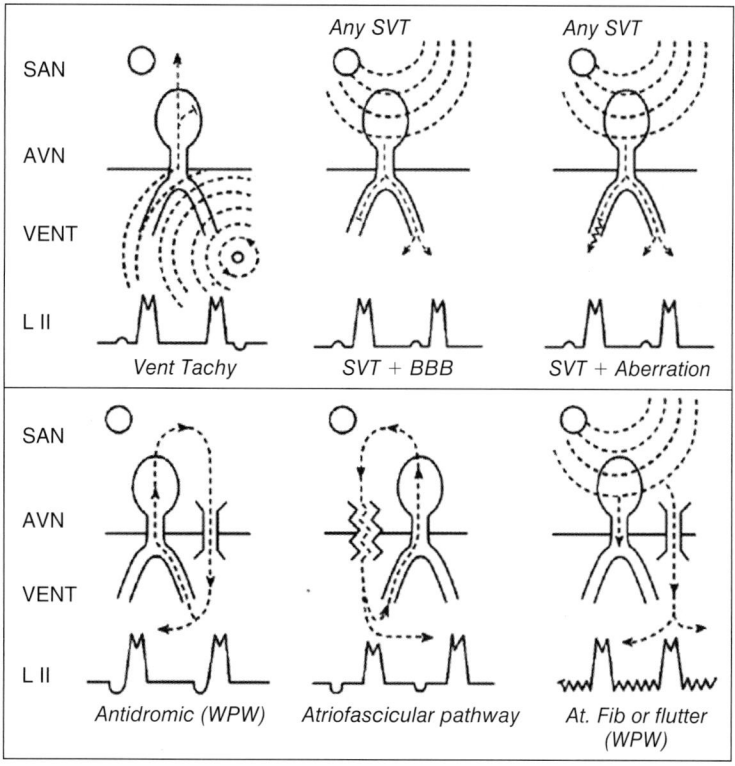

• **Fig. 17.11** Possible mechanisms for "wide" QRS tachycardia.

Differential diagnosis of tachycardia

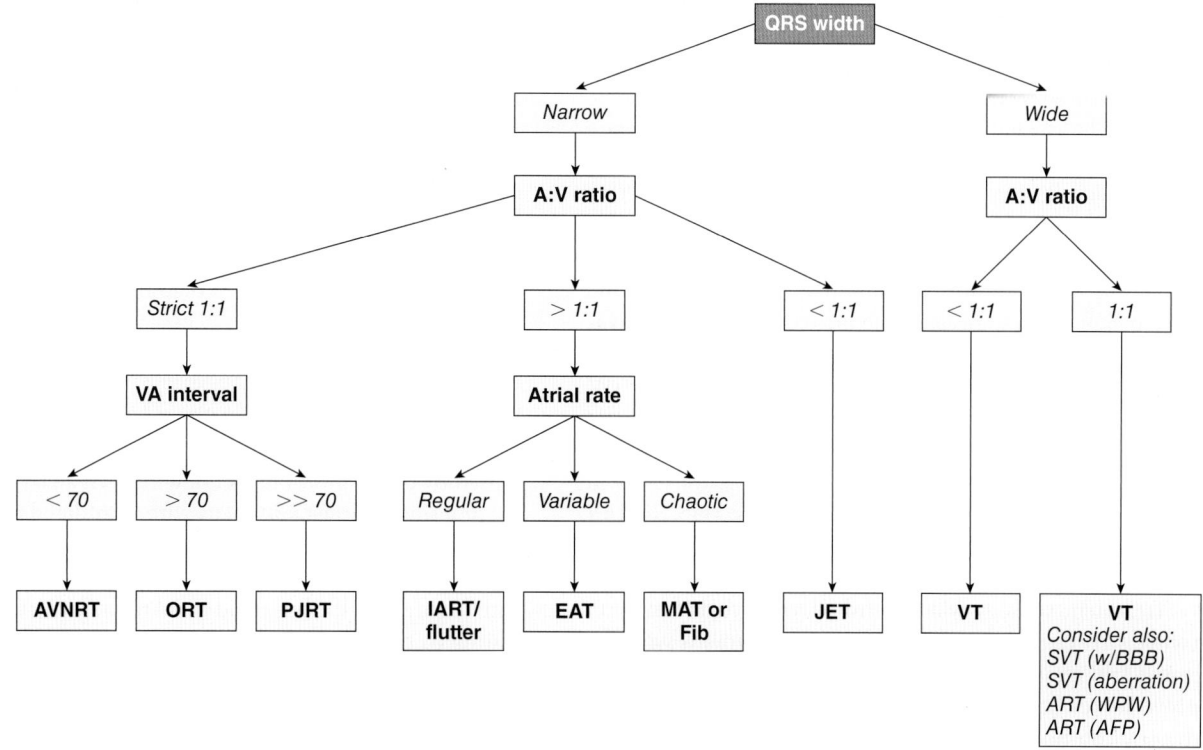

• **Fig. 17.12** Practical scheme for determining the most likely mechanism for a clinical tachycardia based on ECG features.

tachycardias. A formal electrophysiologic study may be needed whenever uncertainty exists.

Management of Supraventricular Tachycardia

The preceding section was meant to serve as a road map for identification of a tachycardia mechanism at the bedside. Treatment strategy is dependent upon an understanding of the pathophysiology of each disorder. The SVTs will be discussed below in the following order: (1) automatic SVTs, (2) atrial muscle reentry, (3) AV nodal reentry, and (4) AP-mediated tachycardias.

Ectopic Atrial Tachycardia

EAT results from enhanced automaticity of a single non-sinus atrial focus. It accounts for less than 10% of SVT cases but is difficult to treat. This arrhythmia can have a variable presentation, ranging from sporadic episodes that produce only mild symptoms of palpitations and dizziness, all the way to incessant tachycardia with congestive heart failure from *tachycardia induced myopathy*. Indeed, it is important not to overlook the possibility of EAT or confuse it with sinus tachycardia when a patient presents with newly diagnosed cardiomyopathy, since this type of ventricular dysfunction can be reversed completely by correcting the rhythm. EAT can occur at any age. When it is seen in infants and young children, there is a reasonable likelihood that it could resolve spontaneously after a few months or years, but if it is seen much beyond age 4 years, it is more likely to be a chronic condition. It may also be seen as a transient disorder following cardiac surgery. The precise etiology of EAT is uncertain.

On ECG, the hallmark of the arrhythmia is an atrial rate that is inappropriately rapid for age and physiologic state, but varies on both a beat-to-beat and a long-term basis to a degree that excludes a reentrant mechanism. The P wave morphology differs from sinus rhythm and depends on the site of the automatic focus, which may be anywhere in the right or left atrium. Because the arrhythmia mechanism is confined to atrial tissue, the ventricular response rate and the PR interval are determined independently by the AV node. First- and second-degree AV block as well as episodic bundle branch aberrancy are common findings (Fig. 17.13). At electrophysiologic study, earliest atrial activation will map to a point distant from the sinus node (Fig. 17.14). This tachycardia cannot be terminated with pacing or DC cardioversion.

Treatment strategy will depend on ventricular function, tachycardia rate, and the patient's age. For patients with depressed function and rapid conduction, symptoms may improve somewhat by lowering the ventricular rate, so acute therapy can initially be directed towards slowing AV nodal conduction with a beta-blocker or calcium channel blocker (assuming hemodynamics are stable enough to tolerate

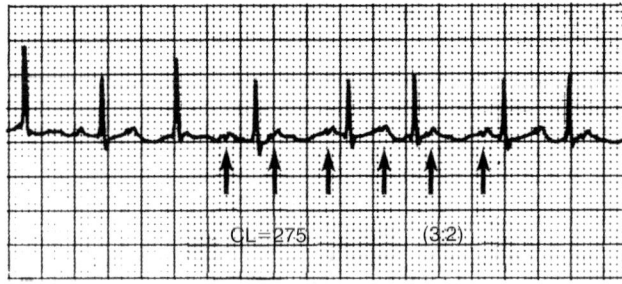
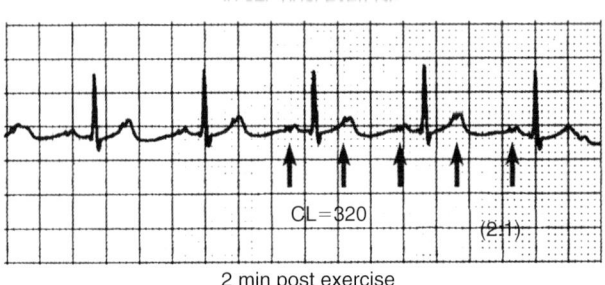

• **Fig. 17.13** Lead II recording from a patient with ectopic atrial tachycardia. The upper strip was obtained after exercise and shows rapid atrial depolarization *(arrows)* at a cycle length *(CL)* of 275 msec, which conducts with a 3:2 ratio. During rest (lower strip), both the atrial rate and A:V ratio are slower.

these agents). Calcium channel blockers rarely have any direct effect on the ectopic focus, although beta-blockers are sometimes effective in slowing the atrial focus in this disorder and may be the only necessary therapy for some patients. Sotalol, amiodarone, phenytoin, ivabradine, and flecainide can be effective in difficult case, but an empiric trial is necessary for each agent.

Aggressive efforts at pharmacologic control are usually made in younger children since the condition could eventually resolve. In older children, medical management with a simple agent like beta-blocker is usually attempted, but if EAT persists despite conservative drug therapy, and/or the patient has evidence of tachycardia-induced myopathy, catheter ablation has now become the most widely accepted therapy.[3] EAT in postoperative patients can usually be controlled medically and tends to be transient.

Multifocal Atrial Tachycardia

MAT (also referred to as *chaotic atrial rhythm*) is a rare disorder encountered mostly in infants that appears to be caused by either multiple foci of enhanced atrial automaticity, or a single ultra-rapid focus with disordered conduction through atrial muscle (so-called *fibrillatory conduction*). The surface ECG demonstrates multiple P wave morphologies with highly variable but rapid atrial rates, sometimes degenerating to patterns indistinguishable from atrial fibrillation. The QRS is usually narrow, but episodic rate-related bundle branch block is common (Fig. 17.15).

Although its exact cause is unknown, MAT is most commonly seen as an idiopathic disorder during infancy[4] that can gradually resolve over the first year or two of life. Very

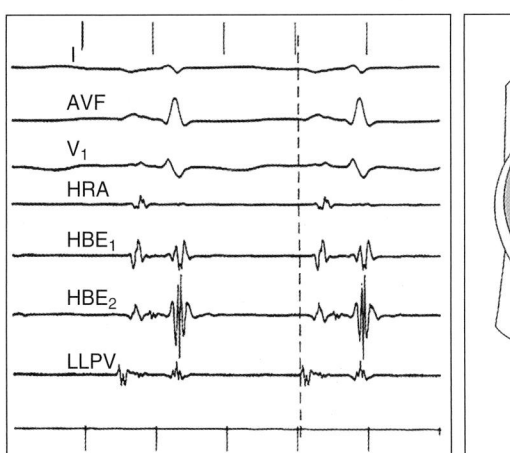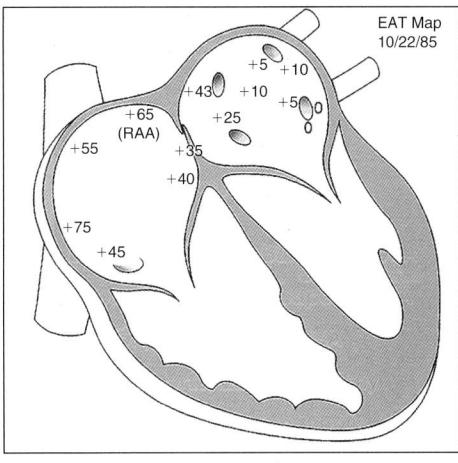

• **Fig. 17.14** Intracardiac mapping of an ectopic atrial focus in the area of the left lower pulmonary vein *(LLPV)*. *EAT*, Ectopic atrial tachycardia; *HBE*, his bundle electrogram; *HRA*, high right atrium; *LLPV*, left lower pulmonary vein.

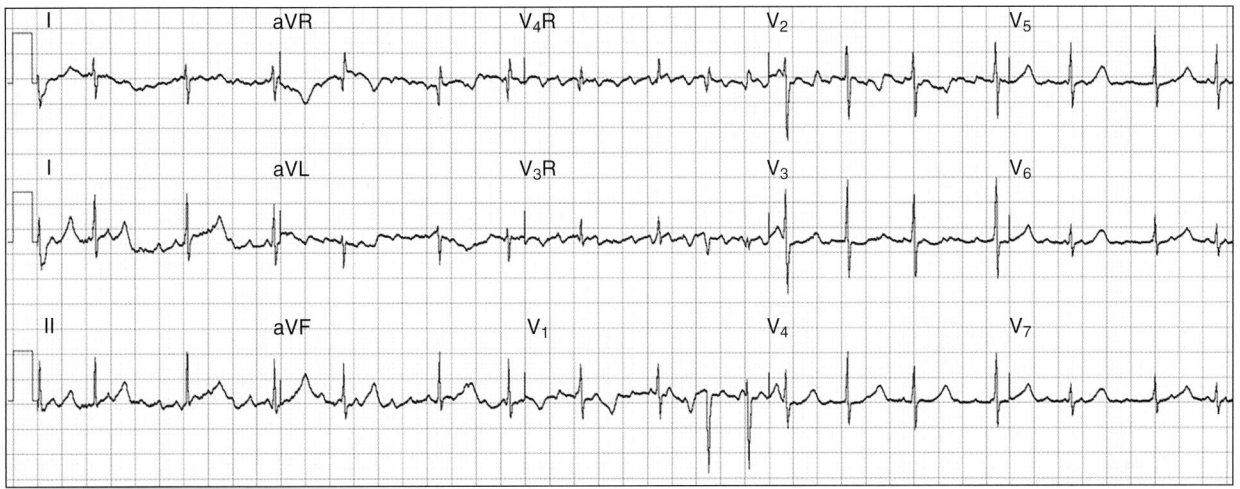

• **Fig. 17.15** Rapid atrial rates and multiple P wave morphologies in an infant with multifocal atrial tachycardia.

rarely it may occur as a transient disorder in the immediate postoperative period after congenital heart surgery.

Treatment is difficult. Beta-blocker may improve the situation to some extent by decreasing the ventricular rate, which may be a reasonable end-point for patients with minimal compromise from the arrhythmia. Partial or complete restoration of sinus rhythm usually requires more potent agents such as sotalol, amiodarone, or flecainide, or some combination of medications. Instances of sudden death have been reported in some infants with MAT and poor rate control, so all cases must be treated aggressively and followed carefully.

Junctional Ectopic Tachycardia

JET likewise appears to be caused by enhanced automaticity, but in this case the focus is within the AV node or the proximal bundle of His. It should not be confused with the normal junctional escape rhythm that may be seen in the setting of sinus node dysfunction or AV block. At times,

junctional rates are only mildly accelerated and are of little hemodynamic significance, but rapid rates (170–300/min) are poorly tolerated (Fig. 17.16).

JET may occur as a congenital disorder with a definite familial tendency,[5] but more commonly is seen as a transient arrhythmia immediately following cardiac surgery for congenital heart defects in very young patients.[6] The postoperative form can cause severe hemodynamic compromise, even when the surgical repair is technically excellent. Prior to the recognition of effective therapies for rapid postoperative JET, the mortality rate was quite high. The congenital form of JET is rare, but it may likewise be associated with serious morbidity and mortality.

The ECG pattern is distinctive. JET is the only form of SVT characterized by AV dissociation with a ventricular rate greater than the atrial rate. True AV block is uncommon, as demonstrated by occasional atrial capture beats when sinus P waves are appropriately timed and by the ability to reestablish AV synchrony by atrial pacing at a rate faster than the rate of the JET focus.

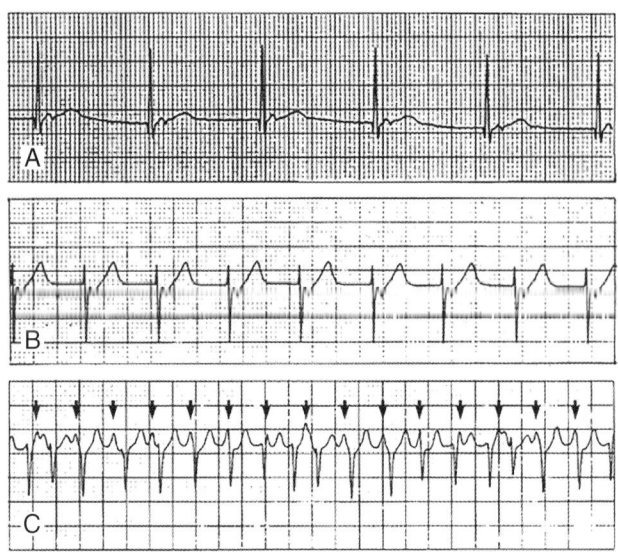

• **Fig. 17.16** The spectrum of junctional rhythm. **(A)** Slow junctional escape rhythm in a patient with sinus node dysfunction at 62 beats/min. **(B)** Mildly accelerated junctional rhythm in a stable postoperative patient of 100 beats/min. **(C)** Rapid junctional ectopic tachycardia at 200 beats/min. Note slower P waves *(arrows)* and instances of "early" QRS due to occasional conduction of atrial depolarization.

For rapid postoperative JET, acute improvement in hemodynamics is best accomplished by both reestablishing AV synchrony and lowering the junctional rate. Synchrony with simple atrial pacing above the JET rate may sometimes be sufficient therapy to stabilize a postoperative patient, but if junctional rates are very rapid, concomitant therapy to directly slow junctional automaticity is necessary. The use of induced hypothermia to 34°C is often effective for this purpose, and for refractory JET the addition of procainamide during hypothermia will slow JET to physiologic rates in most all cases. Intravenous amiodarone has also been reported as effective, as have dexmedetomidine and ivabradine in small series. Postoperative JET will typically resolve completely within 24–48 hours.

The congenital form of JET is a chronic disorder that is capable of causing tachycardia-induced myopathy. Amiodarone is one of the few drugs shown to be broadly effective, though there is growing case material to suggest ivabradine might also be a reasonable option. Catheter ablation of the JET focus with preservation of normal AV conduction is possible in select cases of congenital JET.

Atrial Flutter/Intra-Atrial Reentrant Tachycardia

Atrial flutter involves a single macroreentrant circuit that is usually confined to right atrial tissue. The classic form involves a circuit around the atrial border of the tricuspid valve. It produces the familiar sawtooth flutter wave pattern in ECG leads II, III, and aVF at atrial rates close to 300 beats/min. Atypical atrial circuits are more likely to develop in young patients with atrial scarring from repaired congenital heart disease, and can involve a variety of P wave

appearances with slower atrial rates.[7] To avoid confusion, it has become customary to refer to all forms of a solitary atrial muscle reentry circuit under the umbrella term of *IART.* The essential approach to treatment is identical for all varieties of IART.

The clinical presentation is largely dependent on the ventricular response rate and underlying myocardial function. In the majority of cases, the A:V ratio is > 1, resulting in ventricular rates of 90–160 beats/min, which can be tolerated in the short run. Such patients may complain of palpitations with exertion, weakness, and some shortness of breath, but are usually stable at presentation. Unfortunately, some young patients will experience 1:1 AV conduction, which can lead to far more serious symptoms, including cardiovascular collapse and death. And, regardless of ventricular response rate, patients with long-standing IART can develop atrial thrombi with associated embolic risks.[8] This is clearly a concerning rhythm disorder.

The atrial rate is strictly regular during IART. Sometimes it may be difficult to diagnose on the surface ECG during 2:1 conduction due to superimposition of alternate P waves on the QRS complex (Fig. 17.17). In such cases, the clinical diagnosis can often be made by observing cannon waves in neck veins or on an atrial pressure waveform, or by transiently increasing the degree of AV block with vagal maneuvers or adenosine. If still uncertain, electrogram recording from an esophageal lead (Fig. 17.18 online), an atrial pacing lead, or intracardiac atrial electrode will provide definitive data.

Assuming thromboembolic risks have been dismissed or addressed (as discussed below for atrial fibrillation), a synchronized DC cardioversion under appropriate sedation with relatively low energy (0.25–1.0 J/kg) is almost always successful in terminating IART. Alternatively, if the patient has an atrial pacemaker or an esophageal lead in place, overdrive burst pacing can be performed which will successfully interrupt the atrial reentrant circuit in the majority of patients. If DC shock or overdrive pacing are felt to be impracticable for whatever reason, pharmacologic therapy may be attempted. Digoxin, beta-blocker, or calcium channel blocker can be used to acutely reduce the ventricular response rate in patients with rapid AV conduction, although these agents do not convert IART directly to sinus rhythm. More potent drugs (procainamide, amiodarone, flecainide,

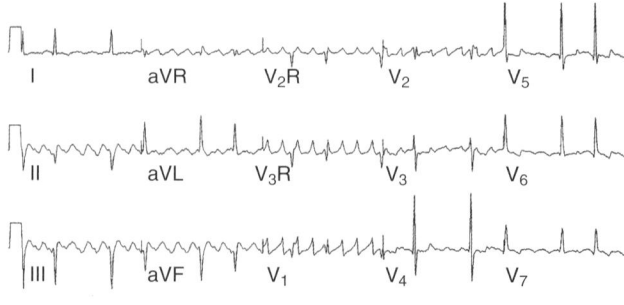

• **Fig. 17.17** Surface ECG showing intra-atrial reentrant tachycardia. Note sawtooth baseline in leads II, III, aVF, and the right chest leads. The ventricular response rate varies from 2:1 to 4:1.

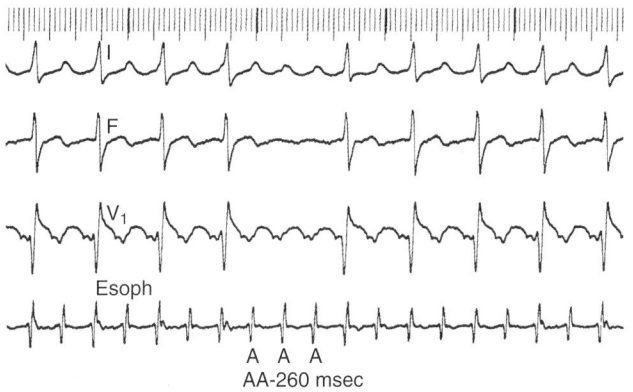

• **Fig. 17.18** Esophageal recording of intra-atrial reentrant tachycardia. The ECG leads display the typical sawtooth baseline when atrioventricular conduction slows in the middle of the recording, but the rhythm could easily be mistaken for sinus tachycardia when conduction is 2:1. The esophageal recording provides unequivocal confirmation of the abnormal atrial rhythm during 2:1 conduction.

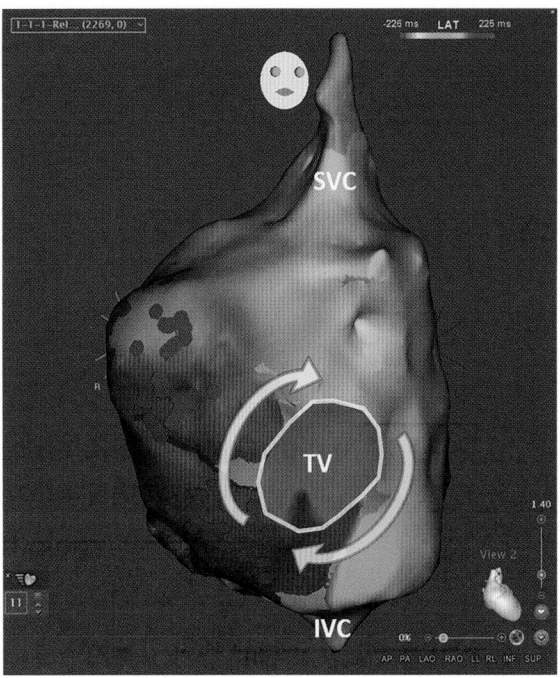

• **Fig. 17.19** Mapping during catheter ablation for intra-atrial reentrant tachycardia in a teenager who has undergone tetralogy repair. The dilated right atrium is shown with locations marked for the tricuspid valve *(TV)* and superior *(SVC)* and inferior vena cava *(IVC)*. Gray dots on the lateral wall indicate areas of scar (likely atriotomy incision). The colors denote atrial activation times (red > green > purple), indicating a circuit propagating clockwise around the TV. An ablation line between the TV and IVC (the so-called cavo-tricuspid isthmus) eliminated this circuit.

and sotalol) can influence atrial conduction properties enough that IART will terminate, although in many cases the atrial rate will merely slow, and cardioversion or overdrive pacing might still be required.

IART in children with normal hearts is exceedingly rare. It can be seen occasionally in a fetus as an idiopathic disorder, sometimes resulting in rapid ventricular rates and hydrops. Transplacental drug therapy with sotalol administered carefully to the mother will sometimes restore sinus rhythm in this setting. Fetal IART rarely recurs following correction after delivery. Far more commonly, problematic IART is seen as a late complication following surgery for congenital heart disease, especially after the Mustard, Senning, and Fontan operations. Thus, long-term management decisions will be influenced not only by IART itself but also by hemodynamic status, the condition of the SA and AV nodes, and whether or not there are concomitant ventricular arrhythmias requiring treatment. Assuming initial symptoms were not too severe, it is often satisfactory to just maintain patients on an AV node blocking drug following conversion of their first episode of IART, which will help prevent a rapid ventricular response should the arrhythmia recur. If IART becomes a recurrent issue, management decisions become more complicated, and consultation with a cardiac electrophysiologist is recommended. The options available include catheter ablation (Fig. 17.19 online), chronic drug therapy with potent agents (e.g., sotalol, amiodarone, flecainide), placement of an atrial antitachycardia pacemaker, or (if the patient is returning to the operating room for other reasons) arrhythmia surgery. None of these can be considered a perfect solution, and all have risks. Final choices for chronic therapy should be made carefully on a case-by-case basis in consultation with an electrophysiologist.

Atrial Fibrillation

Atrial fibrillation is thought to arise from multiple small migratory reentry circuits occurring predominately within the left atrium. Though extremely common in elderly patients, atrial fibrillation is rare in children, possibly because of an atrial size that is inadequate to support multiple circuits. The typical clinical settings for atrial fibrillation in the pediatric age group include congenital heart defects (primarily those involving the mitral and aortic valves), rheumatic heart disease, cardiomyopathy (especially the restrictive type), failing single ventricle circulation, and WPW syndrome. Atrial fibrillation may also be caused by hyperthyroidism in rare cases, and even though the yield is low, this possibility should be investigated in any new patient without obvious underlying heart disease. Occasional teenagers may present with "lone" atrial fibrillation and an otherwise negative evaluation, which may relate to a cryptic underlying SVT involving a different mechanism (e.g., episodic EAT) that triggers the fibrillation as a secondary phenomenon. Finally, there are cases of familial atrial fibrillation where recurrent episodes can begin in teenage years, likely involving some subtle form of channelopathy.

Patients with atrial fibrillation usually experience palpitations, but syncope due to a rapid ventricular response is rare in the absence of WPW syndrome. Those with compromised ventricular function and particularly slow or fast ventricular response rates may experience weakness or congestive heart failure in addition to palpitations.

The ECG reveals low amplitude irregular atrial activity (Fig. 17.20) that at times may be difficult to differentiate

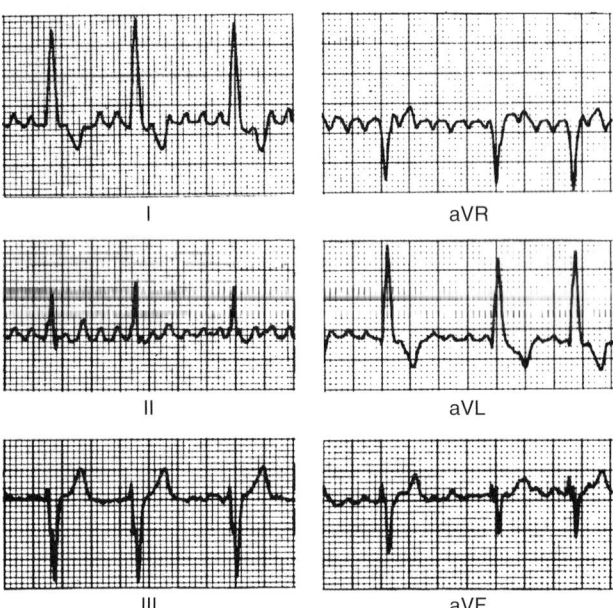

• **Fig. 17.20** Atrial fibrillation that developed in a patient with tricuspid atresia. The ventricular response rate is about 90 beats/min.

from artifact or rapid IART. The ventricular response is highly variable (irregularly irregular) due to chaotic timing of atrial impulses. Intermittent QRS aberration after a long-short conduction interval (*Ashman's phenomenon*) can also be seen (Fig. 17.21).

If the duration of atrial fibrillation is less than about 48 hours, the likelihood of atrial thrombi is minimal, so undivided attention can be directed towards correcting the rhythm. If initial rate control is required, drugs such as beta-blocker or calcium channel blocker can be used (assuming WPW is not present). Atrial fibrillation can then be terminated reliably with DC cardioversion under appropriate sedation, starting with energies of 1–2 J/kg. Alternatively, pharmacologic conversion can be attempted with intravenous agents such as procainamide or amiodarone, or rapid oral loading with sotalol or flecainide.

If the arrhythmia duration is greater than 48 hours or uncertain, the risk of atrial thrombi will cloud all treatment decisions.[8] For a patient with minimal symptoms, it is usually wise to postpone conversion for a minimum of 3 weeks while controlling the rate with an AV node blocking drug and providing anticoagulation with warfarin or another oral agent. At the end of this anticoagulation phase, sinus

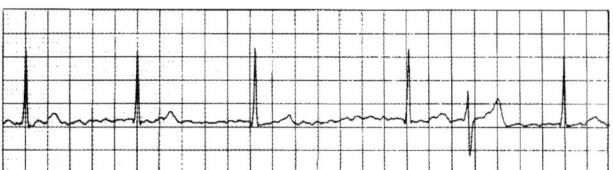

• **Fig. 17.21** Ashman's phenomenon in a patient with atrial fibrillation. There is a relative pause between the third and fourth QRS, followed by closer spacing between the fourth and fifth QRS (which is aberrant). Ashman's aberration typically occurs after such "long-short" intervals.

rhythm can be restored by any of the aforementioned techniques. If, on the other hand, the patient has serious symptoms at presentation, the luxury of prolonged pre-conversion anticoagulation may not be available. If no clots are visible on a careful transesophageal echo, conversion can be performed with reasonably low embolic risk. Following conversion, current guidelines call for continued anticoagulation for 4 weeks after restoration of sinus rhythm. Identical precautions against thromboembolic events are applicable to patients with IART of long or uncertain duration.

Therapy to prevent recurrent atrial fibrillation is similar to that for IART and may be difficult at times. Effective catheter ablation for atrial fibrillation involving isolation of the pulmonary veins from the rest of the left atrium is possible, although it is a somewhat involved procedure with certain risks and frequent need for a second procedure that must all be weighed carefully in the decision process.[9]

Atrioventricular Nodal Reentrant Tachycardia

The reentrant circuit in atrioventricular nodal reentrant tachycardia (AVNRT) involves two discrete conduction pathways within an otherwise normal AV node. One of these, known as the *fast pathway*, conducts with a normal PR interval but has a relatively long refractory period. If a premature atrial beat arrives at the AV node while the fast pathway is still refractory, conduction shifts to the alternate *slow pathway* which has a shorter refractory period and can therefore conduct the impulse, although it does so with a long PR interval. To some extent this is normal physiology, and 30% or more of the general population will demonstrate this so-called *dual AV nodal pathway physiology*. However, when conduction velocity and refractoriness of the two pathways are balanced in just the proper fashion, a reentrant tachycardia can result. The anatomic correlates for the two pathways appear to be small extensions off the compact AV node, with the fast pathway running superior, and the slow pathway inferior and directed towards the tricuspid valve ring. Functional evidence of dual AV nodal physiology is sometimes apparent on a routine ECG as a sudden change in the PR interval, but more often needs to be demonstrated using atrial premature stimuli during electrophysiologic testing (Fig. 17.22). In order for a tachycardia episode to develop in this condition, an appropriately timed premature beat must shift conduction to the slow pathway so the impulse can return to the atrium retrograde via the fast pathway, thereby setting up a *slow-fast* reentry tachycardia. The reverse circuit (*fast-slow* reentry) is also possible but far less common.

AVNRT rarely occurs in infants. It is probable that the electrophysiologic substrate of dual pathways is present from birth, but is simply unmasked with age as both autonomic influences and the characteristics of the AV nodal tissue change with growth. By comparison, AVNRT is the most common mechanism for SVT in patients with normal hearts who first present in adolescence or young adulthood.

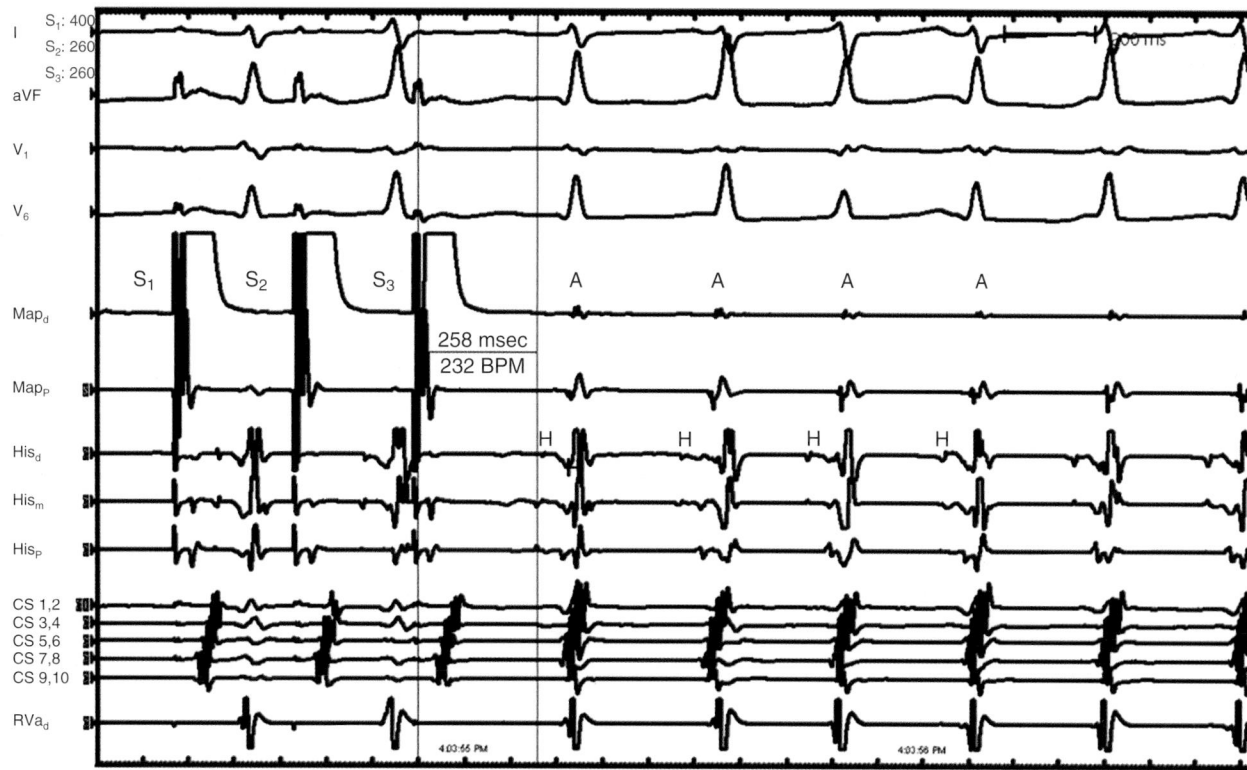

• **Fig. 17.22** Induction of atrioventricular nodal reentrant tachycardia (AVNRT) at electrophysiologic study. The atrium is stimulated with carefully timed premature beats (S1, S2, S3) until the S3 stimulus blocks in the normal fast pathway and conduction shifts to the slow AV nodal pathway, indicated by long delay of 258 msec between S3 and the His bundle deflection *(H)*. This allows retrograde return up the fast pathway setting up slow-fast AVNRT. Note that the retrograde atrial signal *(A)* occurs nearly simultaneous with QRS timing (VA interval < 70 msec).

The tachycardia rate in children with AVNRT is usually 170–230 beats/min. Severe hemodynamic compromise is rare with AVNRT, but feelings of anxiety, chest pain, and dizziness are frequent. The ECG shows a P wave occurring nearly simultaneously with the QRS complex, and often the P wave will not be clearly discernable because of a superimposed QRS, as shown in Fig. 17.22.

In general, any maneuver that enhances vagal tone to slow AV nodal conduction (such as the Valsalva maneuver or elicitation of the diving reflex) may terminate AVNRT. If vagal maneuvers fail, pharmacologic therapy is almost universally successful for acute conversion. Short duration AV node blockade with adenosine is very effective, as is administration of a calcium channel blocker. Though rarely necessary, AVNRT will also terminate with DC cardioversion using very low energy, and can be interrupted promptly with a brief burst of rapid atrial pacing if the need arises.

Patients with infrequent episodes of AVNRT and minimal symptoms can be managed conservatively with the vagal maneuvers described above, trading a few minutes of SVT for possible risks and side effects of more aggressive treatment. On the other hand, patients who suffer from frequent bouts of symptomatic tachycardia will require either chronic medical therapy or catheter ablation. The choice between drugs and ablation depends largely upon patient age and the attitude of the family. Curative ablation, which modifies or eliminates the slow pathway without damaging the normal fast pathway, is now done on a routine basis in children older than about age 4 years, with success rates exceeding 98%. The principal risk during such a procedure is inadvertent fast pathway damage, which could result in high-grade AV block and necessitate pacemaker placement. While this risk is nearly negligible nowadays in experienced hands, particularly since the availability of cryoablation, situations may arise occasionally when chronic medical therapy is chosen. The most reasonable agents for preventing or minimizing AVNRT episodes are beta-blockers and calcium channel blockers.

Twin Atrioventricular Node Tachycardia

This rare condition is seen exclusively in patients with complex heterotaxy syndrome, especially the asplenia (right-atrial isomerism) type. It involves two separate AV nodes and His bundles,[10] usually connected by a so-called *Monckeberg sling*. The most common reentry circuit involves antegrade conduction over one node, across the sling, and retrograde return via the second node. Acute treatment is similar to conventional AVNRT. Successful catheter ablation is possible by eliminating the weaker of the two nodes.

Supraventricular Tachycardia Due To Accessory Pathways

In 1930, Wolff, Parkinson, and White described a syndrome that consisted of a short PR interval, "bundle branch block" on the surface ECG, and paroxysmal tachycardia. Although they were unaware of the electrophysiologic or anatomic basis of this disorder, their report sparked further investigation that ultimately confirmed that WPW syndrome was caused by an AP traversing the AV groove. It is now understood that APs may express themselves through a variety of electrocardiographic patterns and arrhythmias dependent on their conduction properties and location. Three types of APs are commonly recognized (Fig. 17.23):
1. *Conventional AV pathway*
    a) Classic bidirectional AP of WPW syndrome that is capable of both antegrade and retrograde conduction
    b) Unidirectional antegrade-only AP
    c) Unidirectional retrograde-only AP (so-called "concealed" AP)
    d) Extremely slow conducting concealed AP causing incessant SVT known as PJRT
2. *Atriofascicular pathway* (AFP; sometimes erroneously referred to as a Mahaim fiber) with very slow antegrade conduction, which arise near the anterolateral tricuspid valve and travel a long distance along the right ventricular free wall to connect with the right bundle branch.
3. *Fasciculoventricular fiber* (a true Mahaim fiber) running from the His bundle to the crest of the right ventricular septum.

Types 1 and 2 are capable of supporting one or more forms of SVT. Type 3 does not support tachycardia, although it can generate a subtle delta wave on ECG which can be confused with WPW syndrome. There are also extremely rare cases of abnormal connections emanating from the AV node (*nodoventricular or nodofascicular*), which can only be deciphered during formal electrophysiology study, and are well beyond the scope of this chapter.

AV pathways are by far the most common and most relevant to management of young patients. The characteristic WPW pattern on ECG during sinus rhythm is a short PR interval and a slurred initial QRS deflection known as a *delta wave*. These findings reflect the fact that conduction from the atrium to the ventricle via the accessory connection is generally faster than conduction in the AV node. Thus, some segment of the ventricle is *preexcited* by the eccentric spread of activation from the accessory connection. The degree of preexcitation depends on the relative conduction velocities of the AV node and the AP, as well as pathway location.

The axis and morphology of the delta wave can be used to estimate the site of earliest ventricular activation and hence, the location of the accessory connection. Detailed algorithms for this purpose have arisen in response to the experience and demands of catheter ablation for WPW.[11] A simplified ECG algorithm for WPW mapping is shown in Fig. 17.24.

The most common form of SVT in WPW syndrome, known as *orthodromic reciprocating tachycardia (ORT)*, uses the AV node as the antegrade limb, with the AP as the retrograde limb. This circuit generates a narrow QRS complex on ECG since the ventricles are depolarized in the normal fashion over the AV node. While less common than ORT, other forms of tachycardia can also occur in WPW syndrome, including the opposite reentry circuit using the AP as the antegrade limb and the AV node in the retrograde direction, known as *antidromic reciprocating tachycardia*

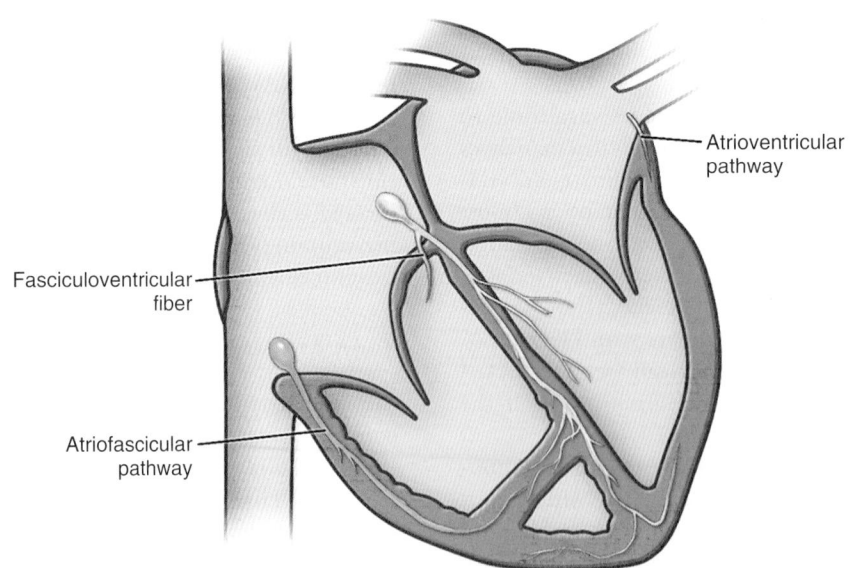

Atrioventricular
pathway

Fasciculoventricular
fiber

Atriofascicular
pathway

• **Fig. 17.23** The three most common types of abnormal electrical connections in the heart: conventional atrioventricular pathways *(purple)*, atriofascicular pathways *(green)*, and fasciculoventricular fibers *(blue)*. Normal conduction tissue is shown in *yellow*. There are several subtypes of atrioventricular pathways distinguished by their conduction characteristics (see text for details).

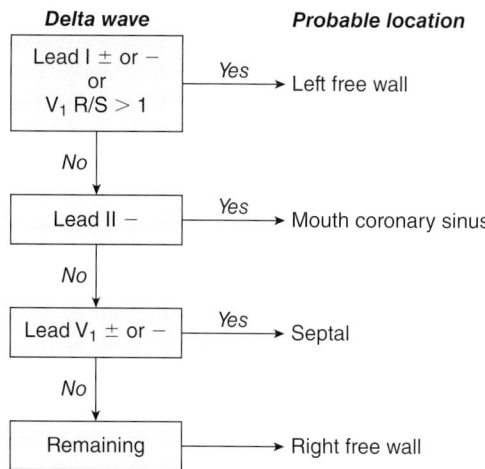

Delta wave   **Probable location**

Lead I ± or − or V₁ R/S > 1 — Yes → Left free wall

No ↓

Lead II − — Yes → Mouth coronary sinus

No ↓

Lead V₁ ± or − — Yes → Septal

No ↓

Remaining → Right free wall

• **Fig. 17.24** Simplified scheme for predicting gross location of an accessory pathway in Wolff-Parkinson-White syndrome based on the standard 12-lead ECG. The polarity of the delta wave and certain gross features of the preexcited QRS help define the approximate site for the ventricular insertion of the pathway. (see reference #11: Arruda MS, McClelland JH, Wang X, et al. Development and validation of an ECG algorithm for identifying accessory pathway ablation site in Wolff-Parkinson-White syndrome. *J Cardiovasc Electrophysiol.* 1998;9:2–12, for a more refined localization strategy.)

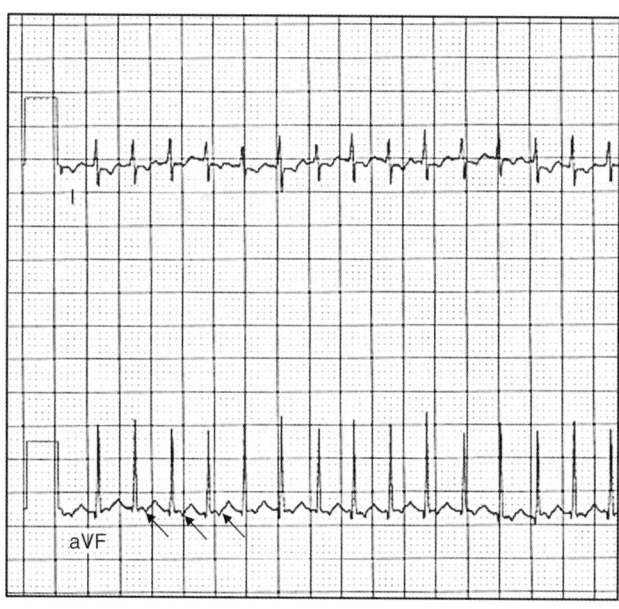

• **Fig. 17.25** Orthodromic reciprocating tachycardia in a 1-month-old showing regular narrow QRS and retrograde P wave *(arrows)* with a ventriculoatrial interval of 100 msec.

(ART). The ECG picture of ART will differ markedly from ORT since the ventricles are depolarized exclusively by the AP, resulting in a wide QRS tachycardia that can be hard to distinguish from VT at first glance. Finally, some patients with WPW may experience episodic atrial fibrillation, which is certainly the most dangerous tachycardia involving APs. During such episodes, the ventricles can be activated in the antegrade direction by both the AV node and AP. The ECG will therefore contain an irregular mixture of narrow, wide, and intermediate QRS complexes, which in some patients may conduct at rates that are rapid enough to cause degeneration into ventricular fibrillation (VF).

Concealed pathways, which conduct only in the retrograde direction and do not generate a delta wave on ECG, can participate in ORT but are incapable of supporting antidromic tachycardia or preexcited conduction of atrial fibrillation.

Orthodromic Reciprocating Tachycardia in WPW

Tachycardia due to ORT is the most common presentation for WPW in young patients. Episodes may begin as early as fetal life, but many patients will remain entirely symptomatic until adolescence or adulthood. Severe hemodynamic compromise is rare in ORT unless the duration is protracted. Common symptoms include palpitations, anxiety, chest discomfort, dizziness, and dyspnea. The most concerning scenario involves ORT in young infants who may have undetected tachycardia for hours to days, sometimes resulting in congestive heart failure and even cardiovascular collapse at presentation.

The surface ECG during ORT typically displays a narrow QRS morphology with a regular rate (Fig. 17.25). Transient rate-related left or right bundle branch block may occur, particularly at the moment of tachycardia initiation. If the bundle branch block occurs ipsilateral to the side of the AP, the tachycardia cycle length usually increases because of the added conduction time in the ventricular muscle portion of the tachycardia circuit (Fig. 17.26 online). When this finding is observed, it can assist in identifying the location of the AP as either right- or left-sided. The natural initiating events for ORT can include APBs, JPBs, or VPBs. The usual requirement for initiation is block of antegrade conduction in the AP plus enough delay in the AV node to allow the AP and atrium to be excitable when the reentrant wavefront reaches them.

During electrophysiologic study, initiation of ORT can usually be achieved with a critically timed atrial premature stimulus that blocks antegrade in the AP and encounters appropriate delay in the AV node. Thus, the atrial premature stimulus must occur at an interval shorter than the refractory period of an accessory connection. Intracardiac recordings during ORT demonstrate an A:V ratio of 1:1, and an interval from the earliest deflection of the QRS to the rapid deflection of the P wave (the VA interval) greater than 70 msec. Once ORT is confirmed, the location of the accessory connection may be mapped by identifying the site of earliest retrograde atrial activation during ORT (Fig. 17.27). Left-sided pathways can be mapped with the benefit of a multielectrode catheter in the coronary sinus, whereas right-sided and septal pathways are localized during point-by-point mapping along the edge of the tricuspid valve. Further discussion of AP mapping will follow in Chapter 18.

Because the AV node is the antegrade limb of the tachycardia circuit in ORT, the therapeutic maneuvers used for

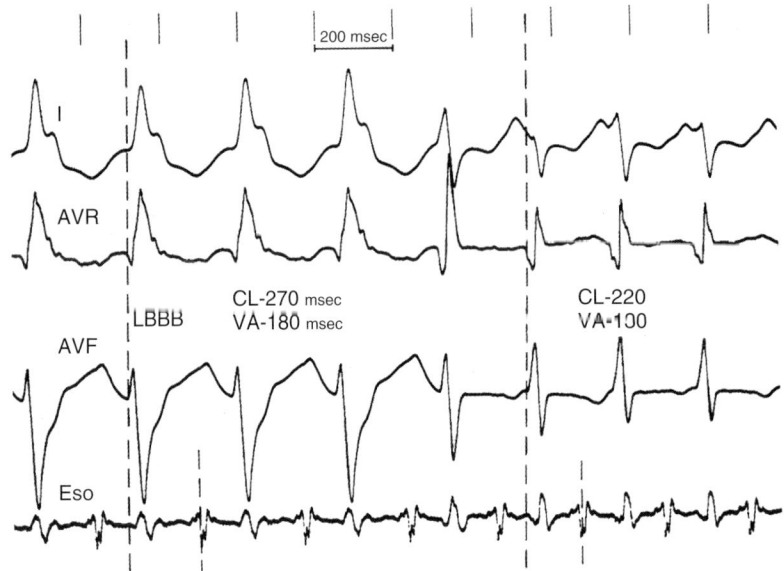

• **Fig. 17.26** A change from left bundle branch block *(LBBB)* to a normal QRS complex during orthodromic tachycardia causing a 50-msec decrease in the cycle length *(CL)*, and a shortening of the ventriuloatrial *(VA)* interval from 180 msec to 130 msec, confirming the diagnosis of a left-sided accessory pathway. Accurate determination of atrial timing is possible with the benefit of an esophageal recording lead *(Eso)*.

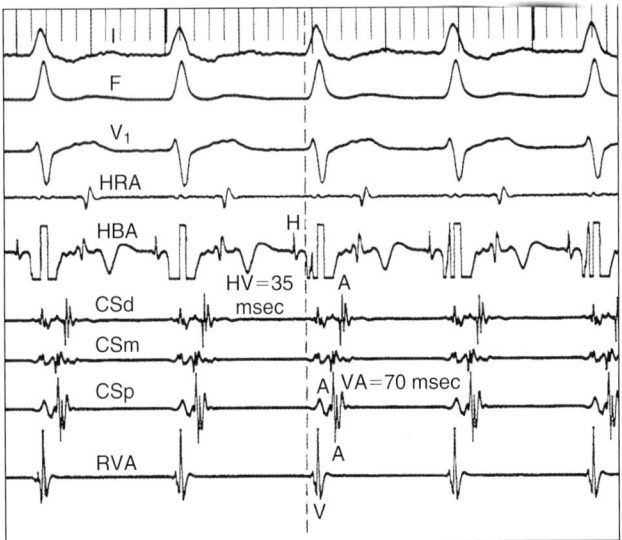

• **Fig. 17.27** Mapping of accessory pathway location during an episode of orthodromic reciprocating tachycardia at electrophysiology study. The QRS complex is normal on the surface ECG, and the H-V interval is normal, confirming anterograde conduction through the atrioventricular node. Retrograde conduction back to the atrium occurs over the accessory pathway. Atrial activation is earliest on the middle coronary sinus electrode *(CS)*, preceding atrial timing on both the HBE lead and the high right atrial *(HRA)* lead. This corresponds to a left posterior position for the accessory pathway.

acute conversion of ORT parallel those already mentioned for AVNRT. This begins with a Valsalva maneuver or facial application of an ice bag to transiently increase vagal tone. If this proves unsuccessful, an intravenous line can be placed and a rapid dose of adenosine can be given. Intravenous procainamide can be considered if adenosine fails or if ORT recurs promptly. If at any time during this treatment cascade the patient begins to develop hemodynamic intolerance of ORT, more deliberate therapy with DC cardioversion or transesophageal atrial overdrive pacing can always be instituted. Naturally, if an infant with longstanding ORT has congestive failure and hypotension at first presentation, urgent intervention with DC cardioversion or transesophageal pacing should be considered as initial therapy rather than squandering time with drug trials.

Patient age, severity of presenting symptoms, antegrade conduction properties of the AP, and AP location must all be taken into account when long-term therapy is being planned for ORT in patients with WPW. As many as 30% of infants with ORT from an AP will have spontaneous resolution of the disorder before their first birthday, and this encourages a policy of reliance on pharmacologic options throughout the first year or so of life.

The drugs used most commonly as initial therapy for WPW during infancy include beta-blocker, flecainide, sotalol, and amiodarone. Much beyond infancy, flecainide is considered one of the only safe drug options. The reason for this caveat relates to the risk of rapid preexcited atrial fibrillation. While atrial fibrillation is exceptionally rare in infants with WPW, it certainly can occur in older children, and many drugs have potential to enhance conduction across an AP. Flecainide is one of the few exceptions. Fortunately, long-term medical therapy is rarely needed in the current era since catheter ablation has become the favored approach to WPW in young patients, with a success rate of 92%–99% depending on pathway location, and very low risks in experienced hands. The complication rate seem to be higher in children under 15 kg in body weight,[12] so most centers are content to continue medical therapy until children are about 4 years old before recommending elective ablation assuming no serious symptomatology has occurred.

Antidromic Reciprocating Tachycardia in WPW

This tachycardia, in which the reentry circuit is the opposite of ORT, accounts for less than 1% of pediatric SVT cases. Because activation of the ventricle occurs entirely via the AP, the QRS complex is wide and abnormal, demonstrating maximal preexcitation (Fig. 17.28). Retrograde conduction from the ventricles to the atria occurs through the AV node (or in rare cases, a second AP), yielding a retrograde P wave axis of about −120 degrees.

Initiation of antidromic reentry requires that antegrade conduction blocks in the AV node while it continues in the AP. For this to occur, the antegrade refractory period of the AP must be shorter than that of the AV node. Maintenance of the tachycardia then requires that the retrograde refractory period of the AV node be less than the tachycardia cycle length. The relative infrequency of antidromic tachycardia seems to be due to difficulty in meeting these conditions. When antidromic tachycardia does occur, the His bundle deflection occurs near the end or after the QRS complex. Retrograde atrial activation, demonstrating a pattern of AV nodal origin, occurs after the His deflection and before the next ventricular activation.

As with ORT, tachycardia maintenance is dependent on conduction through both the AV node and the AP. Consequently, if the diagnosis of antidromic tachycardia is absolutely firm, conversion can be achieved with a protocol identical to that described for ORT. If the episode is the first presentation of a regular wide complex tachycardia in a patient without a prior ECG in sinus rhythm, the arrhythmia will need to be treated as described for VT until proven otherwise. It is difficult and probably hazardous to make the diagnosis of ART unless a patient already has a well-established diagnosis of WPW. If there is any irregularity

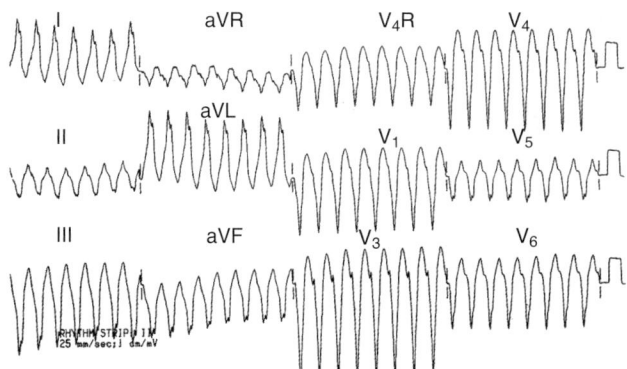

• **Fig. 17.28** Surface ECG of antidromic tachycardia. The initial QRS deflections were identical to the delta wave pattern later seen in preexcited sinus rhythm, strongly suggesting that these complexes represent maximal preexcitation. Subsequent electrophysiologic study confirmed antidromic reciprocating tachycardia involving a right, posterior accessory pathway, although in the acute setting, it would be difficult to eliminate ventricular tachycardia from the differential diagnosis.

whatsoever in the rate or QRS morphology, preexcited atrial fibrillation must be considered and the patient treated accordingly (see below).

Pharmacologic management of ART is similar to that for ORT in patients with WPW syndrome. Beta-blockers, as well as flecainide, sotalol, or amiodarone, are all satisfactory choices for treatment in infants, with focus shifted to flecainide at older ages. However, because virtually all patients with antidromic tachycardia have relatively rapidly conducting APs, ablation has now become the preferred option for all but the very youngest patient. Not only could ablation be curative, it might also eliminate iatrogenic morbidity that sometimes accompanies treatment of wide QRS tachycardia in a facility unfamiliar with the patient's condition.

Preexcited Atrial Fibrillation in WPW

Whenever an AP is present, every beat of atrial origin may activate the ventricles through the AV node, the AP, both, or neither. Thus, during any rapid atrial tachycardia, the rate and pattern of ventricular activation depend on the conduction times and the refractory period of both the AV node and AP(s). The normal protection of the ventricles from rapid conduction of atrial arrhythmias by the AV node is diminished by the presence of an AP. A rapid ventricular rate degenerating to VF in response to atrial fibrillation is a potential cause of sudden death in patients with WPW.[13] Patients with WPW syndrome are clearly more prone to episodic atrial fibrillation than the general population. There is little doubt that the AP contributes directly to this tendency, because elimination of pathway conduction with ablative therapy effectively prevents recurrence of atrial fibrillation in most all cases. An episode of ORT with abrupt and repetitive atrial depolarization at rapid rates is felt to be the most likely trigger for the atrial fibrillation.

A number of risk factors have been identified as contributing to deterioration of the ventricular rhythm during atrial fibrillation: (1) the presence of multiple APs, (2) a very short AP refractory period allowing rapid antegrade conduction, and (3) disorganized ventricular contraction and resultant hypotension due to the extreme irregularity of the rapid ventricular rhythm. A rapid ventricular response to atrial fibrillation in the electrophysiology laboratory is reasonably predictive of those who will experience spontaneous syncope or sudden death. Young patients with WPW who have been resuscitated from VF tend to have *shortest preexcited R-R intervals* (SPRRI) during atrial fibrillation or rapid atrial pacing of 250 msec or less (Fig. 17.29).

The two goals in the acute treatment of atrial fibrillation in WPW are to reduce the ventricular response rate and terminate the atrial fibrillation. If significant hemodynamic compromise is present, synchronized DC cardioversion will accomplish both goals with the lowest risks and quickest results. If the patient is not severely compromised, medical therapy can be considered. Procainamide administered intravenously is the safest drug in this setting, because it can slow conduction over the AP(s) and may also terminate

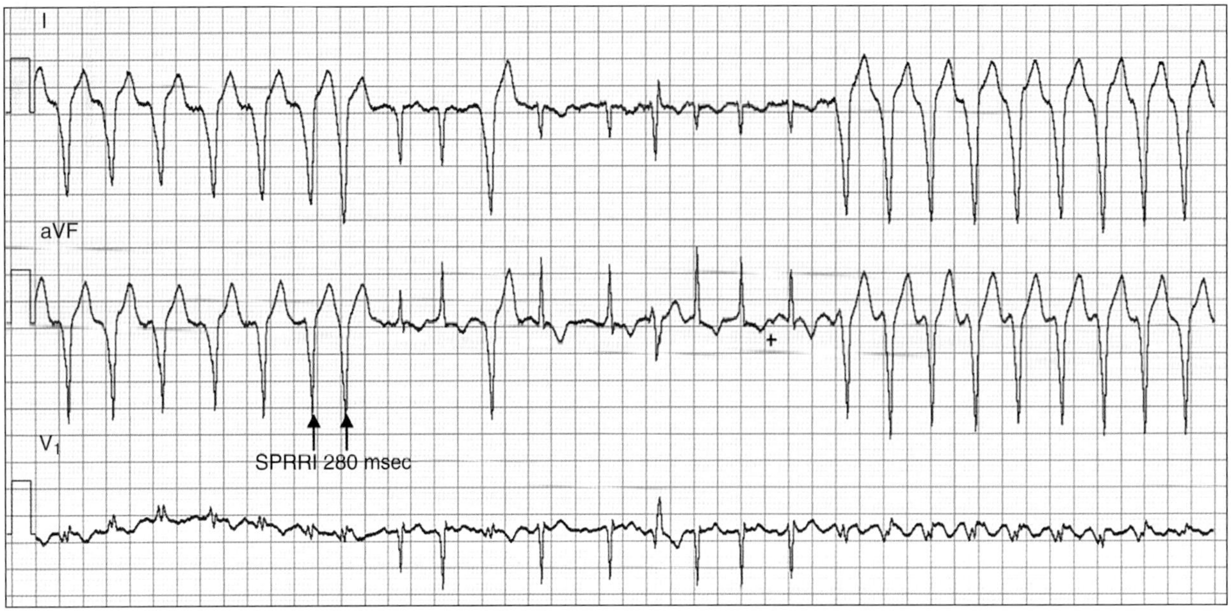

• **Fig. 17.29** Three-lead rhythm strip showing atrial fibrillation in a teenager as the first presentation of Wolff-Parkinson-White syndrome. Note the variable and wide-QRS (mostly preexcited, some conduction over atrioventricular node, some fused) and the irregular pattern of conduction. The shortest preexcited RR interval (*SPRRI*) in this case was 280 msec.

atrial fibrillation directly. Nearly every other drug in the intravenous antiarrhythmic armamentarium has the potential to enhance AP conduction during preexcited atrial fibrillation, with the net result being faster ventricular rate and potential degeneration to VF. Adenosine, digoxin, and calcium channel blockers are the biggest culprits in this regard and need to be avoided at all costs. However, even beta-blockers, sotalol, and amiodarone have the potential to enhance AP conduction and are now considered contraindicated. Generally speaking, catheter ablation should be the proper next step after acute stabilization. However, if the ventricular response during an episode of atrial fibrillation was documented to be slow, and there are legitimate age/size issues or other concerns that make catheter ablation an unattractive option at the moment, then and only then would one consider deferring ablation in favor of temporary medical therapy with an agent such as flecainide.

Some rare cases of WPW syndrome can involve an unusual AP with antegrade-only conduction. Although ORT cannot occur in this setting, ART and preexcited atrial fibrillation are still possible.

Orthodromic Tachycardia Involving a Concealed Accessory Pathway

The syndrome described by Wolff, Parkinson, and White consisted of a delta wave on the ECG and paroxysmal tachycardia. Because the delta wave depends on the ability of an AP to conduct antegrade, only patients with antegrade conduction in their AP have true WPW syndrome. However, orthodromic tachycardia is not dependent on antegrade conduction. When ORT occurs without evidence of ventricular preexcitation in sinus rhythm, the AP

is said to be *concealed* or *unidirectional retrograde*. This has only minimal significance for the presence and management of the ORT, but important implications regarding the risk of sudden death, because rapid antegrade conduction of atrial fibrillation is not possible.

The clinical, electrocardiographic, and electrophysiologic manifestations of ORT involving a concealed AP are identical to those of ORT in the setting of WPW, except that the PR interval and QRS complex are normal during sinus rhythm on ECG, and remain so during changes in atrial rate and various atrial pacing maneuvers. Why some APs are concealed and others have manifest preexcitation is an intriguing question. The site of antegrade block for concealed APs typically occurs at the ventricular insertion, and probably relates to dilution of the relatively small current density in the AP relative to the large ventricular muscle mass, leading to a so-called *impedance mismatch*.

Initial conversion of tachycardia is also identical to that of ORT with WPW. However, the fact that no risk exists for preexcited atrial fibrillation makes the recommendations for long-term management more relaxed. Patients can be safely treated in a fashion similar to AVNRT, including use of beta-blocker and calcium channel blockers. If this is not sufficient, flecainide, sotalol, or amiodarone could be considered as short-term therapy, but young patients who fail multiple drug trials, and most all older children, should be considered candidates for catheter ablation.

Permanent Form of Junctional Reciprocating Tachycardia

A certain subset of concealed AP is characterized by remarkably slow conduction velocity, and this peculiar physiology sets up the conditions for nearly incessant form of reentry known as PJRT (also referred to as *Coumel's tachycardia*). Because the activation wavefront is so delayed within the AP, atrial muscle and the AV node always have ample time to recover from their refractory period, which eliminates any opportunity for the circuit to extinguish. The end result is an ECG picture of incessant tachycardia at modest rates, with a dramatically long VA interval and a rather normal PR interval. The clinical label attached to this disorder is PJRT. Though uncommon, accounting for only 1%–3% of SVT cases in children, the striking difficulty in controlling PJRT, coupled with the profound clinical impact of incessant tachycardia upon ventricular function, make it quite noteworthy.

The relatively slow rates of PJRT rarely cause acute symptoms, but congestive heart failure can eventually arise from the incessant metabolic demand placed on the myocardium by chronically elevated rates. Patients tend to present during infancy or childhood, and only rarely past early adolescence. Similar to EAT, the tachycardia-induced myopathy is reversible once sinus rhythm has been restored.

With rare exception, the AP in PJRT is usually found in the posteroseptal region of the heart. Retrograde conduction into this area will yield an inverted P wave in ECG leads II, III, and aVF with an axis of approximately –120 degrees, while slow conduction in the AP leads to the very long VA interval (Fig. 17.30). The tachycardia may stop for a few beats from time to time, but promptly reinitiates with either sinus tachycardia or a single premature beat. Subtle variation in conduction velocity through both the AV node and the PJRT pathway in response to changes in sympathetic state can result in tachycardia rates that range on a gradual basis from 120 to 200 beats/min in the same patient. Anterograde conduction is always through the AV node during tachycardia, resulting in normal QRS morphology. On electrophysiologic study, the atrial excitation pattern during PJRT usually reveals early activation near the mouth of coronary sinus. A discrete potential representing conduction within the AP can be identified with careful mapping.

The acute treatment protocol outlined for the more typical forms of ORT is probably a reasonable starting point for

PJRT. The problem with such a protocol is that the tachycardia is likely to recur as soon as the terminating stimulus is removed. Thus, vagal maneuvers, adenosine, atrial pacing, and DC cardioversion may terminate PJRT for as little as one beat. If the diagnosis was not entertained at initial contact, it becomes painfully obvious following frustrating attempts at acute conversion. Effective suppression of PJRT is usually only possible with a long-acting medication or catheter ablation.

Many different drugs have been tested for PJRT. Occasionally, control can be achieved with a relatively benign agent such as beta-blocker, but more potent drugs are required for the majority of patients. Flecainide stands out as being perhaps the most effective agent for this condition,[14] though sotalol or amiodarone may also be used. Some infants who present with PJRT as newborns can experience spontaneous AP resolution in the first year or so of life similar to conventional APs, so medical management is usually the preferred approach in the very young. However, beyond infancy, PJRT is now treated with catheter ablation at most all centers, especially if there is any evidence of ventricular dysfunction.

Atriofascicular Pathways

These unusual APs arise from the anterolateral aspect of the right AV groove and travel along the free wall of the right ventricle to terminate near the moderator band.[15] The atrial end involves tissue with AV nodal properties, and the ventricular end approximates or joins the right bundle branch, leading to their designation as an AFP. The conduction pattern is exclusively antegrade. These APs were misunderstood for many years. An older model envisioned a connection between the compact AV node or proximal His bundle and the right ventricle referred to as a *Mahaim fiber*, and this teaching remained in vogue until detailed mapping data from ablation procedures revealed the true nature of the pathway.

As in the WPW syndrome, early ventricular activation can result in the electrocardiographic appearance of a delta wave with an abnormal QRS. However, AFPs have very slow conduction due to the nodal-like tissue at their atrial end, resulting in a fairly normal PR interval (Fig. 17.31). Another feature in common with WPW is a dynamic balance between normal conduction over the His-Purkinje network and abnormal preexcitation over the AFP, which varies according to the refractory characteristics and conduction velocity of the two limbs and is also modulated by the timing of the atrial depolarization. This results in a wide array of electrocardiographic appearances and ultimately can predispose to reentry arrhythmias.

AFPs are rare in both the pediatric and adult populations, although AFPs (as well as conventional APs) seem to occur in a high percentage of patients with Ebstein anomaly (see Chapter 34). The presenting complaint is usually palpitations in an otherwise healthy patient.

The surface ECG in sinus rhythm is variable and often normal. The preexcitation pattern can wax and wane,

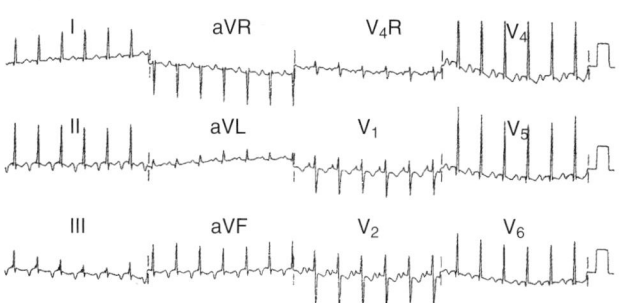

• **Fig. 17.30** ECG showing the permanent form of junctional reciprocating tachycardia. Note the slow tachycardia rate of 150 beats/min, the retrograde P wave axis of –100 degrees, the extremely long VA interval, and the normal P-R interval. The tachycardia was nearly incessant in this 10-year-old girl.

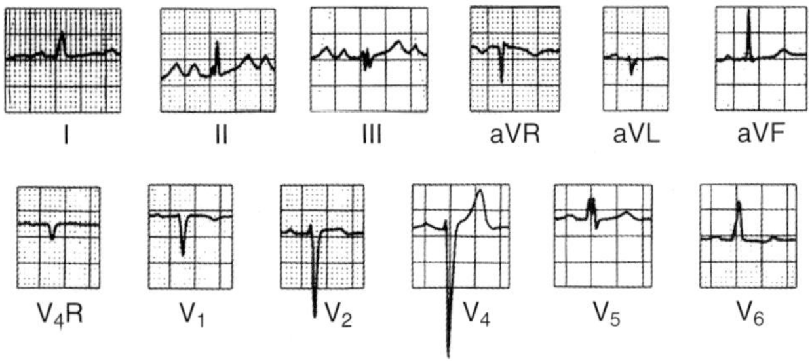

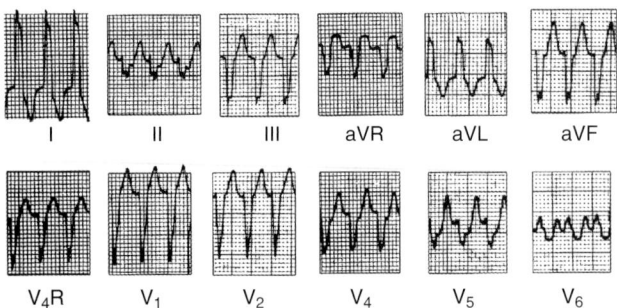

• **Fig. 17.31** ECG from a patient with an atriofascicular pathway proven at intracardiac electrophysiologic study. Note the delta waves in many leads but a normal P-R interval.

depending on sinus rate or the presence of premature beats. Electrophysiologic study may ultimately be necessary to unmask AFP conduction or to distinguish it from a standard AV pathway. Because AFPs preexcite the right ventricle, the delta wave and ventricular activation are directed right to left, sometimes mimicking left bundle branch block.

The reentry circuit in this disorder is antidromic, with forward conduction over the AFP and return over the normal His-Purkinje system and AV node (Fig. 17.32), resulting in a wide QRS tachycardia with retrograde atrial activation. Atrial fibrillation may also occur on rare occasions, with the AFP generating variably preexcited ventricular complexes. However, rapidly conducted atrial fibrillation is not an issue owing to the slow conduction potential of these pathways.

The diagnostic keys during electrophysiologic study include demonstration of a short or negative HV interval for a preexcited beat but with gradual lengthening of the AV time in response to premature stimuli (unlike WPW where the AV time remains fairly constant). During antidromic tachycardia, earliest ventricular activation occurs on the anterior surface of the right ventricle away from the AV groove, and earliest retrograde atrial activation occurs near the His bundle catheter. With careful mapping, one can record discrete potentials from the AFP itself.

In an emergency setting, AFP reentry can appear similar to VT or antidromic tachycardia in the WPW syndrome on the surface ECG, so the diagnosis is often made only after conversion of the initial episode. It may be necessary to

employ an emergency treatment strategy similar to that used for VT at first presentation. If the diagnosis is unquestionably firm in a given patient, simply using a drug that blocks the AV node limb of the circuit (such as adenosine or verapamil) can terminate tachycardia. Chronic therapy can involve either medications (similar to WPW syndrome) or catheter ablation.

Management of Ventricular Tachycardia

Tachycardias originating from myocytes or Purkinje cells below the bifurcation of the bundle of His are grouped under the heading of VT. Generally speaking, VT carries a more serious prognosis that SVT. This difference arises not only from the hemodynamic disadvantage of the fast ventricular rate but, more importantly, from the fact that VT often occurs in abnormal myocardium with sub-optimal function and/or some form of channelopathy, which may be vulnerable to degeneration into VF. Some specific forms of VT in young patients can be relatively benign, but this conclusion can only be reached after underlying pathology has been carefully excluded. In the acute setting, all VT must be taken seriously.

By convention, VT is defined as three or more consecutive ectopic beats of ventricular origin on an ECG. The term *non-sustained* is applied to short self-terminating episodes, whereas the term *sustained* implies an episode lasting longer than 30 seconds and/or causing hemodynamic instability. The QRS complex during VT appears wide and abnormal with a P wave that is either dissociated or arises from passive retrograde conduction. Whenever VA dissociation is present, there may be competition between the ventricular arrhythmia and episodic antegrade conduction over the AV node such that *fusion beats* may be noted (Fig. 17.33A).

Several varieties of VT can be distinguished by the appearance of the QRS during tachycardia. The term *monomorphic* is applied to a uniform QRS morphology (Fig. 17.33B), *bidirectional* denotes two alternating QRS types, *polymorphic* indicates a widely varying QRS (Fig. 17.33C), and *torsades de pointes* describes a specific pattern of positive and negative oscillation of the QRS direction which seems to twist around the isoelectric line of the ECG (Fig. 17.33D).

Intracardiac electrophysiologic study is indicated for some patients in order to rule out atypical SVT as the true mechanism for the arrhythmia, or to gain insight into VT mechanism and focus of origin to help plan therapy or guide catheter ablation. In years past, electrophysiologic studies were also performed to evaluate the response to serial antiarrhythmic drug trials, but this role has declined considerably in the era of the implantable cardioverter defibrillator (ICD) and catheter ablation.

Acute Treatment of Ventricular Tachycardia

Sustained VT should be treated as an emergency. Arterial blood pressure and perfusion should be assessed quickly

• **Fig. 17.32** Sustained wide-QRS tachycardia in a patient with an atriofascicular pathway confirmed at electrophysiology study. In the emergency setting, this tracing can be difficult to distinguish from ventricular tachycardia.

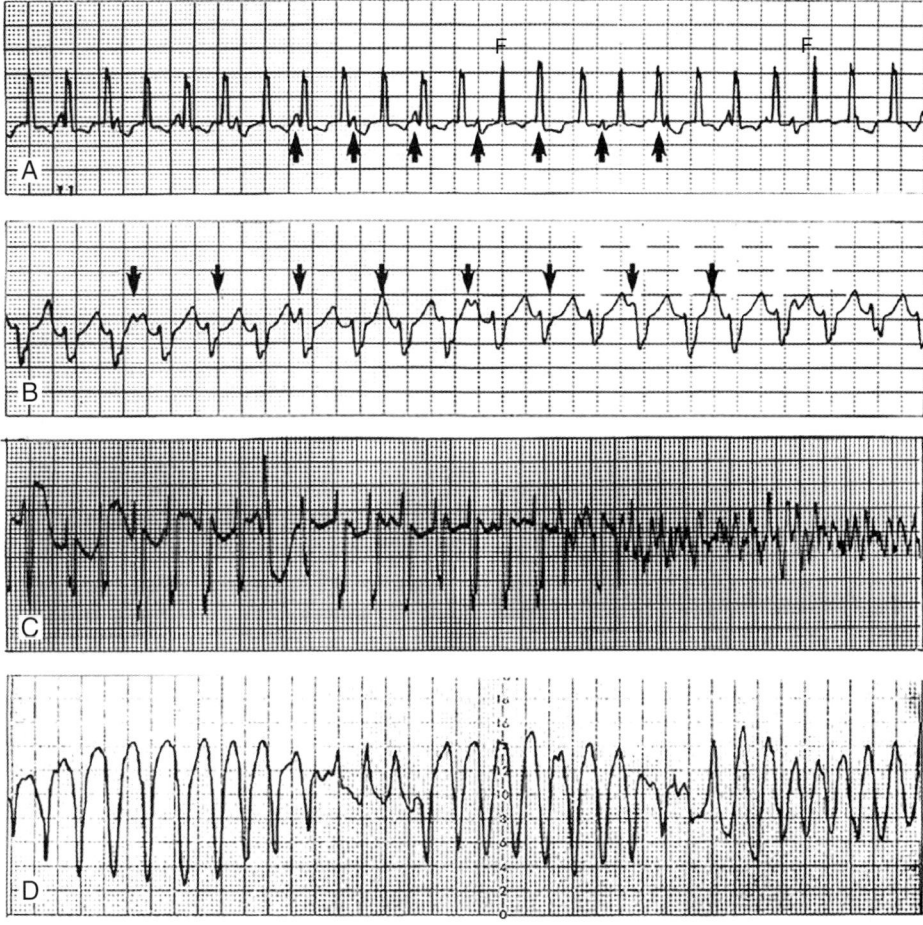

• **Fig. 17.33** Example of ventricular tachycardia (VT). **(A)** Monomorphic VT from an infant with incessant tachycardia, showing dissociated P waves *(arrows)* and fusion beats *(F)*. **(B)** Monomorphic VT from a teenager with myocarditis, again showing A-V dissociation. **(C)** Polymorphic VT from a postoperative patient, degenerating to ventricular fibrillation in the latter portion of the strip. **(D)** Torsades de pointes from a patient with long QT syndrome.

and a 12-lead ECG recorded. A brief history should be obtained from the patient or accompanying family member with particular attention to medications, possible toxic exposures, and known familial arrhythmias.

Any patient who is unresponsive and/or severely hypotensive should be treated with immediate DC shock of 1–2 J/kg. The energy can be synchronized to the QRS if the VT is well organized and has sufficient amplitude, but an unsynchronized discharge is required for VF or rapid polymorphic VT. If an initial shock is unsuccessful, the energy can be increased for additional shock trials while standard resuscitation measures are being carried out according to established guidelines until the patient is stabilized.

If the patient is awake and stable, or if electrical conversion is unsuccessful, intravenous drug therapy should be initiated. Lidocaine, administered as a bolus and followed by a continuous infusion, remains the safest first-line agent. Second-line choices depend somewhat on the electrocardiographic appearance and the cause of the VT. For monomorphic VT, intravenous procainamide, esmolol, or amiodarone can all be considered. However, if VT is of the torsades de

pointes variety or occurs in the setting of antiarrhythmic drug toxicity, esmolol and/or magnesium are more appropriate agents (see Chapter 20).

As a general rule, adenosine or verapamil are avoided in the emergency treatment of a new patient with wide QRS tachycardia, with two possible exceptions. First, if the tachycardia is strictly <u>regular</u>, and if the QRS is strictly <u>monomorphic</u>, and if <u>VA dissociation is absent</u>, then there is a chance the episode is due to SVT with rate-related aberration or preexistent bundle branch block. Under these conditions only, a cautious trial of adenosine can be attempted, and if successful, diagnostic thinking can shift toward a supraventricular mechanism with QRS aberration. The second exception involves a specific form of VT that is strictly <u>regular</u>, strictly <u>monomorphic</u>, and has a relatively sharp onset QRS with a distinctive pattern of <u>right bundle branch block and a superior axis</u>. There may or may not be VA dissociation. This indicates a potential mechanism of left ventricular septal reentrant VT (so-called *Belhassen's tachycardia*), which is often responsive to verapamil.[16] These two exceptions should be reserved for cardiologists who have solid experience with tachycardia management. Novices should assume a wide QRS tachycardia is a potentially serious form of VT and treat accordingly until proven otherwise.

Chronic Management of Ventricular Tachycardia

When choosing a long-term treatment plan for VT, the following must be taken into account: (1) the patient's symptoms (or lack thereof), (2) the presence and degree of underlying cardiac pathology, (3) the rate, duration, and morphology of VT, (4) suspected VT mechanism, (5) family history, and (6) the natural history of the specific disorder. Careful evaluation of cardiac structure and function is an important part of the decision process. All patients should undergo echocardiography, and some may require cardiac catheterization and MRI studies. Subtle pathology such as arrhythmogenic ventricular dysplasia, coronary anomalies, cardiac tumors, and myopathy may only be uncovered with these techniques. If cardiac structure and function are judged to be normal, asymptomatic patients with infrequent isolated beats or even slow non-sustained salvos of ventricular ectopy might be followed closely without therapy, whereas symptomatic patients (whether or not cardiac pathology is demonstrated) are usually treated. Unfortunately, this leaves a large and complex gray zone of patients with varied degrees of cardiac pathology who exhibit high-grade ventricular ectopy but have not yet experienced a malignant event. The clinician must constantly balance side effects of drug therapy, including negative inotropic properties and paradoxical worsening of rhythm status (referred to as *proarrhythmia*), as well as potential complications with ablation or an ICD, against the ultimate risk of a malignant arrhythmia. Consultation with a cardiac electrophysiologist is recommended to assist with these difficult decisions.

Specific Forms of Ventricular Tachycardia in Children

VT is uncommon in children, and its causes are diverse. Unlike VT related to ischemic heart disease in adult patients where treatment protocols are driven and refined by enormous clinical experience, no single condition is sufficiently common in children to permit development of authoritative treatment recommendations. The views expressed here reflect our current institutional policy, but will be subject to change as new data become available.

Benign Transient VT in Infancy

Relatively slow episodes of non-sustained monomorphic VT (sometimes referred to as *idioventricular rhythm*) can be observed in some infants with an otherwise normal heart. It appears to be due to focal automaticity arising from the ventricular outflow region. It is likely related to idiopathic outflow tract VT seen in older patients (discussed below),

at least in terms of mechanism. However, this infant variety tends to resolve over the first year or so of life, and there are no firm data to suggest it recurs in later years. The rates tend to be just slightly above underlying sinus rhythm and do not result in hemodynamic compromise. Treatment is usually unnecessary.[17] Beta-blockers, which are frequently effective in suppressing or reducing this disorder, are sometimes prescribed if VT is present throughout a large percentage of the day.

Rapid Incessant VT in Infancy

This rare and malignant condition involves VT at rapid rates (>200 beats/min), and is often so protracted that ventricular function may become compromised and/or VF may occur. It is usually monomorphic, but different VT morphologies can be seen in the same patient from episode to episode. The VT is typically of left ventricular origin, likely involving His-Purkinje tissue (Fig. 17.34). Its cellular mechanism is poorly understood, but it exhibits many features typical for an automatic focus in that it may fail to respond to DC shock or overdrive pacing. Some young children have undergone successful surgical excision and catheter ablation for uncontrollable VT, and the diseased tissue frequently exhibits pathologic features that suggest hamartomas of Purkinje cell origin. If the tumor is discrete and solitary, surgery or catheter ablation could be curative, but tumors are sometimes present in a diffuse infiltrative process known as *histiocytoid cardiomyopathy*,[18] which is far more difficult to treat. No single antiarrhythmic medication is universally effective in this condition, and potent combinations (e.g., amiodarone plus flecainide plus beta-blockers) are often required to suppress VT. If the patient is not severely compromised and has reasonable ventricular function at presentation, chronic pharmacologic treatment can be used with close follow-up, and this disorder may actually resolve spontaneously over time in some cases. However, in patients with advanced ventricular dysfunction or cardiac arrest, urgent catheter and/or surgical ablation may need to be considered in combination with aggressive medical therapy.

Idiopathic Outflow Tract VT

Relatively benign forms of VT are seen occasionally in children and young adults without demonstrable cardiac pathology. The most common of these involves a focal automatic mechanism arising from the ventricular outflow track. This VT is monomorphic and characterized by relatively slow rates (140–190 beats/min), with a QRS morphology of left bundle branch block and an axis of about +90 degrees on surface ECG (Fig. 17.35). Severe symptoms are uncommon, and some patients are totally unaware of this arrhythmia. However, a few may have nearly incessant VT that can eventually lead to a tachycardia-induced myopathy with congestive symptoms. Furthermore, it is sometimes difficult to distinguish outflow tract VT from the more concerning VT that may arise in patients with true pathology. Symptoms such as syncope, or very

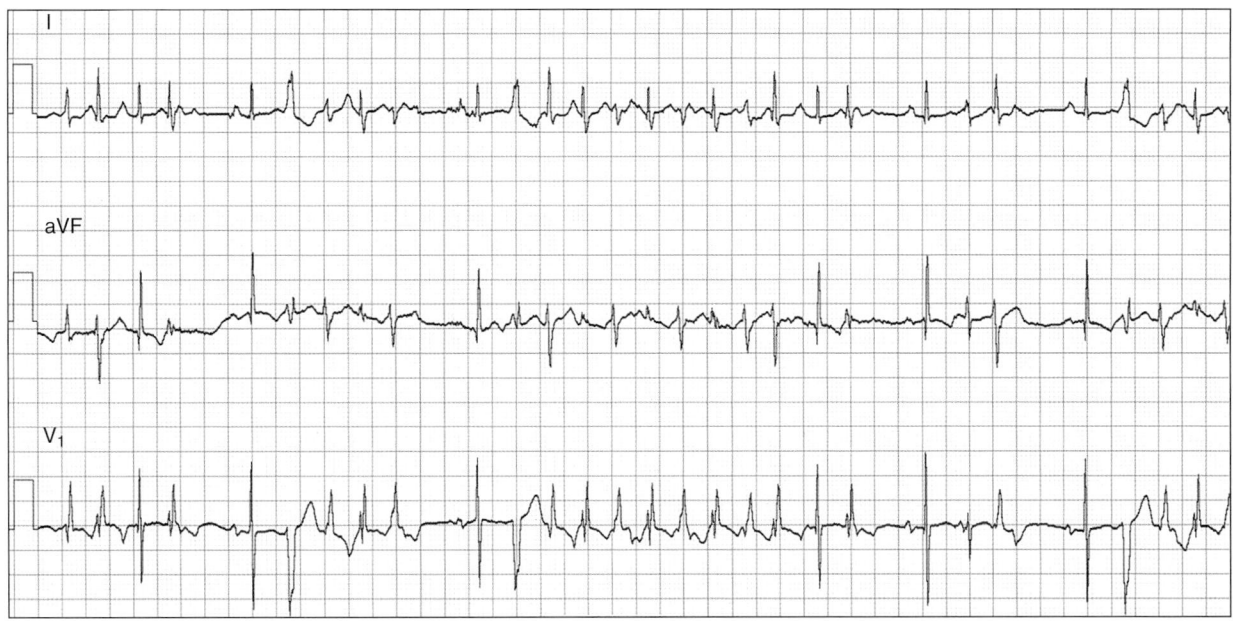

• **Fig. 17.34** Intermittent salvos of rapid ventricular tachycardia in an infant that was nearly incessant and refractory to all medication trials, associated with severe ventricular dysfunction. Control ultimately required multiple ablations procedures as well as medications.

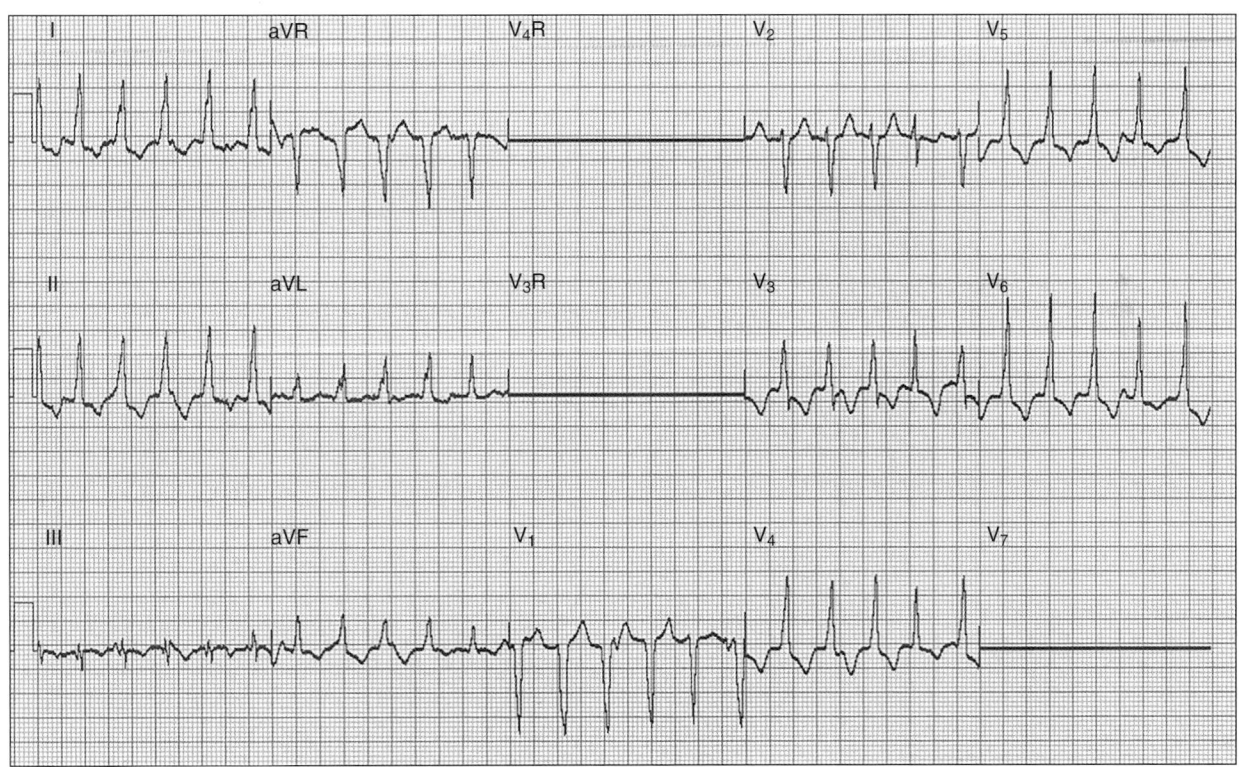

• **Fig. 17.35** Automatic focal ventricular tachycardia in a teenager at a rate of 160 beats/min with a QRS pattern suggesting origin in the right ventricular outflow tract.

rapid VT rates, would tend to favor a more pathologic condition. All patients presenting with this form of VT should have an echocardiogram performed to evaluate ventricular function, and magnetic resonance imaging may be considered if there is a concerning family history or any ECG findings suggesting an underlying myopathy. Assuming all testing is normal and the patient is entirely asymptomatic with well-preserved ventricular function, some of these patients can be followed safely without specific therapy, and VT may resolve spontaneously over time in some cases. If symptoms occur, or the VT is present throughout large portions of the day, treatment with a beta-blocker or calcium channel blocker can be considered, which suppresses or at least reduces VT in many young patients. Any youngster with depressed ventricular function will usually undergo an attempt at catheter ablation of the VT focus. Foci can arise from either the right ventricular outflow tract or the aortic root. Ablation is highly successful for this disorder as long as the VT remains sufficiently active during the mapping process to permit careful localization.[19]

Left Ventricular Septal VT

A second form of relatively benign VT is an interesting reentrant circuit along the left ventricular septum that appears to involve the posterior fascicle of the left bundle branch.[16] It goes by several clinical labels, including *Belhassen's tachycardia*, or *left posterior fascicular tachycardia.* This VT is abrupt in onset, operates at very regular rates in the range of 130–200 beats/min, and has the ECG appearance of right bundle branch block with a superior QRS axis (Fig. 17.36). It is the only form of VT in children that responds reliably to a calcium channel blocker. In fact, this unanticipated drug sensitivity is responsible for yet another clinical label of *verapamil-sensitive VT* that is often attached to this condition. Assuming underlying cardiac pathology has been removed from consideration, long-term verapamil or diltiazem therapy can be used quite successfully to prevent recurrences of VT. Alternatively, elective catheter ablation can be performed by placing lesions along the left ventricular septal surface, guided by the recording of a sharp potential from a Purkinje fiber. The permanent success rate for catheter ablation of Belhassen's VT is better than 90% in young patients.[19]

Long QT Syndrome

A prolonged QTc interval on the ECG is a marker for diffuse abnormalities of ventricular repolarization, which in turn may predispose to recurrent VT of the torsades de pointes type. A prolonged QT may be seen as a congenital disorder, or it may be acquired from exposure to certain drugs, toxins, or electrolyte disturbances.

The congenital forms of long QT deserve the most emphasis here. Our understanding of these membrane channelopathies has expanded dramatically thanks to identification of specific genetic defects in afflicted families and an improved understanding of ion channel function. Whereas only two forms of heredity LQTS were originally recognized based upon gross phenotype (the Romano-Ward syndrome, and the Jervell and Lange-Nielsen syndrome), there are now known to be more than 15 distinct gene abnormalities involved in this condition. In simplistic terms, the heterozygous condition for any one of these defects can be viewed as causing the Romano-Ward phenotype (normal hearing and LQTS), whereas the homozygous condition for any one defect, or the heterozygous condition for any two defects in combination, can be viewed as causing the Jervell and Lange-Nielsen phenotype (congenital deafness and a particularly severe form of LQTS). Knowing the genotypic form of LQTS can help confirm the diagnosis, permit screening within families, and provide prognostic information to tailor therapy. However, some discordance still exists between genotype and phenotype, and the number of unique family mutations or spontaneous mutations which contribute to these gene defects is vast. Furthermore, not all detected gene mutations are disease-producing, and some that are can have variable penetrance. The clinical diagnosis and management of LQTS must involve a careful synthesis of both genotype and phenotype to optimize care (see Chapter 20 for more details).

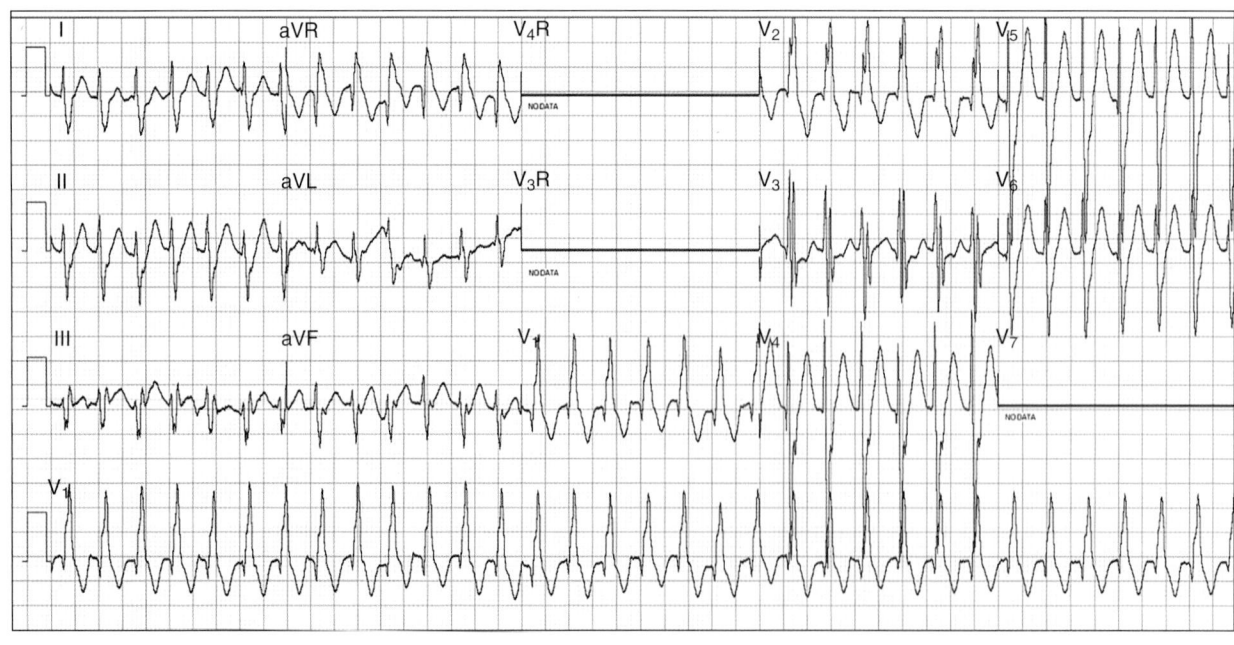

• **Fig. 17.36** Left ventricular septal ventricular tachycardia (Belhassen's VT) in a 12-year-old.

The symptoms of LQTS may surface at any age and usually involve episodic dizziness, palpitations, syncope, "seizures," and even cardiac arrest. While some VT episodes may stop spontaneously, a prolonged episode can be fatal. Clinical events may sometimes be confused with a primary seizure disorder or benign vasovagal syncope. For this reason, it is recommended that an ECG be obtained as a routine part of the work-up for any young patient with unexplained syncope or a first seizure-like episode. LQTS is also felt to be involved in some cases of sudden infant death syndrome. All first-degree blood relatives should have screening ECG performed (regardless of symptom status) whenever an index case is identified, and if a disease-producing mutation is found on genotype analysis, family members can be tested for that same mutation.

The diagnosis depends upon demonstration of a QT interval that is prolonged beyond the normal range when corrected for heart rate (>450 msec for males and >460 msec for females). Certain morphologic features of the T wave (notching or low amplitude), as well as certain clinical features (VT with auditory stimuli or swimming), have been found to correlate with specific gene defects (Fig. 17.37 online). The ECG findings can be combined with the patient's symptoms and family history to generate a clinical risk score,[20] which can be particularly useful when the ECG is borderline or equivocal.

Currently, one must rely on patient symptoms and ambulatory monitoring to gauge effects of therapy. Most often, initial treatment involves high-dose beta blockade. Sinus bradycardia and variable AV block can be seen with some forms of LQTS and may necessitate permanent pacemaker placement both to relieve bradycardia and to reduce VT that may be conditioned by slow ventricular rates. Cases that remain refractory to these measures could be considered for surgery to interrupt the left cervical sympathetic ganglion, and/or ICD implant. Consultation with an electrophysiologist is recommended to determine the optimal therapeutic approach for a specific patient and their family members.

Catecholaminergic Polymorphic VT

As the name implies, catecholaminergic polymorphic VT (CPVT), this unusual disorder is associated with VT at times of exercise or stress.[21] The tachycardia can be monomorphic, but more often has a distinctive bidirectional appearance with two alternating QRS morphologies (Fig. 17.38). The rates are highly variable; sometimes just slightly faster than sinus, while at other times fast enough to

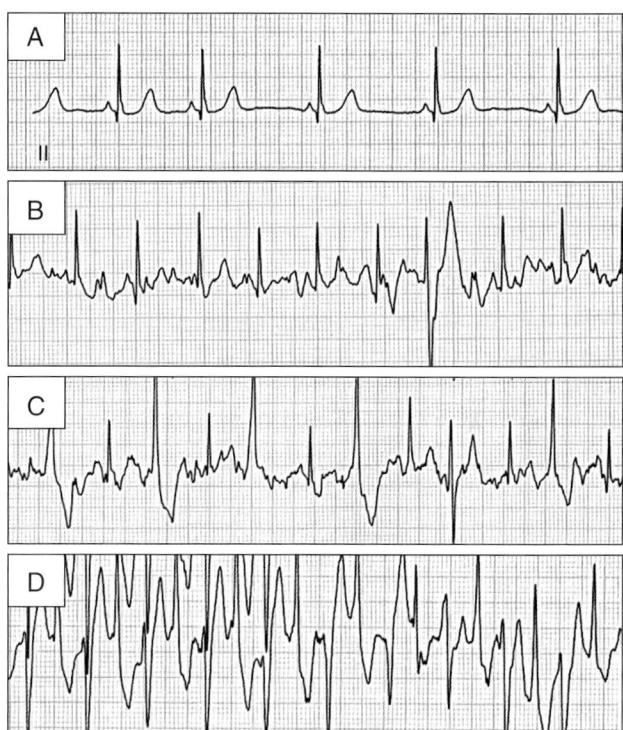

• **Fig. 17.38** Bidirectional ventricular tachycardia (VT) in a teenager with catecholaminergic polymorphic VT during exercise testing. **(A)** Baseline sinus rhythm. **(B)** Ventricular ectopic beat of one morphology in early exercise. **(C)** Appearance of a second form of ventricular ectopy mid-exercise. **(D)** Bidirectional VT.

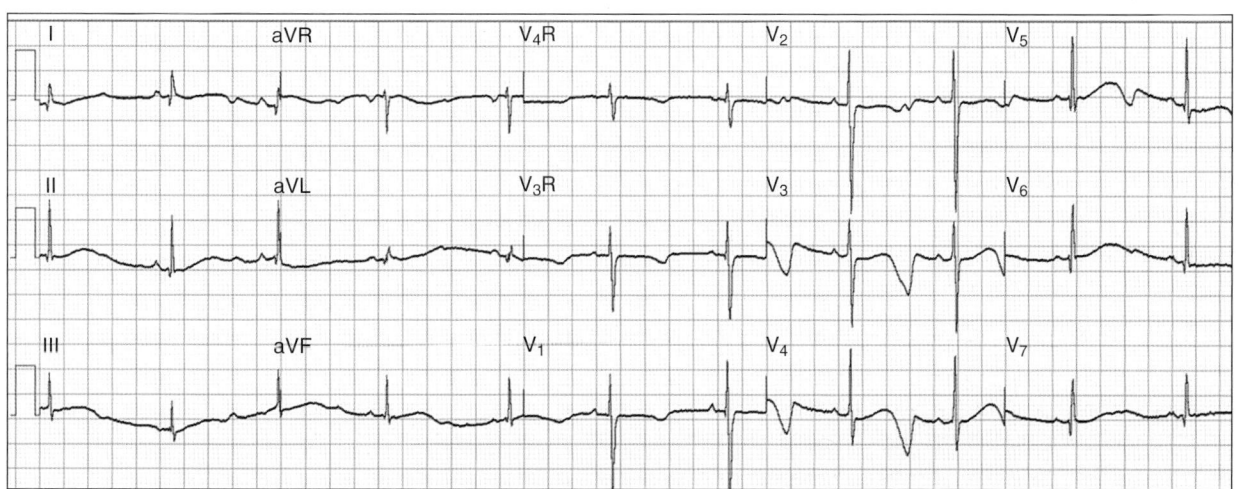

• **Fig. 17.37** ECG from a patient with congenital deafness and long QT syndrome who experienced multiple episodes of torsade de pointes with syncope. The T wave is notched and markedly prolonged. The corrected QT interval at this heart rate exceeded 0.55 msec.

degenerate into VF. Some patients with CPVT may also demonstrate additional tachycardias of atrial and junctional origin. This disorder is another form of channelopathy, usually related to a hereditary defect in the cardiac *ryanodine receptor* which is involved with calcium handling in the sarcoplasmic reticulum. A less common type is related to a defect in the calsequestrin 2 gene (see Chapter 20). Both mutations appear to act by affecting calcium release from the sarcoplasmic reticulum. Regardless of underlying cellular defect, CPVT is unpredictable and potentially fatal. Treatment can begin using high-dose beta-blocker with implant of an internal loop recorder to monitor treatment response. Flecainide has also been identified as another effective pharmacologic treatment in many cases. If concern persists, surgery to interrupt the left cervical sympathetic ganglion can be performed. In the current era, ICD implant is seldom recommended since the catecholamine surge from device shocks can precipitate a recurrent *VT storm*.

A similar appearing bidirectional VT can also be seen in severe digoxin toxicity, as well as *Andersen-Tawil syndrome* (a rare form of LQTS whose phenotype sometimes involves periodic paralysis of skeletal muscle), though the cellular mechanisms differ from CPVT.

Brugada syndrome

Less common than LQTS is the membrane channelopathy referred to as Brugada syndrome.[22] The QTc is usually normal or just mildly increased in this condition, but the ECG reveals variable right ventricular conduction delay and unusual ST elevation in leads V1 through V3 (Fig. 17.39).

These findings can fluctuate in some patients to the point that their ECG appears nearly normal at times. Provocative challenges with antiarrhythmic drugs such as procainamide have been used to bring out the ECG abnormalities when the diagnosis is suspected but uncertain. Episodic VT occurs which can be fatal. A sodium channel defect has been implicated as the cause of most cases of Brugada syndrome, and the pattern of inheritance suggests an autosomal dominant disorder. Symptoms usually do not appear before adulthood, but some highly symptomatic children have been encountered, with VT flare-ups especially common during febrile illnesses. Implant of an ICD is recommended in most cases of symptomatic Brugada syndrome. No specific drug has been demonstrated to be effective in preventing sudden death once symptoms begin, although some recent reports suggest quinidine may show promise to minimize ICD shocks.

VT in Congenital Heart Disease

Ventricular arrhythmias can be seen as a late complication of congenital heart disease. The lesion most frequently associated with VT is tetralogy of Fallot,[23] but VT may occur with other defects, including congenital aortic stenosis and many other conditions if advanced ventricular dysfunction develops. Monomorphic VT due to macroreentry appears to be the predominant mechanism for ventricular arrhythmias in tetralogy patients. In most instances, patients who experience sustained VT demonstrate reproducible initiation of their arrhythmia with programmed stimulation during electrophysiology study. Mapping of VT typically

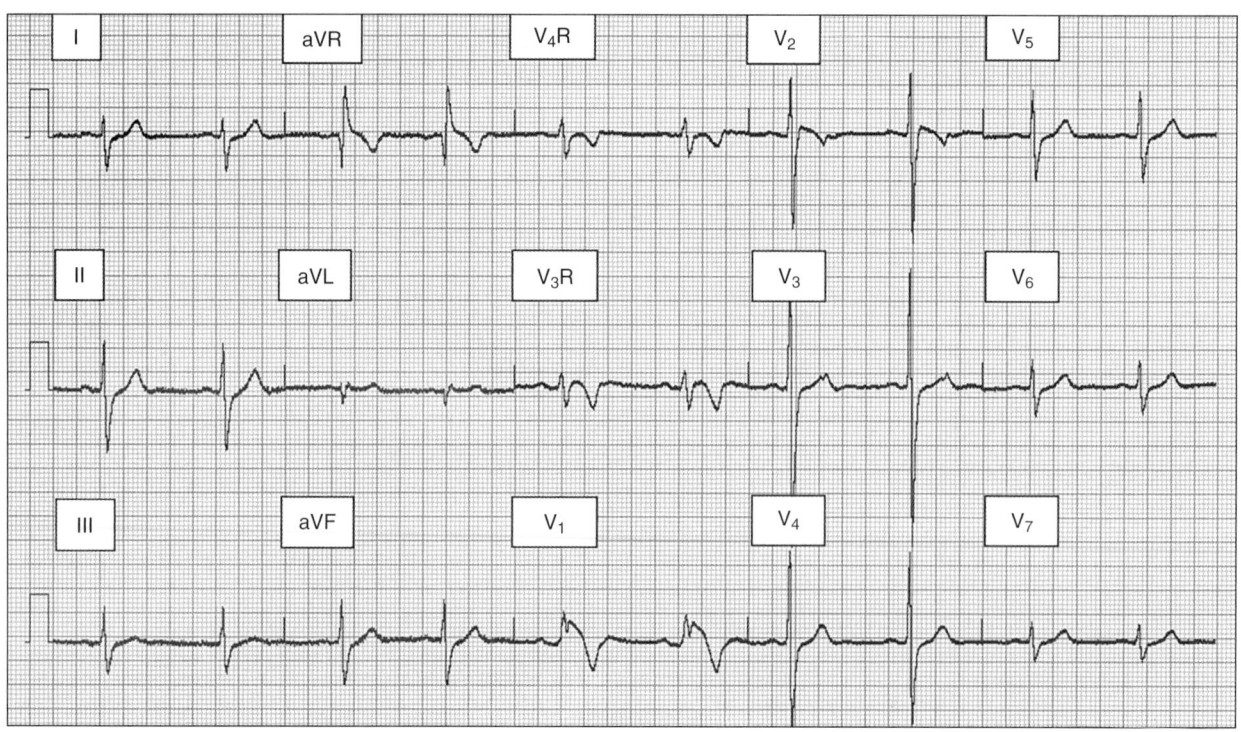

• **Fig. 17.39** ECG from a young patient with Brugada syndrome during a febrile illness, showing the right ventricular conduction delay and dramatic ST abnormalities in the right precordial leads.

reveals a circuit in the right ventricular outflow track with a critical corridor involving the conal septum, though other circuits are possible (Fig. 17.40A and B online).

Although it is universally agreed that patients with sustained VT and symptoms require therapy, decisions are difficult in the absence of symptoms in patients with lower-grade ventricular arrhythmias. Multiple studies have attempted to define predictive models for sustained VT and sudden death among the tetralogy population. Some of the more notable noninvasive risk-factors include: older age at follow-up, older age at repair, prior large palliative shunts, right ventricular failure, left ventricular dysfunction, prolonged QRS duration, and non-sustained VT on ambulatory monitoring. Unfortunately, none of these provide perfect predictive accuracy, and most decisions (ranging from no therapy to ICD implant) are still made on a case-by-case basis. Many centers, including our own, rely on electrophysiologic studies to help guide therapy. Induction of VT with ventricular stimulation at electrophysiology study appears to identify high-risk patients with reasonable accuracy, while a negative protocol suggests a very low risk of malignant events.[24] Aggressive therapy can thus be directed towards those most likely to benefit based on these test results.

Treatment of VT in congenital heart disease may involve correction of residual hemodynamic defects, suppressive drug therapy, ICD implant, catheter ablation, surgical ablation, or some combination of these measures. Surgery to insert a pulmonary valve coupled with cryoablation of scarred areas in the right ventricular outflow tract has recently been advocated in older tetralogy patients with severe regurgitation, although data remain mixed on long-term outcomes from this intervention. No specific antiarrhythmic drug is likely to be protective in all cases. Experience with mexiletine, phenytoin, and beta-blockers suggests efficacy in suppressing ventricular ectopy by Holter monitor criteria, but parallel data with programmed stimulation and long-term clinical outcome are incomplete. Catheter ablation has been used successfully in many patients, but VT recurrences are still too common to support ablation as exclusive therapy in a high-risk patient. In the current era, ICD implant appears to be the safest management strategy for VT in high-risk patients with congenital heart defects.

VT in Cardiomyopathies

The management of ventricular arrhythmias in the setting of cardiomyopathy remains a major challenge. These conditions are unpredictable, and neither ambulatory monitoring nor electrophysiologic study seem capable of removing the uncertainty surrounding the issue of VT and sudden death. Furthermore, attempts at empiric drug suppression of ectopy may worsen compromised ventricular function through negative inotropic effects, or result in unanticipated proarrhythmia. Thus, therapeutic emphasis in recent years has shifted steadily towards ICD implant whenever a patient is viewed as potentially high-risk for VT or VF. The true challenge, of course, is generating an accurate risk-stratification scheme for these conditions.

Hypertrophic cardiomyopathy.

Hypertrophic cardiomyopathy (HCM) is perhaps the most difficult in this regard since so many patients are entirely asymptomatic until malignant VT occurs. No single drug has been found to be broadly protective against VT for this population. The clinical variables that are currently viewed as potential predictors of sudden death in young patients with HCM include: (1) a history of syncope, (2) non-sustained VT on Holter, (3) family history of HCM with sudden death, (4) failure to augment blood pressure with exercise, and (5) dramatic septal thickness.[25] Data are mixed

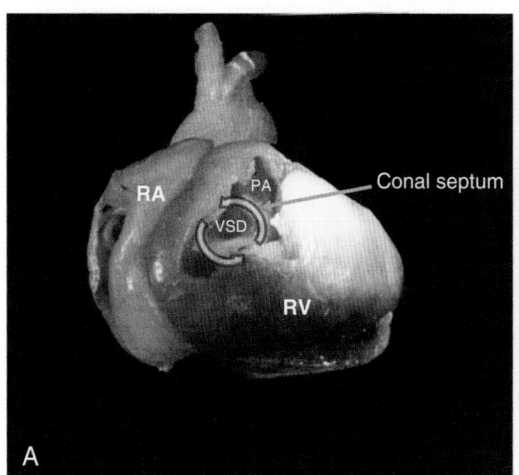
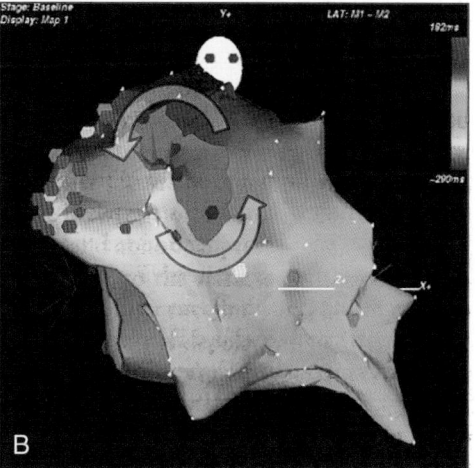

• **Fig. 17.40** **(A)** Pathology specimen from an infant with unrepaired tetralogy of Fallot (who expired from unrelated causes) highlighting the most common potential circuit for ventricular tachycardia in this anatomy through the conal septum around the ventricular septal defect *(VSD)*. **(B)** Mapping at electrophysiology study for an adult patient with tetralogy of Fallot. The reentrant circuit in this case propagated around a right ventricular outflow tract patch *(gray zone)*. Pink dots indicate line of successful catheter ablation. *PA,* Pulmonary artery; *RA,* right atrium; *RV,* right ventricle.

on the predictive accuracy for some of these items, but when all are viewed in aggregate, the negative predictive value for the absence of all risk factors is probably better than 90%. That is to say, if none of these are present, ICD implant would seem unnecessary as a purely prophylactic measure, particularly in a young growing patient where ICD lead complications are so common. How many positive findings are needed to justify an ICD depends somewhat on patient age and size. A single item could perhaps be viewed as sufficient in a fully grown teenager, but not necessarily for a 5-year old where ICD implant and lead maintenance are still technically demanding.

Dilated cardiomyopathy

Dilated cardiomyopathy is likewise associated with unpredictable rhythm status. There is reasonable correlation between ejection fraction (EF) and ventricular arrhythmias in adult patients, with most data suggesting that an EF much less than 35% places the patient at risk for VT or VF, but comparable data in young patients are still lacking. As with HCM, implantation of an ICD has now become the most generally accepted treatment for VT in this setting, though criteria for patient selection still vary widely from center to center. Use of an ICD as a bridge to transplant has become increasingly common in the pediatric age group.

A final myopathy that deserves mention is *arrhythmogenic right ventricular cardiomyopathy*. This familial disease involves fibrofatty degeneration of the right ventricular free wall, sometimes extending to the septum and left ventricle as well, and can be associated with recurrent VT. The ECG is a useful tool for establishing its presence, based on a combination of right ventricular conduction delay, inverted precordial T waves extending out to V_4 or beyond, and a so-

called epsilon wave (Fig. 17.41) in the right precordial leads. In advanced cases, abnormalities of right ventricular size, function, and muscle appearance can be appreciated on magnetic resonance imaging and echocardiography. However, VT may sometimes develop in this condition even before gross structural changes are detectable by these imaging modalities. The VT usually involves macroreentry within the diseased right ventricular tissue. Electrophysiologic testing is fairly reliable in reproducing these arrhythmias, and catheter ablation can also be considered in difficult cases. As with most other forms of cardiomyopathy, ICD implant may ultimately become necessary.

Sinus Node Dysfunction

Although normal values are well established for resting sinus rates in all age groups, individual variation is so dramatic that it is impossible to dictate firm cut-off values as indicative of pathologic bradycardia in children. Much depends on the clinical setting. An awake resting sinus rate of 50 beats/min may be normal for a healthy teenage athlete, but would be strictly abnormal for a similar-aged patient with poor cardiac function.

The electrocardiographic picture for pathologic sinus node behavior is a slow P wave rate, usually with marked sinus arrhythmia, allowing a variety of escape rhythms from low atrial and junctional foci (Fig. 17.42 online). Additionally, the sinus node may display abrupt pauses because of exit block or even complete sinus arrest.

The most common cause of SA node dysfunction in pediatric patients involves direct injury to the node or its arterial supply as a consequence of surgery for congenital heart disease. No open heart procedure, even simple closure of an atrial septal

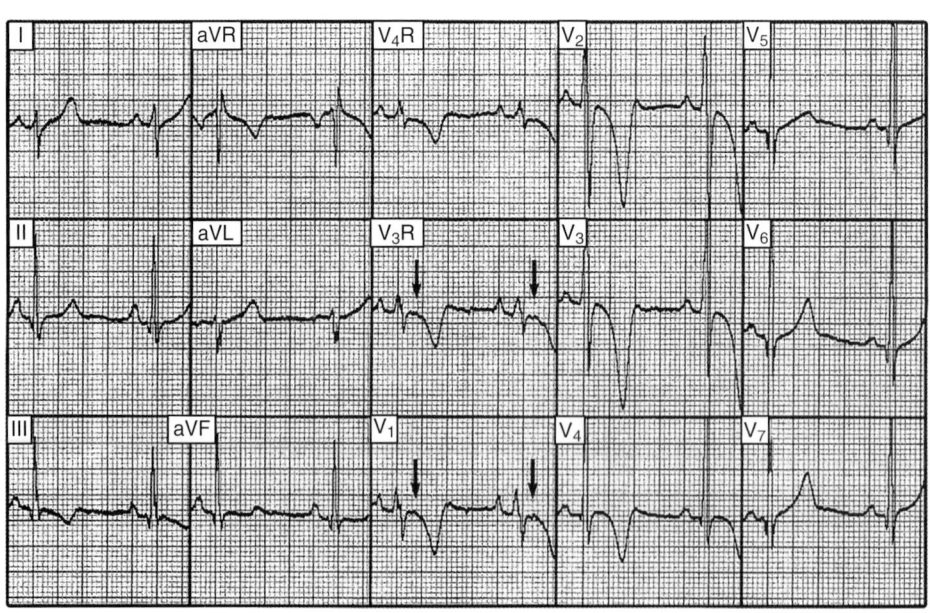

• **Fig. 17.41** ECG from teenager with familial arrhythmogenic right ventricular dysplasia, showing T-wave inversion across the precordium out to lead V3, as well as a sharp epsilon wave in the right precordial leads *(arrows)*.

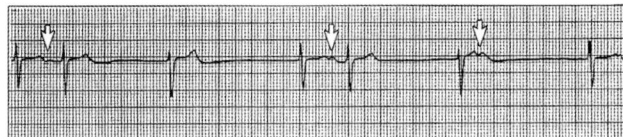

• **Fig. 17.42** Sinus node dysfunction in a patient 10 years after the Mustard operation. The P waves are slow and irregular *(arrows)*, allowing a slow junctional escape rhythm.

defect, is without some risk for SA node dysfunction, although complex atrial baffling procedures such as the Mustard, Senning, and Fontan operations result in the highest incidence. Bradycardia is frequently associated with episodic atrial reentry tachycardia (IART or fibrillation), in which case the clinical label of *tachy-brady syndrome* is applied (Fig. 17.43). The situation may be further complicated by ventricular arrhythmias that can be conditioned by the low rates or arise because of coexistent pathology in ventricular muscle.

Asymptomatic patients with isolated sinus bradycardia of mild–moderate degrees may not require therapy unless there are hemodynamic concerns regarding ventricular contractility or AV valve function. However, any patients with symptoms, profound bradycardia, coexistent tachycardia, or suboptimal hemodynamics should be considered for pacemaker insertion. For those with true tachy-brady syndrome, the simple expedient of correcting bradycardia can reduce atrial tachycardia episodes. If atrial tachycardia episodes remain an issue, suppressive medical therapy or catheter ablation can be considered once the rate is safely supported. In selected patients, a specialized antitachycardia pacemaker can be inserted as therapy for both the brady- and tachy-components of this disorder. Such devices can automatically detect and interrupt IART with short bursts of rapid pacing

in addition to routine antibradycardia function, and may thus eliminate the need for drug therapy in some cases.

Disorders of Atrioventricular Conduction

Abnormalities of AV conduction may involve either the AV node or the proximal His-Purkinje system. They can be subdivided by grades according to the P-QRS relationship on the surface ECG.

First-Degree Atrioventricular Block

In first-degree block, every sinus beat is conducted to the ventricle but with slow conduction velocity that results in a prolonged PR interval on the ECG (Fig. 17.44). Although delay in the AV node proper is the most common cause of first-degree block, intra-atrial delay or His-Purkinje delay may be operative in some cases.

The causes of first-degree block are numerous and include congenital cardiac malformations (atrial septal defects, AV canal defects, congenitally corrected transposition), antiarrhythmic medications, myocardial inflammation or myopathy, infection (Lyme disease, viral myocarditis, endocarditis), hypothyroidism, surgical trauma, and high levels of vagal tone. In general, first-degree AV block is a well-tolerated condition. Management is aimed at identifying any reversible underlying cause, and following the patient closely to be sure the condition does not progress.

Second-Degree Atrioventricular Block

Second-degree block refers to intermittent failure of conduction for a single sinus impulse. It is subclassified as

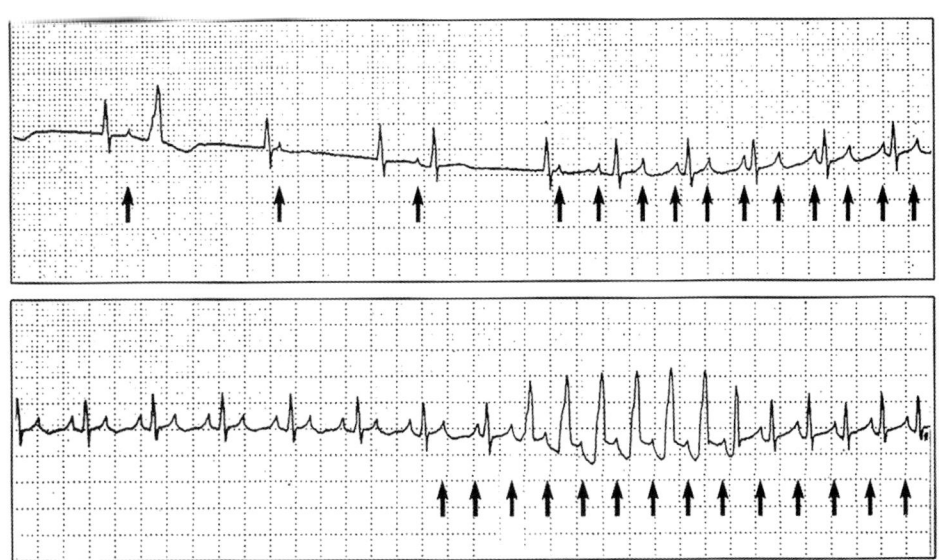

• **Fig. 17.43** Holter monitor recording from a patient with the "tachy-brady syndrome" many years after a Senning operation. The slow rhythm in the upper strip abruptly changes to a rapid, regular atrial rhythm *(arrows)*, which is atrial muscle reentry (intra-atrial reentrant tachycardia). This initially conducts 2:1, but on the lower strip changes to 1:1 conduction. There is transient QRS aberration at the onset of the rapid ventricular response.

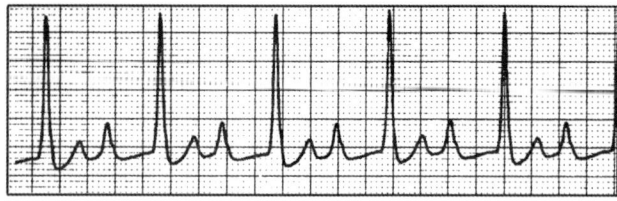

• **Fig. 17.44** First-degree atrioventricular block with a P-R interval of 390 msec.

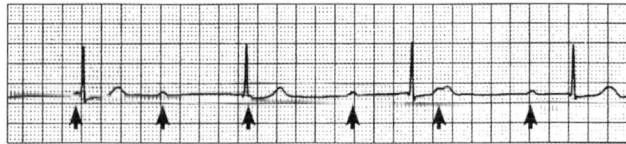

• **Fig. 17.45** Complete heart block showing non-conducted P waves *(arrows)* and a junctional escape rhythm at 37 beats/min.

either the *Mobitz I (Wenckebach)* or *Mobitz II* variety. In the former condition, there is a gradual but progressive increase in the PR interval, culminating in a single non-conducted beat, typically recurring in a sequence that can be described by the ratio of P waves to QRS complexes (2:1 = every other beat blocked, 3:2 = every third beat blocked, etc.). Mobitz I block is usually due to a conduction disorder at the level of the AV node (Fig. 17.5). In Mobitz II block, there is no premonitory conduction delay, but rather an abrupt non-conducted sinus impulse with equal PR intervals for the flanking conducted beats (Fig. 17.5). This disorder usually occurs with disease of the bundle of His and is often associated with a more diffuse disturbance of His-Purkinje conduction, so it is rare to observe true Mobitz II block in a patient without bundle branch block on their ECG.

Mobitz I block is well tolerated and does not always require therapy. It is a normal finding on ambulatory ECG recordings in many healthy adolescents and young adults during sleep. Etiologies are similar to those associated with first-degree block. Although most patients are asymptomatic, in some there may be progression to higher degrees of block, and in rare instances symptomatic bradycardia may also occur. For acute symptoms, treatment with intravenous atropine or isoproterenol usually provides temporary improvement in conduction, but a pacemaker is the safest long-term therapy in symptomatic patients if the underlying cause is not reversible.

Mobitz II block due to His-Purkinje disease is a less predictable situation that usually follows inflammatory or traumatic injury below the level of the AV node. Abrupt progression to complete block may occur in this disorder, necessitating a higher level of concern than with Mobitz I block. Mobitz II block is rare in children. When it occurs as the result of surgical trauma, implantation of a pacemaker is advised.

Third-Degree Atrioventricular Block

In third-degree heart block, electrical communication between the atria and ventricles is completely interrupted. The atria continue to beat at their own rate, while the slower ventricular rhythm is supplied by escape foci in the AV node, His-Purkinje system, or ventricular muscle (Fig. 17.45). The QRS complex is narrow when the escape rhythm arises above the bifurcation of the common His bundle, but will be wide if the escape focus arises lower in

the conducting system or if the patient has concomitant bundle branch block. Third-degree block may be congenital or acquired. The prognosis and therapy vary depending on etiology.

Congenital Complete AV Block

The most common causes of congenital heart block include fetal exposure to maternal antibodies related to connective tissue disease (primarily systemic lupus), and certain congenital cardiac defects (particularly congenitally corrected transposition or AV canal defects). Often, it is first diagnosed *in utero* when a slow fetal pulse is detected on routine obstetrical evaluation. Fetal echocardiography can be performed to rule out structural cardiac defects and to record an M-mode tracing that views simultaneous atrial and ventricular wall motion (Fig. 17.46). Third-degree block is readily diagnosed if the faster atrial motion is completely dissociated from the slow ventricular contraction. If block is seen in the absence of structural defects, maternal testing for antinuclear antibody titers should be performed. It is estimated that as many as 80% of mothers will have serologic evidence of connective tissue disease in this setting.[26] Congenital heart block is usually well tolerated *in utero*, but there are well-described instances of fetal hydrops and even fetal death. Unfortunately, treatment for a distressed fetus is difficult because *in utero* pacing techniques have yet to be perfected. At present, the only recourse for a hydropic infant is early delivery and immediate pacing, but this option is frequently limited by fetal lung immaturity.

In most cases, the fetus adapts to slow heart rates and will usually come to term without difficulty. Delivery should be performed at a high-risk center with pediatric cardiology backup, because abrupt extrauterine decompensation may occur even if the fetus did well *in utero*. Emergency pacemaker placement can stabilize such infants promptly. For

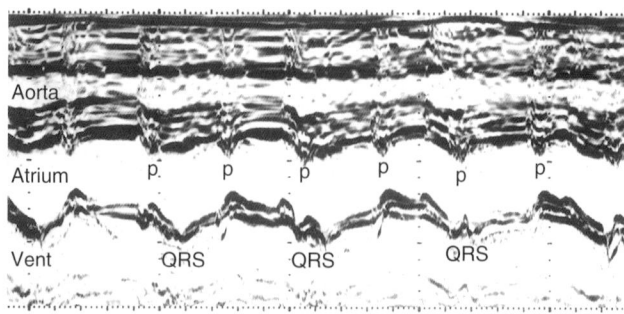

• **Fig. 17.46** M-mode fetal echocardiogram showing complete dissociation of the atrial wall motion *(P)* and ventricular motion *(QRS)* in a fetus with congenital heart block.

the vast majority of newborns with congenital heart block, the transition to extrauterine life is smooth unless complicated by prematurity, lung disease, or anatomic cardiac defects.

Although the short-term prognosis for patients with congenital block is generally good, the long-term outlook is guarded, and most will ultimately require pacemaker insertion. Certainly, any symptomatic patient should be treated promptly with pacing, but pacemaker implant should also be considered in advance of symptoms for patients thought to be at risk for sudden events. Potential risk factors for poor outcome have been sought in multiple studies and include: (1) a resting ventricular rate below 55/min for neonates, (2) a resting ventricular rate below 50/min for older children, (3) prolonged QT interval, (4) wide QRS escape rhythm, (5) ventricular ectopy, and (6) any degree of ventricular dysfunction. It remains uncertain which of these factors is the single best predictor of the need for prophylactic pacer insertion, but given the low risk and high reliability of modern pacer technology, the threshold for recommending the procedure should be low. If none of the above factors are present, it appears reasonable to follow younger patients conservatively if small body size and growth potential could complicate pacemaker implantation and lead maintenance. Ultimately, nearly all patients will likely receive a permanent pacemaker by the time they are fully grown. Even though the prognosis is generally excellent after pacing, some patients can still develop late-onset ventricular dysfunction and require upgrade of their pacing system to a *chronic resynchronization therapy (CRT)* device (see Chapter 19).

Acquired Complete AV Block

The most common etiology for acquired AV block in the pediatric age group is direct injury to the conduction tissues during cardiac surgery or catheterization. In about two-thirds of cases, traumatic AV block is a transient disturbance that needs only to be treated with temporary pacing until normal conduction returns. If improvement is not observed within 10 days, recovery becomes unlikely.

The prognosis for traumatic AV block is poor unless the patient receives a permanent pacemaker. A fatality rate as high as 50% was observed in follow-up of children with postoperative block in the era before pacemaker therapy was routinely available. At present, there does not appear to be any clinical setting where pacemaker implant can be safely deferred for persistent third-degree surgical block.

Complete block can also be acquired from inflammatory processes, metabolic disease, neuromuscular disorders, and infectious diseases (e.g., Lyme disease, viral myocarditis) in the pediatric age group. Unless the block can be reversed by treatment of the underlying cause, pacemaker implant is advisable.

Pharmacologic Therapy for Arrhythmias

The role of antiarrhythmic drugs decreased dramatically following the introduction of catheter ablation and ICD implant. However, medications are still essential tools for rhythm management, especially in the acute setting. Antiarrhythmic drugs are conventionally classified according to their effects on cardiac action potentials, as initially proposed by Vaughan Williams in 1970. As newer agents have been introduced, several variations on the original classification system have emerged[27] to better reflect activity on specific cardiac ion channels. Table 17.2 lists one such updated scheme for the antiarrhythmic formulary. The agents used most frequently in pediatric practice are bold highlighted in the table and are reviewed here with emphasis on cellular effects, indications, and caveats regarding their use

TABLE 17.2 Modified Vaughan Williams Classification of Antiarrhythmic Drugs

	Primary action	Drug
Class 0	*Funny current blocker*	Ivabradine
Class I	*Sodium channel blocker*	*Ia:* **procainamide**, quinidine, disopyramide *Ib:* **lidocaine, mexiletine**, phenytoin *Ic:* **flecainide**, propafenone
Class II	*Autonomically active agents*	*Beta activator:* isoproterenol *Non-selective beta-blocker:* **propranolol, nadolol**, carvedilol, labetalol *B₁-Selective beta-blocker:* **atenolol, esmolol**, metoprolol, bisoprolol *Muscarinic activator:* **digoxin**, pilocarpine *Muscarinic blocker:* atropine *Adenosine receptor activator:* **adenosine** *Adenosine receptor blocker:* aminophylline
Class III	*Potassium channel blocker*	*Nonselective:* **amiodarone**, dronedarone *Selective:* **sotalol**, dofetilide, ibutilide
Class IV	*Calcium channel blocker*	verapamil, diltiazem
Other		Magnesium

in children. Expanded discussion of these topics is available from several comprehensive reviews of antiarrhythmic pharmacology.

We have purposely refrained from making firm dosage recommendations in this chapter, since textbooks are too static to keep up with evolving data. Readers are referred to web-based or hospital-based formularies that are continuously updated with best-practice guidelines for safe administration in the pediatric population. Dosage determinations in young children must be chosen carefully owing to variations in age/size and unique pharmacokinetics, with several agents requiring calculations based on body surface area rather than weight. Furthermore, not all antiarrhythmic drugs are available as a commercial solution or small-dose tablets or capsules. Careful compounding by a trusted pharmacist is frequently needed for young patients, and parents much be coached carefully on proper administration to prevent catastrophic errors. The potential toxicity of the more potent agents demands that these drugs be used with full appreciation of their potential side-effects, including negative inotropy and proarrhythmia.

Class 0. Ivabradine

Ivabradine is a relatively new agent that slows phase 4 depolarization in cells of the sinus node by blocking the inward *funny current*, thereby decreasing the overall sinus rate. It has been used with variable success for inappropriate sinus tachycardia and other automatic supraventricular arrhythmias, including EAT and JET. It is a safe agent without significant negative inotropy and minimal effect on AV node function. It is only available as an oral preparation.

Class Ia: Procainamide

The actions of a class Ia drug involve moderate depression of phase 0 upstroke, a slowing of repolarization, and a prolongation of conduction time in the fast-response cells of atrial muscle, ventricular muscle, His-Purkinje cells, and APs. When these cellular events are translated to the intact heart, the main results are increased duration of the QRS and prolongation of the QT interval in the surface ECG. Procainamide has minimal direct action on slow-response cells in the SA and AV nodes, but may indirectly increase the sinus rate and enhance AV node conduction through anticholinergic side effects. It is administered intravenously as a bolus followed by continuous infusion. Some degree of vasodilation is common during loading and may require volume expansion, but animal models do not demonstrate a direct negative inotropic effect, making it an attractive option for the management of acute postoperative tachycardias. Procainamide is helpful for acute treatment of reentrant arrhythmias involving atrial muscle (e.g., IART or atrial fibrillation), ventricular muscle (e.g., monomorphic VT), and APs (e.g., ORT).

Class Ib: Lidocaine and Mexiletine

The cellular effects of Ib agents are subtle. In therapeutic concentrations, they cause a trivial decrease in the slope of phase 0 of a normal fast-response action potential, although the effect becomes more pronounced under conditions of cell damage, acidosis, or hyperkalemia. In both healthy and injured fast-response cells, the duration of the action potential, and to an even greater degree the refractory period, are shortened. This effect appears primarily in Purkinje fibers and ventricular myocytes and is much less prominent in atrial tissue. Slow-response cells of the normal SA and AV nodes are not affected by Ib agents, and the influence on autonomic tone is negligible. These cellular actions all translate to a surface ECG that is largely unchanged from the pre-drug state, except perhaps for a slight decrease in the QT internal. The Ib drugs are used principally for suppression of ventricular arrhythmias, and can be used safely in the setting of prolonged QT interval.

Lidocaine is the prototype Ib agent. Owing to rapid hepatic metabolism, it is only available for intravenous use as a bolus followed by continuous infusion. Mexiletine is a structural analogue of lidocaine with a prolonged elimination half-life that allows oral administration.

Class Ic: Flecainide

The Ic agents cause marked depression of phase 0 upstroke and profound slowing of conduction in fast-response cells. Their influence on repolarization and action potential duration are minimal, so the refractory period for an individual cell is not typically prolonged. However, in the intact heart, measured effective refractory periods may be increased, particularly in the His-Purkinje system and APs. On the surface ECG, the most notable change is an increase in QRS duration caused by slowing of intraventricular depolarization. The measured QT interval may be prolonged as a consequence of the widened QRS, but the T wave itself is not significantly modified. Some PR prolongation may be seen.

Flecainide is a potent inhibitor of abnormal automaticity and reentry within atrial muscle, ventricular muscle, and APs, but because of its relatively high proarrhythmic potential, use is reserved for patients with good ventricular function, and initiation of therapy usually requires in-hospital monitoring. Flecainide is only available for oral use in the United States. It is highly effective for prevention of tachycardia related to APs (including PJRT), and is used with variable success for atrial arrhythmias such as EAT, IART, and atrial fibrillation. Flecainide has also earned an established role for transplacental management of fetal supraventricular tachyarrhythmias. It is not ordinarily considered a safe agent for treatment of reentrant VT, although it may be quite beneficial in some very specific channelopathic conditions such as CPVT.

Class II: Autonomically Active Drugs

The autonomic nervous system exerts a profound influence on rhythm status, such that modulation of sympathetic and parasympathetic tone is a logical and powerful approach to arrhythmia management. The tools for autonomic modulation are diverse and range from the Valsalva maneuver for interruption of certain forms of SVT, all the way to atropine and isoproterenol for reversal of bradycardia.

Beta-Blockers

The mechanisms by which beta-blockade modifies cardiac arrhythmias are complex. The predominant effect is competitive inhibition of catecholamine binding at cardiac receptors, which reduces both normal and abnormal automaticity and slows AV node conduction. However, direct membrane effects may also occur, including prolonging the duration of the action potential and effective refractory periods, as well as increasing the threshold for VF. These direct cellular actions are most pronounced during chronic administration of moderate to high doses.

Beta-blockers are used to treat a broad spectrum of arrhythmias in children. They are often effective in catecholamine-mediated tachycardias from either abnormal automaticity or triggered activity at both the atrial and ventricular levels. They are less useful for reentry tachycardias but often prove effective if they suppress premature beats that serve as the initiating event for the reentry circuit. Additionally, some forms of reentry SVT may be effectively treated by beta-blockade if the AV node is a necessary part of the circuit and can be sufficiently slowed to prevent rapid conduction.

Propranolol is the prototype beta-blocker. It is *nonselective*, affecting both B_1 (cardiac) and B_2 (bronchial and blood vessel) receptors. Propranolol is commercially available for oral administration in both commercial solution and tablet form. Important limitations include its B_2 blockade properties, which can aggravate reactive airway disease, and its B_1 blockade, which may further depress ventricular function in patients with poor contractility. Nadolol is likewise an oral nonselective beta-blocker that differs from propranolol in requiring less frequent (once daily) dosing.

Esmolol and atenolol are *cardioselective* (B_1 receptor specific) beta-blockers, although some cross-reactivity with B_2 receptors can still occur at high doses. Esmolol is an intravenous agent administered as a bolus followed by continuous infusion. It is unique in its rapid onset and short duration of action, thus lending itself well to emergency management of arrhythmias. Like all other beta-blockers, it is both a negative chronotropic agent and negative inotropic agent. Atenolol is a widely used cardioselective beta-blocker for oral administration in pediatric practice, but must be administered twice daily for optimal effectiveness.

Infants and young children may be prone to hypoglycemia while taking any form of beta-blocker, especially when their regular eating pattern is disturbed. Other non-cardiac side effects may include fatigue and mood disturbances.

Digoxin

Digoxin has some direct electrical effects on the cell membrane, but much of its action at standard doses relates to effects on the autonomic nervous system. The predominant clinical response to this agent (SA-node slowing and depression of AV-node conduction) appears to be due almost exclusively to enhancement of vagal tone. The direct cellular effects on atrial muscle, ventricular muscle, and specialized conduction tissue (including APs) can be best summarized as a mild decrease in the duration of the action potential and shortening of the effective refractory period. The above actions cause predictable changes on the surface ECG that involve mild sinus slowing, slight PR prolongation, and a subtle shortening of the QT interval. Mild depression of the ST segment and flattening of the T wave may occur also.

Digoxin is not considered a very potent antiarrhythmic agent, and is used primarily to slow AV conduction in patients with a primary atrial tachycardia such as IART or fibrillation. More commonly, digoxin is prescribed as adjunctive therapy for heart failure management, typically involving low doses to minimize the chance of toxicity. Recent observations also suggest improved survival when digoxin is prescribed during the interstage period for single ventricle patients, although the precise mechanism behind this beneficial effect is still unclear. Digoxin also has a long history of use in transplacental management of fetal tachycardia where target maternal serum levels need to be at the upper edge of the therapeutic range.

Adenosine

Adenosine is the most familiar antiarrhythmic agent in pediatric practice. It is an endogenous nucleoside found in all cells of the body, but when administered as a rapid intravenous bolus close to the central circulation, it will transiently block AV node conduction and slow SA node automaticity by a direct cellular effect. Adenosine is promptly removed from the circulation by erythrocytes and endothelial cells, resulting in a half-life of less than 10 seconds. It is extremely effective for interrupting narrow QRS tachycardias such as AVNRT and ORT that involve the AV node as part of the circuit. It can also serve as a useful diagnostic agent to transiently block AV nodal conduction and help elucidate the mechanism of certain tachycardias such as IART whenever uncertainty exists. It is an extremely well-tolerated drug. There may be mild hypotension and bradycardia lasting several seconds following a dose, but these effects are of little consequence given such rapid drug elimination. Adenosine may aggravate bronchospasm in patients with reactive airway disease and should be used with caution in this setting. It can also enhance anterograde conduction over APs and should thus never be given to a patient with WPW syndrome who is experiencing a wide QRS tachycardia that might possibly be due to preexcited atrial fibrillation.

Class III: Amiodarone and Sotalol

Drugs that prolong the action potential plateau without affecting phase 0 are grouped in class III. Their dominant electrophysiologic effect is potassium channel blockade, but all class III agents exhibit mixed electrical properties as well as variable effects on the autonomic nervous system.

Amiodarone is the prototype class III agent and is unlike any other antiarrhythmic drug in terms of pharmacokinetics, side effects, and potency. Its electrical effects are felt at all levels of the heart. Most notable is prolongation of action potential duration (and hence refractory period) in all fast-response cells of atrial muscle, ventricular muscle, Purkinje fibers, and APs. Unlike class I agents, it also has direct effects on the SA and AV nodes, decreasing the rate of automatic discharge in the former and slowing conduction in the latter. Amiodarone also possesses alpha- and beta-blocking properties. Widespread changes occur on the ECG, including sinus slowing, PR prolongation, a slight increase in QRS width, and QT prolongation. While real world negative inotropic effects may be mitigated by alpha blockade and vasodilation allowing afterload reduction, animal models show substantial direct negative inotropic effects with intravenous administration, similar to that seen with intravenous sotalol.

Amiodarone is available for both intravenous and oral administration. The intravenous formulation must be used cautiously, especially in infants. Multicenter studies of intravenous amiodarone in children demonstrated a high frequency (>10%) of acute hypotension and cardiovascular collapse. Hemodynamic deterioration is most likely to occur with higher doses, rapid bolus infusion over < 20 minutes, and in patients with borderline hemodynamics at presentation.

Oral amiodarone is very well tolerated from a hemodynamic point of view, and is recognized as one of the few potent antiarrhythmic agents that can be tolerated in patients with poor ventricular function. A major disadvantage of oral administration is the protracted loading phase required before significant drug effect is seen (1–4 weeks).

Serious side effects are possible with either formulation of amiodarone. This drug should not be used for trivial conditions. Proarrhythmia is a concern, as are the multiple noncardiac toxicities, such as corneal microdeposits, thyroid dysfunction, pulmonary interstitial fibrosis, hepatitis, peripheral neuropathy, photosensitive skin rash, and bluish discoloration of the skin. Amiodarone has an elimination half-life longer than 1 month. Thus, steady serum levels are assured with once-daily administration, but drug elimination is very slow should toxicity develop.

Amiodarone is reserved for potentially life-threatening tachyarrhythmia, such as reentrant monomorphic and polymorphic VT, or refractory supraventricular arrhythmias. It also has a second- or third-line role in management of refractory fetal arrhythmias, although the slow onset of action combined with risks of fetal and maternal hypothyroidism limit its use.

Sotalol is the other class III agent in common clinical use. It is available in both oral and intravenous formulations. It acts primarily as a beta-blocker at low doses, but exhibits class III activity at medium-high levels. The oral formulation has proved effective in the treatment of both supraventricular and ventricular arrhythmias in children, although use must be restricted to those with well-preserved ventricular function because of its negative inotropic properties. It also has an established role in transplacental management of fetal supraventricular arrhythmias. Pediatric dosing was studied carefully in 2001 demonstrating that neonates had significantly slower clearance until approximately 9–10 months of age, after which clearance approached adult levels. This has resulted in very rigid dosage guidelines that should be consulted when considering its use in infants.[28]

Intravenous sotalol is now available, but published experience in children is still rather limited. The overall efficacy and safety profile appears to be similar to the oral formulation. Rapid administration can be associated with both exaggerated bradycardia and hypotension.

Class IV: Verapamil and Diltiazem

Verapamil is the most commonly used calcium channel antagonist in pediatric practice. It is available in both oral and intravenous formulations. It acts predominantly on the slow inward current in cells of the SA and AV nodes, causing a decrease in the rate of phase 4 automaticity, a slowing of phase 0 depolarization, and a prolongation of refractoriness and conduction time. Except for a slight decrease in plateau amplitude, its effect on the normal fast-response action potential is negligible. These actions all translate to a surface ECG picture of mild sinus slowing and prolongation of the PR interval, but no noticeable change in the QRS or T wave.

The most common clinical indication for acute intravenous administration is reentry tachycardia that requires the AV node as part of the circuit. Thus, AVNRT and ORT are reasonable indications for this agent. Tachycardia arising from atrial muscle (e.g., EAT, atrial flutter) rarely respond directly to calcium channel blockade, although AV node conduction can be slowed to control the ventricular response rate in such disorders. For idiopathic left ventricular septal tachycardia (Belhassen's VT), the effects of intravenous verapamil in terminating the arrhythmia can be dramatic, although the precise mechanism is still not fully understood.

There are several caveats surrounding the intravenous use of this agent. Most relevant to the pediatric population is the observation that neonates may develop marked hypotension and bradycardia following an intravenous dose. Intravenous verapamil should be avoided in the first 12 months of life, especially now that there are safer alternate techniques for termination of SVT such as adenosine. A second important limitation of verapamil relates to its enhancement of antegrade AP conduction in WPW syndrome. In the setting of preexcited atrial fibrillation, verapamil can increase the ventricular response rate to dangerous levels. Finally, intravenous verapamil should be avoided in patients who are already taking a chronic beta-blocker, due to synergistic negative inotropic effects.

Chronic oral verapamil is used most commonly for tachycardia prevention in patients with AVNRT or ORT due to concealed APs. It is contraindicated in patients with manifest WPW syndrome in the event that atrial fibrillation should occur at some point. It also can be used to manage idiopathic VT in selected patients. In most of these cases, chronic verapamil is employed as a temporary measure while awaiting a suitable time for elective catheter ablation.

Diltiazem is the second most commonly used calcium channel blocker and is available for both oral and intravenous use. Therapeutic considerations are nearly identical to verapamil, except that intravenous diltiazem can be administered as a continuous infusion as opposed to an episodic bolus, making it easier to titrate for rate control in non-preexcited atrial tachycardias such as IART or atrial fibrillation.

Conclusion

Effective arrhythmia management requires a clear understanding of the underlying mechanism, along with appreciation for the risks and benefits of treatment options. This chapter has focused on acute stabilization with an emphasis on ECG diagnosis and pharmacologic therapy. Chapters 18, 19, and 20 will offer a more in-depth discussion of advanced therapies, including transcatheter ablation and implantable devices.

References

1. Walsh EP, Saul JP, Triedman JK, eds. *Cardiac Arrhythmias in Children and Young Adults With Congenital Heart Disease*. Philadelphia: Lippincott Williams & Wilkins; 2001.
2. Blackwell DJ, Schmeckpeper J, Knollmann BC. Animal models to study cardiac arrhythmias. *Circ Res*. 2022;130:1926-1964.
3. Walsh EP, Saul JP, Hulse JE, et al. Transcatheter ablation of ectopic atrial tachycardia in young patients using radiofrequency current. *Circulation*. 1992;86:1138-1146.
4. Salim MA, Case CL, Gillette PC. Chaotic atrial tachycardia in children. *Am Heart J*. 1995;129:831-833.
5. Villain E, Vetter VL, Garcia JM, et al. Evolving concepts in the management of congenital junctional ectopic tachycardia: a multicenter study. *Circulation*. 1990;81:1544-1549.
6. Walsh EP, Saul JP, Sholler GF, et al. Evaluation of a staged treatment protocol for rapid automatic junctional tachycardia after operation for congenital heart disease. *J Am Coll Cardiol*. 1997;29:1046-1053.
7. Sherwin ED, Triedman JK, Walsh EP. Update on interventional electrophysiology in congenital heart disease: evolving solutions for complex hearts. *Circ Arrhythm Electrophysiol*. 2013;6:1032-1040.
8. Meziab O, Marcondes L, Friedman KG, et al. Difference in the prevalence of intracardiac thrombus on the first presentation of atrial fibrillation versus flutter in the pediatric and congenital heart disease population. *J Cardiovasc Electrophysiol*. 2020;31:3243-3250.
9. Sohns C, Nürnberg JH, Hebe J, et al. Catheter ablation for atrial fibrillation in adults with congenital heart disease: lessons learned from more than 10 years following a sequential ablation approach. *JACC Clin Electrophysiol*. 2018;4:733-743.
10. Moore JP, Gallotti RG, Shannon KM, et al. Multicenter outcomes of catheter ablation for atrioventricular reciprocating tachycardia mediated by twin atrioventricular nodes. *JACC Clin Electrophysiol*. 2022;8:322-330.
11. Arruda MS, McClelland JH, Wang X, et al. Development and validation of an ECG algorithm for identifying accessory pathway ablation site in Wolff-Parkinson-White syndrome. *J Cardiovasc Electrophysiol*. 1998;9:2-12.
12. Kugler JD, Danford DA, Deal B, et al. Radiofrequency catheter ablation in children and adolescents: Early results in 572 patients from 24 centers. *N Engl J Med*. 1994;330:1481-1487.
13. Cohen MI, Triedman JK, Cannon BC, et al. PACES/HRS expert consensus statement on the management of the asymptomatic young patient with a Wolff-Parkinson-White pattern. *Heart Rhythm*. 2012;9:1006-1024.
14. Kang KT, Potts JE, Radbill AE, et al. Permanent junctional reciprocating tachycardia in children: a multicenter experience. *Heart Rhythm*. 2014;11:1426-1432.
15. Gandhavadi M, Sternick EB, Jackman WM, Wellens HJJ, Josephson ME. Characterization of the distal insertion of atriofascicular accessory pathways and mechanisms of QRS patterns in atriofascicular antidromic tachycardia. *Heart Rhythm*. 2013;10:1385-1392.
16. Michowitz Y, Belhassen B. New insights on verapamil-sensitive idiopathic left fascicular tachycardia. *J Electrocardiol*. 2018;51:874-878.
17. Van Hare GF, Stanger P. Ventricular tachycardia and accelerated ventricular rhythm presenting in the first month of life. *Am J Cardiol*. 1991;67:42-45.
18. Gharagozloo F, Porter CJ, Tazelaar HD, et al. Multiple myocardial hamartomas causing ventricular tachycardia in young children: combined surgical modification and medical treatment. *Mayo Clin Proc*. 1994;69:262-267.
19. Morwood JG, Triedman JK, Berul CI, et al. Radiofrequency catheter ablation of ventricular tachycardia in children and young adults with congenital heart disease. *Heart Rhythm*. 2004;1:301-308.
20. Priori SG, Napolitano C, Vicentini A. Inherited arrhythmia syndromes: applying the molecular biology and genetic to the clinical management. *J Interv Card Electrophysiol*. 2003;9:93-101.
21. Francis J, Sankar V, Nair VK, Priori SG. Catecholaminergic polymorphic ventricular tachycardia. *Heart Rhythm*. 2005;2:550-554.
22. Marsman EMJ, Postema PG, Remme CA. Brugada syndrome: update and future perspectives. *Heart*. 2022;108:668-675.
23. Atallah J, Gonzalez Corcia MC, Walsh EP, Participating Members of the Pediatric and Congenital Electrophysiology Society. Ventricular arrhythmia and life-threatening events in patients with repaired tetralogy of fallot. *Am J Cardiol*. 2020;132:126-132.
24. Khairy P, Van Hare GF, Balaji S, et al. PACES/HRS expert consensus statement on the recognition and management of arrhythmias in adult congenital heart disease. *Heart Rhythm*. 2014;11:e102-e165.
25. Maron BJ, Rowin EJ, Maron MS. Paradigm of sudden death prevention in hypertrophic cardiomyopathy. *Circ Res*. 2019;125:370-378.
26. Steinberg L. Congenital complete heart block. *Card Electrophysiol Clin*. 2021;13:691-702.
27. Huang CL, Wu L, Jeevaratnam K, Lei M. Update on antiarrhythmic drug pharmacology. *J Cardiovasc Electrophysiol*. 2020;31:579-592.
28. Maghrabi K, Uzun O, Kirsh JA, Balaji S, Von Bergen NH, Sanatani S. Cardiovascular collapse with intravenous amiodarone in children: a multi-center retrospective cohort study. *Pediatr Cardiol*. 2019;40:925-933.

18

Electrophysiology Studies and Transcatheter Ablation

JOHN K. TRIEDMAN AND ELIZABETH DEWITT

KEY LEARNING POINTS

- Electrophysiology (EP) studies with ablation are a primary management strategy for treatment of pediatric arrhythmias due to high success rates and low rate of adverse events.
- Catheter ablation is primarily achieved by targeted thermal injury: heating by radiofrequency energy or freezing with cryothermy.
- EP catheter ablations are performed with minimal fluoroscopy and instead use a variety of methods and technologies

for intracardiac mapping and visualization including electroanatomic mapping, high-density recording, and intracardiac echo.
- The approach to an EP study and ablation, from periprocedural counseling, sedation strategy, vascular access, equipment used, and approach, is highly dependent on the mechanism of arrhythmia and patient-specific factors including age and anatomy.

Introduction

The introduction of transcatheter ablation and the development of both radiofrequency (RF) ablation and cryoablation, in addition to the introduction of electroanatomic mapping, have revolutionized the care of arrhythmias for children and adults with congenital heart disease (CHD). Whereas previously catheter-based electrophysiology studies (EPS) were used primarily for diagnostic purposes and/ or to assess the effect of medical management on inducibility of arrhythmia, they are now a mainstay of therapy in many children with arrhythmias and structurally normal hearts and are a cornerstone of management of arrhythmia in complex CHD.

Historical Experience and Outcomes

Since the introduction of catheter-based RF ablation to pediatrics, the procedure has been remarkably successful. First reports in pediatrics of ablation of accessory pathways (APs) and atrioventricular (AV) nodal reciprocating tachycardias had an acute success rate of 83%.[1] Within a decade, the findings of the Prospective Assessment after Pediatric Cardiac Ablation (PAPCA) trial demonstrated that initial success of ablation of APs and atrioventricular nodal reentrant tachycardia (AVNRT) was between 95% and 98%,

with a rate of AV block reported at 1.3%.[2] In the modern era, the National Cardiovascular Data Registry IMPACT registry (NCDR IMPACT) for pediatric and congenital EPS and ablation demonstrated that the acute success of ablation of AVNRT, concealed or manifest APs remains between 95% and 98%.[3] Ablation for more complex substrates in patients with CHD is more challenging due to the complexity of their anatomic malformations and associated surgical repairs, aberrant location of the normal conduction system, and macroscopic and microscopic fibrosis which may contribute to development of arrhythmia and alter the biophysics of ablation. Nevertheless, ablation is a critically important component of management of these patients.[4,5]

Indications for Electrophysiology Study and Ablation

Indications for EPS and ablation depend on the patient's underlying condition; refractory arrhythmia requiring frequent emergency care, repeated chemical or direct current cardioversion, disruption to activities and decreased quality of life, or desire to avoid long-term suppressive antiarrhythmic medication are common indications. Current guidelines exist from the Pediatric and Adult Congenital Electrophysiology Society (PACES) and Heart Rhythm

Society.[5] The majority of patients coming to the EP lab at Boston Children's Hospital present for evaluation and management of supraventricular tachycardia (SVT). Our informal size threshold for "elective" ablation of Wolff-Parkinson-White (WPW) or SVT is 20–25 kg, with smaller children and infants brought to the lab when medical management alone is insufficient. In older children and teenagers, the safety and efficacy profile of ablation may favor a primary interventional approach as opposed to medical management, though in that circumstance it is important to emphasize in preprocedural counseling that the approach to the case will weigh the arrhythmogenic risk of the substrate versus the anatomical risk of ablation. EPS and ablation of AP-mediated SVT in smaller children with concomitant CHD is sometimes indicated as a preoperative event, in anticipation of loss of simple access to the target site and/or risk of poorly tolerated SVT in the perioperative period (such as for Ebstein anomaly).[6]

Approach to Anesthesia/sedation and Periprocedural Considerations

The anesthetic strategy for EPS and ablation is based on the indication for procedure, patient's age and degree of maturity, and suspected or documented arrhythmia mechanism. General anesthesia is most often used for children undergoing EPS and ablation for reentrant mechanisms such as SVT, WPW, and atrial flutter (AFL). For automatic arrhythmias such as ectopic atrial tachycardia or ventricular premature beats (VPBs), conscious sedation may help ensure that the arrhythmia focus does not extinguish with anesthesia. Heparin is administered after vascular access is obtained, and activated clotted times are checked at least hourly and maintained > 250 seconds for all procedures, and if ablation is performed on the systemic side of the circulation, additional anticoagulation is given after the case.[7] Following the case, patients are admitted to a recovery unit and observed for emergence from anesthesia and

hemostasis, but most patients are able to be discharged the same day.

Equipment

The basic equipment needed to perform EPS and ablation includes an electroanatomic mapping system, additional imaging for catheter localization (typically fluoroscopy), EP recording system, and a cardiac stimulator. For a standard SVT or WPW study, four catheters are placed: a high right atrial mapping/ablation catheter; a His bundle electrogram catheter; a coronary sinus catheter, to provide information regarding the electrical activation of the left heart; and a right ventricular apical catheter to assess RV activation as well as retrograde conduction capabilities. For smaller children, catheters are consolidated to minimize access risks. Arterial access is not typically obtained for most EP studies unless it is required for hemodynamic monitoring or to allow for a retrograde aortic approach to ablation. The typical catheters used for a standard EPS for SVT are summarized in Table 18.1.

Diagnostic Electrophysiology Study

There are three categories of data to be obtained in an EPS: (1) baseline rhythm, (2) functional characteristics, and (3) programmed stimulation with a series of premature beats to initiate tachycardias, as outlined below.

Baseline Rhythm

Resting rhythm is examined to determine conduction times and activation sequence throughout the heart (Fig. 18.1). In normal sinus rhythm, the HRA catheter is the first to register electrical activity by virtue of its close proximity to the sinoatrial node, followed by the low right atrium (first signal on HBE catheter) and then the left atrium on the CS catheter. Conduction time within the AV node may be determined by measuring the *AH interval* of the HBE

TABLE 18.1	Standard Catheter Location and Use for a Four-Wire Electrophysiology Study	
Catheter	**Location**	**Use**
High right atrium/Map	SVC-RA junction or RAA	Assessment of SA and AV nodal function mapping and ablation of arrhythmias
His bundle	Just across tricuspid valve at medial/superior rim	Record atrial, HBE, and RV components; assessment of AV nodal function and AH and HV intervals; evaluation of dual AV nodal physiology
Coronary sinus	Coronary sinus; may require internal jugulation cannulation	Assessment of left-sided atrial and ventricular activation; assessment of latency across CTI in atrial flutter ablations
Right ventricle	RV apex, occasionally RVOT	Assessment of retrograde conduction; evaluation of ventricular arrhythmias and inducibility

AV, Atrioventricular; *CTI*, cavotricuspid isthmus; *HBE*, His bundle electrogram; *RAA*, right atrial appendage; *RV*, right ventricle; *RVOT*, right ventricular outflow tract; *SA*, sinoatrial; *SVC-RA*, superior vena cava- right atrium.

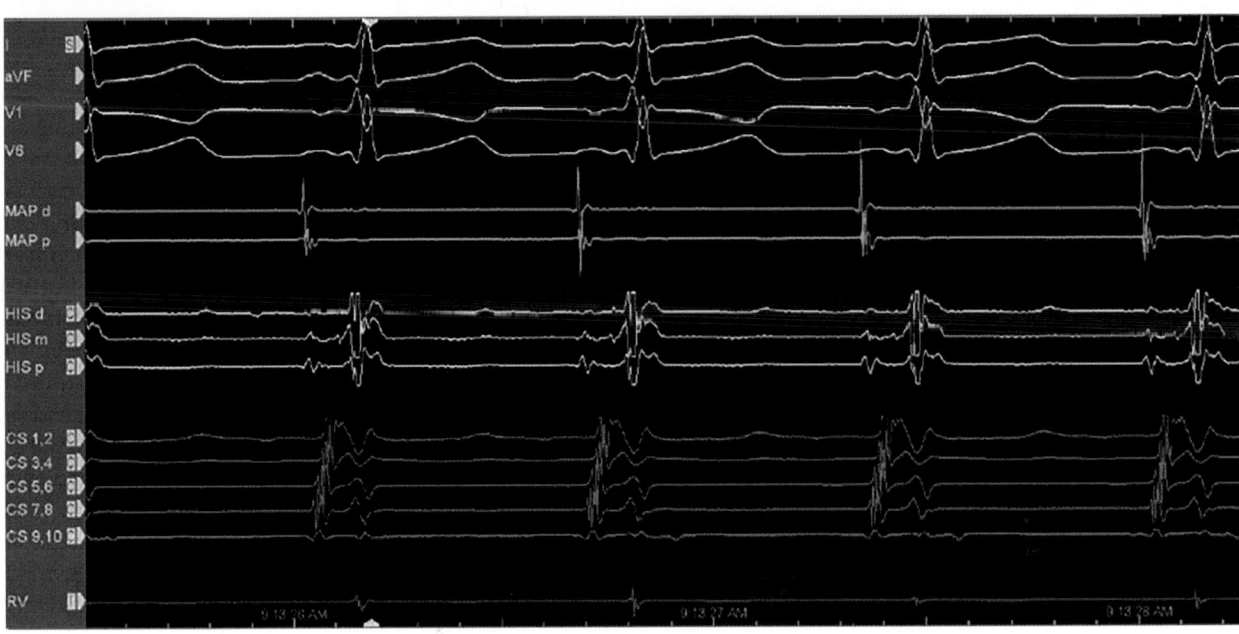

• **Fig. 18.1** Intracardiac tracing of normal sinus rhythm. Standard ECG limb leads are at the top of the slide. *CS,* Coronary sinus; *d,* distal; *m,* mid; *p,* proximal; *RVa,* RV apex.

recording. The normal AH interval varies between 40 and 100 msec in children. The *HV interval,* representing conduction time in the His-Purkinje system, is also recorded by the HBE catheter and should be between 35 and 55 msec in normal children and young adults. Regional ventricular activation times are then assessed. Measurements are indexed against a "V line" at the earliest ventricular activation in any intracardiac or surface lead. In normal activation, the RVA is earliest, ~10 to 35 msec after QRS, with inflow RV (at HBE catheter) and left-sided ventricular signals to follow.

Functional Characteristics

A complete assessment of functional characteristics, as in how the components of the myocardium and specialized conduction system respond to standard pacing maneuvers, will include assessment of the sinus node, the AV node, and atrial and ventricular myocardium. For most children, the most clinically relevant is assessment of the AV node, which will be discussed here. AV nodal conduction is characterized first by single atrial extrastimulus testing (S-AEST) to assess the AH and the HV interval. In AEST, the heart is paced with a drivetrain of typically 8 beats (S1) followed by a progressively earlier beat (S2). The S2 is decreased by 10 ms and the drivetrain is repeated. As the stimulus is moved earlier, a gradual increase in the AH interval is noted. Eventually, a stimulus can be delivered early enough to block at the AV node, defined as the AVN effective refractory period (ERP). AV Wenckebach is also evaluated with atrial pacing at a steady rate (S1) with S1 progressively decreased until there is failure to consistently conduct A to V (AV Wenckebach).

Retrograde AV nodal conduction (V to A) is assessed using single ventricular extrastimuli. Earliest retrograde atrial

activation in the absence of an AP will be on the HBE catheter. Normal retrograde AV nodal conduction is decremental.

The HV interval tends to remain constant with S-AEST, and the QRS complex tends to remain narrow. QRS aberration due to rate-related bundle branch block is sometimes noted in response to early beats, but this is usually a benign finding. Block in the bundle of His with AEST prior to block in the AVN is uncommon in pediatrics and suggestive of His-Purkinje disease.

Cardiac Ablative Technologies

In order to perform an effective cardiac ablation, the electrical activity of an anatomically discrete portion of the myocardium, identified as being critical to the arrhythmia mechanism, must be eliminated or modified. There are several ways in which this could be accomplished, including the use of different forms of energy delivery or locally active drugs or toxins. In current clinical practice, thermal destruction of myocardial tissue is the standard technique used, with catheters available to either heat or freeze tissue. Features relevant to the design of catheters for ablation include their stiffness, both linear and rotational ("torqueability"), and actuation in one or two directions to allow tip flexion and precise mapping and targeting of the myocardium. Typically, ablation is performed during sustained clinical arrhythmia or with pacing maneuvers that engage the arrhythmia substrate so that the therapeutic effect of lesion application can be monitored in real time.

Radiofrequency Ablation

RF ablation causes resistive heating at the contact interface between catheter tip and tissue, which is continuously monitored as impedance. Heat generated at the catheter tip is conducted radially into the myocardium and dissipated by convective heat transfer away from the ablation site by blood flow. Elevation of myocardial temperatures in proximity to the ablation site typically occurs over a period of seconds and is often accompanied by a modest decrease in tissue impedance. Heating results in transient loss of excitability at lower myocardial temperatures, and permanent cellular injury occurs at temperatures of 49°C to 50°C.[8] Cell death is caused by denaturation and coagulation of cellular proteins, and histological examination of RF ablation sites shows a pattern of radial inflammatory necrosis, typically with somewhat ragged edges, infiltration of leukocytes, and ultimate replacement fibrosis. Lesion shape is roughly hemispherical, with convective effects of the blood pool leading to some sparing of endocardial and perivascular tissue.[9]

Regulation of RF application is usually controlled automatically with limits set on power input and temperature measured at the catheter tip. The temperature at the catheter-tissue interface must be kept well below 100°C in order to avoid coagulation or steam formation at the interface, which results in rising impedance and decreased power input; a standard limit derived empirically is 70°C. Conversely, electrical coupling of catheter and tissue, combined with cooling of the ablation site by endocardial blood flow, can result in subendocardial myocardial heating greater than the temperature recorded at the catheter tip. If tissue temperatures exceed 100°C, steam formation can result in "pops" reflecting endocardial and/or epicardial tissue disruption.

Due to the need to control power input within a relatively narrow range to allow for effective electrical coupling, it is often the case that the size of lesions generated by RF ablation can be insufficient in relation to the myocardial substrate to allow for effective ablation. Noting the importance of convective cooling of the catheter tip by the blood pool in determining power input, catheter ablation systems were designed to incorporate internal sources of convection, most commonly as an open system whereby the catheter tip is irrigated with sterile saline to maintain a catheter tip temperature between 30°C and 40°C during ablation. This allows for more efficient power input and a lesion that is larger in size and more deeply centered in the subendocardium.[10]

Cryoablation

The alternative to RF ablation that is currently clinically available is cryoablation. Cryoablation catheters utilize closed refrigerant systems to freeze myocardial tissues, typically achieving catheter tip temperatures of –80°C in 10–20 seconds. While myocardial injury due to freezing is reversible at –30°C, colder temperatures delivered for several minutes result in cell death presumed due to disruption of cellular structures by crystallization. Cryoablation lesions are typically bland and well demarcated compared with RF lesions, and are not typically heavily infiltrated by leukocytes. Cryoablation lesions are similarly subject to the effects of convective heat transfer by blood flow resulting in limitation of lesion size and some sparing of endocardial surfaces and perivascular tissues. In contrast to RF ablation, this is due in cryoablation to the effect of blood flow to rewarm chilled tissue. Lesion size and depth may be dependent in cryoablation on the catheter tip size, with large tips having greater capacity for heat transfer and creating a larger lesion. Additionally, cryoablation is not limited by impedance effects and conditions of low blood flow as RF ablation may be. It also has the advantage in some cases of the property of cryoadhesion (fixation of the catheter by ice during ablation to the underlying tissue), which can be very useful if ablation is to be performed during tachyarrhythmia.[11]

Although both RF ablation and cryoablation create lesions by the physical mechanism of thermal injury, the mechanism of cell death is different in response to heat and cold. There appear to exist different time constants for cellular injury, with RF ablation affecting tissues more rapidly as measured by onset of clinically evident effects. Cryoablation lesions are characterized by relatively slower and more predictable growth, with considerable potential for reversibility of myocardial injury at their advancing edge. This relates to the observation that cell death is avoided altogether at temperatures of –30°C and above, allowing for "cryomapping" using test lesions to avoid injury to critical structures such as the AV node and conversely using time to effect as a marker for accurate targeting of cryolesions such that the arrhythmia substrate is likely to fall within the zone of permanent cellular injury.[12]

There are advantages and applications for both RF ablation and cryoablation in pediatric and congenital EP. For instance, although cryoablation may still be somewhat less effective in long-term ablation cure across all substrates, it is quite remarkable that after extensive clinical use it remains the case that occurrence of inadvertent permanent AV block secondary to cryoablation has not been reported.[13]

A promising experimental technology for catheter ablation called pulsed field ablation is now in advanced clinical trials, and it may open new opportunities for indication-specific use of ablation technology in the near future. Similar to RF ablation, pulsed field ablation uses an electrical field for lesion generation. However, the goal of this high-voltage field is not to generate resistive thermal heating, but instead to cause direct cellular injury and death within the field by membrane electroporation. Differences exist in the dielectric constants of cardiac and extracardiac tissue structures, which may allow for selective targeting of myocardial tissue and avoidance of unintended injury to structures such as the esophagus and epicardial coronary vessels.

Cardiac Mapping Technologies

During ablation, precise and accurate mapping of the targeted arrhythmia substrate is needed, because the dimension of lesions achieved by current methods of ablation is typically quite small and destruction of cardiac tissue not targeted is unnecessary and increases risk of adverse events. Originally catheter ablation was guided entirely by fluoroscopy and signal interpretation, and for large classes of arrhythmia (APs, AVNRT) this approach allowed high rates of procedural success. As interventional EPs have increasingly targeted atrial and ventricular arrhythmias, the need for dense, anatomically accurate and reproducible mapping has increased, as have requirements for precise catheter navigation to allow for construction of complex, confluent linear lesion sets. Since the early 2000s, this has been achieved by electroanatomical mapping (EAM). The primary goals of EAM are: (1) to create an anatomically accurate three-dimensional virtual representation of cardiac structures chambers of interest in real time; (2) to continuously locate EP catheters within that map with high accuracy; and (3) to record, annotate, and display electrical information recorded from catheter electrodes referenced to their locations, and thus provide the user with a map of the myocardial electrical substrate and the activation sequence of the arrhythmia.

Two distinct technologies were developed early on to achieve these goals. One approach used an array of electromagnets to create a reference signal within the patient's thorax that was detected by a dedicated microsensor in the catheter tip, allowing that single point to be located with a very high degree of physical accuracy. The second approach placed an array of skin electrodes, which was used to produce an electrical field within the chest. The measured signal created by this field at different locations within the heart could be processed to determine the relative location of the catheter in multiple axes. In contrast to the first approach, the second could identify the locations of every electrode in the heart simultaneously, but with less physical accuracy due to distortions in the induced fields caused by positioning of the skin electrodes, anatomical variation in thoracic anatomy, and the different electrical properties of thoracic structures other than the heart. The major vendors of EAM platforms now use both of these technologies in a complementary fashion, allowing for well-calibrated, simultaneous, and precise localization of multiple catheters, as they are defined by the positions of their electrodes.

Three additional major advances have considerably enhanced the value of EAM systems as a flexible and effective platform for catheter ablation. The first of these is the advent of multimodal image fusion with EAM. The coordinated presentation of electroanatomical maps with other anatomical imaging allows for the performance of anatomically guided intervention such as antral pulmonary vein isolation in atrial fibrillation, as well as provides an anatomical framework that is complementary to that developed in the process of mapping, and validates it in real time. Adjunct imaging modalities that have been used to enhance mapping include fluoroscopy and cineangiography, cardiac CT, and cardiac MRI. In each case, the key technological issue to be addressed has been the accurate co-registration of the adjunct image with the electroanatomical map so that the

catheter locations depicted in real time are accurately located anatomically. This is achieved with fluoroscopy using digital information derived directly from the fluoroscopy unit, while for CT and MRI images registration is accomplished by use of anatomical landmarks, shape matching algorithms, and manual adjustment when necessary.[14,15]

A second major advance enhancing EAM has been the development of intracardiac echocardiography (ICE), and its digital integration with the mapping system in three dimensions. ICE allows for real-time anatomical visualization of both intracardiac structures of interest for ablation (e.g., pulmonary veins, left atrial appendage, AV grooves), and visualization of EP catheters in relation to these structures, allowing a very precise appreciation of anatomic localization without the need for additional co-registration (Videos 18.1-18.3). ICE can also be used to guide transseptal and transbaffle puncture with a high degree of safety.[15]

A third major advance has been the more recent development of multi-electrode catheter arrays to collect large volumes of data continuously from swaths of the endocardium, markedly enhancing the granular detail of maps which can be created in a short period of time. These arrays can be either grid-like or unstructured (multiple flexible "fronds") and typically have the capacity to record 10–20 bipolar signals simultaneously on a beat-by-beat basis. This requires both considerable signal processing power as well as sophisticated algorithms to reject unreadable signals and quickly and accurately annotate signal activation times in the rest, as well as user interfaces that allow rapid supervision and correction of errors in annotation. These algorithms remain a work in progress but have evolved sufficiently to allow for the rapid acquisition of many thousands of points in each cardiac chamber.

Originally, EAM systems were conceived as a basis for mapping and ablation of complex atrial and ventricular arrhythmias. However, the technology and its use have developed to encompass most ablation procedures, and it is fair to say that EAM has now become the basic platform for ablation procedures, with fluoroscopy now an adjunct imaging modality and many cases being performed without any use of fluoroscopy. The reasons for this are manifold, but certainly include increasing ease of use of the systems and the desire to reduce the use of ionizing radiation in EP procedures in general. Additionally, clinical studies performed in recent years have suggested strongly that outcomes of ablation are favorably affected by the use of EAM.[16,17]

Techniques for Mapping and Ablation of Arrhythmias

Successful application of energy for ablation of tachycardias is contingent on a thorough and specific understanding of the anatomy of the heart and the arrhythmia mechanism, which may be focal or reentrant. Approach is largely dependent on the arrhythmic substrate and will be considered in turn. A full description of techniques of ablation for each of these substrates is beyond the scope of this textbook, but brief descriptions of the general approach for the most common arrhythmia substrates encountered in pediatric and congenital EP are discussed.

Ablation of Reentrant Arrhythmias

Accessory pathways

The precise approach to diagnostic testing, mapping, and ablation for APs depends upon whether a pathway is concealed or manifest and is also influenced by pathway location. Preliminary assessment of antegrade ventricular activation is made in sinus rhythm, as the electrophysiologist may note eccentric ventricular activation in manifest preexcitation. A standard single atrial extrastimulus protocol is then performed. In preexcited patients, this allows for the assessment of accessory pathway effective refractory period (APERP) and shortest preexcited paced cycle length (SPPCL) in addition to the other standard functional assessments. In non-preexcited sinus rhythm, attention should be paid to whether dual AV nodal physiology is also present. Single ventricular extrastimulus testing (VEST) is then performed to assess retrograde pathway conduction. Steady-rate ventricular pacing is performed and adenosine is administered (provided the patient has no significant history of bronchospasm). The VA conduction pattern is observed, with focus on either development of VA block or shifts in the activation pattern that may suggest conduction along single or multiple retrograde pathways.

Often, the next step is attempted to induce SVT with rapid atrial pacing or double or triple AEST. Isoproterenol infusion may be used to increase AV nodal conduction and facilitate arrhythmia induction. In addition to the initiation of SVT, isoproterenol is used to reassess the antegrade conduction properties of manifest APs (APERP, SPPCL-AP) and/or to induce atrial fibrillation to observe pathway conduction (determination of shortest preexcited R-R interval in atrial fibrillation [SPRRI-AF]).

For manifest APs, mapping may be performed in sinus rhythm (targeting the earliest ventricular activation), in SVT, or with ventricular pacing (targeting earliest atrial activation). The latter two strategies are the options for mapping of a concealed AP, wherein mapping targets the earliest atrial activation. Timings are obtained by moving the ablation catheter around the AV groove, seeking a signal with both atrial and ventricular components and a dominant (>2:1) ventricular component. The electroanatomic mapping system is particularly useful for annotating timings to hone in on the precise area of the pathway to facilitate ablation (Fig. 18.2). Once the earliest timing is identified, ablation is performed with the Map catheter to permanently disrupt local electrical conduction across this accessory connection. For septal locations or those close to critical structures (such as coronary arteries), initial mapping may be performed with the EAM-enabled Map catheter prior to switching to a cryoablation catheter for the actual ablation.

Successful ablation of the antegrade component of a manifest AP will be evident by acute loss of preexcitation with ablation. Successful ablation of a concealed AP will be evident by a change in the retrograde activation pattern (abrupt shift to nodal retrograde conduction or VA block), or, if ablating in SVT, by termination of SVT with retrograde block (Fig. 18.3). The latter can produce significant shifts in the cardiac geometry that may lead to movement of the ablation catheter away from the site of success, and can be mitigated by overdrive ventricular pacing once SVT terminates to maintain similar cardiac-catheter relationships. Additional consolidation lesions are placed if safe to do so, with a target of at least 90 seconds of energy at an effective location.[18]

Atrioventricular Nodal Reciprocating Tachycardia

Diagnosis of AVNRT during EPS is made starting with the standard maneuvers as described above. Dual AV nodal physiology, or the presence of both a fast pathway and a slow pathway, is defined as an AH interval "jump" of > 50 ms during S-AEST with a decrease in S2 of 10 ms. Further evidence of dual AV nodal physiology may be demonstrated with steady-rate atrial pacing in which sustained slow pathway conduction, defined as an AH interval > R-R interval, is seen prior to encountering AV Wenckebach. With VEST, retrograde conduction will be midline and decremental, with no shift in VA conduction. In the absence of a concomitant retrograde AP, VA block will typically be seen with administration of adenosine with steady-rate ventricular pacing. Isoproterenol infusion is used to induce AVNRT if it has not been induced, and additional maneuvers (beyond the scope of this text) performed to confirm the mechanism prior to ablation (Fig. 18.4).

Ablation of AVNRT is accomplished by empiric ablation in a standard location in the posterior right AV septum where the slow pathway component of the AV node is most often located. Unlike pathway ablation, where the timings of atrial or ventricular activation are used to infer the precise location of the AP, ablation of AVNRT uses an anatomically guided approach. Rarely, a slow pathway potential may be present, which is a high-frequency signal similar to an HBE but lower in the septum, but this is the exception rather than the rule. With RF ablation in the region of the slow pathway, heat generates junctional automaticity, which, if not excessively rapid, may serve as feedback that the location is likely to be successful. However, care is needed to ensure this feedback is not a sign of excessive injury to the fast pathway. Many centers exclusively employ cryoablation for ablation of AVNRT, which allows for assessment of the AVN function with pacing maneuvers while cryoablation is applied to ensure no damage is incurred. Empiric ablation is continued until it is determined that adequate ablation has been performed, which relies on the reassessment of whether dual AV nodal physiology has been eliminated and whether AVNRT remains inducible.

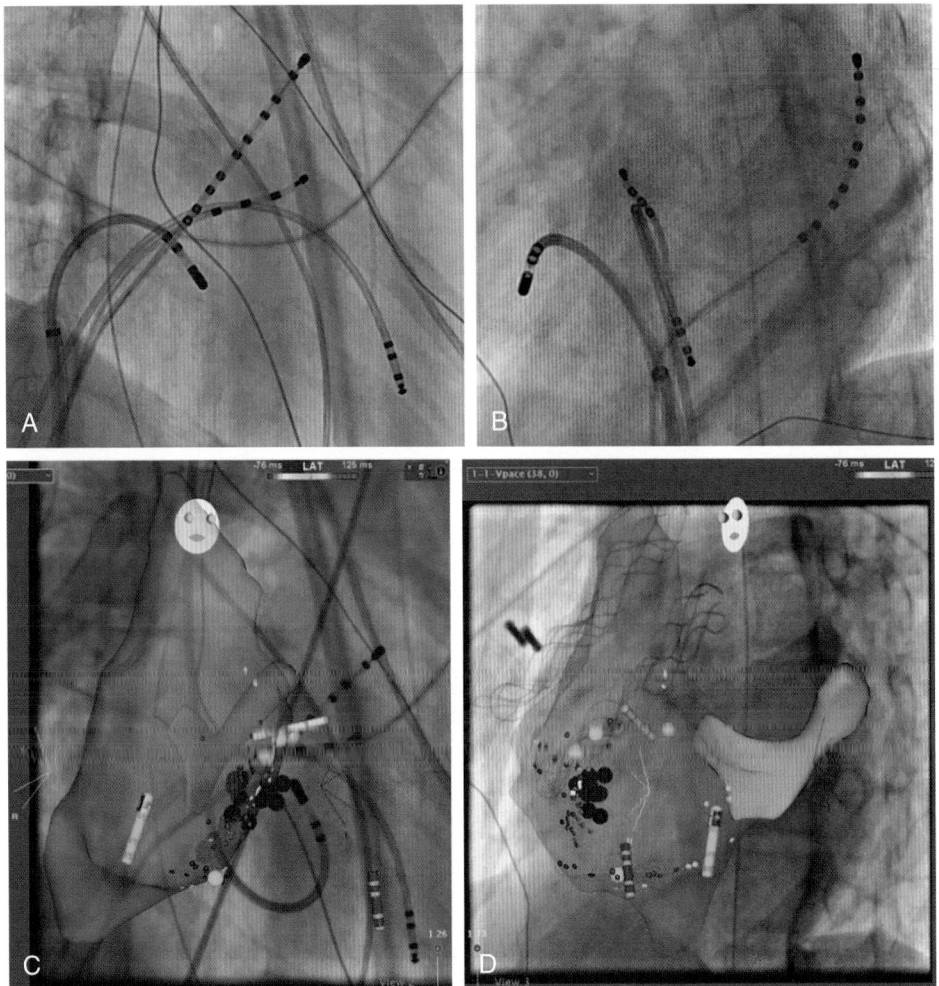

• **Fig. 18.2** Comparison of fluoroscopy and electroanatomic mapping with Biosense Webster Carto 3 Uniview integration. **(A)** Right anterior oblique (RAO) 30 view of standard catheters. **(B)** Left anterior oblique (LAO) 60, caudal 15. The decapolar catheter is in the coronary sinus, with quadripolar catheters at the His and in the RV apex. The Map catheter is on the lateral tricuspid valve annulus from an IVC approach. **(C)** Complimentary RAO view with the electroanatomic shell of the RA and CS. **(D)** The LAO view. In (C), the ablation catheter is seen by fluoro advanced from an SVC approach to achieve ablation. Ablation locations are marked with red dots.

Atrial Flutter and Intra-Atrial Reentrant Tachycardias

As discussed in Chapter 17, macroreentrant atrial tachycardias are independent of the AV node, and include AFL and intra-atrial reentrant tachycardia (IART). Both AFL and IART are more common in adolescents and adults with CHD. Knowledge of the underlying anatomy, the operative details and timing of the surgical repair, and adequate up-to-date imaging, focusing on atrial size and anatomy of any atrial baffles, is essential to effective ablation of these arrhythmias. Despite the potential for complexity, in a large majority of these patients, their macroreentrant atrial circuit will involve the cavotricuspid isthmus (CTI) (or cavomitral isthmus), and while it is prudent to prepare for a more complicated circuit or multiple circuits, effective ablation and termination of tachycardia can often be achieved by ablating across the

CTI. In our own experience at Boston Children's Hospital, in patients with IART/AFL with a two-ventricle repair, 77% of patients taken for ablation had CTI-dependent flutter alone, suggesting that a primary ablative strategy may be a reasonable approach to management (unpublished data).

Diagnosis will often have been made previously due to documented tachycardia or presentation requiring cardioversion back to sinus rhythm. Assuming the patient arrives to the lab in sinus rhythm, rapid atrial pacing or atrial extrastimuli are used to induce the arrhythmia. The induced arrhythmia and ensuing flutter waves are then compared with an ECG of the clinical tachycardia, both in cycle length and morphology/axis, and if consistent, mapping is then performed. In patients with robust AV nodal conduction, infusion of intravenous diltiazem may be needed to allow for stable hemodynamics while extensive mapping is performed. EAM, high-density catheters, and multimodal

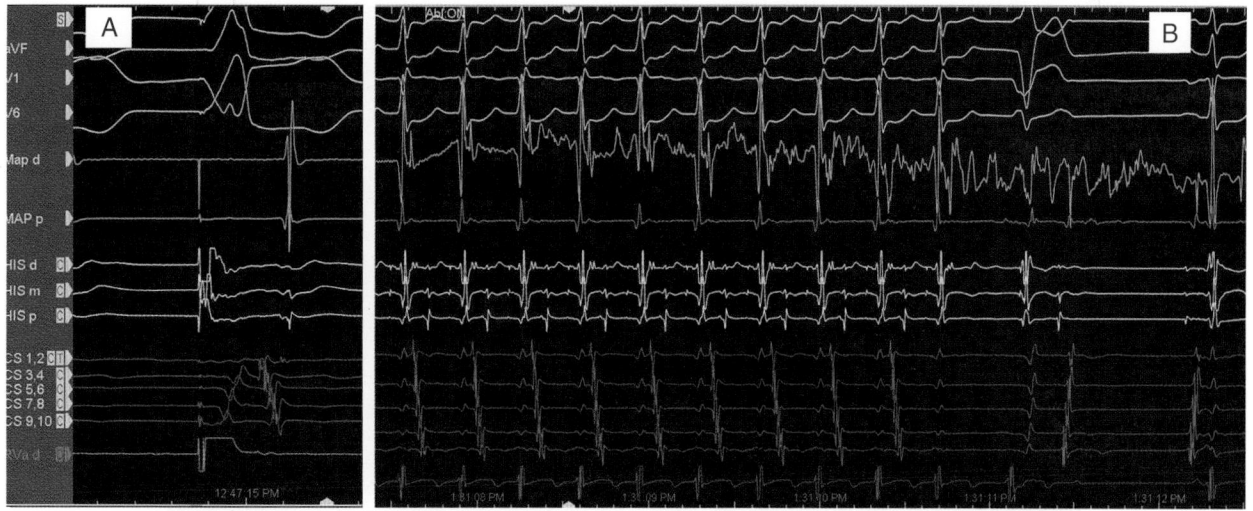

• **Fig. 18.3** **(A)** Assessment of retrograde conduction with ventricular pacing from the RV apical catheter *(RVa)* demonstrates eccentric retrograde conduction, with earliest atrial activation on the distal CS catheter, suggestive of a left-sided accessory pathway. **(B)** Ablation was performed in SVT, with earliest atrial activation noted on the ablation catheter *(Map, green)*. Tachycardiac terminates with a V, suggesting retrograde block has been achieved. On the next ventricular beat, the retrograde pattern has shifted to an earliest A on the His catheter.

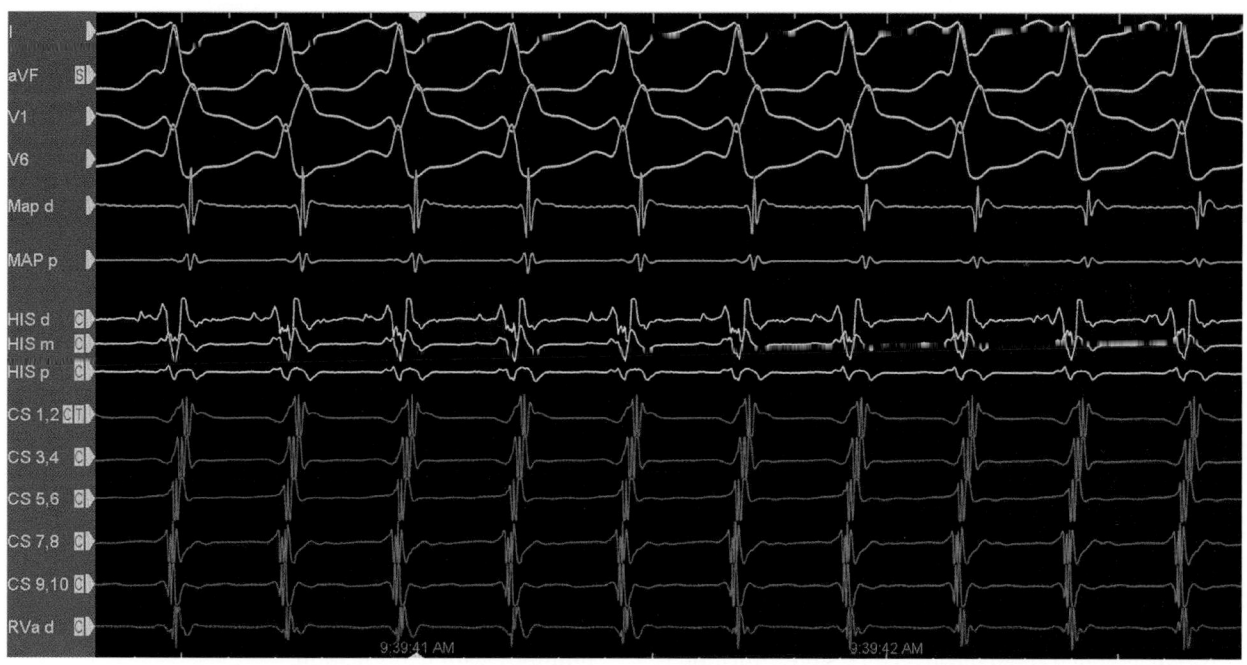

• **Fig. 18.4** Intracardiac tracing of atrioventricular nodal reentrant tachycardia. Note the short VA interval with nearly superimposed atrial and ventricular activation. Standard ECG limb leads are at the top of the slide. *CS,* Coronary sinus; *d,* distal; *m,* mid; *p,* proximal; *RVa,* RV apex.

imaging, as well as intracardiac echo, are essential to efficient and effective ablation in these patients. Endpoints of successful ablation will typically include slowing of atrial cycle length and termination with ablation. Latency may be assessed across the CTI for isthmus-dependent flutters after ablation to demonstrate that effective block has been achieved (Fig. 18.5).

Ectopic Atrial Tachycardia

Ablation of automatic arrhythmias with a focal origin, such as EAT, is conceptually simple. Because the electrical activation of the heart spreads radially from a focal source, the process of identifying a suitable target for ablation involves systematic sampling of electrical activation of the heart

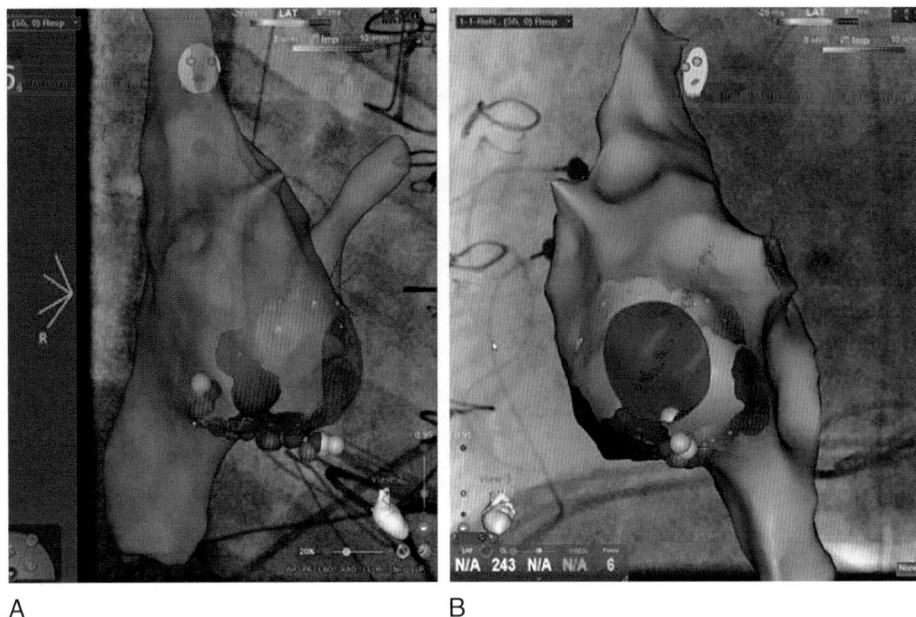

A   B

• **Fig. 18.5** Repaired tetralogy of Fallot with second-degree atrioventricular block, epicardial pacemaker, and atrial flutter. RAO view **(A)** and LAO/caudal **(B)** demonstrates the tricuspid valve annulus with a line of ablation lesions across the cavotricuspid isthmus and electroanatomic map demonstrating block across the isthmus when pacing from the coronary sinus with activation now in the counterclockwise direction.

during the rhythm. The earliest site of electrical activation corresponds to the origin of the abnormal rhythm, and ablation at that site typically results in termination of the tachycardia. This can be done with point-by-point mapping using an ablation catheter, or can be performed with high-density mapping catheters as described for AFL/IART. One of the most challenging aspects of these ablations is the sedation strategy, as in some circumstances automatic tachycardias of this nature may become quiescent as soon as anesthesia is initiated.

Ventricular Premature Beats

Similar to ectopic atrial tachycardia ablation (described above), ablation of VPBs relies upon having spontaneous ectopy for ablation, which is often best accomplished with a strategy of conscious sedation. Spontaneous clinical VPBs can be stored in the EAM system to allow for comparison with pace mapping if spontaneous ectopy stops. Ablation is again performed by seeking the region of the earliest endocardial activation on a mapped VPB. The use of unipolar electrograms to determine source may be helpful to target the earliest activation. As with EAT, with ablation the ectopic source may have transient automaticity prior to extinguishing (Fig. 18.6).

Evaluation of Ventricular Arrhythmias

The use of ventricular stimulation studies has evolved over the decades of interventional EP, with common indications currently including: (1) to assess for inducible ventricular arrhythmias in adult patients with CHD to risk stratify for ICD implantation; (2) to assess preoperative or postoperative risk of ventricular tachycardia (VT) in patients with Ebstein anomaly[6]; and (3) to assess inducibility of arrhythmia after resection of cardiac tumors for risk stratification for ICD implantation.

Protocols for ventricular stimulation vary, and it must be remembered that a point can be reached at which the stimulation becomes so provocative that an induced arrhythmia is nonspecific and bears little resemblance to the clinical tachycardia. At our center, ventricular stimulation studies usually involve the protocol demonstrated in Fig. 18.7. Whenever sustained arrhythmias are induced and result in hemodynamic compromise, the team must react quickly to terminate the condition. For monomorphic VT, this can often be accomplished with a short burst of overdrive pacing in the ventricle, but rapid polymorphic VT or ventricular fibrillation needs to be terminated promptly with defibrillation.

Complications of Electrophysiology Study and Ablation

Overall, in pediatric EP adverse outcomes must be held to a very low level, as risk tolerance in pediatrics is in general very low, post-procedure life expectancy is long, and the majority of ablations performed in this age group are for nonlethal conditions such as SVT. Complications of EPS and ablation can be broadly divided into four categories: direct unwanted damage or injury to the structures of the

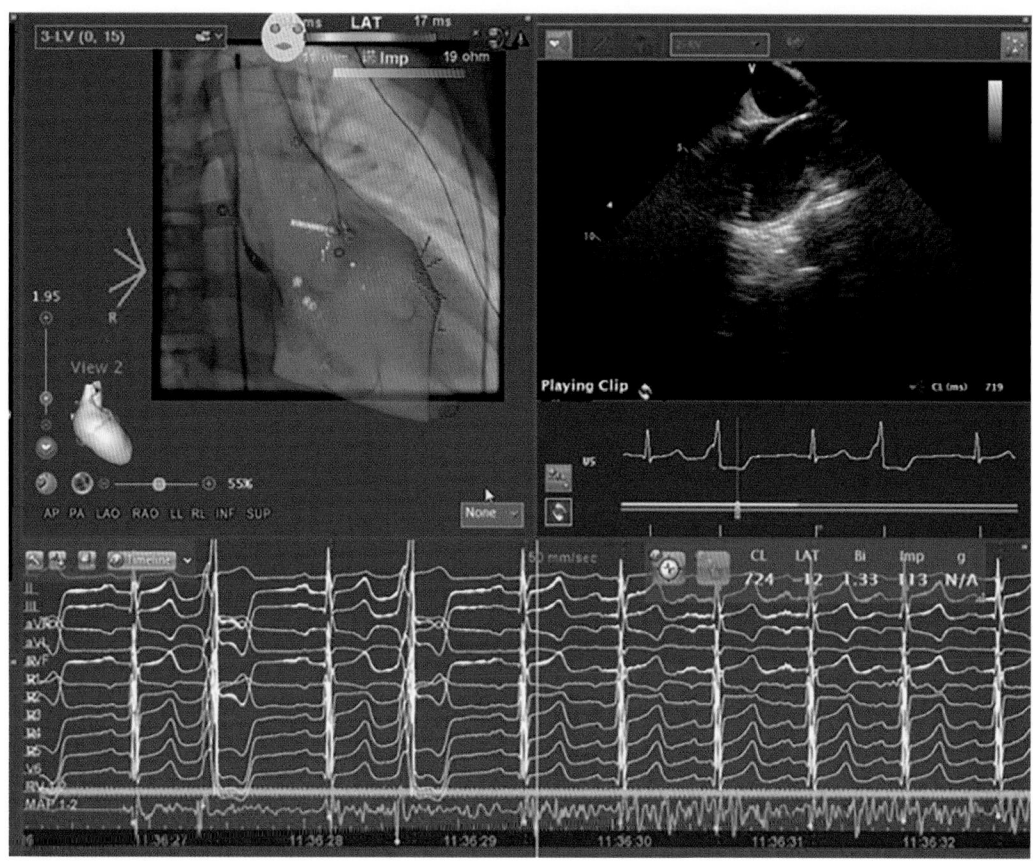

• **Fig. 18.6** Comparison of electroanatomic mapping image with intracardiac echo image demonstrating ablation catheter in the non-coronary cusp of PVC focus in a patient with history of D-TGA with arterial switch as a neonate. Intracardiac echocardiography allows for visualization of distance of the catheter from the coronaries. With ablation, PVCs extinguish as seen in bottom portion of slide.

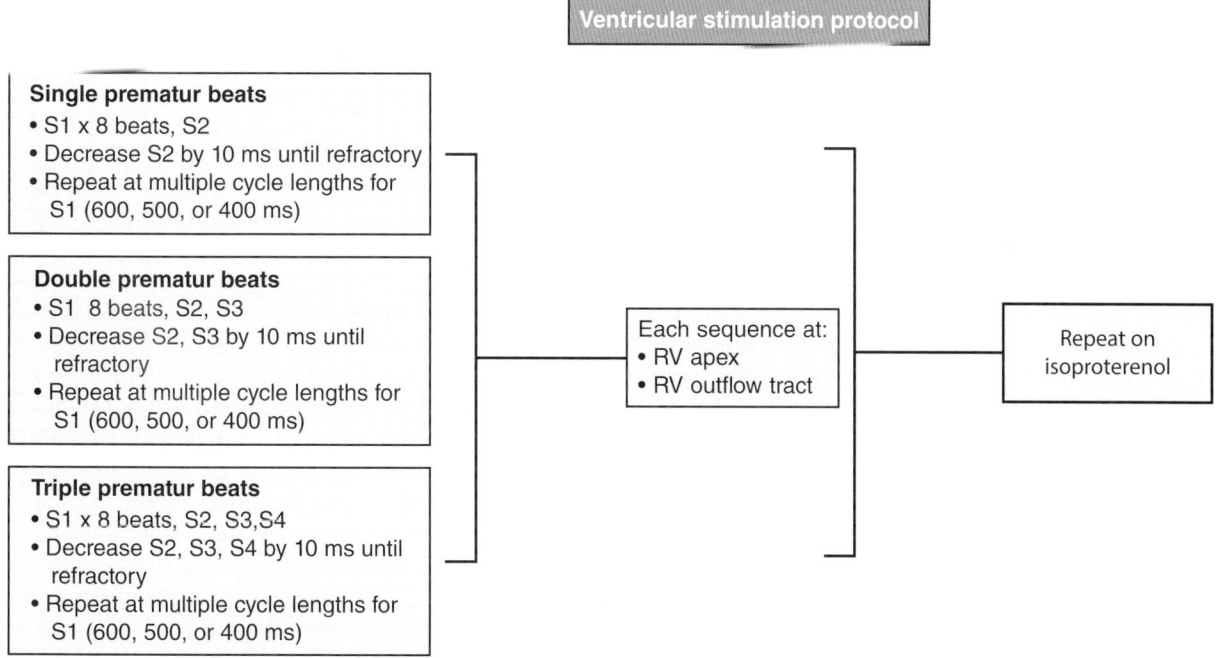

Ventricular stimulation protocol

Single prematur beats
• S1 x 8 beats, S2
• Decrease S2 by 10 ms until refractory
• Repeat at multiple cycle lengths for S1 (600, 500, or 400 ms)

Double prematur beats
• S1 8 beats, S2, S3
• Decrease S2, S3 by 10 ms until refractory
• Repeat at multiple cycle lengths for S1 (600, 500, or 400 ms)

Triple prematur beats
• S1 x 8 beats, S2, S3,S4
• Decrease S2, S3, S4 by 10 ms until refractory
• Repeat at multiple cycle lengths for S1 (600, 500, or 400 ms)

Each sequence at:
• RV apex
• RV outflow tract

Repeat on isoproterenol

• **Fig. 18.7** One example of a ventricular stimulation protocol, versions of which may be employed in the assessment of inducible ventricular arrhythmias/risk of clinical ventricular arrhythmia.

heart, injury to noncardiac structures secondary to direct or indirect effects of ablation, peripheral injuries related to vascular access, and inadvertent creation of proarrhythmic state by ablation. Risk and incidence of adverse outcomes of ablation are importantly dependent in pediatric patients on patient age and body size.

Direct Ablation-Related Injury

By far, the most common major adverse outcome encountered in pediatric ablation is injury to the AV node resulting in AV block. In early registry series, the incidence of AV block for all pediatric ablations was understood to be 1%–2%, but modern data and institutional experience suggest that with current technology and expertise the occurrence of unintended complete AV block attributable to ablation is much lower, in the range of 0.25% from 2010 to 2020 at Boston Children's Hospital.[19,20] The principle risk factor for procedural AV block is location of the ablation substrate, typically an AP, in the midseptal or anteroseptal location, despite the use of a variety of diagnostic and ablative techniques to mitigate this risk. Interestingly, use of cryoablation has never been reported as a cause of permanent complete AV block, and offers certain other advantages, such as cryoadhesion of the catheter tip to underlying tissue, that favor it for use in these ablation sites. It is important to recognize that AV block of varying degrees is a relatively commonly seen phenomenon during ablation of septal arrhythmias. While emergence of AV block during ablation is almost always an indication to stop ablation, in the vast majority of cases the immediate effects of ablation are transient and AV conduction normalizes within seconds to minutes.

Other well-recognized types of direct cardiac injury include cardiac perforation, injury to coronary vessels and pulmonary veins, and damage to indwelling pacemaker leads. Cardiac perforation can occur from EP catheters directly, but is more commonly seen during transseptal puncture, and usually results in pericardial effusion. Injury to epicardial coronary vessels, presumably caused by extension of the ablation lesion into the vascular walls resulting in inflammation and stenosis, has been reported principally with ablations performed in the ostium of the coronary sinus. In this area, the catheter tip may be in close proximity to the distal right coronary artery, and that proximity has been related to the likelihood of vascular injury.[21] Pulmonary veins also are prone to acquired stenosis and atresia after ablation, although there is likely an important role played by the application of multiple lesions in linear circumferential arrays as was done initially in pulmonary vein isolation, when this complication was frequently reported. Alteration of pulmonary vein isolation techniques to locate circumferential lesions in the pulmonary venous antral region has reduced this adverse event, but in pediatric EP it is not rare to encounter an ectopic atrial tachycardia focus arising from a pulmonary vein. Finally, we have noted, and it has anecdotally been reported, that ablation poses a risk to indwelling pacemaker leads, with the possibility of lead dislodgement as well as creation of lead exit block if a lesion extends into the capture "footprint" of an indwelling lead.

Injury to Noncardiac Structures Attributable to Ablation

In general, the thermal effects of ablation are sufficiently limited in dimension that direct extracardiac effects of catheter ablation are rare. The notable exception to this is the rare but catastrophic occurrence of atrioesophageal fistula secondary to more common esophageal injuries caused by ablation of atrial fibrillation. This is because of the proximity of the posterior left atrial wall to the esophagus, and it has prompted many modifications of technique and monitoring that have reduced its prevalence. It is also hoped that advances in ablation technology such as pulsed field array ablation described above may further improve the safety profile of ablation in this anatomical area.[22]

An indirect consequence of ablation is the risk of thromboembolism after ablation. This is presumably due to direct platelet-activating and thrombogenic effects of ablation on the endocardium. The risk of thromboembolic stroke after ablation is thought to be < 1:2000 cases, although anecdotally the occurrence of migraine and transient neurological findings post procedure are likely considerably higher. Given that left-sided, subarterial ablation is an identified risk factor for this adverse event, it is common practice to fully anticoagulate patients undergoing ablation of left-sided structures with monitoring of activated clotting times, either at the beginning of the case or immediately after transseptal puncture. (It should also be noted that many centers, including Boston Children's Hospital, use procedural anticoagulation at the start of all intracardiac EP studies.)

Injuries Related to Vascular Access

Procedural complications to vascular access points are generally not as likely to be life-threatening or irreversible as some of the cardiac adverse events noted above, and most cases of postprocedural bleeding from access can be managed with simple observation. Careful and judicious use of percutaneous vascular closure devices has likely reduced the frequency of postprocedural bleeds and certainly allows for a shortened period of postprocedural observation prior to discharge. However, more serious complications, while uncommon, are not rare and can require careful attention and high index of suspicion to diagnose and treat them. Particular attention must be given to the possibility of retroperitoneal bleeding in patients with back pain, falling hematocrit, and tachycardia in the early post-ablation period. A second uncommon but treatable complication of the late post-procedure period is the development of femoral artery pseudoaneurysm at the site of vascular puncture in patients who have undergone retrograde arterial catheter placement.

Proarrhythmic Complications of Catheter Ablation

An uncommon complication of ablation in children is paradoxical proarrhythmic effect. This typically results from incomplete ablation of a targeted arrhythmia substrate. Recurrence or persistence of slowed conduction in a segment of an arrhythmia circuit affected by intentional or inadvertent ablation, such as an AP or the AV node complex, may slow the cycle length of tachycardia sufficiently to cause a tachycardia that had been paroxysmal to become incessant. It is not thought that ablation has the potential to cause de novo ectopic arrhythmia, but extensive ablation may sometimes result in increased ectopy post-ablation. Similarly, modest acceleration of junctional rhythm may be observed after slow pathway modification for AVNRT. Post-ablation tachycardias may be problematic for management and provoke considerable anxiety, but although some will require additional ablation or medical management, the majority have a transient course.

References

1. Kugler JD, Danford DA, Deal BJ, et al. Radiofrequency catheter ablation for tachyarrhythmias in children and adolescents. *N Engl J Med.* 1994;330:1481-1487.

2. van Hare GF, Carmelli D, Smith WM, et al. Prospective assessment after pediatric cardiac ablation: design and implementation of the multicenter study. *Pacing Clin Electrophysiol.* 2002;25:332-341.

3. Dubin AM, Jorgensen NW, Radbill AE, et al. What have we learned in the last 20 years? A comparison of a modern era pediatric and congenital catheter ablation registry to previous pediatric ablation registries. *Heart Rhythm.* 2019;16:57-63.

4. Hernández-Madrid A, Paul T, Abrams D, et al. Arrhythmias in congenital heart disease: a position paper of the European Heart Rhythm Association (EHRA), Association for European Paediatric and Congenital Cardiology (AEPC), and the European Society of Cardiology (ESC) Working Group on Grown-up Congenital heart disease, endorsed by HRS, PACES, APHRS, and SOLAECE. *Europace.* 2018;20:1719-1720.

5. Philip Saul J, Kanter RJ, Abrams D, et al. PACES/HRS expert consensus statement on the use of catheter ablation in children and patients with congenital heart disease: developed in partnership with the Pediatric and Congenital Electrophysiology Society (PACES) and the Heart Rhythm Society (HRS)Endorsed by the governing bodies of PACES, HRS, the American Academy of Pediatrics (AAP), the American Heart Association (AHA), and the Association for European Pediatric and Congenital Cardiology (AEPC). *Heart Rhythm.* 2016;13:e251-e289.

6. Shivapour JKL, Sherwin ED, Alexander ME, et al. Utility of preoperative electrophysiologic studies in patients with Ebstein's anomaly undergoing the Cone procedure. *Heart Rhythm.* 2014;11:182-186.

7. Hinsley K, Evans-Langhorst M, Porter C, et al. Low molecular weight heparin as an anticoagulation strategy for left-sided ablation procedures. *Congenit Heart Dis.* 2018;13:222-225.

8. Wood M, Goldberg S, Lau M, et al. Direct measurement of the lethal isotherm for radiofrequency ablation of myocardial tissue. *Circ Arrhythm Electrophysiol.* 2011;4:373-378.

9. Glashan CA, Stevenson W, Zeppenfeld K. Lesion size and lesion maturation after radiofrequency catheter ablation for ventricular tachycardia in humans with nonischemic cardiomyopathy. *Circ Arrhythm Electrophysiol.* 2021;14:e009808.

10. Mehta N, Morgaenko K, Sauer W, et al. Impact of variable orientation and flow rates on radiofrequency ablation lesions created by externally irrigated catheters: an ex-vivo study. *J Atr Fibrillation.* 2020;13:2353.

11. Erinjeri JP, Clark TWI. Cryoablation: mechanism of action and devices. *J Vasc Interv Radiol.* 2010;21:S187-S191.

12. Eryazici PLS, Razminia M, D'silva O, et al. Time-limited cryomapping during tachycardia: improved long-term outcomes for cryoablation of AVNRT. *J Interv Card Electrophysiol.* 2016;47:125-131.

13. Wells P, Dubuc M, Klein GJ, et al. Intracardiac ablation for atrioventricular nodal reentry tachycardia using a 6 mm distal electrode cryoablation catheter: prospective, multicenter, North American study (ICY-AVNRT STUDY). *J Cardiovasc Electrophysiol.* 2018;29:167-176.

14. Njeim M, Desjardins B, Bogun F. Multimodality imaging for guiding EP ablation procedures. *JACC Cardiovasc Imaging.* 2016;9:873-886.

15. Restrepo AJ, Dickfeld TM. Image integration using intracardiac echography and three-dimensional reconstruction for mapping and ablation of atrial and ventricular arrhythmias. *Card Electrophysiol Clin.* 2021;13:365-380.

16. Bigelow AM, Smith PC, Timberlake DT, et al. Procedural outcomes of fluoroless catheter ablation outside the traditional catheterization lab. *Europace.* 2017;19:1378-1384.

17. Debreceni D, Janosi K, Vamos M, et al. Zero and minimal fluoroscopic approaches during ablation of supraventricular tachycardias: a systematic review and meta-analysis. *Front Cardiovasc Med.* 2022;9:856145.

18. Dionne A, Gauvreau K, O'Leary E, et al. Risk factors for early recurrence following ablation for accessory pathways: the role of consolidation lesions. *Circ Arrhythm Electrophysiol.* 2020;13:8848.

19. Kugler JD, Danford DA, Houston KA, et al. Pediatric radiofrequency catheter ablation registry success, fluoroscopy time, and complication rate for supraventricular tachycardia: comparison of early and recent eras. *J Cardiovasc Electrophysiol.* 2002;13:336-341.

20. Krause U, Paul T, Bella P della, et al. Pediatric catheter ablation at the beginning of the 21st century: results from the European Multicenter Pediatric Catheter Ablation Registry "EUROPA". *Europace.* 2021;23:431-440.

21. Schneider HE, Stahl M, Schillinger W, et al. Double cryoenergy application (freeze-thaw-freeze) at growing myocardium: lesion volume and effects on coronary arteries late after energy application. Implications for efficacy and safety in pediatric patients. *J Cardiovasc Electrophysiol.* 2019;30:1127-1134.

22. Assis FR, Shah R, Narasimhan B, et al. Esophageal injury associated with catheter ablation for atrial fibrillation: determinants of risk and protective strategies. *J Cardiovasc Electrophysiol.* 2020;31:1364-1376.

19

Pacemakers and Anti-Tachycardia Devices

EDWARD T. O'LEARY AND DOUGLAS Y. MAH

KEY LEARNING POINTS

- Learn what components make up a pacemaker or defibrillator, and how they can be implanted epicardially or endocardially.
- Introduce how pacemakers or defibrillators are programmed.

- Understand when a pacemaker or defibrillator is indicated in the pediatric and congenital heart disease population.
- Learn about the complications that can occur with implanted cardiac rhythm devices.

Pacemakers

Pacemakers are important tools in the treatment of bradycardia. They include: (1) a generator that houses the pacemaker's battery and computer programming; and (2) leads, or wires, that are secured to the myocardium and plugged into the generator. These leads can sense the heart's intrinsic electrical activity and pace the heart by delivering painless electrical impulses. Devices can consist of single-chamber systems (pacing and sensing either the atrium or the ventricle), dual-chamber systems (pacing/sensing both the atrium and ventricle), or cardiac resynchronization therapy (CRT) devices (pacing/sensing the atrium, sensing the ventricle and pacing it in two locations) (Fig. 19.1).

Epicardial Versus Transvenous Devices

Pacemakers can either be *transvenous*, placed within the vascular system and affixed within the atrium or ventricle, or they can be *epicardial*, with leads secured to the external surface of the heart. The generators used in transvenous or epicardial pacing systems are the same but generally placed in different locations—upper chest for transvenous devices, or behind the rectus muscle in epicardial devices (Fig. 19.1).

Infants and young children often receive epicardial systems, as their venous anatomy may not be amenable to the placement of relatively bulky leads. This requires a more invasive approach with either a thoracotomy or sternotomy. Subsequent lead revisions will thus require repeated intrathoracic surgery, a not uncommon occurrence as epicardial

leads (compared with transvenous) have a higher risk for malfunction.[1] Placement of epicardial leads may also make it prohibitive for a patient to receive an MRI. In contrast, transvenous systems are less invasive and increasingly compatible with MRIs. This must be weighed against the higher risk of venous thrombosis from chronic indwelling leads. Transvenous leads also expose patients to more complex lead management[2] and multiple lead extractions over a lifetime.

At our institution, patients weighing under 15 kg often receive epicardial pacing systems. In very small patients (<2.5 kg), the generator is left in the pleural cavity (Fig. 19.2). Once above 2.5 kg, a single-versus dual-chamber pacing system can be debated, with the larger dual-chamber system chosen above 3.5 kg. Over 15 kg, a transvenous pacemaker can be considered. Although placement of transvenous leads is technically feasible under 15 kg, this must be weighed against the higher risk of venous occlusion.[1] Similarly, we tend to wait until 25 kg before offering a transvenous dual-chamber system and 35 kg for CRT devices requiring three leads.

Although a patient may be large enough for a transvenous pacing system, anatomic considerations may preclude their use. Patients with single ventricles often require epicardial devices, as anatomic barriers can prevent the placement of atrial and ventricular leads. Placement of leads within the systemic circulation should also be avoided due to the risk of thromboembolic events. Similarly, residual shunts can result in paradoxical emboli, doubling the risk of systemic thromboembolism despite the use of anticoagulation.[3] It may also be undesirable to place leads through atrial baffles given the increased risk of obstruction, or atrioventricular (AV) valves

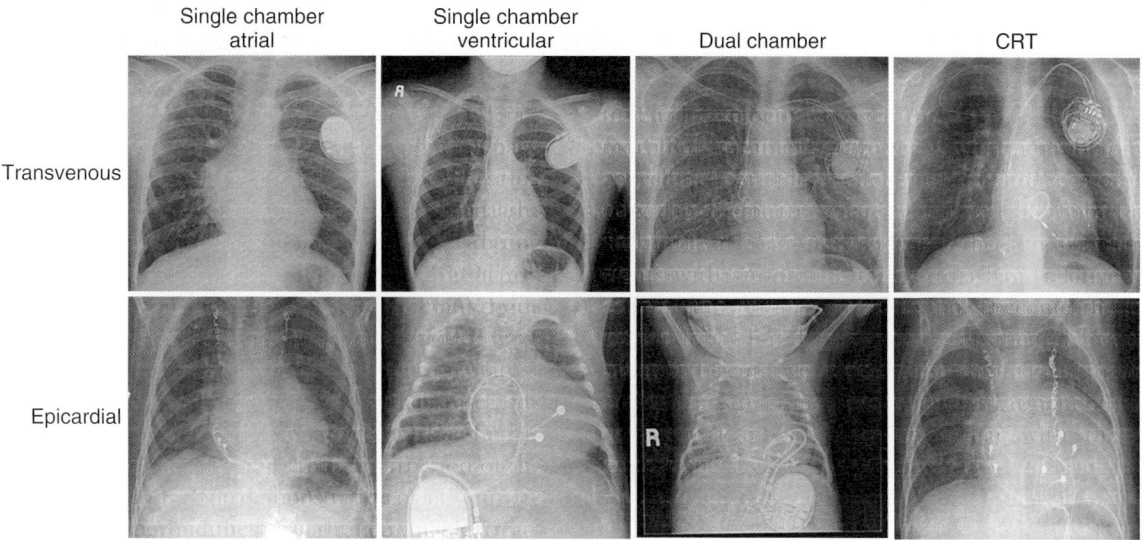

• Fig. 19.1 Representative examples of transvenous and epicardial pacemakers, with single- and dual-chamber configurations, as well as cardiac resynchronization therapy *(CRT)*.

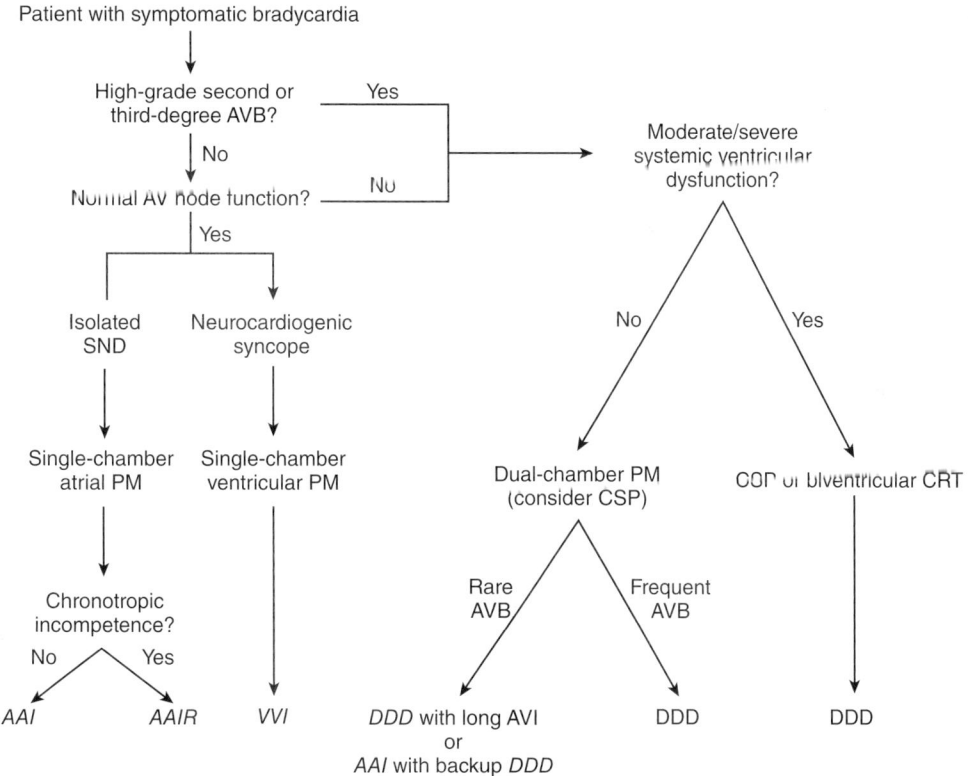

• Fig. 19.2 Decision-making process when determining what type of pacemaker *(PM)* to implant and how it should be programmed based on clinical information. *AV,* Atrioventricular; *AVB,* atrioventricular block; *CRT,* cardiac resynchronization therapy; *CSP,* conduction system pacing; *SND,* sinus node dysfunction.

that are mechanical or stenotic.[4] Transvenous leads can also cause valvar regurgitation that may not be tolerated in patients who are hemodynamically tenuous.

Single- Versus Dual-Chamber Devices

Fig. 19.3 outlines the decision-making process when choosing the type of pacemaker to implant. In patients with structurally normal hearts, single-chamber ventricular pacemakers are well tolerated when they are young. As they get older, they may require the addition of an atrial lead to improve their chronotropic response, especially as they become involved in more demanding activities and competitive sports.[5] The threshold to add an atrial lead in patients with congenital heart disease (CHD) is lower, as some may need the additional cardiac output offered by restoring

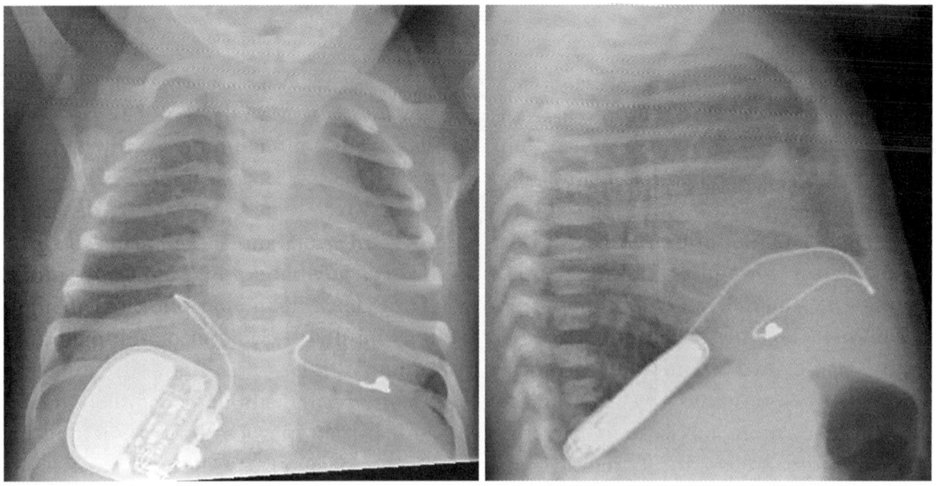

• **Fig. 19.3** Single-chamber ventricular pacemaker with the generator in the right pleural cavity.

synchronized atrial contraction, while others may have AV valve regurgitation that is worsened by the loss of AV synchrony.

Transvenous Systems

When implanting a pacemaker, the position of the ventricular lead deserves thoughtful consideration. Transvenous ventricular leads have traditionally been placed in the right ventricular (RV) myocardium for a secure and easily obtainable pacing site. However, it is now known that chronic RV pacing can result in "pacemaker-induced cardiomyopathy,"[6] which has prompted interest in conduction system pacing. Based on first principles, the optimal ventricular pacing site would engage the native proximal His-Purkinje system to produce the most rapid and synchronous ventricular contraction (Fig. 19.4). Effective His bundle pacing (HBP) maintains ventricular synchrony and function with strikingly narrow paced QRS durations.[7] However, HBP is limited by long-term risk of elevated capture thresholds, ventricular undersensing, atrial oversensing, and lead dislodgement. These issues result in a nontrivial increase in the need for lead revision of premature pulse generator replacement compared with traditional RV apical or septal lead positioning.[8]

To overcome these limitations, the technique of left bundle branch area pacing (LBBAP) was developed where the RV pacing lead is drilled across the ventricular septum to engage the left bundle region (Fig. 19.4). Long-term follow-up studies of LBBAP have demonstrated lower capture thresholds and improved sensing compared with HBP while preserving left ventricular (LV) synchrony and systolic function.[9] Moreover, LBBAP implantation is typically straightforward due to the fan-like distribution of the left bundle branch, resulting in a larger anatomical target zone for lead deployment than HBP. Notably, HBP and LBBAP may not correct distal His-Purkinje disease, which usually requires traditional biventricular pacing.

Epicardial Systems

When placing an epicardial pacing system, the usual approach through a sternotomy allows for easy access to the anterior surface of the RV. Care should be taken to avoid placing the lead on the basal RV and outflow tract, as these sites can have a detrimental impact on LV function and synchrony. RV apical pacing is better, although pacing from the LV apex may be best in preserving LV function in patients with structurally normal hearts.[10]

Cardiac Resynchronization Therapy

Resynchronization therapy seeks to restore synchronous contraction to the ventricle, whether it be due to dyssynchronous pacing from a single ventricular lead or dyssynchronous activation due to bundle branch block or distal His-Purkinje disease. This can be accomplished by adding a second lead to pace the ventricle from a different site, allowing the multiple wavefronts to mimic a more natural contraction of the heart.

Unfortunately, not all patients respond to CRT. Patients with left bundle branch block or systemic LVs tend to respond better than those with right bundle branch block, nonspecific intraventricular conduction delay, or systemic RVs.[11] In the appropriate anatomy, this can be accomplished by cannulating the coronary sinus and placing a transvenous lead within one of its posterior or posterolateral branches, while others will require surgical placement of an epicardial lead. Broadly speaking, the resynchronization of systemic LVs requires the placement of leads in an anterior-posterior orientation, in essence "sandwiching" the LV and mimicking the circumferential contraction of its native activation (Fig. 19.5).

It is less clear how to best resynchronize systemic RVs given the longitudinal contraction of the RV from apex to base. Individual assessment of each patient and evaluation of their electrical and mechanical activation has helped improve our ability to treat these patients with lead locations either in the anterior-posterior direction, apex-base orientation, or other novel configurations[12,13] (Fig. 19.5).

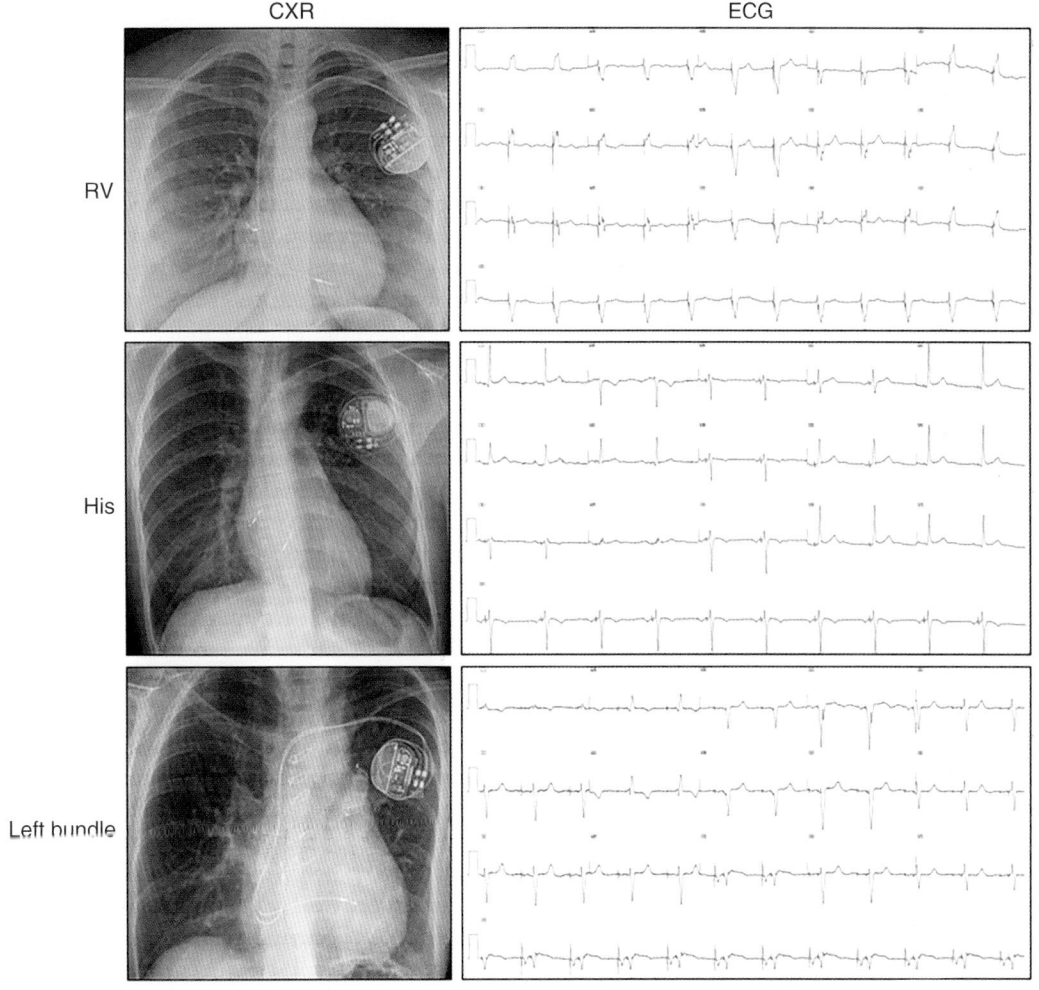

• **Fig. 19.4** Single-site ventricular pacing options: traditional right ventricular *(RV)* septal pacing, His bundle pacing, and left bundle branch area pacing. *CXR,* Chest X-ray; *ECG,* electrocardiogram.

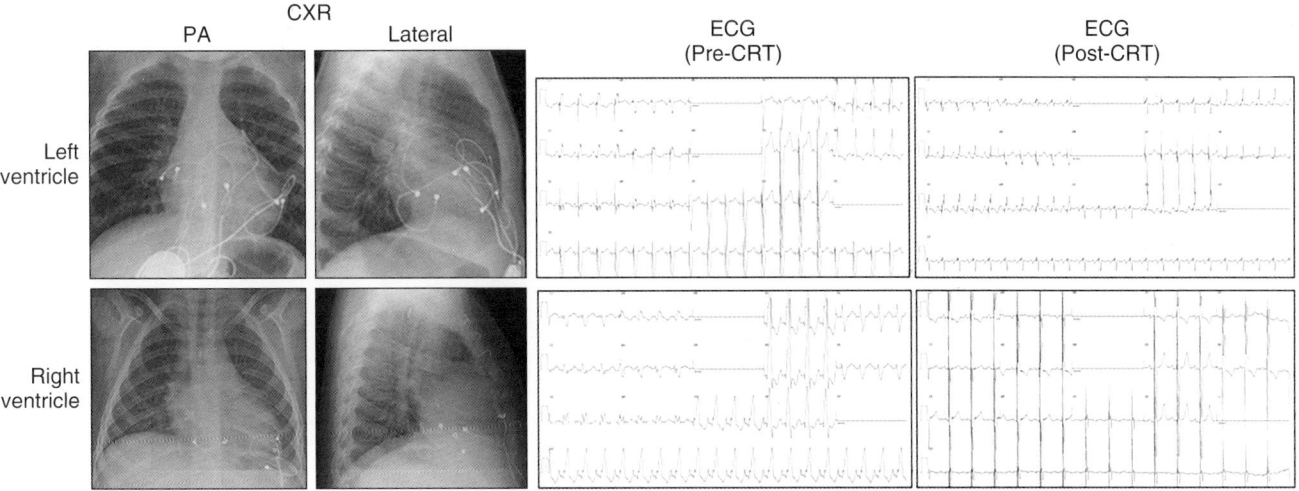

• **Fig. 19.5** Examples of resynchronization in patients with a systemic left and right ventricle. The patient with a systemic left ventricle had complete heart block and developed pacing-induced cardiomyopathy requiring an upgrade to cardiac resynchronization therapy *(CRT).* The patient with a systemic right ventricle had an intrinsic right bundle branch block causing dysfunction, requiring placement of a CRT pacemaker. *CXR,* Chest X-ray; *ECG,* electrocardiogram; *PA,* posterior-anterior.

Leadless Pacemaker

Leadless pacemakers were created to remove the risk of lead malfunctions and infections, with an entire pacemaker encapsulated within a pen-cap sized device that can be delivered transvenously to the RV septum (Fig. 19.6). At the time of publication, these devices have been used primarily for ventricular-demand pacing only, with limited ability to provide AV synchrony in young patients.[14] Their use is further limited in pediatrics, as their delivery mechanism requires a large-caliber sheath. Nevertheless, the technology is promising—further developments will include the ability to implant dual-chamber leadless systems, as well as devices that can adhere to the septum in such a way as to engage the native conduction system.

Indications

An abbreviated summary of the 2021 HRS/ACC/AHA guidelines[15] on indications of permanent pacemaker implantation in pediatric patients is provided in Table 19.1.

Sinus Node Dysfunction

Sinus node dysfunction (SND) manifests as resting sinus bradycardia, intermittent sinus pauses, and/or chronotropic incompetence with exercise. Mechanisms of SND are discussed further in Chapter 17. Regardless of the type of SND, the correlation of symptoms to age-inappropriate bradycardia is a critical factor in considering permanent pacemaker implantation, with no absolute minimum heart rate or maximum pause duration that obligates permanent pacing.

Atrioventricular Block

Postoperative atrioventricular block (AVB) requiring permanent pacemaker implantation complicates ~1% of all CHD surgery. Of those with high-grade and complete postoperative AVB that regain conduction during their ICU course, >85% recover by postoperative day 7 and >95% by postoperative day 10.[16] Permanent pacemaker implantation is recommended for high-grade and complete postoperative AVB that persists beyond 7–10 days. In borderline cases (e.g., return of AV conduction on day 7), lesion-specific risk may assist in clinical decision-making.

The pathophysiology and clinical management of congenital complete AVB (CCAVB) are discussed in Chapter 17. The primary indication for permanent pacemaker implantation in CCAVB is symptomatic bradycardia for age. Other common indications include a wide QRS escape rhythm, complex ventricular ectopy, and ventricular dysfunction. In the absence of symptoms related to bradycardia, permanent pacing should be considered for mean heart rates < 50 beats/min in infants without structural heart disease or < 60–70 beats/min in those with complex CHD. It should be stressed, however, that infants and children with mean heart rates above these cut-off values may still develop symptoms and/or end-organ dysfunction related to bradycardia, in which case permanent pacemaker implantation is still indicated.

Pacemaker Programming

Pacemakers are programmed using a standardized three- to four-letter coding system (Table 19.2). Rate-adaptive pacing treats SND with chronotropic incompetence by detecting physical activity through an accelerometer in the pulse generator that can then adjust the pacing rate according to programmable activity zones.

Single-chamber pacemakers are programmed to provide atrial-demand (*AAI*) or ventricular-demand (*VVI*) pacing, where a pacing stimulus is delivered when no sensed event is

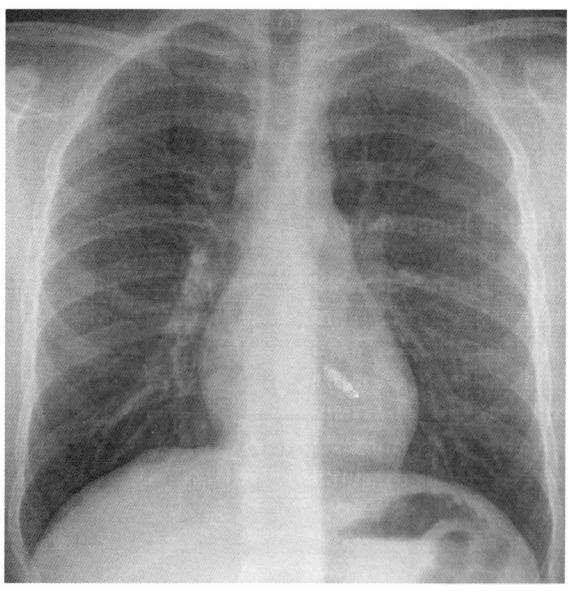

• **Fig. 19.6** Posterior-anterior chest X-ray of a leadless pacemaker implanted on the mid-right ventricular septum.

TABLE 19.1	**Indications for Pacemaker Implantation**

Common Permanent Pacing Indications	
Sinus node dysfunction	• Symptomatic bradycardia for age • Symptomatic bradycardia due to necessary chronic medical therapy • Resting bradycardia < 40 beats/min or prolonged pauses > 3 seconds with complex CHD • Resting junctional bradycardia with impaired hemodynamics attributable to loss of AV synchrony
Postoperative AV block	• High-grade second- or third-degree AV block lasting > 7–10 days following cardiac surgery • Late-onset, high-grade second- or third-degree AV block following cardiac surgery
Congenital complete AV block	• Symptomatic bradycardia for age • Wide QRS escape rhythm, complex ventricular ectopy, or ventricular dysfunction • Asymptomatic infant with mean ventricular rate < 50 beats/min in the absence of CHD, or < 60–70 beats/min in the presence of CHD
Miscellaneous	• Channelopathy with pause-dependent VT or functional 2:1 AV block • Intra-atrial reentrant tachycardia amenable to antitachycardia pacing • Recurrent breath-holding spells or vasovagal syncope refractory to medical therapy and with documented severe bradycardia/asystole • Kearns-Sayre syndrome with any degree of AV block and/or intraventricular conduction delay • Muscular dystrophies with significant first-degree AV block and/or intraventricular conduction delay

AV, Atrioventricular; *CHD,* congenital heart disease; *VT,* ventricular tachycardia.

TABLE 19.2	**Nomenclature for Modes of Cardiac Pacing**		

Position I	**Position II**	**Position III**	**Position IV**
Chamber(s) Paced	*Chamber(s) Sensed*	*Response to Sensed Event*	*Rate Adaptive Pacing*
A: Atrium V: Ventricle D: Atrium and ventricle O: No pacing function	A: Atrium V: Ventricle D: Atrium and ventricle O: No sensing function	I: Pacing inhibited T: Pacing triggered D: Pacing inhibited and/or triggered	R: Rate adaptive pacing on

detected after a defined escape interval (in milliseconds) that corresponds to the programmed lower rate limit (in beats per minute); pacing is inhibited if a sensed intrinsic event preempts the escape interval.

Dual-chamber pacemakers are most commonly programmed *DDD* that allows for maintenance of AV synchrony in patients with high-grade or third-degree AVB. In addition to a lower rate limit, an upper rate limit is also defined which corresponds to the maximum sensed atrial rate that will be tracked to the ventricle; atrial rates above the upper rate limit will produce varying degrees of pacemaker-mediated AVB (also termed upper rate behavior). AV intervals (analogous to a PR interval) are programmed and can be shortened to commit to ventricular pacing or lengthened to encourage native conduction, depending on intrinsic AV node function. A postventricular atrial refractory period (PVARP) is set to avoid pacemaker-mediated tachycardia that can result from atrial sensing of retrograde conducted P waves. Practitioners managing temporary or permanent pacemakers that are programmed *DDD* should be aware of the interplay between the programmed AV intervals, PVARP, and upper rate limit; an inappropriately long AV interval and/or PVARP will restrict the allowable upper rate

limit and may result in 2:1 pacemaker-mediated AVB at physiologic sinus rates, especially in infants.

Asynchronous pacing modes (*AOO, VOO,* or *DOO*) provide constant pacing output at the programmed lower rate limit independent of sensed activity. These are most often selected for pacemaker-dependent patients undergoing surgical procedures that require the use of electrocautery, which produces noise inhibition and poorly tolerated bradycardia or asystole when devices are left in an inhibited mode (*AAI, VVI,* or *DDD*).

Implantable Cardioverter Defibrillators

The primary function of an implantable cardioverter defibrillator (ICD) is to detect and terminate life-threatening arrhythmias, specifically ventricular tachycardia (VT) or fibrillation (VF). An ICD also consists of a generator and leads, with at least one lead having a "coil" that can provide a life-saving shock to the heart. All modern transvenous and epicardial ICDs can function as a pacemaker, though subcutaneous ICDs (S-ICDs) do not have pacing capabilities. Antibradycardia programming is identical to that described in the pacemaker section above.

Types of ICDs

The type of ICD implanted, as with pacemakers, is determined by patient factors including the patient's age and size, venous diameter, and anatomy. Due to their additional functionality, ICD leads and generators are larger than standard pacing leads and generators, limiting their use in smaller children due to risks of venous occlusion and generator erosion.

Epicardial ICDs require the placement of both a pace/sense lead and a defibrillator coil. The coil is placed posteriorly, behind the systemic ventricle, to provide a vector between the coil and the generator to cover the bulk of the ventricular myocardium. At times, this requires placement of a subcutaneous lead in the parasternal region to create a dual coil system that allows for better coverage of the heart (Fig. 19.7). In transvenous systems, single coil leads are preferred. Dual coil leads, with a coil on the RV portion and superior vena caval (SVC) portion of the lead, are generally reserved for patients in whom there is concern that the ventricular portion of the coil does not provide a suitable vector for defibrillation, such as those with right-sided implants (Fig. 19.7). Dual coil leads are not routinely placed, however, as they can be more difficult to extract, with an increased risk of SVC tear and death.[17,18]

S-ICDs are increasingly used, as they do not require hardware to be placed within the venous circulation, negating the risk of endocarditis and need for extraction[19] (Fig. 19.8). S-ICDs, however, do not having pacing capabilities, limiting their use in patients who require chronic pacing. Patients must also be screened in for S-ICDs, as they sense from electrodes along the length of the subcutaneous coil. The QRS complex must satisfy specific parameters to avoid oversensing or undersensing of the native rhythm, resulting in failure to produce a shock or delivering a shock for inappropriate reasons. Lastly, the S-ICD generator is larger, as it needs to provide a higher-joule external shock than transvenous ICDs. This limits its use in smaller children and those with a smaller body habitus.

Indications

ICDs are implanted for primary prevention or secondary prevention of sudden cardiac arrest (SCA) from life-threatening VT/VF. Primary prevention refers to the decision to implant an ICD in a patient deemed at sufficient risk for SCA but with no prior history of aborted SCA, in contrast to secondary prevention whereby an ICD is implanted following aborted SCA. Primary prevention ICD decision-making is more complicated in children due to the wide inter- and intra-group variability in SCA risk among the common pediatric diseases where primary prevention devices are considered. The decision to implant an ICD in a child should be made only after careful consideration of reversible or modifiable causes and in conjunction with in-depth counseling of the patient and family regarding the potential for medical and psychological device-related complications.[20] Table 19.3 is adapted from

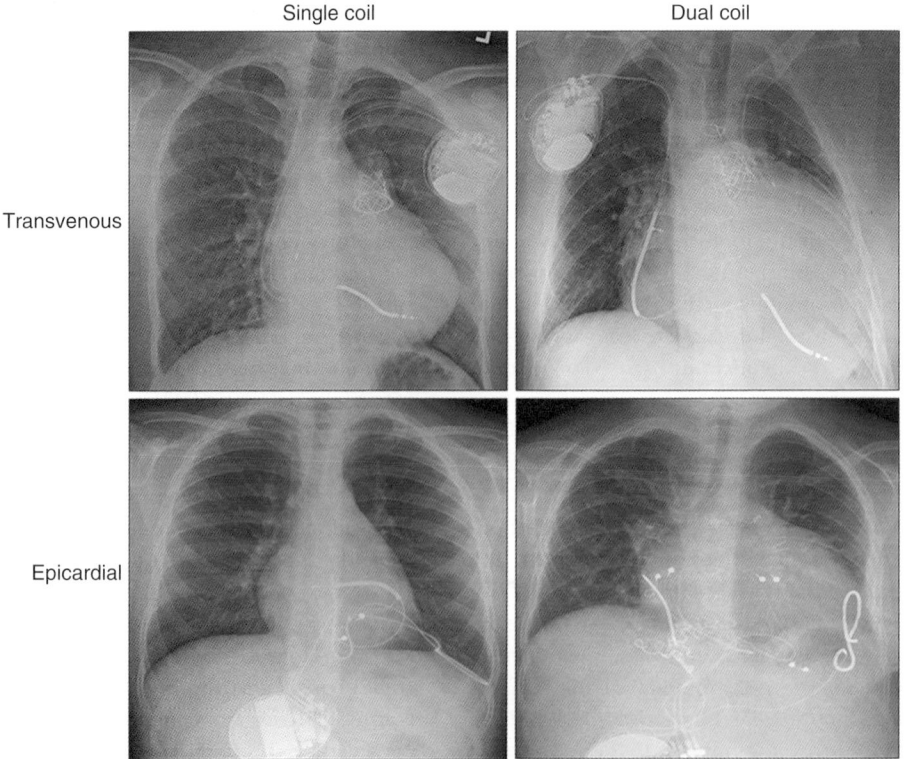

Single coil   Dual coil

Transvenous

Epicardial

• **Fig. 19.7** Representative examples of transvenous and epicardial implantable cardioverter defibrillators, with single- and dual-coil configurations.

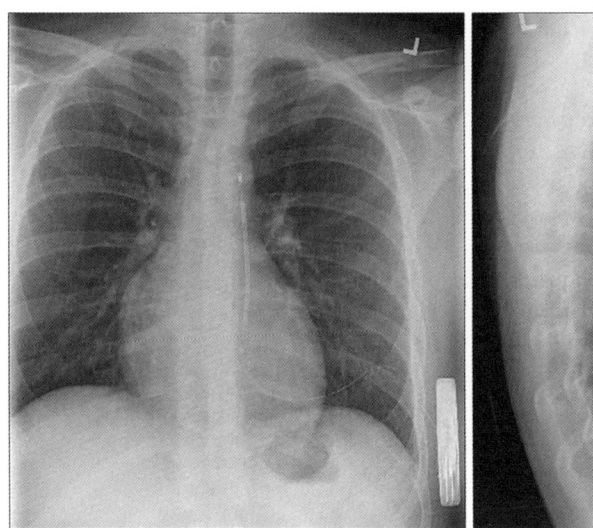
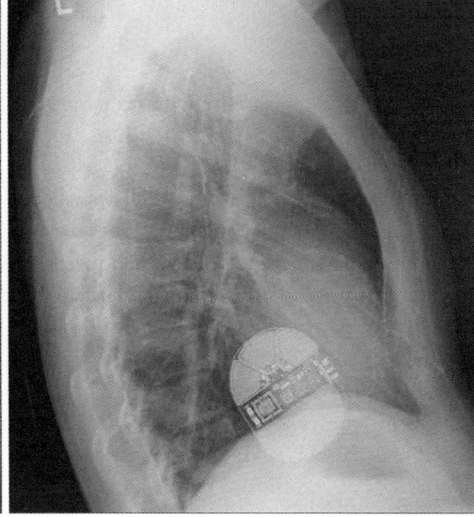

• **Fig. 19.8** Posterior-anterior and lateral chest X-ray of a subcutaneous implantable cardioverter defibrillator.

TABLE 19.3	Indications for Implantable Cardioverter Defibrillator (ICD) Implantation

Common ICD Indications

Channelopathies • *Long QT syndrome (LQTS)* • *Catecholaminergic polymorphic ventricular tachycardia (CPVT)* • *Brugada syndrome*	• LQTS with aborted SCA or refractory arrhythmic symptoms despite beta blockade and/or cardiac sympathetic denervation • CPVT with aborted SCA or arrhythmic syncope despite beta blockade, flecainide, and/or cardiac sympathetic denervation • Brugada syndrome with aborted SCA, or spontaneous sustained VT, or arrhythmic syncope with a spontaneous type 1 Brugada ECG pattern
Cardiomyopathy • *Hypertrophic cardiomyopathy (HCM)* • *Dilated cardiomyopathy (DCM)* • *Arrhythmogenic cardiomyopathy (ACM)*	• HCM with aborted SCA, spontaneous sustained VT, or ≥1 clinical risk factors (e.g., massive LVH, syncope, family history of SCA, LGE on CMR) • DCM with aborted SCA, spontaneous sustained VT, LVEF < 35% despite optimal medical therapy • ACM with aborted SCA, spontaneous sustained VT, arrhythmic syncope, LVEF < 35%, or certain high-risk pathogenic mutations
Congenital heart disease	• Aborted SCA or spontaneous sustained polymorphic VT/VF and elimination of reversible causes • Spontaneous or inducible monomorphic VT not amenable to catheter ablation or surgical repair • Systemic ventricular EF < 35% with sustained VT or arrhythmogenic syncope

CMR, Cardiac magnetic resonance imaging; *EF,* ejection fraction; *LGE,* late gadolinium enhancement; *LVH,* left ventricular hypertrophy; *SCA,* sudden cardiac arrest; *VF,* ventricular fibrillation; *VT,* ventricular tachycardia.

the 2021 HRS/ACC/AHA guidelines and summarizes common pediatric ICD indications according to disease substrate.[12]

ICD Programming

ICDs treat VT/VF by continuously sensing ventricular activity and delivering therapies when specific, programmable criteria are satisfied. Sensed ventricular rates that are faster than defined cut-off values and sustain for defined durations will enter a "treatment" zone, where therapies such as anti-tachycardia pacing (ATP) or defibrillation are delivered, or a "monitor" zone that simply stores the recorded electrograms for future review. Modern ICD generators have advanced algorithms to assist in differentiating VT/VF from sinus tachycardia or atrial tachyarrhythmias, though inappropriate therapies can still occur. Primary prevention ICDs are often programmed conservatively to avoid inappropriate therapies, with very high "treatment" zones (e.g., >220 beats/min) and long detection times. Secondary prevention ICDs are ideally programmed based on the patient's clinical ventricular arrhythmia (if known). ATP delivered prior to defibrillation can be a useful adjunctive treatment for reentrant, monomorphic VT and can reduce the number of painful shocks experienced by the patient.

Complications

Close follow-up of any patient with a pacemaker or ICD is vital. Children have a much higher risk for complications from their device due to their age and size at implant, somatic growth, and overall activity level.[1] Epicardial leads are also more likely to malfunction than their transvenous counterparts, and have the additional potential of causing coronary artery compression and cardiac strangulation.[21]

Defibrillators are more prone to lead malfunctions,[22] and also place patients at risk for inappropriate shocks. This can be due to shocks delivered for sinus tachycardia, T-wave oversensing (resulting in "double counting"), or lead fractures causing the device to sense electrical artifact. Inappropriate shocks have been associated with increased morbidity and mortality,[23] including post-traumatic stress disorder.

Device Follow-up and Remote Monitoring

Proper long-term pacemaker and ICD function requires scheduled in-person device interrogation and remote transmissions to monitor remaining generator battery life, lead performance, and tachyarrhythmia episodes. Stable sensing and capture of all leads should be checked at least annually, especially with ICD leads where sufficient R wave amplitudes are crucial to appropriately detect VT/VF. Lead impedance trends are reviewed and may note the presence of a conductor fracture (high impedance) or insulation breach (low impedance). Stored arrhythmia episodes, such as those in ICD "monitor" zones, should be reviewed and can inform subsequent programming, antiarrhythmic drug titration, and/or catheter ablation targets.

Every pacemaker and ICD has the ability to send a transmission through a transmitter supplied to the patient, or increasingly, through an app on their mobile phone. Transmissions have become more automated as wireless technology has grown, with some devices having the ability to send transmissions every 24 hours if an abnormality is noted. Many devices still require a manual transmission though, with the recommendation that the patient send data every 3 months. Scrutinizing this data can reduce complication rates, facilitate communication, and provide reassurance to patients and their families.[24] Nevertheless, there remains a high rate of noncompliance with remote transmissions, resulting in the loss of rare but actionable data that could prevent more catastrophic complications.[25]

References

1. Fortescue EB, Berul CI, Cecchin F, et al. Patient, procedural, and hardware factors associated with pacemaker lead failures in pediatrics and congenital heart disease. *Heart Rhythm.* 2004;1:150-159.
2. Pham TD, Cecchin F, O'Leary E, et al. Lead extraction at a pediatric/congenital heart disease center: the importance of patient age at implant. *JACC Clin Electrophysiol.* 2022;8:343-353.
3. Khairy P, Landzberg MJ, Gatzoulis MA, et al. Transvenous pacing leads and systemic thromboemboli in patients with intracardiac shunts: a multicenter study. *Circulation.* 2006;113:2391-2397.
4. Khairy P, Landzberg MJ, Lambert J, et al. Long-term outcomes after the atrial switch for surgical correction of transposition: a meta-analysis comparing the Mustard and Senning procedures. *Cardiol Young.* 2004;14:284-292.
5. Karpawich PP, Perry BL, Farooki ZQ, et al. Pacing in children and young adults with nonsurgical atrioventricular block: comparison of single-rate ventricular and dual-chamber modes. *Am Heart J.* 1987;113:316-321.
6. Moak JP, Hasbani K, Ramwell C, et al. Dilated cardiomyopathy following right ventricular pacing for AV block in young patients: resolution after upgrading to biventricular pacing systems. *J Cardiovasc Electrophysiol.* 2006;17:1068-1071.
7. Abdelrahman M, Subzposh FA, Beer D, et al. Clinical outcomes of His bundle pacing compared to right ventricular pacing. *J Am Coll Cardiol.* 2018;71:2319-2330.
8. Vijayaraman P, Naperkowski A, Subzposh FA, et al. Permanent His-bundle pacing: long-term lead performance and clinical outcomes. *Heart Rhythm.* 2018;15:696-702.
9. Su L, Wang S, Wu S, et al. Long-term safety and feasibility of left bundle branch pacing in a large single-center study. *Circ Arrhythm Electrophysiol.* 2021;14:e009261.
10. Janousek J, van Geldorp IE, Krupickova S, et al. Permanent cardiac pacing in children: choosing the optimal pacing site: a multicenter study. *Circulation.* 2013;127:613-623.
11. Zareba W, Klein H, Cygankiewicz I, et al. Effectiveness of cardiac resynchronization therapy by QRS morphology in the multicenter automatic defibrillator implantation trial-cardiac resynchronization therapy (MADIT-CRT). *Circulation.* 2011;123:1061-1072.
12. Mah DY, O'Leary ET, Harrild DM, et al. Resynchronizing right and left ventricles with right bundle branch block in the congenital heart disease population. *JACC Clin Electrophysiol.* 2020;6:1762-1772.
13. Miyazaki A, Sakaguchi H, Kagisaki K, et al. Optimal pacing sites for cardiac resynchronization therapy for patients with a systemic right ventricle with or without a rudimentary left ventricle. *Europace.* 2016;18:100-112.
14. Chinitz L, Ritter P, Khelae SK, et al. Accelerometer-based atrioventricular synchronous pacing with a ventricular leadless pacemaker: results from the Micra atrioventricular feasibility studies. *Heart Rhythm.* 2018;15:1363-1371.
15. Writing Committee Members, Shah MJ, Silka MJ, et al. 2021 PACES expert consensus statement on the indications and management of cardiovascular implantable electronic devices in pediatric patients. *Heart Rhythm.* 2021;18:1888-1924.
16. Weindling SN, Saul JP, Gamble WJ, Mayer JE, Wessel D, Walsh EP. Duration of complete atrioventricular block after congenital heart disease surgery. *Am J Cardiol.* 1998;82:525-527.
17. Segreti L, Di Cori A, Soldati E, et al. Major predictors of fibrous adherences in transvenous implantable cardioverter-defibrillator lead extraction. *Heart Rhythm.* 2014;11:2196-2201.
18. Sunderland N, Kaura A, Murgatroyd F, et al. Outcomes with single-coil versus dual-coil implantable cardioverter defibrillators: a meta-analysis. *Europace.* 2018;20:e21-e29.
19. von Alvensleben JC, Dechert B, Bradley DJ, et al. Subcutaneous implantable cardioverter-defibrillators in pediatrics and congenital heart disease: a Pediatric and Congenital Electrophysiology Society multicenter review. *JACC Clin Electrophysiol.* 2020;6:1752-1761.
20. Webste G, Panek KA, Labella M, et al. Psychiatric functioning and quality of life in young patients with cardiac rhythm devices. *Pediatrics.* 2014;133:e964-e972.
21. Mah DY, Prakash A, Porras D, et al. Coronary artery compression from epicardial leads: more common than we think. *Heart Rhythm.* 2018;15:1439-1447.

22. Atallah J, Erickson CC, Cecchin F, et al. Multi-institutional study of implantable defibrillator lead performance in children and young adults: results of the Pediatric Lead Extractability and Survival Evaluation (PLEASE) study. *Circulation.* 2013;127:2393-2402.

23. Moss AJ, Schuger C, Beck CA, et al. Reduction in inappropriate therapy and mortality through ICD programming. *N Engl J Med.* 2012;367:2275-2283.

24. Dechert BE, Serwer GA, Bradley DJ, Dick M II, LaPage MJ. Cardiac implantable electronic device remote monitoring surveillance in pediatric and congenital heart disease: utility relative to frequency. *Heart Rhythm.* 2015;12:117-122.

25. Leoni L, Padalino M, Biffanti R, et al. Pacemaker remote monitoring in the pediatric population: is it a real solution? *Pacing Clin Electrophysiol.* 2015;38:565-571.

20

Inherited Arrhythmia Syndromes and Arrhythmogenic Cardiomyopathies

DOMINIC J. ABRAMS AND VASSILIOS BEZZERIDES

KEY LEARNING POINTS

- A prolonged corrected QT interval on the electrocardiogram can be intrinsic or acquired (secondary to certain medication or electrolyte disturbances). The intrinsic forms (long QT syndrome [LQTS]) are inherited genetic disorders that can be a cause of recurrent syncope or sudden cardiac death due to a form of ventricular tachycardia known as *torsades de pointes*.
- Treatment for LQTS begins with beta blockade but can escalate to cardiac sympathectomy, or occasionally requires placement of an implantable defibrillator.
- Certain unusual cardiac repolarization abnormalities (Andersen-Tawil syndrome, Timothy syndrome) represent

- unique phenotypes and require different therapy than conventional LQTS.
- Catecholaminergic polymorphic ventricular tachycardia presents with recurrent syncope at times of physical or emotional stress, and can be a cause of sudden cardiac death. Remarkably, the electrocardiogram at rest is entirely normal. Detection hinges on recording of exercise-induced arrhythmias.
- Arrhythmogenic cardiomyopathy typically involves the right ventricle, but left ventricular and biventricular forms also exist.

Introduction

The inherited arrhythmia syndromes and arrhythmogenic cardiomyopathies (ACMs) represent a group of largely monogenic disorders with varied penetrance and expressivity that manifest in varying ways during childhood. Although potentially considered two separate entities, there is significant overlap, specifically due to the ability of specific genes to cause various electrophysiologic or structural disorders (e.g., SCN5A) and the early arrhythmic manifestations of specific cardiomyopathies that can precede the typical electrocardiographic, histologic, and structural features of the disorder. In this chapter we will review the clinical features, investigations, and genetic etiology of different conditions. An overview of the cardiomyocyte action potential, associated ion channels, and specific disorders is displayed in Fig. 20.1.

Inherited Arrhythmia Syndromes

Long QT Syndrome

Long QT syndrome (LQTS) is caused by genetically encoded abnormalities in cardiac ion channels responsible for cardiac depolarization and repolarization. Although prior reports exist, the first classical description of the syndrome was by Jervell and Lange-Nielsen in the late 1950s who described four Norwegian children with an autosomal recessive form of LQTS characterized by recurrent syncope, sudden cardiac death (SCD), and profound sensorineural deafness.[1] ECG recordings taken from affected children showed severe QT prolongation associated with a broad-based T wave, with further post-exertional QT prolongation. Romano and Ward subsequently described affected individuals displaying similar symptoms in a pattern consistent with autosomal dominant inheritance and varied penetrance.[2,3] The genetic basis for the three most common types of LQTS (LQTS 1–3) was elucidated in the mid-1990s, and genetic testing now represents an important component of the overall investigative strategy in managing families with the disorder.[4-6]

LQTS may be present in various ways, including symptoms, cascade screening of families, and incidental ECG finding and most recently secondary findings on exome sequencing performed for noncardiac indications. Classic symptoms include arrhythmic syncope, cardiac arrest, and SCD. Arrhythmic events may have specific triggers

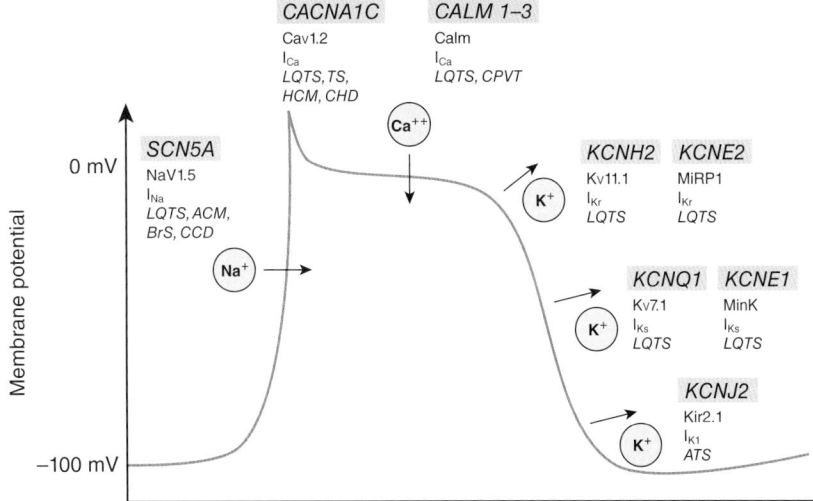

• **Fig. 20.1** The cardiac action potential is shown with the major ionic determinant for each phase; phase 0, sodium (Na$^+$); phase 1-2 calcium (Ca^{++}), and phase 3-4 potassium (K$^+$). The genetic etiology of differing conditions is shown with the associated protein, current and clinical conditions. Long QT syndrome (*LQTS*) resulting from prolongation of the action potential may occur either from excessive sodium or calcium inward conductance and hence prolonged depolarization or reduced outward potassium conductance leading to delayed repolarization. Genetically encoded abnormalities in specific channel components or associated proteins affect cardiomyocyte function and are associated with various conditions including LQTS, arrhythmogenic cardiomyopathy (*ACM*), Brugada syndrome (*BrS*), catecholaminergic polymorphic ventricular tachycardia (*CPVT*), Andersen-Tawil syndrome (*ATS*), Timothy syndrome (*TS*), hypertrophic cardiomyopathy (*HCM*), congenital heart disease (*CHD*), and cardiac conduction disease (*CCD*).

including exercise and specifically swimming in LQTS type 1, auditory stimulation in LQTS type 2, and at rest in LQTS type 3.[7]

The condition may also be diagnosed by the identification of genetic variants on sequencing following sudden death, with further validation in surviving family members. Patients often experience multiple episodes of syncope, and delayed diagnosis remains common with patients frequently misdiagnosed with seizure disorders due to witnessed epileptiform movements during syncopal episodes.[8]

LQTS types 1 and 2 are caused by delayed repolarization resulting from structural or functional abnormalities of cardiomyocyte potassium channels. The respective genes (*KCNQ1* and *KCNH2*) encode the potassium channel proteins $K_V7.1$ and $K_V11.1$, which regulate cellular repolarization via the slow (I_{Ks}) and rapid (I_{Kr}) delayed rectifier currents. The less common LQTS type 3 results from excessive activity of the depolarizing late sodium current (I_{Na}) or a decreased activation threshold secondary to functional abnormalities in the cardiac sodium channel $Na_V1.5$, encoded by the gene *SCN5A*.[9] See Table 20.1 for further details.

ECG remains the cornerstone of diagnosis. The QT interval is measured using the tangent technique in either lead II or V5 and corrected for heart rate using Bazett's formula ($QTc = QT/\sqrt{RR}$). A borderline corrected QT interval of greater than 450 ms in males or 460 ms in females should make one suspicious of a problem and prompt manual remeasurement and investigation of potential causes (such as medications or electrolyte abnormalities). A corrected QT interval of greater than 470 ms in males and 480 ms in females is always considered pathologically prolonged.[9] Abnormal repolarization is often reflected in varying T wave with different patterns of repolarization evident with the three types of LQTS and represent an important component of the diagnosis in the absence of overt QT prolongation.[10] The exercise test is an invaluable tool in unmasking repolarization abnormalities, as many individuals who are genetically predisposed to LQTS have normal corrected QT intervals at rest, especially asymptomatic family members. The patient should exercise to maximal capacity, and the corrected QT interval is measured each minute during the period. Paradoxical QT prolongation is typically seen early during recovery in LQTS type 1 and later during recovery in LQTS type 2.[9]

The hallmark arrhythmia of LQTS is *torsades de pointes*, an inherently unstable tachycardia believed to represent reentrant wave fronts that rotate through the ventricular myocardium, frequently splitting and colliding leading to spontaneous termination in up to 80% of cases. This explains the relative frequency of recurrent arrhythmic syncope compared with cardiac arrest in symptomatic individuals.

The nonselective beta-blockers nadolol or propranolol are the first-line treatment for all forms of LQTS and have demonstrated significant efficacy in reducing arrhythmic events in symptomatic individuals.[11] To what degree these are beneficial in asymptomatic patients with a normal resting QT interval remains unclear; however, current guidelines recommend they may be beneficial and appear to be a pragmatic option for most individuals.[12] Long-term compliance is, however, a major issue. Left cardiac

TABLE 20.1 Types of Long QT Syndrome (LQTS) Classified by Genetic and Molecular Findings

LQTS Type	Gene	Protein	Current	Evidence for Causing LQTS[†]
LQT1	KCNQ1	Kv7.1	IKs ↓	Definitive
LQT2	KCNH2	KV11.1	IKr ↓	Definitive
LQT3	SCN5A	Nav1.5	INa ↑	Definitive
LQT4	Ankyrin-B	Ankyrin	Na$^+$/K$^+$ ATPase and ?	Definitive
LQT5	KCNE1	MinK	IKs ↓	Limited for cLQTS, strong for aLQTS
LQT6	KCNE2	MiRP1	IKr ↓	Disputed for cLQTS, strong for aLQTS
LQT7	KCNJ2	Kir2.1	IK1 ↓	Limited for cLQTS, definitive for Anderson-Tawil syndrome
LQT8	CACNA1C	CaV1.2	ICa-L ↑	Moderate for LQTS, definitive for Timothy syndrome
LQT9	CAV3	Caveolin3	INa ↑	Limited
LQT10	SCN4B	SCNβ4subunit	INa ↑	Disputed
LQT11	AKAP-9	Yotiao	IKs ↓	Disputed
LQT12	SNTA1	Syntrophin-α1	INa ↓	Disputed
LQT13	KCNJ5	Kir3.4	IKACh ↓	Disputed
LQT14	CALM1	Calmodulin	Calcium signaling disorder	Definitive
LQT15	CALM2	Calmodulin	Calcium signaling disorder	Definitive
LQT16	CALM3	Calmodulin	Calcium signaling disorder	Definitive
LQT17	TRDN	Triadin	Calcium signaling disorder	Strong

ICa, Calcium current; IKACh, G-protein coupled potassium current; IKi, inward rectifying potassium current; IKr, rapidly activating potassium current; IKs, slowly activating potassium current; INa, sodium current.

↑ Gain of function.
↓ Loss of function.

[†] PMID: 31983240

sympathetic denervation was initially restricted to highly symptomatic individuals with multiple arrhythmic episodes, although as experience has grown, this is now being used earlier in management and has become a first-line alternative to long-term beta-blockade in selected patients.[13] Early in the overall experience, implantable cardioverter defibrillators (ICDs) were used frequently in LQTS, although as complication rates are high and many patients can be successfully managed with other strategies, only a small minority of individuals with LQTS in the current era have an indication for either a primary or even secondary prevention ICD. Patients with LQTS should avoid any other medications that can further prolong the QT interval by further inhibition of cardiomyocyte potassium channel function. Due to the recognized association of exercise as an arrhythmic trigger in LQTS (especially type 1), patients were initially restricted from strenuous exercise, although subsequent studies showed a low event rate in well-managed patients, and many individuals with LQTS now participate safely in various forms of competitive athletics.[9]

Genetic testing is an important component of the overall investigative strategy, although LQTS is a clinical diagnosis and therefore genetic testing should be used to support clinical findings, rather than as a diagnostic tool in the absence of a robust clinical phenotype. Genetic testing is typically performed in the proband after detailed counseling and consent, and in family members together with clinical evaluation if a pathogenic variant is identified. Evaluation of multiple family members using both clinical and genetic testing remains a very powerful tool to validate genetic findings in the family.

Andersen-Tawil Syndrome

Andersen-Tawil syndrome (ATS) is an autosomal dominant, multisystem disorder characterized by a clinical triad of cardiac arrhythmia, periodic paralysis, and craniofacial-skeletal developmental anomalies. Initially considered a form of LQTS (LQTS type 7), the different electrocardiographic pattern and noncardiac features led to the recognition of this as a separate entity. Cardiac features include U waves, polymorphic ventricular premature beats, and both polymorphic and bidirectional tachycardia.

ATS is associated with variants in the gene *KCNJ2*, encoding the K$^+$ channel Kir2.1, which underlies the inward rectifying current I$_{K1}$, contributing to cellular excitability in the heart, brain, and skeletal muscle. In cardiomyocytes, abnormal Kir2.1 function and reduction in the I$_{K1}$ leads to delayed afterdepolarizations and triggered arrhythmia, explaining the arrhythmic phenotype seen in ATS.[14]

Timothy Syndrome

Timothy syndrome (previously referred to as LQTS type 8) is another multisystem disorder characterized by QT prolongation and T-wave morphological abnormalities, with structural and congenital cardiac anomalies well recognized. Other features include pulmonary hypertension, hypoglycemia, syndactyly, distinctive facial features, and neuropsychological disability. Timothy syndrome relates to a specific variant (G406R) in the gene *CACNA1C*, which encodes the alpha subunit of the L-type voltage-dependent calcium channel (Ca$_V$1.2).[15] Other variants in *CACNA1C* can be associated with LQTS, hypertrophic cardiomyopathy, and congenital heart disease, with all three seen associated with one specific amino acid substitution (R518C) in a single family.[16]

Catecholaminergic Polymorphic Ventricular Tachycardia

Catecholaminergic polymorphic ventricular tachycardia (CPVT) is a disorder of cellular calcium dysregulation, characterized clinically by atrial arrhythmias and polymorphic and bidirectional ventricular tachycardia (VT) induced by physical or emotional stress.[17] CPVT has an estimated prevalence of 1:10,000, although this is based on no empiric data. There appear to be no significant differences in presentation or outcome between sexes. CPVT is typically diagnosed in childhood or early adolescence, although like LQTS diagnostic delay is well recognized. A genetic diagnosis of CPVT can be made on postmortem genetic testing following SCD.[18]

CPVT is an autosomal dominant condition associated with variants in the gene encoding the cardiac ryanodine receptor (*RYR2*), which regulates calcium release from the sarcoplasmic reticulum. Genetic variants in *RYR2* cause structural and functional changes in the cardiac ryanodine receptor leading to inappropriate diastolic calcium release, after depolarizations and triggered arrhythmias. There is a high rate of *de novo* variants, reflecting the malignant nature of the disease and genetic fitness.[17] Homozygous or compound heterozygous variants in calsequestrin 2 (*CASQ2*), the main cellular calcium buffer, cause an autosomal recessive form of CPVT, although more recently autosomal dominant CASQ2-mediated disease has been recognized.[19]

Treatment strategies include pharmacological therapy to suppress the catecholaminergic stimulation of beta-receptors (nonselective beta-blockers nadolol and propranolol)[11] and flecainide, which has various cellular effects including a direct inhibitory effect on overactive ryanodine receptors.[20] Left cardiac sympathetic denervation also has an important antiadrenergic role.[21] The use of ICD has diminished significantly over the last decade, as the unique adrenergic features and arrhythmia mechanism, the high burden of atrial arrhythmia, and the young age of CPVT onset have contributed to significant device-related morbidity and mortality, including fatal arrhythmic storms.[22] The long-term incidence of life-threatening events remains unacceptably high, with estimates exceeding 50% in probands by 15 years of follow-up despite standard treatments, which has promoted the development of new biological and gene therapies to address the underlying genetic and molecular abnormalities.

Calmodulinopathies

Three distinct genes (*CALM1*, *CALM2*, and *CALM3*) encode for an identical 149 amino acid calmodulin protein (CaM), which is highly conserved across species. CaM is a cytoplasmic Ca^{2+}-binding protein which interacts with multiple other cellular proteins including the L-type Ca^{2+} channel and RyR2, having an inhibitory role on both. Loss of normal interaction of CALM with the L-type Ca^{2+} channel leads to excessive calcium conductance into the cell; affected individuals have severe QT prolongation and a high rate of symptoms including cardiac arrest in infancy and early life. Conversely, loss of CaM inhibition of the cardiac ryanodine receptor (RyR2) causes diastolic calcium leak, manifest clinically as CPVT.[23]

J-Wave Syndromes

The J-wave syndromes include Brugada syndrome (BrS) and early repolarization syndrome (ERS), represented by elevation of the J point in the anterior precordial or inferolateral leads, respectively.

BrS is well recognized but very rare in childhood and may lead to ventricular arrhythmia and cardiac arrest. The molecular basis of the disorder is related to decreased inward sodium current and can be associated with genetic variants in the cardiac sodium channel gene *SCN5A*; however, a polygenic etiology is increasingly recognized. The ECG features and associated arrhythmic risk may be precipitated by fever in children and can be mistaken for febrile "seizures."[24] Treatment is directed toward avoidance of environmental triggers (fever, pharmacological agents that may further inhibit the sodium current), appropriate risk stratification, and prevention of sudden death with ICDs in high-risk cases. The role of quinidine to suppress ventricular arrhythmias continues to be evaluated.

Early repolarization is a common ECG finding in young patients, although it has been implicated in polymorphic

VT and ventricular fibrillation. The role of ERS in pediatric cardiac arrest and sudden death is unclear.

Arrhythmogenic Cardiomyopathies

ACM is defined as an arrhythmogenic heart muscle disorder not explained by ischemic, hypertensive, or valvular heart disease. Arrhythmic manifestations include atrial fibrillation, conduction disease, VT, or ventricular fibrillation, and may occur prior to the onset of electrocardiographic, structural, or histopathological changes.[25]

Initially identified as a disease of the right ventricle and termed arrhythmogenic right ventricular dysplasia or cardiomyopathy (ARVD/ARVC), it is now clear that both left dominant and biventricular subtypes exist, and now include variants previously considered dilated cardiomyopathy with a high arrhythmic burden. As experience with the condition has increased, so has an understanding of the genetic and molecular etiology, with emerging evidence of genotype-phenotype correlation.

The three types of ACM can be classified as follows[26]:

1. Classical or right-sided ACM (referred to subsequently as ARVC), defined as isolated right ventricular (RV) disease or left ventricular (LV) involvement in the presence of notable RV enlargement and/or dysfunction.

   This was first reported in 24 patients with T-wave inversion in the right precordial leads and associated ST-segment post-excitation (epsilon) waves, VT with a left bundle morphology, and RV dilatation. Historically the condition is believed to have four distinct phases, which may or may not occur in sequential fashion.[27,28] The first, a "concealed" phase prior to the onset of classical electrocardiographic, histological, and structural changes, characterized by intermittent exacerbations of disease activity, which may be associated with life-threatening ventricular arrhythmias in an otherwise quiescent disease process. Patients may be considered to have CPVT due to the inducible polymorphic VT on exercise testing. Subsequent stages include a second, overt arrhythmic phase characterized by macroreentrant circuits facilitated by the presence of diffuse myocardial fibrosis with functional and structural RV remodeling, and a third phase associated with further RV dysfunction and failure. A small minority progress to a fourth stage of biventricular dilatation and congestive heart failure, although this is increasingly recognized in adult patients.

   The diagnosis is made clinically using the 2010 International Task Force Criteria (TFC),[29] and typically changes on both the resting (T-wave inversion and terminal activation delay) or ambulatory ECG (premature ventricular beats) precede any structural changes identifiable on cardiac imaging. The genetic etiology of ARVC is very dominated by truncating variants in plakophilin-2 (PKP2), the gene encoding the desmosomal protein of the same name, and, to a

much lesser degree, other desmosomal proteins, desmocollin-2 (DSC2) and desmoglein-2 (DSG2). Autosomal recessive variants in plakoglobin (JUP) cause a severe cardiocutaneous syndrome, but this is almost exclusively limited to the Greek island of Naxos.

Treatment is primarily targeted at arrhythmia management using various pharmacological agents including beta-blockers and flecainide, and protection against SCD with ICDs. A risk prediction model has been devised for ARVC, best applied to patients over 14 years of age (www.arvcrisk.com).[30] Electrophysiology studies to guide radiofrequency ablation is indicated in those with recurrent VT, but typically requires pericardial access to perform epicardial mapping and ablation, reflecting disease pathophysiology. Correlation has been made between excessive exercise and ARVC related to PKP2.[31]

2. Left dominant ACM, with prominent LV manifestations in the setting of relatively mild right-sided disease.

   Parallel to the genetic discovery that plakoglobin was responsible for Naxos syndrome, genetic studies in a family from Ecuador identified a homozygous variant in desmoplakin (DSP) associated with a similar cardiocutaneous phenotype (Carvajal syndrome) although with predominantly LV involvement. Left dominant ACM has now been reported in numerous individuals and families, associated with ventricular arrhythmias and varying degrees of LV dysfunction. DSP is the dominant desmosomal gene, although the mechanism behind development of a fundamentally different phenotype is unclear. An important aspect of the cardiac phenotype is myocardial inflammation, characterized by chest pain, ST elevation on ECG, and troponin release, which occurs in 15%–20% of individuals with varying DSP variants, and is often recurrent.[32] Alternative diagnostic criteria have been proposed that reflect predominant LV involvement.

   Converse to ARVC, structural features precede those on the electrocardiogram, and the earliest evidence of an emerging phenotype is typically LV sub-epicardial delayed enhancement evident on cardiac MRI.[28] Ventricular premature beats detected on ambulatory ECG are also an early finding. Many patients with DSP-mediated ACM have a subtle cutaneous phenotype characterized by plantar keratoderma and tightly curled, brittle hair.[33]

   In line with the overarching concept of ACM, the spectrum of left dominant disease now includes disease associated with other non-desmosomal genes including desmin (DES), lamin A/C (LMNA), phospholamban (PLN), cardiac sodium channel (SCN5A), filamin-C (FLNC), RNA-binding motif protein 20 (RBM-20), and TMEM-43.[25] Similar to ARVC, treatment is directed toward rhythm management and prevention of SCD, with an increased emphasis on heart failure management.

3. Biventricular ACM, characterized by equal, bilateral involvement with no apparent predilection for either ventricle.

Biventricular ACM typically represents end-stage disease with significant ventricular dysfunction, evolving in the latter stages of either ARVC or left dominant ACM. However, patients may present early in life with biventricular disease as the primary manifestation, which can be differentiated from dilated cardiomyopathy by the presence of RV failure and arrhythmia burden. The diagnosis is often confirmed on histological evaluation of myocardial tissue ascertained at the time of ventricular assist device implantation or transplant. Accurate diagnosis allows for appropriate investigation of family members. There appears to be no specific genetic predisposition with both desmosomal and non-desmosomal genes implicated.

References

1. Jervell A, Lange-Nielsen F. Congenital deaf-mutism, functional heart disease with prolongation of the Q-T interval, and sudden death. *Am Heart J.* 1957;54:59-68.
2. Romano C, Gemme GPR. Aritme cardiache rare del' eta pediatrica. *Clin Pediatr.* 1963;45:656.
3. Ward O. A new familial cardiac syndrome in children. *J Ir Med Assoc.* 1964;54:103-106.
4. Wang Q, Shen J, Splawski I, et al. SCN5A mutations associated with an inherited cardiac arrhythmia, long QT syndrome. *Cell.* 1995;80:805-811.
5. Wang Q, Curran ME, Splawski I, et al. Positional cloning of a novel potassium channel gene: KVLQT1 mutations cause cardiac arrhythmias: refined genetic and physical localization of LQT1. *Nat Genet.* 1996;12:17-23.
6. Curran ME, Splawski I, Timothy KW, Vincent GM, Green ED, Keating MT. A molecular basis for cardiac arrhythmia: HERG mutations cause long QT syndrome. *Cell.* 1995;80:795-803.
7. Schwartz PJ, Priori SG, Spazzolini C, et al. Genotype-phenotype correlation in the long-QT syndrome: gene-specific triggers life-threatening arrhythmias. *Circulation.* 2001;103:89-95.
8. MacCormick JM, McAlister H, Crawford J, et al. Misdiagnosis of Long QT syndrome as epilepsy at first presentation. *Ann Emerg Med.* 2009;54:26-32.
9. Krahn AD, Laksman Z, Sy RW, et al. Congenital long QT syndrome. *JACC Clin Electrophysiol.* 2022;8:687-706.
10. Zhang L, Timothy KW, Vincent GM, et al. Spectrum of ST-T-wave patterns and repolarization parameters in congenital long-QT syndrome: ECG findings identify genotypes. *Circulation.* 2000;102:2849-2855.
11. Ackerman MJ, Priori SG, Dubin AM, et al. Beta-blocker therapy for long QT syndrome and catecholaminergic polymorphic ventricular tachycardia: are all beta-blockers equivalent. *Heart Rhythm.* 2017;14:e41-e44.
12. Priori SG, Wilde AA, Horie M, et al. HRS/EHRA/APHRS expert consensus statement on the diagnosis and management of patients with inherited primary arrhythmia syndromes: document endorsed by HRS, EHRA, and APHRS in May 2013 and by ACCF, AHA, PACES, and AEPC in June 2013. *Heart Rhythm.* 2013;10:1932-1963.
13. Niaz T, Bos JM, Sorensen KB, Moir C, Ackerman MJ. Left cardiac sympathetic denervation monotherapy in patients with congenital long QT syndrome. *Circ Arrhythm Electrophysiol.* 2020;13:e008830.
14. Tristani-Firouzi M, Jensen JL, Donaldson MR, et al. Functional and clinical characterization of KCNJ2 mutations associated with LQT7 (Andersen syndrome). *J Clin Invest.* 2002;110:381-388.
15. Splawski I, Timothy KW, Sharpe LM, et al. Ca(V)1.2 Calcium channel dysfunction causes a multisystem disorder including arrhythmia and autism. *Cell.* 2004;119:19-31.
16. Gakenheimer-Smith L, Meyers L, Lundahl D, et al. Expanding the phenotype of CACNA1C mutation disorders. *Mol Genet Genomic Med.* 2021;9:1-8.
17. Priori SG, Napolitano C, Memmi M, et al. Clinical and molecular characterization of patients with catecholaminergic polymorphic ventricular tachycardia. *Circulation.* 2002;106:69-74.
18. Lahrouchi N, Raju H, Lodder EM, et al. Utility of post-mortem genetic testing in cases of sudden arrhythmic death syndrome. *J Am Coll Cardiol.* 2017;69:2134-2145.
19. Lahat H, Pras E, Olender T, et al. A missense mutation in a highly conserved region of CASQ2 is associated with autosomal recessive catecholomine induced polymorphic ventricular tachycardia in Bedouin families from Israel. *Am J Hum Genet.* 2001;69:1378-1384.
20. Watanabe H, Chopra N, Laver D, et al. Flecainide prevents catecholaminergic polymorphic ventricular tachycardia in mice and humans. *Nat Med.* 2009;15:380-383.
21. De Ferrari GM, Dusi V, Spazzolini C, et al. Clinical management of catecholaminergic polymorphic ventricular tachycardia the role of left cardiac sympathetic denervation. *Circulation.* 2015;131:2185-2193.
22. Van Der Werf C, Lieve K V, Bos JM, et al. Implantable cardioverter-defibrillators in previously undiagnosed patients with catecholaminergic polymorphic ventricular tachycardia resuscitated from sudden cardiac arrest. *Eur Heart J.* 2019;40:2953-2961.
23. Crotti L, Spazzolini C, Tester DJ, et al. Calmodulin mutations and life-threatening cardiac arrhythmias: insights from the International Calmodulinopathy Registry. *Eur Heart J.* 2019;40:2964-2975.
24. Peltenburg PJ, Blom NA, Vink AS, et al. In children and adolescents from Brugada syndrome-families, only SCN5A mutation carriers develop a type-1 ECG pattern induced by fever. *Circulation.* 2020;142:89-91.
25. Towbin JA, McKenna WJ, Abrams DJ, et al. 2019 HRS expert consensus statement on evaluation, risk stratification, and management of arrhythmogenic cardiomyopathy. *Heart Rhythm.* 2019;16:e301-e372.
26. Sen-Chowdhry S, Syrris P, Ward D, Asimaki A, Sevdalis E, McKenna WJ. Clinical and genetic characterization of families with arrhythmogenic right ventricular dysplasia/cardiomyopathy provides novel insights into patterns of disease expression. *Circulation.* 2007;115:1710-1720.
27. Cardiomyopathy D, Corrado D, Fontaine G, Marcus FI, Mckenna WJ. Arrhythmogenic right ventricular dysplasia/cardiomyopathy: need for an international registry. *Circulation.* 2000;101:e101-e106.
28. DeWitt ES, Chandler SF, Hylind RJ, et al. Phenotypic manifestations of arrhythmogenic cardiomyopathy in children and adolescents. *J Am Coll Cardiol.* 2019;74:346-358.

29. Marcus FI, McKenna WJ, Sherrill D, et al. Diagnosis of arrhythmogenic right ventricular cardiomyopathy/dysplasia: proposed modification of the task force criteria. *Circulation.* 2010;121: 1533-1541.

30. Cadrin-Tourigny J, Bosman LP, Nozza A, et al. A new prediction model for ventricular arrhythmias in arrhythmogenic right ventricular cardiomyopathy. *Eur Heart J.* 2019;40:1850-1858.

31. James CA, Bhonsale A, Tichnell C, et al. Exercise increases age-related penetrance and arrhythmic risk in arrhythmogenic right ventricular dysplasia/cardiomyopathy-associated desmosomal mutation carriers. *J Am Coll Cardiol.* 2013;62: 1290-1297.

32. Smith ED, Lakdawala NK, Papoutsidakis N, et al. Desmoplakin cardiomyopathy, a fibrotic and inflammatory form of cardiomyopathy distinct from typical dilated or arrhythmogenic right ventricular cardiomyopathy. *Circulation.* 2020;141:1872-1884.

33. Hylind R, Beauséjour-Ladouceur V, Plovanich ME, et al. Cardiocutaneous features of autosomal dominant desmoplakin-associated arrhythmogenic cardiomyopathy. *Circ Genom Precis Med.* 2020;13:719-721.

Specific Congenital Heart Defects

21
Atrial Septal Defects

LISA BERGERSEN

KEY LEARNING POINTS

- Atrial septal defects (ASDs) include any defect in the atrial septum, typically resulting in atrial shunting, either as isolated defects or in combination with more complex forms of congenital heart disease.
- Physiology is primarily characterized by left-to-right shunting, right ventricular volume overload, and increased pulmonary blood flow.
- Patients with ASDs are often asymptomatic; however, those with symptomatic or moderate to large ASDs may be

- considered for either surgical or transcatheter device closure, dependent on defect morphology and available technologies.
- The primary reason to close an ASD is to prevent later development of volume load complications such as pulmonary vascular disease and atrial dysrhythmias.
- In the case of patent foramen ovale, the primary reason for closure is to prevent ischemic stroke.

Definition

Atrial septal defects (ASDs) include an opening anywhere in the atrial septum and range in diameter from millimeters to a virtual absence of the septum (Fig. 21.1). Atrial defects may be single or multi-fenestrated. This chapter will cover defects that result in atrial level shunts including:

- Secundum ASD
- Patent foramen ovale (PFO)
- Partial anomalous pulmonary vein connection
- Sinus venosus defects
  - Superior vena caval sinus venosus defect
  - Inferior vena caval sinus venosus defect
  - Scimitar syndrome
  - Unroofed coronary sinus

Primum ASD or *ostium primum*, large single atrial defects involving the septum primum are of endocardial origin and are discussed in the chapter on complete atrioventricular (AV) canal (see Chapter 31) (Fig. 21.1). *Common atrium* is defined by the absence of the septum primum, septum secundum, and the AV canal septum and is usually associated with heterotaxy syndrome (see Chapter 32).

Prevalence

Because of the absence of symptoms and significant murmurs, many patients with typical significant atrial defects are still seen for the first time in childhood, even adulthood.

Atrial defects are the second most common form of congenital heart disease in children,[1] and the most common form identified in adults.[2] The prevalence of atrial defects is estimated at 1.6 per 1000 live births,[3] with the incidence in recent studies varying from 0.5 to 1.0 per 1000 live births,[4,5] far exceeding the 0.073 per 1000 rate in very ill infants reported in earlier years.[1] This large increase is likely due to the more widespread use of echocardiography, which identifies many smaller defects unaccompanied by symptoms or murmurs.

Embryology

Early fetal hearts comprise one common atria that then septates, known as the *ostium* primum, or first hole. Atrial septation embryologically involves three structures: the septum primum, septum secundum, and AV canal septum. The septum primum is first to appear in the developing atria and consists of a venous valve that grows from the junction between the inferior vena cava (IVC) and the right atrium toward the septum secundum (Fig. 21.2). The latter is a crescent-shaped muscular ridge that forms in the superior-posterior aspect of the common atrium as an invagination between the developing atria. This forms the *ostium secundum*, or second hole, that is present as the septum primum grows toward the septum secundum. As they come together, the *fossa ovalis* is formed, with a small gap left between the *septum primum* and *septum secundum* known as the foramen

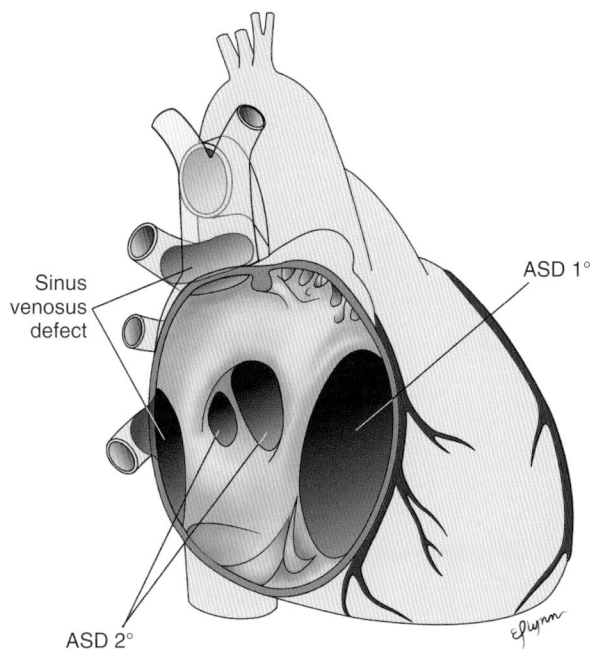

• **Fig. 21.1** Diagram of the atrial septum showing several types of atrial septal defects. An ostium primum defect *(ASD1°)* is located immediately adjacent to the mitral and tricuspid valves. Ostium secundum defects *(ASD2°)* are located near the fossa ovalis in the center of the septum. Sinus venosus defects are located in the area derived from the embryologic sinus venosus. (From Fyler DC, ed. *Nadas' Pediatric Cardiology*. Philadelphia: Hanley & Belfus; 1992.)

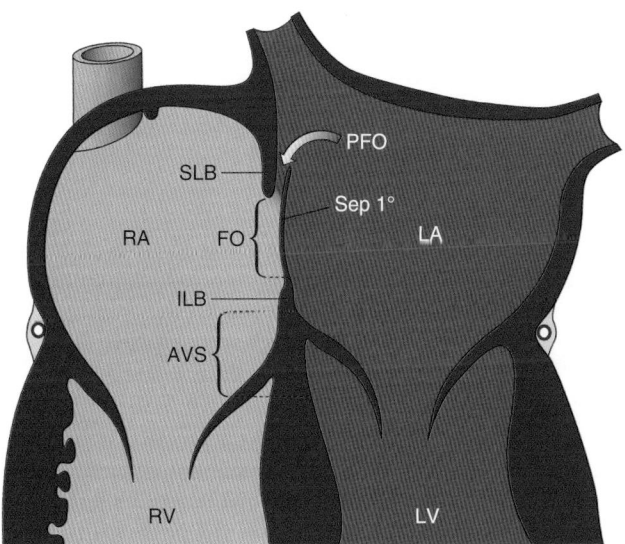

• **Fig. 21.2** Diagram of atrial septal components, showing patent foramen ovale *(PFO, arrow)*, septum primum *(Sep 1°)*, left atrium *(LA)*, left ventricle *(LV)*, fossa ovalis *(FO)*, superior *(SLB)* and inferior *(ILB)* limbic bands, atrioventricular septum *(AVS)*, right atrium *(RA)*, and right ventricle *(RV)*.

ovale, which is bordered on the left by septum primum and by the superior limbic band of the fossa ovalis (septum secundum) on the right (Fig. 21.2). The AV canal septum is formed, at least in part, by the superior and inferior endocardial cushions and contributes to septation of the outlet portion of the atria and the inlet portion of the ventricles. The tissue that separates the right pulmonary veins from the

superior vena cava (SVC) and from the posterior aspect of the right atrium is termed sinus venosus septum.

During fetal life, right-to-left flow occurs through the foramen ovale because right atrial pressure exceeds left atrial pressure. After birth, the atrial pressures reverse as the lungs aerate, pulmonary vascular resistance decreases, and systemic vascular resistance increases with elimination of placental circulation. As a result, the septum primum opposes the superior limbic band of the fossa ovalis and the foramen ovale narrows.

Anatomy

Secundum Atrial Defect

A secundum atrial defect in the fossa ovalis is the most common cause of an atrial-level shunt (excluding PFO) and is most frequently due to a deficiency of the septum primum. A secundum ASD can be a single defect or be multi-fenestrated. Rarely, a secundum defect results in a deficiency of the septum secundum. Their size is generally defined by diameter as trivial (<3 mm), small (3 to <6 mm), moderate (6–8 mm), or large (>8 mm). However, the relative size of the defect to the patient size may be more clinically relevant.

Patent Foramen Ovale

When the foramen ovale, a normal interarterial connection *in utero*, persists after birth, it is known as a PFO. A PFO is seen in almost all newborns and with decreasing frequency throughout life. Only in rare conditions, such as hypoplastic left heart syndrome, will a newborn not have a PFO.

Partial Anomalous Pulmonary Venous Connection

Partial anomalous pulmonary venous connection is a connection between one or more (but not all) of the pulmonary veins with a systemic vein. Partial anomalous pulmonary veins are relatively common, usually complicating other cardiac abnormalities. An associated interatrial communication is not considered integral to the anomaly, but is often present. There are several anatomic variations (Fig. 21.3). The most common type is anomalous connection of the left upper pulmonary vein to the left innominate vein. One or more of the left pulmonary veins can connect directly to the right SVC, the coronary sinus, or the hemiazygos vein.

Anomalous drainage of one or more pulmonary veins to the right atrium results from leftward malposition of septum primum, at times in conjunction with deficiency or absence of the superior limbic band. The normally connecting pulmonary veins drain anomalously. This anomaly has been demonstrated in patients with heterotaxy syndrome with polysplenia.

Sinus Venosus Defects

Sinus venosus defect is a communication between one or more of the right pulmonary veins and the cardiac end

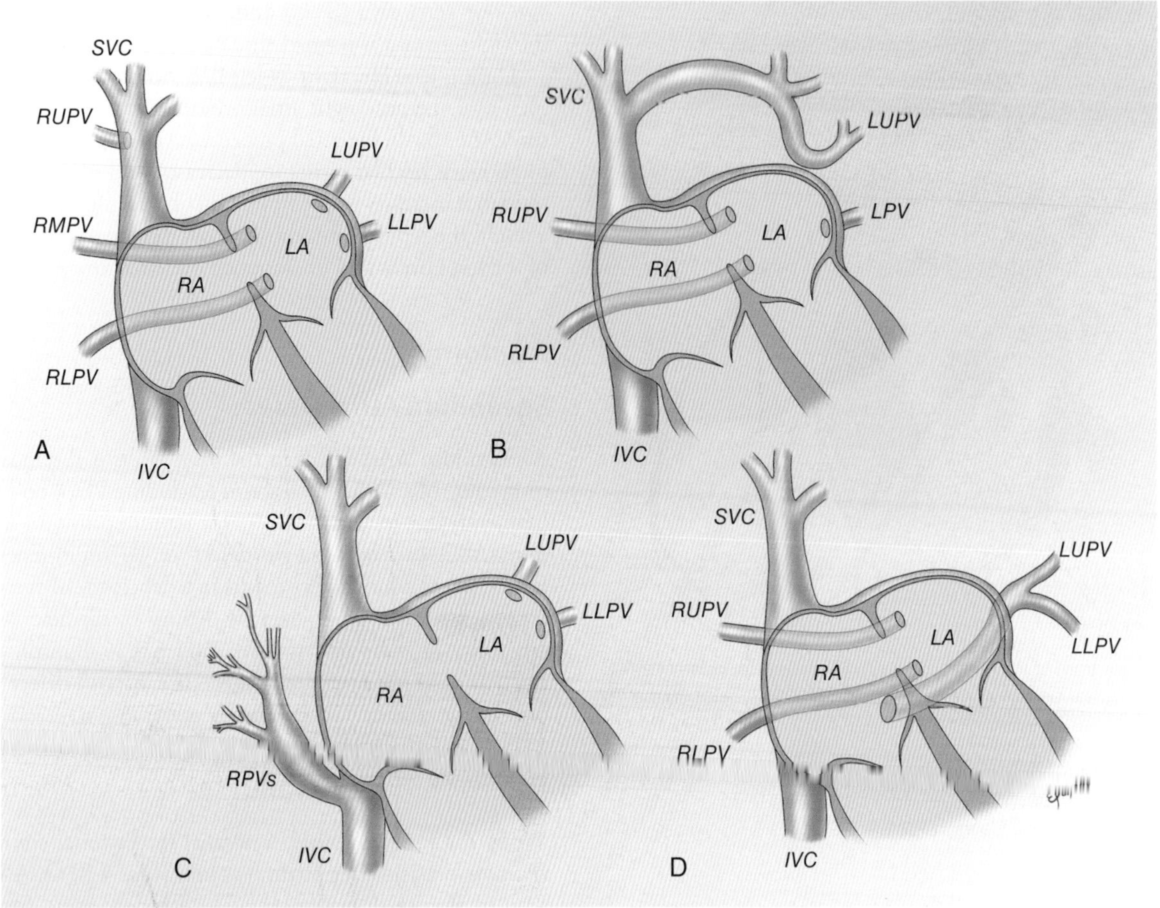

• **Fig. 21.3** Diagram of several connections of anomalous pulmonary veins to the systemic venous circulation. **(A)** Drainage of the right upper veins *(RUPV)* to the superior vena cava *(SVC)*. **(B)** Drainage of the left upper veins *(LUPV)* through the left vertical vein to the innominate vein. **(C)** Drainage of lower right-sided veins *(RPVs)* into the inferior vena cava *(IVC; scimitar syndrome)*. **(D)** Drainage of left pulmonary veins *(LPVs)* into the coronary sinus.

of the vena cava or the posterior wall of the right atrium (Fig. 21.1). Anatomically, it is not an ASD because it does not allow direct communication between the left and right atria, but rather the interatrial communication is through one or more of the pulmonary veins.

Superior Vena Caval Sinus Venosus Defect

This caval defect is most commonly located between the right upper pulmonary vein and the cardiac end of the SVC (called the SVC type), the defect being due to the absence of the anterior wall of the right upper pulmonary vein and the posterolateral wall of the cardiac end of the SVC. The deficiency of the sinus venosus septum can extend peripherally to involve secondary branches of the right pulmonary veins, resulting in the appearance of several pulmonary veins draining into the SVC. The left atrial orifice of the right upper pulmonary vein is usually patent, allowing for an interatrial communication through it. In addition, blood from the right upper pulmonary vein flows to the right atrium through the defect in the sinus venosus septum. When the left atrial orifice of the right upper pulmonary vein is atretic, there is no interatrial communication, and

the anatomic appearance is that of partially anomalous pulmonary venous connection of the right upper pulmonary vein to the SVC.

Inferior Vena Caval Sinus Venosus Defect

Rarely, the caval defect involves the right lower or middle pulmonary veins and the middle or superior aspects of the right atrium. This type of sinus venosus defect is called the IVC type, although direct involvement of the IVC is either extremely rare or not present. For that reason, the term *sinus venosus of the right atrial type* is preferred. These rare defects, adjacent to the orifice of the IVC, are often associated with anomalous return of the right lower pulmonary veins.[6]

Scimitar Syndrome

Anomalous connection of some or all of the right pulmonary veins to the IVC is termed scimitar syndrome. The term derives from the appearance of the anomalous right pulmonary vein on chest x-ray, which has the curving appearance of the Turkish sword. Other elements of the syndrome include hypoplasia of the right lung, secondary

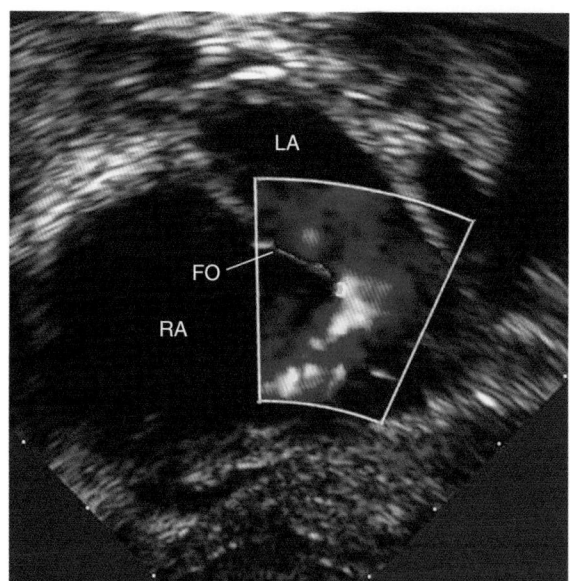

• **Fig. 21.4** Echocardiogram of coronary sinus septal defect outlined by color flow Doppler. *FO,* Foramen ovale; *LA,* left atrium; *RA,* right atrium.

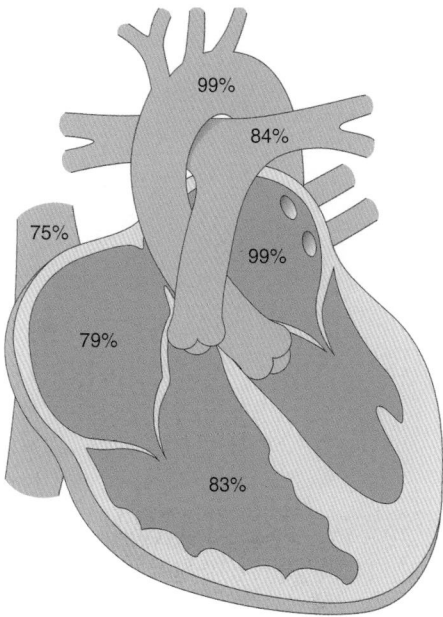

• **Fig. 21.5** Isolated secundum atrial septal defect with saturation measurements. (From Bergersen L, ed. *Congenital Heart Disease: The Catheterization Manual.* New York: Springer; 2009.)

dextrocardia, and arterial supply of parts of the right lung by collateral arterial blood vessels, usually from the descending aorta.

Unroofed Coronary Sinus

Unroofed coronary sinus or *coronary sinus septal defect* is a rare type of interatrial communication in which the septum between the coronary sinus and the left atrium is either partially or completely unroofed, leading to a left-to-right shunt through the coronary sinus orifice (Fig. 21.4). The orifice of the coronary sinus in this anomaly is usually large as a result of the left-to-right shunt, resulting in a sizeable defect in the inferior aspect of the atrial septum near the entry of the IVC. The association of a coronary sinus septal defect and persistent left SVC is termed *Raghib syndrome.*[7] When the coronary sinus is completely unroofed, the left SVC enters the left superior corner of the left atrium, anterior to the orifice of the left upper pulmonary vein and posterior to the left atrial appendage.

Physiology

Isolated atrial level defect physiology is primarily defined by left-to-right shunting, right ventricular volume overload, and increased pulmonary blood flow. Left-to-right shunting at the atrial level results in a "step up" in saturations from the SVC to the right atrium (Fig. 21.5). The amount of shunting through a large atrial defect is determined by the relative right and left ventricular compliance. Early in infancy, the right ventricle is less compliant; therefore, left-to-right shunting is minimal. As the right ventricle becomes more compliant with age, the shunting increases, with moderate to large shunts exceeding a Qp:Qs of 1.5:1. In the case of a superior venal

caval sinus venosus defect, which is often small, shunting usually does not exceed 2:1 Qp/Qs. In some patients, the left-to-right shunt can be phasic, varying with systole and diastole, leading to a small right-to-left shunt detectable by color flow Doppler, occasionally manifesting in a slightly lower than normal average arterial oxygen saturation. Left ventricular compliance decreases as a normal part of aging, which may be exacerbated by systemic hypertension, and may increase left-to-right shunting. This could account for the adult diagnosis of an atrial defect, sometimes in unfortunate circumstances complicated by the new diagnosis of atrial tachyarrhythmias, pulmonary vascular obstructive disease, or congestive heart failure.

Clinical Manifestations

Children with an atrial defect are usually discovered at a few years of age, and occasionally in the neonatal period. The lack of symptoms and the lack of a readily audible murmur account for the delay in discovering these patients. Generally, the defect is uncovered during routine examination of an otherwise well child, such as at the first preschool examination.

In some instances, patients with an ASD or PFO, without other cardiac abnormality, are cyanotic, particularly during exercise. This is considered to be an extreme version of the small right-to-left shunt measurable in almost all patients with an ASD and perhaps aggravated by an unusually large eustachian valve often found in these patients. Closing the atrial defect is curative (Fig. 21.6). In addition, some small infants and older adults present with symptoms secondary to pulmonary overcirculation (see Course).

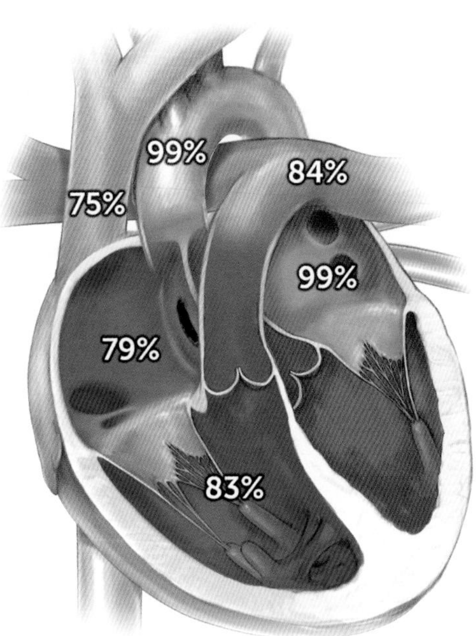

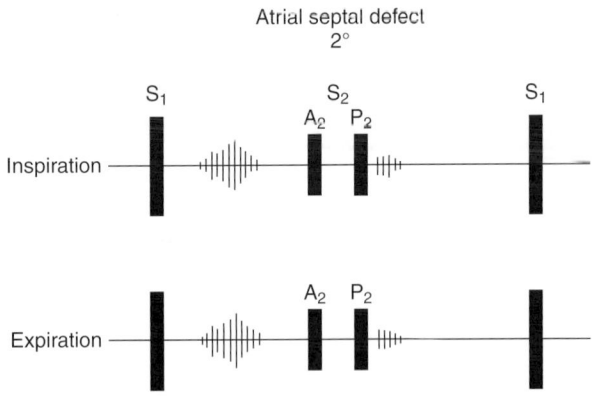

Atrial septal defect
2°

• **Fig. 21.7** Auscultatory findings resulting from an atrial septal defect. The second heart sound (*S2*) is widely split and does not vary with respiration. There is a minimal systolic murmur of the ejection type. Often there is an early diastolic rumble that arises from excess flow across the tricuspid valve and seems to occur early in diastole, in part, because of the widely split second heart sound. *A2,* Aortic valve closure; *P2,* pulmonic valve closure; *S1,* first heart sound. (From Fyler DC, ed. *Nadas' Pediatric Cardiology.* Philadelphia: Hanley & Belfus; 1992.)

• **Fig. 21.6** Catheterization data in a 30-year-old woman with huge atrial secundum septal defect. There is right-to-left shunting at the atrial level and normal pulmonary artery pressure. This atrial defect was surgically closed with a patch, with now normal postoperative physiologic data. %, oxygen saturation; *AO,* Aorta; *LA,* left atrium, *LV,* left ventricle; *PA,* pulmonary artery; *RA,* right atrium; *RV,* right ventricle.

Diagnostic Techniques

Physical Examination

With a large shunt, there can be a palpable left parasternal predominance due to an enlarged right ventricle. The first heart sound is characteristically loud at the left lower sternal border (in the presence of a normal or short P-R interval on the electrocardiogram). The second heart sound at the left upper sternal border is widely split due to delayed emptying of the volume-loaded right ventricle. In addition, the time between the first and second heart sound is fixed unaffected by respiration (Fig. 21.7), as the resulting shunt equalizes the respiratory influence on both right and left ventricular output. In the case of partial anomalous pulmonary venous connections without an associated atrial defect, the second sound may be well split but is not fixed relative to respiration.

The intensity of the pulmonary component is almost always normal, reflecting normal pulmonary pressure and resistance. Detection of a loud P2 should raise concerns regarding the development of pulmonary vascular disease. Murmurs are typically not loud and may even be absent. However, there is usually an ejection systolic murmur (grade 2 at most) at the left upper sternal border due to increased flow across the pulmonary valve, even in the presence of a normal valve. Also, there is frequently a harder to detect early diastolic flow rumble (grade 1 or 2), often of high frequency, at the left lower sternal border due to increased flow across the tricuspid valve.

Electrocardiography

Incomplete right bundle branch block is a common finding in patients with ASD and identification on electrocardiogram, although in many cases a normal finding in combination with other findings can be an indication to consider an ASD evaluation in an otherwise healthy patient. Additional findings such as electrocardiographic evidence of atrial enlargement or right ventricular enlargement/hypertrophy may be signs of large left-to-right shunts.

Chest X-Ray

Chest X-ray is not currently used as a diagnostic tool for suspected isolated atrial defects, but incidental findings such as evidence of cardiomegaly or increased pulmonary vascular markings when obtained for other indications may bring patients with large left-to-right shunt to attention for further evaluation. In this scenario, the SVC shadow may be absent on the right of the spine on the plain chest film related to right atrial enlargement and clockwise rotation of the heart and/or cardiomegally may be present. Scimitar syndrome can be readily recognized on the plain chest X-ray because there is hypoplasia of the right lung, the heart shadow is shifted to the right, and the visible right pulmonary veins create a silhouetted curve (the scimitar appearance) toward the IVC (Fig. 21.8).

Echocardiography

Echocardiography is the primary imaging modality used for evaluation and diagnosis of ASDs. The atrial septum and the adjacent systemic and pulmonary veins are imaged from several acoustic windows for any abnormal communication. Color flow Doppler mapping is used to image blood flow direction and velocity. In addition, attention is given to

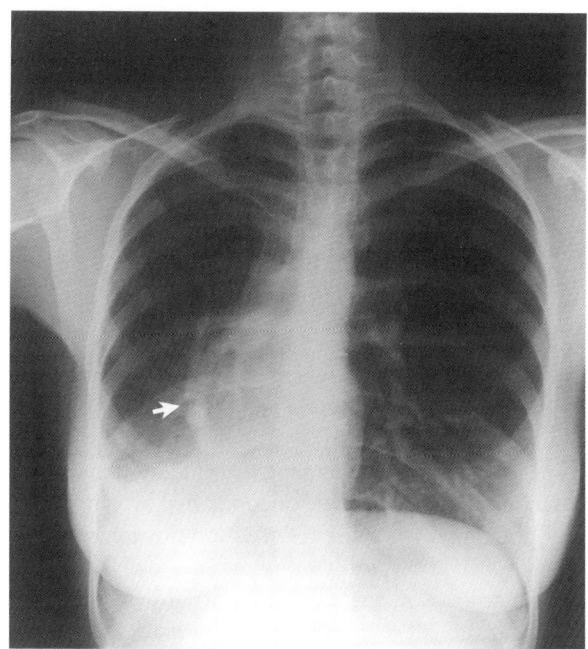

• **Fig. 21.8** X-ray of an asymptomatic 15-year-old patient with scimitar syndrome showing the anomalous pulmonary vein *(arrow)* draining to the inferior vena cava. Note the dextrocardia because of hypoplasia of the right lung and the corresponding increase in size of the left lung.

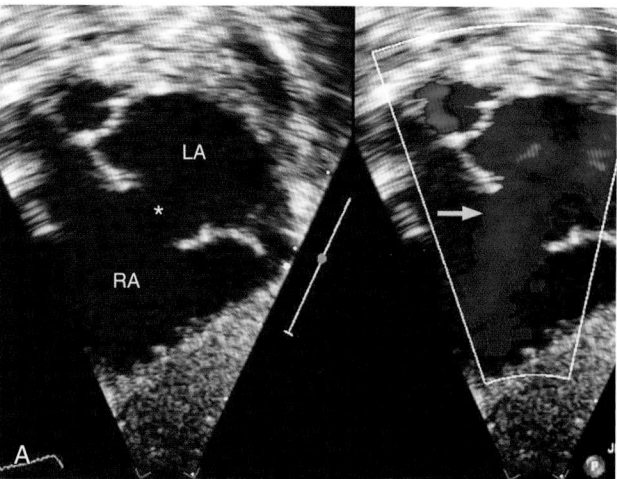

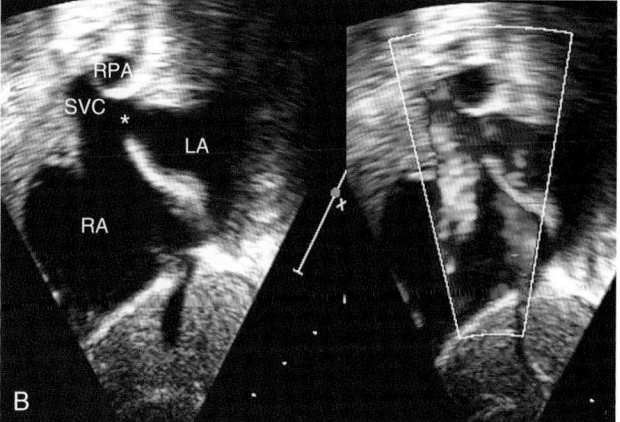

• **Fig. 21.9** Echocardiographic imaging of atrial defects. **(A)** Secundum atrial septal defect in the center of the fossa ovalis *(*)*. Note the left-to-right flow imaged by color Doppler *(arrow)*. **(B)** Superior vena cava *(SVC)*-type sinus venosus defect located above the fossa ovalis between the SVC and the right upper pulmonary vein as it enters the left atrium *(LA)*. *RA,* Right atrium; *RPA,* right pulmonary artery. (Reprinted from The Lancet, 383, Tal Geva, Jose D Martins, Rachel M Wald, Atrial septal defects, 1921-32, 2014, with permission from Elsevier.)

evidence of excess volume load on the right heart structures as a result of the left-to-right shunt. The right atrium, right ventricle, and pulmonary arteries are typically enlarged, and the interventricular septum flattens during diastole as a result of the increased flow. Although echocardiographic measurements of the magnitude of the left-to-right shunt have been reported to correlate with invasive techniques, this parameter is not routinely evaluated in clinical practice, in part because of uncertainties about its accuracy and reproducibility.

The atrial septum is best imaged from the subxiphoid window because the ultrasound beam is perpendicular to the atrial septum (Fig. 21.9). Even a thin septum primum is visible from this view, and the likelihood of false dropouts is minimized. In contrast, a false dropout in the mid-portion of the fossa ovalis is common when imaging from the apical view because the ultrasound beam is parallel to the septum. The parasternal short axis and the right parasternal border (parasagittal) views are also helpful. Particular attention should be paid to the location and size of the defect, to its relationship with adjacent structures such as the venae cavae, pulmonary veins, and AV valves, and to the presence of additional defects. In patients who are candidates for transcatheter device closure of the defect, septal rims and total septal length are measured.

In addition to color flow Doppler mapping, contrast echo using agitated saline can be helpful in detecting an atrial-level shunt. When a PFO is suspected, injection of agitated saline during a Valsalva maneuver (which causes an increase in right atrial pressure) can demonstrate passage of contrast into the left side of the heart, indicating a right-to-left shunt across the foramen. In the setting of a superior vena caval sinus venosus defect, echocardiographic evaluation demonstrates right heart volume overload characteristics, but with no obvious defect visible in the central atrial septum. Meticulous examination is required to visualize this superior defect (Fig. 21.9). Although some have real anomalous return of right upper pulmonary veins to the SVC, for the most part, it is the defect location that makes this more apparent than real.[6] When an unroofed coronary sinus is suspected, injection of agitated saline through an intravenous line placed in the left arm can substantiate the diagnosis by demonstrating appearance of contrast in the left atrium before it appears in the right atrium (Fig. 21.4).

Transesophageal echocardiography provides an excellent window for imaging of the atrial septum and atrial ends of the systemic and the pulmonary veins and is routinely used for guidance during transcatheter closure of ASDs. Some centers prefer intracardiac echocardiography for the latter. Intraoperative transesophageal echocardiography is seldom used in our center in patients with isolated secundum ASD, but is frequently used in patients undergoing closure of sinus defects and other complex interatrial communications.

Magnetic Resonance Imaging

Magnetic resonance imaging (MRI) can offer anatomic information in cases where echocardiography is incomplete or inconclusive. In addition, shunt calculations can obviate the need for more invasive diagnostic tests for diagnostic purposes. The goals of the MRI examination include both anatomic and functional information. Anatomic features such as atrial defect location, size, and its relationship to key neighboring structures can assist in determination of the suitability for transcatheter versus surgical closure. By obtaining pulmonary and systemic flow measurements, the hemodynamic burden, as described by the pulmonary-to-systemic flow ratio (Qp:Qs), can be calculated. Additional quantitative measurements include the right ventricular size and function. In suspected cases of a sinus venosus defect and anomalous pulmonary venous connection, MRI is particularly helpful because patient size and acoustic windows do not limit its diagnostic capabilities (Fig. 21.10).

Management

Preprocedural Evaluation

A preprocedural echocardiogram will help determine the optimal intervention for closure. Key elements of the imaging evaluation should include accurately measuring the defect size and rims, determining degree of left-to-right shunting, identifying any other cardiac defects, and assessing for pulmonary hypertension. Defects may be closed

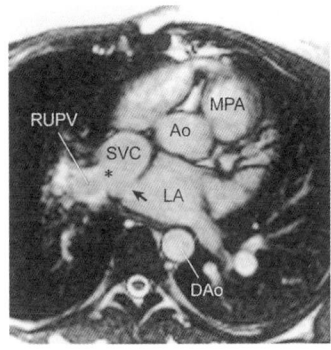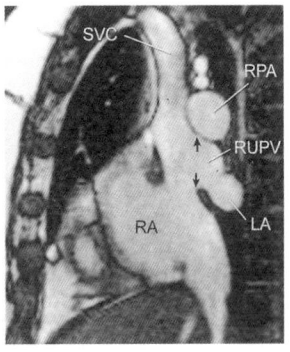

A   B

• **Fig. 21.10** Gradient echo cine magnetic resonance images of sinus venosus defect. **(A)** An image in the axial plane showing the sinus venosus defect (*) as an area of unroofing of the wall between the right upper pulmonary vein *(RUPV)* and the superior vena cava *(SVC)*. The arrow points to the left atrial orifice of the RUPV, which allows communication between the left atrium *(LA)* and the RUPV and SVC. **(B)** An image in the sagittal plane showing the sinus venosus defect *(arrows)*.

surgically or via transcatheter device placement methods depending on the type of ASD and the presence of other cardiac defects. Technological advancements have created more options for percutaneous closure and will continue to evolve with novel devices. Currently, percutaneous closure can be offered for closure of secundum ASDs, as detailed below, but not in patients with sinus venosus, primum, or coronary sinus ASD.

Secundum ASD

In patients with good acoustic windows and unambiguous delineation of the atrial septal and venous anatomy, transthoracic echocardiography is usually the only diagnostic tool necessary for management planning. After diagnosis of a secundum ASD is made or confirmed by echocardiography, the patient may be referred for closure, which can be accomplished surgically or by catheter-delivered device. The primary reason for closing an atrial defect is to prevent the future development of pulmonary vascular disease. In addition, closure may reduce the incidence and severity of supraventricular dysrhythmias (particularly atrial fibrillation), although it does not eliminate this problem even when performed in childhood[8] and has been shown to have a diminishing effect in patients over 40 years of age and recurrence of arrhythmias in long-term follow-up (>5 years).[9-11]

For practical purposes, defects measuring 8 mm or larger with evidence of a significant left-to-right shunt, greater than 1.5:1, should be closed when identified, even in very young patients, because such a defect will likely not close spontaneously and may in fact get larger.[5] However, it is reasonable to follow smaller defects in young patients, who are generally asymptomatic, for a few years because many defects are likely to close spontaneously, particularly those smaller than 3 mm.[5] Then after some years of follow-up, if echocardiographic evidence of shunting persists and the defect is 5 mm or larger, intervention can be considered.

Surgical Intervention

In 1952, the first reported successful open heart repair under direct vision was an ASD repair in a 5-year-old girl using hypothermia and inflow occlusion by Lewis and Taufic. Current approaches to surgical ASD repair require cardiopulmonary bypass. While surgical closure traditionally required a median sternotomy, most isolated surgical ASD repairs are completed using minimally invasive heart surgeries. This can be done via partial sternotomy, mini thoracotomy, or most recently via robotically assisted heart surgery.[12] With these advancements, patients are at lower risk for complications and bleeding events, and have a shorter hospital stay after surgery (3 days)[12] (see Chapter 62).

Cardiac Catheterization

Device closure at catheterization was initially described in 1976,[13] and in those few original patients after 27 years of follow-up, occlusion remained effective, although atrial arrhythmias did occur. With advancements in available devices, delivery equipment, and technique, percutaneous closure has become a common approach to closure of secundum ASDs. The first FDA-approved device was the Amplatzer Septal Occluder (ASO).[14] New technologies continue to become available, such as bioresorbable occlusion devices, which are currently in clinical trials. Isolated ASD closures are considered relatively low-risk transcatheter procedures, and patients can often be discharged the same or following day.[15]

If catheterization is undertaken, special care is required when obtaining the right superior vena caval oxygen saturation for shunt calculation purposes. Considerable reflux of left atrial highly saturated blood occurs up the SVC when a large shunt is present. Thus, an uncontaminated venous sample should be obtained high in the vena cava, even from the left innominate vein. We do not use inferior vena caval samples, considering them unreliable because of contamination by both reflux and very high renal vein values. If catheterization data in a patient with pulmonary hypertension suggest a defect might be safely closed, temporary device occlusion may be tested at that study. Transcatheter ASD device placement procedures are now done primarily using ultrasound guidance, either transesophageal or intracardiac echocardiography, with minimal fluoroscopy and no angiography.

Patent Foramen Ovale

With increasing use of and technologic improvements in echocardiographic equipment, the PFO has become a common observation, especially in young patients. Because there is little, if any, shunting and thus no volume overload evidence on the right heart chambers, it has been by and large considered a finding of no significance. Although echocardiographically it is closed in most children by 18 months of age, persistent patency in some 20% of patients older than 90 years has been noted at autopsy.[16] With the introduction of echocardiographic "bubble studies" and color flow Doppler, right-to-left atrial shunting, especially with Valsalva maneuvers (which elevate right atrial pressure), became evident. This finding was soon noted to be common in patients with neurologic insults suggestive of an embolic etiology.[17] There is thus widespread interest in management of such patients with this combination of lesions. Treatment strategies, including foramen closure surgically or by catheter-delivered devices, are being used that have reduced but not completely eliminated the neurologic events.[17]

Partial Anomalous Pulmonary Venous Connection

As an isolated defect, partial anomalous pulmonary veins does not usually cause symptoms and pulmonary hypertension is rare. Abnormal entry of a single small pulmonary vein does not require surgical intervention. The anomalous veins pose the practical problem of what to do when the chest has been opened to repair an atrial defect. For the most part, these anomalous veins can be corrected, but the surgical difficulty, the likelihood of success, and the probable benefits should be weighed carefully before proceeding. Small pulmonary veins entering the left innominate vein may be ligated without a problem or left alone. Pulmonary veins entering the IVC in older patients can be baffled successfully to the left atrium. In neonates and infants, however, this may be very difficult, and such an attempt in this age group may result in severe obstruction or complete occlusion of the created channel. In those with much or all of the left pulmonary veins returning to the left innominate vein, the connecting vertical vein is usually large and long enough to detach from the innominate vein and anastomose to the left atrium. In each case, tailoring the response to the anatomy is required.

Sinus Venosus Defect

All sinus venosus patients are referred to surgery. In older patients, surgery has been very successful using patch defect closure through a trans caval approach.[18] In very young patients, especially when right upper pulmonary venous return is anomalous to the SVC, there is not much room available for a baffle. To circumvent this problem, the SVC is transected superior to the anomalous veins and the distal caval end anastomosed to the right atrial appendage. The atrial defect is then closed in such a way that the proximal vena cava and anomalous veins drain to the left atrium.[19] In older patients, this operation has been quite successful.[19] In our own experience (mean surgical age, 4 years), although dysrhythmias have not been evident, obstruction at the SVC–right atrial anastomosis has occurred in some and has been managed successfully by balloon dilation and stent placement (Fig. 21.11). In the setting of an IVC sinus venosus defect, appropriate single patch will close the defect with the veins on the correct side, the patch assuming the normal position of the atrial septum.

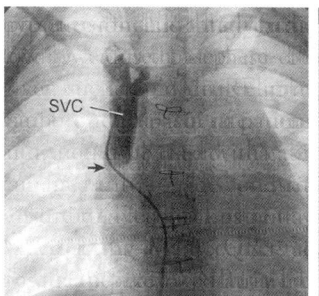 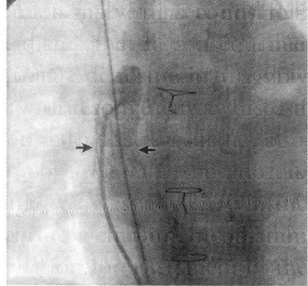

A   B

• **Fig. 21.11** Cineangiogram in the superior vena cava *(SVC)* of 7-year-old patient showing **(A)** virtual occlusion of SVC–right atrial anastomosis *(arrow)* done as part of repair of sinus venosus atrial defect and **(B)** now wide-open anastomosis following balloon dilation and stent *(arrows)* placement.

Scimitar Syndrome

Sometimes, the physiologic advantage of surgical correction of scimitar syndrome is not obvious in the adult because the amount of blood shunting through the small right lung may be small (less than 1.5/L). In those detected in infancy, symptoms, heart failure, ASD, pulmonary sequestration, and hypertension are common, and some 25% have pulmonary vein stenosis. Transcatheter occlusion techniques have been helpful in eliminating the arterial blood supply for pulmonary sequestrations. For those undergoing surgical repair, postoperative obstruction to pulmonary venous return is very common in infants, and diminished right lung flow is present in almost all.[20] Newer surgical techniques that involve baffling rather than reimplantation of the anomalous right pulmonary vein have demonstrated improved results with less postoperative obstruction.[21]

Unroofed Coronary Sinus

Surgical repair of unroofed coronary sinus is tailored to the anatomy present. If a left SVC is present, it is redirected to the right atrial side either through ligation, if an adequate innominate vein is present or through an intra–left baffle or tunnel to the right atrium. If there is no left SVC and the coronary sinus defect is huge, then the orifice of the coronary sinus is closed. Whether the coronary venous blood flow drains into the left atrium or is redirected to the right is of little practical consequence.

Follow-up of Patients After Closure

Overall, it is remarkable how frequently exercise tolerance improves in patients considered asymptomatic before surgery. It is also quite striking how many patients continue to remain undiagnosed for many decades, with many reports comprising hundreds of such patients.[5] Residual patch leaks are uncommon, and most patients are clinically better. Echocardiographically, right ventricular volumes decrease but do not reach normal values in many, especially in those operated on at older ages.[5,8,10] Late appearance of pulmonary vascular obstructive disease or congestive heart failure after repair is virtually unknown, although if some is present preoperatively, it may progress.[22]

Course

The natural course of ASD, except for the largest openings and those associated with other cardiac defects, is relatively benign.[5] Many patients with significant defects survive for several decades before developing symptoms. It is likely that acquired diseases of adulthood (coronary artery problems, systemic hypertension) often elevate left ventricular end-diastolic pressure, leading to a rise in the left atrial value, which in turn increases the left-to-right shunting. Mitral valve prolapse (see Chapter 33) is a curious finding seen among some patients with ASD, without known practical

consequence. Improvement in the degree of prolapse after repair of the atrial defect suggests that mitral valve prolapse may be caused by the atrial defect itself.[23] Late problems include congestive heart failure, atrial fibrillation, and rarely pulmonary vascular obstructive disease.

Although most infants with an ASD are asymptomatic, a few develop congestive heart failure and growth failure requiring closure in the first year of life. Most often, but not always, these infants have large left-to-right shunts in early infancy because there are additional defects, such as ventricular septal defect, patent ductus arteriosus, coarctation, myocardial dysfunction, an anatomically small left ventricle, or systemic hypertension. In some infants, the high incidence of ASD-associated extracardiac anomalies[1] accounts for the growth failure and a number of these infants with early difficulty will undergo spontaneous closure of the defect. This might suggest that many of these "defects" are actually dilated patent foramina ovalia that became incompetent because of elevated left atrial pressure for whatever reason and later, with resolution of the underlying left-sided problem, the foramen ovale closes.

Older patients may develop pulmonary vascular disease. In general, this unfortunate occurrence is rare before the age of 20 years and in the past occurred in 5% to 10% of adults with ASD who had not undergone surgical repair, though in rare instances can occur in children[22,24,25] (Fig. 21.12). This incidence is likely to be quite less in the future because most

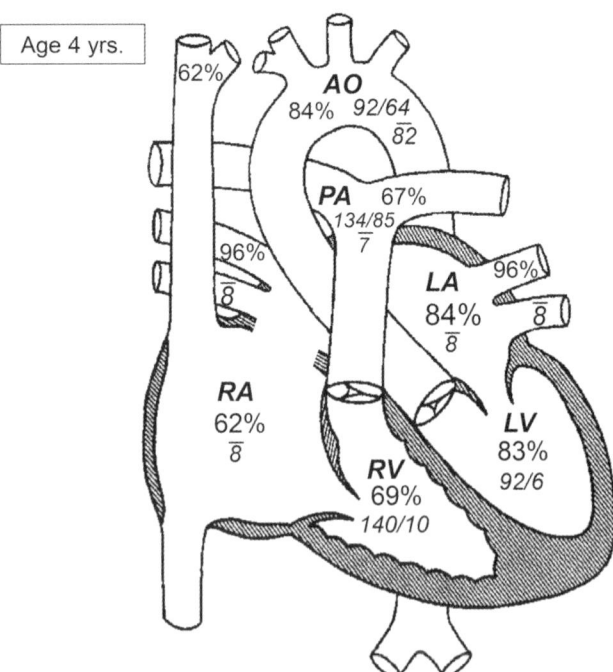

• Fig. 21.12 Catheterization data in a 4-year-old girl with Down syndrome, a very large atrial defect, right-to-left shunting across this defect *(arrows)*, suprasystemic right ventricle *(RV)* and pulmonary artery *(PA)* pressures, and severe pulmonary vascular obstructive disease unresponsive to oxygen and vasodilators. She died 22 months later. *AO*, Aorta; *RA*, right atrium; *LA*, left atrium; *RV*, right ventricle; *LV*, left ventricle; *PA*, pulmonary artery; *%*, oxygen saturation.

atrial defects are now being closed on discovery, thus preventing the development of pulmonary vascular disease. Catheterization with evaluation of response to oxygen and nitric oxide is advisable in all such patients. Any underlying causes such as obstructive airway disease, sleep apnea, high altitude, or drugs require careful investigation because these are reversible.

Without closure, the natural course of an atrial defect may lead to atrial dysrhythmias, particularly as patients age. With catheterization and surgery altering the natural course, we are noticing a lower incidence of these arrhythmias, and sometimes improvement in existing atrial arrhythmias.[8-11]

In the setting of an isolated PFO, multiple other clinical manifestations have been observed including cryptogenic stroke, migraine and vascular headaches, decompression sickness and air embolisms, as well as platypnea-orthodeoxia syndrome.[26]

Acknowledgment

The author would like to thank and acknowledge Drs. John F. Keane, Tal Geva, and Donald C. Fyler for their contributions to a previous version of this chapter.

References

1. Fyler DC, Buckley LP, Hellenbrand WE, et al. Report of the New England Regional Infant Cardiac Program. *Pediatrics*. 1980;65:376.
2. Shuler CO, Tripathi A, Black GB, Park YM, Jerrell JM. Prevalence of treatment, risk factors, and management of atrial septal defects in a pediatric Medicaid cohort. *Pediatr Cardiol*. 2013;34:1723-1728.
3. van der Linde D, Konings EE, Slager MA, et al. Birth prevalence of congenital heart disease worldwide: a systematic review and meta-analysis. *J Am Coll Cardiol*. 2011;58:2241-2247.
4. Mai CT, Isenburg JL, Canfield MA, et al. for the National Birth Defects Prevention Network. National population-based estimates for major birth defects, 2010-2014. *Birth Defects Res*. 2019; 111:1420-1435.
5. Geva T, Martins JD, Wald RM. Atrial septal defects. *Lancet*. 2014;383:1921-1932.
6. Van Praagh S, Kakou-Guikahue M, Kim HS, et al. Atrial situs in patients with visceral heterotaxy and congenital heart disease: Conclusions based on findings in 104 postmortem cases. *Coeur*. 1988;19:484-502.
7. Raghib G, Ruttenberg HD, Anderson RC, et al. Termination of left superior vena cava in left atrium, atrial septal defect, and absence of coronary sinus: a developmental complex. *Circulation*. 1965;31:906-918.
8. Roos-Hesselink JW, Meijboom FJ, Spitaels SE, et al. Excellent survival and low incidence of arrhythmias, stroke and heart failure long-term after surgical ASD closure at young age: a prospective follow-up study of 21-33 years. *Eur Heart J*. 2003;24:190-197.
9. Chubb H, Whitaker J, Williams SE, et al. Pathophysiology and management of arrhythmias associated with atrial septal defect and patent foramen ovale. *Arrhythm Electrophysiol Rev*. 2014;3:168-172.
10. Abrahamyan L, Dharma C, Alnasser S, et al. Long-term outcomes after atrial septal defect transcatheter closure by age and against population controls. *JACC Cardiovasc Interv*. 2021;14: 566-575.
11. O'Neill L, Floyd CN, Sim I, et al. Percutaneous secundum atrial septal defect closure for the treatment of atrial arrhythmia in the adult: a meta-analysis. *Int J Cardiol*. 2020;321:104-112.
12. Vida VL, Zanotto L, Zanotto L, et al. Minimally invasive surgery for atrial septal defects: a 20-year experience at a single centre. *Interact Cardiovasc Thorac Surg*. 2019;28:961-967.
13. King T, Thompson S, Steiner C, et al. Secundum atrial septal defect: Nonoperative closure during cardiac catheterization. *JAMA*. 1976;235:2506-2509.
14. Berger F, Ewert P, Bjornstad PG, et al. Transcatheter closure as standard treatment for most interatrial defects: experience in 200 patients treated with the Amplatzer septal occluder [see comment]. *Cardiol Young*. 1999;9:468-473.
15. Quinn BP, Yeh M, Gauvreau K, et al. Procedural risk in congenital cardiac catheterization (PREDIC3T). *J Am Heart Assoc*. 2022;11:e022832.
16. Hagen PT, Scholz DG, Edwards WD. Incidence and size of patent foramen ovale during the first 10 decades of life: An autopsy of 965 normal hearts. *Mayo Clin Proc*. 1984;59:17-20.
17. Mac Grory B, Ohman EM, Feng W, et al. Advances in the management of cardioembolic stroke associated with patent foramen ovale. *BMJ*. 2022;376:e063161.
18. Nicholson IA, Chard RB, Nunn GR, et al. Transcaval repair of the sinus venosus syndrome. *J Thorac Cardiovasc Surg*. 2000;119:741-744.
19. Gustafson RA, Warden HE, Murray GF. Partial anomalous pulmonary venous connection to the superior vena cava. *Ann Thorac Surg*. 1995;60:S614-S617.
20. Najm HK, Williams WG, Coles JG, et al. Scimitar syndrome: twenty years' experience and results of repair. *J Thorac Cardiovasc Surg*. 1996;112:1161-1169.
21. Geggel RL, Gauvreau K, Callahan R, Feins EN, Baird CW. Scimitar syndrome: a new multipatch technique and incidence of postoperative pulmonary vein obstruction. *JTCVS Tech*. 2020; 4:208-216.
22. Steele PM, Fuster V, Cohen M, et al. Isolated atrial septal defect with pulmonary vascular obstructive disease: long term follow-up and prediction of outcome after surgical correction. *Circulation*. 1987;76:1037-1042.
23. Schreiber TL, Feigenbaum H, Weyan AE. Effect of atrial septal defect repair on left ventricular geometry and degree of mitral valve prolapse. *Circulation*. 1980;61:888-896.
24. Besterman E. Atrial septal defect with pulmonary hypertension. *Br Heart J*. 1961;23:587.
25. Zaver AG, Nadas AS. Atrial septal defect—secundum type. *Circulation*. 1965;32:24.
26. Giblett JP, Williams LK, Kyranis S, Shapiro LM, Calvert PA. Patent foramen ovale closure: state of the art. *Interv Cardiol*. 2020;15:e15.

22

Ventricular Septal Defects

JAMI LEVINE

KEY LEARNING POINTS

- Ventricular septal defects (VSDs) are one of the most common congenital heart diseases and the most common diagnosis in healthy newborns in the first year of life. Defects vary considerably in both size and anatomic location within the ventricular septum.
- Both genetic and environmental factors have been implicated in the creation of VSDs. There is an association with abnormalities of chromosome number as well as single gene defects but for most, when genetics are a factor, the inheritance is multifactorial. Though there is an increased risk for VSD occurrence in those with a first-degree relative who has a VSD, the risk remains quite low.
- The likelihood of developing symptoms related to VSD will be determined by the size and location of the VSD as well any

other factors that affect the ease with which blood can shunt from one ventricle to the other. The goal of care is to avoid any chance that the VSD is causing permanent changes to the pulmonary vascular bed in addition to minimizing congestive symptoms to allow for adequate nutrition and growth.
- Some VSDs are associated with outflow tract obstruction or aortic valve prolapse; anatomic changes that once present may worsen over time and drive treatment decisions.
- Less than 25% of isolated VSDs require closure. Closure should be considered in the first year of life if the right ventricular pressure is above half systemic or it growth is inadequate due to symptoms of pulmonary overcirculation. Most of the time, intervention will be surgical, but transcatheter device closure is an option for some.

Definition

A ventricular septal defect (VSD) is a deficiency in the ventricular septum, the solid wall that separates the deoxygenated blood in the right ventricle (RV) from the oxygenated blood in the left ventricle (LV). The presence of a VSD allows blood to cross from one ventricle to the other. The physiologic significance will depend on the relative resistance to flow on the two sides of the ventricular septum as well as the size and location of the defect.

Prevalence

VSDs are one of the most common congenital heart defects identified in infancy, with most studies suggesting that isolated VSDs occur at the rate of 5000–5500/100,000 births[1 3]; however, the true prevalence has been difficult to estimate accurately, largely related to ascertainment bias. Historically, estimates were derived using databases of individuals referred for evaluation secondary to symptoms or abnormal physical exam findings. Because not all defects are symptomatic and some resolve before detection, prevalence was likely underestimated. In the current era, some have estimated prevalence utilizing full population screening instead. Unfortunately, the populations amenable to this

type of screening may have other sources of bias. For example, VSD prevalence in fetuses and in preterm infants may underestimate prevalence because these are subjects known to have difficult imaging windows and elevated pulmonary vascular resistance, making small VSDs easy to miss.

Embryology

The ventricular septum forms when a few distinct embryologic components coalesce to form a solid wall that separates the ventricular mass into two chambers by the end of the 7th week of gestation. There is debate about how best to describe and label the components that make up the septum, but a common conceptualization considers the septum to be constructed from three major components: the trabecular muscular septum, the atrioventricular (AV) canal septum, and the outlet septum. Some consider the outlet septum to then be subdivided into a membranous component and a conal-septal component. Our group currently uses a variation which divides the septum into five components (Fig. 22.1A and B). Defects in the septum occur secondary to failure of component formation or incomplete fusion of components with each other or the ventricular free wall. A more detailed discussion of the embryology can be found in Chapter 2.

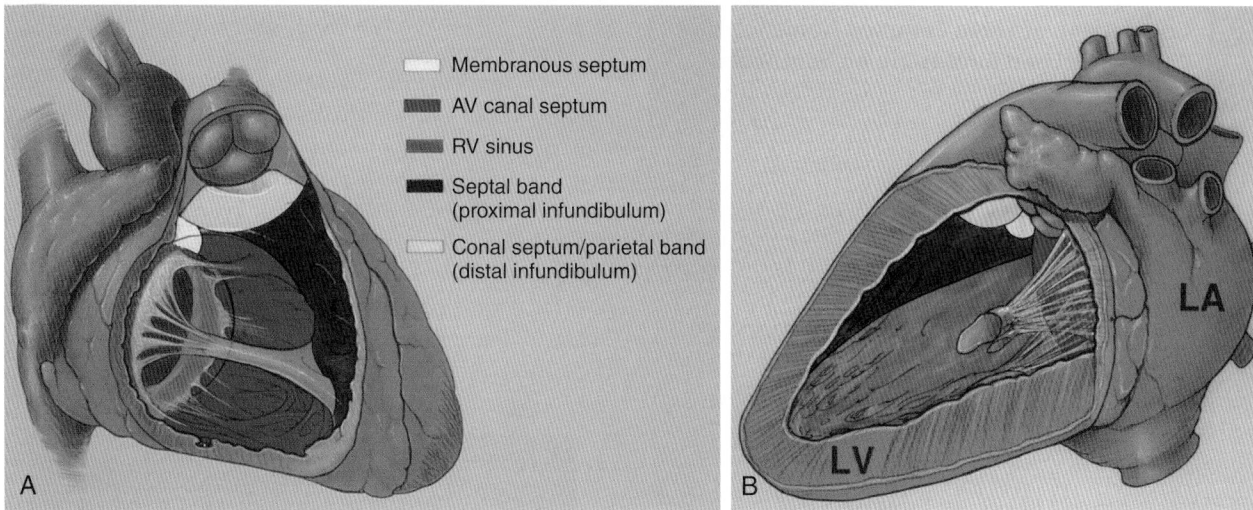

Membranous septum

AV canal septum

RV sinus

Septal band (proximal infundibulum)

Conal septum/parietal band (distal infundibulum)

• **Fig. 22.1** Ventricular septal morphology. (A) View from the right ventricle *(RV)* side of the septum. (B) View from the LV side of the septum. The conal septum sits just apical to the pulmonary valve and the membranous septum sits just apical to the aortic valve. The atrioventricular canal septum surrounds the posterior and septal portions of the tricuspid and mitral valve annuli. In this classification, the trabecular muscular component is divided into two segments: the RV sinus and the septal band. (Generously shared and reproduced with permission by Dr. Tal Geva.)

Etiology

Both environmental and genetic factors are important for the evolution of VSDs on a population scale, but in each individual patient, one or the other may dominate as the etiology for VSD formation.[4-6]

The importance of genetic factors is highlighted by the increased risk for VSD occurrence in individuals with certain genetic syndromes. Those at increased risk include individuals with abnormalities of chromosome number (e.g., trisomy 13, 18, 21) as well as some with single-gene defects (e.g., Holt-Oram syndrome).[5] Further evidence of the existence of genetic influences comes from familial data that show that the risk for having a VSD rises to 2–3% if there is a first-degree relative (parent or sibling) with a VSD. Risk is lower if the affected relative is a second- or third-degree relative, though may still be slightly higher than the risk in the general population. This is typical for what one would expect in multifactorial inheritance. Proof that environmental factors also play an important role comes from the observation that there is an increased incidence of VSDs associated with a wide variety of *in utero* exposures. Well-known examples include an increased risk for VSD in fetal alcohol syndrome, fetal exposure to lithium, and infants of diabetic mothers.

Morphology/Classification

VSDs are "named" according to their location in the septum. There is much debate regarding the best terminology and multiple classification systems have been proposed, including the recent publication of by the International Society for Nomenclature of Paediatric and Congenital Heart Disease whose goal is to create more unified terminology for use in

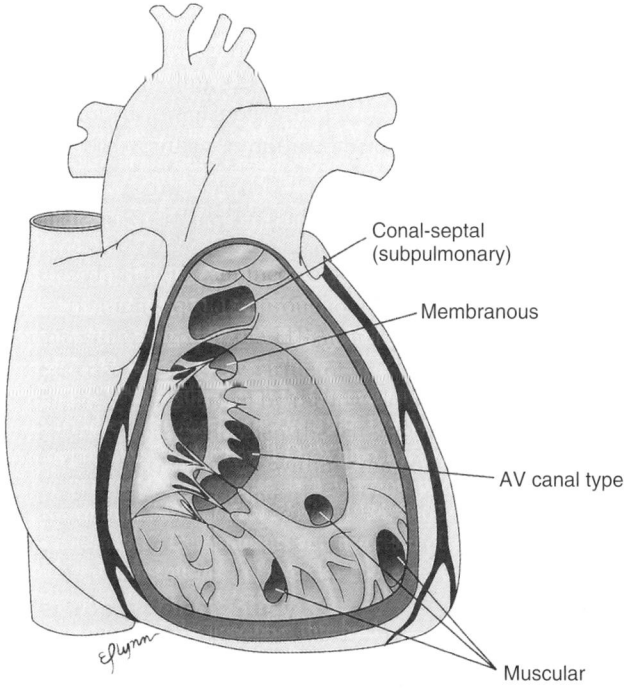

Conal-septal (subpulmonary)

Membranous

AV canal type

Muscular

• **Fig. 22.2** Ventricular septal defect (VSD) nomenclature. View of the septum from the right ventricle, illustrating different VSD types. Note that conoventricular (malalignment type) VSDs are not shown. *AV,* Atrioventricular.

pediatric heart disease.[7] The terminology currently in use in our institution[8] is illustrated in Fig. 22.2.

Table 22.1 compares the most commonly used paradigms.

Membranous VSDs involve a deficiency in the thin portion of the septum that lies just apical to the aortic valve (Fig. 22.3). Though the membranous septum is a relatively anterior portion of the septum, the defects often extend

TABLE 22.1	Comparison of Three Common Nomenclature Constructs Used for Describing Ventricular Septal Defects		
BCH (Van Praagh)	ISNPCHD	Anderson	
AV canal type	Inlet (not including those with complete AV canal defect)	Perimembranous inlet	
Membranous	Central perimembranous	Perimembranous	
Conoventricular (malalignment)	Outlet with malalignment	Perimembranous with malignment	
Conal-septal (subpulmonary)	Outlet	Doubly committed subarterial	
Muscular (designate location)	Trabecular muscular	Muscular (designate location)	

AV, Atrioventricular; *BCH,* Boston Childrens Hospital; *ISNPCHD,* International Society for Nomenclature of Paediatric and Congenital Heart Disease.

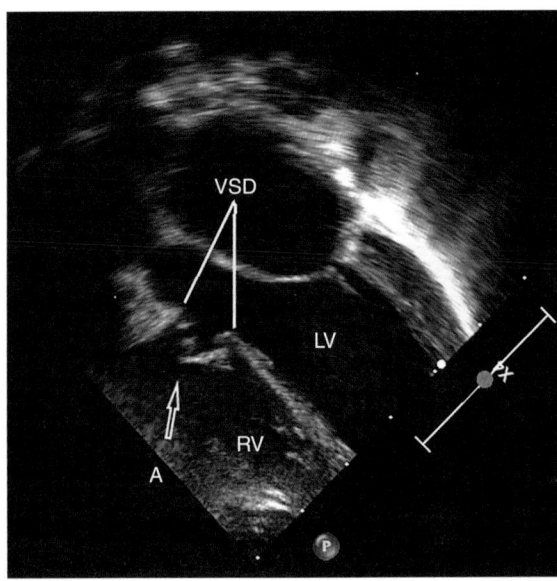

• **Fig. 22.3** Membranous ventricular septal defect (VSD). Echocardiographic image from apical window, angled anteriorly to highlight the left ventricular outflow tract. A large VSD sits just below the aortic valve *(straight lines)*. *Arrow* indicates an aneurysm of accessory tissue. *A,* Aneurysm; *LV,* left ventricle; *RV,* right ventricle.

posteriorly such that a portion may lie behind tricuspid valve attachments on the RV side of the septum. These valve attachments can become an important factor in determining the flow pattern through the defect. The membranous septum shares a border with all of the other components and defects can occur due to a lack of fusion with any of them. It is not unusual for membranous VSDs to be contiguous with defects involving these neighboring components

(e.g., a membranous VSD that extends into the muscular or AV canal septum).

Conoventricular VSDs are located within the "Y" of the septal band of the ventricular septum. They are often secondary to abnormal positioning of the conal septum such that it is no longer in the same plane as the muscular septum, often called a malalignment type of conoventricular defect. When the conal septum is deviated anteriorly/rightward, it may encroach on the RV outflow tract and can be associated with subvalvar pulmonary stenosis and/or hypoplasia of the pulmonary valve or main pulmonary artery (Fig. 22.4). A common example is tetralogy of Fallot. When

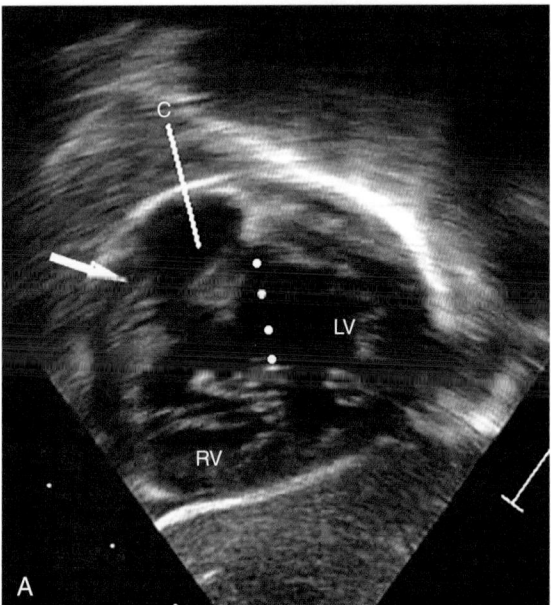

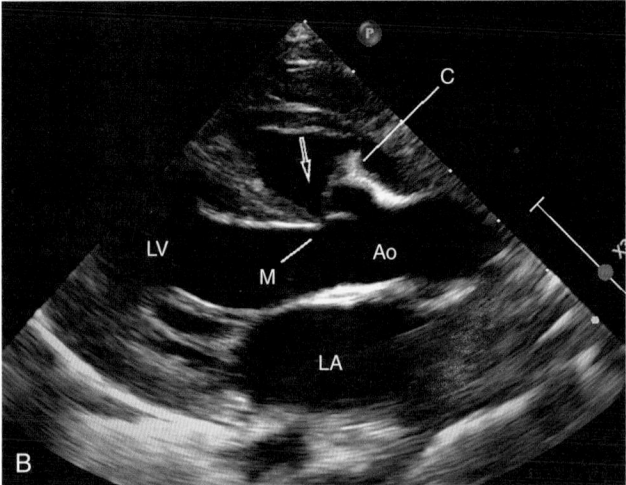

• **Fig. 22.4** Conoventricular ventricular septal defect (VSD) with anterior malalignment. (A) Subcostal short-axis image. The *dotted line* denotes the normal plane of the ventricular septum. Rightward and anterior/deviation of conal septum has narrowed the right ventricular outflow tract *(arrow)* and created a VSD. (B) Parasternal long-axis image. The muscular septum is normally positioned. The anterior deviation of the conal septum has "pulled" the aortic root anteriorly *(arrow)* causing it to override the crest of the muscular septum. *Ao,* Aortic root; *C,* conal septum; *LA,* left atrium; *LV,* left ventricle; *M,* crest of muscular septum; *RV,* right ventricle.

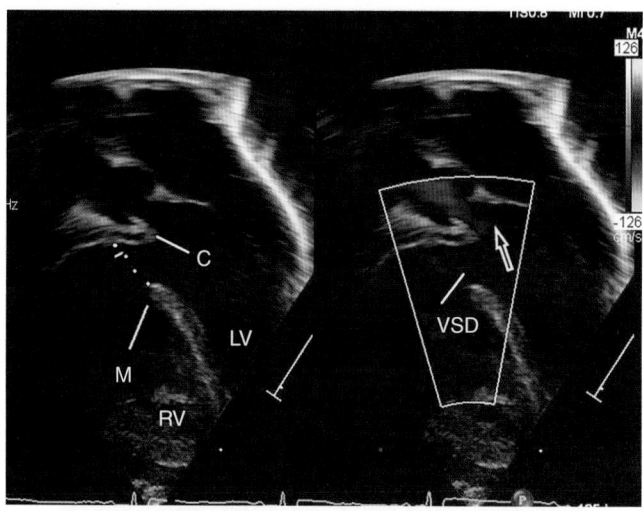

• **Fig. 22.5** Conoventricular ventricular septal defect *(VSD)* with posterior malalignment. Apical image highlighting the left ventricular outflow tract. The *dotted line* denotes the normal plane of the ventricular septum. The conal septum is deviated to the left and posteriorly, narrowing the area under the aortic valve *(arrow)* and creating a VSD. *C,* Conal septum; *LV,* left ventricle; *M,* crest of muscular septum; *RV,* right ventricle.

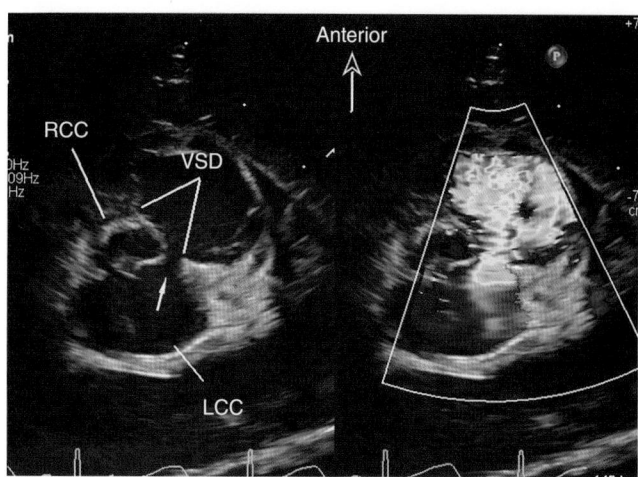

• **Fig. 22.6** Conal-septal ventricular septal defect *(VSD)*. Parasternal short-axis image of the aorta and right ventricular outflow tract. Absence of the conal septum results in a large VSD; flow is restricted by prolapse of the right coronary cusp. The color panel and the *arrow* highlight that the functional defect is significantly smaller than the anatomic defect. Note the discrepancy in the appearance of the right and left coronary cusps due to the prolapse. Typically, these would be uniform in size and appearance. *LCC,* Left coronary cusp; *RCC,* right coronary cusp.

the conal septum is deviated posteriorly/leftward, it encroaches instead on the left ventricular outflow tract. This may be associated with aortic valve hypoplasia, aortic arch hypoplasia, and/or aortic arch obstruction (Fig. 22.5). This may be seen in patients with interrupted aortic arch and VSD.

The conoseptal portion of the ventricular septum is located anterior to the membranous septum, just below the right coronary cusp of the aortic valve and immediately to the right of the pulmonary valve. Defects in this part of the septum are relatively rare overall, though they are much more common in Asian populations.[9] Complete absence of the conal septum leaves behind a large defect that is often confluent with the pulmonary valve annulus (Fig. 22.6). We typically use the term conal-septal or subpulmonary VSD to describe this type of defect. When the conal septum is present but there is a defect within it, we use the term intraconal VSD. These can be of any size, and usually are not confluent with the pulmonary valve annulus (Fig. 22.7).

AV canal VSDs are located in the basal portion of the septum at the crux of the heart. They are apical and inferior to the tricuspid and mitral valves. The hallmark of this type of VSD is that there is no muscular tissue separating the defect from the valve annuli (Fig. 22.8). These are frequently associated with other abnormalities of the AV canal and will be discussed in more detail in Chapter 31.

Muscular VSDs can be gaps within the large muscular portion of the ventricular septum or at the junction of the septum with the LV free wall. They can be of any size and their shape and appearance are quite variable (Figs. 22.9 and 22.10). They are often further named according to their location within the septum. In our institution, we usually identify their location in the anterior-posterior plane as well as in the apex-to-base plane. Muscular defects are often

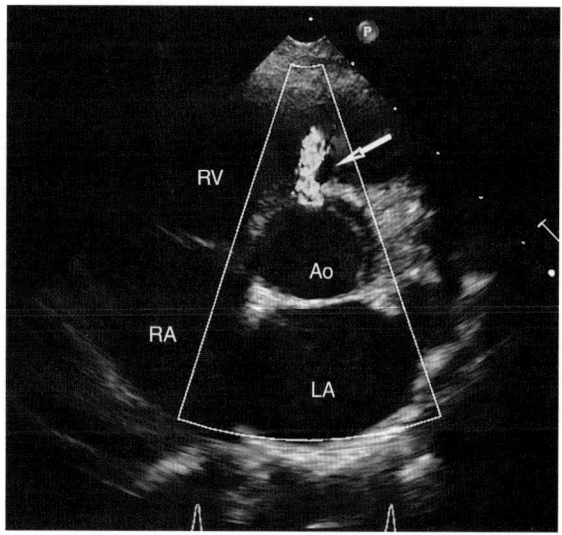

• **Fig. 22.7** Intraconal ventricular septal defect (VSD). Parasternal short-axis image of a small intraconal VSD *(arrow)* directly under the right coronary cusp of the aortic valve. Flow is directed anteriorly, typical for this type of VSD. *Ao,* Aortic root; *LA,* left atrium; *RA,* right atrium; *RV,* right ventricle.

single but may be multiple. When multiple defects are present, they can be clustered together or widely spread through the muscular septum.

Gerbode defect: This is an unusual variation of a septal defect that is not really a VSD. It is a defect in the very small segment of tissue that has LV on one side and right atrium on the other. When present, the shunt is from LV to right atrium.

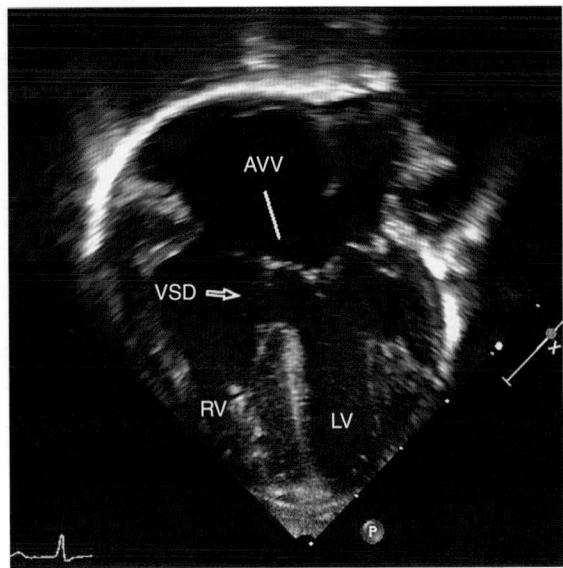

• **Fig. 22.8** Atrioventricular canal ventricular septal defect *(VSD)*. Apical image of the crux of the heart. A large VSD *(arrow)* sits just below the atrioventricular valves and no muscular tissue separates the defect from the valves. A large primum atrial septal defect is visible just above the valve. *AVV*, Atrioventricular valve; *LV*, left ventricle; *RV*, right ventricle.

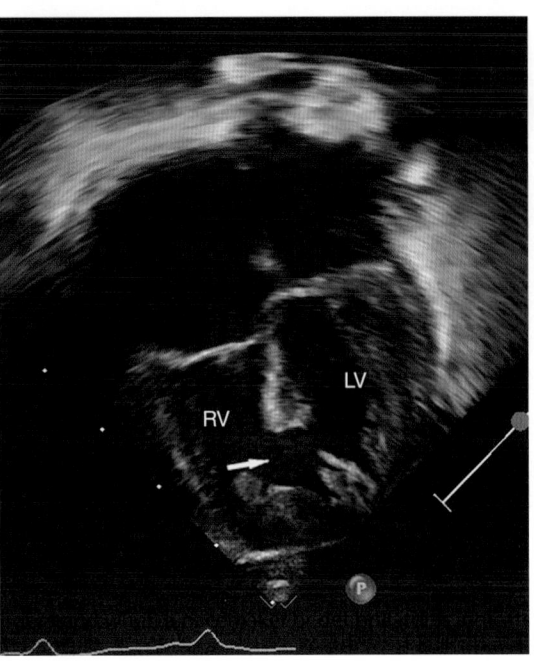

• **Fig. 22.10** Apical muscular ventricular septal defect (VSD). Apical image showing a large VSD *(arrow)* in the lower half of the septum. *LV*, Left ventricle; *RV*, right ventricle.

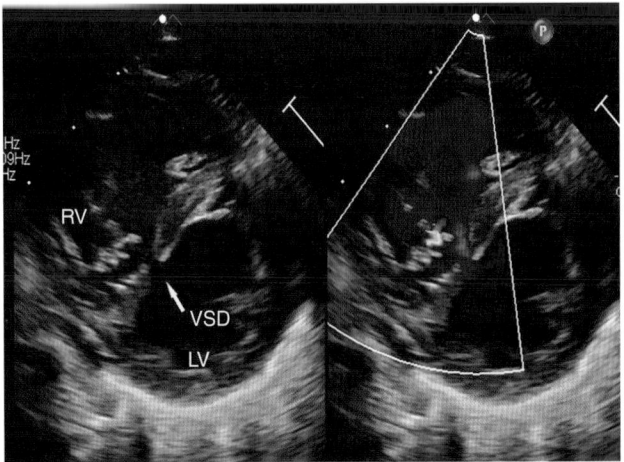

• **Fig. 22.9** Mid-muscular ventricular septal defect *(VSD)*. Parasternal short-axis image of a small mid-muscular VSD *(arrow)*. The defect splits into multiple smaller jets as it passes through trabeculations and valve tissue in the RV. *LV*, Left ventricle; *RV*, right ventricle.

All VSDs are similar with regard to their physiological effects. On the other hand, they vary tremendously with respect to their potential to become less physiologically important over time, the likelihood of being associated with other cardiac malformations, and their propensity to impact neighboring structures.

Physiology

Normally with ventricular contraction, blood in the RV crosses the pulmonary valve to enter the pulmonary circulation and blood in the LV crosses the aortic valve to enter the systemic circulation (Fig. 22.11). Like all fluids, blood

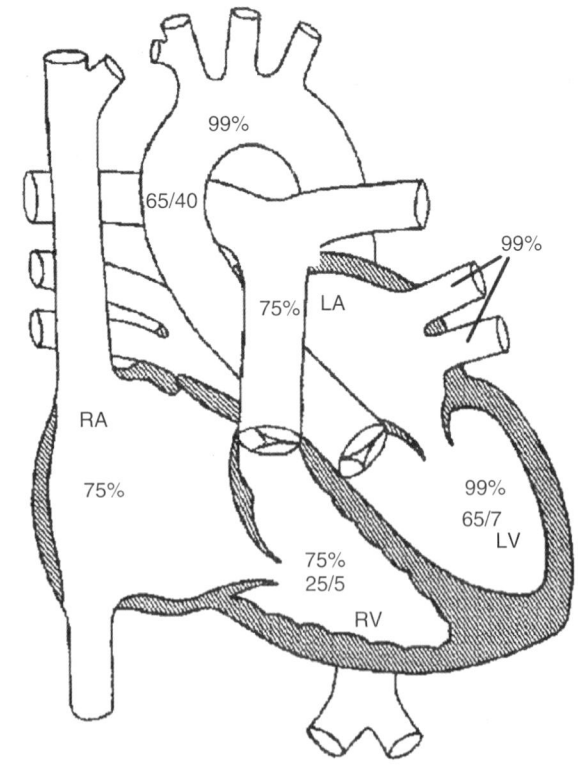

• **Fig. 22.11** Normal newborn hemodynamics. When the ventricular septum is intact, the deoxygenated blood in the right heart cannot mix with the oxygenated blood in the left heart and intraventricular pressures can differ on the two sides of the septum. *LA*, Left atrium; *LV*, left ventricle; *RA*, right atrium; *RV*, right ventricle.

follows the path of least resistance. When a VSD is present, blood in the ventricles now has the opportunity to cross the septum instead of crossing the appropriate semilunar valve. The direction of the shunt across the VSD and the physiologic importance will depend on the relative difference in the resistance to flow along these two potential pathways— the trans-septal path and the path across the semilunar valve. The resistances in turn will be determined by a complicated combination of factors including: VSD anatomy and size, semilunar valve size and function, great artery size, and the pulmonary and systemic vascular resistances.[10-13]

Fetus

In the fetus, the pulmonary and systemic vascular beds have similar levels of resistance and the RV pressure is similar to the LV pressure (see Chapter 4). Under these conditions, if a VSD is present, there may be very little flow that crosses it. With contraction, the ejected blood meets with similar resistance in the normal antegrade path and the abnormal trans-septal path to the opposite ventricle. Because of this, defects can be difficult to see in fetal imaging and the direction of ventricular level shunting, if present, is unpredictable.

Infants/Young Children

After birth, with expansion of the lungs and the loss of the placenta, the resistance in the pulmonary vascular bed begins to fall and the resistance in the systemic vascular bed rises. This takes hours to days to evolve. In the first hours after birth, the physiology is similar to that in the fetus, typically with little or no shunting across the VSD (Fig. 22.12). Over the next few days, however, there will be a developing "resistance gradient" that favors flow toward the lungs. Now with ventricular contraction, blood in the LV finds a lower resistance path out of the heart if it crosses the VSD to enter the RV than if it follows the normal antegrade pathway to the systemic circulation. The differences in resistance are small enough that most of the blood ejected from the LV still crosses the aortic valve and the magnitude of the left-to-right shunt across the VSD may be small. Normally pulmonary vascular resistance continues to decrease over the first few months of life and left-to-right shunting across the VSD will increase as the resistances on the two sides of the septum become more discrepant. Ultimately, there may be enough additional blood flow entering the pulmonary vasculature to cause symptoms of pulmonary congestion. The term "pulmonary overcirculation" is often used to describe this phenomenon. As flow to the lungs increases, so does return from the lungs to the left side of the heart, causing dilation of the left-sided structures. VSD size is one of the most important factors in determining the volume of left-to-right shunting.[10-13] Small defects tend to have small shunts because of the narrow path that they provide for egress from one ventricle to the other; therefore, those with small VSDs rarely have symptoms related to pulmonary

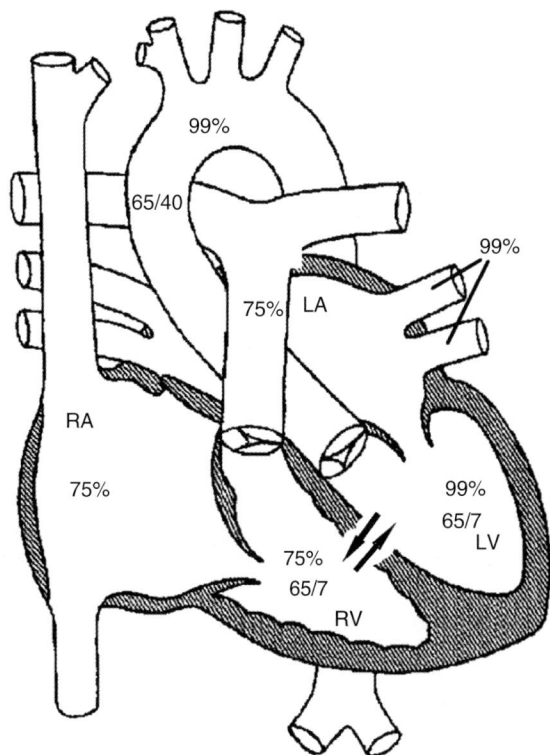

• **Fig. 22.12** Hemodynamics in newborn with ventricular septal defect (VSD). Normally high pulmonary vascular resistance in newborns leads to minimal shunting, bidirectional shunting, or rarely, right-to-left shunting across a VSD in the first few days of life. *LA,* Left atrium; *LV,* left ventricle; *RA,* right atrium; *RV,* right ventricle.

congestion. The larger the defect, the more likely one is to develop symptoms of overcirculation (Fig. 22.13A and B).

Any anatomic or physiologic change that affects the balance of resistance on the right and left side of the septum may also impact shunt volume and direction. Mechanical obstruction at the level of the RV outflow tract, pulmonary valve, or pulmonary arteries, will act to increase resistance to flow through the right heart and this will decrease left-to-right shunting through the VSD. A common example is in those with a VSD and pulmonary valve stenosis. The pulmonary stenosis acts to "protect" the lungs from excessive blood flow so patients are less likely to be symptomatic. Alternatively, mechanical obstruction on the left side of the heart such as aortic valve stenosis, aortic arch hypoplasia, or aortic arch obstruction can exacerbate left-to-right shunting across the defect, leading to earlier and more severe symptoms. In the young patient with coarctation of the aorta and a medium-sized VSD, increased resistance to flow across the aortic arch may lead to more VSD shunting than expected, resulting in symptoms of overcirculation in addition to the symptoms of arch obstruction. This can make it difficult to know if both the arch obstruction and the VSD require intervention or if correcting the arch obstruction alone will reduce trans-septal shunting to acceptable levels.

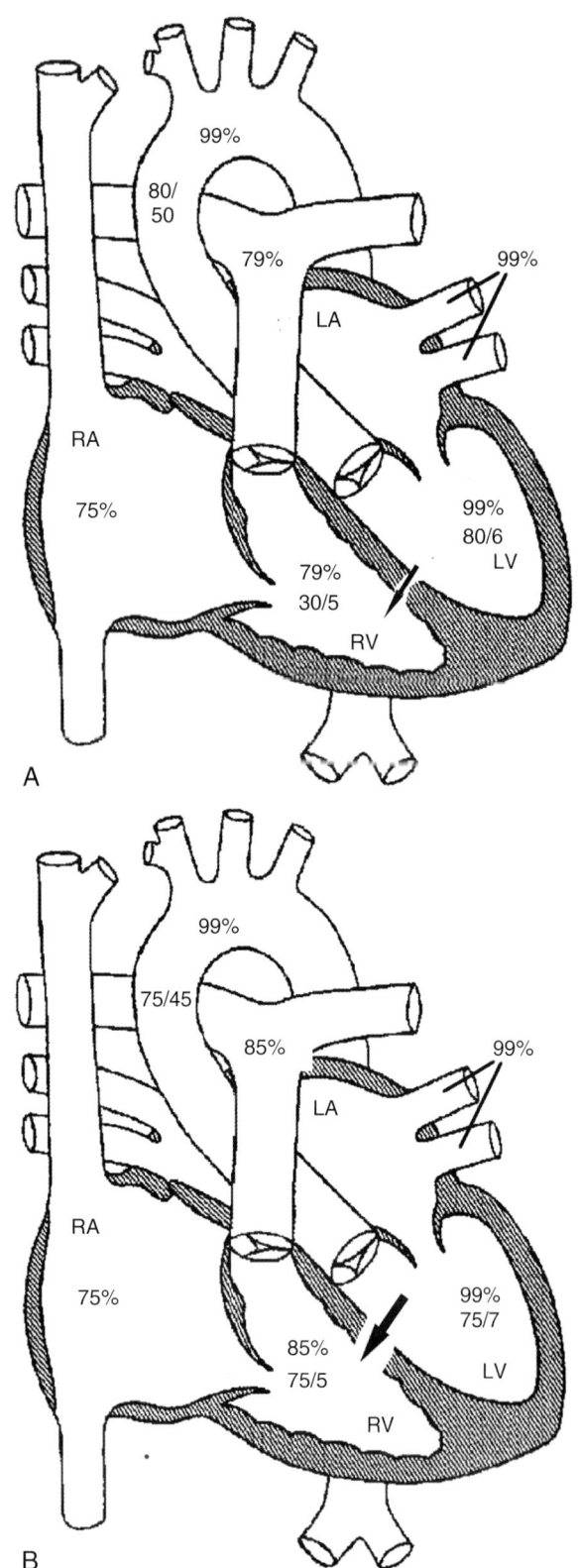

A

B

• **Fig. 22.13** Hemodynamics in a 6-month-old with ventricular septal defect (VSD). (A) Small VSDs allow for no more than small increases in right ventricular pressure and oxygen saturation as shunt volume is typically less than a Qp:Qs of 2:1. (B) Large VSDs allow for equalization of ventricular pressures and overcirculation; pulmonary artery saturations are much higher than right atrial saturations due to a Qp:Qs of > 2:1. *LA*, Left atrium; *LV*, left ventricle; *RA*, right atrium; *RV*, right ventricle.

Extracardiac conditions can also be a factor. Lung disease, chest masses, pleural effusion, and skeletal anomalies can lead to increases in pulmonary vascular resistance and therefore decreased trans-septal shunting. Likewise, elevations in systemic vascular resistance due to systemic hypertension or use of vasoconstricting drugs may lead to increased trans-septal shunting.

In a small number of patients, pulmonary vascular resistance does not fall appropriately after birth due to abnormalities in the vascular bed. In these patients, the VSD may not produce symptoms and the importance of the VSD to the patient's long-term health may be underestimated.

Older Children

In the short term, moderate and large left-to-right shunts typically cause symptoms that are treatable and reversible, but there can be important and irreversible changes in those with longstanding large shunts. Shunt volume is often expressed as the ratio of flow to the lungs (Qp) compared with flow to the body (Qs). When the Qp:Qs is > 2:1, there is at least a moderate shunt. When the Qp:Qs is > 3:1, most would consider the shunt to be large. When the lungs have been exposed to moderate or more shunting for a prolonged period of time, the pulmonary vascular bed may begin to remodel in an effort to increase vascular resistance and decrease pulmonary overcirculation. This leads to decreased compliance of the distal pulmonary vessels and this process may be irreversible, resulting in a condition known as pulmonary vascular obstructive disease. This condition was relatively common before the availability of congenital heart surgery, but due to improved diagnosis and treatment, the incidence of new cases is relatively rare in the current era. Therapeutic options are available to help mitigate symptoms from pulmonary vascular obstructive disease and slow the progression of vascular changes, but this can be a condition that is very difficult to treat and may be associated with a shortened life span as well as decreased quality of life.[14-17] Data suggests that VSDs rarely cause irreversible changes in pulmonary vascular resistance in the first 2 years of life, though there are important exceptions, such as infants with trisomy 21. In this group, irreversible changes in resistance have been reported in infants as young as 6 months.

When an individual develops pulmonary vascular obstructive disease, the trans-septal shunt will decrease and symptoms will be more tolerable. Eventually, as the vascular compliance continues to decrease, the Qp:Qs may normalize and there will be no symptoms. Over time, however, the resistance in the lungs will be high enough that the shunt may actually reverse and deoxygenated blood from the RV will now shunt towards the LV, leading to hypoxia. This physiological condition is called Eisenmenger's syndrome (Fig. 22.14). In the current era, it is much less common for large VSDs to escape early detection and the incidence of Eisenmenger's syndrome appears to be falling.

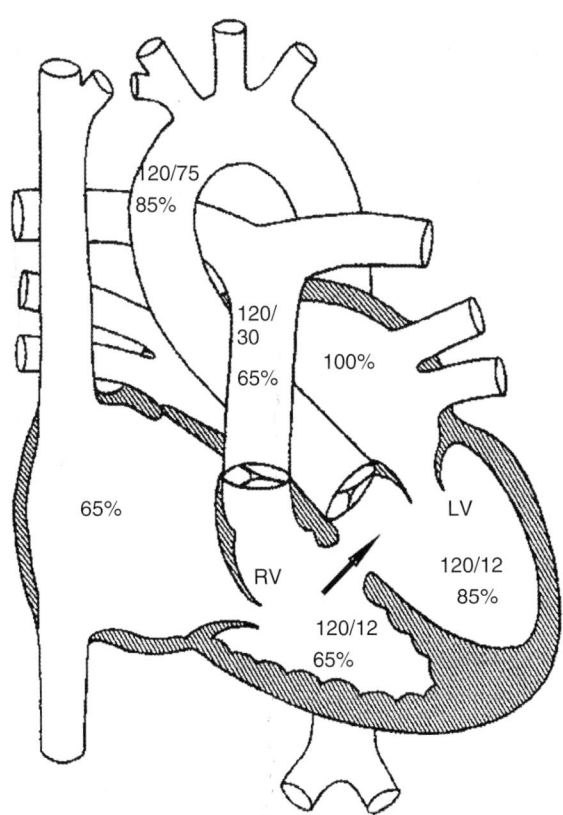

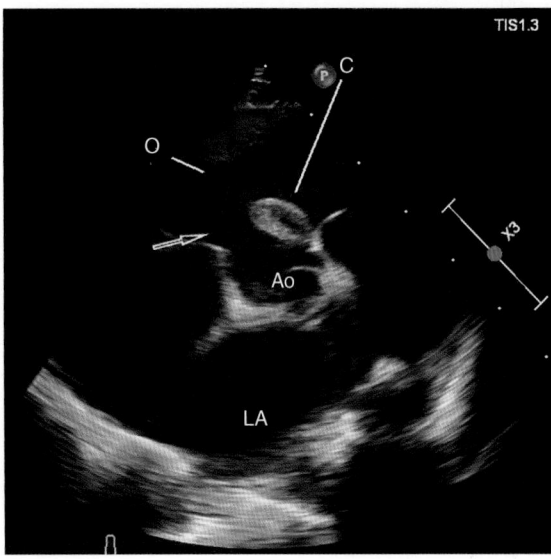

• **Fig. 22.15** Double-chambered right ventricle. Parasternal short-axis image highlights a hypertrophied conal septum, which narrows the area of the os infundibulum *(O)*, causing a pressure gradient. A cono-ventricular ventricular septal defect *(arrow)* is also present. *Ao,* Aortic root; *C,* conal septum; *LA,* left atrium.

• **Fig. 22.14** Hemodynamics in a 20-year-old with large ventricular septal defect (VSD)-Eisenmenger physiology. Prolonged exposure to large VSDs may lead to pulmonary vascular obstructive disease and ultimately right-to-left shunting across the VSD, resulting in reduced systemic saturations. *LA,* Left atrium; *LV,* left ventricle; *RA,* right atrium; *RV,* right ventricle.

Associated Anatomic Disease

VSDs can be seen both in isolation and in association with other cardiac malformations. Many complex congenital heart defects include a VSD as an integral part of the malformation, such as tetralogy of Fallot, double outlet RV, and truncus arteriosus. For other heart defects, a VSD is a frequent additional finding but not necessarily an integral part of the malformation. For instance, about 50% of individuals with coarctation of the aorta will have an associated VSD. In these patients, the defect can be of any size and anatomic type and may or may not be of hemodynamic significance.

There are a small group of pathologic findings that are highly associated with VSDs but are unlikely to be present at birth. Instead, these anatomic changes evolve over time. Most notable are double-chambered RV, subaortic membrane, and aortic valve prolapse.

Double-Chambered Right Ventricle

In some patients, the muscle at the entrance to the infundibular portion of the RV outflow tract, known as the os infundibulum, becomes hypertrophied (Fig. 22.15). This

can cause obstruction to flow from the sinus of the RV into the infundibulum of the RV. This obstruction may evolve while the VSD is present or after VSD closure. When a VSD is present, it typically enters the portion of the RV that is below the level of obstruction, so the narrowing at the os infundibulum acts to discourage LV-to-RV shunting. The portion of the RV below the os infundibulum is under higher pressure than the area beyond the obstruction, hence the term double chamber.[18]

Subaortic Obstruction

VSDs are associated with a few different anatomic variants of LV outflow tract obstruction. As discussed already, posterior malalignment VSDs may be associated with outflow tracts that are narrowed due to anatomic "crowding" by the conal septum. Subaortic membranes are very different. Subaortic membranes are predominantly associated with membranous VSDs and as with double-chambered RV, can be present while the VSD is open or may evolve after VSD closure.[19] They may present as an isolated thin membrane that crosses the LV outflow tract from the septal surface to the anterior mitral valve leaflet (Fig. 22.16) or they can be associated with a prominent fibromuscular septal ridge (Fig. 22.17). In some, obstruction will be mild and static and will not require intervention. In others, there can be progressive LV outflow tract obstruction. Surgical intervention is typically advised if there are symptoms of reduced cardiac output or if progressive obstruction is causing disadvantageous remodeling of the left ventricular myocardium as it compensates for the increased workload. A final concern is that subaortic membranes can impact aortic valve function. For some, the membrane may be attached to the ventricular

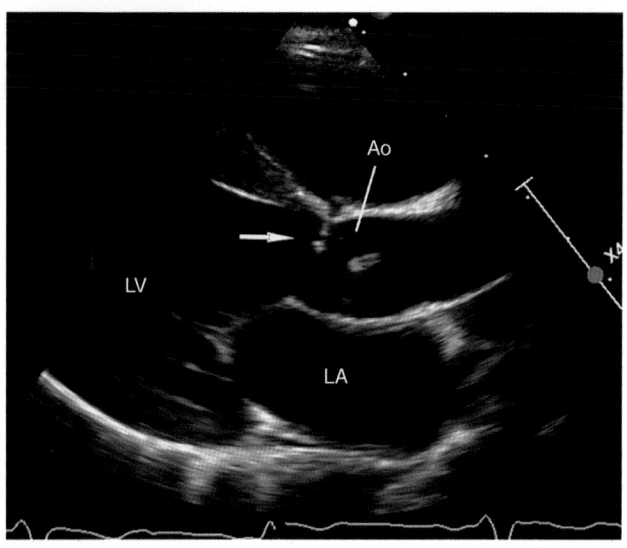

• **Fig. 22.16** Discrete subaortic membrane. Parasternal long axis view of a discrete subaortic membrane (*arrow*) in close proximity to the anterior leaflet of the aortic valve. The associated small membranous ventricular septal defect is not visible in this frame. *Ao,* Aortic root; *LA,* left atrium; *LV,* left ventricle.

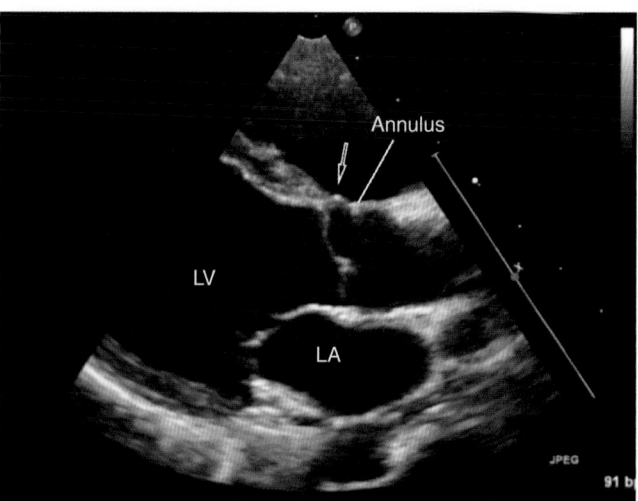

• **Fig. 22.18** Aortic valve prolapse. Parasternal long-axis image with the plane of the aortic annulus marked. A portion of the aortic valve is imaged below the annular plane and a small amount of valve tissue protrudes through the ventricular septal defect into the right ventricle (*arrow*). *LA,* Left atrium; *LV,* left ventricle.

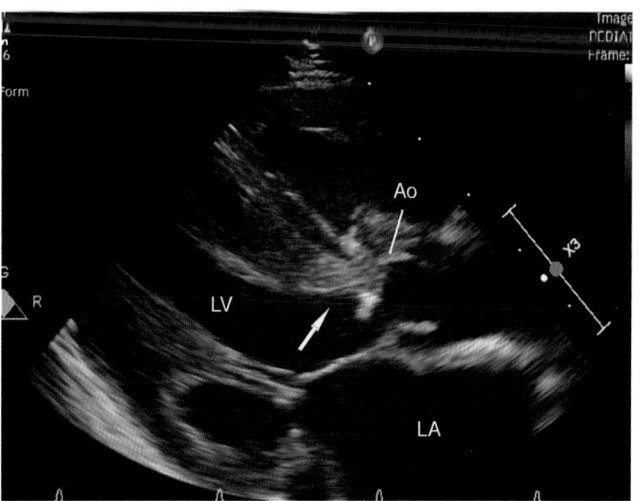

• **Fig. 22.17** Fibromuscular ridge. Parasternal long axis view of a sub-aortic membrane associated with a prominent muscular ridge (*arrow*). The muscular ridge narrows the left ventricular outflow tract and the membrane narrows it further. *Ao,* Aortic root; *LA,* left atrium; *LV,* left ventricle.

surface of one or more of the aortic valve cusps, impacting the normal motion of the valve. For others, the abnormal flow pattern created by the obstruction may impact valve mobility. Either way, abnormalities of valve motion can lead to valve dysfunction and progressive aortic regurgitation over time. Occasionally, surgical intervention is undertaken in a patient with mild obstruction because of the need to improve or preserve the aortic valve function. These types of subaortic obstruction can be difficult to surgically treat in a durable way; fibromuscular ridges are difficult to completely resect without damaging the conduction system and discrete membranes can recur after successful removal.

Aortic Valve Prolapse

Shunting across membranous and conal-septal VSDs can create a current in the LV outflow tract that has the potential to "drag" the aortic valve leaflets out of position. This is called the Venturi effect and it can ultimately cause the right and/or non-coronary cusps to prolapse below the level of the aortic annulus. In some, the leaflets will protrude into or through the VSD. The presence of aortic valve tissue in the defect may make the VSD shunt volume smaller and reduce symptoms of overcirculation, but the trade-off is that it may also disrupt aortic valve geometry enough to impact valve competency (Fig. 22.18). Mild aortic regurgitation will be well tolerated but more than mild aortic regurgitation can be symptomatic and progressive.[12,19,20] As in those with subaortic membranes, there are times when surgical intervention will be considered to protect or improve valve function even if there is no hemodynamically significant shunt across the VSD.

Clinical Signs and Symptoms

Physical Examination

The most important elements of the exam for evaluation of someone with a VSD will include characterization of the heart murmur, heart sounds, and assessment of precordial impulse in addition to the evaluation for evidence of overcirculation, including respiratory symptoms, suboptimal nutrition, and organomegaly.

Murmur

Whether or not one can hear an audible murmur will depend on the amount of flow crossing the defect as well as the pressure drop across the septum. If there is little flow or no significant pressure drop across the VSD, there may be no audible murmur. As pulmonary resistance falls and shunting increases, murmurs become easier to hear. In isolated VSDs, the smaller the defect, the greater the pressure drop. More restrictive defects have a higher pitched murmur that can be very loud, while larger defects produce a murmur that is lower in frequency and may be softer. Larger defects are associated with a holosystolic murmur, whereas smaller defects may be heard only in early systole. This is because the defect may close during systole as the muscle around it contracts. Those with large shunts may also have a diastolic murmur secondary to increased flow across the mitral valve. The evaluation of murmurs in those with a VSD will be less straightforward if there are other lesions present which can also create an audible murmur such as outflow tract obstruction or semilunar valve stenosis. The murmurs of these associated lesions may mask the sound of a ventricular level shunt.

Heart Sounds

In large defects, there is often equalization of pressures between the ventricles, and this will produce a single second heart sound instead of the typical splitting of S2.

Precordial Impulse

Large shunts are frequently associated with a prominent precordial impulse. Alternatively, very small shunts may create a localized, palpable thrill. These are more commonly noticed when the VSD is located in one of the more anterior regions of the heart, near the chest wall.

Respirations

In those with pulmonary congestion, tachypnea is typical and associated retractions may be present. Oxygen saturations are usually normal, but in some there may be enough congestion in the lung tissue to cause reduced oxygen saturations as well. In patients with Eisenmenger's physiology or those in whom the VSD is associated with a delayed fall in pulmonary resistance, respirations may be normal but oxygen saturations might be reduced secondary to shunting from RV to LV. In those with small VSDS, no respiratory symptoms should be present.

Additional Physical Findings

In those with large shunts that are not adequately controlled, one expects to find other evidence on exam that the circulation is overworked and there is total body volume overload. These findings will vary, depending on each patient's compensatory mechanisms, but frequent additional findings when there is a large shunt include organomegaly, tachycardia, and reduced growth parameters.

Physical findings often vary with age.[10-13]

Newborns

In the newborn period, left-to-right shunting is usually mild and well tolerated. Newborns are rarely symptomatic from overcirculation, so the most common clinical sign of a VSD is a heart murmur. If there is little flow due to the normal elevated pulmonary resistance of the newborn, there may be no audible murmur. As pulmonary resistance falls and shunting increases, murmurs become more audible.

Infants

In most, the pulmonary vascular resistance will fall considerably by 3 months of age. With this fall in resistance, left-to-right shunting across the VSD will increase, and the risk for developing the signs and symptoms of pulmonary overcirculation will also increase. In small VSDs, this is not a concern. The fall in resistance may make the murmur more prominent but will not result in excessive pulmonary blood flow.

In moderate or large VSDs, there can be considerable flow through the VSD by 3 months of age. As a result, the lungs become congested and symptoms tend to follow. The exam will often reveal a low or medium pitched holosystolic murmur as well as a single S2 and a prominent precordial impulse. There may be tachycardia. Typically blood pressures will be normal and pulses will be full. The liver is often enlarged and the edge will be palpable below the right costal margin. Respiratory rate may be elevated and there may be subcostal as well as intercostal retractions at rest. The most common observation by parents is that their infant is tachypneic and has decreased ability to feed comfortably. They may note increased diaphoresis and tiring during feeds. Eventually this will result in diminished nutrition and impaired weight gain and growth. There are rare infants in whom the normal fall in pulmonary resistance does not take place. In these situations, a large VSD may go undetected.

Older Children

Small VSDs may persist into childhood and will be audible on exam but should not cause any symptoms as the children grow into adulthood. Because VSDs are typically audible in infancy and/or symptomatic, it is rare for a hemodynamically important VSD to present in older childhood. When there is late presentation, it is often related to the presence of a murmur but occasionally presenting symptoms may be due to the sequalae of pulmonary vascular disease, including decreased activity tolerance and hypoxia. It is very unusual for older children to present with symptoms of pulmonary congestion.

Diagnosis

Electrocardiography

Electrocardiography is rarely diagnostic but will show changes if there has been alteration in chamber size. In those with pulmonary overcirculation, left-sided voltages may rise as the LV dilates. In older patients with elevated pulmonary vascular resistance due to Eisenmenger's syndrome, one would expect instead to see a rise in right-sided voltages secondary to RV dilation and/or hypertrophy. Those with AV canal–type VSDs often have a superior QRS axis.

Chest X-Ray

The appearance of the heart and lungs will depend on the shunt volume. In those with a small shunt, the cardiac silhouette and lung fields should be normal. In those with a moderate or large shunt, one expects to see an increase in heart size due to left ventricular volume overload and an increase in pulmonary vascular markings, consistent with pulmonary congestion.

Echocardiography

Echocardiography is currently the cornerstone of diagnosis and is an excellent modality for evaluating the anatomic details that will determine prognosis. It is key in making early treatment decisions and may be used intermittently for following physiology.

Anatomic Evaluation

Risks, prognosis, and therefore management decisions will be determined by VSD size and anatomy as well as the presence or absence of associated cardiac defects. To that end, the initial echocardiogram should include a complete anatomic survey with extra focus on the detailed anatomic features of the VSD and neighboring structures.

Physiologic Evaluation

Small VSDs rarely affect overall physiology and will not need frequent reevaluation. Larger defects will require intermittent evaluation. The echocardiographic features that will be most important in the assessment of long-term risk and/ or need for intervention will be estimates of the RV pressure and the LV volume.

The RV pressure can be calculated by subtracting the VSD gradient from the LV pressure. The LV pressure is estimated from the cuff blood pressure. It should be the same as the systolic blood pressure (as long as there is no aortic valve or arch obstruction). The VSD gradient is measured with spectral Doppler across the defect to evaluate flow velocity. If RV pressure is less than half of LV pressure, this is reassuring in that the risk for developing pulmonary vascular obstructive disease will be low. When RV pressure is more than half systemic, there is still risk for evolving permanent pulmonary vascular changes.

The LV volume can be measured by many methods. We favor an estimate of LV volume that is calculated by the equation 5/6 (area × length). This can be made with a good quality apical four-chamber view and a parasternal short axis view (Fig. 22.19A and B). A rough "rule of thumb" is that a left ventricular end diastolic volume z score of + 2.5 or higher suggests a ventricular shunt (Qp:Qs) of at least

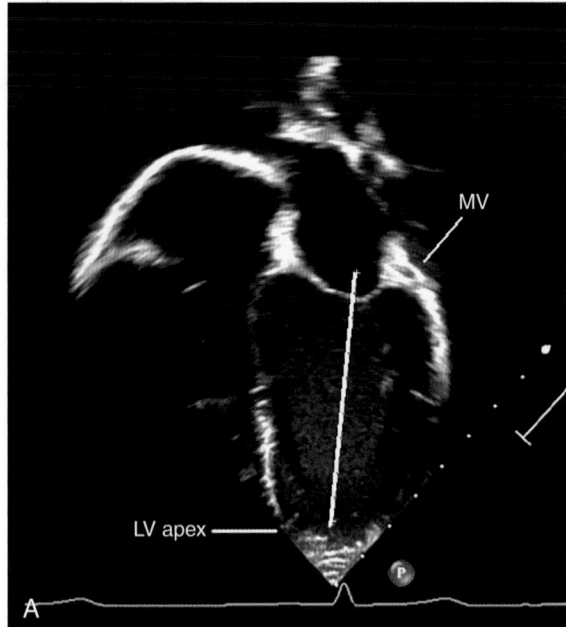

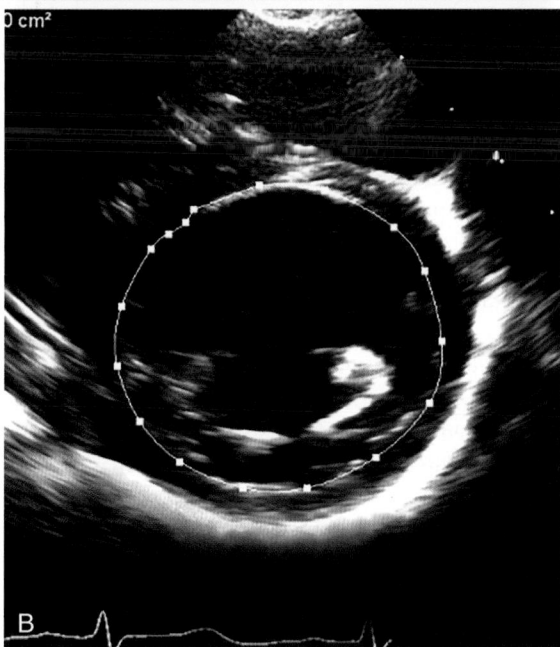

• **Fig. 22.19** Measurement of left ventricular volume. (A) Left ventricular length is measured at end diastole in the apical view. It is the distance from the mitral valve *(MV)* annulus to the apical endocardium. (B) Left ventricular area is assessed at end diastole in the parasternal short-axis view by tracing the mid-ventricle endocardial surface *(dotted line)*. *LV,* Left ventricle.

2:1 and this typically correlates with symptoms of overcirculation. Though echocardiography allows for excellent non-invasive estimates of RV pressure and LV size, when there is clinical concern that echocardiographic measurements may not accurately reflect the patient's hemodynamics, other modalities for investigation of shunt volume and RV pressure should be considered.

Evaluation of Impact on Neighboring Structures

As noted earlier, some VSDs can be associated with progressive ventricular outflow tract obstruction and/or aortic valve prolapse. Depending on the type of VSD, surveillance echocardiograms may be done throughout childhood to monitor for these complications and, if present, to assess for hemodynamically significant progression.

Postoperative Evaluation

Following intervention to close the VSD, echocardiography will be used to assess the success of the intervention. In addition to documenting VSD closure, studies will focus on assessment of valve and ventricular function. Over time, intermittent evaluation will document whether or not right ventricular pressure and left ventricular size return to expected levels.

Catheterization

Cardiac catheterization remains the gold standard for the hemodynamic assessment of VSDs. In the current era, non-invasive methods of estimating shunt volume and RV pressure have improved and catheterization is used less often than it once was. There are situations, however, in which catheterization is needed for hemodynamic assessment and/or therapeutic intervention.

Hemodynamic Evaluation

Direct measurement of RV and pulmonary artery pressure is done with extreme accuracy utilizing a fluid-filled catheter attached to a calibrated pressure transducer, and this remains the most accurate way to evaluate for evolving pulmonary hypertension.

Shunt volume is also best evaluated by catheterization. As noted earlier, the magnitude of the shunt is expressed as the ratio of pulmonary flow to systemic flow, Qp:Qs. Left to-right shunts result in oxygenated blood crossing into the RV. This causes increased oxygen saturation in the pulmonary artery in comparison with the saturation in the right atrium and the difference between them will be proportional to the quantity of the shunt (Fig. 22.14). Blood samples from each location in the heart are withdrawn from the catheter and the oxygen saturations are easily measured. The changes in saturation between locations can be used to derive the Qp:Qs. Saturation data can also be used in combination with assessments of oxygen consumption, to derive the pulmonary vascular resistance (measured in woods units), a critical piece of data for planning a safe treatment strategy (see Chapter 13 for further discussion of catheterization techniques).

Anatomic Evaluation

Angiography involves capturing fluoroscopic images of the heart after the delivery of a bolus of dye through the catheter and into the chamber of interest. It can be used to evaluate the anatomy of the VSD as well as the anatomy of the outflow tracts and the distal pulmonary vasculature.

Tapering of the distal pulmonary vessels is important evidence for the presence of pulmonary vascular obstructive disease and angiography is currently the best modality available for this assessment.

Therapeutic Evaluation

Catheterization is an excellent tool for the evaluation of vasodilator therapy and its effect on pulmonary vascular resistance. In patients with known or suspected pulmonary vascular obstructive disease, this is a very important adjunct to care. Once baseline measurements are obtained, an intravenous or inhaled pulmonary vasodilator is administered and repeat measures of intracardiac pressures, oxygen saturations, and pulmonary vascular resistance are obtained. The response to therapeutic manipulations during catheterization can then be used to help design out-patient therapeutic regimens.

Therapeutic Intervention

For some, the VSD can be closed with a device delivered via catheterization. Patient selection is critical for a successful procedure as not all VSDs are amenable to this approach.

Magnetic Resonance Imaging/Computed Tomography

The role for magnetic resonance imaging (MRI) and computed tomography (CT) is evolving rapidly. MRI can be used to estimate Qp:Qs as an alternative to cardiac catheterization, when appropriate. This is done by calculating the volume of flow crossing the pulmonary valve and comparing it with the volume of flow crossing the aortic valve. The software algorithms that evaluate flow are quite good and can closely approximate catheter data as long as there are no complicating factors such as arrhythmias, significant valve disease, or other sources of blood flow to the lungs. These modalities are also excellent for the assessment of left atrial and ventricular size, particularly in situations where echocardiography has failed, due to restrictive imaging windows. Finally, the ability to see anatomic details of septal defects is improving rapidly. In unusual defects and in patients with poor echocardiographic images, this can be a great help to the surgeon, as these technologies offer both 2D and 3D datasets that can be manipulated after acquisition to give excellent multiplane views of VSD size, shape, and borders.

Prognosis

Overall, the prognosis for isolated VSDs is excellent, though about 15–20% will ultimately require an intervention to close the defect. The overall goal of treatment is to minimize the risk for the development of pulmonary vascular obstructive disease as well as to control symptoms of overcirculation while deciding if an intervention will be needed. The timing of intervention will vary, depending on many factors, including clinical symptoms, VSD anatomy, and personal characteristics that may increase or decrease the risks involved. In all cases, the prolonged presence of more than mild left heart dilation or elevated RV pressure (half systemic) through the first 6–12 months of life should signal a need to consider intervention. Each type of VSD has some unique characteristics that will need to be considered in the decision-making process.

Membranous

Membranous VSDs vary widely in size. Sometimes the anatomic size of the defect does not correlate with the functional size because of the presence of accessory or aneurysmal tissue that restricts flow (Fig. 22.20). The presence of aneurysmal tissue can alter the prognosis in that it can be so restrictive that the VSD is no longer hemodynamically significant. In some, the tissue will completely close the defect. Because aneurysmal tissue can become more restrictive over time, there is a tendency to observe those who have aneurysmal tissue surrounding their membranous VSD for longer. The hope is that the aneurysmal tissue will reduce the shunt enough that surgical intervention can be avoided. Membranous defects can also become smaller due to prolapse of aortic valve tissue into the defect.[19] This can also lead to enough reduction in flow to avoid surgical intervention. On the other hand, if the prolapse leads to significant aortic regurgitation, surgery may instead be needed to repair the aortic valve. Finally, membranous VSDs can be associated with progressive development of double-chamber RV or subaortic obstruction. Because of the risk for these late changes, even if the VSD becomes physiologically insignificant or closes entirely, we typically advise intermittent, echocardiographic evaluation to assess for these late changes.

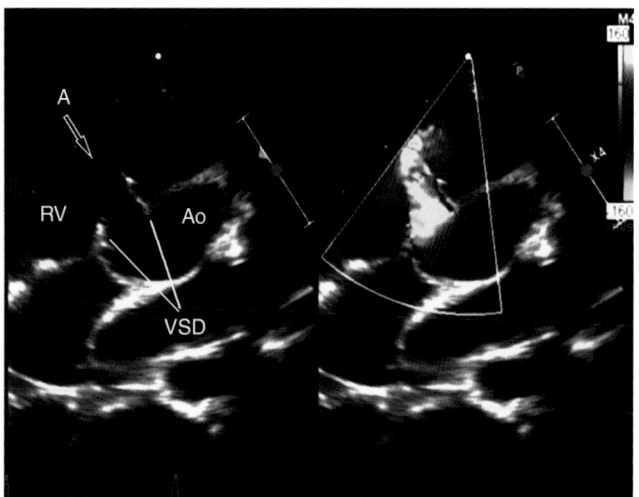

• **Fig. 22.20** Aneurysmal narrowing of membranous ventricular septal defect (VSD). Parasternal short-axis image of a large VSD surrounded by aneurysmal tissue *(arrow)*. The color panel shows that the aneurysm is restricting shunt volume by narrowing the path from the left to the right ventricle. *A,* aneurysmal tissue; *Ao,* Aortic root; *RV,* right ventricle.

Conoventricular

Conoventricular VSDs are usually large and have little or no potential to become smaller without intervention. Because of this, they typically require surgical intervention in the first year of life, often in the first 6 months of life. The timing may depend on the presence or absence of other cardiac malformations, but in general, intervention is driven by the presence of symptoms of overcirculation. When isolated, we tend to operate on these by about 3–6 months of age. As surgical intervention has a high rate of technical success and a low risk for poor outcome, our philosophy has been to avoid prolonged medical treatment and the risks of poor growth by correcting the defect early in life.

Conal-Septal

Conal-septal VSDs can vary in size. This type of defect has a particularly high rate of associated aortic valve prolapse, and this is the only mechanism by which a large defect can get smaller.[9] In some, the prolapse can close the defect or make it small enough to ignore. As in membranous VSDs, if valve competency is maintained, no intervention is needed. It is difficult to predict which patients will develop prolapse and of those, which are at risk for significant aortic regurgitation. Prolapse can cause significant distortion of the valve without disrupting function. On the other hand, sometimes mild distortion is associated with progressive aortic regurgitation. When progressive aortic regurgitation is identified, surgery to improve valve function is undertaken, even if the VSD is small. When there is no prolapse, defect size alone will determine the need for surgery. Our philosophy has evolved over the last few decades. We currently recommend careful observation of these patients for signs and symptoms of overcirculation, sustained pulmonary hypertension, and/or progressive aortic regurgitation. If none develop, we do not typically recommend surgical intervention.

Muscular

Muscular VSDs are a very heterogeneous group. The prognosis will depend on the number and size of the defects. The muscular portion of the septum has the potential to hypertrophy and remodel, and this can alter the size and geometry of VSDs over time. When muscular defects appear to be small in the early months of life, they will stay small or slowly close as the muscular septum matures. Larger defects may not close, but may get small enough that they are no longer physiologically important and surgical intervention will not be needed. If a muscular defect stays large, then like other VSDs, intervention will be needed.

Atrioventricular Canal

AV canal defects are rarely isolated findings. They can be of any size and are usually associated with all or some of the following: cleft mitral valve, atrial septal defect primum, and tricuspid and mitral regurgitation. The overall prognosis will be based on the combination of the VSD size and the presence or absence of these associated components. If the VSD is moderate or large, than similar to other VSDs one would expect symptoms of overcirculation and ultimately a high risk for developing irreversible pulmonary hypertension if left untreated.

Endocarditis

Endocarditis risk is increased in those with a history of VSD, even if the VSD is closed. In the current era, this is a rare event.[21] Those with isolated VSD are no longer among the group for whom subacute bacterial endocarditis prophylaxis is recommended.

Treatment

Treatment strategy in the first year of life is aimed at control of symptoms to optimize growth and development while minimizing the risk of developing pulmonary vascular obstructive disease. The keys to the plan of care will be intermittent assessment of growth, physical findings, valve function, and RV pressure.

Small VSDs

No treatment is needed for small VSDs unless there are issues related to aortic valve prolapse or outflow tract obstruction.

Moderate or Large VSDs

The goal in devising a care plan for those with a hemodynamically significant VSD is first deciding if there is any chance that the VSD will get smaller over time. When there is no chance for the VSD to get smaller over time and there is no protection for the lungs, the RV pressure will remain elevated and so will the pulmonary artery pressure. Under these circumstances, a procedure to close the VSD or restrict pulmonary blood flow should be considered by 3–6 months of age. Surgical results are excellent for most types of VSDs with very low mortality as well as a low rate of short- and long-term complications.[22-24] The risk-to-benefit ratio does not improve after 3 months, so there is little value in waiting until the patient is older to intervene.

If there is a chance that the VSD can get smaller on its own, there is often interest in observing for an extended period of time to allow for growth and maturation. When that is the case, the following strategies can be considered to control symptoms and allow for a longer period of observation. These same therapies may be considered if there is interest in delaying surgery because the patient has elevated surgical risk, but with time will become a better surgical candidate.

The treatment plan can include one or some combination of the following therapies: medication, high-caloric diet, assisted feeding, and temporary restriction of flow across the main pulmonary artery.

Medication

The medications most commonly used to treat congestive symptoms are diuretics. These are safe and effective in small children and infants. In our institution, we have the most experience with Lasix, but others may also be used safely. Other medications that have been used with variable success include Digoxin and afterload reducing agents, such as ACE inhibitors.

Nutrition

Infants may struggle to grow due to decreased ability to feed comfortably in combination with increased metabolic needs. When infants struggle to feed due to congestive symptoms, there are two ways to increase caloric intake. The first is by increasing the caloric density of the breast milk or formula from the baseline of 20 calories/ounce. There are a number of recipes and products that have been used; often caloric density is increased in a step-wise fashion until an acceptable level of growth is achieved. We have gone as high as 30–32 calories/ounce in some, though not all infants will tolerate such high-caloric density. A second avenue for increasing calories is to deliver some or all of the nutrition via a nasogastric or gastric tube. This strategy allows for regular feeding and caloric intake that is not dependent on appetite. This is typically not necessary in the otherwise healthy infant, but in those with more complicated medical issues, this may be an important adjunct to improve nutrition.

Restricting Pulmonary Blood Flow

In some instances, it is desirable to delay surgery to allow for growth and maturation and medication/calories alone are insufficient. When this is the case, one can restrict flow through the main pulmonary artery by placing a device that narrows the diameter of the main pulmonary artery and acts as a mechanical barrier on the RV side of the circulation. This can be done surgically with an external band that is placed in the mid portion of the main pulmonary artery or more recently, by placing an internal restrictive device in the main or branch pulmonary arteries via a catheter. This will increase the resistance to flow to the lungs and decrease left-to-right shunting across the VSD. When no longer needed, the band can be removed surgically or sometimes it can be dilated with a catheter so that it is no longer restrictive.

There are some defects that fall in the gray zone with regard to intervention. The LV may be mildly dilated but the RV pressure is low and the patient is growing well without symptoms. For this group, it makes sense to hold off on intervention and give nature more time. This strategy will include reevaluation of RV pressure and LV size at regular intervals to make sure that there are no changes that may impact long-term health. Typically, if the LV volume z score is below +2.5, surgery can be put off indefinitely. If LV volumes are increasing with age or if RV pressure begins to rise, then intervening to close the VSD should be considered.

Intervention for VSD Closure

Once there is a commitment to intervention, the options for how to proceed include surgery, device closure in the catheterization or a hybrid procedure, called perventricular device closure.

Surgical Intervention

Surgery is done through a midline sternotomy on cardiopulmonary bypass. Surgical results in the current era are excellent. Most large defects are closed with a patch. Patches are cut to size from either tightly woven synthetic material such as Dacron or Goretex or they can be made from pericardium that is removed from the patient's heart at the start of the procedure and treated with glutaraldehyde. The surgical visualization of the VSD will depend on the VSD anatomy. Membranous VSDs may be closed through the tricuspid valve or the aortic valve. Most conoventricular VSDs will be approached the same way, though for some, like those associated with tetralogy of Fallot, the approach will be through the right ventricular outflow tract as this will be opened as part of the complete repair. Conal-septal defects are often approached through the pulmonary valve. The approach for muscular VSDs will depend on the location of the defect. For apical defects, the approach may be through an apical ventriculotomy. For defects that are closer to the base of the heart and/or the anterior portion of the septum, visualization will be better through the tricuspid valve or one of the semilunar valves. In long-term follow-up, late complications are infrequent, but when present include arrhythmias, heart block, and residual VSDs. Less commonly, there can be valve and ventricular dysfunction.

Nonsurgical Closure of VSDs

There are some VSDs that can be closed with a device delivered by catheter, either through the systemic venous system (usually the femoral vein) or the perventricular approach. This approach involves opening the chest to expose the surface of the heart and then puncturing the myocardium to deliver the device, usually with fluoroscopic and/or echocardiographic guidance.[25] These catheter-based interventions have been done successfully in both muscular- and membranous-type defects as well as residual defects at the margins of surgically placed patches. The technique is still relatively new in comparison with surgical closure, and the medium- and long-term outcomes are unknown. Patient selection, and therefore technical results, are improving, and there may be wider application of these options in the future. At the present time, the vast majority of VSDs are still addressed surgically.

References

1. Fyler DC, Buckley LP, Hellenbrand WE, Cohn HE, Kirklin JW, Nadas AS. Report of the New England regional infant cardiac program. *Pediatrics*. 1980;65:376.

2. Hoffman JIE, Kaplan S. The incidence of congenital heart disease. *J Am Coll Cardiol*. 2002;39:1890-1900.

3. Du ZD, Roguin N, Barak M, Bihari SG, Ben-Elisha M. High prevalence of muscular ventricular septal defect in preterm neonates. *Am J Cardiol*. 1996;78:1183-1185.

4. Ferencz C, Loffredo CA, Correa-Villansenor AC, McGee CA. *Genetic and Environmental Risk Factors of Major Cardiovascular Malformations: The Baltimore-Washington Infant Study: 1981-1989*. Armonk, NY: Futura; 1997.

5. Pierpont M, Brueckner M, Chung WK, et al. Genetic basis for congenital heart disease: revisited: a scientific statement from the American Heart Association. *Circulation*. 2018;138:e653-e711.

6. Driscoll DJ, Michels VV, Gersony WM, et al. Occurrence risk for congenital heart defects in relatives of patients with aortic stenosis, pulmonary stenosis, or ventricular septal defect. *Circulation*. 1993;87:114-120.

7. Lopez L, Houyel L, Colan SD, et al. Classification of ventricular septal defects for the eleventh iteration of the International Classification of Diseases—striving for consensus: a report from the International Society for Nomenclature of Paediatric and Congenital Heart Disease. *Thorac Surg*. 2018;106:1578-1589.

8. Van Praagh R, Geva T, Kreutzer J. Ventricular septal defects: how shall we describe, name and classify them? *J Am Coll Cardiol*. 1989;14:1298-1299.

9. Tohyama K, Satomi G, Momma K. Aortic valve prolapse and aortic regurgitation associated with subpulmonic ventricular septal defect. *Am J Cardiol*. 1997;79:1285-1289.

10. Gabriel HM, Heger M, Innerhofer P, et al. Long term outcome of patients with ventricular septal defect considered not to require surgical closure during childhood. *J Am Coll Cardiol*. 2002;39:1066-1071.

11. Long-term follow-up of congenital aortic stenosis, pulmonary stenosis, and ventricular septal defect. *Circulation*. 1993;87(suppl 2):I1-I126.

12. Ellis JH, Moodie DS, Sterba R, Gill CJ. Ventricular septal defect in the adult: natural history and unnatural history. *Am Heart J*. 1987;114:115-120.

13. Hoffman JIE, Rudolph AM. The natural history of ventricular septal defects in infancy. *Am J Cardiol*. 1965;16:634-653.

14. Hoffman JIE, Rudolph AM, Heymann MA. Pulmonary vascular disease with congenital heart lesions: pathologic features and causes. *Circulation*. 1981;64:873-877.

15. Diller GP, Gatzoulis MA. Pulmonary vascular disease in adults with congenital heart disease. *Circulation*. 2007;115:1039-1050.

16. Rabinovitch M, Keane JF, Norwood WI, Castaneda A, Reid L. Vascular structure in lung tissue obtained at biopsy correlated with pulmonary hemodynamic findings after repair of congenital heart defects. *Circulation*. 1984;69:655-667.

17. Galie N, Humbert M, Vachiery JL, et al. 2015 ESC/ERS Guidelines for the diagnosis and treatment of pulmonary hypertension: the joint task force for the Diagnosis and Treatment of Pulmonary Hypertension of the European Society of Cardiology (ESC) and the European Respiratory Society (ERS): endorsed by: Association for European Paediatric and Congenital Cardiology (AEPC), International Society for Heart and Lung Transplantation (ISHLT). *Eur Respir J*. 2015;37:67-119.

18. Simpson WF, Sade RM, Crawford FA, Taylor AB, Fyfe DA. Double-chambered right ventricle. *Ann Thorac Surg*. 1987;44:7-10.

19. Eroglu AG, Oztunc F, Saltik L, Bakari S, Dedeoglu S, Ahunbay G. Evolution of ventricular septal defect with special reference to spontaneous closure rate, subaortic ridge and aortic valve prolapse. *Pediatr Cardiol*. 2003;24:31-35.

20. Rhodes LA, Keane JF, Keane JP, et al. Long follow-up (to 43 years) of ventricular septal defect with audible aortic regurgitation. *Am J Cardiol*. 1990;66:340-345.

21. Gersony WM, Hayes CJ, Driscoll DJ, et al. Bacterial endocarditis in patients with aortic stenosis, pulmonary stenosis or ventricular septal defect. *Circulation*. 1993;87:121-126.

22. Anderson BR, Stevens KN, Nicolson SC, et al. Contemporary outcomes of surgical ventricular septal defect closure. *J Thorac Cardiovasc Surg*. 2013;145:641-647.

23. Scully BB, Morales DL, Zafar F, McKenzie ED, Fraser Jr CD, Heinle JS. Current expectations for surgical repair of isolated ventricular septal defects. *Ann Thorac Surg*. 2010;89:544-549.

24. Roos-Hesselink JW, Meijboom FJ, Spitaels SE, et al. Outcome of patients after surgical closure of ventricular septal defect at young age: longitudinal follow-up of 22-34 years. *Eur Heart J*. 2004; 25:1057-1062.

25. Dongxu Li, Xu Zhou, Mengsi Li, Qi An. Comparisons of per-ventricular device closure, conventional surgical repair, and transcatheter device closure in patients with perimembranous ventricular septal defects: a network meta-analysis. *BMC Surg*. 2020;20:115.

23

Anomalies of the Ductus Arteriosus

JULIA GARCIA-MANCEBO AND JOHN N. KHEIR

KEY LEARNING POINTS

- The ductus arteriosus is a normal fetal vascular structure connecting the pulmonary artery and aorta. In term infants, it typically closes by 48 hours of life. Persistent patent ductus arteriosus (PDA) is more common in preterm infants and in patients born at altitude.
- Many children with an isolated PDA are asymptomatic and identified by physical exam findings, including a murmur and bounding pulses. A hemodynamically significant PDA may cause congestive heart failure, failure to thrive, and pulmonary hypertension.
- The classic murmur is described as "machinelike" with a continuous crescendo–decrescendo murmur that peaks at the second heart sound and is loudest at the second left intercostal space.

- Echocardiography is the examination of choice. The preferred views are the parasternal short-axis and the suprasternal view, localizing the descending aorta and pulmonary artery such that the PDA appears between the great vessels. Color flow mapping will help identify a PDA even if small.
- The optimal timing and method of closure remains a subject of debate. If the PDA is considered responsible for congestive heart failure, cardiogenic shock, endocarditis, or other sequelae of a hemodynamically significant shunt, timely closure is recommended. Closure can be performed with pharmacotherapy, surgery, or interventional catheterization.

Definition

The ductus arteriosus (DA) is a normal fetal vessel connecting the pulmonary and systemic circulations. This essential vascular structure allows oxygenated blood from the placenta to bypass the high-resistance pulmonary circulation and to contribute to systemic perfusion. In full-term newborns, functional closure typically occurs within 48 hours after delivery. Failure of this vessel to close beyond the third postnatal day is referred to as patent ductus arteriosus (PDA) and is considered abnormal.

Prevalence

PDA is the third most frequent congenital heart defect after ventricular and atrial septal defects. The reported incidence has increased from 0.138 in the 1970s to 1.004 per 1000 live births based on a systematic review in 2019.[1,2] Greater use of echocardiography and improved techniques for early detection may explain this trend. At Boston Children's Hospital, the number of patients in the last 20 years (2002–2021) requiring treatment for PDA has decreased, especially among the preterm infants (Table 23.1 and Fig. 23.1A and B). This is related in part to changes in clinical practice favoring expectant management.

PDA is more common in preterm infants, especially <28 weeks' gestational age (GA), with an incidence of over 50%.[3] Maternal rubella was thought to be the cause of seasonal variation, which was noted before immunization was widely introduced. Similarly, children born at elevation are at increased risk of PDA compared with those born at sea level, with the incidence increasing proportionate to birth altitude; this suggests that ductal patency may be affected by ambient oxygen fraction.[4] There are genetic contributors, with PDA more prevalent as either an isolated cardiac malformation or in combination with other defects in patients with trisomy 21, 22q11.2 deletion, Noonan syndrome, Cantú syndrome, and Cornelia de Lange syndrome among others.[5] The female-to-male ratio is reported to be as high as 2:1.

Anatomy

In normal cardiovascular development, the proximal portions of the sixth pair of embryonic aortic arches form the proximal segment of the pulmonary arteries. The distal portion of the left sixth embryonic arch persists as the DA connecting the origin of the left main pulmonary artery to the aorta, just distal to the left subclavian artery. This metamorphosis is complete by 8 weeks of fetal life.

TABLE 23.1	Boston Children's Hospital Experience 2002–2021			
Age at Procedure	Thoracotomy	VATS	Catheterization	Total
<1 month	603	0	7	610
1–12 months	192	46	41	279
1–5 years	7	39	192	238
6–10 years	0	4	56	60
>10 years	0	6	46	52
Total	802	95	342	1239

The overall 30-day mortality rate following the procedure was 1.5%, all in premature babies in the thoracotomy group. None of the mortalities were deemed procedure related.

Patent Ductus Arteriosus (PDA) From 2002 to 2021, there were 1239 patients (56% female) with a primary diagnosis of PDA that required intervention. Among these were 708 (57%) premature babies up to 3 months of age. Closure management of PDA included surgery (thoracotomy, video-assisted thoracic surgery [VATS]) or by catheter-delivered devices.

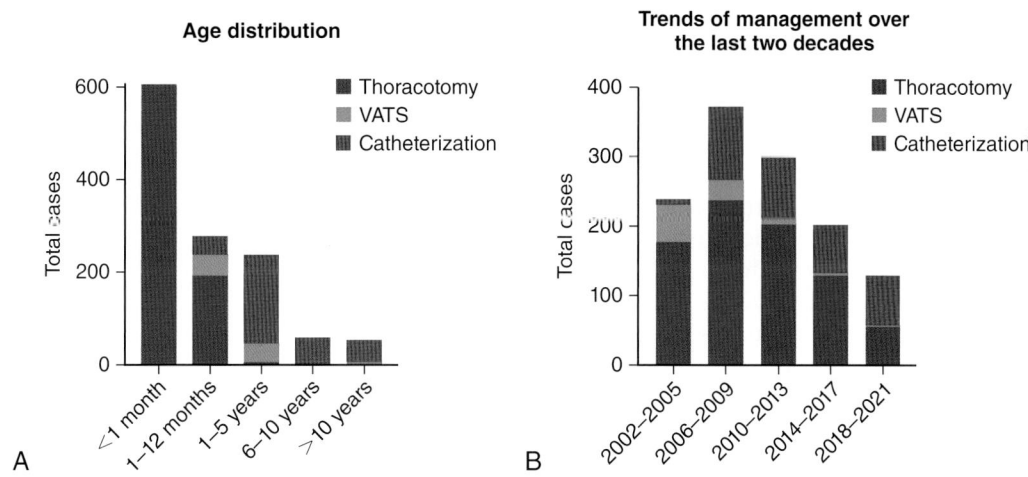

• **Fig. 23.1** (A) Patent ductus arteriosus (PDA) closure techniques by age distribution. Thoracotomy remains the primary technique in small infants, especially in premature babies, while closure with interventional procedures is the predominant approach in older children. (B) The number of patients with PDA requiring invasive treatment has decreased over time. Improvements in transcatheter methods have resulted in an increasing proportion of closures by this method. *VATS,* Video-assisted thoracic surgery.

During fetal life, the DA is as large as the ascending aorta and diverts the majority of right ventricular output to the descending aorta (Fig. 23.2); it is therefore an essential structure for normal fetal development. Fetal patency of the DA is controlled by many factors, the most important being low fetal oxygen tension and cyclooxygenase-mediated products such as prostaglandin and prostacyclin. The reciprocal relationship between the effects of oxygen and prostaglandins varies with maturity; oxygen is more effective in promoting ductal closure in the mature infant and less in the immature. Normally, the DA closes within hours of birth. Closure begins at the pulmonary end and often leaves behind a remnant on the aorta known as a ductus diverticulum. This mechanism is complex and is affected by the interaction of pulmonary and systemic arterial oxygen tensions, serum prostaglandin concentration, genetic predetermination, and other unknown factors.

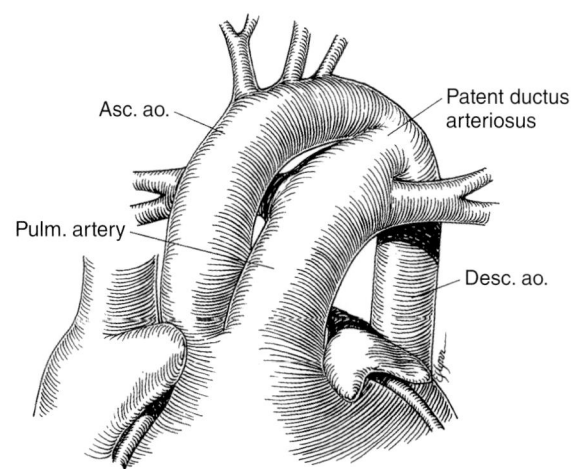

• **Fig. 23.2** Anatomic drawing of a large persistent patent ductus arteriosus. (From Fyler DC, ed. *Nadas' Pediatric Cardiology.* Philadelphia: Hanley & Belfus, 1992.)

After birth, the abrupt increase in oxygen tension inhibits ductal smooth muscle potassium channels, resulting in an influx of calcium and muscular constriction. Prostaglandin and prostacyclin levels fall following removal of placenta from the circulation. These factors cause the DA to constrict, obliterating the lumen. Functional closure usually occurs within 48 hours in term neonates. Over the following weeks, the endothelium proliferates resulting in a fibrous band that creates a permanent seal, thereafter known as the ligamentum arteriosum.[6] In premature infants, the process of ductal closure is the same but delayed, sometimes for weeks or months.

Unless managed with continuous prostaglandin or a catheter-based intervention, the DA usually becomes restrictive or closes completely in the first days of life even when the circulation depends on left-to-right (e.g., pulmonary valve atresia) or right-to-left (e.g., interrupted aortic arch) shunting for survival. Ductal closure or constriction may be induced by administration of corticosteroids or indomethacin to the mother, or by administration of indomethacin, ibuprofen, or acetaminophen to the neonate.

In some cases, a PDA persists in a variety of sizes and configurations that have implications for management. In the setting of a right aortic arch, the ductus usually remains left sided and only rarely arises in a mirror image, entering the right pulmonary artery. Bilateral ductus is rare. In pulmonary atresia, the ductus is nearly always tortuous and small; in these patients, *in utero* flow across the ductus is from the aorta to the pulmonary artery and therefore constitutes a small fraction of the normal fetal circulation. The ductus can be absent in some cases, most often in the setting of conotruncal anomalies (e.g., truncus arteriosus). The histopathology of PDA is different from that found in a normal DA, suggesting that persistent patency may be a primary anomaly and not a secondary effect.

Physiology

When an infant takes its first breaths after birth, pulmonary arteriolar resistance falls abruptly. The DA reverses flow and begins to shunt from left to right. In a matter of hours, the vessel may be functionally closed. If the DA remains widely patent, the hemodynamic impact in an otherwise normal cardiovascular system is determined by the magnitude of the shunt, which in turn depends on the size of the ductus and the relative resistance of the systemic and pulmonary circulations. The length, diameter, and tortuosity of the PDA impact shunt burden.

Generally, as pulmonary resistance falls, left-to-right (i.e., aortic to pulmonary) shunting increases. A persistent runoff from the aorta to the pulmonary artery causes excessive pulmonary blood flow, dilation of pulmonary veins and left atrium, and left ventricular volume loading (Fig. 23.3); this causes an increase in left ventricular stroke work, end-diastolic pressure, and may result in ventricular hypertrophy.[6] When the ductal shunt is extreme, left atrial dilation may "spring" open the foramen ovale, allowing left-to-right

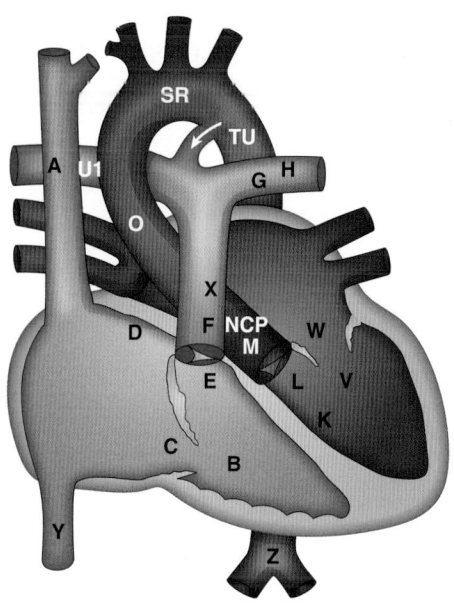

• **Fig. 23.3** Diagram of the hemodynamics in a patient with a patent ductus arteriosus and moderate pulmonary hypertension. Note the low pulmonary venous oxygen that results from a combination of an oxygen diffusion gradient in the alveolus due to extravasated lung water, due to excess pulmonary flow and hydrostatic pressure, congestive heart failure, and pulmonary infection. Note also the wide systemic arterial pressure differences owing to the diminished volume of the systemic circulation in diastole. *AO,* Aorta; *LA,* left atrium; *LV,* left ventricle; *PA,* pulmonary artery; *PV,* pulmonary vein; *RA,* right atrium; *RV,* right ventricle; *SVC,* superior vena cava.

atrial shunting and right ventricular volume loading. Unrestricted aortic-to-pulmonary flow increases myocardial oxygen demand (i.e., cardiac work needs to be supranormal to provide a full cardiac output to the systemic circulation) and decreases flow to the systemic circulation, which may result in end-organ malperfusion. Increased pulmonary blood flow and pressure cause fluid extravasation into the alveoli (i.e., pulmonary edema), which requires increased lymphatic absorption to compensate. Pulmonary edema decreases lung compliance and increases work of breathing. If a PDA persists, particularly when it is unrestrictive, pathologic pulmonary vascular remodeling may become irreversible, although this is rare in the first year of life. In cases of primary or secondary pulmonary hypertension, ductal flow may be right to left (i.e., pulmonary artery to descending aorta).

Clinical Manifestations

Physical Examination

PDA in a full-term infant or child produces symptoms and signs proportionate to the size of the shunt. When restrictive, the only abnormality may be the presence of a soft murmur. When the ductus is large, symptoms of congestive heart failure or pulmonary hypertension may be present.

Peripheral arterial pulsations provide important first clues to the presence and physiology of a PDA. Normally, the arterial impulse against the examiner's finger is maximal during systole, but the artery remains palpably distended throughout diastole. The presence of a large PDA allowing continuous left-to-right shunting will result in an "emptier" systemic circulation during diastole, thereby creating the sensation of bounding pulses; the larger the left-to-right shunt, the more prominent the peripheral arterial pulsations will be.

Most children are discovered to have a murmur within days or weeks of birth. The murmur is not characteristically continuous in the early weeks of life, but it is recognized as a systolic murmur. If the PDA is large, symptoms of congestive heart failure (e.g., tachypnea, dyspnea, intercostal or subcostal retractions, hepatomegaly, or growth failure) may alert clinicians to a cardiac problem. These infants are not cyanotic unless there is pulmonary edema or reasons for abnormally elevated pulmonary vascular resistance.

Classically, in the older child, there is a crescendo systolic murmur, peaking in intensity at aortic closure and continuing into diastole as a high-frequency, decrescendo diastolic murmur (Fig. 23.4), often referred to as a "machinery murmur." Usually, though not invariably, the diastolic component of the murmur extends the entire length of diastole. Often, there are coarse sounds (clicks or "shaking dice" noises) during systole, which contribute to the machinery quality. The murmur is loudest at the second left intercostal space; maximal intensity anywhere else should cause doubt that the murmur emanates from a PDA. When shunt burden is substantial, there may be an apical diastolic rumble from excessive mitral valve flow that is difficult to differentiate from the transmitted sounds of the loud continuous murmur. In the small infant, it is uncommon to hear the diastolic component of the murmur even if the PDA is large. In older infants with a large PDA and equilibration of aortic and pulmonary pressures, there may be only a systolic murmur, usually recognizable because of its location, its crescendo quality, and occasionally a click.

The presence of a continuous murmur of crescendo–decrescendo quality, loudest at the time of the second sound, with systolic clicks, and located in the second left intercostal space should be interpreted as resulting from a PDA. Other defects that may mimic these findings include the following[7]:

1. The most common is an aortopulmonary (AP) window; however, the AP window is usually so large that an audible continuous murmur is unusual.
2. A venous hum is usually louder when the patient is sitting rather than lying down, and it may be louder to the right of the sternum. Hums have an evanescent quality, changing with respiration as well as position.
3. A fistula between a coronary artery and a cardiac chamber may produce a continuous murmur of crescendo–decrescendo quality, which is usually not loudest at the second left intercostal space. The murmur may be louder in systole or diastole, depending on the hemodynamics (see Chapter 42).
4. A ruptured sinus of Valsalva to the right chambers also produces a continuous murmur, which most often is also loudest at the second left interspace, but this is a new-onset murmur, not previously heard, and it is normally symptomatic including chest pain, dyspnea, fatigue, and syncope. These signs must prompt an echocardiogram to facilitate the diagnosis.
5. Tetralogy of Fallot with pulmonary atresia and collateral circulation produces continuous murmurs heard across the front and back of the chest. If there are sufficient collaterals, the patient may not be visibly cyanotic.

Electrocardiography

The electrocardiogram is normal when there is a small PDA. It demonstrates left ventricular hypertrophy with a larger PDA due to volume overload. Combined ventricular hypertrophy and right atrial enlargement may be present when there is a large PDA and pulmonary hypertension. When pulmonary vascular disease dominates the clinical picture, there may be only right ventricular hypertrophy.

Chest Radiograph

The aorta, left ventricle, left atrium, pulmonary vessels, and main pulmonary arteries are enlarged in proportion to the amount of left-to-right shunt and may alter the cardiac silhouette and position of the left mainstem bronchus on the plain chest radiograph. Classic findings of a large PDA include cardiomegaly, increased pulmonary vascular markings, and hyperinflation of the lungs with flattened diaphragms. Older patients who have developed pulmonary hypertension and subsequent right-to-left shunting may demonstrate pruning of the peripheral vasculature with oligemic lung fields.

Echocardiography

Echocardiography is the examination of choice to confirm and characterize a PDA. On two-dimensional echocardiography, the PDA is easily visualized, and shunting is demonstrated with color flow mapping (Fig. 23.5) even in the presence of a small shunt. The preferred views are the

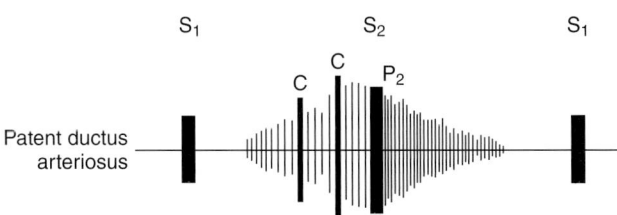

• **Fig. 23.4** Diagram of the machinery murmur of patent ductus arteriosus. Typically, the murmur is maximally loud at the time of the second heart sound (S₂); clicking noises (C) in systole contribute to the machinery sound. (From Fyler DC, ed. *Nadas' Pediatric Cardiology*. Philadelphia: Hanley & Belfus, 1992.)

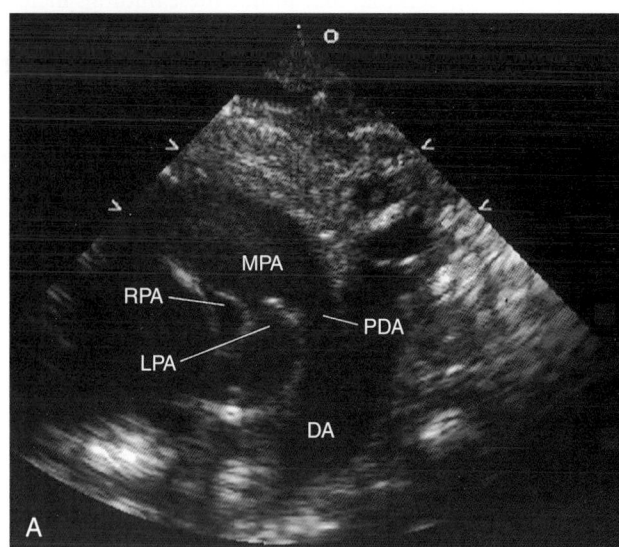

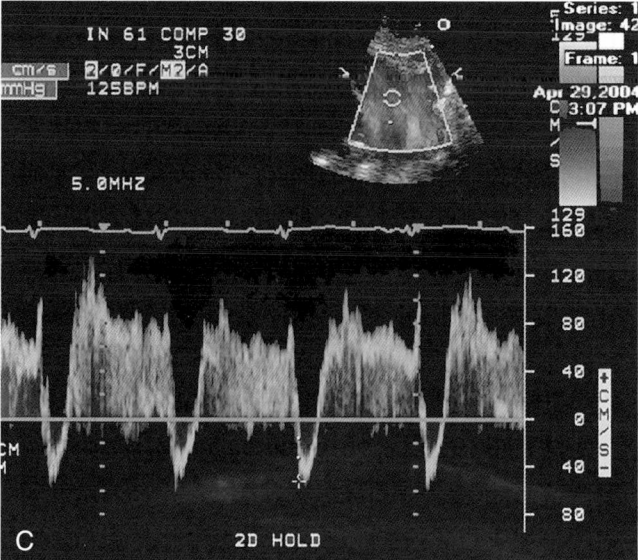

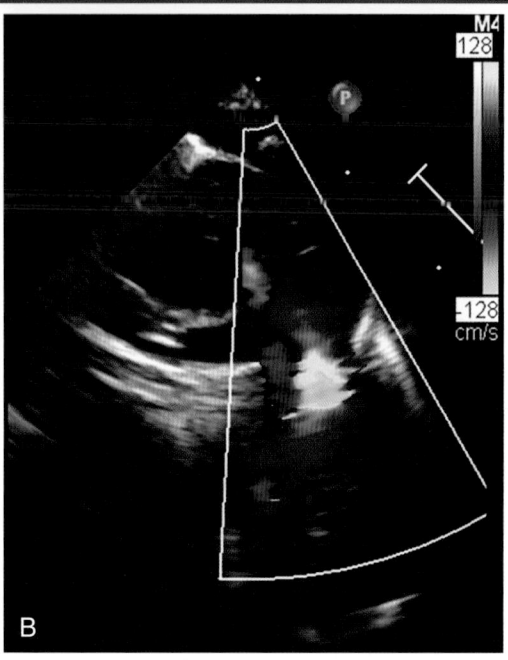

• **Fig. 23.5** (A) High left parasternal view of a large patent ductus arteriosus *(PDA)* between the proximal descending aorta *(DA)* and the main pulmonary artery *(MPA)*. The anatomic relationship of the PDA arising above left pulmonary artery *(LPA)*, which is superior to the right pulmonary artery *(RPA)* origin, is shown. (B) Color flow Doppler mapping confirms the presence of flow as the red color jet of the PDA flow is seen to enter the MPA. (C) Spectral Doppler is used to show the timing and velocity of flow across the PDA. In this case, there is mostly low-velocity left-to-right flow (signal above the baseline indicates a positive Doppler shift reflecting flow toward the transducer) with transient right-to-left flow in early systole (negative Doppler shift).

parasternal short-axis and the suprasternal view, localizing the descending aorta and pulmonary artery such that the PDA appears between these great vessels. If the ductal flow is significant, enlargement of the left atrial and ventricular chambers is evident. In many patients, incompetence of the foramen ovale allowing left-to-right shunting is evident on color flow Doppler. Estimations of pulmonary artery pressure may be made using the velocity of the tricuspid regurgitation jet, if present, and by continuous wave color Doppler. Although there is usually a pressure gradient between the aorta and pulmonary artery, absence of a gradient may reflect pulmonary hypertension. In these circumstances a PDA can be difficult to localize, but findings such as septal flattening, unexplained ventricular hypertrophy, and high-velocity pulmonary or tricuspid regurgitation should prompt further investigation.

Cardiac Catheterization

Cardiac catheterization for diagnostic purposes has not been used for many decades except to study pulmonary vascular resistance when a long-standing PDA is present. It is, however, very commonly used for interventional closure as described below.

Course

After the first successful closure of a ductus by Dr. Gross in 1938,[8] surgical management of this lesion became so widespread that a real natural history picture was no longer available. In a retrospective review by Campbell in 1968,[9] high infant mortality, spontaneous closure, endocarditis, heart failure, and pulmonary vascular obstructive disease were described, with a mortality rate of 60% by age 60 years. At present, it is reasonable to suggest that in areas of the world with high healthcare resource utilization, diagnosis is being made at a younger age and when indicated, virtually all cases are being closed either surgically or by interventional catheterization.

In the United States, it is now extremely rare to encounter a patient with vascular obstructive disease from PDA; however, it can occur by age 2 years in an untreated large lesion. In such a patient, the characteristic murmur may be absent, the peripheral pulses may not be bounding, and the heart may not be very large. The electrocardiogram may show pure right ventricular hypertrophy. On chest radiograph, a large main pulmonary artery may be visible (Fig. 23.6). If the degree of pulmonary vascular disease is uncertain, cardiac catheterization should be considered to measure pulmonary resistance in room air, with supplemental oxygen, and with a vasodilator such as inhaled nitric oxide, both with the ductus open and with it temporarily balloon-occluded. If the resistance value is fewer than 8.0 Wood units in room air and if there is a significant decrease with the previously mentioned maneuvers, then, especially in the very young, closure by device may be undertaken at that time or by surgery shortly thereafter. Without surgery, survival for several decades with vascular obstructive disease may occur. Differential cyanosis is common in older, affected patients. There may be minimal, if any, cyanosis of the lips and fingers because fully saturated blood comes to these sites from the left ventricle, whereas clubbing and obvious cyanosis of the toes result from the right-to-left shunting through the PDA into the descending aorta. This shunt of desaturated blood also results in increased renal erythropoietin and hemoglobin production, with surprisingly high levels of the latter in the face of minimal upper body desaturation.

An untreated PDA is a favored site for infective endocarditis. The chance of developing endocarditis has been estimated at 0.45% per year.[9] Closure of the ductus eliminates this possibility.

In the past, late spontaneous closure of a small patent ductus, largely based on auscultation, was noted on a few occasions; since the advent of echocardiography and color flow, this is now rarely encountered.

Management

The goal of management of uncomplicated PDA is to interrupt the left-to-right shunt. Indications for intervention include elimination of congestive heart failure and promotion of growth in the small infant, prevention of infective endocarditis, and prevention of pulmonary vascular disease. For practical purposes, every isolated PDA should be closed.

Closure can be accomplished with minimal risk using a variety of techniques. Pharmacotherapy with indomethacin, ibuprofen, or acetaminophen has been associated with renal and gastrointestinal complications in some cohorts but is generally considered a low-risk initial strategy in neonates.[10]

Interventional catheterization techniques for PDA closure are increasingly common (Table 23.1 and Fig. 23.1B).[11] In the current era, this approach may be done on an outpatient basis and avoid the risks of the traditional surgical approach. It is technically easier to do when the PDA is restrictive, long, and has an ampulla at the aortic end. The technique continues to evolve. Currently, coils are frequently used in small lesions, while occlusion devices are considered for moderate and large PDA. A catheter or sheath is advanced across the ductus from either of the great vessels and the closure device is positioned within the lumen of the PDA (Fig. 23.7). Complete closure rates generally exceed 95%.[12] Catheter-based closure in infants (<1 year of age) is an active area of research with regards to feasibility and safety.[13]

Age and size do not preclude surgical management. The surgical approach is most commonly via thoracotomy with exposure of the PDA, ligation, and division and has excellent results at all ages and sizes. Video-assisted thoracoscopic surgery and robotic-assisted surgery may be used for this lesion. Successful closure of PDA via surgical techniques is reported to be 95–100%, with low mortality (<3%). Compared with interventional catheterization, however, surgical ligation has been associated with higher resource use, longer duration of postoperative admission, and higher in-hospital mortality in some circumstances.[14] Ductal ligation has been followed by later appearance of a left-to-right shunt because of either incomplete ligation or recanalization. Dividing the ductus and oversewing the stumps prevents recanalization; however, the difficulties and dangers of

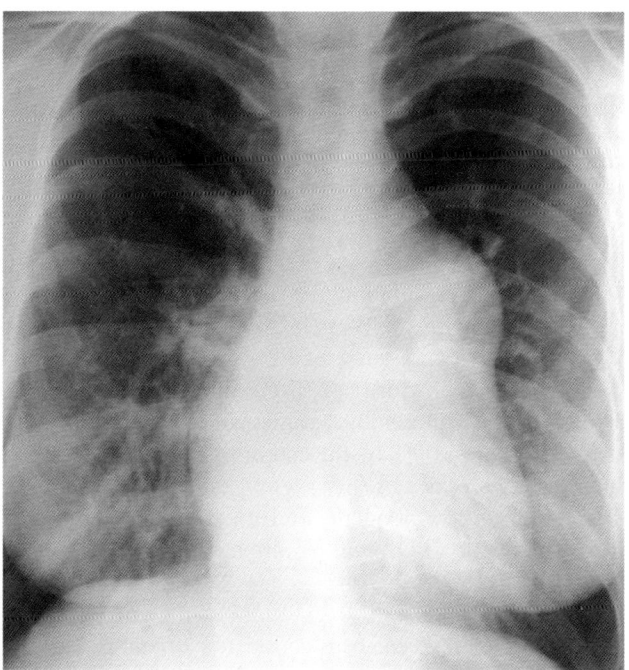

• **Fig. 23.6** Chest radiograph in a young woman with a large patent ductus arteriosus and advanced pulmonary vascular disease. This patient died within a year after this picture was taken. Note the very large main pulmonary artery and the near normal size of the heart. (From Fyler DC, ed. *Nadas' Pediatric Cardiology*. Philadelphia: Hanley & Belfus, 1992.)

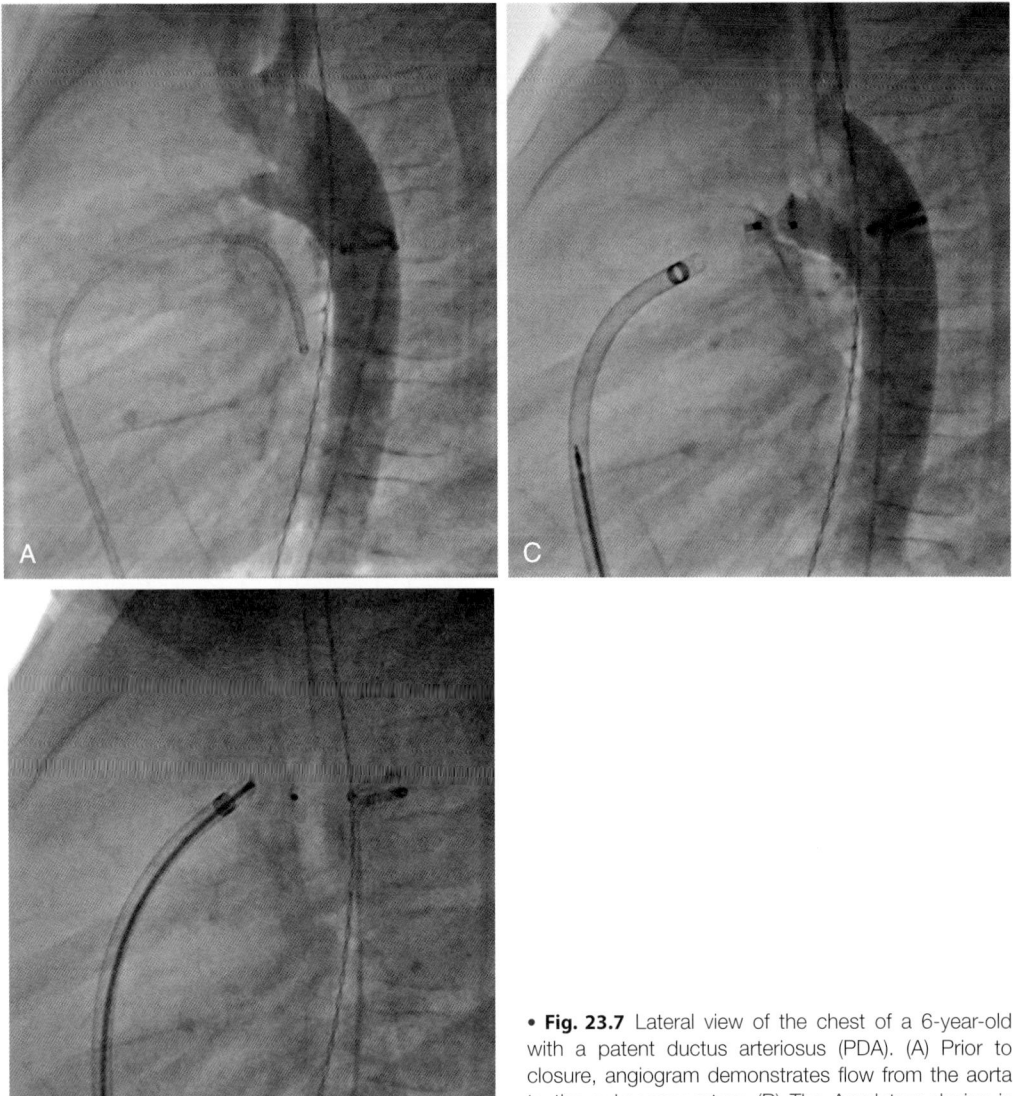

• **Fig. 23.7** Lateral view of the chest of a 6-year-old with a patent ductus arteriosus (PDA). (A) Prior to closure, angiogram demonstrates flow from the aorta to the pulmonary artery. (B) The Amplatzer device is confirmed in the correct position. (C) Angiogram demonstrates device occlusion of PDA.

division, although small, are nonetheless sufficient that some surgeons favor ligation.

Close monitoring and follow-up are necessary for infants with PDA. Effective closure should be confirmed, screening for potential complications of interventions should be performed, and early and midterm follow-up is encouraged. Long-term evaluation has generally been considered unnecessary for corrected PDA, although as we learn more about the lifelong implications of congenital heart disease, even in those patients repaired as infants, that perspective may change.

Variations

Ductus Arteriosus in Premature Infants

Prevalence
Functional closure of the DA occurs in 90% of full-term newborns within a couple of days of life. In premature infants, ductal closure may be delayed, but will occur in almost all neonates ≥30 weeks' GA by day 4. In younger GA infants, the incidence of PDA beyond this time increases, but two-third of preterm infants weighing 1000–1500 g will exhibit spontaneous ductal closure by day 7 and almost 90% by the end of their first year. Among infants ≤27 weeks' GA (or weighing <1000 g), spontaneous closure is less frequent, and one out of four infants discharged with a PDA will require intervention.[15]

Anatomy
PDA in the preterm infant is considered a result of vascular immaturity, as the preterm ductus is structurally different from mature vessels. The intima in the mature ductus is thickened and irregular with mucoid material sometimes referred to as intimal cushions, which are absent in the preterm ductus. Additionally, the preterm PDA has fewer layers of smooth muscle, which may deter postnatal ductal constriction.

Physiology

The level of pulmonary vascular resistance is less in preterm infants than in full-term babies. This favors left-to-right shunting in the presence of PDA. The presence of hypoxemia due to lung disease promotes continued patency of the ductus. Increased pulmonary blood flow and pressure may cause pulmonary hemorrhage. In addition, ductal steal from the systemic circulation may reduce intestinal flow predisposing infants to necrotizing enterocolitis, or cause fluctuations in cerebral blood flow contributing to intraventricular hemorrhage and other neurologic morbidities.[3] Pulmonary venous oxygen desaturation and pulmonary hypertension were consistent features in premature infants with PDA undergoing cardiac catheterization in earlier eras.

Clinical Manifestations

The murmur in premature infants is usually atypical, rarely being more than a systolic murmur, and not necessarily crescendo. Indeed, any systolic murmur in a very small premature baby should be considered indicative of a PDA until proven otherwise. Rarely, a premature infant may have a known PDA with no audible murmur. Prominence of the peripheral pulses is a good indication that the PDA may be pathophysiologic.

Characterizing hemodynamic significance of a PDA in preterm infants can be challenging, but growing consensuses agrees that a comprehensive appraisal of the cardiovascular status incorporating echocardiography can provide hemodynamic information that either complements what is clinically suspected or delivers novel physiologic insight.[16,17] Several clinical and echocardiographic elements are considered to define hemodynamic significance: (1) PDA shunt volume assessment and its impact on the systemic and pulmonary circulations; (2) myocardial systolic and diastolic function; and (3) antenatal and perinatal characteristics that may mitigate or exacerbate the consequences of a shunt.[18] Evidence suggests that this approach provides an accurate predictive definition of hemodynamic significance with a link to morbidity.[19]

Management

Non-interventional conservative management of PDA may be beneficial in selected patients.[20] Medical management includes ventilatory support and fluid restriction. Oxygen therapy may facilitate PDA closure in some cases, but it should be balanced with the increased risk of morbidities such as retinopathy of prematurity. Pharmacotherapy with indomethacin, ibuprofen, and/or acetaminophen has been shown to be effective.[3,21-23]

While there is no one set of clinical or echocardiographic features that necessitate PDA closure, a thorough appraisal of all factors may result in an improved risk prediction. This in turn facilitates a more accurate and targeted selection of infants more likely to benefit from invasive treatment. Definitive PDA closure should be considered in preterm babies with hemodynamically significant shunts determined by a combination of echocardiographic and clinical variables

(e.g., tachycardia, tachypnea, respiratory support, abdominal symptoms, or other signs of organ dysfunction), when adjusted by individual risk factors for adverse events, including GA and other comorbidities.[24] Surgical ligation is associated with a higher risk profile and therefore risks and benefits should be weighed if medical treatment is not successful or is contraindicated.[25] Catheterization-based closure is increasingly common in preterm infants, with newer devices approved for patients as small as 700 g.[26]

Course

It is not clear whether a PDA increases the overall mortality rate in neonates as studies offer conflicting data. The mortality associated with surgical closure has improved significantly over time and the morbidities associated with interventional procedures are diminishing rapidly.

Aneurysm of the Ductus Arteriosus

Aneurysm of the DA can occur after infective endarteritis, surgical closure, or transcatheter occlusion. A variation of the normal ductus diverticulum, the remnant of the ductus at the point of attachment of the aorta, can become aneurysmal.[27] In up to 20% of these cases, an underlying genetic condition is present (e.g., Ehlers-Danlos syndrome, Marfan syndrome, trisomy 21 or trisomy 13). Most of them have a benign course and remain asymptomatic, but there is a potential risk of local compression of adjacent structures or clot formation, with subsequent increased risk of emboli or infection. Surgical resection may be indicated.

Maternal Rubella

Rubella infection in the first trimester of pregnancy is a leading cause of vaccine-preventable birth defects worldwide. Congenital rubella syndrome is typically associated with cataracts, hearing impairment, developmental delay, and congenital heart disease, oftentimes PDA or peripheral pulmonary artery stenosis.

Acknowledgment

We thank Philip T. Levy, MD, for his expert contributions to the section on Clinical Manifestations and Management of the preterm infant with PDA.

References

1. Fyler DC, Buckley LP, Hellenbrand WE, et al. Report of the New England regional infant cardiac program. *Pediatrics*. 1980;65:398.
2. Liu Y, Chen S, Zühlke L, Black GC, et al. Global birth prevalence of congenital heart defects 1970-2017: updated systematic review and meta-analysis of 260 studies. *Int J Epidemiol*. 2019;48:455-463.
3. Hamrick SEG, Sallmon H, Rose AT, et al. Patent ductus arteriosus of the preterm infant. *Pediatrics*. 2020;146:e20201209.

4. Zheng JY, Tian HT, Zhu ZM, et al. Prevalence of symptomatic congenital heart disease in Tibetan school children. *Am J Cardiol.* 2013;112:1468-1470.

5. Pierpont ME, Brueckner M, Chung WK, et al. American Heart Association Council on Cardiovascular Disease in the Young; Council on Cardiovascular and Stroke Nursing; and Council on Genomic and Precision Medicine. Genetic Basis for Congenital Heart Disease: Revisited: A Scientific Statement From the American Heart Association. *Circulation.* 2018;138:e653-e711.

6. Crockett SL, Berger CD, Shelton EL, Reese J. Molecular and mechanical factors contributing to ductus arteriosus patency and closure. *Congenit Heart Dis.* 2019;14:15-20.

7. Ginghină C, Năstase OA, Ghiorghiu I, Egher L. Continuous murmur: the auscultatory expression of a variety of pathological conditions. *J Med Life.* 2012;5:39-46.

8. Gross RE, Hubbard JP. Surgical ligation of a patent ductus arteriosus. Report of the first successful case. *JAMA.* 1939;112:729-731.

9. Campbell M. Natural history of persistent ductus arteriosus. *Br Heart J.* 1968;30:4.

10. Ferguson JM. Pharmacotherapy for patent ductus arteriosus closure. *Congenit Heart Dis.* 2019;14:52-56.

11. O'Byrne ML, Millenson ME, Grady CB, et al. Trends in transcatheter and operative closure of patent ductus arteriosus in neonatal intensive care units. analysis of data from the Pediatric Health Information Systems Database. *Am Heart J.* 2019;217: 121-130.

12. Baruteau AE, Hascoët S, Baruteau J, et al. Transcatheter closure of patent ductus arteriosus: past, present and future. *Arch Cardiovasc Dis.* 2014;107:122-132.

13. Backes CH, Rivera BK, Bridge JA, et al. Percutaneous patent ductus arteriosus (PDA) closure during infancy: a meta-analysis. *Pediatrics.* 2017;139:e20162927.

14. Kuntz MT, Staffa SJ, Graham D, et al. Trend and outcomes for surgical versus transcatheter patent ductus arteriosus closure in neonates and infants at US Children's Hospitals. *J Am Heart Assoc.* 2022;11:e022776.

15. Clyman RI, Couto J, Murphy GM. Patent ductus arteriosus: are current neonatal treatment options better or worse than no treatment at all? *Semin Perinatol.* 2012;36:123-129.

16. Afif EK, James AT, Corcoran JD, et al. A patent ductus arteriosus severity score predicts chronic lung disease or death before discharge. *J Pediatr.* 2015;167:1354-1361.e2.

17. Van Laere D, Van Overmeire B, Gupta S, et al. Application of NPE in the assessment of a patent ductus arteriosus. *Pediatr Res.* 2018;84:46-56.

18. Kluckow M, Lemmers P. Hemodynamic assessment of the patent ductus arteriosus: beyond ultrasound. *Semin Fetal Neonatal Med.* 2018;23:239-244.

19. Fink D, El-Khuffash A, McNamara PJ, Nitzan I, Hammerman C. Tale of Two patent ductus arteriosus severity scores: similarities and differences. *Am J Perinatol.* 2018;35:55-58.

20. Clyman RI, Liebowitz M, Kaempf J, et al. PDA-TOLERATE trial: an exploratory randomized controlled trial of treatment of moderate-to-large patent ductus arteriosus at 1 week of age. *J Pediatr.* 2019;205:41-48.e6.

21. Kluckow M, Jeffery M, Gill A, Evans N. A randomized placebo-controlled trial of early treatment of the patent ductus arteriosus. *Arch Dis Child Fetal Neonatal Ed.* 2014;99:F99-F104.

22. Mitra S, Florez ID, Tamayo ME, et al. Association of placebo, indomethacin, ibuprofen, and acetaminophen with closure of hemodynamically significant patent ductus arteriosus in preterm infants: a systematic review and metaanalysis. *JAMA.* 2018;319:1221-1238.

23. Bardanzellu F, Neroni P, Dessì A, Fanos V. Paracetamol in patent ductus arteriosus treatment: efficacious and safe? *BioMed Res Int.* 2017;2017:1438038.

24. Sung SI, Chang YS, Kim J, Choi JH, Ahn SY, Park WS. Natural evolution of ductus arteriosus with noninterventional conservative management in extremely preterm infants born at 23-28 weeks of gestation. *PLoS One.* 2019;14(2):e0212256.

25. Su BH, Lin HY, Chiu HY, Tsai ML, Chen YT, Lu IC. Therapeutic strategy of patent ductus arteriosus in extremely preterm infants. *Pediatr Neonatol.* 2020;61:133-141.

26. Sathanandam SK, Gutfinger D, O'Brien L, et al. Amplatzer Piccolo Occluder clinical trial for percutaneous closure of the patent ductus arteriosus in patients ≥700 grams. *Catheter Cardiovasc Interv.* 2020;96:1266-1276.

27. Jan SL, Hwang B, Fu YC, Chai JW, Chi CS. Isolated neonatal ductus arteriosus aneurysm. *J Am Coll Cardiol.* 2002;39:342-348.

24

Coarctation of the Aorta and Interrupted Aortic Arch

HENRY CHENG

KEY LEARNING POINTS

- In the presence of four cardiac chambers on fetal ultrasound and a patent ductus arteriosus (PDA), both coarctation of the aorta and interrupted aortic arch (IAA) can be underdiagnosed *in utero*.
- Coarctation of the aorta and IAA can lead to compromised systemic perfusion and cardiovascular collapse in the neonatal period as the PDA closes.
- The clinical diagnoses of coarctation of the aorta and IAA are often dependent on the state of the PDA. The presence of

a PDA can lead to delayed diagnoses of these lesions in the neonatal period.
- Surgery is the intervention of choice for coarctation of the aorta and IAA.
- Patients with coarctation of the aorta and IAA need lifelong cardiovascular follow-up to monitor for recurrent obstruction as well as associated cardiovascular disease, such as hypertension.

Coarctation

Definition

Coarctation of the aorta is an obstruction in the descending aorta located almost invariably opposite the insertion of the ductus arteriosus (Fig. 24.1). Coarctation of the aorta occurs with a prevalence of approximately 4.4/10,000 live births.[1]

Embryology/Genetics

In the normal fetus, the left fourth arch forms the transverse part of the aortic arch, and the right fourth arch normally regresses. The pulmonary arteries are derived in part from the sixth arches; the distal sixth arch on the left forms the ductus arteriosus (DA) while that on the right regresses.

The precise cause of coarctation remains unknown but is thought to be due either to an abnormal (reduced) flow pattern in the aortic arch *in utero* or to extension of the ductal tissue into the wall of the aorta. In the former, lesions that lead to decreased flow in the ascending aorta, such as ventricular septal defect (VSD) or obstruction at the mitral, subaortic, or aortic valve level, result in hypoplasia of the transverse arch and aortic isthmic area.[2] With regard to the ductal tissue theory, it is thought that constriction after

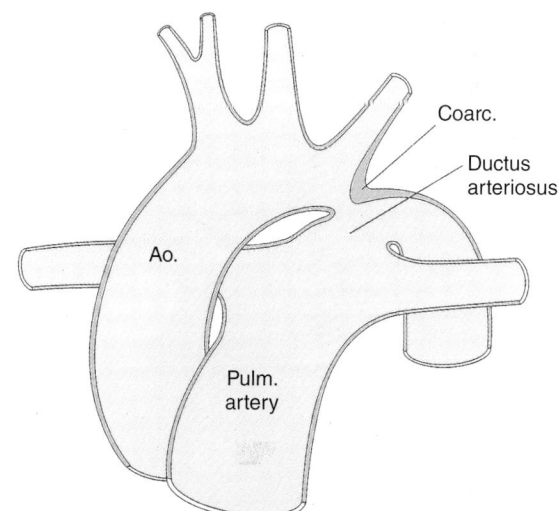

• **Fig. 24.1** Coarctation of the aorta. (From Nadas AS, Fyler DC [eds]. *Nadas' Pediatric Cardiology*. Philadelphia, PA: Hanley and Belfus, 1992.)

birth of aberrant ductal tissue extending into the aortic wall results in obstruction.[3] The observation that coarctation of the aorta is seen in close relatives and is also associated with certain syndromes (such as Turner syndrome) suggests a genetic etiology of disease.[4]

Diagnosis

Despite improvements in prenatal detection rates of many types of congenital heart disease (CHD), coarctation of the aorta remains one of the most challenging diagnoses to make in the fetal or neonatal period.[5,6] Fetal echocardiography can identify signs of aortic arch obstruction, but the presence of a normal four-chamber view often complicates prenatal detection. Clinical presentation and diagnosis of coarctation is dependent on the state of the DA. As the DA closes, patients present with signs of arch obstruction (e.g., decreased femoral pulses, four limb systolic blood pressure differences), which may progress to cardiogenic shock. The presence of a patent ductus arteriosus (PDA) can mask arch obstruction, and thus coarctation has one of the highest proportions of delayed diagnoses of all critical CHD.[7] Prostaglandin E1 infusion is used to maintain the PDA, which provides blood flow to the lower body and is an essential therapy for the neonate with coarctation presenting in shock.

Echocardiography is the primary tool for definitively diagnosing coarctation and provides additional diagnostic information such as presence of a PDA, size of the aorta/aortic arch (including ascending aorta, transverse arch, isthmus, and descending aorta), ventricular systolic function, and associated congenital heart lesions, most commonly bicuspid aortic valve (Fig. 24.2).

Coarctation may be diagnosed later in life, typically when a patient is found to have upper extremity hypertension. In these circumstances, collateral flow involving the intercostal, internal mammary, and scapular vessels provides perfusion to the lower body. The interconnecting arteries of the collateral circulation are present at birth, enlarging to accommodate the need for increased distal flow as needed. Because of extensive collateral circulation, it is possible to have severe obstruction of the aorta with only a small difference in blood pressure at rest between the arms and legs. The collateral vessels become larger and more tortuous with time, and the intercostals can ultimately erode the undersurface of the ribs seen as rib notching on chest radiograph (Fig. 24.3). In these situations, patients may present with clinical signs such as systemic hypertension, murmur, decreased lower extremity pulses, or heart failure.[8]

Surgical Intervention

Surgery remains the primary intervention for treatment of coarctation. In addition to preventing the acute complications noted above, early repair reduces the long-term adverse sequelae including systemic (upper extremity and cerebral) hypertension with resulting left ventricular hypertrophy and coronary artery and cerebral vascular disease. Surgery in most cases consists of resection with end-to-end or extended end-to-end anastomosis via left thoracotomy without cardiopulmonary bypass. After mobilization of the aortic arch and thoracic descending aorta, the diseased aortic segment and ductal tissue are resected, and an anastomosis is performed (Fig. 24.4A and B).[10] When there is significant arch hypoplasia proximal to the area of coarctation, a more extensive arch reconstruction on cardiopulmonary bypass may be needed and approached via median sternotomy.[11]

Surgical patient outcomes are excellent, with perioperative mortality of ~1%–2% and recurrent arch obstruction < 10%.[10,12] Need for intervention for recurrent arch obstruction has been associated with younger age at surgery, an aberrant

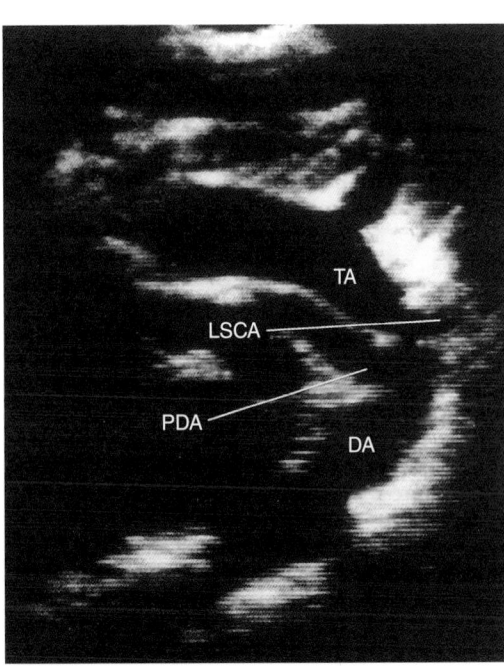

• **Fig. 24.2** Echocardiogram image showing coarctation of the aorta. *DA,* Descending aorta; *LSCA,* left subclavian artery; *PDA,* patent ductus arteriosus; *TA,* transverse arch.

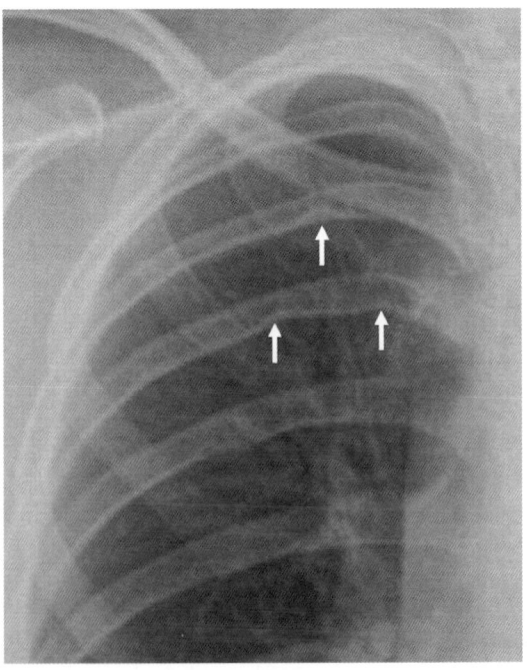

• **Fig. 24.3** Chest X-ray showing rib notching secondary to collateral vessels eroding ribs in a patient with coarctation of the aorta.[9] (From Ijland MM, Tanke RB. Aortic coarctation. *Circulation.* 2009;120:1294–1295.)

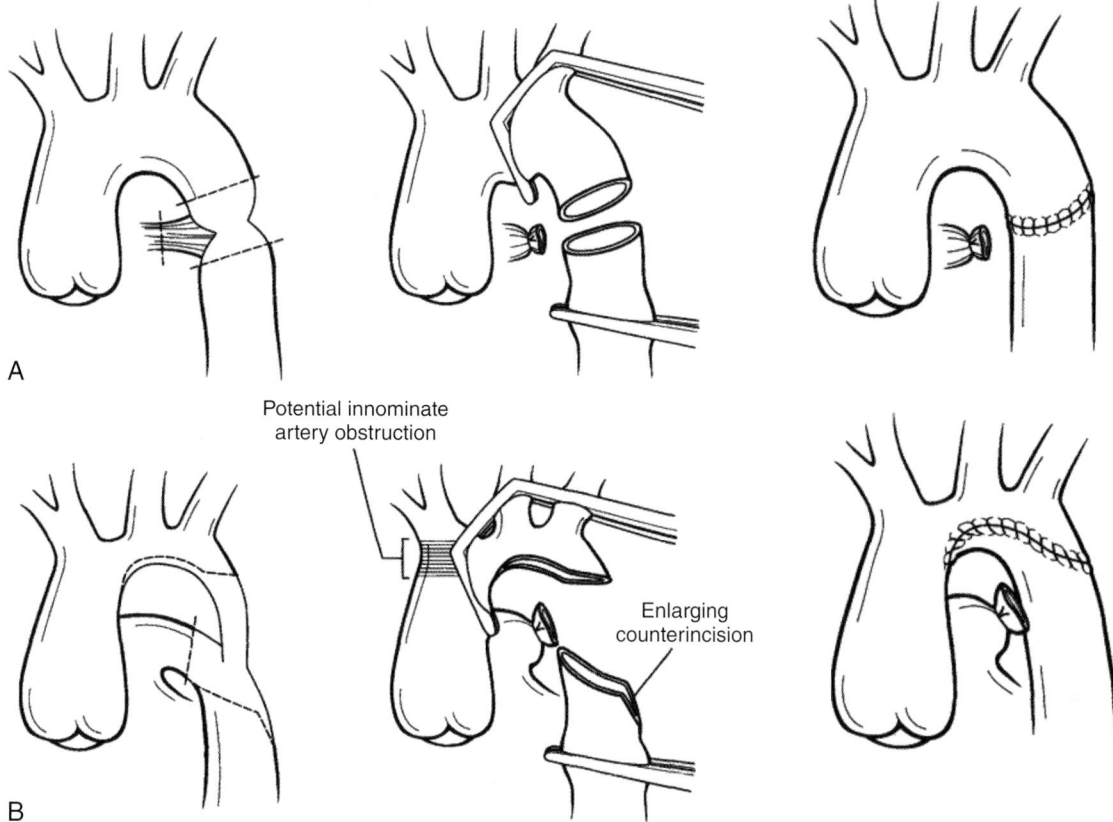

• **Fig. 24.4** Repair of coarctation of the aorta using end-to-end anastomosis (A) and extended end-to-end anastomosis (B). (Surgical figures from Jaquiss RDB. Coarctation of the aorta: end-to-end anastomosis. *Oper Tech Thorac Cardiovasc Surg.* 2002;7:2–10.)

right subclavian artery, diffusely hypoplastic aortic arch, persistent upper and lower blood pressure gradient postoperatively, and postoperative Doppler gradient by echocardiography.[10] Later age at repair, however, particularly after age 9 years, has been associated with persistent post-repair hypertension.[13,14]

Catheter-Based Intervention

Whereas surgical management is the preferred management in the newborn, catheter-based intervention may be indicated in infants when risk factors for surgery exist, such as significant end-organ injury and/or severe ventricular dysfunction. In such cases, catheter-based balloon dilation or stenting of the coarctation can serve as a temporizing procedure until definitive surgical correction can be performed.[15] Isolated coarctation presenting later in childhood and adulthood is often amenable to percutaneous intervention, with excellent results reported.[16] Controversy remains surrounding the use of primary catheter-based interventions in the clinically stable neonate.[17]

Postoperative Care/Follow-Up

Patients with coarctation of the aorta need lifelong cardiovascular care despite definitive intervention on the anatomic obstruction. Long-term follow-up in this population demonstrates elevated rates of systemic hypertension, recurrent arch obstruction, need for additional cardiovascular interventions, and decreased survival.[13]

Interrupted Aortic Arch

Definition

Interruption of the aortic arch (IAA) describes a point of atresia or absence of a segment of the aortic arch. IAA is rare, accounting for approximately 1.3% of all CHD with a prevalence of 2/100,000 live births.[18]

IAA is associated with a wide range of congenital heart defects, including aortopulmonary window, truncus arteriosus, transposition of the great arteries, posterior malalignment VSD, and single ventricle heart disease.[19] For the purposes of this discussion, we will focus on two ventricle heart disease with two normally related great arteries.

Classification of IAA is based on the site of the aortic arch interruption: type A, interruption distal to the left subclavian artery origin; type B, interruption between the left carotid and left subclavian artery origins; and type C, interruption between the innominate and left carotid artery origins (Fig. 24.5).[20] The most common is type (B ~70%–80%), followed by type A (~10%–20%), and the least common is type C (<5%).[21,22] An interventricular communication is

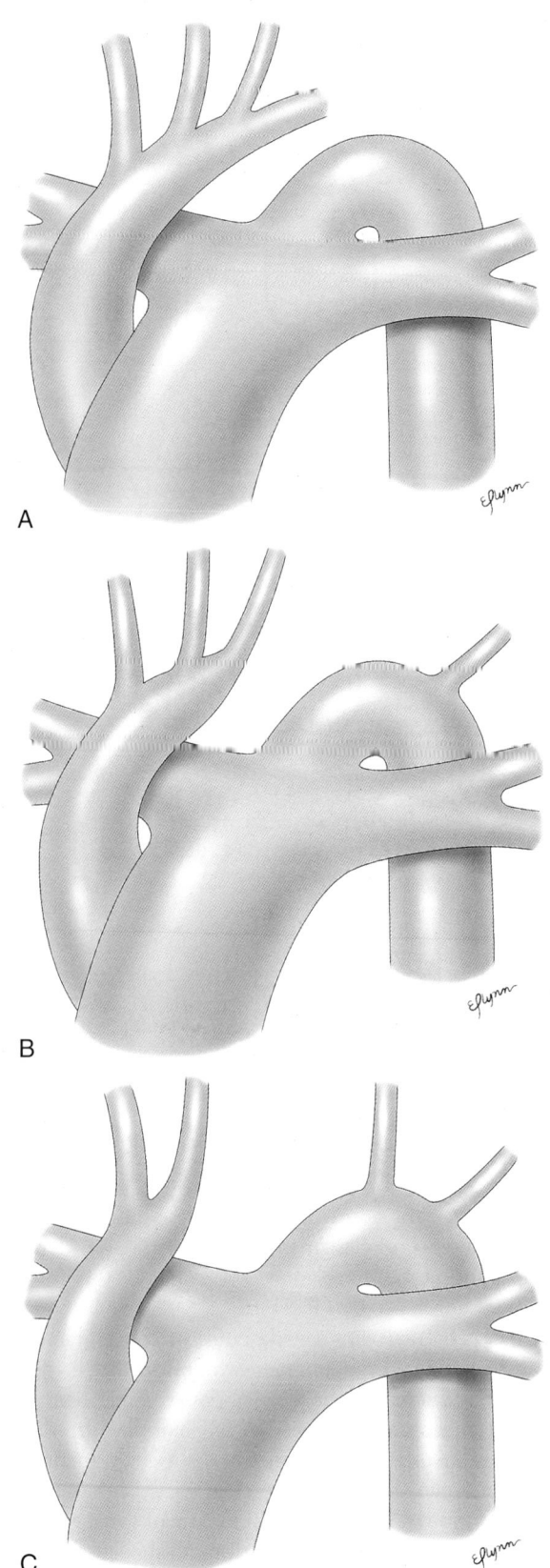

A

B

C

• **Fig. 24.5** Classification of interrupted aortic arch. (From Nadas AS, Fyler DC [eds]. *Nadas' Pediatric Cardiology*. Philadelphia, PA: Hanley and Belfus, 1992.)

present in nearly all patients with two ventricles. A conoventricular VSD is present in the vast majority (>70%) of patients with IAA, frequently with posterior malalignment of the infundibular septum relative to the trabecular septum.[19,23] Aortic stenosis is common (valvar, subvalvar, or both) as are bicuspid aortic valve and an aberrant origin of the right subclavian artery from the descending aorta.[21]

Embryology/Genetics

The left fourth arch in the embryo forms the transverse aortic arch from the left carotid to the ductal insertion. Abnormalities in the formation of this area are thought to be responsible for at least two of the types of interrupted arch (types B and C) and perhaps type A. An alternative explanation for type A involves decreased flow across the arch and hence across the isthmus. In conjunction with right-to-left flow via the DA to the descending aorta, this leads to absence of the isthmus. Deletion of chromosome 22q11 is strongly linked to IAA (~50%), especially type B (>70%).[24]

Diagnosis

Patients with IAA are almost always diagnosed by imaging in the fetal or clinically in the neonatal period. Similar to coarctation of the aorta, the DA is required to supply blood to the lower half of the body. As with other conotruncal defects with four chambers seen on fetal ultrasound, IAA can be difficult to diagnose *in utero*. The association of VSDs with IAA, however, can result in an increased *in utero* detection rate.[5] Fetal detection rates vary widely, with rates as low as 2% in large population-based studies and up to 24% at a quaternary pediatric referral center.[7,25] The presence of a PDA can preclude diagnosis of IAA and can lead to delayed diagnosis in the postnatal period. Differential cyanosis may be present before PDA closure as the patient's condition deteriorates and pulmonary venous blood is no longer fully saturated.[7] Severe cardiogenic shock develops as the DA closes. Prostaglandin E1 infusion is used to maintain a PDA and provide lower extremity blood flow.

Echocardiography is utilized to diagnose type of IAA, VSD type, aortic arch dimensions, aortic valve morphology/size/function, left ventricular outflow tract, ventricular systolic function, and additional associated anomalies (Fig. 24.6).

Surgical Intervention

The preferred surgical treatment for many patients with IAA is a single-stage biventricular repair with arch reconstruction and VSD closure. Deep hypothermia with circulatory arrest or hypothermic regional cerebral perfusion is typically used for the arch reconstruction. After resection of ductal tissue, the ascending and descending aorta are anastomosed with the aid of a patch along the anterior aspect of the anastomosis. Following the aortic repair/augmentation, intracardiac repairs are performed (Fig. 24.7).[26] Perioperative mortality

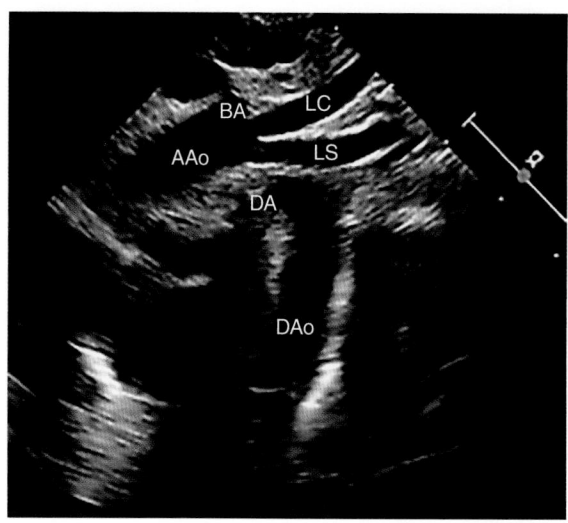

• **Fig. 24.6** Suprasternal echocardiogram showing an interruption of the aortic arch distal to the subclavian artery. *AAo,* Ascending aorta; *BA,* brachiocephalic artery; *DA,* ductus arteriosus; *DAo,* descending aorta; *LC,* left carotid artery; *LS,* left subclavian artery. (From KW, Anderson RH, Spicer DE, Morales DLS. Coarctation and interrupted aortic arch. In: Wernovsky G, Anderson RH, Kumar K, et al. [eds] *Anderson's Pediatric Cardiology,* 4th edn. Elsevier;2020:843–864.e6.)

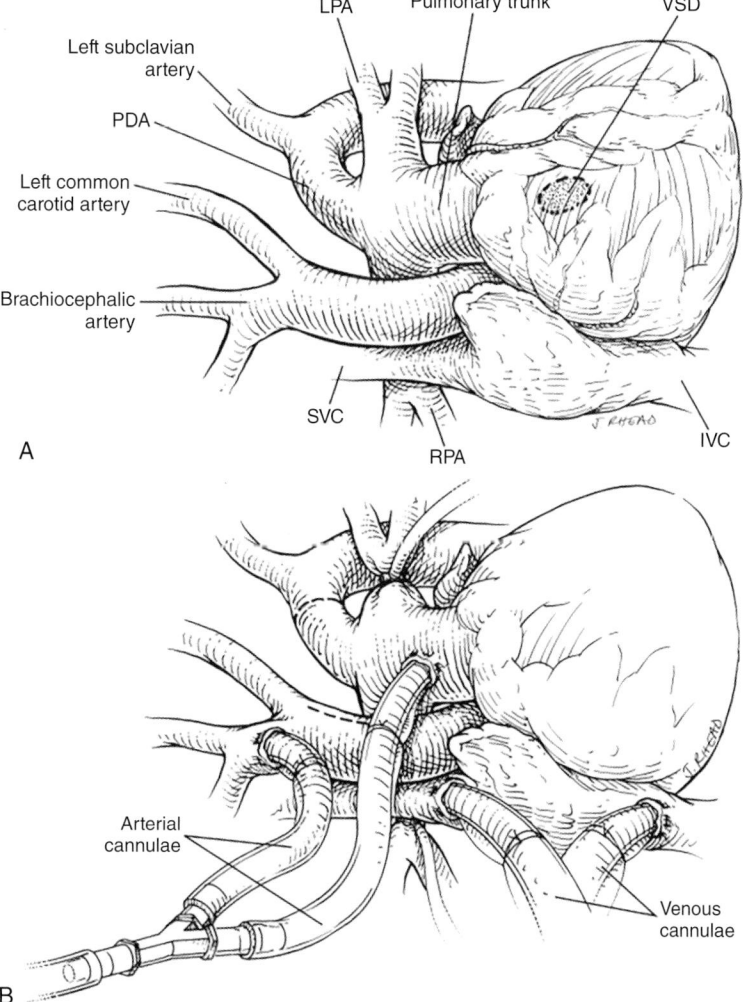

• **Fig. 24.7** Primary repair of interrupted aortic arch using continuous cardiopulmonary bypass (CPB). **(A)** Cardiac exposure is through a standard median sternotomy, and preparation and dissection are similar to that used for repair of hypoplastic left heart. This figure shows type B aortic arch interruption, with patent ductus arteriosus *(PDA)* and ventricular septal defect *(VSD).* **(B)** Two separate arterial cannulae are used, one introduced into the brachiocephalic artery and the other into the pulmonary trunk. Venous cannulation is performed into superior *(SVC)* and inferior venae cavae *(IVC)* through standard purse strings. After beginning CPB, branch pulmonary arteries are temporarily occluded. Moderate hypothermia and standard cardioplegic myocardial protection are used. *Dashed lines* show points of transection of distal ductus arteriosus and incision in posterolateral aspect of the ascending aorta.

Continued

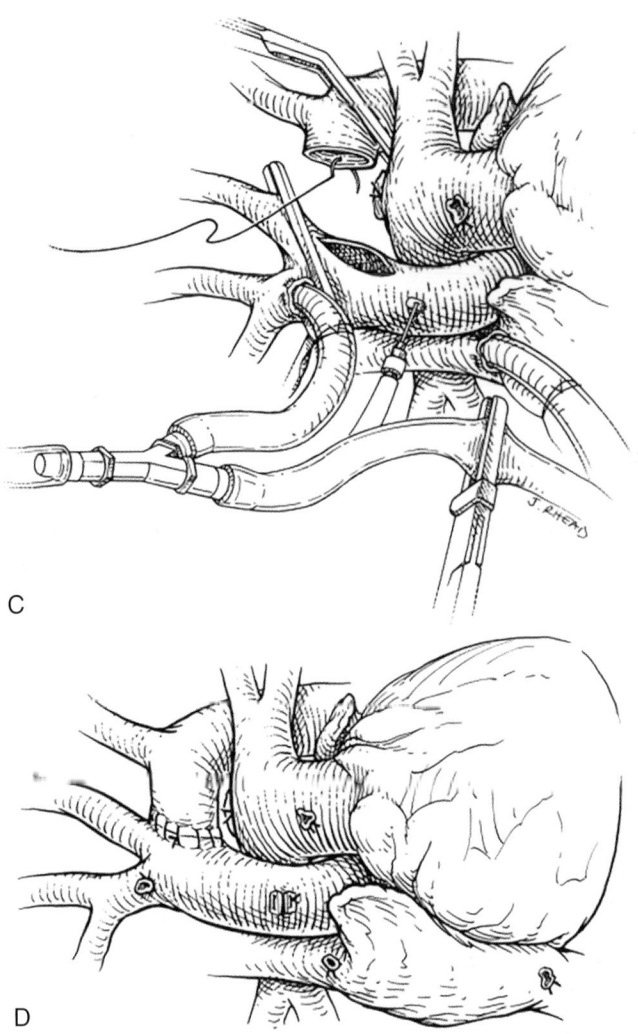

C

D

• **Fig. 24.7, cont'd** **(C)** Cardioplegia has been introduced through a catheter in mid-ascending aorta. Proximal aortic clamp is positioned to allow continued flow through brachiocephalic and left carotid arteries. Arterial cannula in pulmonary trunk has been removed and ductus arteriosus ligated and divided. All the ductus tissue has been removed from distal aorta. Incision in posterolateral aspect of ascending aorta has been made. Running suture anastomosis is begun at posterior aspect of circumference of descending aorta. **(D)** Completed arch repair. Aortic clamps have been removed and patient separated from CPB (see text for details of methodology for ventricular septal defect closure). *LPA,* left pulmonary artery; *RPA,* right pulmonary artery. (From Kouchoukos NT, Blackstone EH, Hanley FL, Kirklin JK. Chapter 48: coarctation of the aorta and interrupted aortic arch. In: Kouchoukos NT, Blackstone EH, Hanley FL, Kirklin JK, eds. *Kirklin/Barratt-Boyes Cardiac Surgery,* 4th edn. Saunders:2013:1717–1779.)

for neonatal patients undergoing repair of isolated IAA with only an associated ASD or VSD is approximately 4%.[27]

Some patients with IAA have significant left ventricular outflow tract obstruction (LVOTO) at the subvalvar and valvar levels caused by posterior deviation of the conal/infundibular septum, left ventricular muscle bundles, or abnormal aortic valve morphology (e.g., unicuspid, bicuspid, hypoplastic valve).[21] Patients with significant LVOTO that would result in significant obstruction of LV to systemic outflow may undergo a Yasui procedure. The Yasui procedure consists of creation of an intraventricular baffle to divert the LV outflow across the VSD to the native pulmonary valve, aortic arch reconstruction with a Damus-Kaye-Stansel pulmonary artery to ascending aorta connection,

and placement of a right ventricle to pulmonary artery conduit (Fig. 24.8).[28] Perioperative mortality associated with the Yasui procedure is now relatively low, with centers reporting perioperative mortality ranging from 0–6%.[29,30]

The decision to undergo a single-staged biventricular repair versus a Yasui procedure incorporates many factors, including a patient's size, degree of LVOTO, and size of left heart structures. One guideline proposed for determining whether to pursue a single-stage biventricular repair versus a Yasui procedure incorporates the preoperative aortic valve annulus size. An aortic valve annulus size (in mm) less than the patient's weight in kilograms is felt to be associated with early LVOTO and therefore suggests that a Yasui procedure should be performed. Patients with an aortic valve annulus

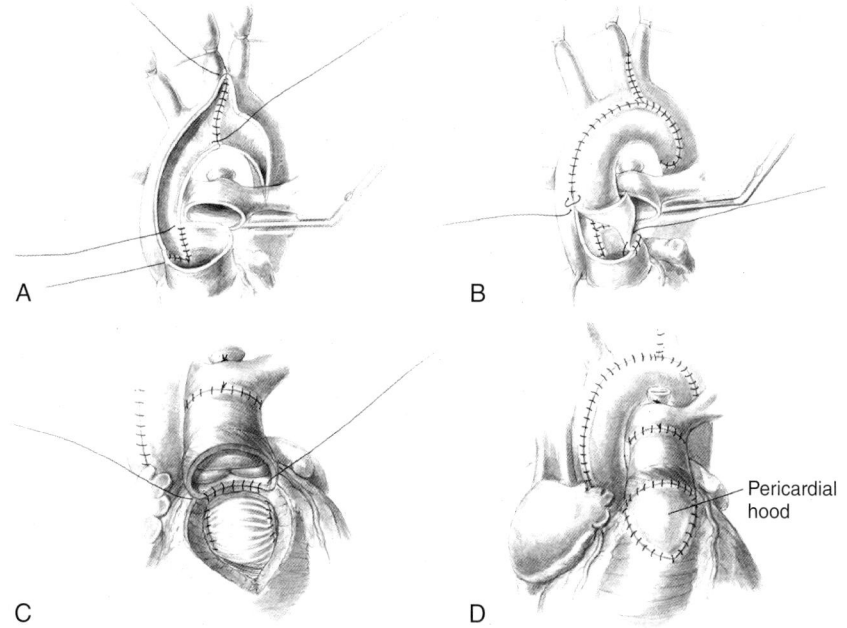

• **Fig. 24.8** The Yasui procedure severe left ventricular outflow tract obstruction, with an interrupted aortic arch and a ventricular septal defect (VSD). **(A)** Repair of interrupted aortic arch combined with a Damus-Kaye-Stansel (DKS). **(B)** Completion of the aortic arch repair and DKS with a patch. **(C)** The VSD patch baffle is shown connecting the left ventricle to the DKS root. A pulmonary homograft is being used to establish right ventricle to pulmonary artery continuity. **(D)** The completed reconstruction. (Reproduced with permission from Kanter K.)[11]

size (in mm) greater than the patient's weight in kilograms + 1 is likely suitable for single-stage biventricular repair.[31]

Postoperative Care/Follow-Up

The long-term incidence of LVOTO requiring intervention is reported to be 14%–38%.[21] Factors associated with the development of postoperative LVOTO include smaller LVOT size (aortic annulus, aortic root, sinotubular junction), aberrant origin of the right subclavian artery, use of a pulmonary homograft or polytetrafluoroethylene interposition graft for aortic arch repair, and the presence of a small- or medium-sized VSD.[21]

Long-term follow-up is needed in patients with IAA; studies have shown 10-year survival ranging from 67% to 85%.[32,33]

References

1. Botto LD, Correa A, Erickson JD. Racial and temporal variations in the prevalence of heart defects. *Pediatrics*. 2001;107:e32.
2. Morrow WR, Huhta JC, Murphy Jr DJ, McNamara DG. Quantitative morphology of the aortic arch in neonatal coarctation. *J Am Coll Cardiol*. 1986;8:616-620.
3. Talner NS, Berman MA. Postnatal development of obstruction in coarctation of the aorta: role of the ductus arteriosus. *Pediatrics*. 1975;56:562-569.
4. Parker LE, Landstrom AP. Genetic etiology of left-sided obstructive heart lesions: a story in development. *J Am Heart Assoc*. 2021;10:e019006.
5. Quartermain MD, Pasquali SK, Hill KD, et al. Variation in prenatal diagnosis of congenital heart disease in infants. *Pediatrics*. 2015;136:e378-e385.
6. Lytzen R, Vejlstrup N, Bjerre J, et al. The accuracy of prenatal diagnosis of major congenital heart disease is increasing. *J Obstet Gynaecol*. 2020;40:308-315.
7. Wren C, Reinhardt Z, Khawaja K. Twenty-year trends in diagnosis of life-threatening neonatal cardiovascular malformations. *Arch Dis Child Fetal Neonatal Ed*. 2008;93:F33-F35.
8. Meller SM, Fahey JT, Setaro JF, Forrest JK. Multi-drug-resistant hypertension caused by severe aortic coarctation presenting in late adulthood. *J Clin Hypertens*. 2015;17:313-316.
9. Ijland MM, Tanke RB. Aortic coarctation. *Circulation*. 2009; 120:1294-1295.
10. Mery CM, Guzman-Pruneda FA, Trost Jr JG, et al. Contemporary results of aortic coarctation repair through left thoracotomy. *Ann Thorac Surg*. 2015;100:1039-1046.
11. Gray WH, Wells WJ, Starnes VA, Kumar SR. Arch augmentation via median sternotomy for coarctation of aorta with proximal arch hypoplasia. *Ann Thorac Surg*. 2018;106:1214-1219.
12. Wright GE, Nowak CA, Goldberg CS, Ohye RG, Bove EL, Rocchini AP. Extended resection and end-to-end anastomosis for aortic coarctation in infants: results of a tailored surgical approach. *Ann Thorac Surg*. 2005;80:1453-1459.
13. Brown ML, Burkhart HM, Connolly HM, et al. Coarctation of the aorta: lifelong surveillance is mandatory following surgical repair. *J Am Coll Cardiol*. 2013;62:1020-1025.
14. Canniffe C, Ou P, Walsh K, Bonnet D, Celermajer D. Hypertension after repair of aortic coarctation—a systematic review. *Int J Cardiol*. 2013;167:2456-2461.
15. Stegeman R, Breur J, Heuser J, et al. Primary coronary stent implantation is a feasible bridging therapy to surgery in very low

birth weight infants with critical aortic coarctation. *Int J Cardiol.* 2018;261:62-65.

16. Holzer R, Qureshi S, Ghasemi A, et al. Stenting of aortic coarctation: acute, intermediate, and long-term results of a prospective multi-institutional registry—Congenital Cardiovascular Interventional Study Consortium (CCISC). *Catheter Cardiovasc Interv.* 2010;76:553-563.

17. Bhatt AB, Lantin-Hermoso MR, Daniels CJ, et al. Isolated coarctation of the aorta: current concepts and perspectives. *Front Cardiovasc Med.* 2022;9.617666.

18. Report of the New England Regional Infant Cardiac Program. *Pediatrics.* 1980;65:375-461.

19. Jonas RA, Quaegebeur JM, Kirklin JW, Blackstone EH, Daicoff G. Outcomes in patients with interrupted aortic arch and ventricular septal defect: a multiinstitutional study. Congenital Heart Surgeons Society. *J Thorac Cardiovasc Surg.* 1994;107:1099-1109; discussion 1109-1113.

20. Backer CL, Mavroudis C. Congenital Heart Surgery Nomenclature and Database Project: patent ductus arteriosus, coarctation of the aorta, interrupted aortic arch. *Ann Thorac Surg.* 2000; 69:S298-S307.

21. Korsuize NA, van Wijk A, Haas F, Grotenhuis HB. Predictors of left ventricular outflow tract obstruction after primary interrupted aortic arch repair. *Pediatr Cardiol.* 2021;42:1665-1675.

22. Jegatheeswaran A, McCrindle BW, Blackstone EH, et al. Persistent risk of subsequent procedures and mortality in patients after interrupted aortic arch repair: a Congenital Heart Surgeons' Society study. *J Thorac Cardiovasc Surg.* 2010;140:1059-1075.

23. Freedom RM, Bain HH, Esplugas E, Dische R, Rowe RD. Ventricular septal defect in interruption of aortic arch. *Am J Cardiol.* 1977;39:572-582.

24. Marino B, Digilio MC, Persiani M, et al. Deletion 22q11 in patients with interrupted aortic arch. *Am J Cardiol.* 1999;84: 360-361.

25. Vogel M, Vernon MM, McElhinney DB, Brown DW, Colan SD, Tworetzky W. Fetal diagnosis of interrupted aortic arch. *Am J Cardiol.* 2010;105:727-734.

26. Kaza AK, Thiagarajan RR. Left ventricular outflow tract obstruction: coarctation of the aorta, interrupted aortic arch, and borderline left ventricle. *Pediatr Crit Care Med.* 2016;17: S315-S317.

27. Sanchez Mejia AA, Cambronero N, Dongarwar D, et al. Hospital outcomes among infants with interrupted aortic arch with simple and complex associated heart defects. *Am J Cardiol.* 2022;166:97-106.

28. Abarbanell G, Border WL, Schlosser B, Morrow G, Kelleman M, Sachdeva R. Preoperative echocardiographic measures in interrupted aortic arch: which ones best predict surgical approach and outcome. *Congenit Heart Dis.* 2018;13:476-482.

29. Kanter KR, Kirshbom PM, Kogon BE. Biventricular repair with the Yasui operation (Norwood/Rastelli) for systemic outflow tract obstruction with two adequate ventricles. *Ann Thorac Surg.* 2012;93:1999-2005; discussion 2005-2006.

30. Nakano T, Kado H, Tatewaki H, et al. The Yasui operation for patients with adequate-sized ventricles and ventricular septal defect associated with obstructions of the aortic arch and left ventricular outflow tract. *Eur J Cardiothorac Surg.* 2014;45: e166-e172.

31. Riggs KW, Tweddell JS. How small is too small? Decision-making and management of the small aortic root in the setting of interrupted aortic arch. *Semin Thorac Cardiovasc Surg Pediatr Card Surg Annu.* 2019;22:21-26.

32. Fulton JO, Mas C, Brizard CP, Cochrane AD, Karl TR. Does left ventricular outflow tract obstruction influence outcome of interrupted aortic arch repair? *Ann Thorac Surg.* 1999;67:177-181.

33. Schreiber C, Eicken A, Vogt M, et al. Repair of interrupted aortic arch: results after more than 20 years. *Ann Thorac Surg.* 2000;70:1896-1899; discussion 1899-1900.

25

Pulmonary Stenosis

MICHAEL J. LANDZBERG

KEY LEARNING POINTS

- Valvar pulmonary stenosis (PS) is among the most common congenital heart defects; its severity is readily and reliably characterized by physical examination, electrocardiography, and echocardiogram.
- Patients with a low peak resting gradient < 36 mm Hg (peak transvalvar Doppler velocity < 3 m/sec) with normal right ventricular systolic performance are unlikely to suffer consequence over their lifetime.
- Therapy for significant non-dysplastic valvar PS (typically balloon valvuloplasty) is highly effective and safe. Patients

should be followed after valve dilation due to potential pulmonary valve regurgitation.
- Diastolic consequences of significant pulmonary valve stenosis may occasionally appear as oxygen-unresponsive hypoxemia in the setting of Patent Foramen Oval (PFO) or Atrial Septal Defect (ASD).
- Critical PS in a newborn can be life-threatening with severe cyanosis unless ductal patency is maintained.

Definition

Obstruction to the outflow from the right ventricle (RV), whether within the body of the RV, at the pulmonary valve (PV), or in the pulmonary arteries, is described as "pulmonary stenosis" (PS). Often these obstructions occur with other major cardiac abnormalities, but for this chapter discussion will be limited to patients with normal biventricular anatomy and an intact ventricular septum, with a focus on stenosis at the valvar level.

Prevalence

PS is a common lesion, typically occurring in some 7–10% of patients with congenital heart disease. The incidence of valvar stenosis has been reported at 0.6–0.8 per 1000 live births,[1] and when associated with other congenital cardiac lesions, it may occur in as many as 50% of all patients with congenital heart disease; sex-specific incidence is split nearly evenly.

Anatomy

Valvar PS is characterized by fused or absent commissures. In most patients, the valve is a mobile, dome-shaped structure with an orifice that may be tiny and sometimes eccentric (Fig. 25.1). The jet of blood through the valve

usually causes poststenotic dilation, most often involving the main and left main pulmonary arteries, either because that is the direction of the jet or due to association with bicuspid aortic valve and presumed shared abnormalities of connective tissue in the ascending great arteries[2] (Fig. 25.2). When there is severe valvar stenosis, there is RV hypertrophy, including infundibular muscle, which may contribute to the obstruction.

Dysplastic valves consisting of thickened, irregular, immobile tissue, often with hypoplasia of the valve annulus, and a small, short main pulmonary artery are much less common.[3] Rarely, acquired pulmonary valvar stenosis can be associated with carcinoid syndrome and deposition, or rheumatic disease and inflammation.

Subvalvar obstruction, also uncommon, is usually muscular and in most cases appears to be caused by displacement of the moderator band. The latter is often associated with a membranous ventricular septal defect, spontaneous closure of which results in isolated outflow obstruction. In very rare instances, the obstruction is ringlike and near the PV, resembling subaortic stenosis. In some patients, the subpulmonary obstruction is progressive.[4]

Peripheral pulmonary stenosis (PPS) may take several forms. These include single discrete obstructive lesions at a central pulmonary origin, multiple bilateral stenoses at distal branch origins with poststenotic dilation, and unilateral or bilateral diffuse hypoplasia of long segments of

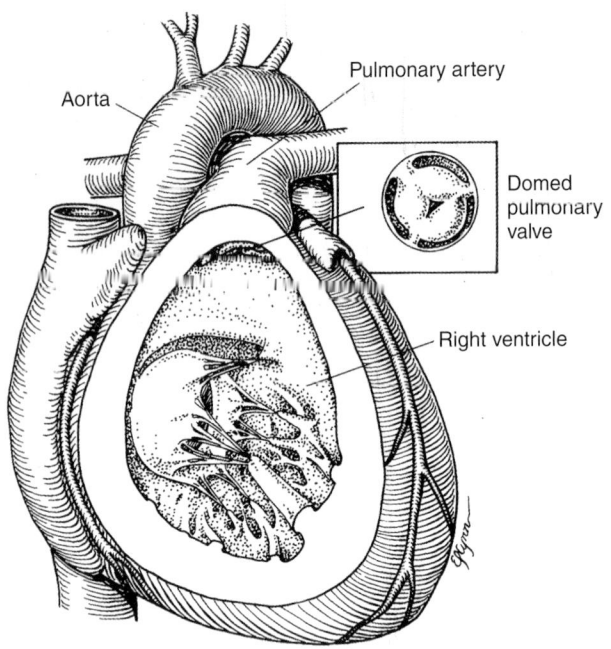

• **Fig. 25.1** Drawing of valvar pulmonary stenosis. Note the domed pulmonary valve and poststenotic dilation.

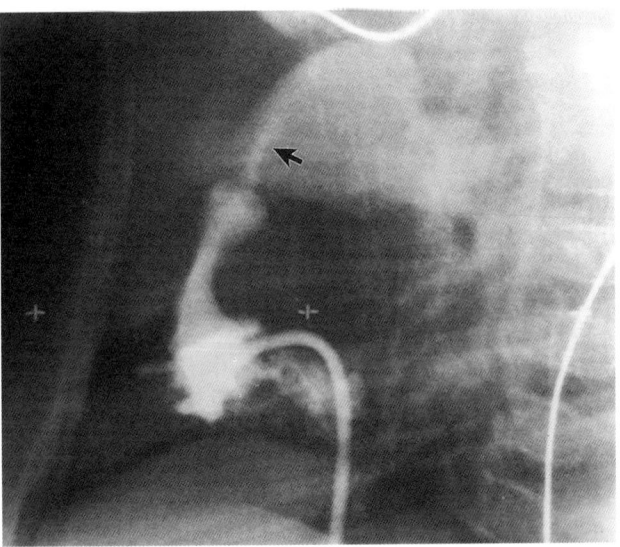

• **Fig. 25.2** Right ventricular angiogram in a patient with valvar pulmonary stenosis. Note the jet of contrast through the domed valve *(arrow)* and the poststenotic dilation.

a pulmonary artery (Fig. 25.3). Various combinations of these lesions are encountered in patients with the maternal rubella syndrome,[5] Alagille syndrome,[6] Williams syndrome (often with aortic supravalvular obstruction in addition),[7] and sometimes Noonan's syndrome[8]; on rare occasion, isolated PPS can be identified in adults,[9] though confounding diagnoses of postinfectious obstruction, chronic thromboembolic pulmonary hypertension, rheumatologic inflammation, and sarcoma should be ruled out.

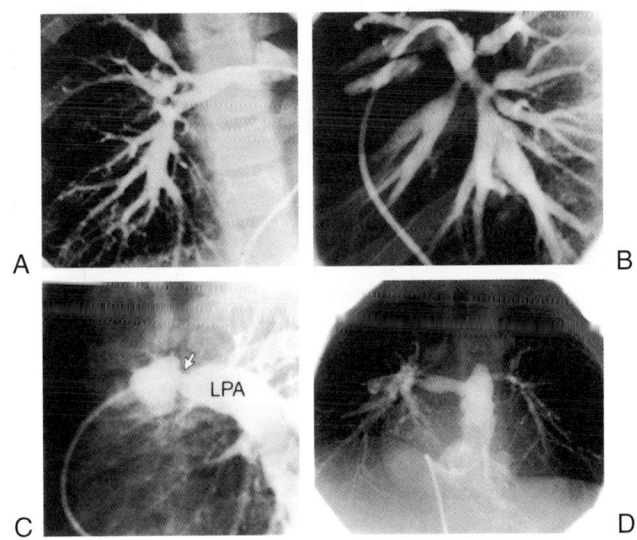

• **Fig. 25.3** Several angiograms of patients with various forms of peripheral pulmonary stenosis (PPS). **(A)** Diffuse PPS anteroposterior view. **(B)** Diffuse PPS lateral view. **(C)** Discrete left pulmonary artery *(LPA)* stenosis. **(D)** Diffuse hypoplasia of LPA.

Physiology

To provide adequate cardiac output, the RV pressure must be elevated sufficiently to overcome PS. With exercise, the requirement for cardiac output is increased, and RV pressure rises proportionately until the capacity of the RV muscle is surpassed. To estimate the severity of the obstruction, it is important to know the amount of blood being pumped across the valve as well as the pressure required. For this reason, estimates of the severity of obstruction require a reproducible measurement of blood flow. Consequently, a well-documented pressure gradient, measured noninvasively or invasively with the patient in a calm, relaxed state (ideally not anesthetized), is used for categorizing the severity of PS (Fig. 25.4). The point between the RV and the pulmonary artery at which the pressure drops is the point of anatomic obstruction (Fig. 25.5).

Chronic elevation of the RV pressure results in concentric RV hypertrophy and a less compliant RV. Greater right atrial pressures are required to fill the ventricle and relative right and left atrial pressures may be reversed; if an atrial septal defect exists or a foramen ovale persists, right-to-left shunting results.

Deformity and malfunctioning of the left ventricle may occur in proportion to the degree and duration of RV hypertension, and while other causes of left ventricular function are frequently sought, left ventricular systolic dysfunction most often improves with relief of the RV hypertension.

Valvar Pulmonary Stenosis

Among all congenital heart lesions, uncomplicated valvar PS beyond the neonatal period, and in contrast to valvar aortic stenosis, is one of the easiest lesions to deal with. Physical

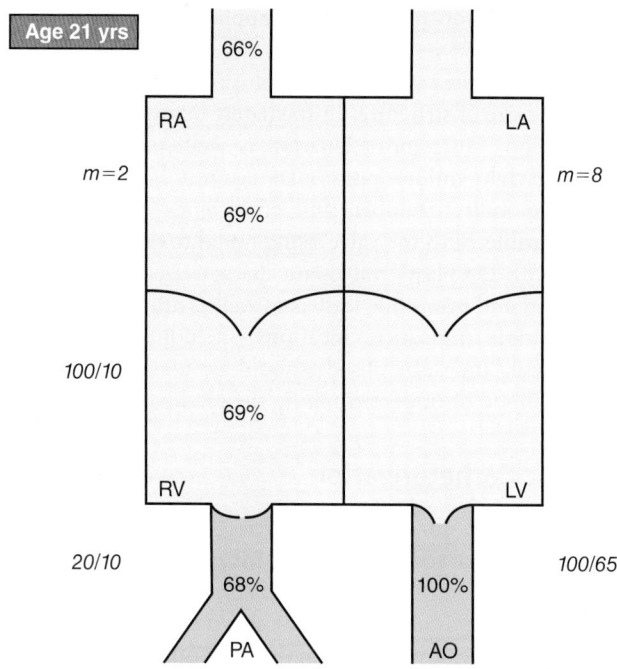

Age 21 yrs

66%

RA   LA

m=2   m=8

69%

100/10

69%

RV   LV

20/10   100/65

68%   100%

PA   AO

• **Fig. 25.4** Physiologic diagram of a 21-year-old patient with valvar pulmonary stenosis. Note the normal pulmonary artery pressure with systemic level right ventricular pressure.

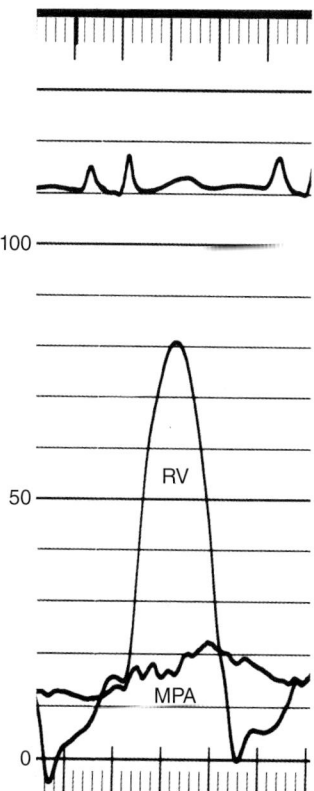

100

50

RV

MPA

0

• **Fig. 25.5** Simultaneous right ventricular *(RV)* and main pulmonary artery *(MPA)* pressures in a 12-year-old patient with valvar pulmonary stenosis with a peak–peak gradient of 60 mm Hg.

findings are diagnostic, and the degree of obstruction can be effectively ascertained based on these, on electrocardiographic data, and on echocardiographic information, either alone or in combination.[10] Gradient measurement echocardiographically is often comparable to that at catheterization, and endocarditis is extremely rare. Obstruction relief, whether by balloon dilation or surgery, is invariably successful for non-dysplastic valves, and is followed by normal, or substantively improved, exercise tolerance.[11]

Clinical Manifestations

Characteristically, children with uncomplicated valvar PS and an intact septum grow well and are asymptomatic. This cardiac defect is discovered on routine auscultation, usually at birth, because of the murmur. This systolic murmur is loudest at the second left intercostal space and is ejection in type, with the maximal intensity being at midsystole or later (Fig. 25.6). The later the peak intensity of the murmur, the greater the obstruction. Often, there is a systolic thrill in the same area. The first heart sound is easily audible because the murmur is ejection, in contrast to the muffled first sound with the pansystolic murmur in a patient with ventricular septal defect. The second heart sound is split, proportionate to the severity of the obstruction: the greater the obstruction, the longer the RV takes to empty and the wider the splitting. The second component (pulmonary) is decreased in intensity in proportion to the pressure in the pulmonary artery: the lower the pressure, the softer the second component of the second heart sound (and with maximal obstruction, it may be inaudible). Usually, there is a loud variable ejection click early in systole; without a click, other diagnoses should be considered. The smaller the interval between the first sound and the click, the more severe the stenosis. A wave pulsations in the neck veins are not unusual, though clinical right-sided congestive heart failure is uncommon in the young. When there are prominent A waves, a fourth heart sound may be audible. A small infant with maximal obstruction may have a minimal murmur, sometimes overlooked, with accompanying cyanosis.

Adults may present with RV lift and fourth heart sound, with preserved pulmonary component of the second heart sound (if valvar PS is well tolerated) or with soft or absent P2 in the presence of increasing immobility of the valve

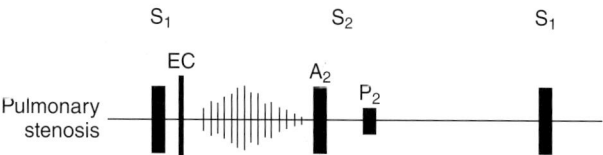

• **Fig. 25.6** Diagrammatic presentation of the murmur in a patient with valvar pulmonary stenosis. *A₂,* Aortic component of the second heart sound; *EC,* ejection click; *S₁,* first sound; *S₂,* second sound. (From Avery ME, First LP [eds]. *Pediatric Medicine.* Baltimore: Williams & Wilkins, 1989.)

leaflets. With increasing age, signs of right-sided congestive heart failure may be more common.

Electrocardiography

The electrocardiogram shows right-axis deviation and RV hypertrophy in proportion to the amount of obstruction (Fig. 25.7). The R wave in the right chest leads is commensurate with RV pressure and a superior (negative) T wave in lead avF indicates very severe obstruction.[10] There may be P pulmonale (see Chapter 8).

Chest X-Ray

Except in cases of maximal obstruction in early infancy, the heart size is normal or only slightly enlarged. Poststenotic dilation of the main and left main pulmonary artery is usually visible. In the cyanotic patient, the pulmonary vasculature is decreased. Occasionally, in a patient with maximal obstruction, the RV may be grossly dilated (seen as cardiomegaly on the conventional chest X-ray). Adults may present with PV calcification.

Echocardiography and MRI

Measurement of the pressure gradient across the outflow tract by Doppler echocardiography (maximum instantaneous velocity) is quite reliable,[12] being about 10% greater than the peak-to-peak gradient measured at cardiac catheterization. While transvalvar pressure gradients can be estimated by magnetic resonance imaging (MRI), comparative accuracy and current need for prolonged calm state during image acquisition makes clinical application of such measure uncertain.[13]

The size of the pulmonary annulus is readily identifiable, as are the size of structures immediately before and after the obstruction. Poststenotic dilation is well seen, as are the proximal right and left pulmonary arteries.

The mobility, number, and consistency of leaflets are clearly visible, with the valve being noted to dome in systole (Fig. 25.8). Dysplastic valves are characterized by markedly thickened and immobile leaflets as well as annular hypoplasia. Multiple transducer locations, including parasternal, para-apical, and subxiphoid, should be used to minimize the likelihood of underestimating the gradient.

Cardiac Catheterization

Catheterization for many years has been used only as a therapeutic procedure since the introduction of balloon dilation for management of this lesion.[14,15] This procedure can be carried out at any age, but elective studies, for safety and technical reasons, are often deferred until age 1 year. At the study, the diameter of the outflow tract at the level of the hinge points of the pulmonary leaflets is measured at end diastole from the lateral projection of a ventricular angiogram. A balloon usually 120% of this value is introduced and inflated across the stenotic valve.

Management

When gradient relief is indicated, balloon dilation is the treatment of choice; surgical valvotomy is rarely used. In earlier years, a peak ejection gradient (with preserved RV systolic performance) of at least 50 mm Hg across these mobile stenotic valves was used as the indication for dilation. In the setting of low cardiac output, lower gradient may be considered as indication for dilation, with goals of improving RV afterload. As experience grew and excellent results were achieved with minimal risk, indication for valve dilation crept to lower valve gradient of 30 mm Hg or more in the setting of normal cardiac output. Exercise restriction or endocarditis prophylaxis are not recommended for persons with lower gradients, either *de novo* or post intervention, in the setting of preserved RV systolic function. American College of Cardiology/American Heart Association clinical care guidelines for adults with congenital heart disease now classify valvar PS into mild (peak gradient < 36 mm Hg, i.e., peak velocity < 3 m/sec), moderate (peak gradient 36–64 mm Hg; i.e., peak velocity 3–4 m/sec), and severe (peak gradient 64 mm Hg; peak velocity > 4 m/sec; mean gradient > 35 mm Hg).[16] In adults with moderate or severe valvar PS, indications (recommendation class Ib) for valvar intervention (typically balloon valvuloplasty, with surgical valvotomy reserved for those patients who are either ineligible for balloon dilation or in whom such has failed) include otherwise unexplained symptoms of heart failure, cyanosis from interatrial right-to-left communication, and/or exercise intolerance. Class IIa "reasonable" indication for intervention

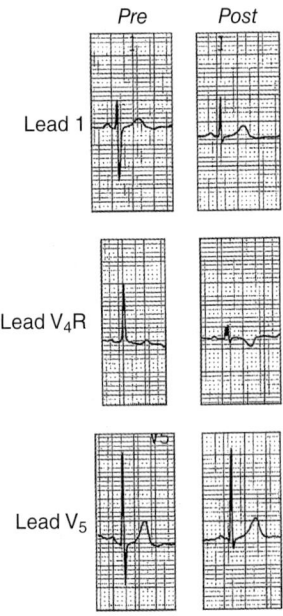

• **Fig. 25.7** Electrocardiogram in a patient with severe valvar pulmonary stenosis showing prehypertrophy at age 5 years before dilation and after QRS axis shift, and regression of hypertrophy at age 6 years after gradient reduction of 76 mm to 6 mm by balloon dilation.

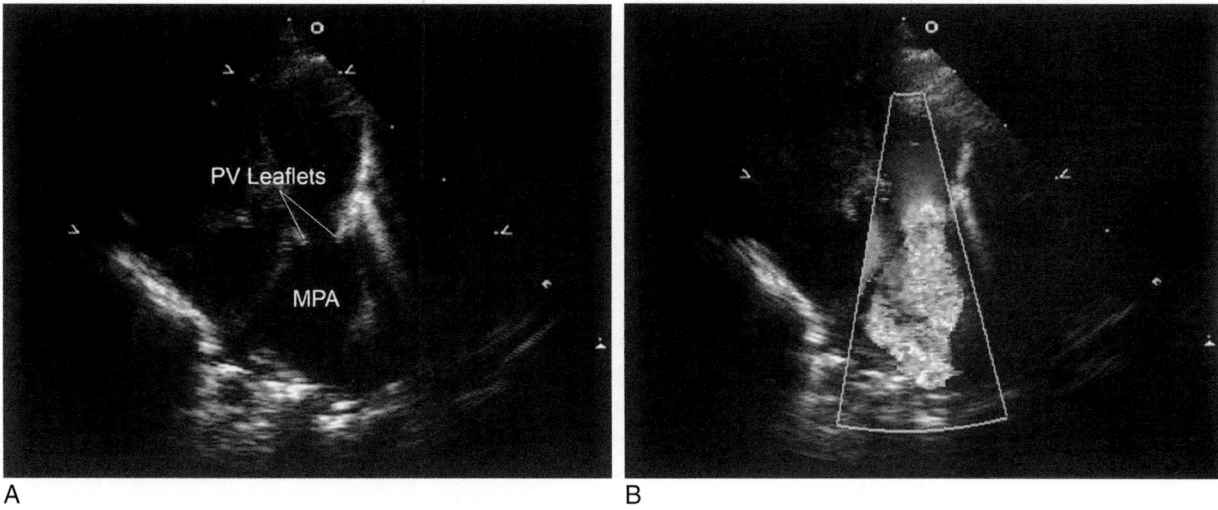

A   B

• **Fig. 25.8** **(A)** Parasternal long-axis view of the right ventricular outflow tract demonstrating a doming pulmonary valve with thickened leaflets *(PV)* and a dilated main pulmonary artery *(MPA)*. **(B)** Continuous-wave Doppler recording through the valve. The peak velocity is 4.3 m/sec, indicating a peak pressure gradient of about 75 mm Hg.

is allowed for asymptomatic adults with severe valvar PS. Intervention for cardiovascularly asymptomatic women with moderate-severe PS who are considering pregnancy may reduce risks of right heart failure and atrial arrhythmia during pregnancy; balloon pulmonary valvuloplasty may be performed during pregnancy if symptoms of heart failure occur, though timing and periprocedural support should be coordinated between maternal-fetal medicine, anesthesiology, and adult congenital heart disease specialists.

In the past, among surgical patients with very severe obstruction, some were encountered with so-called suicidal

ventricles due to severe subvalvar obstruction, which was accentuated by acute relief of the valvar stenosis; use of beta-blockade surrounding intervention has mitigated acute consequence of such residual muscular subvalvar obstruction, which tends to resolve in time, without clinical sequelae.

Course

In medically managed patients, mild obstruction in most remains unchanged, whereas moderate or more obstruction does progress in some[17] (Fig. 25.9), more commonly in the

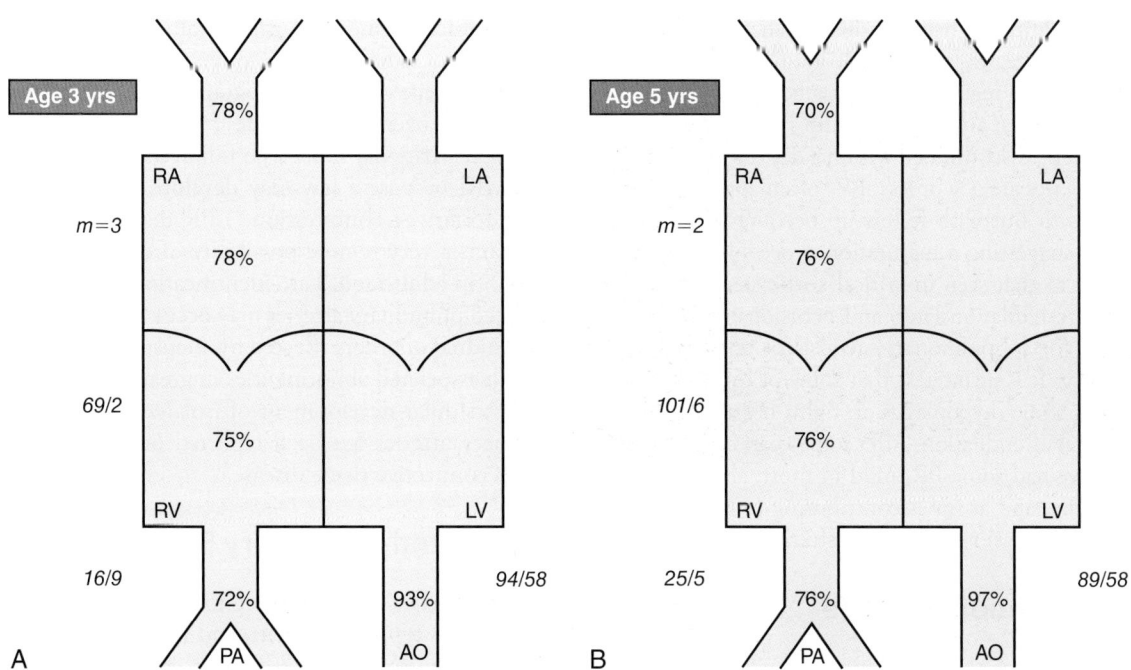

A   B

• **Fig. 25.9** Catheterization date showing progression of peak–peak gradient from 47 mm Hg **(A)** to 76 mm Hg **(B)** over a 2-year-period in patient with valvar pulmonary stenosis (same patient as in Fig. 25.7).

young and occasionally in the elderly or those with heavily calcified valves.[18] In those managed surgically, results were excellent, with some 97% being in New York Heart Association class 1 after more than 20 years of follow-up, only 4% requiring a second procedure for persistent or recurrent stenosis, and with endocarditis being a very rare complication. Increasing reintervention for pulmonary regurgitation (PR) has been noted approximating the 20-year mark after surgical intervention.[18] In balloon dilation experience, now with similar duration follow-up, outcomes appear similar.[19] Development of PR has been associated with earlier age at intervention and technically with higher balloon-annulus ratio; likewise, increasing PR fraction has been demonstrated to correlate with increasing RV volumes and decreased exercise capacity.[19] Guidelines for intervention (surgical or transcatheter) for isolated PR after intervention for valvar PS in adults reserve PV replacement (class I recommendation) for symptomatic patients with moderate or greater PR with RV dilation or RV dysfunction.[16]

Critical Valvar Pulmonary Stenosis in the Neonate

Maximal PS in the neonate is a life-threatening problem. Most of these children are blue due to right-to-left atrial shunting, have systemic level or greater RV pressure, are "duct dependent," and require prostaglandin E_1 and intubation. The tricuspid valve and RV size are normal in most, with some degree of hypoplasia in the others. Tricuspid regurgitation is common. The PV orifice is severely obstructed and even atretic in a few; occasionally while functionally echocardiographically atretic, it is found at catheterization to be patent. Relief of obstruction is urgently required in these neonates, and while surgery was initially the primary treatment, balloon dilation has become the procedure of choice. In most cases, gradient reduction is excellent, tricuspid regurgitation is relieved, right-to-left atrial shunting ceases, and prostaglandin E_1 and mechanical ventilation can be discontinued within a day. Early mortality rates in most series are 4% or less. PVs often appear dysplastic to begin with but with follow-up become thinner and more pliable, suggesting a maturation process in these tiny babies similar to that seen in critical aortic stenosis. A few patients require redilation later, and occasional patients require surgery for subpulmonary stenosis or an obstructive dysplastic valve. It is of interest that some of these neonates initially have some hypoplasia of right heart structures, which improves after dilation. After some years of follow-up, about half have had some PR, mild in most, although progressive in some, and at times contributing to late valve replacement[20]; on occasion, coronary fistulae may be present.

Dysplastic Pulmonary Valve

These are uncommon; they are seen in about 7% of patients with Noonan's syndrome.[21] Anatomically, the normally attached leaflets are very thickened and obstructive and are

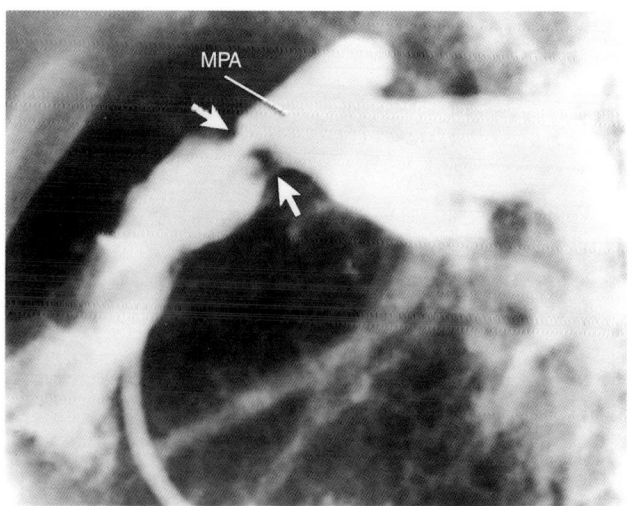

• **Fig. 25.10** Lateral view right ventricular cinegram showing dysplastic pulmonary valve *(arrows)* and short main pulmonary artery *(MPA)*.

clearly visible echocardiographically and on angiography (Fig. 25.10). Although surgical leaflet excision and transannular patch placement are necessary in many, balloon dilation is effective in some. Thus, if neither annular nor main pulmonary artery hypoplasia is significant, initial attempt at balloon dilation might be considered reasonable.

Pulmonary Regurgitation

As a congenital lesion, isolated PR may be associated with dilated pulmonary arteries, and is a rare entity. This combination is referred to as idiopathic dilation of the pulmonary artery.

In childhood, patients are asymptomatic and are discovered either during a murmur evaluation (mild PR) or if a chest X-ray is obtained for some other reason. The anomaly is identifiable on echocardiography or MRI. While remaining stable over many decades,[22] at times even beyond age 70 years, patients should be followed by echocardiography or MRI because a few may develop respiratory symptoms due to airway compression,[23] PR may increase, and there remains a very remote possibility of dissection and sudden death in adulthood. Late identification of isolated PR with dilated pulmonary arteries may occur in association with, or in kindred of others effected by, bicuspid aortic valve disease (with associated abnormalities in great vessel connective tissue)[2]; similar development of isolated PR and dilated pulmonary arteries has been reported on occasion in persons with connective tissue disease.

Peripheral Pulmonary Stenosis

Mild PPS is a common diagnosis; in children an ejection murmur is typically present, and if the obstruction is bilateral, the murmur is found to be equally loud all over the chest. The discovery of an ejection murmur of minimal intensity heard equally loud in all parts of the chest is virtually diagnostic of PPS, and if the electrocardiogram is normal, the severity can be said to be mild. Fortunately, these obstructions often regress[24] and thus, for clinical purposes, are largely a curiosity. Most patients with PPS require little or no intervention. These lesions are often seen in patients with Williams and Noonan's syndromes. However, consequences of severe bilateral PPS may be devastating, allowing for development of RV restrictive physiology, RV systolic failure, or pulmonary vascular disease and resistance elevation in pulmonary arterial segments not "protected" by the presence of proximal stenoses. Treatment consists of dilation with conventional high pressure or cutting balloons with or without stent placement; surgical management may be undertaken in those with central lesions not amenable to catheter-based techniques. Baseline abnormalities of pulmonary blood flow to effected segments and restoration of blood flow after interventions may be observed and followed via radionuclide lung perfusion scanning (or at times when obstructions are more central, with cardiac MRI flow measures).

*The authors express their gratitude to John F. Keane, MD, both for his foundational efforts for this chapter in prior editions as well as for his sentinel contributions to the understanding and treatment of valvar heart disease.

References

1. Hoffman IE, Kaplan S. The incidence of congenital heart disease. *J Am Coll Cardiol.* 2002;39:1890-1900.
2. Martin LJ, Hinton RB, Zhang X, et al. Aorta measurements are heritable and influenced by bicuspid aortic valve. *Front Genet.* 2011;2:61.
3. Becu L, Somerville J, Gallo A. "Isolated" pulmonary valve stenosis as part of more widespread cardiovascular disease. *Br Heart J.* 1976;38:472-482.
4. Pongiglione G, Freedom RM, Cook D, et al. Mechanism of acquired right ventricular outflow tract obstruction in patients with ventricular septal defect: an angiocardiographic study. *Am J Cardiol.* 1982;50:776-780.
5. Rowe RD. Cardiovascular disease in the rubella syndrome. In: Keith JD, Rowe RD, Vlad P, eds. *Heart Disease in Infancy and Childhood.* 3rd ed. New York: Macmillan; 1979:3-13.
6. Alagille D, Odievre M, Gautier M, et al. Hepatic ductular hypoplasia associated with characteristic facies, vertebral malformations, retarded physical, mental, and skeletal development and cardiac murmur. *J Pediatr.* 1975;86:63-71.
7. Williams JCP, Barrett-Boyes BG, Lowe JB. Supravalvar aortic stenosis. *Circulation.* 1961;24:1311-1318.
8. Noonan JA, Ehmke DA. Associated non-cardiac malformations in children with congenital heart disease. *J Pediatr.* 1963;63:468-470.
9. Kreutzer J, Landzberg MJ, Preminger TJ, et al. Isolated peripheral pulmonary artery stenoses in the adult. *Circulation.* 1996; 93:1417-1423.
10. Ellison RC, Freedom RM, Keane JF, et al. Indirect assessment of severity in pulmonary stenosis. *Circulation.* 1977;56:14-20.
11. Devanagondi R, Peck D, Sagi J, et al. Long-term outcomes of balloon valvuloplasty for isolated pulmonary valve stenosis. *Pediatr Cardiol.* 2017;38:247-254.
12. Lima CO, Sahn DJ, Valdez-Cruz LM, et al. Noninvasive prediction of transvalvar pressure gradient in patients with pulmonary stenosis by quantitative two-dimensional echocardiographic Doppler studies. *Circulation.* 1983;67:866-871.
13. Nguyen TQ, Hansen KL, Bechsgaard T, et al. Non-invasive assessment of intravascular pressure gradients: a review of current and proposed novel methods. *Diagnostics.* 2018;9:5.
14. Kan JS, White RF, Mitchell SE, et al. Percutaneous balloon valvuloplasty: a new method for treating congenital pulmonary valve stenosis. *N Engl J Med.* 1982;307:540.
15. Chen CR, Cheng TO, Huang T, et al. Percutaneous balloon valvuloplasty for pulmonic stenosis in adolescents and adults. *N Engl J Med.* 1996;335:21-25.
16. Stout KK, Daniels CJ, Aboulhosn JA, et al. 2018 AHA/ACC guideline for the management of adults with congenital heart disease: executive summary: a report of the American College of Cardiology/American Heart Association task force on clinical practice guidelines. *J Am Coll Cardiol.* 2019;73:1494-1563.
17. Rowland DG, Hammill WW, Allen D, et al. Natural course of isolated pulmonary valve stenosis in infants and children utilizing Doppler echocardiography. *Am J Cardiol.* 1997;79:344-349.
18. Earing MG, Connolly HM, Dearani JA, et al. Long-term follow-up of patients after surgical treatment for isolated pulmonary valve stenosis. *Mayo Clin Proc.* 2005;80:871-876.
19. Harrild DM, Powell AJ, Tran TX, et al. Long-term pulmonary regurgitation following balloon valvuloplasty for pulmonary stenosis risk factors and relationship to exercise capacity and ventricular volume and function. *J Am Coll Cardiol.* 2010;55: 1041-1047.
20. Poon LK, Menahem S. Pulmonary regurgitation after percutaneous balloon valvuloplasty for isolated pulmonary valvar stenosis in childhood. *Cardiol Young.* 2003;13:444-450.
21. Burch M, Sharland M, Shinebourne E, et al. Cardiologic abnormalities in Noonan syndrome: phenotypic diagnosis and echocardiographic assessment of 118 patients. *J Am Coll Cardiol.* 1993;22:1189-1192.
22. Rose C, Wessel A. Three-decade follow-up in pulmonary artery ectasia: risk assessment strategy. *Ann Thorac Surg.* 2002;73: 973-975.
23. Veldtman GR, Dearani JA, Warnes CA. Low pressure giant pulmonary artery aneurysms in the adult: natural history and management strategies. *Heart.* 2003;89:1067-1070.
24. Nomura Y, Nakamura M, Kono Y, et al. Risk factors for persistence of pulmonary arterial branch stenosis in neonates and young infants. *Pediatr Int.* 2001;43:36-41.

26

Tetralogy of Fallot

KEVIN G. FRIEDMAN, EDWARD P. WALSH, AND TAL GEVA

KEY LEARNING POINTS

- Tetralogy of Fallot (TOF) is the most common cyanotic congenital heart lesion.
- There is a spectrum of disease in TOF ranging from pink TOF (minimal pulmonary outflow obstruction) to complete pulmonary atresia. Additional variations include TOF with absent pulmonary valve and TOF with complete atrioventricular canal defect. Evaluation and management plans must be adjusted according to the underlying pathophysiology.

- Severe hypercyanotic "spells" need to be treated promptly and aggressively to prevent neurologic damage. True spells are relatively rare in neonates, although mild-moderate drops in saturations can occur with crying.
- The typical age for repair of TOF in the current era is about 3 months.
- Acute surgical results are generally excellent, but careful follow-up is necessary into adulthood to detect and monitor late problems such as progressive right ventricular failure and arrhythmias.

Definition

Tetralogy of Fallot (TOF) is the most common form of cyanotic congenital heart disease. It is characterized by infundibular pulmonary stenosis (PS), a conoventricular septal defect, dextroposition of the aorta (such that the aortic root overrides the crest of ventricular septum), and right ventricular (RV) hypertrophy. This complex of lesions was described in detail by Dr. Etienne-Lous Arthr Fallot in 1888.[1] There is a spectrum of disease ranging from a normal-sized pulmonary valve annulus with minimal PS ("pink TOF") to TOF with complete pulmonary atresia (PA). Rarer variants include TOF with absent (or dysplastic) pulmonary valve, and TOF with associated common atrioventricular canal defect.

Prevalence and Genetics

TOF has an incidence of 3.26 per 10,000 live births, or about 1300 new cases per year in the United States, and accounts for 7%–10% of all congenital heart disease.[2,3] Approximately 20% of cases occur as part of a clear clinical syndrome. Mutations in several genes have now been identified in TOF: chromosome 22q11 microdeletion in DiGeorge syndrome, *NKX2.5* (which accounts for 4% of TOF), *GATA4* mutations, JAG1 in Alagille syndrome (in which the incidence of TOF is high); *TBX5* in Holt-Oram syndrome; and *FOXC2* in hereditary lymphedema-distichiasis.[4] Deletion of human

TBX1 appears to be the basis for the 15% of TOF attributable to chromosome 22q11.2 microdeletion. TOF can occur in trisomy 21, 18, and 13, which together account for 10% of TOF cases.[5] There is a well-described recurrence risk in families affected by TOF. One study evaluated the risk of congenital heart disease in family members of patients with tetralogy (excluding those with 22q11 deletion) and found that the frequency of congenital heart defect was 3% in siblings, 0.5% in parents, 0.3% in grandparents, 0.2% in uncles or aunts, and 0.6% in first cousins.[6]

Pathology

TOF is one of several cardiac malformations that have defective embryonic neural crest migration resulting in abnormal conotruncal development. Van Praagh et al.[7] observed that the severity of subpulmonary stenosis is directly correlated with the degree of aortic override and have proposed that the primary problem in TOF is underdevelopment of the pulmonary infundibulum, with the other features being secondary.

The surgical anatomy of TOF has been well described.[8] The ventricular septal defect (VSD) is typically large, unrestrictive, and subaortic, and characterized by anterior deviation/malalignment of the conal septum relative to the underlying muscular septum (Fig. 26.1). Rarely, it is restrictive or may become so due to partial occlusion by overlying tricuspid valve tissue. A cardinal feature of TOF is anterior deviation of the

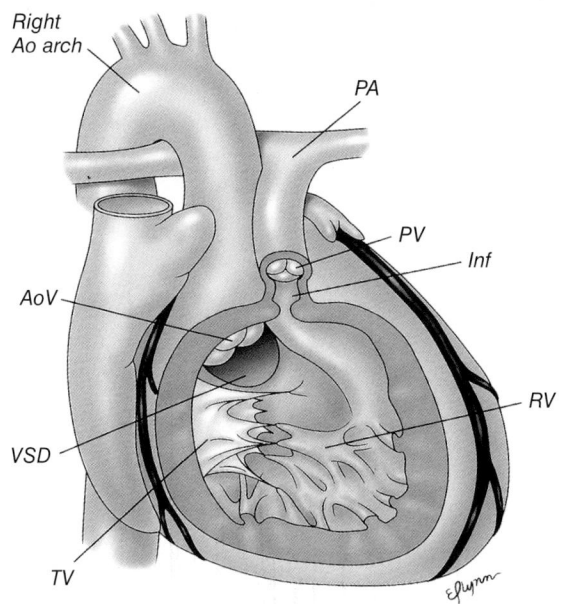

• **Fig. 26.1** Drawing of the cardiac anatomy of tetralogy of Fallot with pulmonary stenosis, viewed through the right ventricle *(RV)*. Features include a conoventricular septal defect *(VSD)*, through which the aortic valve *(AoV)* is seen; subpulmonary infundibular *(Inf)* narrowing; hypoplastic pulmonary valve *(PV)*; hypoplastic pulmonary arteries *(PA)*; and normal tricuspid valve *(TV)*. A right aortic *(Ao)* arch, present in many cases, is also shown.

conal septum and infundibular hypoplasia that constitute the anatomic substrate for subpulmonary obstruction. The degree of subpulmonary stenosis varies, ranging from very mild in some patients to critically severe in others, and the degree of obstruction often increases with age in unrepaired patients.

Frequently, there are multiple levels of RV and pulmonary obstruction in TOF, consistent with the hypothesis that obstruction to blood flow in the embryonic heart may impair the development of more distal cardiovascular structures.[7] Furthermore, outflow obstruction may become increasingly severe, during both fetal and postnatal development. The pulmonary valve itself is often abnormal, bicuspid, and can have a variable degree of annular hypoplasia as well as thickened, fused, and doming leaflets. The main and branch pulmonary arteries may be hypoplastic, particularly in TOF with PA, and may have discrete peripheral stenoses. This contrasts with isolated valvar PS and PA with intact ventricular septum, in both of which the pulmonary arteries are typically well developed (see Chapters 25 and 37). Large aortopulmonary collateral arteries may be present but are most typical of TOF with PA.

The overriding aortic root is typically dilated in TOF. In some cases, aortic valve regurgitation may develop over time. Several other anatomic abnormalities of clinical relevance may be associated with TOF. Many patients have a patent foramen ovale, but some have a true secundum atrial septal defect (ASD) meriting closure at surgery. Approximately 5% have one or more additional VSDs involving the muscular septum that may also require closure at the time of TOF repair. About 25% of patients have a

right aortic arch, most often with mirror-image branching. Importantly for planning the surgical repair, approximately 5%–10% of patients have a coronary artery anomaly in which all or part of the left anterior descending territory is supplied by a large branch of the right coronary artery that crosses over the right ventricular outflow tract (dual left anterior descending coronary artery or left coronary from the right coronary artery). These coronary anomalies may complicate and even preclude the infundibulotomy that is part of the standard repair, warranting alternative surgical approaches (e.g., RV to PA conduit) Finally, other associated anomalies such as abnormal connections of the systemic and pulmonary veins have been reported.

In addition to the previously mentioned features common to all forms of TOF, there are three unique subgroups: (a) TOF with PA, (b) TOF with absent pulmonary valve, and (c) TOF with common atrioventricular canal. These subgroups are considered separately in the following subsections of this chapter.

TOF With Pulmonary Atresia

Among patients with TOF, 5%–10% have atresia rather than stenosis of the pulmonary valve, with no antegrade pulmonary blood flow (Fig. 26.2). In most cases, this is a congenital problem, although it may be acquired postnatally in rare circumstances. Progression of PS to atresia *in utero* has been reported. The atresia may be limited to the pulmonary valve (membranous atresia), or it may additionally involve the subpulmonary infundibulum (muscular or long-segment atresia). Further, there is a spectrum of hypoplasia and atresia of the central pulmonary arteries,

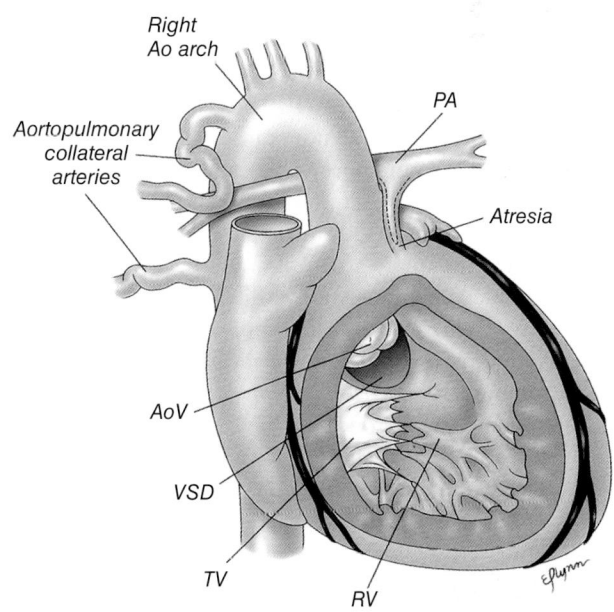

• **Fig. 26.2** Drawing of the cardiac anatomy of tetralogy of Fallot with pulmonary atresia (abbreviations as in Fig. 26.1). There is atresia of the pulmonary outflow tract, and the pulmonary arteries are markedly hypoplastic. The proximal segments of two aortopulmonary collateral arteries are also represented.

occurring either from the same embryopathy that causes valvar atresia, or possibly acquired as a consequence of the lack of blood flow. The main pulmonary artery may be present and supplied retrograde through the ductus arteriosus. However, in many instances the main pulmonary artery is entirely absent, and the branch pulmonary arteries are diminutive with multiple stenoses. In these cases, pulmonary blood flow is typically supplied by aortopulmonary collaterals. There may be discontinuities of the right and left pulmonary arteries and of individual lobar branches or, rarely, both mediastinal branch pulmonary arteries are absent.

Together with pulmonary artery hypoplasia, aortopulmonary collateral arteries are a hallmark of TOF with PA. During early embryogenesis, these vessels connect the aortic arches and the dorsal aorta with the developing lungs. They normally involute once the central pulmonary arteries develop. In TOF with PA, systemic-to-pulmonary collateral vessels arise directly from the aorta or its primary or secondary branches. They appear in association with deficient physiologic pulmonary perfusion and serve a compensatory role, increasing pulmonary blood flow and, hence, systemic arterial oxygenation; however, the vasculogenic mechanisms that underlie their development are not entirely known.

Right aortic arch, dilation of the ascending aorta, and aortic valve regurgitation are more common in TOF with PA than other forms of tetralogy.[9]

TOF With Absent Pulmonary Valve

In this rare anatomic variant, the pulmonary valve leaflets are vestigial or rudimentary (some prefer the term dysplastic to absent). As a result, the RV outflow is effectively unguarded, with free pulmonary regurgitation and often pronounced dilation of the right ventricle and central pulmonary arteries (Fig. 26.3). Indeed, in many cases, there is massive aneurysmal dilation involving the main and right and left pulmonary arteries. The precise etiology of this vasculopathy is unknown, but it may arise from an inherent abnormality of the pulmonary artery wall, volume overload *in utero*, or both. The ductus arteriosus is characteristically absent in these patients, a feature that may also contribute to abnormal pulmonary artery flow and development.[10] In cases with severe pulmonary artery dilation, the bronchi can be obstructed due to external compression by the dilated central pulmonary arteries and abnormally branching segmental pulmonary arteries that appear to intertwine with the intraparenchymal bronchi.[11] There may also be developmental abnormalities intrinsic to the airways themselves. Of note, absent pulmonary valve syndrome also occurs in isolation (i.e., not associated with TOF).

TOF With Common Atrioventricular Canal

In 2–3% patients with TOF, there is coexisting common atrioventricular canal. This combination of malformations is seen more frequently in trisomy 21. The conoventricular septal defect extends far posterior into the inlet septum, and

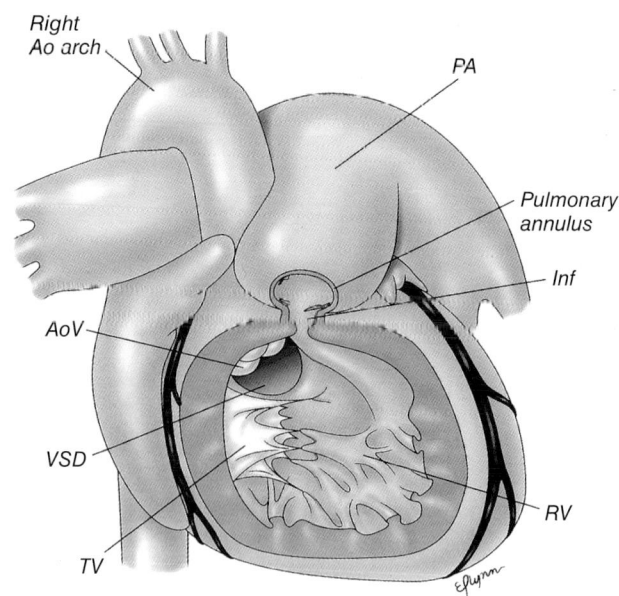

• **Fig. 26.3** Drawing of the cardiac anatomy of tetralogy of Fallot with absent pulmonary valve (abbreviations as in Fig. 26.1). The vestigial pulmonary valve leaflets leave the pulmonary outflow essentially unguarded. The pulmonary annulus is typically small, but there is marked dilation of the main and branch pulmonary arteries.

there is a primum ASD and a common atrioventricular valve. In addition to requiring more extensive surgical repair, these patients bear other risks associated with the potential for atrioventricular valve regurgitation that affect the timing of repair and the postoperative management.

Physiology

Patients with TOF can be cyanotic because of right-to-left shunting at the ventricular level. Cyanosis occurs when the right ventricular outflow tract obstruction is severe enough to result in resistance to pulmonary blood flow that exceeds systemic vascular resistance. Under these circumstances, deoxygenated blood in the right ventricle shunts across the VSD into the left ventricle and from there to the systemic circulation. Right-to-left shunting may also occur at the atrial level if the diastolic pressure in the hypertrophic right ventricle and right atrium exceeds left atrial pressure. In those rare cases in which the VSD is restrictive, the RV pressure can become suprasystemic and represents an added clinical risk. The volume of the ventricular right-to-left shunt, and hence the degree of cyanosis, is directly proportional to the severity of RV outflow obstruction. When the subpulmonary infundibulum is severely hypoplastic or the pulmonary valve severely stenotic, there is little antegrade pulmonary blood flow, and most of the RV output exits through the VSD. Thus, systemic output is maintained, but at the expense of an cyanosis due to right-to-left shunting across the VSD. In contrast, when RV outflow obstruction is mild, there is little or no right-to-left shunt. Patients with mild right ventricular outflow tract obstruction typically have normal systemic arterial oxygen saturation (pink

TOF). In these patients with mild PS, there is left-to-RV shunting and in some cases, pulmonary overcirculation and heart failure with physiology similar to patients with isolated VSDs.

Superimposed on fixed anatomic RV outflow obstruction, dynamic factors may serve to further compromise pulmonary blood flow, increase right-to-left shunting, and worsen cyanosis in TOF. Dynamic muscular constriction or spasm of the subpulmonary infundibulum will have this effect, as will an increase in pulmonary vascular resistance (e.g., a crying infant), or a decrease in systemic vascular resistance. Catecholamine stimulation of RV mechanoreceptors has also been postulated to increase right-to-left shunting.[12] One or more of these dynamic factors is thought to underlie the physiology of hypercyanotic spells. Conversely, maneuvers that increase systemic vascular resistance will limit right-to-left shunting. Older children with unrepaired TOF often assume a characteristic squatting position to increase systemic vascular resistance and decrease right-to-left shunting.

TOF With Pulmonary Atresia

In the presence of PA and no anterograde pulmonary blood flow, the entire RV output (systemic venous return) necessarily exits to the aorta. Pulmonary blood flow derives solely from systemic-to-pulmonary artery communications—including patent ductus arteriosus, bronchial arteries, aortopulmonary collaterals, or a combination of these—and comprises mixed arterial and venous blood. These are left-to-right shunts and, therefore, constitute a volume load on the left ventricle. In many instances, these vessels are restrictive, and thus pulmonary artery pressures remain low; however, collateral perfusion may produce excessive flow and pulmonary hypertension in isolated lung segments.

TOF With Absent Pulmonary Valve

In the absence of functional pulmonary valve leaflets, there is free pulmonary regurgitation that represents a volume load both on the right ventricle and on the central pulmonary arteries. The stroke volume of the right ventricle may be markedly increased to compensate for a large regurgitant fraction and result in significant right ventricular dilation. Ejection of this increased stroke volume into the proximal pulmonary arteries may contribute to their characteristically severe dilation. When the pulmonary arteries are severely dilated and compress the bronchial tree, there is segmental air trapping and difficulty with ventilation that can be life-threatening in severe cases.

TOF With Common Atrioventricular Canal

The physiology in these patients is substantially the same as that in patients with TOF alone. However, there may be regurgitation of the common atrioventricular valve, either congenital or acquired, adding volume load to one or both ventricles.

Clinical Manifestations

The neonate or infant with TOF may initially come to attention because of a murmur, with or without cyanosis, or increasingly because of fetal echocardiographic diagnosis. The murmur is produced by turbulent flow across a narrowed right ventricular outflow tract rather than across the unrestrictive VSD, and so is present at birth. It is typically a harsh, long, crescendo–decrescendo systolic ejection murmur well heard along the left sternal border and transmitted into the lung fields. The second heart sound is often single, comprising only the aortic component, and accentuated owing to the more anterior dextroposed aorta. When RV hypertrophy is severe, there is often a RV parasternal lift. The degree of cyanosis is a function of the severity of RV outflow obstruction and may not be apparent in the neonate. The remainder of the newborn cardiovascular examination is usually normal.

The clinical symptoms of the infant are directly related to the amount of pulmonary blood flow. In infants with severe PS, parents may report variable blueness at rest that becomes more apparent with crying. The degree of PS and resultant cyanosis tend to increase with age. However, even with significant cyanosis, many infants may remain otherwise well, without respiratory distress, feeding intolerance, or lethargy. In contrast, in pink TOF with little or no outflow obstruction, a substantial ventricular level left-to-right shunt is present resulting in pulmonary overcirculation and in symptoms and signs of heart failure. Parents may report symptoms similar to those with VSDs including tachypnea, sweating with feeds, poor oral feeding, and difficulty with weight gain.

Hypercyanotic spells, known colloquially as "tet spells," are a hallmark of TOF. In a typical spell, the child becomes distressed and inconsolable. Crying and agitation are associated with deeper cyanosis. Spells are self-aggravating; if unabated, the deepening hypoxemia appears to exacerbate the distress, and more distress brings even more profound cyanosis. Auscultation during the spell reveals a diminished or even absent murmur due to reduction in flow across the right ventricular outflow tract. Holding the infant with the knees brought up tight to the chest, simulating squatting, has been noted empirically to bring relief in some instances. In severe cases, the spell terminates with unconsciousness and, rarely, convulsions. If the hypoxemia is extreme, permanent neurologic sequelae and even death may ensue. True hypercyanotic spells are rare in neonates, although mild-moderate degrees of cyanosis may occur with crying.

Certain clinical features classically associated with TOF appear only beyond infancy and, therefore, are rarely seen in contemporary practice, in which repair in infants is now the rule. Older children with unrepaired TOF experience discomfort and air hunger associated with cyanosis, particularly with excitement or exertion, and find that this is relieved when they assume the squatting position, which increases systemic vascular resistance and diminishes ventricular right-to-left shunting. Chronic cyanosis is associated with clubbing of the nail beds of the fingers and toes and may also cause delayed physical growth and diminished cognitive function.

TOF With Pulmonary Atresia

The clinical presentation of TOF with PA is distinct to the extent that there is no systolic outflow murmur. Instead, there may be continuous murmurs audible in the chest and particularly over the back, indicative of aortopulmonary collateral flow or a ductus arteriosus. The degree of cyanosis in these infants is a function of the extent of collateralization. They may be very blue if there are few or no collaterals and the ductus arteriosus is closed, or they may be relatively pink to the point of congestive failure if there are extensive collaterals with excessive pulmonary blood flow. With PA, hypercyanotic spells are less common but can occur, presumably due to shifts in the relative pulmonary and systemic vascular resistances affecting collateral flow rather than infundibular spasm (which would have no effect). Up to 40% of TOF patients with PA have chromosomal abnormalities, particularly chromosome 22q11.2 microdeletion (DiGeorge syndrome) and associated clinical manifestations.[13]

TOF With Absent Pulmonary Valve

Additional clinical manifestations of TOF with absent pulmonary valve are due to the presence of severe pulmonary regurgitation and airways disease. Approximately half of these patients present with severe, even critical, respiratory compromise in the neonatal period, with signs of lower airway obstruction on examination. Ventilation may be worse in the supine (as compared with prone) position because of greater bronchial compression by the aneurysmal pulmonary arteries.[14] In other patients, however, respiratory compromise may be mild or even absent. Further, the clinical severity appears not to correlate reliably with the degree of pulmonary artery enlargement, suggesting that intrinsic bronchial abnormalities may be a more important determinant. Characteristically, on cardiac auscultation there is a prominent early to mid-diastolic decrescendo murmur of free pulmonary regurgitation, best heard along the left sternal border, in addition to the typical systolic outflow murmur (i.e., a "to-and-fro" systolic–diastolic murmur).

TOF With Common Atrioventricular Canal

The clinical presentation and auscultatory findings in the setting of common atrioventricular canal are the same as those in simple TOF. Trisomy 21 with associated features is more common.

Electrocardiography

The electrocardiogram in TOF characteristically shows evidence of RV hypertrophy that increases with age, attributable to chronic pressure overload. Right-axis deviation and right atrial enlargement are also present in many cases. If there is a large left-to-right shunt, as in pink TOF, or in the presence of a large ductus arteriosus or excessive aortopulmonary collateral flow, there may also be left atrial enlargement and biventricular hypertrophy. There are no additional distinctive electrocardiographic features associated with TOF with PA or absent pulmonary valve. With common atrioventricular canal, there is a superior QRS axis, typical of endocardial cushion defects (see Chapter 8).

Chest Radiography

The chest radiograph of the infant with TOF typically shows normal visceral situs, levocardia, normal heart size, variable degree of decreased pulmonary vascularity, and, in some cases, a right aortic arch. If there is a large left-to-right shunt as in pink TOF, or in the presence of a large ductus arteriosus or excessive aortopulmonary collateral flow, the heart may instead be enlarged and pulmonary vascularity increased. The apex of the heart is often elevated owing to RV hypertrophy. This feature, in combination with a relatively concave contour along the left upper heart border due to main pulmonary artery hypoplasia or atresia, gives the cardiac silhouette a so-called boot shape (*coeur en sabot*), although this may not be apparent in the infant with a prominent thymus. Absence of a thymus shadow in the newborn may indicate associated chromosome 22q11.2 microdeletion (DiGeorge syndrome).

In TOF with PA, the pulmonary vascular markings may vary in regions with greater or lesser collateral blood flow. Otherwise, there are no additional distinctive chest radiographic features associated with PA. In TOF with absent pulmonary valve, the heart size may be increased due to RV dilation caused by the volume overload of free pulmonary regurgitation. Very large main and branch pulmonary arteries may be evident. Signs of bronchial compression may be seen, including segmental or overall hyperinflation. There are no distinctive chest radiographic features associated with common atrioventricular canal and TOF.

Echocardiography

Prenatal diagnosis of TOF may be made readily by fetal echocardiography (Fig. 26.4). The large malalignment conoventricular septal defect, deviated conal septum, and overriding aorta are seen as early as the later portion of the first trimester on two-dimensional imaging. Later in gestation, the central pulmonary arteries may appear hypoplastic, often progressively so on serial examinations. Doppler interrogation of the ductus arteriosus may show retrograde flow (i.e., from aorta to pulmonary artery) if right ventricular outflow tract obstruction is severe.

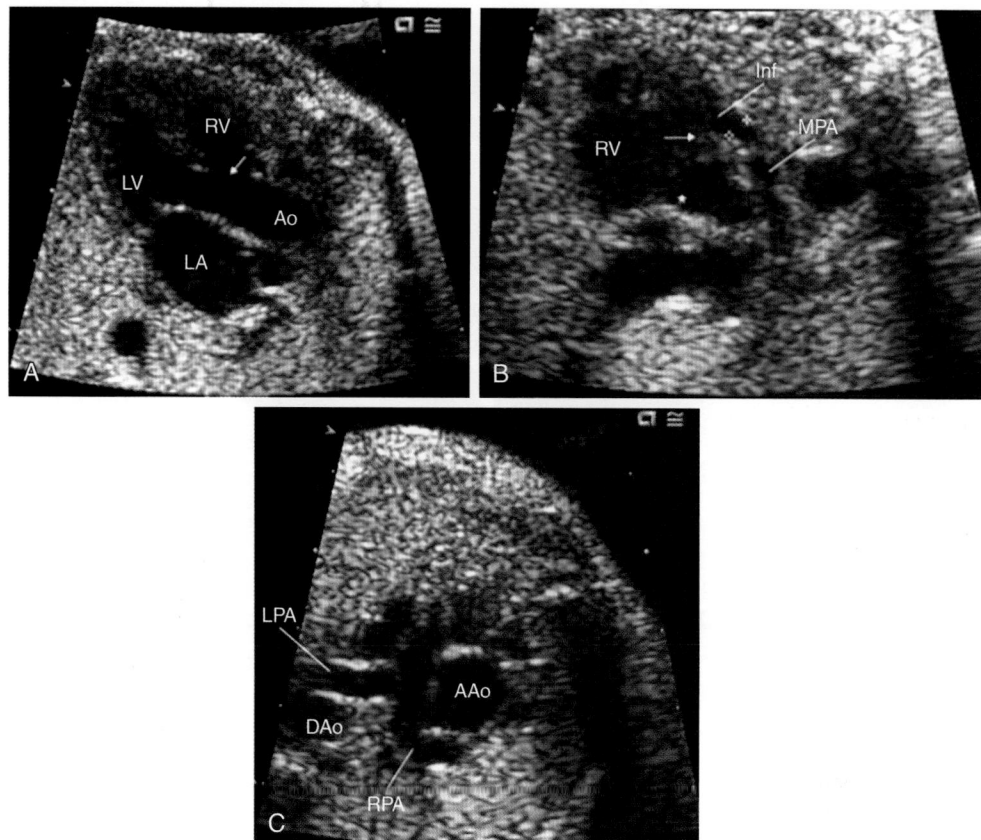

• **Fig. 26.4** Fetal echocardiogram in tetralogy of Fallot with pulmonary stenosis. **(A)** Long-axis view of the left ventricular outflow tract demonstrating a dilated aortic root that overrides a large conoventricular septal defect *(arrow)*. **(B)** Image showing anteriorly deviated conal septum *(arrow)*. The right ventricular infundibulum *(Inf)* and main pulmonary artery *(MPA)* are hypoplastic. The small dots mark the dimension of the proximal ox infundibulum of the right ventricular outflow tract. **(C)** Transverse view of the fetal chest showing borderline hypoplastic main and branch pulmonary arteries in continuity and the dilated ascending aorta *(AAo)*. *Ao,* Aorta; *DAo,* descending aorta; *LA,* left atrium; *LPA,* left pulmonary artery; *LV,* left ventricle; *RPA,* right pulmonary artery; *RV,* right ventricle.

Postnatally, echocardiography can identify all the characteristic anatomic features of TOF in most cases (Fig. 26.5). These include the malaligned conoventricular septal defect, the anterior deviation of the conal septum, the level(s) of right ventricular outflow tract obstruction, and the dextroposed, overriding aorta. A complete echocardiogram is usually sufficient to provide all clinically important structural and functional information relevant to planning the surgical repair or, if indicated, palliation, including the following:
• The size and extent of the VSD, including the rare restrictive defect
• The location and size of additional muscular VSDs, if present
• The levels of right ventricular outflow obstruction, including the severity of infundibular stenosis, the presence or absence of more proximal intracavitary muscle bands, and the degree of pulmonary valve abnormality, including annular hypoplasia (indexed to body-surface area with z-scores)
• The pulmonary artery anatomy, including possible hypoplasia and stenoses of the main or proximal branch pulmonary arteries that may also need to be addressed at operation

• The size and competency of the aortic valve
• The coronary artery anatomy, particularly the presence of a left anterior descending coronary from the right or other important branch of the right coronary crossing the infundibulum that must not be divided and, therefore, may constrain or preclude placement of an outflow patch (Fig. 26.6)
• The presence of certain other associated defects that may require surgical attention, such as an ASD or a patent ductus arteriosus
• The presence of certain other anatomic variants that may impact the surgical approach, such as a right aortic arch or a left superior vena cava to coronary sinus

Echocardiography is also a valuable tool for surveillance and diagnosis after surgical repair of TOF. In the early postoperative period, it is useful for the identification of residual VSDs, residual right ventricular outflow tract obstruction, and ventricular systolic dysfunction. In long-term follow-up, it is helpful in the assessment of recurrent right ventricular outflow tract obstruction, pulmonary regurgitation, proximal branch pulmonary artery stenosis, aortic regurgitation, and ventricular size and systolic dysfunction.

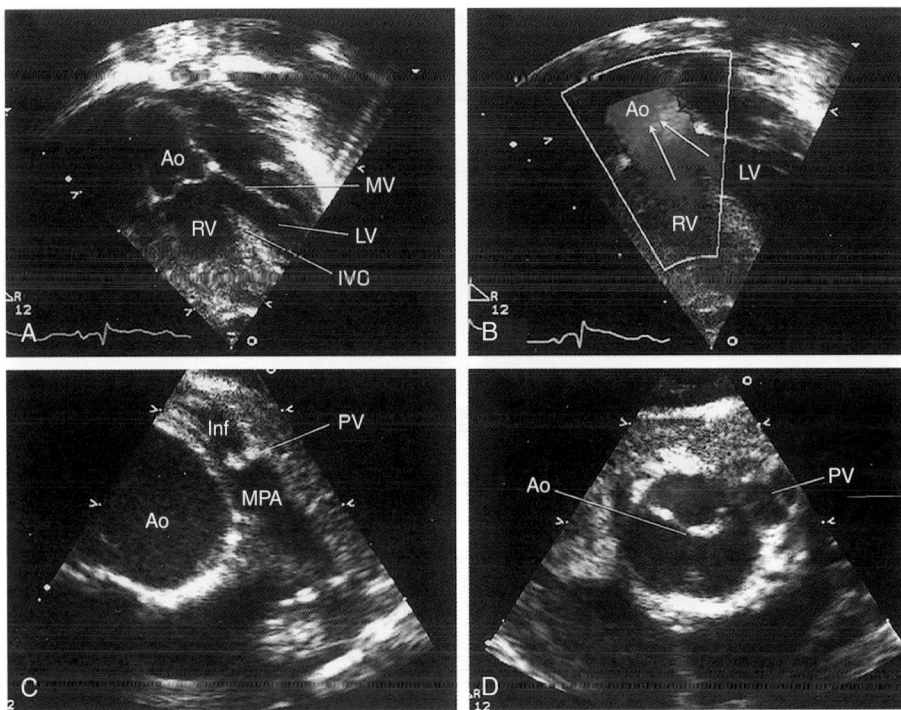

• **Fig. 26.5** Echocardiogram of an infant with tetralogy of Fallot (TOF). **(A)** Modified apical four-chamber view showing the conoventricular septal defect and dextroposed aorta (Ao) overriding the crest of the muscular interventricular septum (IVS) and related substantially to the right ventricle (RV). Note the absence of subaortic conus, with retained fibrous continuity between the aortic valve and mitral valve (MV), distinguishing TOF, with preserved left ventricle (LV)-to-aorta continuity, from double-outlet right ventricle. **(B)** Color Doppler mapping corresponding to the image in panel A, demonstrating systolic flow (blue) from both the left and right ventricles into the aorta (arrows). **(C)** Parasternal short-axis view demonstrating the hypoplastic subpulmonary infundibulum (Inf) and small, dysplastic pulmonary valve (PV), small main pulmonary artery (MPA), and large aorta. **(D)** Parasternal short-axis view demonstrating the hypoplastic pulmonary valve and large aortic valve.

TOF With Pulmonary Atresia

In addition to the features listed earlier, PA is recognized by two-dimensional imaging and by Doppler analysis demonstrating the absence of right ventricle-to-pulmonary artery flow. The length of the atretic segment is seen, ranging from very short membranous atresia of the valve alone to longer-segment atresia that also involves part or all of the main pulmonary artery. The branch pulmonary arteries may be visible if good sized when supplied by a ductus arteriosus as opposed to aortopulmonary collaterals. However, they are often severely hypoplastic and may not be detectable by echocardiography. Aortopulmonary collaterals may be identified with characteristic continuous flow pattern on color flow Doppler mapping. Imaging may show the origins of sizable collaterals, but smaller vessels are not typically resolved, nor are the distal connections to the pulmonary arteries. Thus, in TOF with PA, echocardiography alone is not sufficient to demonstrate key aspects of pulmonary artery anatomy and blood supply, and cardiac catheterization and/or cardiac CT is required to fully delineate the collateral and branch pulmonary anatomy.

TOF With Absent Pulmonary Valve

The key cardiovascular features of the absent pulmonary valve syndrome are readily apparent on the echocardiogram

(Fig. 26.7). On two-dimensional imaging, the pulmonary valve leaflets are rudimentary or vestigial and the main and bilateral branch pulmonary arteries are severely dilated. Doppler analysis shows severe pulmonary regurgitation. The bronchi and their relationship to the pulmonary arteries cannot be demonstrated by echocardiography, so other imaging modalities (such as CT or MRI) may be required.

TOF With Common Atrioventricular Canal

Imaging shows extension of the VSD to involve the inlet septum, the contiguous primum ASD, and the common atrioventricular valve (see Chapter 31). Doppler analysis reveals the degree of atrioventricular valve regurgitation

Cardiac Catheterization

For decades, catheterization was a standard component of the diagnostic evaluation of TOF before surgical repair. However, over the last 20-30 years with the improvement in the quality of echocardiography, there has been a shift away from catheterization for preoperative evaluation of patients with TOF, apart from those with hypoplastic branch or discontinuous pulmonary arteries and/or concern for multiple aortopulmonary collaterals.

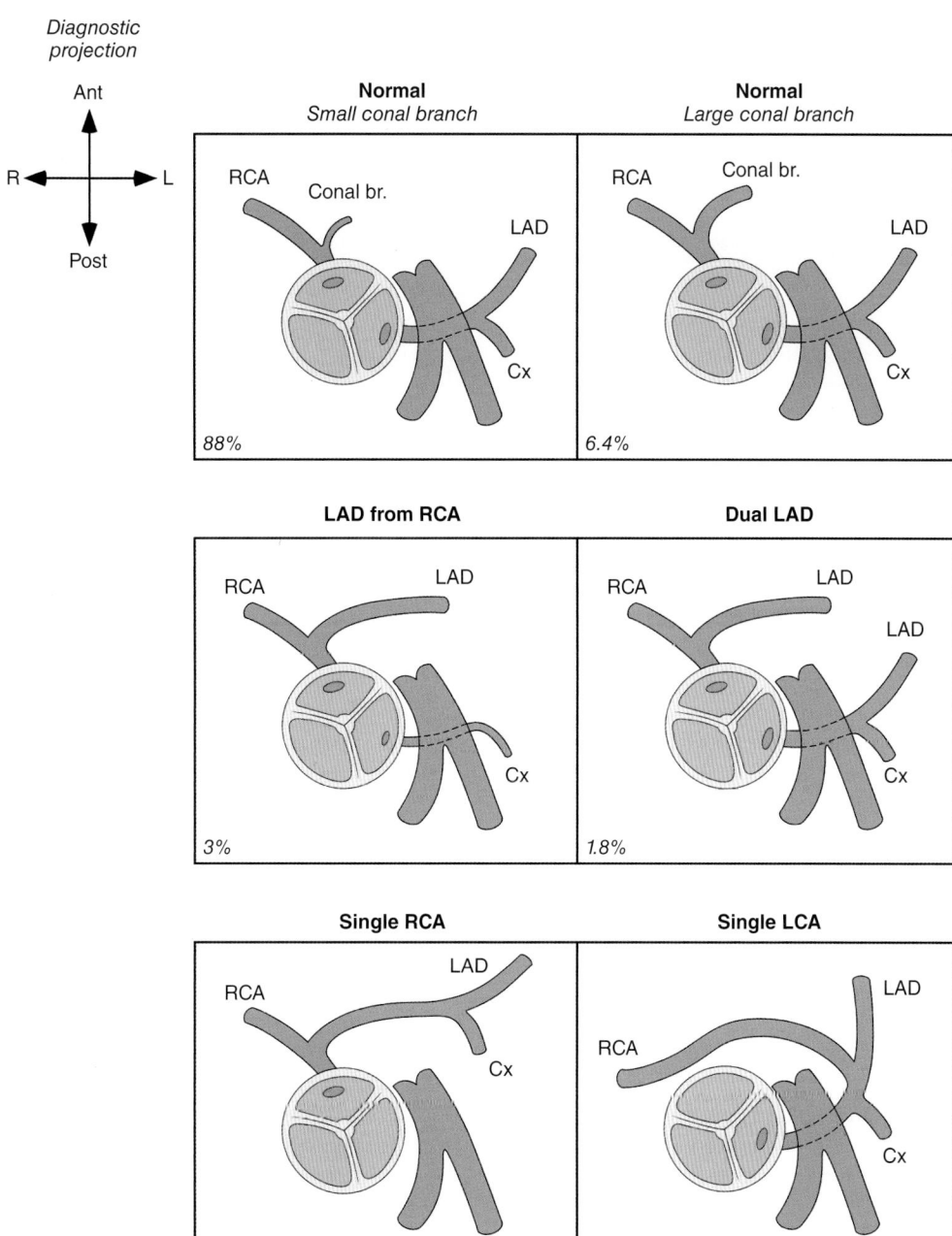

Diagnostic projection

Ant

R ◄———► L

Post

Normal
Small conal branch

RCA   Conal br.   LAD

Cx

88%

Normal
Large conal branch

RCA   Conal br.   LAD

Cx

6.4%

LAD from RCA

RCA   LAD

Cx

3%

Dual LAD

RCA   LAD

LAD

Cx

1.8%

Single RCA

RCA   LAD

Cx

0.3%

Single LCA

RCA   LAD

Cx

0.2%

• **Fig. 26.6** Diagram of the coronary artery patterns in tetralogy of Fallot. *Ant,* Anterior; *br,* branch; *Cx,* circumflex; *L,* left; *LAD,* left anterior descending coronary artery; *LCA,* left coronary artery; *Post,* posterior; *R,* right; *RCA,* right coronary artery.

In those few cases in which catheterization is undertaken, conventional oximetry and hemodynamic measurements are obtained (see Chapter 13). Angiography is performed with a series of contrast injections in the right ventricle, pulmonary artery, left ventricle, and aortic root, as needed, in projections suited to profile key anatomic features including the right ventricular outflow tract, pulmonary arteries, potential additional VSDs, and coronary arteries.

Aside from diagnostic indications, catheterization may be undertaken for interventional purposes in some cases of TOF. Large aortopulmonary collateral arteries that may be relatively inaccessible at surgery can be occluded using embolization coils at catheterization before or after the repair. Significant peripheral pulmonary artery stenoses can be dilated using balloon catheters and, when resistant to dilation alone, stented.[15] Balloon dilation of a stenotic pulmonary valve may be useful as a palliative step to increase pulmonary blood flow in certain patients in whom reparative surgery is delayed[16] and to gain access for preoperative pulmonary artery rehabilitation in patients with severe PS and diminutive pulmonary arteries.[15]

Catheterization may also be indicated after surgical repair. In the early postoperative period, it may be needed to evaluate hemodynamically significant residual lesions, such

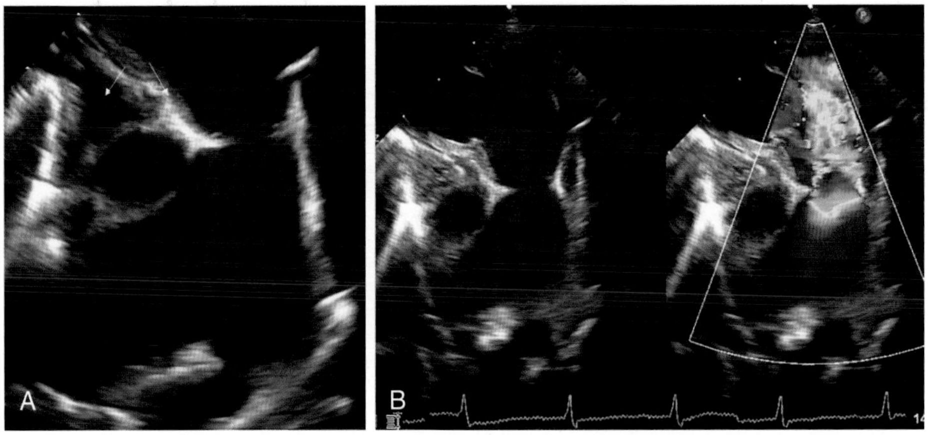

• **Fig. 26.7** Echocardiogram of an infant with tetralogy of Fallot with absent pulmonary valve. **(A)** Parasternal short-axis view showing the vestigial pulmonary valve leaflets *(PV)* and markedly dilated main *(MPA)*, right *(RPA)*, and left *(LPA)* pulmonary arteries. **(B)** Color Doppler mapping corresponding to the image in panel A, demonstrating turbulent diastolic flow (multicolor) through the regurgitant pulmonary valve into the right ventricular outflow tract, toward the apex of the scan sector.

as right ventricular outflow tract obstruction and residual VSDs in patients who are unstable or otherwise unable to wean from support. Catheter interventions may also be indicated in selected postoperative patients for balloon dilation of the pulmonary valve in patients with valvar PS after valve-sparing repair, balloon dilation of distal pulmonary artery stenoses, or coil embolization of residual aortopulmonary collaterals.

TOF With Pulmonary Atresia

Although catheterization is only rarely required in standard TOF, it remains essential in for evaluation and treatment of TOF with PA (Fig. 26.8). Diagnostic angiography is needed to show the detailed anatomy of the pulmonary arteries, including their arborization within the lungs, and to delineate all sources of pulmonary blood flow. Key features to be identified include the size and continuity or discontinuity of the central pulmonary arteries, stenosis or atresia involving lobar and segmental branches, and the origins and courses of all aortopulmonary collaterals and their connections to the true pulmonary arteries. Pulmonary vein wedge injections, in addition to contrast injections in the systemic arteries and collaterals, may be required to visualize all lung segments. Cardiac CT and MRI have been increasingly used to evaluate aortopulmonary collateral and branch pulmonary artery anatomy, but catheterization remains the gold standard for evaluating which lung segments are supplied by aortopulmonary collaterals versus anterograde flow from central pulmonary arteries versus both anterograde flow and collateral supply ("dual supply").

Interventional catheterization is a mainstay of therapy, along with surgery, for patients with TOF with PA. In selected patients with membranous PA, it may be possible at catheterization to perforate the valve mechanically with a guidewire, or by radiofrequency perforation, followed by balloon dilation of the valve to establish antegrade pulmonary blood flow from the right ventricle. Once right ventricle-to-pulmonary artery continuity has been created, either at catheterization or more commonly surgery, percutaneous balloon angioplasty and stenting are employed for rehabilitation of the hypoplastic and stenotic pulmonary arteries characteristic of this disease.[17] Vascular coils are delivered to occlude aortopulmonary collaterals. Often, narrowed segments of conduits can be dilated and stented, relieving RV hypertension and delaying the need for surgical conduit revision for months or years.

Catheterization is important in the long-term management of repaired TOF with PA, not only for ongoing pulmonary artery rehabilitation but also for the evaluation and treatment of right ventricle-to-pulmonary artery conduit obstruction and timing of VSD closure. In severe forms of TOF with PA and major aortic pulmonary collaterals, the VSD is often left open during infancy due to high pulmonary vascular resistance. Pulmonary vascular resistance and Qp:Qs from cardiac catheterization provide vital information for determining timing of VSD closure in patients undergoing pulmonary rehabilitation.

Other Studies

Cardiac MRI can provide extensive anatomic and functional data, but is rarely needed in infancy. It is, however, a vital tool for the evaluation of older children and adults with repaired TOF.[18] In patients in whom echocardiography is limited by poor acoustical windows, excellent anatomic and functional data can still be obtained noninvasively by MRI. Moreover, MRI provides quantification of RV mass, volume, ejection fraction, pulmonary regurgitant fraction, branch pulmonary artery flow distribution, and myocardial scar tissue burden (Fig. 26.9). In older postoperative patients, this data allows for precise monitoring of RV size and function as well as evaluation of pulmonary arteries, pulmonary regurgitation fraction, and other anatomic details. Cardiac MRI measurements of RV size and function are now routinely used in determining which

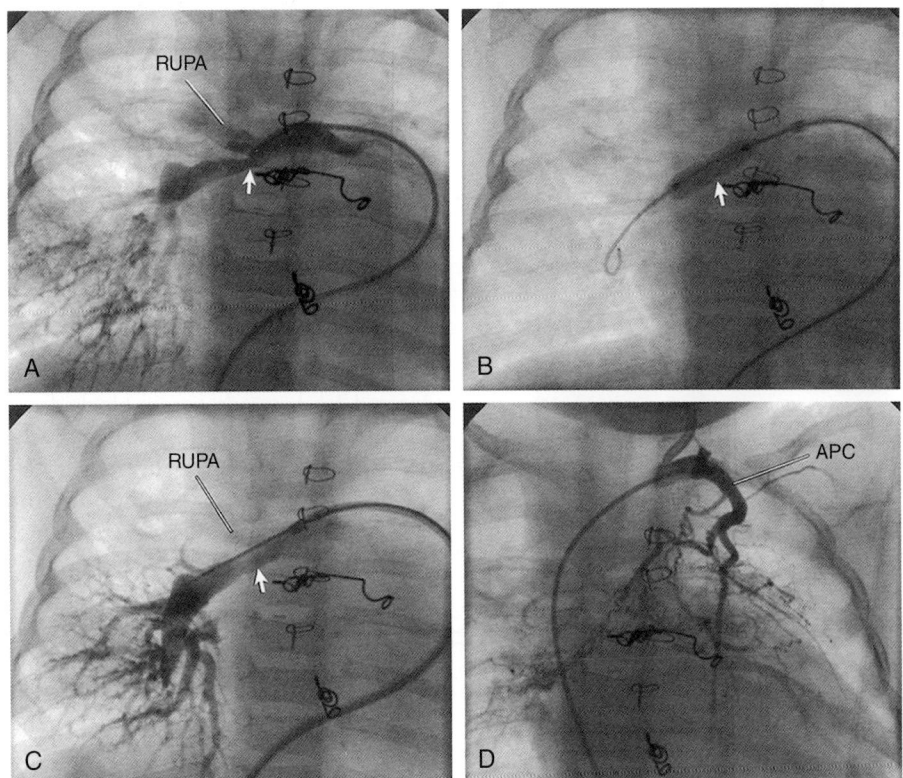

• **Fig. 26.8** Angiograms of a patient with tetralogy of Fallot with pulmonary atresia who had undergone surgery for placement of a right ventricle-to-pulmonary artery conduit, and prior catheterization for vascular coil embolization of aortopulmonary collaterals. **(A)** Right pulmonary arteriogram, via a venous catheter (inferior vena cava to right atrium to right ventricle to conduit to pulmonary artery), showing a discrete stenosis *(arrow)* just distal to the takeoff of the right upper pulmonary artery *(RUPA)* branch. **(B)** Balloon catheter showing a "waist" at the point of narrowing *(arrow)*. **(C)** Repeat right pulmonary arteriogram showing increased caliber of the right pulmonary artery stenosis *(arrow)*. **(D)** Angiogram demonstrating an aortopulmonary collateral artery *(APC)* arising from the left innominate artery in this patient with a right aortic arch (note course of retrograde arterial catheter); the collateral was then coil-occluded (not shown).

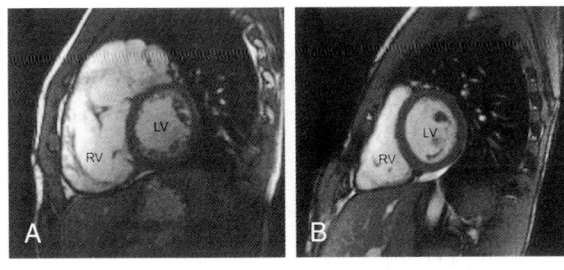

• **Fig. 26.9** Magnetic resonance ventriculography late after repair of tetralogy of Fallot. **(A)** Parasagittal image showing marked dilation of the right ventricle *(RV)* with a normal-sized left ventricle *(LV)*. **(B)** Parasagittal image showing a normal RV for comparison.

patients would benefit from pulmonary valve replacement.[18] Cardiac CT is used in older patients with repaired TOF when MRI safety is a concern due to presence of older generation pacemakers or implanted defibrillators.

Nuclear lung perfusion scanning (e.g., using technetium-99m–labeled microaggregated albumin) is also used in patients with TOF, especially those with PA and hypoplastic pulmonary arteries, for evaluation of pulmonary blood flow distribution to the right and left lungs. This information, typically obtained before and after pulmonary balloon angioplasty, is useful as a measure of the immediate success of the intervention. Followed serially, it can also provide evidence of recurrence of stenosis on one side or the other.

TOF With Pulmonary Atresia

MRI or CT imaging can provide detailed information on sources of pulmonary blood flow, including aortopulmonary collaterals (Fig. 26.10).

TOF With Absent Pulmonary Valve

MRI or CT imaging can provide excellent images of the dilated pulmonary arteries (Fig. 26.11), obstructed airways, and their interrelationships. However, in current practice, the echocardiographic images are usually sufficient for diagnosis and surgical planning.

Management and Course

Most neonates with TOF are initially only mildly-moderately cyanotic, or even acyanotic, and require no specific medical therapy before their surgical repair. Rare newborns with critical

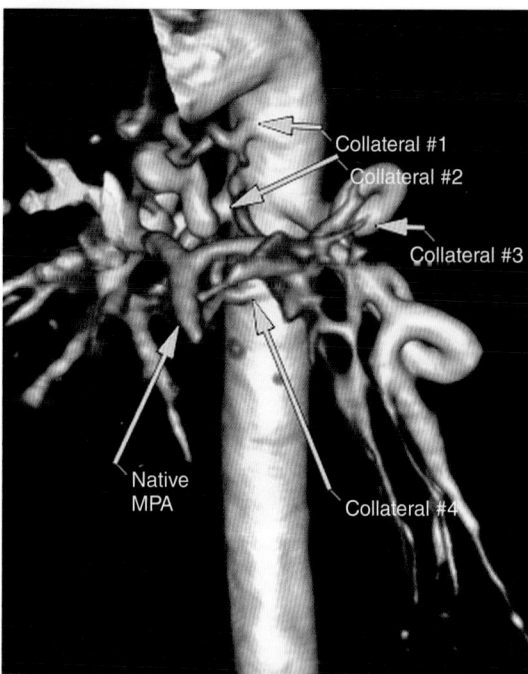

• **Fig. 26.10** Computed tomography angiogram of tetralogy of Fallot with pulmonary atresia. Three-dimensional reconstruction of a magnetic resonance angiogram in virtual left lateral projection showing diminutive main pulmonary artery (MPA) and branch pulmonary arteries as well as four aortopulmonary collaterals arising from the aorta (Ao).

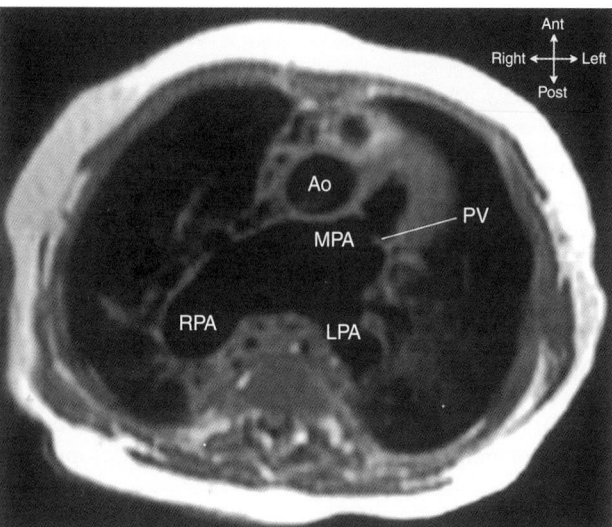

• **Fig. 26.11** Magnetic resonance image of a patient with tetralogy of Fallot with absent pulmonary valve, showing an axial cut through the vestigial pulmonary valve (PV) and markedly dilated main (MPA), right (RPA), and left (LPA) pulmonary arteries, compared with the more normal-caliber aorta (Ao).

RV outflow obstruction may be dependent on the ductus arteriosus for pulmonary blood flow and require prostaglandin infusion to maintain ductal patency pending surgical or catheter intervention. Patients with pink TOF, however, with little right ventricular outflow tracts obstruction and pulmonary overcirculation, may develop heart failure and require treatment with anticongestive medications prior to repair.

Patients who have a hypercyanotic spell are potentially at risk for severe neurologic sequelae and even death and, therefore, merit urgent attention. The spelling patient should be placed in the knee–chest position to simulate squatting and should be consoled to the extent possible. If outside the hospital, an ambulance should be called. Responding emergency medical personnel, whether in the field or in the hospital, should provide supplemental oxygen and intravenous fluid to expand the intravascular volume and increase pulmonary blood flow. Morphine should be administered immediately to relieve distress and air hunger; this may break the spell in some cases. Propranolol may be infused for beta-adrenergic blockade, thought to relax infundibular spasm. If the spell persists, an alpha-adrenergic agonist such as phenylephrine may be infused to increase the systemic vascular resistance, favoring pulmonary blood flow. Tracheal intubation and mechanical ventilation, extracorporeal membrane oxygenation, or emergency palliative surgery may be necessary to rescue the rare patient who has refractory spells. Drugs that produce systemic vasodilation can precipitate spells and are to be avoided in patients with TOF. Spells may be precipitated by sedation, such as for echocardiography or catheterization; therefore, vigilance for the development of signs such as deepening cyanosis, progressive arterial oxygen desaturation, hyperpnea, or metabolic acidosis is important. Patients who have had one or more spells and are awaiting surgery may be maintained on propranolol, which may help to prevent recurrent spells.

Before repair, infants with TOF tend to become more cyanotic with time owing primarily to progressive infundibular stenosis and increased ventricular right-to-left shunting. Chronic hypoxemia is correlated with cognitive impairment in large cohort studies (see Chapter 55). Older children with unrepaired or palliated TOF may have additional complications associated with chronic cyanosis and polycythemia, including stroke, brain abscess, and gallstones. Those patients with large surgical systemic-to-pulmonary artery shunts or persisting large aortopulmonary collaterals may develop pulmonary vascular obstructive disease (see Chapter 56). These problems are rare in contemporary practice in which infant repair is standard.

Since 1954, when surgical repair of TOF was first attempted,[19] the recommended age for elective repair of TOF has declined steadily, and is now typically about 3 months for infants born at full term with uncomplicated anatomy.[20] Repair in early infancy has been made possible by advances in surgical technique and postoperative management. Infant repair allows early restoration of normal circulatory physiology, thereby minimizing long-term risks associated with chronic cyanosis and RV hypertrophy and hypertension. Operative repair of TOF is approached through a median sternotomy, on cardiopulmonary bypass. Both transatrial and transventricular approaches are described.[21] For the ventricular approach, a longitudinal incision is made in the free wall of the infundibulum, with extension proximally to the level of the conal septum. Distally, this incision is extended to just below the pulmonary valve annulus (non-transannular) if the annulus is adequate sized (typically pulmonary valvar annulus z-score > −2.5), or across the annulus (transannular) and anterior wall of the main pulmonary artery to the bifurcation in cases when pulmonary valve is not adequate. The incision may be further extended across one or both origins of the right and left pulmonary arteries if they are also narrowed. Thickened and obstructing pulmonary valve leaflets and obstructing RV muscle bundles are resected. The VSD is visualized and repaired through the infundibulotomy. An outflow tract patch, is sewn into the infundibulotomy to augment the circumference of the right ventricular outflow tract anteriorly. Associated lesions, including patent ductus arteriosus, additional muscular VSDs, and ASDs, are also addressed during the operation. The patent foramen ovale or small ASD is sometimes left open to permit the right atrium to decompress, at the expense of some systemic arterial oxygen desaturation, if there is right-to-left atrial shunting due to a non-compliant, hypertrophied right ventricle in the early postoperative period.

Certain patients with TOF may require different surgical timing or management for a variety of reasons. Infants with PA and good sized branch pulmonary arteries supplied by a patent ductus can undergo full neonatal repair or palliation with patent ductus arteriosus stent or Blalock-Taussig-Thomas shunt. Neonates or infants who develop cyanosis, or hypercyanotic spells, are generally referred immediately for repair. Repair may be postponed if certain aspects of the anatomy are unsuitable, including patients with complex muscular VSDs or coronary artery anomalies. In cases in which reparative surgery is deferred, interim palliation, usually with an aortopulmonary shunt, is necessary it there is cyanosis or hypercyanotic spells.

Outcomes after complete repair of TOF are generally excellent. Actuarial data on patients repaired in the late 1950s and 1960s indicate that nearly 90% were alive 30 years after surgery, excluding early postoperative deaths.[22] For patients repaired in more recent decades, the early mortality is 3% or less.[20] Despite excellent survival in the modern era, a number of problems may develop and represent important management issues usually beginning around the third decade of life with increasing frequency in older age (see Chapter 57).

Clinically important residual VSDs, either residual patch margin defects or muscular defects, are often identified and closed early after repair. Recurrent right ventricular outflow tract obstruction may develop during childhood at one or more levels and require surgical revision to relieve significant RV hypertension. Muscle bundles may grow to obstruct the os infundibulum in 3% of patients repaired in infancy. In patients with valve-sparing repairs, the pulmonary valve annulus and leaflets may become narrowed/stenotic as the child grows. Patients with significant pulmonary artery hypoplasia at initial presentation may develop additional sites of peripheral pulmonary artery stenosis over time. Progressive aortic root dilation and aortic valve regurgitation develop in some patients, and has been found to

correlate with longer time between palliation and complete repair, as well as with PA, right aortic arch, and male sex.

Patients with repaired TOF are at risk for RV dilation and hypertrophy, systolic and diastolic dysfunction, arrythmias, exercise intolerance, heart failure symptoms, and premature death as they age into the third and fourth decades of life. Contributors to this risk vary among patients but include RV volume load from pulmonary regurgitation, pressure load from residual outflow obstruction, surgical incision/ventriculotomy, RV outflow tract patch, myocardial fibrosis/scarring, and post–cardiopulmonary bypass ischemia-reperfusion injury. Transatrial rather than transventricular repair has been advocated to avoid RV incision, but this may be at the expense of residual outflow obstruction in some patients.[21] A number of patients with RV dysfunction also have measurable left ventricular dysfunction, an apparent consequence of adverse ventricular interaction. Patients with RV dysfunction may remain relatively asymptomatic for years, but may eventually develop impaired exercise capacity[23] and right heart failure.

Pulmonary valve replacement has been shown to be associated with favorable RV remodeling when performed in a timely fashion before irreversible myocardial dysfunction occurs. Pulmonary valve replacement produces short-term improvement in symptoms, better subjective exercise tolerance, and lower rates of premature death. However, despite restoration of pulmonary valve competence, the potential for recovery of RV function may be limited, particularly if valve replacement is delayed until RV dysfunction is present.[18] Therefore, careful longitudinal surveillance of ventricular size and function and other anatomic and physiologic parameters is essential in patients with repaired TOF.

Bacterial endocarditis can occur in patients with TOF. Antibiotic prophylaxis is recommended at times of predictable risk for 6 months after corrective surgery or transcatheter implant of prosthetic material until sutures and other artificial surfaces have endothelialized. Prophylaxis may also be considered longer term in patients who have prosthetic heart valves in place, or who still have residual defects at the site or adjacent to the site of a prosthetic device or material (see Chapter 50).

Patients with TOF, even those with excellent hemodynamic results from surgery, remain at risk for late-onset atrial and ventricular arrhythmias. The arrhythmogenic substrates involve macroreentrant circuits generated by abnormal pressure/volume loads, surgical scars, and certain specific features of TOF anatomy. Rhythm disturbances typically do not become manifest until the third decade of life or beyond, suggesting that a period of degenerative tissue remodeling in necessary before these circuits become well established. The most common atrial arrhythmia in TOF patients is intra-atrial reentrant tachycardia (IART). It is estimated that 20% or more of the tetralogy population will develop IART by adulthood. It remains a source of high morbidity, including the risk of thromboembolic complications. The potential reentrant circuits include conventional atrial flutter (rotating around the tricuspid valve orifice), as well as reentry on the lateral right atrial free wall (rotating around an atriotomy scar). These circuits are relatively resistant to spontaneous or pharmacologic conversion, and usually necessitate electrical cardioversion or overdrive pacing for termination. The results of pharmacologic therapy for prevention of recurrent IART have been disappointing, owing to both lack of efficacy and drug intolerance. Accordingly, catheter ablation has been adopted widely as the preferred approach. During such procedures, tachycardia is induced with pacing maneuvers and the activation pattern is mapped (see Chapters 17 and 18), after which strategic ablation lines are created to interrupt the circuits. The standard lesion set for patients with tetralogy usually involves a line between the inferior vena cava and tricuspid valve (the so-called cavotricuspid isthmus) and a second line from the lower edge of the atriotomy scar down to the inferior vena cava. Results have been encouraging with acute success in over 90%, although recurrence is possible necessitating a second procedure.[24]

Ventricular tachycardia (VT) and sudden cardiac death (SCD) in TOF have been under intense investigation since the 1970s. It has become clear that the intrinsic anatomy of the RV in this condition involves structural features that can support monomorphic macroreentry circuits near the outflow tract, and that surgical scaring reinforces this potential (Fig. 26.12).[25] Patients with tetralogy can also develop more disorganized polymorphic VT, especially when ventricular function is poor. Although VT and SCD are uncommon during childhood and adolescence, the risk rises as high as 5%–10% per decade of follow-up by adulthood. Risk factors for VT and SCD in this population include patient age, surgical timing/technique, measures of hemodynamic status,

electrocardiographic findings, and noninvasive rhythm monitoring. For all noninvasive parameters, the positive predictive accuracy for any single measure is only modest. This uncertainty has led to increased reliance at many centers on invasive electrophysiologic studies incorporating programmed ventricular stimulation for patients perceived to be at high risk. Inducible VT correlates strongly with all-cause mortality at 5-year follow-up, while a negative study is reassuring.[26] Treatment for VT in patients with tetralogy centers on catheter ablation and implantable cardioverter defibrillators. If there are correctable hemodynamic problems that require surgery (e.g., pulmonary valve replacement), consideration can also be given to surgical cryoablation in the operating room.

Like patients with congenital heart disease in general (see Chapter 55), those with TOF have lower median intelligence quotient than control populations and higher psychosocial morbidity.[27] The factors that underlie neurodevelopmental morbidity may include both associated genetic syndromes and acquired abnormalities that ensue from chronic hypoxemia, hemodynamic instability, and surgery, including cardiopulmonary bypass.

TOF With Pulmonary Atresia

The initial medical management of the newborn with TOF with PA varies according to the sources and amounts of pulmonary blood flow. At one extreme, infants with inadequate aortopulmonary collaterals may depend on a ductus arteriosus for pulmonary blood flow and require prostaglandin infusion to maintain ductal patency pending surgical or catheter intervention. Most infants have adequate collaterals and maintain acceptable arterial oxygen saturations between 80% to low 90% without treatment. At the other extreme, rare patients may have excessive aortopulmonary collateral flow, and this may increase further as pulmonary arteriolar resistance decreases, even to the extent that anticongestive medicines may be needed.

The definitive management of TOF with PA includes a combination of interventional catheterization and surgical techniques that establish antegrade pulmonary blood flow from the right ventricle, rehabilitate the pulmonary arteries, and eventually close the VSD. Fundamental to this strategy is the understanding that postnatal growth of the hypoplastic pulmonary arterial tree can be promoted by maximizing antegrade flow, minimizing competing collateral flow, and eliminating stenoses.

The precise management is dictated by the individual anatomy in each patient, largely the severity of pulmonary artery hypoplasia, and extent of collateralization. It is possible in some patients to achieve a one-stage surgical repair, but many require a staged approach.[17] All patients should undergo catheterization to define the pulmonary artery anatomy and all sources of pulmonary blood flow. If there are excessive aortopulmonary collaterals that deliver competing flow with dual supply to lung segment, coil embolization of

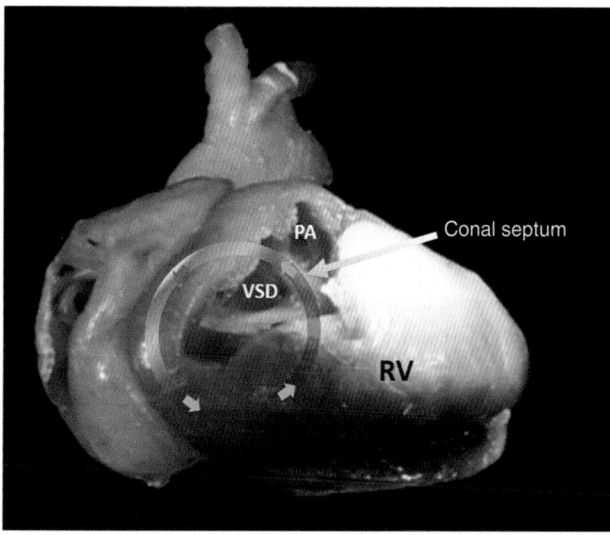

• **Fig. 26.12** Autopsy specimen of infant's heart with tetralogy of Fallot, tracing a potential reentrant circuit for ventricular tachycardia in the right ventricle *(RV)* that is dependent upon conduction through the conal septum. The conal septum represents a protected corridor for conduction between the malalignment ventricular septal defect *(VSD)* and the stenotic pulmonary artery *(PA)*, and is known to be a common substrate for ventricular tachycardia in this condition.

these vessels may be undertaken. This is particularly useful for those collaterals that are inaccessible at surgery.

Possibilities for creating continuity between the right ventricle and pulmonary arteries include perforation and dilation at catheterization if there is membranous atresia limited to the valve, or a transannular outflow patch may be placed at surgery. If there is long-segment atresia or absent main pulmonary artery segment, a right ventricle-to-pulmonary artery homograft conduit is placed.

If the native pulmonary arteries supply only a limited number of bronchopulmonary segments, it is imperative to surgically recruit additional segments supplied solely by collateral vessels into the reconstructed pulmonary arterial tree. This is accomplished by unifocalization of aortopulmonary collateral vessels, during which collaterals are detached from the aorta and anastomosed to the central pulmonary arteries.

Once right ventricle-to-pulmonary artery continuity has been achieved, patients with diminutive pulmonary arteries usually require catheterizations for balloon dilation of pulmonary artery narrowings. Vascular stents are delivered to segments of elastic narrowing for which dilation alone is not adequate. These interventions decrease RV hypertension, increase flow to distal pulmonary segments, and improve the match between ventilation and perfusion.

The timing of closure of the VSD in TOF with PA depends on adequacy of pulmonary arterial tree. Once the ventricular defect is closed, the pulmonary arteries must have adequate capacity to receive all systemic venous return from the right ventricle. If the total cross-sectional area of the pulmonary arteries is too small, RV failure and low cardiac output will ensue.[17] In patients born with relatively good sized pulmonary arteries, it may be possible to close the VSD at the time of initial right ventricular outflow tract reconstruction. In patients with diminutive pulmonary arteries, VSD closure is delayed. The development of left-to-right shunting through the VSD (i.e., Qp:Qs > 1) is often used as an indicator that it can safely be closed. A fenestration may intentionally be placed in the VSD patch to allow decompression of the right ventricle in cases where there is concern for significant residual RV hypertension.[17]

Patients with TOF with PA palliated with a right ventricle-to-pulmonary artery conduit typically require one or more additional operations as they grow in size. Right ventricle-to-pulmonary artery conduits are fixed in diameter and tend to calcify over time. Obstructed right ventricle-to-pulmonary artery homograft conduits can be dilated and stented, often permitting surgical conduit revision to be postponed for months or years and potentially reducing the total number of such operations that the patient will ultimately have to undergo. Typically, this is undertaken when the RV pressure approaches systemic arterial pressure. Patients with TOF with PA are at risk for persistent or recurrent peripheral pulmonary artery stenosis and even acquired atresia of lobar and segmental branches. Patients with TOF with PA are at higher risk for progressive aortic root dilation and aortic regurgitation than those with PS.

TOF With Absent Pulmonary Valve

The initial medical management of TOF with absent pulmonary valve depends on the degree of the accompanying airway disease.[14] Some neonates present with severe bronchial obstruction and require immediate tracheal intubation, mechanical ventilation, prone ventilation, and early surgical repair. In the most severe cases, adequate ventilation may not be achieved even with mechanical support, resulting in death due to respiratory failure. Patients with little or no airway obstruction may require no additional support in the neonatal period and go on to elective repair later in infancy. The surgical repair of TOF with absent pulmonary valve, in addition to VSD closure and RV outflow reconstruction, often involves reduction of the aneurysmal mediastinal pulmonary arteries to relieve bronchial compression.[14] Approaches include plication or excision of portions of the walls of these vessels, reducing their circumference, or complete removal of dilated segments and replacement with conduit. Surgeons may also place an artificial pulmonary valve in the reconstructed outflow to control pulmonary regurgitation and, thereby, limit the vascular pulsatility, volume load, and ongoing dilation of the vessels that may further compromise the airways. The efficacy of placing a pulmonary valve as part of the initial surgical palliation of TOF with absent pulmonary valve is uncertain.

Even after surgical repair, including reduction of the aneurysmal central pulmonary arteries, some patients continue to have significant bronchial obstruction. As these patients grow, however, pulmonary function generally tends to improve as pulmonary artery pressures fall and the maturing tracheobronchial tree develops less compressible walls and larger caliber.

TOF With Common Atrioventricular Canal

The medical management of TOF with common atrioventricular canal is similar to uncomplicated tetralogy. The surgical repair involves conventional right ventricular reconstruction, as described earlier, with closure of the atrioventricular septal defect and division and resuspension of the common atrioventricular valve (see Chapter 31). Of particular note is the risk for atrioventricular valve incompetence after canal repair and the extent to which this may compound other residual problems in tetralogy. Postoperative tricuspid valve regurgitation adds to the volume overload of the right ventricle, already overloaded by pulmonary regurgitation, accelerating RV dilation, and dysfunction. Similarly, mitral regurgitation adds volume load to the left ventricle which may be more vulnerable due to adverse ventricular interactions, prior cardiopulmonary bypass, and/or other residual hemodynamic lesions.

References

1. Fallot A. Contribution à l'anatomie pathologique de la maladie bleue (cyanose cardiaque). *Mars Med.* 1888;25:77-138.

2. Ferencz C, Rubin JD, McCarter RJ, et al. Congenital heart disease: prevalence at livebirth. The Baltimore-Washington Infant Study. *Am J Epidemiol.* 1985;121:31-36.

3. National Center for Health Statistics, Birth Data, 2004. Available at: http://www.cdc.gov/nchs/births.htm.

4. Morgenthau A, Frishman WH. Genetic origins of tetralogy of Fallot. *Cardiol Rev.* 2008;26:86-92.

5. Ferencz C, Loffredo CA, Correa-Villasenor A, et al. *Genetic and Environmental Risk Factors of Major Cardiovascular Malformations: The Baltimore-Washington Infant Study 1981–1989.* Armonk, NY: Futura; 1997.

6. Digilio MC, Marino B, Giannotti A, Toscano A, Dallapiccola B. Recurrence risk figures for isolated tetralogy of Fallot after screening for 22q11 microdeletion. *J Med Genet.* 1997;34:188-190.

7. Van Praagh R, Van Praagh S, Nebesar RA, et al. Tetralogy of Fallot: underdevelopment of the pulmonary infundibulum and its sequelae. *Am J Cardiol.* 1970;26:25-33.

8. Anderson RH, Allwork SP, Ho SY, et al. Surgical anatomy of tetralogy of Fallot. *J Thorac Cardiovasc Surg.* 1981;81:887-896.

9. Niwa K, Siu SC, Webb GD, et al. Progressive aortic root dilatation in adults late after repair of tetralogy of Fallot. *Circulation.* 2002;106:1374-1378.

10. Emmanoulides GC, Thanopoulos B, Siassi B, et al. "Agenesis" of ductus arteriosus associated with the syndrome of tetralogy of Fallot and absent pulmonary valve. *Am J Cardiol.* 1976;37:403-409.

11. Rabinovitch M, Grady S, David I, et al. Compression of intrapulmonary bronchi by abnormally branching pulmonary arteries associated with absent pulmonary valves. *Am J Cardiol.* 1982;50:804-813.

12. Kothari SS. Mechanism of cyanotic spells in tetralogy of Fallot—the missing link? *Int J Cardiol.* 1992;37:1-5.

13. Digilio MC, Marino B, Grazioli S, et al. Comparison of occurrence of genetic syndromes in ventricular septal defect with pulmonic stenosis (classic tetralogy of Fallot) versus ventricular septal defect with pulmonic atresia. *Am J Cardiol.* 1996;77:1375-1376.

14. Heinemann MK, Hanley FL. Preoperative management of neonatal tetralogy of Fallot with absent pulmonary valve syndrome. *Ann Thorac Surg.* 1993;55:172-174.

15. Kreutzer J, Perry SB, Jonas RA, Mayer JE, Castañeda AR, Lock JE. Tetralogy of Fallot with diminutive pulmonary arteries: preoperative pulmonary valve dilation and transcatheter rehabilitation of pulmonary arteries. *J Am Coll Cardiol.* 1996;27:1741-1747.

16. Sluysmans T, Neven B, Rubay J, et al. Early balloon dilatation of the pulmonary valve in infants with tetralogy of Fallot: risks and benefits. *Circulation.* 1995;91:1506-1511.

17. Rome JJ, Mayer JE, Castaneda AR, et al. Tetralogy of Fallot with pulmonary atresia. Rehabilitation of diminutive pulmonary arteries. *Circulation.* 1993;88:1691-1698.

18. Valente AM, Geva T. How to image repaired tetralogy of Fallot. *Circ Cardiovasc Imaging.* 2017;10:e004270.

19. Lillehei CW, Varco RL, Cohen M, et al. The first open heart corrections of tetralogy of Fallot: a 26-31 year follow-up of 106 patients. *Ann Surg.* 1986;204:490.

20. Pigula FA, Khalil PN, Mayer JE, del Nido PJ, Jonas RA. Repair of tetralogy of Fallot in neonates and young infants. *Circulation.* 1999;100:57.

21. Edmunds Jr LH, Saxena NC, Friedman S, et al. Transatrial repair of tetralogy of Fallot. *Surgery.* 1976;80:681-688.

22. Nollert G, Fischlein T, Bouterwek S, et al. Long-term survival in patients with repair of tetralogy of Fallot: 36-Year follow-up of 490 survivors of the first year after surgical repair. *J Am Coll Cardiol.* 1997;30:1374-1383.

23. Wessel HU, Paul MH. Exercise studies in tetralogy of Fallot: a review. *Pediatr Cardiol.* 1999;20:39-47.

24. Mah DY, Alexander ME, Cecchin F, Walsh EP, Triedman JK. The electroanatomic mechanisms of atrial tachycardia in patients with tetralogy of Fallot and double outlet right ventricle. *J Cardiovasc Electrophysiol.* 2011;22:1013-1017.

25. Zeppenfeld K, Schalij MJ, Bartelings MM, et al. Catheter ablation of ventricular tachycardia after repair of congenital heart disease: electroanatomic identification of the critical right ventricular isthmus. *Circulation.* 2007;116:2241-2252.

26. Khairy P, Van Hare GF, Balaji S, et al. PACES/HRS expert consensus statement on the recognition and management of arrhythmias in adult congenital heart disease. *Heart Rhythm.* 2014;11:e102-e165.

27. Shampaine EL, Nadelman L, Rosenthal A, et al. Longitudinal psychological assessment in tetralogy of Fallot. *Pediatr Cardiol.* 1989;10:135-140.

27

Double-Outlet Right Ventricle

DANIEL L. HAMES AND ADITYA K. KAZA

KEY LEARNING POINTS

- Double-outlet right ventricle (DORV) is present when the trunks of both great arteries arise completely or predominantly from the right ventricle. Discontinuity between the mitral valve and the adjacent semilunar valve is often present.
- A ventricular septal defect (VSD) is usually (but not always) present. The VSD may be subaortic, subpulmonary, doubly committed (both subaortic and subpulmonary), or remote/noncommitted.
- Most patients with double-outlet right ventricle have some degree of pulmonary stenosis. Most commonly the aorta and pulmonary artery are side by side with the former rightward (d-malposition), but they may also be in a d-transposition

configuration with the pulmonary artery posterior/leftward of the aorta.
- The hemodynamics for a particular patient depends on the relationship between the VSD and the great arteries, the relative outflow tract obstruction, and the relative systemic-to-pulmonary artery resistance. Clinical manifestations may vary depending on the underlying hemodynamics and range from cyanosis to congestive heart failure to a combination of both.
- Surgical management can include both biventricular and single-ventricle strategies depending on the underlying anatomy. Considerations include the size of the ventricles, location and size of the VSDs, degree of pulmonary stenosis, and associated lesions.

Definition

Double-outlet right ventricle (DORV) is present when the trunks of both great arteries arise completely or predominantly from the morphologic right ventricle.[1]

Prevalence

Reported incidences of DORV in infants range from 0.06 to 0.2/1000 live births.[2,3]

The diagnosis of DORV depends greatly on how much one or the other great vessel overrides the right ventricle. The criteria for this diagnosis have varied over the years. Determining which ventricle the great artery relates to may be difficult and can subsequently make it challenging to distinguish DORV from tetralogy of Fallot or d-transposition of the great arteries. Consequently, there is likely variation in the prevalence of this disease from center to center and within one center over time.

Pathology

DORV is a heterogenous cardiac anomaly used to describe the position of the great arteries in association with a variety

of cardiac defects including ventricular septal defects, tetralogy of Fallot, transposition of the great arteries, single ventricle, or atrioventricular (AV) valve atresia. There is a gradation of defects ranging from subaortic ventricular septal defect with subpulmonary or pulmonary stenosis, which can mimic tetralogy of Fallot. In the absence of pulmonary stenosis, the defect can behave like a large VSD. There is a similar range of clinical problems extending from subpulmonary VSD with varying degrees of overriding of the pulmonary artery which can present like transposition of the great arteries. Another anatomic spectrum ranges from a single right ventricle with a hypoplastic left ventricle, to a DORV with a small left ventricle that is, nevertheless, of sufficient size to permit a two-ventricle repair.

Discontinuity between the mitral valve and the adjacent semilunar valve is often present and is thought by some to be essential to diagnosis of DORV. Conal musculature is usually seen under both great arteries but may be absent under one or both. In cases without bilateral conal tissue, there is usually continuity between the adjacent great artery and the tricuspid valve; most of these children have mitral atresia.

Anatomic and physiologic considerations in DORV include the position and size of the VSD as well as its relationship to the semilunar valves, presence or absence of pulmonary outflow tract obstruction, the relationship of the great arteries, and associated anomalies.

Ventricular Septal Defect

DORV can be classified based on VSD location in relation to the great arteries.[4] A VSD is usually (but not always) present, providing the only outlet for the left ventricle. When no VSD is present, pulmonary venous blood reaches the right ventricle by shunting left to right through an atrial septal opening.[5,6] In relation to the great arteries, the VSD may be subaortic (most common), subpulmonary (second most common), doubly committed (both subaortic and subpulmonary), or remote/noncommitted (muscular, AV canal type) (Fig. 27.1).[5-11] The subaortic and subpulmonary defects rarely lie immediately below the corresponding semilunar valve without intervening conal tissue. The position of the VSD in relation to the great arteries is related to the distribution of conal tissue with deviations in conal tissue preferentially aligning the VSD with one of the great vessels. The distribution of conal tissue may also contribute to subaortic stenosis or pulmonary stenosis.[7] As in most other complex groups of cardiac anomalies, some ventricular defects tend to get smaller with time.

Pulmonary Stenosis

Most patients with DORV have some degree of pulmonary stenosis, which is usually associated with a subaortic VSD. Pulmonary atresia is rare but also possible. The stenosis is usually subvalvar and is derived from conal tissue. The extreme degrees of aortic override seen in tetralogy of Fallot can resemble the anatomy seen in DORV. While this can make it difficult to distinguish between the two defects, the presence of mitral-aortic valvar continuity establishes the diagnosis of tetralogy of Fallot. Absence of aortic-mitral continuity characterizes DORV.

Relation of the Great Arteries

Most commonly, the aorta and pulmonary artery are side by side with the former on the right (d-malposition).[6] They may also be in a d-transposition configuration with the pulmonary artery posterior and leftward to the aorta. In these cases, it may be difficult to distinguish if the diagnosis is DORV or transposition in the presence of a VSD, especially when pulmonary atresia is present. When there is a subpulmonary ventricular defect that delivers left ventricular blood to the pulmonary artery, the hemodynamics and the anatomy resemble those of transposition of the great arteries, and the latter is diagnosed if there is mitral-pulmonary valvar continuity.

The **Taussig-Bing anomaly** is a specific variation of this problem in which the hemodynamics and usual anatomy of transposed great arteries are present, but both arteries arise from the right ventricle. There is a subpulmonary VSD, no pulmonary stenosis, and absence of mitral-pulmonary valve continuity. The level of the semilunar valves is the same and the great vessels are parallel.[8,9]

Other Associated Anomalies

Virtually every other cardiac anomaly can be found associated with DORV. Any malfunction of the AV or semilunar valves may be present, with various types of pulmonary stenosis being the most common. A variety of outflow valve and subvalvar obstructions, interrupted aortic arch, and coarctation of the aorta are seen. Hypoplasia or stenosis of the aortic valve is often encountered when there is coarctation of the aorta, although subvalvar aortic stenosis may be seen in the absence of coarctation. A defect of the common AV canal is frequently present, with its associated mitral and tricuspid valve abnormalities (Table 27.1).

Mitral atresia, mitral stenosis, and straddling AV valves are common. Some babies with mitral atresia and a hypoplastic left ventricle do surprisingly well because there may be no aortic valve obstruction and normal sized aorta receives usual amounts of blood flow from the right ventricle. Superior-inferior (upstairs-downstairs) ventricles are often associated with the origin of both great arteries from the upper right ventricle. Inverse ventricles are common, as are visceral heterotaxy, polysplenia, and asplenia.

Physiology

The hemodynamics for a particular patient depends on the relationship between the VSD and the great arteries, the relative outflow tract obstruction, and the relative systemic-to-pulmonary artery resistance. DORV without outflow obstruction mimics the physiology seen in large VSDs. Patients with a subaortic VSD and pulmonary stenosis develop physiology similar to that seen in tetralogy of Fallot. Patients with a subpulmonary VSD display transposition physiology.

Clinical Manifestations

Depending on the physiology, the child may have problems of cyanosis, congestive heart failure, or both. Patients with a subaortic VSD without pulmonary stenosis will develop symptoms of congestive heart failure as pulmonary vascular resistance falls, similar to a large VSD. With pulmonary stenosis, there will be a degree of cyanosis that may get worse with time, similar to tetralogy of Fallot. Patients with a subpulmonary VSD and transposition physiology may present with poor systemic output if there is a degree of subaortic or aortic arch obstruction. Clinical presentation may also depend on the presence of associated anomalies including single or hypoplastic ventricle, AV valve abnormalities, and obstructed or unobstructed total anomalous pulmonary venous connection.

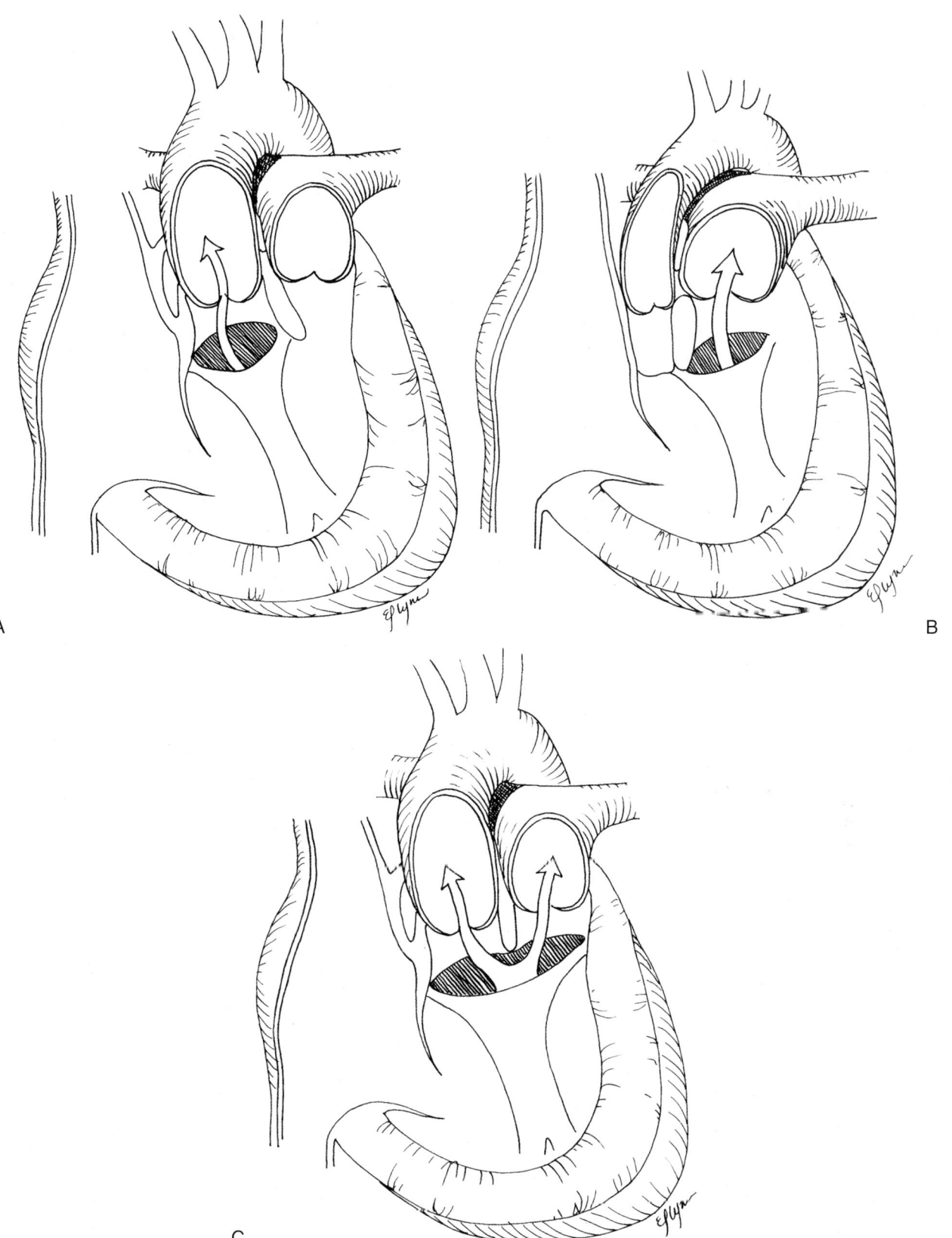

• **Fig. 27.1** Three drawings of double-outlet right ventricle. **(A)** Subaortic ventricular septal defect. **(B)** Subpulmonary ventricular septal defect. **(C)** Doubly committed ventricular septal defect related equally to both great arteries. Not shown are ventricular septal defects of the atrioventricular canal type or one or more muscular ventricular defects that may be associated with the above anomalies or exist as the sole communication between the left and right ventricles. (From Keane JF. *Nadas' Pediatric Cardiology*, 2nd Ed. Elsevier, Philadelphia; 2006.)

TABLE 27.1   Boston Children's Hospital experience 2003–2020

There were 516 patients who were categorized as having double-outlet right ventricle (DORV; compared with 300 patients during 1988–2002). Of 516 patients, 55 had a diagnosis of "single ventricle" with single right ventricle and DORV. There were 140 cases that carried a diagnosis of hypoplastic left ventricle with DORV, but this included all gradations of hypoplastic left ventricle.

Associated Diagnoses	DORV N = 321	Hypoplastic Left Ventricle With DORV N = 140	Single Ventricle With DORV N = 55
Pulmonary stenosis	155	58	19
Pulmonary atresia	59	21	10
Complete atrioventricular canal			
Balanced	53	0	0
Unbalanced	48	60	10
Total anomalous pulmonary venous connection	41	20	13
L-Transposition of the great arteries	60	16	4
Hypoplastic aorta	26	23	12
Coarctation*	30	10	10
Aortic stenosis**	25	19	2
Mitral atresia	3	37	11

Surgical Procedures			
Operative Procedure	DORV N = 305	Hypoplastic Left Ventricle With DORV N = 130	Single Ventricle With DORV N = 51
Fontan	20	63	28
Bidirectional Glenn[a]	10	15	11
Arterial-pulmonary shunt[b]	13	12	11
Pulmonary artery band[c]	8	6	1
Arterial switch operation with VSD closure	40	4	1
With aortic arch repair	21	1	0
VSD closure with RVOT augmentation[d]	68	9	1
Rastelli[d]	84	15	0
VSD closure[d]	20	3	0
Nikaidoh[d]	11	1	0

Repair Pathway			
	DORV N = 305	Hypoplastic Left Ventricle With DORV N = 130	Single Ventricle With DORV N = 51
Primary biventricular repair	120	10	0
Primary single-ventricle palliation	45	95	49
Staged or conversion from single ventricle to biventricular repair	132	23	2
1.5 ventricle repair	7	2	0

RVOT, right ventricular outflow tract; *VSD,* ventricular septal defect.
*Includes interrupted aortic arch.
**Includes both aortic and subaortic stenosis.
[a]Includes cases with bidirectional Glenn and pulmonary artery band or arterial-pulmonary shunt.
[b]Includes cases with pulmonary artery band as well as stage 1 procedure.
[c]Includes cases with arterial switch operation, aortic arch repair, and bidirectional Glenn.
[d]Includes cases with atrial baffle procedures.

Electrocardiography

There is no characteristic electrocardiographic pattern. However, virtually patients have a pattern compatible with right ventricular hypertrophy.

Chest Radiography

There is similarly no characteristic chest radiograph. The size of the heart and the prominence of the pulmonary vasculature are dependent on the underlying physiology and hemodynamics and may range from a relatively small heart with decreased pulmonary vascularity to a large heart with increased pulmonary vascular markings.

Echocardiography

Echocardiography is the primary tool used to diagnose DORV. The diagnosis is made with visualization of both great arteries, either completely or predominantly, aligned with the right ventricle (Fig. 27.2). Bilateral conus may be present but is not necessary to make the diagnosis.[5] Given the large number of anatomic variations and associated intracardiac lesions, a thorough examination, including Doppler interrogation, of all segments of the heart is mandatory. Of importance are the VSD position relative to the great arteries, the degree of outflow tract obstruction, the relationship of the great arteries, and the relative size of each ventricle.

Cardiac Catheterization

With detailed anatomic information provided by echocardiography and Doppler estimations of obstructive lesions and regurgitant valves, cardiac catheterization is not always necessary, particularly in infants. Catheterization may be indicated where anatomic and physiologic uncertainties exist and to evaluate pulmonary resistance in older patients. Catheterization is also helpful in evaluating hemodynamics in patients who underwent prior palliative procedures prior to consideration of a two-ventricle repair. The information obtained from the echocardiogram may suggest the best positioning of the patient to demonstrate the origins of the great vessels and the location of the ventricular defects (Fig. 27.3). Catheterization may also be indicated in patients with pulmonary outflow tract obstruction for stent placement in the patent ductus arteriosus as a palliative intervention and alternative to a surgical arterial to pulmonary shunt. This may allow the child to grow and leave the hospital prior to surgical intervention.

Cardiac Magnetic Resonance Imaging

Advanced cardiac imaging with cardiac magnetic resonance imaging (MRI) can be helpful in operative planning and determination of candidacy for a biventricular repair. Cardiac

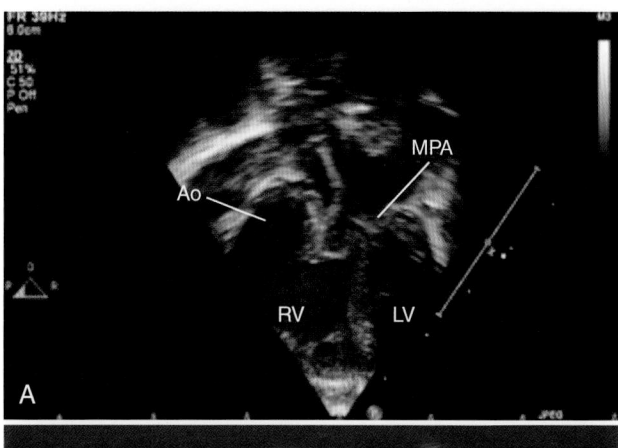

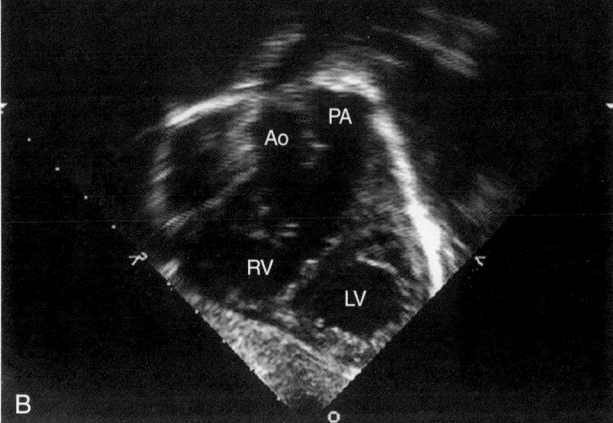

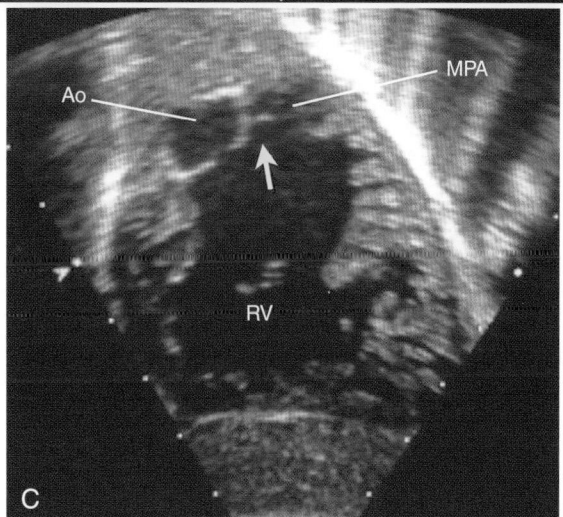

• **Fig. 27.2** Subxyphoid echocardiogram of **(A)** double-outlet right ventricle with subaortic ventricular septal defect (VSD) with both the aorta *(Ao)* and main pulmonary artery *(MPA)* arising from the right ventricle *(RV)*; **(B)** Taussig-Bing type of double-outlet right ventricle *(RV)*. The apex of the left ventricle *(LV)* is seen with both the aorta *(Ao)* and pulmonary artery *(PA)* arising from the RV, each from a subarterial infundibulum; and **(C)** doubly committed VSD. (B, From Keane JF. *Nadas' Pediatric Cardiology*, 2nd Ed. Elsevier, Philadelphia; 2006.)

MRI can be useful in further delineation of intracardiac and extracardiac (including systemic and pulmonary venous connections) anatomy, left ventricular size, and visualization of the pathway from the left ventricle to the aortic valve (Fig. 27.4).

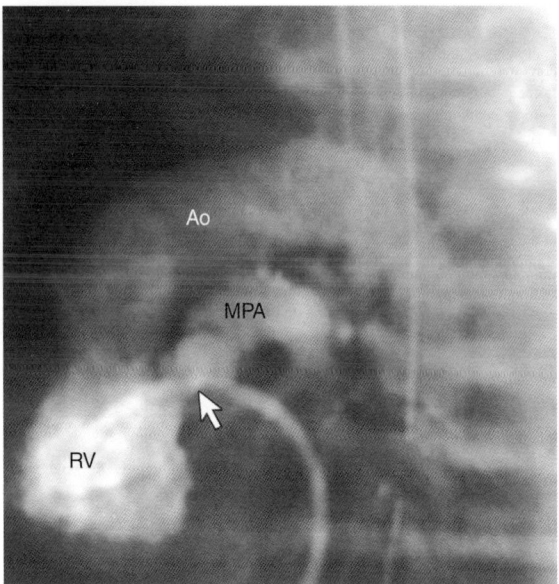

• **Fig. 27.3** Lateral right ventricular *(RV)* angiogram in a 1-day-old baby with a double-outlet right ventricle and subpulmonary stenosis *(arrow)*. Note that both great vessels arise from the RV with the aorta *(Ao)* anterior to the main pulmonary artery *(MPA)*. (From Keane JF. *Nadas' Pediatric Cardiology*, 2nd Ed. Elsevier, Philadelphia; 2006.)

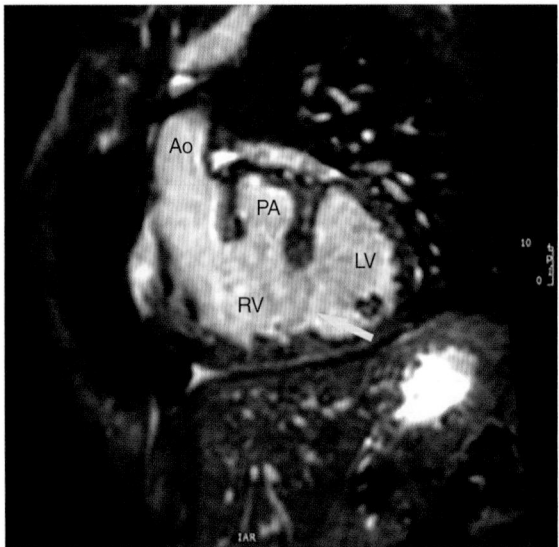

• **Fig. 27.4** Cardiac magnetic resonance image of infant with double-outlet right ventricle with large atrioventricular canal type ventricular septal defect *(yellow arrow)* and side-by-side great arteries. This patient underwent main pulmonary artery banding due to lack of pulmonary stenosis and unrestrictive pulmonary blood flow. Note the bilateral conus under both aorta and pulmonary artery. *Ao,* Aorta; *LV,* left ventricle; *PA,* pulmonary artery; *RV,* right ventricle.

Management

The initial management decisions surrounding DORV are dependent on evaluating the many potential associated lesions. The major considerations include:

1. Are there two adequately sized ventricles to accomplish a biventricular repair?

2. Where is (are) the VSD(s)? Is it of adequate size and can it be baffled to the future systemic great artery?
3. If pulmonary stenosis is present, can it be repaired or is a conduit necessary?
4. Can any associated lesions be repaired?

With an unrestrictive subaortic VSD and d-malposed great vessels, an intraventricular tunnel repair baffling the left ventricle to the aorta and closing the VSD is all that is necessary.[10,11] Patients without pulmonary stenosis may require pulmonary artery banding to prevent the development of congestive heart failure and allow for growth prior to definitive repair. Patients with pulmonary stenosis may require augmentation of the right ventricular outflow tract or a right ventricle-to-pulmonary artery conduit placement depending on the degree of pulmonary stenosis. Enlargement of the VSD to augment the pathway from the left ventricle to the systemic great artery may also be necessary.[12-14] Additionally, some patients may require atrial baffling to direct venous return depending on atrial situs.

If the defect is subpulmonary (Taussig-Bing anomaly), then baffling the left ventricle to the pulmonary artery together with an arterial switch operation repairs the lesion.[15,16] Aortic arch repair may also be necessary if there is aortic arch obstruction.[17] Patients felt not to be candidates for an arterial switch operation because of either pulmonary stenosis or concerns about the development of left ventricular outflow tract obstruction may be managed with aortic translocation and biventricular outflow tract reconstruction (Nikaidoh procedure).[18] Some doubly or noncommitted ventricular defects have been baffled to the systemic great artery with or without an arterial switch.[19-21]

At the single ventricle end of the spectrum, a modified stage 1 operation is often the initial surgery with a Fontan procedure in the future. This approach is also an option in those in whom the VSD location is a contraindication to baffling, such as in the inlet septum. A temporary modified Blalock-Taussig-Thomas shunt or cardiac catheterization for stent placement in the patent ductus arteriosus may be the initial procedure in some with pulmonary stenosis or atresia.

Patients with complex anatomy such as multiple VSDs or non-committed defects, total anomalous pulmonary venous connection, small left ventricular size, or complex AV valve anatomy may undergo a staged approach to a biventricular repair over a series of operations[14] (Fig. 27.5). Alternatively, patients may be managed with a one-and-a-half ventricle repair with two ventricles and superior cavopulmonary anastomosis left in place. The staged approach allows for patient growth to mitigate the risk of left ventricular outflow tract obstruction with the left ventricle to aorta pathway, optimization of the AV valve, and growth of a hypoplastic ventricle. Intraoperative conduction system mapping during surgical repair may be useful in localizing the conduction system to lower the risk of postoperative heart block.[22]

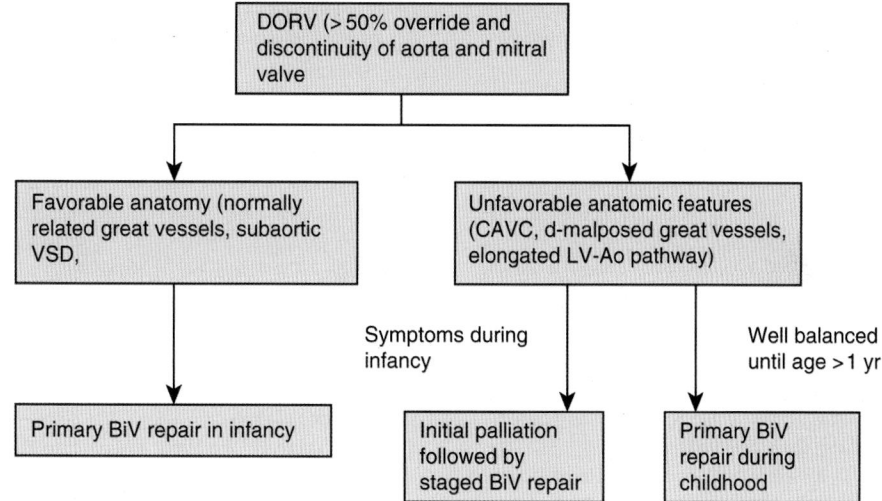

• **Fig. 27.5** Algorithm used at Boston Children's Hospital to determine whether or not a patient should undergo a primary or staged biventricular (BiV) repair. CAVC, Complete atrioventricular canal; DORV, double-outlet right ventricle; VSD, ventricular septal defect. (From Oladunjoye O, Piekarski B, Baird C, et al. Repair of double outlet right ventricle: Midterm outcomes. J Thorac Cardiovasc Surg. 2020;159:260.)

Course

Mortality and reintervention rates vary based on underlying anatomy and surgical repair. In a series of patients from our institution undergoing biventricular repair between 2000 and 2017, transplant-free survival at 3 years was 89%. Freedom from surgical reintervention at 3 years was 65%.[14] Indications for reintervention included left ventricular outflow tract obstruction, right ventricular outflow obstruction, AV or semilunar valve disease, and residual VSD. Others have reported similar survival rates in the first decade after repair[11,13,23] and reintervention rates.[13,23] In simple uncomplicated patients, 96% survival at 15 years has been reported with lower rates in complicated patients.[10]

Double-Outlet Left Ventricle

Double-outlet left ventricle is said to be present when both great arteries arise completely or predominantly from the morphologic left ventricle.

It is a very rare anomaly with most reports isolated to case series. Associated lesions include VSDs, pulmonary stenosis, tricuspid valve anomalies, and right ventricular hypoplasia.[24] Most patients have situs solitus of the atria and viscera and AV concordance.[25] We have seen 13 such patients from 2003 to 2020. Nine patients had pulmonary stenosis and three had pulmonary atresia. Four patients had tricuspid atresia.

Management depends on the specific anatomy with both biventricular and single-ventricle repairs being reported. In our series, eight of the patients underwent biventricular repair and the remaining five underwent single-ventricle palliation. In a separate series of 16 patients undergoing repair, 7 underwent a biventricular repair.[24]

References

1. Walters HL, Mavroudis C, Tchervenkov CI, et al. Congenital heart surgery nomenclature and database project: double outlet right ventricle. *Ann Thorac Surg.* 2000;69:249-263.
2. Shuler CO, Black GB, Jerrell JM. Population-based treated prevalence of congenital heart disease in a pediatric cohort. *Pediatr Cardiol.* 2013;34:606-611.
3. Ailes EC, Gilboa SM, Honein MA, et al. Estimated number of infants detected and missed by critical congenital heart defect screening. *Pediatrics.* 2015;135:1000-1008.
4. Lev M, Bharati S, Meng CCL, et al. A concept of double-outlet right ventricle. *J Thorac Cardiovasc Surg.* 1972;64:271-281.
5. Ebadi A, Spicer DE, Backer CL, et al. Double-outlet right ventricle revisited. *J Thorac Cardiovasc Surg.* 2017;154:598-604.
6. Sridaromont S, Feldt RH, Ritter DG, et al. Double outlet right ventricle: hemodynamic and anatomic correlations. *Am J Cardiol.* 1976;38:85-94.
7. Kurosawa H, Van Mierop LHS. Surgical anatomy of the infundibular septum in transposition of the great arteries with ventricular septal defect. *J Thorac Cardiovasc Surg.* 1986;91: 123-132.
8. Van Praagh R. What is the Taussig-Bing malformation? *Circulation.* 1968;38:445-449.
9. Yacoub MH, Radley-Smith R. Anatomic correction of the Taussig-Bing anomaly. *J Thorac Cardiovasc Surg.* 1984;88:380-388.
10. Brown JW, Ruzmetov M, Okada Y, et al. Surgical results in patients with double outlet right ventricle: a 20-year experience. *Ann Thorac Surg.* 2001;72:1630-1635.
11. Belli E, Serraf A, Lacour-Gayet F, et al. Biventricular repair for double outlet right ventricle: results and long term follow up. *Circulation.* 1998;98:II360-II365.
12. Li S, Ma K, Hu S, et al. Surgical outcomes of 380 patients with double outlet right ventricle who underwent biventricular repair. *J Thorac Cardiovasc Surg.* 2014;148:817-824.
13. Villemain O, Belli E, Ladouceur M, et al. Impact of anatomic characteristics and initial biventricular surgical strategy on outcomes in various forms of double-outlet right ventricle. *J Thorac Cardiovasc Surg.* 2016;152:698-706.

14. Oladunjoye O, Piekarski B, Baird C, et al. Repair of double outlet right ventricle: midterm outcomes. *J Thorac Cardiovasc Surg.* 2020;159:254-264.

15. Takeuchi K, McGowan Jr FX, Moran AM, et al. Surgical outcome of double outlet right ventricle with subpulmonary VSD. *Ann Thorac Surg.* 2001;71:49-53.

16. Wetter J, Sinzobahamvya N, Blaschczok HC, et al. Results of arterial switch operation for primary total correction of the Taussig-Bing anomaly. *Ann Thorac Surg.* 2001;77:41-46.

17. Fricke TA, Thungathurthi K, Naimo PS, et al. Arterial switch operation in patients with Taussig-Bing anomaly and aortic arch obstruction. *Ann Thorac Surg.* 2022;114:834-840.

18. Secse L, Turbendian HK, Thibault D, et al. Utilization and outcomes of the Nikaidoh, Rastelli, and REV procedures: an analysis of The Society of Thoracic Surgeons Congenital Heart Surgery Database. *Ann Thorac Surg.* 2022;114:800-808.

19. Uemura H, Yagihara T, Kadohama T, et al. Repair of double outlet right ventricle with doubly-committed ventricular septal defect. *Cardiol Young.* 2001;11:415-419.

20. Lacour-Gayet F, Haun C, Ntalakoura K, et al. Biventricular repair of double outlet right ventricle with non-committed ventricular septal defect (VSD) by VSD rerouting to the pulmonary artery and arterial switch. *Eur J Cardiothorac Surg.* 2002;21:1042-1048.

21. Li S, Ma K, Hu S, et al. Biventricular repair for non-committed ventricular septal defect. *Eur J Cardiothorac Surg.* 2015;48:580-587.

22. Feins EN, O'Leary ET, Hoganson DM, et al. Intraoperative conduction mapping in complex congenital heart surgery. *JTCVS Tech.* 2022;12:159-163.

23. Bradley TJ, Karamlou T, Kulik A, et al. Determinants of repair type, reintervention, and mortality in 393 children with double-outlet right ventricle. *J Thorac Cardiovasc Surg.* 2007;134:967-973.

24. Imai-Compton C, Elmi M, Manlhiot C, et al. Characteristics and outcomes of double outlet left ventricle. *Congenit Heart Dis.* 2010;5:532-536.

25. Van Praagh R, Weinberg PM, Srebro JP. Double outlet left ventricle. In: Adams FH, Emmanoulides GC, Riemenschneider TA, eds. *Moss' Heart Disease in Infants, Children and Adolescents.* 4th ed. Baltimore: Williams & Wilkins; 1989;461-485.

28

Aortic Outflow Abnormalities

DAVID W. BROWN, KSHITIJ MISTRY, AND ADITYA K. KAZA

KEY LEARNING POINTS

- Valvar aortic stenosis is the most common form of left ventricular outflow tract obstruction. The most common valve morphology is a bicommissural or bicuspid aortic valve, which is associated with both congenital and acquired aortic stenosis.
- Patients with congenital valvar aortic stenosis often have progressive obstruction and are at increased risk for infectious endocarditis and sudden death. Most children and adolescents with aortic stenosis are asymptomatic, underscoring the importance of regular clinical follow-up.
- Subaortic stenosis is rare in infants, and is most often an acquired and progressive lesion in the pediatric age group.

- Surgery is usually the definitive therapy, although recurrence is a common problem.
- Supravalvar aortic stenosis is often associated with abnormalities in the elastin gene, a characteristic finding of Williams syndrome; this may be associated with more extensive arteriopathy. The definitive treatment is surgical correction.
- Aortic regurgitation is caused by many disorders and complicates many types of congenital heart disease. Symptoms of significant aortic regurgitation are rare, and intervention is indicated for progressive left ventricular dilation and/or dysfunction.

Introduction

Left ventricular outflow tract obstructive lesions account for approximately 6% of congenital heart disease in children. Obstruction can occur at subvalvar, valvar, and supravalvar levels. While these may occur in combination in some patients, clinically these lesions are distinct, with different etiologies, natural history, and treatment strategies. Thus, in this chapter we will consider each of these individually, recognizing that combination left ventricular outflow tract obstructions may occur in some and clinical management may need to incorporate multiple considerations.

Valvar Aortic Stenosis

Valvar aortic stenosis is by far the most common form of left ventricular outflow tract obstruction, accounting for 70–80% of cases. Reported incidence of valvar aortic stenosis range from 0.04 to 0.38 per 1000 live births, and more than 75% of affected patients are male. In most cases, it is associated with a congenitally deformed valve, particularly a bicommissural/bicuspid one (two leaflets rather than three), although unicommissural variants may occur and a minority of children with valvar aortic stenosis have a tricuspid valve.

Pathology

Anatomically, the normal aortic valve has three leaflet cusps (tricuspid) and three commissures (tricommissural). Interestingly, cusp sizes are rarely equal (less than 16%), enlargement of the right or noncoronary being the most common observation. In young patients, a congenitally deformed and usually noncalcified mobile valve is almost always present, whereas almost half of elderly patients with valvar aortic stenosis have very thick, calcified, immobile tricuspid valves. In children, the most common aortic valve anomaly is a **bicuspid (bicommissural) valve**, which has been shown in multiple studies to have an incidence in the general population of 1%–2%.[1,2] Familial clustering has also been observed; recent studies have shown that 35% of patients with bicuspid aortic valve will have at least one affected immediate family member.[3,4] In young patients, the right/left (intercoronary) commissure is most frequently absent (60–70%, Fig. 28.1A), with right/noncoronary commissural absence the next most common (35–40%, Fig. 28.1B), and absence of the left/non-commissure a rarity (less than 2%).[5] The two leaflets are sometimes unequal in size such that the valve orifice may be quite eccentric, even in the absence of obstruction; leaflet thickness is also variable, but calcification is rare in children and adolescents.[6,7]

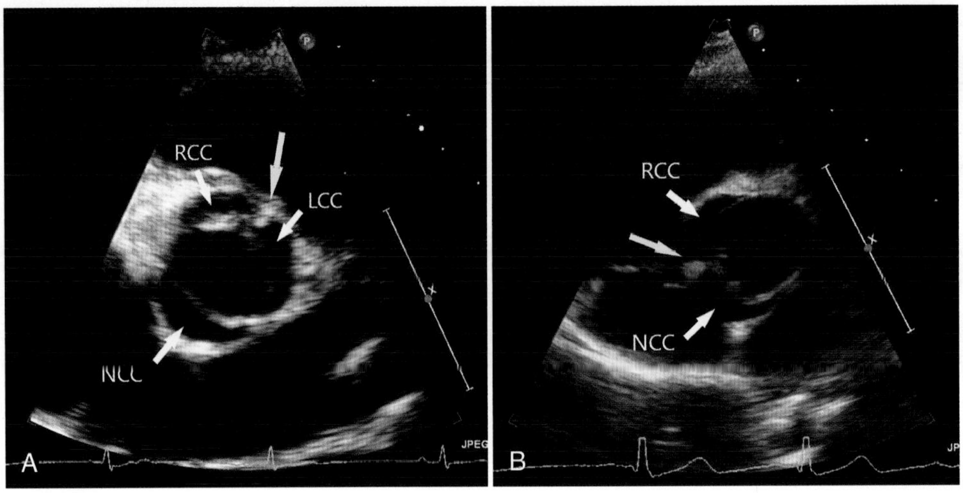

• **Fig. 28.1** Bicuspid aortic valve variants. **(A)** Parasternal short-axis echocardiogram view demonstrates a bicommissural aortic valve with fusion of the right/left aortic commissure; note the raphe present at the site of the fused commissure *(yellow arrow)*. **(B)** Similar parasternal view of a bicommissural aortic valve with fusion of the right/noncoronary commissure, with a similar raphe present *(yellow arrow)*. *LCC,* Left coronary cusp; *NCC,* noncoronary cusp; *RCC,* right coronary cusp.

While isolated regurgitation without prior medical or surgical intervention is unusual in young patients, stenosis is common and progressive in about 28% of cases.[7] Among pediatric patients with at least mild aortic stenosis, progression is generally the rule although the rate of progression varies considerably. More rapid progression may be seen in infants, particularly in the first few months of life. Progression is likely related to increasing adhesion of remaining commissure margins and leaflet thickening. Valve morphology has been shown to be associated with different pathologies; those with absence of the right/noncoronary commissure more often have significant valvar disease (aortic stenosis or regurgitation), and those with absence of the right–left commissure more often have associated coarctation of the aorta.[8] Among those with a bicuspid aortic valve, approximately 6% have associated coarctation of the aorta; conversely, as many as 30–40% of patients with coarctation have a bicuspid aortic valve.[5] A dilated ascending aorta is commonly associated with a bicuspid aortic valve and may occur in the presence of a normally functioning valve[4]; other associated congenital cardiac lesions include ventricular septal defect (VSD), patent ductus arteriosus, and mitral valve abnormalities.

Physiology

With most cases of valvar aortic stenosis, cardiac adaptation occurs to maintain normal systemic blood pressure and cardiac output in the face of an obstructive aortic valve; this occurs at the cost of increased left ventricular systolic pressure and total cardiac work. Left ventricular wall thickness is often increased to maintain normal left ventricular wall stress. Due to a hypertrophied, hypertensive left ventricle, there is increased myocardial oxygen demand along with a concomitant decrease in coronary perfusion pressure and diastolic filling time (due to the

stenotic orifice). This myocardial oxygen supply and demand imbalance may be exacerbated by exercise, anemia, and other conditions including those that are associated with an increased heart rate, such as hyperthyroidism; at some point, this imbalance may result in subendocardial ischemia and infarction. This pathophysiology likely underlies the observed association between severe aortic stenosis and cases of sudden cardiac death.[9]

Physiologic Assessment

For the last several decades, the invasive measurement of the peak-to-peak gradient across a stenotic aortic valve has been used as the gold standard assessment of disease severity. As some of the most comprehensive natural history studies occurred during an era when catheterization data was the key diagnostic assessment tool, most of our clinical management strategies use this hemodynamic gradient as a basis for treatment. At catheterization in the sedated patient, this peak–peak ejection gradient is measured preferably from two catheters, one on either side of the aortic valve, or alternatively during withdrawal of a single catheter from ventricle to aorta while simultaneously measuring cardiac output. If the left ventricular pressure is compared with a simultaneous distal arterial pressure (such as a femoral artery), the gradient may be underestimated because the latter systolic value is often higher than the central aortic pressure; this phenomenon is known as the *standing wave effect* (Fig. 28.2).

More recently with the remarkable improvements in echocardiographic technology, measurement of obstruction is now routinely performed using Doppler techniques. It is important to remember that when using Doppler, the maximum velocity of blood across the stenotic orifice is being assessed, and then using the modified Bernoulli equation a maximum instantaneous gradient is estimated. Thus, while

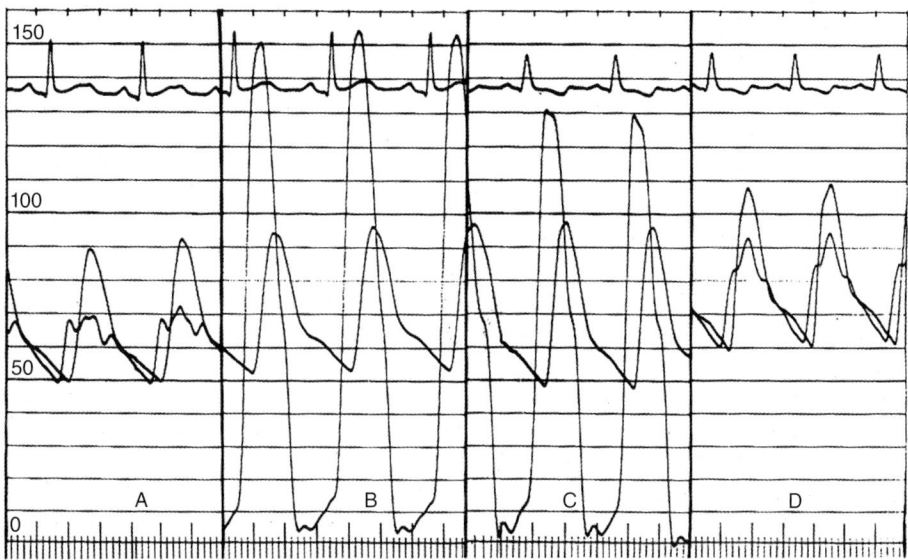

• **Fig. 28.2** Pressure recordings in a patient with valvar aortic stenosis. The numeric scale on the left is in millimeters of mercury (mm Hg). **(A)** Comparison of the pressure recorded from the ascending aorta with that in the femoral artery. Note that the pressure tracing is delayed in the femoral artery and is 20 mm Hg higher in the femoral artery than in the ascending aorta, an example of the standing wave effect. **(B)** Comparison of the femoral artery pressure with the left ventricular pressure. Note that the gradient of pressure across the valve measures 60 mm Hg but underestimates the true gradient (80 mm Hg) by 20 mm Hg. **(C)** Comparison of the femoral artery pressure and the left ventricular pressure after balloon dilation of the aortic valve. Note that the pressure gradient is now smaller, the left ventricular systolic and end-diastolic pressures lower, and the arterial pulse pressure higher. The electrocardiogram now shows bundle branch block, a transitory phenomenon. **(D)** Comparison of the ascending aorta and femoral artery pressures after dilation. Note that the pulse contour of the ascending aorta has changed: the pulse pressure is greater and the pressures are higher than in panel A. (From Fyler DC, ed. *Nadas' Pediatric Cardiology*. Philadelphia: Hanley & Belfus, 1992.)

there is a tendency for this Doppler value to be used as the equivalent of the catheterization-derived peak–peak gradient, this is an erroneous assumption; indeed, investigators have shown this comparison to be unreliable, with instances of overestimation and underestimation being common.[10] These differences occur for a variety of reasons including differences in sedation, loading conditions, heart rate, variations in acoustic window used, and adjustments for poststenotic pressure recovery. Our own experience including use of Doppler mean values is similar, with the most reliable correlations noted between the maximum instantaneous gradient from apical four-chamber views and the mean Doppler gradient from high parasternal imaging planes.[11] The latter is thought by some investigators to be reliable in adults. Nevertheless, the Doppler instantaneous gradient measurement is a valuable parameter for use in serial follow-up studies and should be used in conjunction with other variables such as fractional shortening (hyperdynamic function is the usual finding in children), wall stress, and thickness (see Chapter 9).

With significant aortic stenosis, the systemic arterial pressure is characterized by a smaller-than-normal pulse pressure. The small pulse of aortic stenosis (*pulsus parvus*) has stimulated many attempts to determine the severity of the aortic stenosis from the arterial pressure wave. Although this idea is solidly based in science and may be useful to a degree in adults, it is not reliable in children.

Clinical Manifestations

Congenital aortic stenosis can occur at any time from the fetal period through young adulthood. For the typical pediatric case, the child with valvar aortic stenosis (even those with moderate-severe stenosis) is asymptomatic and is growing and developing normally but is discovered to have a heart murmur during a routine physical examination. Discovery of unexpected aortic stenosis in teenagers occurs occasionally, and the required examination of students participating in sports uncovers a few new patients each year. Rarely, a child complains of typical angina pectoris with exercise; in toddlers and small children, this symptom is not well articulated, yet sometimes a child is observed who suddenly stops and clutches the anterior chest during exercise. Fainting, very rare, is another ominous finding in these children; nevertheless, exercise intolerance is not a common symptom. Infants as noted above can often have rapidly progressive disease and may present with heart failure in the first several months of life; those with the most severe type called *critical aortic stenosis* may present with cardiogenic shock with closure of the ductus arteriosus, which prior to closure allowed the right ventricle to help support the circulation. Fetal valvar aortic stenosis has been well described in the literature and can often progress to the hypoplastic left heart syndrome, described in more detail in Chapter 16.

On physical examination outside of infancy, the child is well developed and well nourished. The peripheral pulses may be small and the measured pulse pressure less than normal. Often there is a systolic thrill in the suprasternal notch; with more severe stenosis, a thrill may also be felt at the second right intercostal space. On auscultation, a constant systolic ejection click usually precedes the crescendo–decrescendo systolic murmur. The murmur is loudest at the second right interspace and is typically harsh; it transmits well into the neck (Fig. 28.3). Because ventricular systole is prolonged proportionate to the severity of aortic stenosis, the aortic component at the second heart sound is delayed, producing a narrowly split second heart sound, sometimes with the aortic closure appearing after pulmonary closure (reverse splitting) similar to what is demonstrated with left bundle branch block.

Because aortic regurgitation is commonly associated with aortic stenosis, there may be an early diastolic regurgitant murmur as well (Fig. 28.4). Aortic regurgitation is often directed caudally and best appreciated from the lower left sternal border.

Electrocardiography

The electrocardiogram is not a reliable indicator of obstruction severity other than (a) being almost always normal when the catheterization measured gradient is less than 25 mm Hg, and (b) abnormalities including increased left ventricular voltages, decreased right anterior forces, and T wave changes being more likely when the gradient is at least 50 mm Hg (Fig. 28.5). In conjunction with physical examination findings, it has some use in identifying lesser

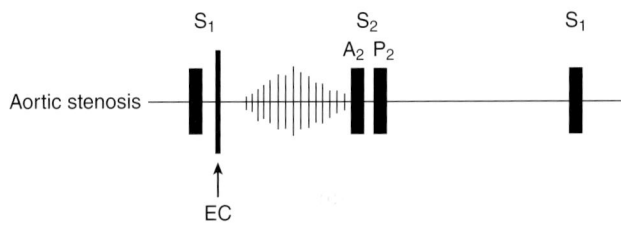

• **Fig. 28.3** Diagram of the ejection murmur of valvar aortic stenosis. Note the early systolic ejection click *(EC)* characteristic of valvar aortic stenosis. The crescendo–decrescendo murmur reaches peak intensity in mid-systole. (From Fyler DC, ed. *Nadas' Pediatric Cardiology*. Philadelphia: Hanley & Belfus, 1992.)

gradients, although the murmur intensity heavily influences the clinical assessment.

Chest X-Ray

The heart size (except in small infants in congestive heart failure) is usually normal; because of poststenotic dilation or dilation associated with a bicuspid aortic valve, the ascending aorta is often visible especially in the older patient.

Echocardiography

The number, mobility, and thickening of aortic leaflets; size of the ascending aorta; and maximum instantaneous gradient across the valve are all readily achievable. Ventricular function, wall stress, and hypertrophy information is also available (see Chapter 9). Leaflet thickness, mobility, and annular diameter at the hinge points are best evaluated in the long-axis view, whereas commissural anatomy is best seen in the short-axis view. In diastole, most aortic valves appear to be trileaflet (or tricuspid), just like on angiography. If a commissure is present, the valve leaflets separate all the way to the valve annulus, but if commissural fusion is present, separation is incomplete, and a raphe can be seen connecting the more peripheral aspects of the adjacent leaflets (Fig. 28.1A and B). Three-dimensional imaging of the valve leaflets can be helpful in further defining the leaflet sizes and shapes and for preprocedural planning.

Absence of the right–left commissure is more common than the right coronary–non-coronary commissure, whereas absence of the left coronary–noncoronary commissure is extremely rare.[5]

Regurgitation is seen best in parasternal long and short-axis views, using color flow Doppler mapping. Quantification of the regurgitation degree is very useful and is based on the diameter of the flow jet at the level of the valve seen by color flow Doppler mapping (called the *vena contracta*), the size of the left ventricle, and the Doppler flow pattern in the descending aorta. The instantaneous gradient is evaluated using pulsed or continuous-wave Doppler examination, with the transducer located in the apex, the right sternal border, or the suprasternal notch (recognizing that values may well be different in the same patient), and using sedation in the very young.

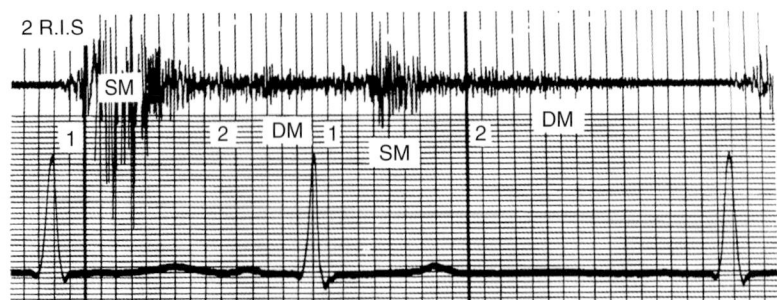

• **Fig. 28.4** Phonocardiogram of the murmurs present in a patient with valvar aortic stenosis and regurgitation. Note the diamond-shaped systolic murmur peaking in early to mid-systole and the high-frequency, lower-intensity murmur throughout diastole. *1,* First heart sound; *2,* second heart sound; *2RIS,* second right intercostal space; *DM,* diastolic murmur; *SM,* systolic murmur. (From Fyler DC, ed. *Nadas' Pediatric Cardiology*. Philadelphia: Hanley & Belfus, 1992.)

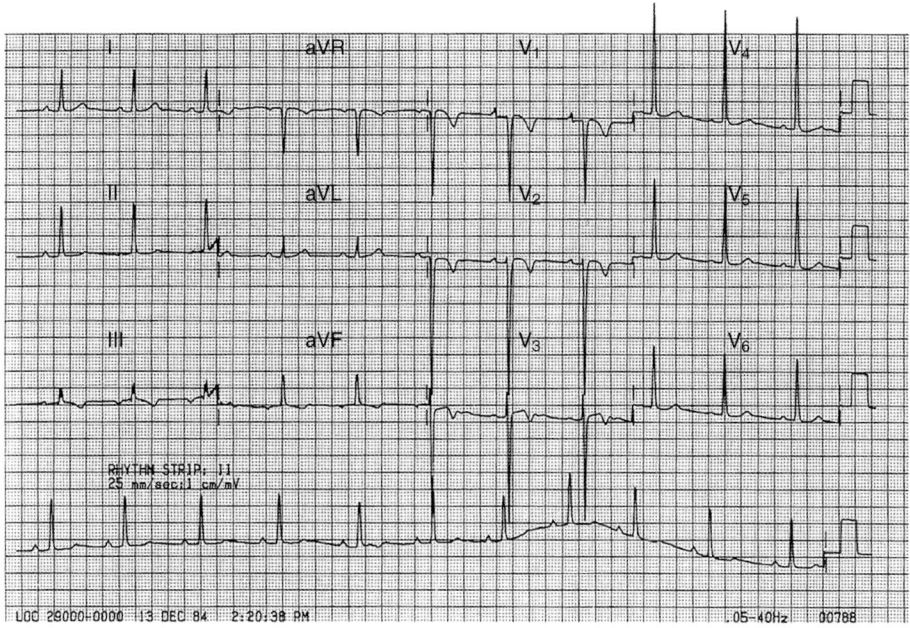

• **Fig. 28.5** Electrocardiogram from a 10-year-old boy, with peak–peak gradient of 107 mm across the aortic valve, showing marked left ventricular hypertrophy by voltage criteria and the significantly diminished anterior forces (V_1, V_2) commonly seen in pressure overload lesions.

Stress Testing

Maximal exercise testing can be a useful procedure, particularly in asymptomatic patients. Because symptoms such as angina or syncope as well as changes in the ST segment and T wave are indications for intervention, exercise testing in patients who already have these changes does not add useful information. In asymptomatic patients with normal, borderline, or suspicious findings, especially in those thought to have little obstruction who want to engage in strenuous exercise or competitive athletics, a stress test may be very valuable. Significant obstruction may be present with exertion if ST segment and T wave changes occur; however, the false-positive rate (ST changes with less severe stenosis) in children and young adults with exercise testing may be as high as 40%, so these require cautious interpretation.

Cardiac Catheterization

Due to the availability and accuracy of noninvasive evaluation, cardiac catheterization for the patient with isolated valvar aortic stenosis is now rarely undertaken for hemodynamic evaluation only. Nearly always the intention is for potential intervention, namely balloon aortic valve dilation. The indications for cardiac catheterization include the following:

1. An echocardiographic maximum instantaneous pressure gradient of 60 mm Hg or more is an indication for cardiac catheterization and probable dilation of the valve.
2. Given a lesser echo-Doppler gradient in an asymptomatic child who has no changes in the ST segment and T wave, the decision to catheterize is based on the presence/amount of left ventricular hypertrophy on echocardiography, the intensity of the murmur, and the desire to demonstrate the effects of exercise testing for a

given patient (such as potential clearance for sports participation).

3. A fainting episode in a patient who has aortic stenosis requires serious consideration of cardiac catheterization. Clearly, if the echo-Doppler evaluation indicates mild obstruction, a search for other causes of syncope is needed; but none being found, fainting, in the presence of aortic stenosis, is a signal for further study and potential therapy. Episodes of feeling dizzy or faint without actual syncope are also encountered and similarly require careful evaluation.
4. Anginal pain that is convincing has the same significance as syncope.
5. Changes in the ST segment and T wave, either on routine follow-up electrocardiograms or during stress tests, generally merits cardiac catheterization.
6. Because ventricular ectopy further complicates the delivery of cardiac output through an obstructive valve, and may otherwise be a signal of left ventricular impairment, the tendency to obtain hemodynamic data and possibly intervene is increased when ectopy is present. The peak–peak pressure gradient across the valve is a precise measure of the degree of obstruction, provided the cardiac output is not depressed.

Cardiac output is routinely measured in these patients, either by the Fick method using oximetry or by thermodilution techniques. The measured gradient determines whether a balloon angioplasty should be carried out and is usually done if the peak–peak gradient is more than 40 mm Hg (in the setting of normal cardiac output) and aortic regurgitation, if present, is mild at most. The end-diastolic pressure, if elevated, can be another factor included in the decision to balloon dilate those with borderline gradients for intervention. Contrast injected in the mid-ascending aorta in the anteroposterior and lateral views outlines the aortic valve, degree of aortic regurgitation if any, and the jet of unopacified blood being ejected through the valve from the left ventricle. Anatomic valve information is also provided; for example, in those with absence of the intercoronary commissure, the most common bicuspid valve anomaly, the conjoined cusp in the lateral view is visible as a continuous band of contrast undivided by a commissure when the valve is open in systole (Fig. 28.6). For measurement of the valve annulus for proposed valve dilation, this is done from a long axial oblique projection with contrast injection in the left ventricle.

Management

In marked contrast to pulmonary valvar stenosis (see Chapter 25), which is easily diagnosed, quantitated, and treated and is essentially free of endocarditis, valvar aortic stenosis is a difficult entity to treat and requires lifelong attention. It is progressive, may be associated with catastrophic incidents such as sudden death, is likely to require repeated interventions, and is a common site for endocarditis.[9] Calcification with age is common, and regurgitation may become a significant problem, as may left ventricular dysfunction, all problems related to its location in the systemic circuit.

Excluding infants in heart failure, it is reasonable to use the severity categories of peak–peak catheterization gradients as outlined in the original Natural History Study as guides to management.[7,9] These groups consisted of those with gradients of less than 25 mm Hg, 25–49 mm Hg,

50–79 mm Hg, and greater than 80 mm Hg—all require strict endocarditis prophylaxis. For those with a stable gradient of less than 25 mm Hg and normal electrocardiogram and stress test, no restriction on physical activities is reasonable. For those with a 25- to 49-mm Hg gradient and normal electrocardiogram and stress test, strenuous competitive level activities should be considered carefully. Annual evaluations should be done for both groups. For all others, that is with gradients greater than 50 mm Hg, intervention is indicated. In earlier years, before balloon valvotomy, a surgical valvotomy was always done for a gradient of 80 mm Hg or more, with management strategy varying between institutions for values ranging from 50 to 79 mm Hg. In the latter, however, better results at follow-up were evident in those managed surgically.[7] Thus, when balloon valvotomy became available as an alternative to surgery (mid-1980s), a peak–peak gradient of 50 mm Hg or more, in the absence of more than mild aortic regurgitation, became an indicator for intervention. In many institutions in the United States and other countries, balloon aortic valvotomy replaced surgery as the initial procedure in these patients.

By and large, balloon aortic valvotomy has been quite effective as initial treatment strategy, with an acute peak–peak gradient reduction of at least 50% typical. However, aortic regurgitation is common after this procedure, and although mild in most cases, moderate or greater regurgitation occurs in 14%, more commonly in older patients. In a large study of 509 children and adolescents with congenital aortic stenosis from our own institution undergoing the procedure at a median of 2.4 years of age, overall survival rate at 5, 10, and 20 years was 95%, 93%, and 88%, respectively. Survival rate free from any aortic valve reintervention was 89%, 72%, 65% and 27% at 1, 5, 10, and 20 years, respectively.[12] Results from surgical series of mixed ages have generally demonstrated similar short- and long-term results,[13,14] although with the refinement of surgical techniques there is renewed interest in surgical relief of aortic stenosis, particularly when other associated lesions may require a surgical approach.

In terms of balloon equipment, considerable improvement has continued such that arterial access problems are considerably less than they were 10-15 years ago. The effectiveness of balloon dilation is remarkable when one considers that a balloon is being inflated across the usually eccentrically located orifice of a valve whose leaflets vary in both thickness and commissural fusion. Clearly, the weakest site in the orifice "rim" will be the first to tear or separate, whether it be commissure or a leaflet at its free margin edge or its attachment site to the aorta. Indeed, the latter is a frequent observation at later surgery for regurgitation, the detachment frequently being anteriorly located. Nevertheless, balloon dilation remains the initial treatment of choice for significant valvar stenoses given the reasonable results, very short hospital stay, and absence of both a sternotomy scar and cardiopulmonary bypass. Balloon dilation, however, is largely ineffective in adults, in whom valves are by then often deformed and calcified. Surgical valve repair or

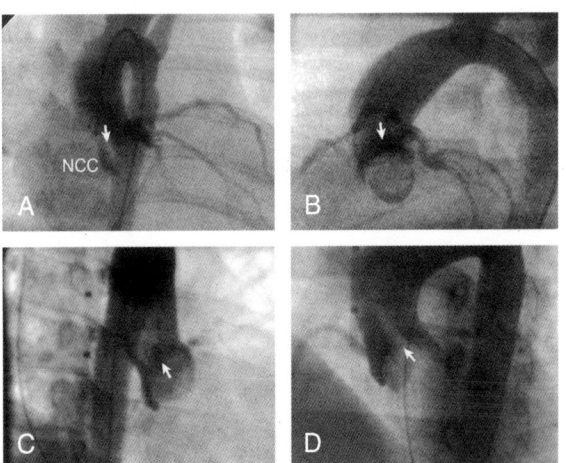

• **Fig. 28.6** Biplane aortic cineangiograms, during ventricular systole, in two children with bicuspid stenotic valves: (1) Absent R-L commissure: **(A)** Frontal projection showing presence of right non-coronary cusp (NCC) commissure *(arrow)*. **(B)** Lateral projection showing absence of R-L commissure, identified by solid bar of contrast *(arrow)* extending the entire width of the common cusp. (2) Absent N-R commissure: **(C)** Right anterior oblique projection showing solid bar of contrast *(arrow)* extending across the common cusp. **(D)** Long axial oblique projection showing presence of right–left commissure *(arrow)*; absence of the non–left cusp commissure is extremely rare.

replacement is usually necessary, especially if accompanied by moderate or more regurgitation.

Clinical Course

The likelihood that progressive obstruction will have occurred by late adult life is high, even in those with a less than 25-mm Hg gradient to begin with. In the pediatric years, significant progression in the Natural History Study occurred in one-third of all patients managed medically.[7] The 25-year survival rate for all patients was 85%, 92% for those with initial gradients of less than 50 mm Hg, and 80% for those greater. By 25 years, only 60% of medically managed patients remained intervention free, and 60% of the surgically treated patients had undergone reoperation. Sudden death was a rare event, occurring in 25 (5%) patients during the study period. Of these, 75% were postoperative patients, all with significant obstruction, regurgitation, or both; one younger than age 10 years was catheterization related; most were older than 20 years; and one-fourth were related to endocarditis. This was, of course, a population studied and operated on between 1958 and 1979, since when surgical and other techniques have improved greatly.

Residual or recurrent obstruction with at most mild regurgitation in pediatric years can be managed by surgical valvotomy or balloon dilation, the latter being both repeatable and effective although the risk of significant aortic regurgitation becomes greater with repeat procedures (Fig. 28.7). In later years, valve repair or replacement becomes necessary in many using a variety of repair techniques, prosthetic devices, or the patient's transplanted pulmonary valve (Ross procedure). The latter requires replacement of the transplanted pulmonary valve, typically by a homograft from right ventricle to pulmonary artery. Results with the Ross operation have varied considerably across reporting centers, with generally good long-term autograft durability

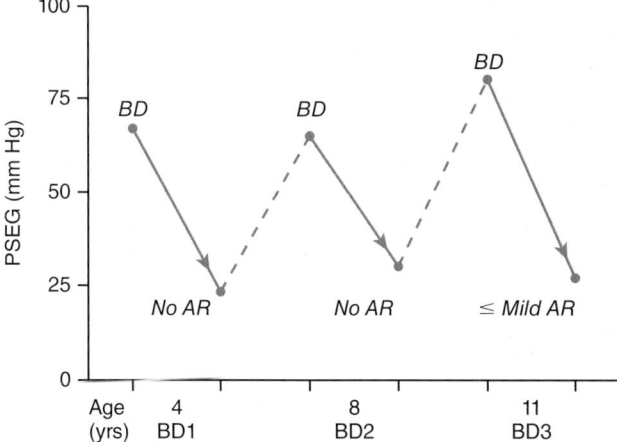

• **Fig. 28.7** Balloon dilation *(BD)* performed on three occasions in a patient with recurrent obstruction at ages 4, 8, and 11 years for peak–peak gradients of at least 70 mm Hg, each followed by reduction to about 25 mm Hg with only mild, at most, regurgitation after the final procedure. *AR,* aortic regurgitation|; *PSEG,* peak systolic ejection gradient.

but high rates of right ventricular outflow tract reintervention, particularly in the young.[15] Prosthetic devices with mechanical leaflets requiring anticoagulation are avoided when possible in women approaching childbearing age.

Exercise intolerance is not a common symptom and is rarely a factor in deciding management questions. In contrast, stress tests do uncover patients who are prone to arrhythmias and changes in the ST segment and T wave during maximal exercise, an observation that should be taken seriously.[16] Rhythm abnormalities, at rest or on exercise, are encountered and are taken as a sign of ventricular dysfunction, and sometimes influence the decision to intervene. Abnormalities in ventricular function tests, volume measurements, shortening fractions, and other indices (see Chapter 9) should be taken seriously, particularly if a pattern of deterioration is documented in the course of follow-up.

Exercise restriction for patients with aortic stenosis has evolved over time to be less conservative than in prior decades, although still recommended for those with more severe obstruction. Evidence in favor of this practice includes the association with sudden death in those with severe aortic stenosis observed in natural history studies,[9] as well as the finding that large registry studies of athletes with sudden death have often included a small number of patients with undiagnosed aortic stenosis.[17] Balancing these observations is more recent evidence that sudden death in those with appropriately treated aortic stenosis is very rare,[18] along with increasing appreciation for the many physiologic and socioemotional benefits of sports participation and vigorous exercise in all patients with congenital heart disease. Current guidelines thus recommend exercise restriction for those with moderate or worse disease, although in clinical practice these are not always strictly adhered to by clinicians.

Summary recommendations for the older child/adolescent with valvar aortic stenosis:

- Regular cardiology follow-up, typically annually, including electrocardiogram and echocardiogram is essential. Follow-up is a lifetime commitment and, for most patients, requires visits to the cardiologist when there are, in fact, no symptoms or limitations.
- Those with hemodynamic gradients > 50 mm Hg should be treated due to the high risk of ventricular arrhythmias, heart failure, and sudden death. Those with hemodynamic gradients < 25 mm Hg are at lower risk and can be followed regularly. Those with hemodynamic gradients 25–50 mm Hg are at intermediate risk and merit close monitoring for symptoms or any changes in clinical testing.
- Symptoms including chest pain with exercise and syncope are rare, but serious, and may merit further evaluation including catheterization even with suspected mild disease.
- Formal exercise testing should be considered for those with more than mild obstruction by echocardiography, and even in the absence of ST and T wave changes on electrocardiogram, particularly in those desiring clearance for athletic participation.

- Infective endocarditis remains a potential threat, although antibiotic prophylaxis to prevent it is not recommended except for patients with a prior history of endocarditis or in those with prosthetic aortic valves.

Neonatal Aortic Stenosis

Neonates with critical valvar aortic stenosis constitute a special group with maximal aortic valve obstruction. A murmur may have been noticed at birth and, indeed, the diagnosis of aortic stenosis may have already been made by fetal echocardiography (fetal aortic stenosis is reviewed in detail in Chapter 16). Congestive failure develops in the first weeks of life and, very rapidly, a life-threatening situation evolves. It is important to remember that some of these infants initially in the first few days of life look clinically well and seem to be tolerating some obstruction even with what seems a moderate, at most, instantaneous gradient of less than 30 mm Hg. Such gradients may increase rapidly within weeks, perhaps related to left ventricular function becoming hyperdynamic and lesions such as patent ductus and muscular ventricular defects spontaneously closing (Fig. 28.8).

The valves in these infants are notable, sometimes appearing as gelatinous blobs of tissue unrecognizable as

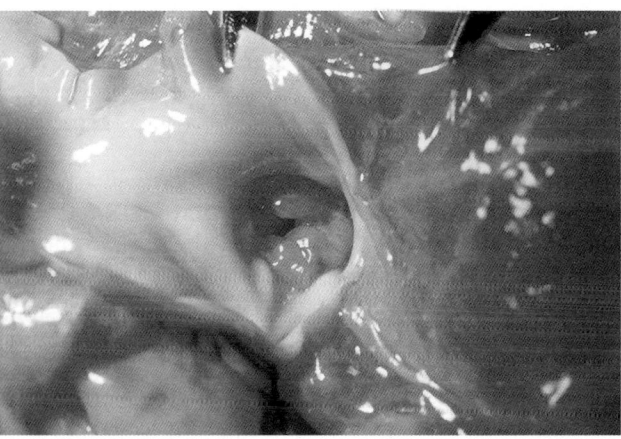

• **Fig. 28.9** Autopsy picture of a nodular primitive-looking critically obstructive valve in a 4-week-old baby who died suddenly at home, undiagnosed. Such valves with survival can mature to become typically bicuspid structures.

leaflets (Fig. 28.9). The left ventricle may be hypoplastic, and for some infants, it is too small to be compatible with life. A newborn ventricle that can accommodate a maximal volume of 20 mL is borderline in its ability to support life. Because of left ventricular failure, acquired mitral regurgitation, and gross elevation of left atrial pressures, the foramen ovale becomes incompetent, and atrial left to right shunting adds to the problems, further aggravating congestive heart failure. Shunting right to left through the ductus arteriosus is helpful in this situation because it allows the right ventricle to contribute some systemic cardiac output that does not have to pass through the aortic valve. Thus, in the most critical situation, administration of prostaglandin E_1 opens the ductus, thereby augmenting cardiac output and stabilizing the infant.

On physical examination, the infant is in congestive heart failure, sometimes in shock, and is ashen and pulseless. Most have an apical ejection click and a systolic murmur. The intensity of the ejection murmur depends on left ventricular function status and indeed may be absent in those with extremely poor function. Many have a murmur of mitral regurgitation due to ventricular dysfunction. The electrocardiogram shows right or left ventricular hypertrophy with changes in the ST segment and T wave (Fig. 28.10). The chest x-ray shows an enlarged heart with pulmonary edema on echocardiography. On echocardiography, the obstructed, usually very thickened aortic valve is well seen, as is any mitral regurgitation, atrial left-to-right shunting, right-to-left shunting at the ductal level, and any aortic arch abnormality. The degree of stenosis can be estimated and related to left ventricular function. Importantly, the adequacy of left ventricular volume can be determined as to whether it is of sufficient size to supply a systemic cardiac output.

Catheterization in these infants, often intubated and being administered prostaglandin E_1, since the late 1980s has been carried out as a therapeutic procedure, that is, for balloon dilation. From a historical standpoint,

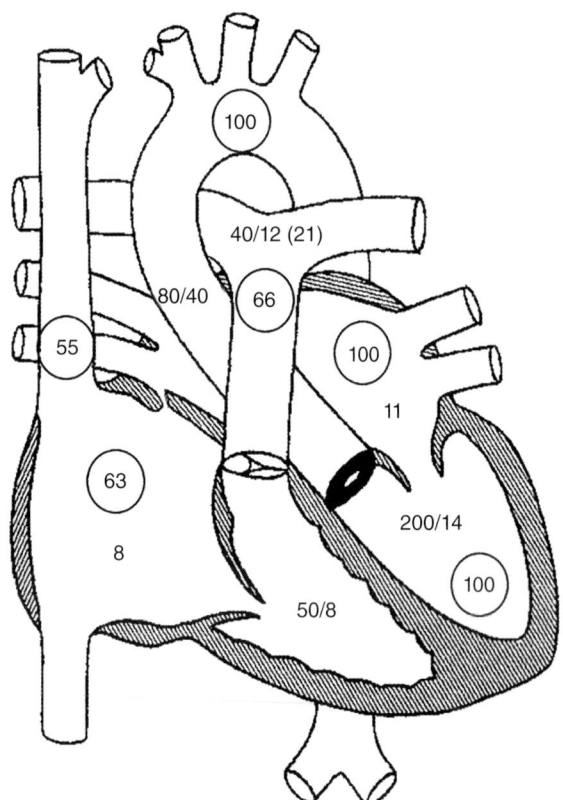

• **Fig. 28.8** Catheterization data in a 40-day-old boy showing a peak–peak ejection gradient of 120 mm Hg. An echocardiographic study at age 2 days revealed a maximum instantaneous gradient of 30 mm Hg and normal ventricular function. Oximetry data represented in *circles*, pressure data in millimeters of mercury (mm Hg).

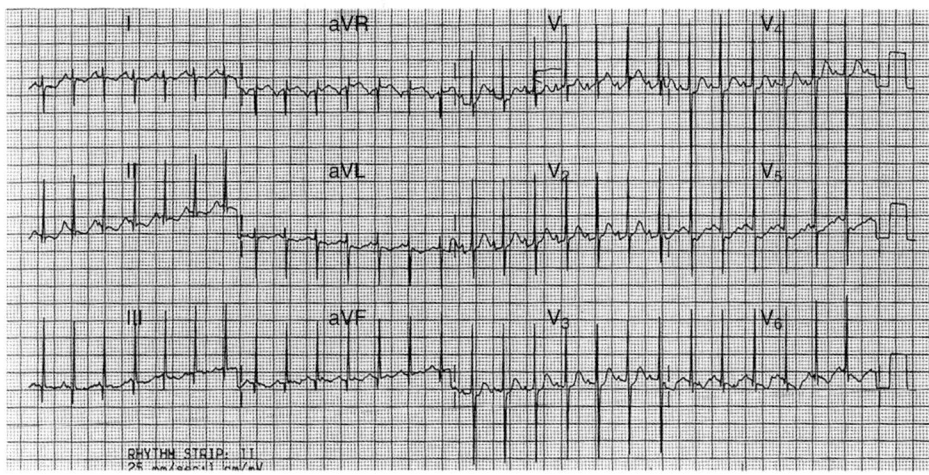

• Fig. 28.10 Electrocardiogram from a 10-day-old boy with critical aortic valvar stenosis with a peak–peak systolic ejection gradient of 90 mm Hg showing left ventricular hypertrophy with strain, especially in leads V$_5$ and V$_6$.

surgical valvotomy was introduced in the 1960s because medical management previously had a universally fatal outcome. Within a decade, it was apparent that only a limited valvotomy, that is, modestly enlarging the orifice, was necessary to achieve excellent early clinical results, including significantly decreasing the incidence of severe aortic regurgitation, often a result of the early extensive valvotomies. It was also noted that at later repeat surgical valvotomy, the originally immature nodular and myxomatous-appearing valves had usually evolved into valves with a more typical bicuspid appearance. Balloon dilation was later introduced as an alternative management strategy in the late 1980s, and using the surgical approach of limited valvotomy, smaller balloons with an average balloon-to-annular ratio of 0.8 were used with satisfactory results. Balloon technology has improved considerably over the years, with much lower profiles and sizes becoming available. With balloon dilation, the major immediate changes at catheterization indicating success are significant decreases in left ventricular systolic, diastolic, and atrial pressures and peak–peak gradient (about 50%) (Fig. 28.11). These are followed by rapid extubation, an excellent clinical course, significant improvement in mitral regurgitation, and disappearance of atrial-level shunts.

The survival rate for treatment of neonatal aortic stenosis with balloon valvotomy is at least 75% at 8 years, with about one-third requiring redilation for obstruction; some 10–15% have significant (moderate or worse) regurgitation. In some, initially hypoplastic aortic annuli and left ventricular chambers on echocardiography normalize during follow-up. With further refinements in surgical techniques, some centers have reported similar outcomes with surgical valvotomy in this setting,[13,14] although due to the increased morbidity and recovery time associated with surgery many centers prefer balloon valvotomy as the initial approach for patients without associated defects requiring surgery.

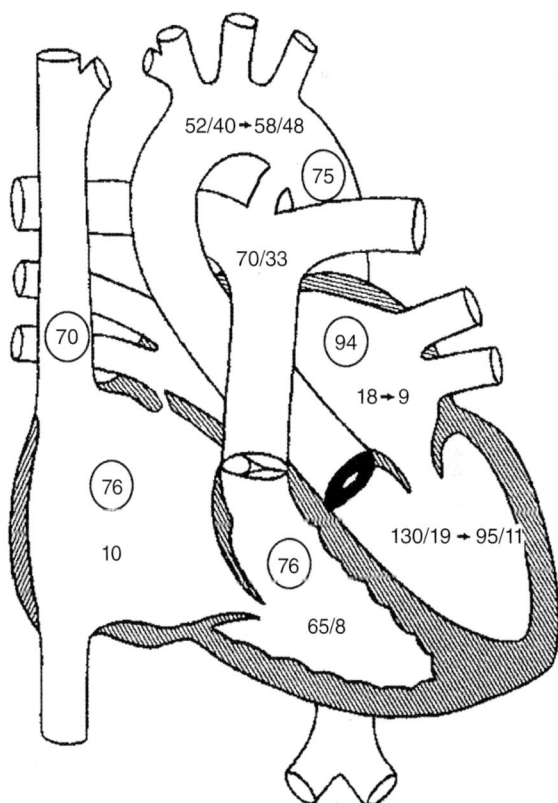

• Fig. 28.11 Catheterization data in an 11-day-old neonate with critical aortic valvar obstruction who underwent balloon dilation through an umbilical arterial retrograde approach, showing marked immediate reduction *(numbers with arrows)* in gradient, left ventricular systolic and diastolic, and left atrial pressures in millimeters of mercury (mm Hg). Baseline oximetry data is shown in *circles*.

Subaortic Stenosis

Definition

Obstruction to outflow from the left ventricle beneath the aortic valve in the presence of two adequate-sized ventricles is called subaortic stenosis.

Prevalence

Subaortic stenosis is rarely recognized in the newborn period but is common in infancy and childhood. It is often associated with other lesions, such as VSD, coarctation of the aorta, interrupted aortic arch, double-chambered right ventricle, and atrioventricular canal. Isolated subaortic stenosis is the second most common form of left ventricular outflow tract obstruction, accounting for some 10–14% of patients, and similar to valvar stenosis, more common in males.

Pathology

There are four distinct types of subvalvar aortic stenosis (Fig. 28.12).
- Discrete type
  The most common form is a discrete, thin, fibromuscular ridge or membrane located at a variable distance beneath the aortic valve, sometimes so close to the valve that the obstructing tissue is difficult to distinguish from the valve itself. Indeed in some cases, this tissue has been noted to progressively involve the undersurface of the aortic valve leaflets, causing reduced leaflet mobility and valve dysfunction. Although the term membranous subaortic stenosis is occasionally used, this can be misleading because the obstructing tissue usually has some thickness and a fibromuscular component is often present. The opening may be eccentric. The part of the obstruction situated beneath the left coronary cusp, which is frequently attached to the anterior leaflet of the mitral valve, causes the characteristic fluttering and thickening of that leaflet as seen on echocardiography and angiography. Over time, likely due to the high-velocity jet of blood across the subvalvar obstruction, thickening and distortion of the aortic valve leaflets may be observed, leading to aortic regurgitation. The obstruction itself is variable in that a complete circumferential ring is not always present. Indeed by echocardiography, a small non-obstructive localized protuberance from the region of the membranous septum is frequently identified as an early precursor to subsequent obstruction. Downstream cardiac

defects that obstruct blood flow, such as interrupted aortic arch and severe coarctation, are common and sometimes are associated with a membranous VSD or a mitral valve deformity. Severe subvalvar obstruction is rare in neonates: however, progression during childhood is well recognized, this was also noted decades ago in Newfoundland dogs.
- Tunnel type
  The rarer fibromuscular tunnel has greater length, often affecting 1 cm or more of the outflow tract. Because of its length, or perhaps contributing to it, the anterior leaflet of the mitral valve is often involved, a feature of some significance at the time of surgical correction.
- Hypertrophic subaortic stenosis
  Cardiomyopathy of the idiopathic hypertrophic variety often produces clinically important subaortic obstruction, often solely due to muscle but sometimes involving the anterior leaflet of the mitral valve. This type of obstruction is reviewed in detail elsewhere (see Chapter 48).
- Accessory endocardial cushion tissue
  Rarely, tissue presumed to be derived from the embryologic endocardial cushions may obstruct the left ventricular outflow tract. It may be attached to a pedicle or act as a sail or sheet across the outflow tract, moving with cardiac contraction and the flow of blood.
  Subaortic stenosis is commonly associated with a wide range of other cardiac defects, particularly VSD and coarctation.

Pathogenesis

The etiology of the obstruction remains unknown, but anatomic abnormalities of the outflow tract, such as separation of aortic and mitral valve annuli, acute angulation of ventricular septal and ascending aortic axes, and aortic override have been described in these patients. This anatomic substrate and resulting turbulent flow through the left ventricular outflow tract is thought to lead to endothelial sheer stress, fibrosis and a vicious cycle of worsening obstruction, left ventricular hypertrophy, and hyperdynamic left ventricular function.

Physiology

The physiologic abnormalities are comparable to those seen in valvar aortic stenosis, except that subaortic stenosis is almost never severe enough to cause congestive heart failure in infancy, at least as an isolated lesion. Concentric left ventricular hypertrophy as a response to worsening outflow obstruction is typical, along with usually hyperdynamic systolic function. The associated aortic regurgitation is rarely severe in children preoperatively, and indeed moderate or worse regurgitation (some 14% of all patients) is largely confined to those who have had surgical or balloon angioplasty procedures for associated valvar disease.

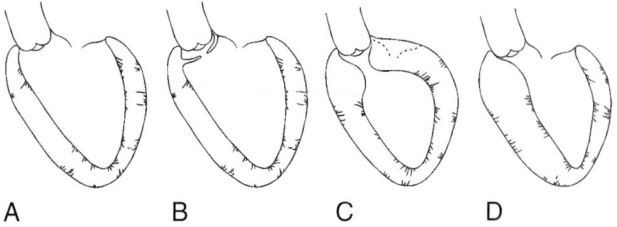

A   **B**   **C**   **D**

• **Fig. 28.12** Drawings illustrating three types of subaortic stenosis: **(A)** normal; **(B)** membranous; **(C)** fibromuscular tunnel; **(D)** hypertrophic cardiomyopathy with subaortic obstruction. (From Fyler DC, ed. *Nadas' Pediatric Cardiology*. Philadelphia: Hanley & Belfus, 1992.)

Clinical Manifestations and Physical Examination

Isolated subaortic stenosis produces a stenotic systolic murmur that often has a characteristic "shrieking" quality at the mid left sternal border. Sometimes a precordial thrill may also be present with severe obstruction, in the same location. Usually, there is no systolic click, unless a bicuspid aortic valve is also present; some patients have an early diastolic blowing murmur of aortic regurgitation, often best appreciated at the left lower sternal border. Unlike valvar aortic stenosis, the peripheral pulses are rarely thought of as small, and congestive heart failure resulting from isolated subaortic stenosis is virtually non-existent.

Electrocardiography

The electrocardiogram usually shows left ventricular hypertrophy in proportion to the degree of obstruction. Mild obstruction often produces no abnormality, whereas severe obstruction results in left ventricular hypertrophy with changes in the ST segments and T waves.

Chest X-Ray

The isolated form of subaortic stenosis is not characterized by cardiac enlargement or enlargement of the ascending aorta. Finding an abnormality on the chest x-ray is unusual unless there are associated defects.

Echocardiography

Echocardiography is the standard diagnostic tool for subaortic stenosis, using two- and three-dimensional imaging along with spectral and color Doppler. The anatomy of the lesion is clearly outlined (Fig. 28.13), as is ventricular function. The amount of ventricular muscle hypertrophy is usually proportional to the degree of obstruction, the latter measured as a maximum instantaneous gradient. Fluttering of the left coronary cusp due to the jet across the obstruction is usual, as is leaflet thickening. The maximum and mean instantaneous Doppler gradient by echocardiography correlate reasonably well with catheterization gradients, with some of the same measurement differences discussed with valvar stenosis; however, care must be taken to ensure that with continuous wave Doppler any mitral regurgitation is not contaminating the assessment (a common problem in patients with hypertrophic cardiomyopathy). Aortic regurgitation, which tends to evolve over time and is usually mild or less, is evident on color flow Doppler. Any associated lesions are also outlined.

Cardiac Catheterization

Cardiac catheterization provides a reliable measurement of the peak–peak pressure gradient across the outflow tract of the left ventricle in the sedated patient (Fig. 28.14). This gradient is generally less, sometimes by as much as 50%, than instantaneous gradients of less than 50 mm Hg. Because anatomic information is readily available by echocardiography, the only reason for catheterization is for gradient measurement for management decisions; often catheterization is helpful in determining the relative contributions if multiple levels of left ventricular outflow tract obstruction are present. The ventricular end-diastolic pressure is also sometimes helpful in guiding management decisions. Subaortic stenosis is not relieved by balloon dilation and thus is not performed for this purpose. If angiography is carried out, a right anterior oblique with 20 degrees of caudal angulation (Fig. 28.15) and simultaneous long-axis oblique views provide excellent visualization. The degree of aortic regurgitation may be demonstrated by angiography to complement the echocardiographic assessment.

Management

In the patient with uncomplicated discrete membranous obstruction, surgical treatment is more definitive than in the patient with valvar aortic stenosis. Balloon dilation, on the other hand, is ineffective. Thus, because obstruction is

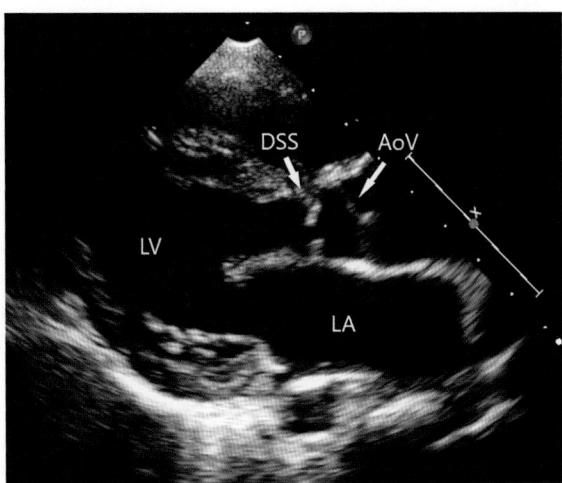

• **Fig. 28.13** Parasternal long-axis echocardiogram of discrete subaortic stenosis *(DSS)* located several millimeters below the aortic valve *(AoV)*. *LA,* Left atrium; *LV,* left ventricle.

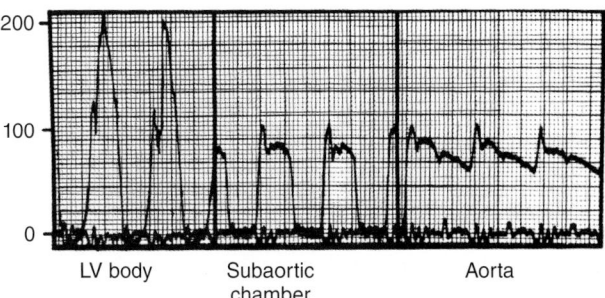

• **Fig. 28.14** Pressure recorded during withdrawal of a catheter from the left ventricle to the aorta in a patient with subaortic stenosis. Note that as the catheter passes the obstructed area, the left ventricular pressure falls; only when it is withdrawn across the aortic valve does a typical arterial pressure contour appear. Sometimes, the space between the subvalvar obstruction and the aortic valve is so small that this type of tracing cannot be recorded. (From Fyler DC, ed. *Nadas' Pediatric Cardiology*. Philadelphia: Hanley & Belfus, 1992.)

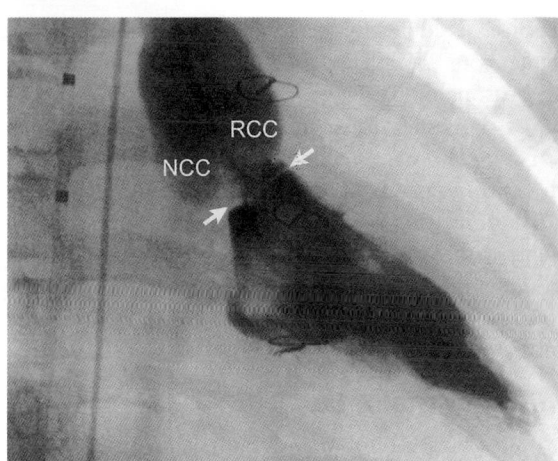

• **Fig. 28.15** Left ventricular cineangiogram in a 9-year-old boy in a right anterior oblique view showing a discrete subaortic membrane *(arrows)*. This had developed since he underwent surgical valvuloplasty 6 years earlier. *NCC,* Non-coronary cusp; *RCC,* right coronary cusp.

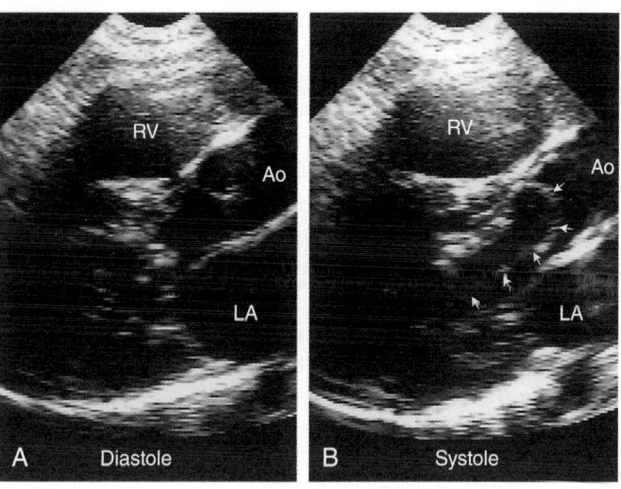

• **Fig. 28.16** Parasternal long-axis echocardiogram of the left ventricular outflow tract at end-diastole (A) and mid-systole (B) showing atypical subaortic stenosis secondary to accessory atrioventricular valve tissue that billows into the ascending aorta during ejection (arrows). *Ao,* Aorta; *LA,* left atrium; *RV,* right ventricle.

progressive in many, and because aortic regurgitation at some point is common, surgical treatment is recommended for a lower peak–peak gradient than for valvar obstruction (30 versus 50 mm Hg). Because the echocardiographically measured Doppler instantaneous gradient commonly exceeds the peak–peak value obtained at catheterization (often due to differences in level of sedation and heart rate), it is reasonable to assume that a catheterization value of 30 mm Hg is similar to a maximum instantaneous value of 50 mm Hg. Thus, a Doppler maximum instantaneous value exceeding this is typically used as an indicator for surgery. Because obstruction recur in some 20% postoperatively,[19] patients with instantaneous gradients less than 50 mm Hg without other indicators can be followed medically. Aortic regurgitation commonly develops over time, although usually mild in most cases; however, the appearance of mild aortic regurgitation is often considered an additional indicator for surgery to prevent progression to more significant regurgitation.

Surgical techniques have changed over the years from simple membrane excision alone to more extensive resection, including stripping of any associated tissue from the undersurface of the aortic leaflets and septal myectomy. Occasionally, in the past, excision of tissue from the anterior leaflet of the mitral valve resulted in perforation of that structure, and septal muscle excision resulted in VSD creation, and/or conduction difficulties including complete heart block. The likelihood of complete heart block in most reported series for an initial operation is approximately 5%, and increases with repeat operations. Mortality following surgery for subaortic stenosis is very low. In those with more diffuse tunnel-like obstructions, more extensive procedures, such as trigone release, Ross and Konno or modifications thereof, may be necessary.

Subaortic obstruction due to accessory endocardial tissue is a very rare entity. Currently, this entity is identified by echocardiography. Associated cardiac lesions such as complete atrioventricular canal, tetralogy of Fallot, and coarctation occur in some. Echocardiographically, the most common appearance is that of a parachute-like structure appearing in the outflow tract during systole (Fig. 28.16). The degree of obstruction is quite variable. Anatomically, this accessory tissue often has a number of attachments to the mitral valve leaflets, conal septum, or even the papillary muscles. At surgery, the lesion is typically removed through the aortic valve with elimination of obstruction. In certain cases, a combined transaortic and mitral approach may be necessary to address this obstructive lesion.

Clinical Course

Although discrete obstruction is known to progress in many young patients, a substantial number of patients with mild obstruction remain stable for decades with evidence of slow progression in late life. Adult series have demonstrated a relatively slow rate of progression relative to children. Aortic regurgitation in unoperated patients, although common, is rarely of a significant degree even into adult life; indeed, significant regurgitation almost always occurs only in those who have undergone a procedure (angioplasty or surgery) or who have had endocarditis.[20] Postoperatively, among series extending over decades, recurrent obstruction occurs in about 20%, often requiring more extensive procedures. Such a scenario is more likely when obstruction is of the tunnel variety. Other documented risk factors for recurrence in pediatric patients include younger age at initial operation, higher preoperative maximum instantaneous gradient, close proximity to the aortic valve annulus, and the presence of associated aortic valve stenosis.[19]

Summary recommendations for the older child/adolescent with subaortic stenosis

- For patients with maximum instantaneous Doppler gradient < 50 mm Hg and no more than trivial aortic regurgitation, surgery is often deferred with close follow-up.
- Those with more severe obstruction or with mild or worse aortic regurgitation usually merit a surgical approach.
- Those with maximum instantaneous gradients < 30 mm Hg may be followed conservatively; due to the tendency for progression, regular follow-up is required.

Supravalvar Aortic Stenosis

Definition

Supravalvar aortic stenosis denotes obstructive constriction of the ascending aorta above the aortic valve. This anomaly is commonly associated with Williams syndrome, and other vascular lesions such as coarctation, coronary artery or renal artery stenoses, and peripheral pulmonary stenosis may also be present.

Prevalence

Supravalvar aortic stenosis is the least common form of left ventricular outflow tract obstruction, accounting for approximately 10% of cases.[1] Many patients have Williams syndrome (also known as Williams-Beuren syndrome), a complex developmental disorder usually caused by a microdeletion of chromosome 7q11.23 (see Chapter 6). This region includes the elastin gene, which is thought to be the pathogenesis of the observed arteriopathy. Various familial forms of elastin arteriopathy have been reported, usually inherited in an autosomal dominant pattern and without Williams syndrome features, with most demonstrating various mutations in the elastin gene.[21] Supravalvar aortic stenosis has also been reported as a sporadic problem without a family history, which may represent patients with new mutations in the elastin gene.

The majority of patients have discrete constriction with an obstructing ring of thickened aortic wall, sometimes asymmetric, situated above the aortic valve and the sinuses of Valsalva. The edge of the obstructing tissue may impinge on a sinus of Valsalva as noted, compromising flow to the coronary ostia. Occasionally, the coronary occlusion is complete, a leaflet of the distorted aortic valve adhering to the obstructing collar of tissue. When the aortic lumen is compromised, there is proportionate left ventricular hypertension and hypertrophy. The obstruction is commonly localized, but in about 20%, it extends diffusely into the ascending aorta (Fig. 28.17). The aortic leaflets are often thickened and distorted, sometimes adherent to the aortic wall, but although aortic regurgitation is common, it is rarely severe.

Some patients have other vascular obstructions as noted. Peripheral pulmonary stenosis with hypoplasia of the pulmonary arteries occurs in 30%, coarctation of the aorta in 15%, renal artery stenosis in 5%; obstructions may also occur in branches of the aorta. In those with Williams syndrome, some 85% have cardiovascular anomalies, with supravalvar aortic stenosis in 71%, peripheral pulmonary stenosis in 38%, and mitral regurgitation in about 20%, sometime progressive.[22] Abdominal coarctation of the aorta has been described and may lead to renal vascular involvement. These obstructions in the aorta can be acquired and are often progressive. Indeed, all these peripheral phenomena may be seen in the absence of supravalvar aortic stenosis and are sometimes readily recognized as part of Williams syndrome.

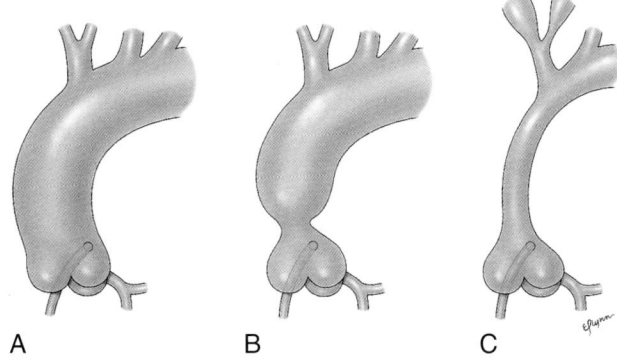

- **Fig. 28.17** The anatomic types of supravalvar aortic stenosis: **(A)** normal; **(B)** and **(C)** two forms of supravalvar stenosis. The difference between these two forms is in the length of the obstruction, which sometimes involves virtually all the ascending aorta. Note the obstructions in the innominate and common carotid arteries as they arise from the aortic arch. Other obstructions, such as coarctation of the aorta, renal artery stenosis, and pulmonary artery stenosis, are found in some patients. (From Fyler DC, ed. *Nadas' Pediatric Cardiology*. Philadelphia: Hanley & Belfus, 1992.)

Physiology

The physiology is comparable to that of valvar aortic stenosis except that coronary blood flow is usually under increased pressure, being proximal to the aortic obstruction. Exceptions to this include patients with associated coronary ostial stenosis, or less commonly, due to entrapment of a coronary sinus from lumen narrowing and leaflet attachments to the supravalvar ridge. In these situations, the demands of a hypertrophied ventricle, with coronary ostial or pre-coronary obstruction, are likely to result in a marked mismatch of myocardial demand and perfusion. Some patients with supravalvar aortic stenosis are thus high risk for procedural care (e.g., with induction of anesthesia for catheterization or surgery), with the group of patients with biventricular outflow tract obstruction being notoriously prone to adverse cardiovascular events.[23] Sudden death has also been reported in this high-risk group, although sudden death may occur even in those with Williams syndrome even in the absence of outflow tract obstruction.

Clinical Manifestations and Physical Exam

Patients with Williams syndrome have typical elfin facies, dental problems, hypercalcemia, short stature, intellectual disability, and often a friendly, cheerful personality. Patients in whom this diagnosis is suspected should be evaluated for possible supravalvar aortic stenosis. Otherwise, supravalvar stenosis is discovered in these patients because of a basilar murmur, sometimes associated with a thrill. There may be a family history of supravalvar aortic stenosis. These children tend to grow poorly; they may have exercise intolerance and, occasionally, angina with effort. Syncope has been reported.

On physical examination, other than evidence of Williams syndrome, patients have a systolic murmur over the base of the heart and in the suprasternal notch, the latter often associated with a shudder or thrill. There may be hypertension if coarctation of the aorta or renal artery stenosis is present. Murmurs suggesting peripheral pulmonary stenosis may be audible, as may the murmur of minimal aortic insufficiency. Hypercalcemia is seen in patients with Williams syndrome in early infancy.

Electrocardiography

If the obstruction in the ascending aorta is severe, there will be left ventricular hypertrophy. Prolongation of the QTc occurs in approximately 14% of patients with Williams syndrome, and may contribute to the risk of sudden death reported in these patients. Familial forms of elastin arteriopathy in the absence of Williams syndrome typically do not demonstrate prolonged QTc.

Chest X-Ray

The heart may be somewhat enlarged due to left ventricular hypertrophy, but a chest x-ray is rarely helpful in this diagnosis.

Echocardiography

The diagnosis is identified at echocardiography. The anatomy of the aortic valve leaflets, the sinuses of Valsalva, the coronary arteries, and the supravalvar obstructing collar can be visualized and Doppler estimations of the pressure gradient across the obstructed area made. The supravalvar narrowing is most readily imaged in a parasternal long-axis view (Fig. 28.18), the appearance of the lesion being generally much less impressive than the measured gradient. Wall thickening at the site of obstruction is generally apparent. The aortic valve leaflets may appear thickened and may move abnormally despite absence of commissural fusion. The left ventricular myocardial thickness is generally indicative of the degree of obstruction.

The aortic arch and brachiocephalic vessels should be imaged because coarctation and stenosis of the brachiocephalic arteries commonly accompany supravalvar aortic stenosis. Occasionally, the origin of a coronary artery is stenosed or, rarely, obstructed by a coronary leaflet as previously described.

Magnetic Resonance Imaging and Cardiac Computed Tomography

Both of these imaging techniques provide superior anatomic details (see Chapter 10), but not often necessary because of

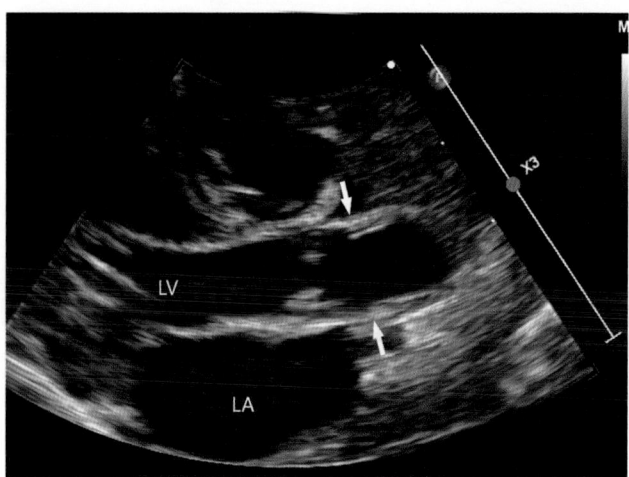

• **Fig. 28.18** Parasternal long-axis echocardiogram of the left ventricle (LV), atrium (LA), and proximal ascending aorta demonstrating typical hourglass-shaped supravalvar aortic stenosis (arrows) just above the sinuses of Valsalva. Note the classic "train track" appearance of the ascending aortic wall which is markedly thickened.

the excellent echocardiographic images. However, cardiac CT in particular may provide additional imaging of the origins and proximal course of the coronary arteries, as well as excellent demonstration of any associated lesions of the head and neck vessels, abdominal aorta, and branches.

Cardiac Catheterization

In the uncomplicated patient, in whom all anatomic details are clearly evident on non-invasive studies, cardiac catheterization is unnecessary (Figs. 28.19 and 28.20). If, however, an associated lesion such as significant distal peripheral pulmonary stenosis is suspected, catheterization is undertaken to dilate (with or without stents) these pulmonary lesions because they are generally inaccessible surgically. This combined approach of pulmonary artery dilation and surgical relief of supravalvar aortic stenosis offers better long-term survival than surgery alone in those with the severest elastin arteriopathy.[24] It should be emphasized, however, that catheterization of patients with severe bilateral outflow obstruction may be quite dangerous with significant risk of cardiovascular events. Occasionally, stenoses of individual aortic arch branches can also be managed by dilating and stenting these obstructions.

Management

Surgery for supravalvar aortic stenosis is often undertaken for gradient levels that are lower than that for valvar aortic stenosis, due to the tendency for obstruction to progress in many and the usually excellent outcomes from surgery for the localized type of obstruction. With symptoms or a hemodynamic gradient of more than 30 mm Hg, particularly when the lesion is discrete, surgical repair using a variety of techniques is undertaken. The most successful approach with best long-term freedom from reoperation is the three-patch technique augmenting each sinus across the sinotubular junction.

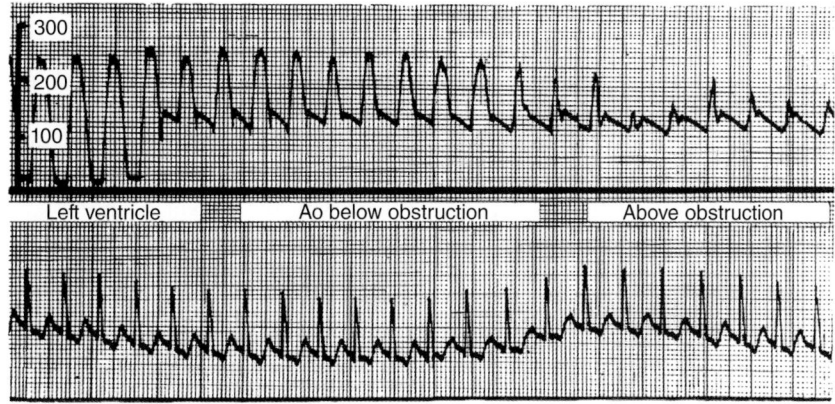

• **Fig. 28.19** Pressure tracing recorded in a patient with supravalvar aortic stenosis during withdrawal of a catheter from the left ventricle to the ascending aorta. Note that there is no change in systemic pressure as the catheter passes the valve and an arterial pressure trace appears. Further withdrawal shows a drop from a higher to a lower arterial pressure. (From Fyler DC, ed. *Nadas' Pediatric Cardiology*. Philadelphia: Hanley & Belfus, 1992.)

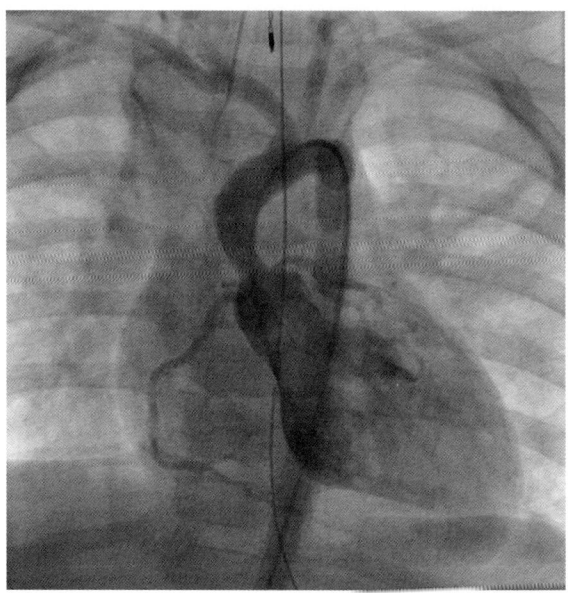

• **Fig. 28.20** Catheter angiogram of the ascending aorta in this 6-month-old with supravalvar aortic stenosis, in the frontal projection. Note the hourglass deformity and relative hypoplasia of the ascending aorta.

Additional considerations at time of surgery include need for augmenting obstructed coronary ostia, relieving arch obstruction, and setting up transverse arch graft to help augment the obstructed descending thoracic aorta at a later time. Surgical mortality continues to improve, currently under 4% in most recent series.

Clinical Course

Further obstructions may develop even though there has been successful surgical relief of the supravalvar obstruction. Coarctation of the aorta, renal artery stenosis, or obstructions of the branches of the aortic arch may develop or recur. Each new problem is evaluated on its own merits and managed independently. The incidence of required reoperation with the more recent three-patch technique is around

10% at 5 years.[25] It is of interest that moderate or lower degrees of peripheral pulmonary stenosis in some of these patients improve spontaneously particularly after infancy.

Summary recommendations for the older child/adolescent with supravalvar aortic stenosis:

- Upon diagnosis, clinical evaluation for Williams syndrome and other abnormality of the elastin gene should be considered.
- Supravalvar aortic stenosis is often progressive, and close clinical follow-up is required. Careful diagnostic evaluation for more extensive arteriopathy is important, particularly prior to any cardiac procedures given the associated risks.
- Surgical correction should be undertaken for hemodynamic pressure gradients over 30 mm Hg.
- Outcomes after surgical relief of supravalvar stenosis are generally good, although reintervention may be required for other associated lesions.

Aortic Regurgitation

Definition

The reflux of blood from the ascending aorta into the left ventricle during diastole is described as aortic regurgitation or aortic insufficiency.

Prevalence

Aortic regurgitation is found in association with almost all known pediatric cardiac problems, although rarely identified as a sole clinical finding. From an echocardiographic standpoint, the incidence of aortic regurgitation in a normal heart in childhood has been reported as 0%, increasing to 3–8% in adults. Of all heart valves in normal patients, the aortic valve is the least associated with regurgitation, followed by the mitral valve, and then the tricuspid and pulmonary valves in which the majority of patients will have minor degrees of regurgitation.

Pathology

There is no specific pathology for aortic regurgitation because there are multiple causes. There may be dilation of the valve ring, as seen in patients with tetralogy of Fallot (see Chapter 26) or in those with Marfan syndrome. In the latter, there is also often enlargement of all three leaflet cusps. The valve may be congenitally abnormal, such as bicuspid, or due to severe underdevelopment of the right coronary leaflet. The regurgitation may result from an intervention for stenosis such as balloon angioplasty or surgery. Incompetence of a normal valve may result from the jet effect in patients with subaortic stenosis or because of deformity or adherence of a cusp to a supravalvar obstructing ridge. It may follow prolapse of a cusp into a VSD or perforation of a leaflet due to endocarditis. Rheumatic fever remains a major cause in some countries but is rare in the United States.

Physiology

When there is aortic regurgitation, the amount of blood that is refluxed must be pumped forward in addition to that supplying the appropriate cardiac output. The left ventricular volume is thereby enlarged in direct proportion to the amount of regurgitated blood. With increased amounts of regurgitation, the left ventricular volume increases, ultimately resulting in a dilated heart. In an effort to normalize wall stress in the setting of a dilated ventricle, the heart responds with compensatory hypertrophy, referred to as *eccentric hypertrophy* (increased mass, but with normal mass:volume ratio). The runoff from the aorta to the left ventricle results in a wide pulse pressure, the systolic pressure becoming higher as the diastolic pressure becomes lower with increasing regurgitation.

Ultimately, over many years, increasing aortic regurgitation can lead to a failure of compensatory eccentric hypertrophy and elevated wall stress, systolic and diastolic dysfunction, and congestive heart failure.

Clinical Manifestations and Physical Exam

A high-frequency, early diastolic blowing murmur, usually best heard along the left sternal border, is virtually diagnostic of aortic regurgitation (Figs. 28.20 and 28.21). The frequency of the murmur (the blowing quality) is higher with

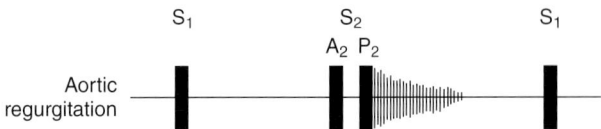

• **Fig. 28.21** Schematic drawing of the murmur of aortic regurgitation. Note the decrescendo, early diastolic murmur that begins after the second heart sound. S_1, first heart sound; S_2, second heart sound composed of A_2 (aortic closure) and P_2 (pulmonary closure). (From Fyler DC, ed. *Nadas' Pediatric Cardiology*. Philadelphia: Hanley & Belfus, 1992.)

aortic regurgitation than with pulmonary regurgitation. The murmur is quite difficult to discover, let alone distinguish, when there are continuous murmurs from other causes such as patent ductus arteriosus, collateral circulation, shunt operations, and other lesions. The murmur is heard well in a small child lying down, but among teenagers, it is easier to hear with the patient sitting up and leaning forward. It is best heard with the diaphragm of the stethoscope at the left sternal border, usually at the third interspace. An Austin Flint murmur due to relative mitral stenosis produced by the aortic regurgitant jet may be audible at the apex in mid-diastole when incompetence is significant.

In the past, the discovery of isolated aortic regurgitation was synonymous with the diagnosis of rheumatic heart disease; this is no longer the case. Still, this possibility should be considered for each patient with isolated aortic regurgitation, and any history or family history suggesting rheumatic fever should be carefully reviewed.

With increasing degrees of aortic regurgitation, the peripheral pulses become more prominent as the pulse pressure increases. Associated with this wide pulse pressure is a wonderful cacophony of physical findings and signs, including capillary pulsations; de Musset's (head bobbing), Duroziez's, Traube's, Müller's, and Quincke's signs; and Corrigan's (water hammer) pulse. Generally, with routine observation of the carotid pulsations, the pediatrician sees the wide pulse pressure before he or she feels it. Confirmation of the wide pulse pressure by blood pressure measurement documents the somewhat elevated systolic pressure and low diastolic pressure.

The hyperdynamic left ventricular impulse is displaced down and leftward, sometimes reaching the anterior axillary line at the sixth interspace. The hyperactive impulse conveys the impression of forceful ejection of large amounts of blood.

Electrocardiography

With increasing left ventricular volume overload, there is increased left ventricular voltage on the electrocardiogram (Fig. 28.22), and in the extreme form, there may be depression of the ST segment and T-wave inversion.

Chest X-Ray

The heart size is directly proportional to the amount of aortic regurgitation, or it may be grossly enlarged through the dilation of congestive heart failure superimposed on a large regurgitant volume. The dilated ascending aorta is usually visible.

Echocardiography

The regurgitant flow across the aortic valve is readily detected by color Doppler interrogation (Figs. 28.23 and 28.24). Indeed, this sensitive technique frequently identifies aortic regurgitation without an audible murmur. In addition to providing valvar and ascending aorta anatomic information, the former often better delineated on three-dimensional imaging, estimates of the regurgitation severity are possible

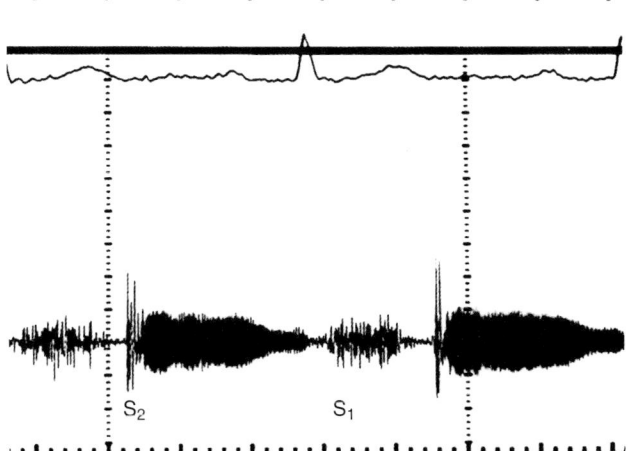

• **Fig. 28.22** Phonocardiogram in a patient who suddenly developed a loud, high-frequency murmur of aortic regurgitation because of a perforation in an aortic valve leaflet. (From Fyler DC, ed. *Nadas' Pediatric Cardiology.* Philadelphia: Hanley & Belfus, 1992.)

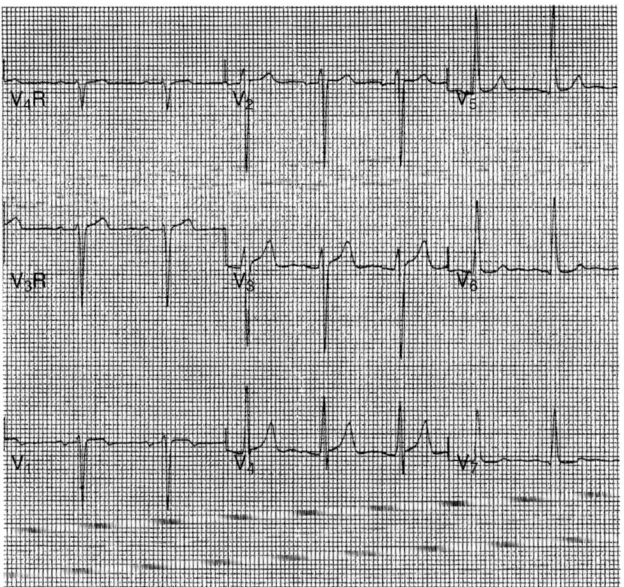

• **Fig. 28.23** Electrocardiogram showing left ventricular hypertrophy by voltage criteria (V leads at half standard) in a 19-year-old with bicuspid valve and severe aortic regurgitation.

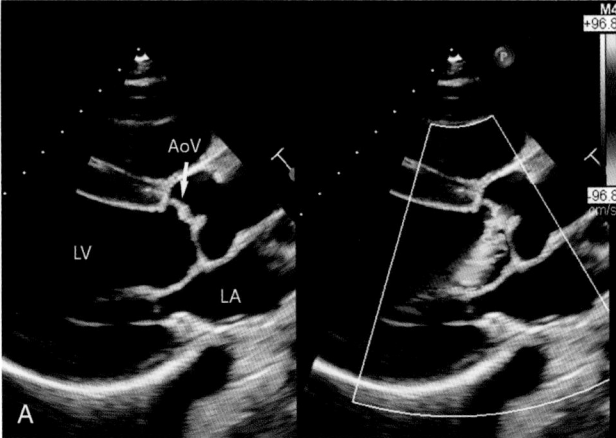

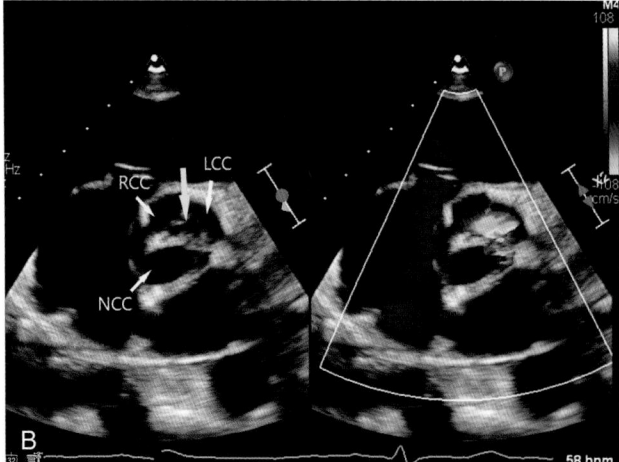

• **Fig. 28.24** Parasternal long- and short-axis echocardiogram images of a 18-year-old patient with bicuspid aortic valve and moderate-severe aortic regurgitation. In (A) long-axis view, note the large jet of regurgitation directed posteriorly; short-axis view (B) demonstrates the large coaptation gap *(yellow arrow)* through which the regurgitation emanates. *AoV,* Aortic valve; *LA,* left atrium; *LCC,* left coronary cusp; *LV,* left ventricle; *NCC,* noncoronary cusp, *RCC,* right coronary cusp.

based on jet dimension, ventricular volumes, and descending aorta runoff information. Very importantly, especially for management guidance, sophisticated ventricular function parameters (end-diastolic and systolic sizes, fractional shortening, wall stress, left ventricular muscle mass) are now readily available (see Chapter 9). Cardiac MRI may provide additional information in those with poor acoustic windows and yields accurate data on degree of aortic regurgitation (regurgitant fraction) as well as precise ventricular volumes and systolic function.

Cardiac Catheterization

Cardiac catheterization is not required in the evaluation of a patient with aortic regurgitation. However, because most

of these children have other defects, cardiac catheterization may be used to provide more physiologic information or to interventionally manage an additional compounding lesion such as a patent ductus arteriosus. Evaluation, if necessary, of the degree of aortic regurgitation during cardiac catheterization is accomplished by the injection of contrast material above the aortic valve (the catheter not in contact with the valve) and observing the amount that enters the ventricle.

Management

Any patient with known aortic regurgitation who has syncope or anginal chest pain or who has developed congestive heart failure is a candidate for surgery, although such symptoms are rare. Progressive enlargement and decreasing function, at rest, of the left ventricle on serial echocardiographic studies are surgical indications (Fig. 28.25). The appearance of ventricular dysrhythmias, an event of ominous significance, is another indication for surgery. In asymptomatic patients with significant regurgitation but with stable,

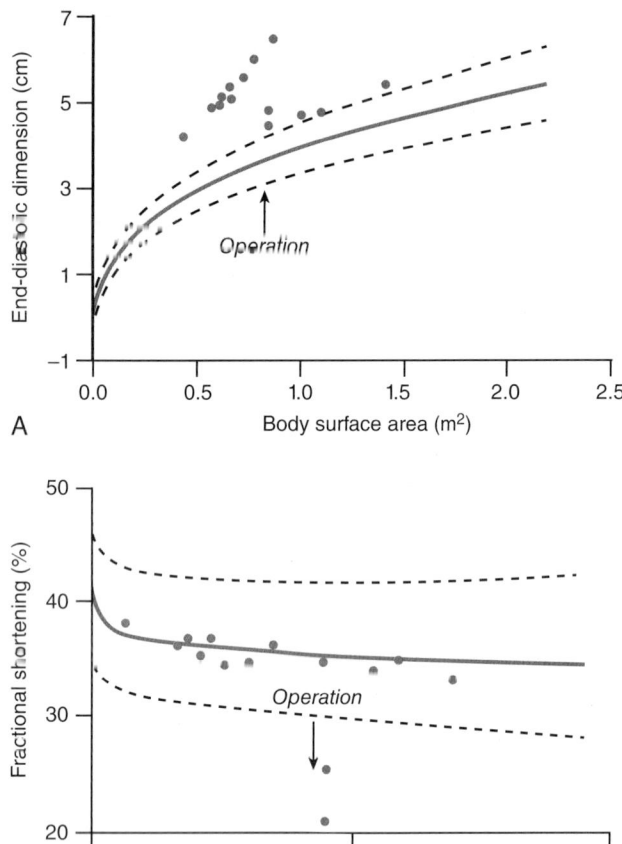

• **Fig. 28.25** Serial echocardiographic measurements showing **(A)** indexed left ventricular end-diastolic volumes and **(B)** fractional shortening before and after surgical valvuloplasty at age 9 years for severe aortic regurgitation after balloon angioplasty for stenosis. Note the dramatic immediate decrease in both parameters postoperatively with recovery of the latter during follow-up. (Courtesy of Dr. Steven Colan.)

modestly increased end-diastolic volumes and normal function, medical management with afterload reduction is a reasonable temporizing measure. There is little published evidence in the pediatric age group for the use of vasodilators, although ACE inhibitor therapy has been associated with reduction in left ventricular size and regurgitation fraction in one study.[26] Biomarkers that are elevated in the setting of stressed cardiac muscle such as B-type natriuretic peptide may provide additional information, but are rarely used in determining timing of intervention.

Whenever possible, surgeons undertake valve repair, which is sometimes dramatically successful, particularly in those with a perforated or prolapsed leaflet. In addition, many with a bicuspid valve or a hypoplastic leaflet or torn valve from balloon angioplasty can be satisfactorily palliated by a valvuloplasty procedure.[27] Newer surgical techniques include the "bicuspidization" technique, which involves using native valve tissue and creating two leaflets from a dysfunctional three leaflet valve, and the Ozaki technique of complete leaflet replacement. Case series in pediatric patient groups have reported encouraging results with both of these

techniques.[28] The Ross operation is another option (see previous discussion in this chapter with aortic valve stenosis). Biologic and mechanical valve replacements are additional options for the patient with the failed valve repair, although the biologic valves have a relatively high failure rate with degeneration and progressive calcification, particularly in the pediatric patient population.

Clinical Course

In young patients, relief of severe aortic regurgitation is commonly followed immediately by marked reduction in both end-diastolic volume and shortening fraction, the latter normalizing with time (Fig. 28.25).

Summary recommendations for the older child/adolescent with aortic regurgitation:

- Patients with aortic regurgitation should have regular clinical follow-up to monitor for symptoms (rare) and for progression of regurgitation with echocardiography. Cardiac MRI may provide additional diagnostic information.
- Medical management consists of vasodilator therapy, which may slow the rate of progression of left ventricular dilation and eventual dysfunction.
- Indications for surgical valve repair or replacement include signs/symptoms of heart failure, ischemia with exertion, or worsening left ventricular systolic function. Progressively increasing left ventricular size/volume is another relative indication.

References

1. Hoffman JI, Kaplan S. The incidence of congenital heart disease. *J Am Coll Cardiol.* 2002;39:1890-1900.
2. Tutar E, Ekici F, Atalay S, Nacar N. The prevalence of bicuspid aortic valve in newborns by echocardiographic screening. *Am Heart J.* 2005;150:513-515.
3. Huntington K, Hunter AG, Chan KL. A prospective study to assess the frequency of familial clustering of congenital bicuspid aortic valve. *J Am Coll Cardiol.* 1997;30:1809-1812.
4. Galian-Gay L, Carro Hevia A, Teixido-Tura G, et al. Familial clustering of bicuspid aortic valve and its relationship with aortic dilation in first-degree relatives. *Heart.* 2019;105:603-608.
5. Fernandes SM, Sanders SP, Khairy P, et al. Morphology of bicuspid aortic valve in children and adolescents. *J Am Coll Cardiol.* 2004;44:1648-1651.
6. Basso C, Boschello M, Perrone C, et al. An echocardiographic survey of primary school children for bicuspid aortic valve. *Am J Cardiol.* 2004;93:661-663.
7. Wagner HR, Ellison RC, Keane JF, Humphries OJ, Nadas AS. Clinical course in aortic stenosis. *Circulation.* 1977;56: I47-I56.
8. Fernandes SM, Khairy P, Sanders SP, Colan SD. Bicuspid aortic valve morphology and interventions in the young. *J Am Coll Cardiol.* 2007;49:2211-2214.
9. Keane JF, Driscoll DJ, Gersony WM, et al. Second natural history study of congenital heart defects: results of treatment of patients with aortic valvar stenosis. *Circulation.* 1993;87: I16-I27.

10. Barker PC, Ensing G, Ludomirsky A, Bradley DJ, Lloyd TR, Rocchini AP. Comparison of simultaneous invasive and noninvasive measurements of pressure gradients in congenital aortic valve stenosis. *J Am Soc Echocardiogr.* 2002;15:1496-1502.

11. Vlahos AP, Marx GR, McElhinney D, Oneill S, Goudevenos I, Colan SD. Clinical utility of Doppler echocardiography in assessing aortic stenosis severity and predicting need for intervention in children. *Pediatr Cardiol.* 2008;29:507-514.

12. Brown DW, Dipilato AE, Chong EC, Lock JE, McElhinney DB. Aortic valve reinterventions after balloon aortic valvuloplasty for congenital aortic stenosis intermediate and late follow-up. *J Am Coll Cardiol.* 2010;56:1740-1749.

13. Siddiqui J, Brizard CP, Galati JC, et al. Surgical valvotomy and repair for neonatal and infant congenital aortic stenosis achieves better results than interventional catheterization. *J Am Coll Cardiol.* 2013;62:2134-2140.

14. Hill GD, Ginde S, Rios R, Frommelt PC, Hill KD. Surgical valvotomy versus balloon valvuloplasty for congenital aortic valve stenosis: a systematic review and meta-analysis. *J Am Heart Assoc.* 2016;5:e003931.

15. Nelson JS, Pasquali SK, Pratt CN, et al. Long-term survival and reintervention after the Ross procedure across the pediatric age spectrum. *Ann Thorac Surg.* 2015;99:2086-2094; discussion 2094-2095.

16. Driscoll DJ, Wolfe RR, Gersony WM, et al. Cardiorespiratory responses to exercise of patients with aortic stenosis, pulmonary stenosis, and ventricular septal defect. *Circulation.* 1993;87:I102-I113.

17. Maron BJ, Doerer JJ, Haas TS, Tierney DM, Mueller FO. Sudden deaths in young competitive athletes: analysis of 1866 deaths in the United States, 1980-2006. *Circulation.* 2009;119:1085-1092.

18. Brown DW, Dipilato AE, Chong EC, et al. Sudden unexpected death after balloon valvuloplasty for congenital aortic stenosis. *J Am Coll Cardiol.* 2010;56:1939-1946.

19. Pickard SS, Geva A, Gauvreau K, et al. Long-term outcomes and risk factors for aortic regurgitation after discrete subvalvular aortic stenosis resection in children. *Heart.* 2015;101:1547-1553.

20. van der Linde D, Roos-Hesselink JW, Rizopoulos D, et al. Surgical outcome of discrete subaortic stenosis in adults: a multicenter study. *Circulation.* 2013;127:1184-1191, e1-4.

21. Hayano S, Okuno Y, Tsutsumi M, et al. Frequent intragenic microdeletions of elastin in familial supravalvular aortic stenosis. *Int J Cardiol.* 2019;274:290-295.

22. Bruno E, Rossi N, Thuer O, et al. Cardiovascular findings, and clinical course, in patients with Williams syndrome. *Cardiol Young.* 2003;13:532-536.

23. Hornik CP, Collins RT II, Jaquiss RD, et al. Adverse cardiac events in children with Williams syndrome undergoing cardiovascular surgery: an analysis of the Society of Thoracic Surgeons Congenital Heart Surgery Database. *J Thorac Cardiovasc Surg.* 2015;149:1516-1522.e1.

24. Stamm C, Friehs I, Moran AM, et al. Surgery for bilateral outflow tract obstruction in elastin arteriopathy. *J Thorac Cardiovasc Surg.* 2000;120:755-763.

25. Fricke TA, d'Udekem Y, Brizard CP, et al. Surgical repair of supravalvular aortic stenosis in children with Williams syndrome: a 30-year experience. *Ann Thorac Surg.* 2015;99:1335-1341.

26. Alehan D, Ozkutlu S. Beneficial effects of 1-year captopril therapy in children with chronic aortic regurgitation who have no symptoms. *Am Heart J.* 1998;135:598-603.

27. Bacha EA, Satou GM, Moran AM, et al. Valve-sparing operation for balloon-induced aortic regurgitation in congenital aortic stenosis. *J Thorac Cardiovasc Surg.* 2001;122:162-168.

28. Baird CW, Cooney B, Chavez M, et al. Congenital aortic and truncal valve reconstruction using the Ozaki technique: short-term clinical results. *J Thorac Cardiovasc Surg.* 2021;161:1567-1577.

29

D-Transposition of the Great Arteries

KIMBERLY I. MILLS, DAVID W. BROWN, AND JOHN E. MAYER JR.

KEY LEARNING POINTS

- Untreated D-transposition of the great arteries (D-TGA) is a highly lethal condition without early catheterization and surgical interventions.
- The adoption of the early arterial switch approach to surgical treatment of D-TGA and D-TGA with ventricular septal defect has resulted in improved survival and preservation of cardiac rhythm and ventricular function compared with atrial level repairs.

- More complex forms of D-TGA, including aortic arch or pulmonary pathway obstructions, are amenable to surgical treatment but are associated with higher early and late risks.
- Long-term follow-up of patients with D-TGA is mandatory, as uncertainty continues regarding the fate of the neoaortic valve and the coronary arteries after the arterial switch procedure.

Definition

D-transposition of the great arteries (D-TGA) describes reversal of the anatomic position of the great arteries. Normally, the aorta is located posterior and rightward and the pulmonary artery anterior and leftward; in D-transposition, the aorta is anterior and rightward whereas the pulmonary artery is posterior and leftward. In normally related great arteries, the aorta relates directly to the left ventricle and the pulmonary artery to the right ventricle, while in transposition there is ventriculoarterial discordance while maintaining atrioventricular (AV) concordance. The subject of this chapter is confined to TGA associated with D-looping of the ventricles. L-looping and other forms of transposition associated with single ventricle or heterotaxy are found in their respective chapters (see Chapters 30 and 32).

In most infants with D-TGA, there is an intact ventricular septum. In those with ventricular septal defects (VSDs), the defects range in size from insignificant to large, sometimes in combination with pulmonic stenosis or pulmonary atresia. Other possible associated cardiac anomalies are coarctation or interruption of the aorta, pulmonary valve stenosis, subpulmonary stenosis, or mitral valve disease. The appropriate classification for a patient with transposition is not always possible as the spectrum of disease may range from double-outlet right ventricle (both great arteries arising from the right ventricle) to transposition with a VSD or transposition with some ventricular hypoplasia compared to those with a single ventricle.

Prevalence

D-TGA is the second most common neonatal congenital cardiac defect. D-TGA accounts for 3% of all congenital heart disease and nearly 20% of cyanotic heart disease.[1]

Embryology

The definitive embryologic explanation for D-TGA remains unknown; however, a widely accepted theory implicates abnormal development of the subarterial conus bilaterally. During normal cardiac formation, there is initially a common arterial trunk arising from the right ventricle. This common arterial trunk and its subvalvar conus undergo a spiraling septation process. Both the subaortic conus and subpulmonary conus are present initially with both great arteries situated above the right ventricle. At approximately 30–34 days into gestation, the subaortic conus starts to resorb in conjuction with the truncal septation process, while the aorta migrates inferiorly and posteriorly to lie directly over the left ventricle. Simultaneously, the subpulmonary conus persists so that the pulmonary artery remains stationary over the right ventricle. In D-TGA, it is the subpulmonary conus that resorbs, leading to reversal of the normal arterial migration with the pulmonary artery moving inferiorly and posteriorly to result in the pulmonary valve coming into fibrous continuity with the mitral valve. Because not all forms of D-TGA can be explained simply by this theory, an alternate explanation suggests a failure of the embryonic truncus arteriosus to septate normally.

To date, no genetic abnormality has been identified to explain the existence of D-TGA. Recurrence in the same family is virtually unrecognized and the risk of congenital heart disease in siblings is no higher than the general population. Furthermore, D-TGA is rarely associated with genetic syndromes such as trisomy 21. D-TGA is associated with fewer extracardiac anomalies (<10%) than are most other congenital cardiac defects. Finally, there is evidence of a higher incidence of D-TGA with gestational diabetes resulting in large-for-gestational-age neonates, with advanced maternal age, and with maternal exposure to antiepileptics.

Anatomy

In D-TGA, the aorta arises from the right ventricle, being most often positioned directly in front of the pulmonary artery in a lateral view, and slightly to the right of the pulmonary artery in the anteroposterior view (Fig. 29.1). The pulmonary artery arises behind the aorta from the left ventricle, a position that allows preferential ejection from the left ventricle into the right pulmonary artery and probably accounts for the large right pulmonary artery and increased flow to the right lung. There is a subaortic conus as well as pulmonary and mitral valve fibrous continuity. Because most of these infants are discovered at birth or shortly afterward, the foramen ovale and ductus arteriosus are often patent. True atrial septal defects are uncommon.

Among infants with an intact ventricular septum, dynamic outflow tract obstruction from the left ventricle is common. This obstruction appears to be caused by bowing

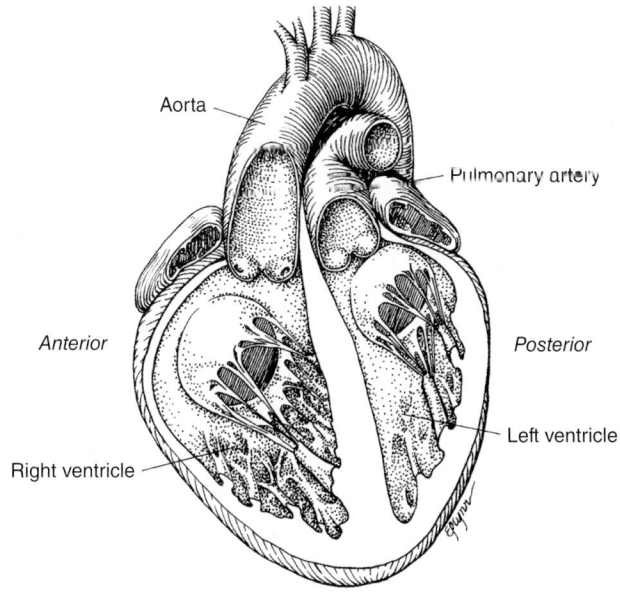

• **Fig. 29.1** Transposition of the great arteries, lateral view. The aorta arises anteriorly from the right ventricle; the pulmonary artery arises posteriorly from the left ventricle. As diagrammed, there is no communication shown between the pulmonary and systemic circulations, a situation not compatible with life. For survival there must be communication between the two circuits, usually as a patent ductus arteriosus, ventricular defect, or atrial opening. (From Fyler DC, eds. *Nadas' Pediatric Cardiology*. Hanley & Belfus Inc. Philadelphia; 1992.)

of the ventricular septum to the left because of a higher right ventricular pressure than the subpulmonary left ventricle. The resulting proximity of the mitral valve and ventricular septum can cause obstruction. These dynamic gradients disappear with surgical anatomic correction. However, a patient may rarely have anatomic subvalvar or valvar pulmonary stenosis, a challenging management problem.

VSDs are present at birth in 50% of the infants with D-TGA. However, spontaneous closure in the first year of life reduces the number of children with VSDs by one-third. VSDs may be located anywhere in the ventricular septum. There does not appear to be a difference in the type of VSDs from that in infants without D-TGA. Additional cardiac anomalies are more common in children with D-TGA with VSDs as opposed to those with an intact ventricular septum. These additional cardiac anomalies include pulmonary stenosis, pulmonary atresia, overriding or straddling AV valve, coarctation of the aorta, and interruption of the aorta. Right ventricular outflow tract obstruction is rare, except in cases where there is coarctation or interruption of the aortic arch.

The coronary anatomy in TGA is important, since anomalies of the coronary arteries are associated with mortality following the arterial switch procedure (Fig. 29.2).[2] A simple rule that accounts for all variations of coronary anatomy is that the coronaries arise from the sinuses of Valsalva that face the pulmonary artery and follow the shortest route to their ultimate destination. If the great arteries lie in an anteroposterior position, the right-facing sinus typically gives rise to the right coronary artery, whereas the left coronary artery arises from the left-facing sinus. Important to note, the proximal course of the coronary arteries may follow an intramural path without interposed adventitia, which is critical knowledge for surgical correction during an arterial switch procedure. Improvements in surgical technique have resulted in no added mortality for common coronary variants for patients with D-TGA following an arterial switch repair. However, patients with a single coronary or those that follow an intramural course continue to confer a higher mortality rate.[2]

Abnormalities of the tricuspid and mitral valves are frequent but are seldom of major importance unless there is AV valve straddling. Infants with a VSD of the endocardial cushion type may have an overriding or straddling tricuspid valve. When septal chordal attachments extend into the left ventricle, the valve is said to be straddling, and when the tricuspid valve allows direct flow into the left ventricle, without straddling chordae, it is described as overriding. With an overriding or straddling tricuspid valve, some right atrial blood is delivered into the left ventricle, resulting in less flow through the right ventricle that may result in ventricular hypoplasia.

Physiology

With D-TGA, the deoxygenated systemic venous blood passes through the right heart to reach the aorta, while the oxygenated pulmonary venous blood passes through the left heart and returns to the lungs. Survival is dependent on

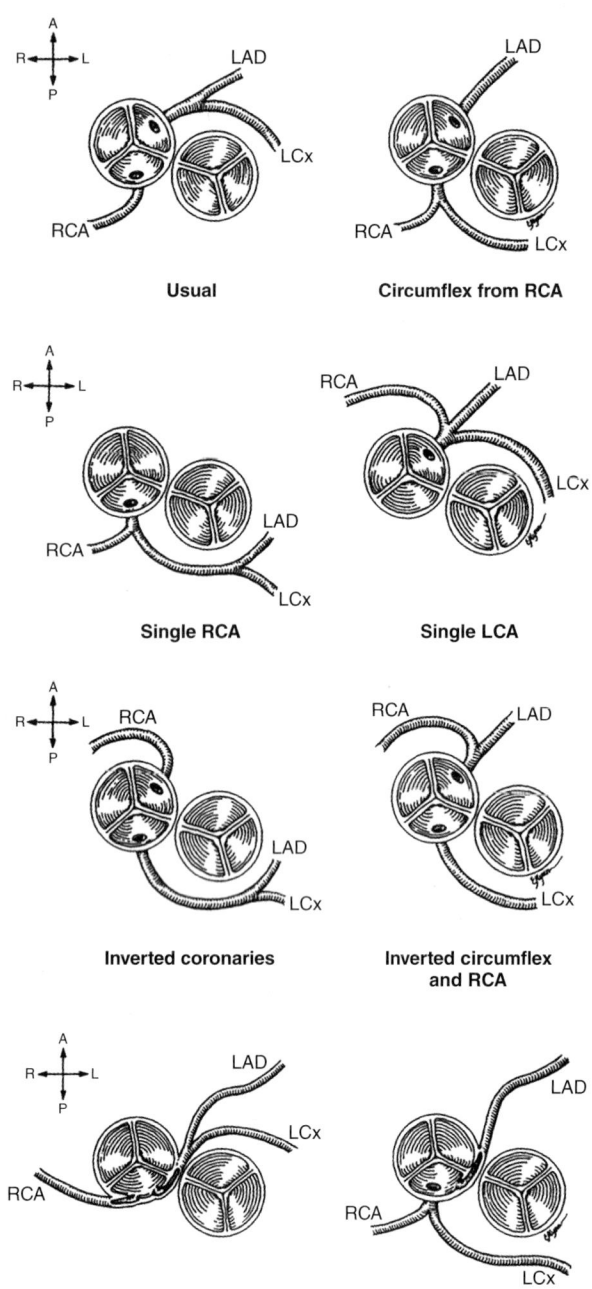

• **Fig. 29.2** Coronary artery patterns in D-transposition of the great arteries. The "usual" or most common pattern observed is noted in the top left panel, with the right coronary arising from the rightward facing sinus and the left main coronary from the leftward facing sinus, giving rise to the left anterior descending and circumflex coronary branches. *RCA*, right coronary artery; *LAD*, left anterior descending; *LCA*, left coronary artery; *LCx*, left circumflex; *RCA*, right coronary artery; *LCA*, left coronary artery. (From Pasquali SK, Hasselblad V, Li JS, et al. Coronary artery pattern and outcome of arterial switch operation for transposition of the great arteries: a meta-analysis. *Circulation.* 2002;106:2575–2580, with permission.)

adequate mixing between these two parallel circulations. Those with an intact ventricular septum are able to survive in the short term because of flow through the ductus arteriosus into the pulmonary circuit and mixing at the atrial level through a dilated foramen ovale (Fig. 29.3). For the

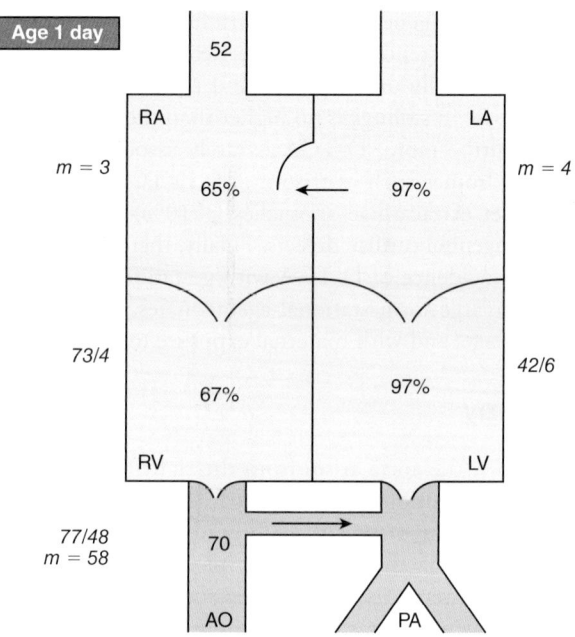

• **Fig. 29.3** Hemodynamic diagram of the circulation with transposition of the great arteries with intact ventricular septum. This infant survives because of flow through the ductus arteriosus to the lungs and return of equal flow from the left atrium to the right through a sprung foramen ovale. It is believed that, at birth, an excess of blood is supplied to the pulmonary circuit by the patent ductus arteriosus, thereby raising the left atrial pressure sufficiently to force open the foramen ovale, and thereby allowing compensatory pulmonary-to-systemic flow. *AO,* Aorta; *italics,* pressure in mm Hg; *LA,* left atrium; *LV,* left ventricle; *PA,* pulmonary artery; *RA,* right atrium; *RV,* right ventricle; *%,* percent oxygen saturation. (From Fyler DC, eds. *Nadas' Pediatric Cardiology.* Hanley & Belfus Inc. Philadelphia; 1992.)

required atrial shunt to occur, the flap of the foramen ovale must become incompetent. At birth, increased flow through the pulmonary circuit results in elevated left atrial pressures that are decompressed through an incompetent foramen ovale into the right atrium. Increasing the ductal left-to-right shunt, as witnessed with an infusion of prostaglandin E, increases flow into the pulmonary circuit, which must in turn be compensated for by increased flow toward the systemic circuit via the foramen ovale.[3]

If the incompetent foramen ovale cannot accommodate the increased blood flow, the pulmonary circuit will become overloaded (Fig. 29.4). Enlarging the atrial opening by balloon atrial septostomy or surgical creation of an atrial defect allows for increased mixing between the two circulations, with improved arterial oxygenation. Rarely, a patient is born with a large atrial defect allowing equal bidirectional shunting with good survival even without a patent ductus arteriosus or balloon atrial septostomy. These patients can be recognized because of the equilibration of atrial pressures and the lack of other shunts. Administering supplemental inspired oxygen has little effect on the systemic arterial oxygen saturation.

Infants with VSDs tend to have a larger volume of shunting with higher systemic arterial saturations. The defect

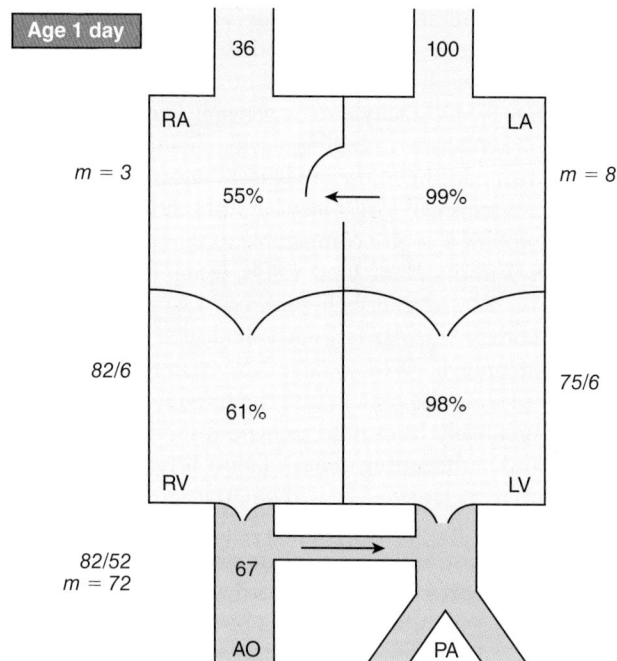

• **Fig. 29.4** Hemodynamic diagram of a newborn infant with transposition of the great vessels and intact ventricular septum, who has received prostaglandins E1. The pulmonary blood flow is excessive, the left atrial pressure is higher than the right, and there is pulmonary hypertension. Compare with Fig. 29.5. *AO,* Aorta; *italics,* pressure in mm Hg; *LA,* left atrium; *LV,* left ventricle; *PA,* pulmonary artery; *RA,* right atrium; *RV,* right ventricle; *%,* percent oxygen saturation. (From Nadas AS, Fyler DC, eds. *Nadas' Pediatric Cardiology.* Philadelphia, PA: Hanley and Belfus; 1992.)

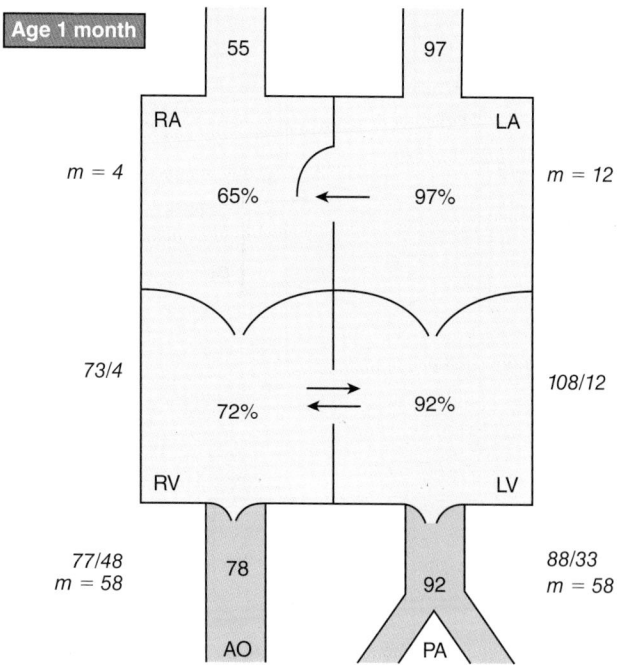

• **Fig. 29.5** Hemodynamic diagram of a patient with transposition of the great arteries and ventricular septal defect. Note that blood flows toward the lungs via the ventricular defect and from the lungs via both a sprung foramen ovale and the ventricular defect. The arterial oxygen saturation (78%) is compatible with growth. *AO,* Aorta; *italics,* pressure in mm Hg; *LA,* left atrium; *LV,* left ventricle; *PA,* pulmonary artery; *RA,* right atrium; *RV,* right ventricle; *%,* percent oxygen saturation. (From Nadas AS, Fyler DC, eds. *Nadas' Pediatric Cardiology.* Philadelphia, PA: Hanley and Belfus; 1992.)

allows shunting toward the pulmonary circuit with return to the systemic circuit via the foramen ovale given the elevated left atrial pressure (Fig. 29.5). Since VSDs may close spontaneously over time, survival may be dependent entirely on a shunt at the foramen level, since the ductus arteriosus may no longer be patent. On the other hand, a large ventricular defect provides good mixing, but the unrestrictive pulmonary blood flow may result in early heart failure with minimal cyanosis and places the patient at risk for developing pulmonary vascular obstructive disease.

The physiologic effect of pulmonary stenosis depends on the presence of a VSD. In infants with an intact ventricular septum, the outflow of the left ventricle may be obstructed by dynamic subpulmonary stenosis as a result of right ventricular hypertension causing leftward malposition of the ventricular septum. Close apposition of the septum to the mitral valve accentuates the obstruction. The obstruction is rarely severe and tends to resolve following the arterial switch procedure.

True valvar pulmonic stenosis is rare, although bicuspid pulmonary valve is an uncommon but well-described variant. Fixed anatomic pulmonary stenosis, usually subvalvar, is more common in the presence of a VSD (Fig. 29.6). The restriction of pulmonary blood flow coupled with a VSD is likely to result in fewer symptoms of heart failure and allows adequate growth. Consequently, these infants first present to the cardiologist at a somewhat older age than most of the babies with D-TGA and intact ventricular septum.

In D-TGA with an intact ventricular septum, the level of left ventricular pressure required to overcome pulmonary resistance decreases within hours of birth and is less than half of the right ventricular pressure by the end of the first week. This is associated with remodeling and failure of the left ventricle to thicken with increasing age. Because the arterial switch procedure requires the left ventricle to function at systemic pressure immediately following surgery, most centers carry out arterial switch operations within the first week of life. The same approach is undertaken with infants who have small- to moderate-sized VSDs as well. The left ventricle of infants with a large VSD functions at systemic pressure, making the arterial switch procedure feasible, as the left ventricle remains prepared by exposure to systemic pressures, and surgical intervention can be planned beyond the first week. In the modern era, however, given improvements in the management of bypass and perioperative care, most centers choose to repair patients with D-TGA and large VSDs in the neonatal period. Recent data suggests a reduction in major postoperative morbidities and resource utilization, represented as cost savings, if the arterial switch procedure is undertaken around the third day of life.[4] Furthermore, impaired brain growth and neurodevelopment have been described when definitive repair occurs beyond the second week of life.

Non-reparative surgical interventions on a single lesion in D-TGA may disturb the precarious balance of circulation

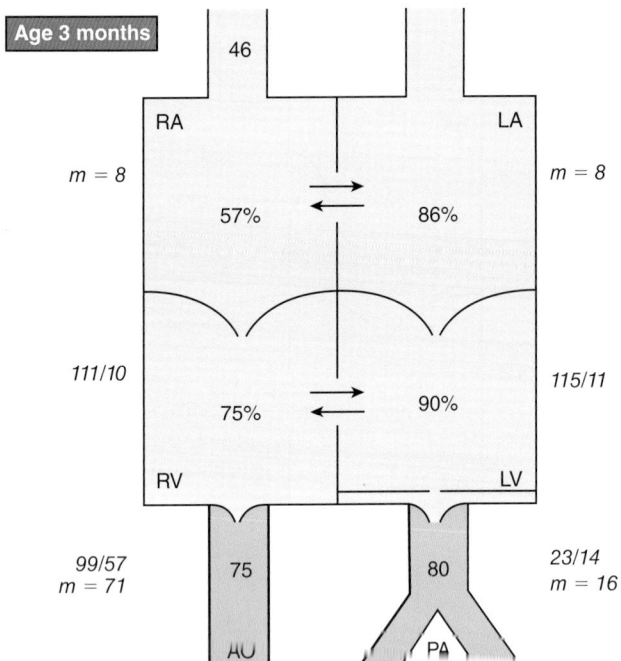

Age 3 months

RA m = 8 57% 46 86% LA m = 8

111/10 75% 90% 115/11

RV LV

99/57 m = 71 75 80 23/14 m = 16

AO PA

• **Fig. 29.6** Hemodynamic diagram of a patient with transposition of the great arteries, ventricular septal, defect and subpulmonary stenosis. The balance of the circulation is similar to that shown in Fig. 29.5; however, there is normal pulmonary arterial pressure. The pulmonary stenosis prohibits excess pulmonary blood flow; therefore, left atrial pressures are lower. *AO*, Aorta; *italics*, pressure in mm Hg; *LA*, left atrium; *LV*, left ventricle; *PA*, pulmonary artery; *RA*, right atrium; *RV*, right ventricle; *%*, percent oxygen saturation. (From Nadas AS, Fyler DC, eds. *Nadas' Pediatric Cardiology*. Philadelphia, PA: Hanley and Belfus; 1992.)

between the systemic and pulmonary circuits. Thus, the patient with D-TGA and intact ventricular septum in heart failure related to a large patent ductus arteriosus often does poorly with division of the ductus. Similarly, correction of an interrupted aortic arch or coarctation of the aorta may upset the balance between the two circuits, particularly if the intercircuit communications are marginal. By contrast, a straddling or overriding AV valve improves mixing. While more difficult to repair surgically, these deformities promote higher saturation and therefore a more stable preoperative clinical course than those infants without such deformities.

Pulmonary vascular disease is more frequent and occurs earlier in patients with D-TGA, whether or not a VSD is present. Infants with D-TGA and an associated VSD are at higher risk for developing pulmonary vascular disease than infants with identical-sized VSDs without D-TGA. The additional feature that promotes earlier pulmonary vascular disease is elusive, but may be related to perturbations in systemic Po_2, Pco_2 and pH, as well as elevated pulmonary blood flow, oxygen saturation, and pressure.[5]

Clinical Manifestations

Infants born with D-TGA are predominantly male and often are born at normal birth weight or large for gestational age. Cyanosis in the first day of life suggests the possibility

of D-TGA, and if the ventricular septum is intact, the infant may become severely cyanotic within hours of birth. Cyanosis is often less pronounced in infants with D-TGA and a large VSD. Tachypnea is generally present without prominent retractions. Feeding may be prolonged, with the neonate tiring in the midst of vigorous efforts.

Infants with small VSDs may get little additional mixing and may follow a course comparable to that of infants with no VSD. With medium-sized VSDs, recognition of cyanosis may be delayed and tachypnea can vary depending on the pulmonary vascular resistance or degree of pulmonary stenosis if present. With a large VSD, clinically apparent cyanosis may not be present and the respiratory status may progress gradually from mild tachypnea to marked respiratory distress in the setting of heart failure similar to that seen in infants with large VSD without transposition. Infants with a straddling or overriding tricuspid valve are likely to follow this course as well. An infant with a VSD and coarctation of the aorta or an interrupted aortic arch may have marked heart failure within days of birth.

Physical Examination

Usually neonates with D-TGA and intact ventricular septum are visibly cyanotic and tachypneic with normal to mildly increased work of breathing. The cyanosis does not improve with the administration of oxygen (i.e., failed hyperoxia test). Murmurs are not a prominent feature unless there is a pressure gradient across the left ventricular outflow tract (LVOT). Most observers find that the pulmonic component of the second heart sound is difficult to discern with the posterior position of the pulmonic valve relative to the aorta.

In D-TGA and VSD, neonates are often less cyanotic but more tachypneic with increased work of breathing. A murmur is likely to be present in patients with a small- or moderate-sized VSD within a few days after birth once the pulmonary vascular resistance has dropped. Growth failure and feeding intolerance are more frequent than in patients with D-TGA and intact ventricular septum.

Electrocardiography

In most newborns with D-TGA, the electrocardiographic findings are normal. However, right ventricular hypertrophy develops later on if unrepaired. Among infants with an overriding or straddling tricuspid valve, there is left dominance and often a leftward superior axis (Fig. 29.7).

Chest Radiography

The chest radiograph is virtually normal within a few days of birth. In those with a large VSD, cardiomegaly and increased pulmonary vascularity are present. A right aortic arch can be appreciated in 1% of patients with an intact ventricular septum, 3% of those with a VSD, and in 10% of patients with a VSD and pulmonary stenosis or atresia.

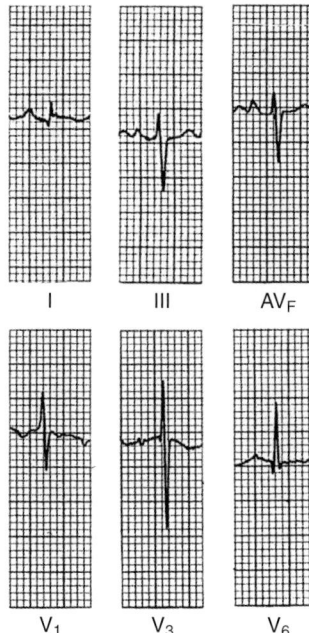

• **Fig. 29.7** Electrocardiogram of a patient with a straddling tricuspid valve. Often when there is an overriding or straddling tricuspid valve, there is hypoplasia of the right ventricle and excessive blood flow through the left ventricle compared with the right. The electrocardiogram may show a leftward-superior axis and left ventricular hypertrophy. (From Nadas AS, Fyler DC, eds. *Nadas' Pediatric Cardiology*. Philadelphia, PA: Hanley and Belfus; 1992.)

Echocardiography

The diagnosis of D-TGA is made by echocardiography. Prenatal detection of D-TGA has improved, particularly after imaging of the ventricular outflow tracts was added to the requirements for the standard obstetrical screening ultrasound in 2013; however, the prenatal detection rate still remains below 50%.[6] Therefore, postnatal echocardiography is both diagnostic and confirmatory in neonates with D-TGA. Subcostal and long-axis imaging demonstrate the left ventricle giving rise to a posterior great artery that then branches into a right and left pulmonary artery (Fig. 29.8A and B). The aorta arises anteriorly from the right ventricle in the short axis or parasagittal plane with rightward orientation of the transducer (Fig. 29.8C). Sweeping leftward from this position demonstrates the posterior pulmonary artery related to the left ventricle. The atrial septum is best visualized from the subcostal four-chamber and sagittal views (Fig. 29.9A–C). Atrial shunting is easily demonstrated using color flow Doppler interrogation. Atrial septal restriction is suggested by deviation of the septum primum into the right atrium as well as a pressure gradient between the atria estimated by Doppler interrogation of the region or by increased velocity of color flow Doppler.

The size, location, and number of VSDs should be addressed using subxiphoid, apical, and parasternal views. The subcostal and parasternal short-axis views are excellent for visualizing

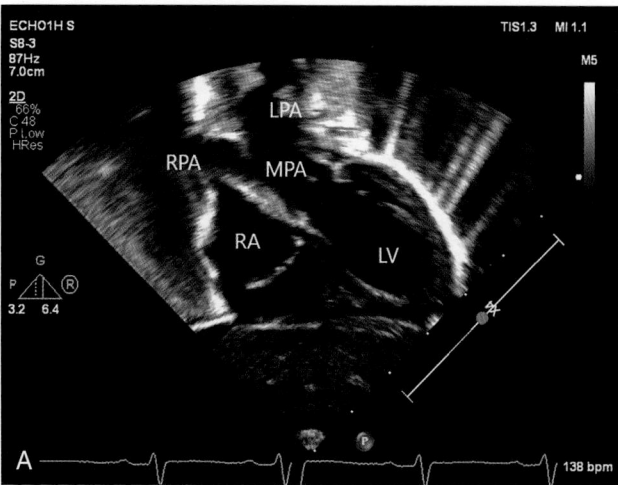
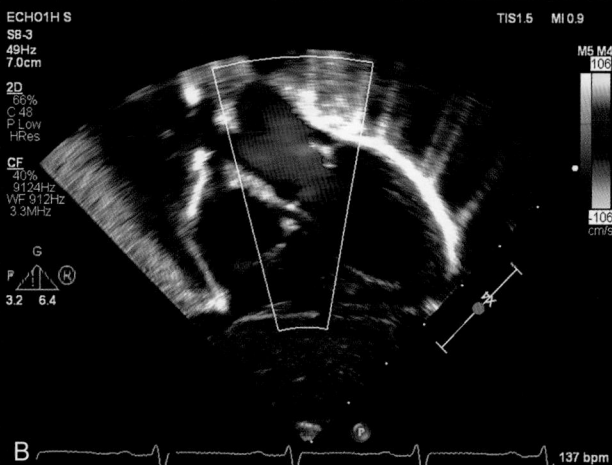
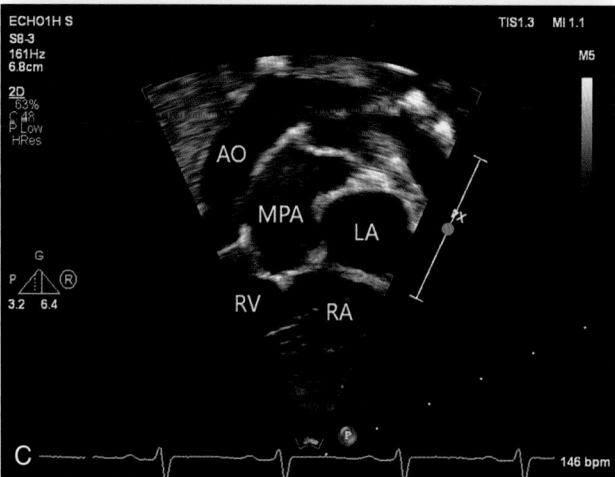

• **Fig. 29.8** D-loop transposition of the great arteries seen in **(A)** subxiphoid long-axis view showing the bifurcating pulmonary artery aligned with the left ventricle by two-dimensional imaging and **(B)** same view with color Doppler, demonstrating antegrade flow *(blue)* from the left ventricle to the main and branch pulmonary arteries. **(C)** Subxiphoid short-axis view demonstrating the aorta, including the aortic arch, aligned with the right ventricle. Note the parallel course of the great vessels, which is a hallmark of transposition. *AO,* Aorta; *LPA,* left pulmonary artery; *LV,* left ventricle; *MPA,* main pulmonary artery; *RA,* right atrium; *RPA,* right pulmonary artery; *RV,* right ventricle.

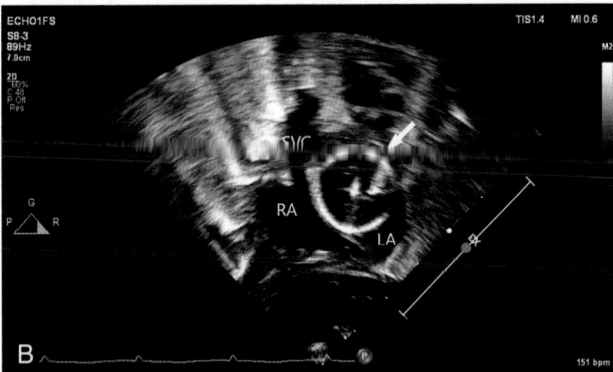

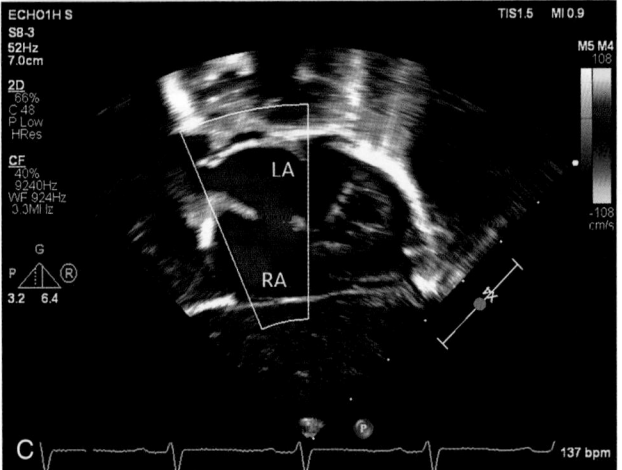

• **Fig. 29.9** Subxiphoid view of the interarterial septum in an infant with D-transposition of the great arteries. **(A)** Before balloon atrial septostomy. Note the thin septum primum bulging into the right atrium and the tiny interatrial communication. **(B)** During septostomy. Note the expanded balloon *(arrow)* nearly completely filling the left atrium. **(C)** After septostomy, note the large jet of flow left to right *(red flow)* across the atrial septum. *FO,* Foramen ovale; *LA,* left atrium; *RA,* right atrium; *SVC,* superior vena cava.

peri-membranous and AV canal defects with enhancement using color flow Doppler mapping. Anterior muscular defects are best identified using parasternal short-axis views with color flow Doppler imaging. Posterior and apical muscular defects can be seen best by scanning in the apical four-chamber, short-axis subcostal, and short-axis parasternal views.

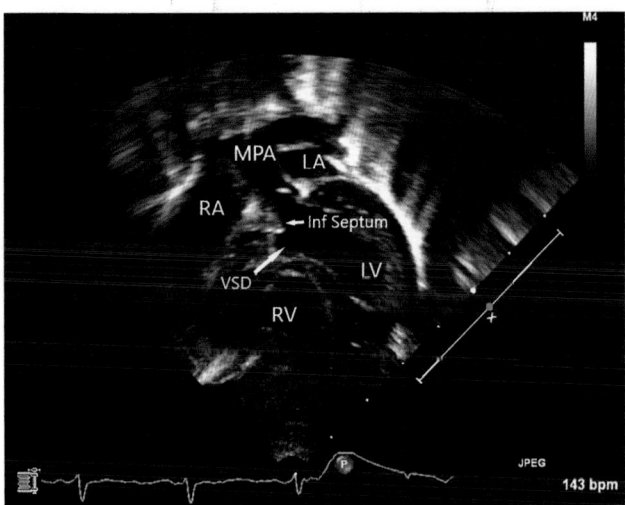

• **Fig. 29.10** Left ventricular outflow tract in a patient with D-transposition of the great arteries, a posterior malalignment ventricular septal defect, and subpulmonary stenosis. Note the posterior malalignment of the infundibular septum *(Inf Septum),* which protrudes below the pulmonary valve into the left ventricular outflow tract. *LA,* left atrium; *LV,* left ventricle; *MPA,* main pulmonary artery; *RA,* right atrium; *RV,* right ventricle; *VSD,* ventricular septal defect.

The LVOT should be examined carefully in parasternal long- and short-axis, apical long-axis, and subxiphoid long-axis views to exclude obstruction (Fig. 29.10). The morphology of the pulmonary valve should be determined in a parasternal short-axis view. Causes of LVOT obstruction include posterior malalignment of the infundibular septum, posterior bowing of the interventricular septum (dynamic subpulmonary stenosis), valvar stenosis, subvalvar membrane, accessory AV valve tissue, and a hypertrophied muscle of Moulaert (an anterolateral band of muscle in the left ventricle). The gradient across the outflow tract can be estimated using Doppler interrogation from the apical long-axis or subxiphoid short-axis views.

Occasionally in the presence of a basal VSD, the AV valve attachments may interfere with repair of the defect. Usually, abnormal attachment of the tricuspid valve to the infundibular septum can be seen in the subxiphoid short-axis views. Abnormal mitral attachments are best visualized in the parasternal short-axis, subxiphoid short-axis, and apical views.

Accurate identification of the coronary artery anatomy is critical in the setting of D-TGA. Multiple views are necessary to provide a composite pattern of the coronary branches.[7] Using the parasternal short-axis view, the left main coronary artery and its bifurcation can be seen with clockwise rotation of the transducer, and the proximal right coronary artery is noted best with counterclockwise rotation (Fig. 29.11A–B). The bifurcation of the left main coronary artery can also be seen well using a parasternal long-axis view with angling toward the left shoulder. Often an apical or subxiphoid four-chamber view is useful for demonstrating a coronary artery passing posterior to the pulmonary root in cases of single right coronary artery or origin of the left circumflex

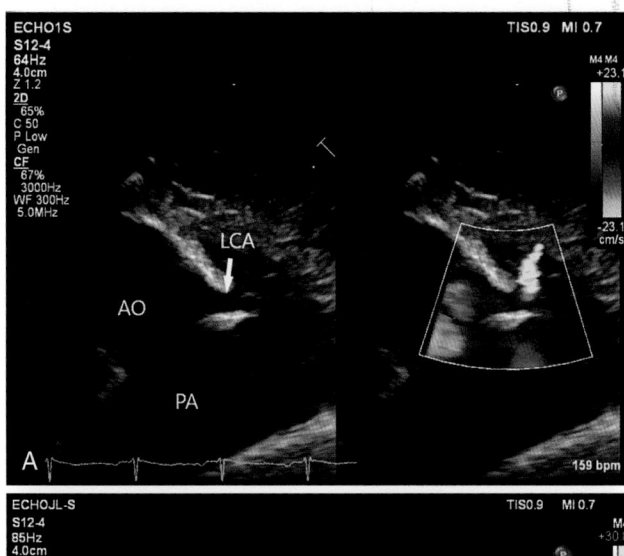

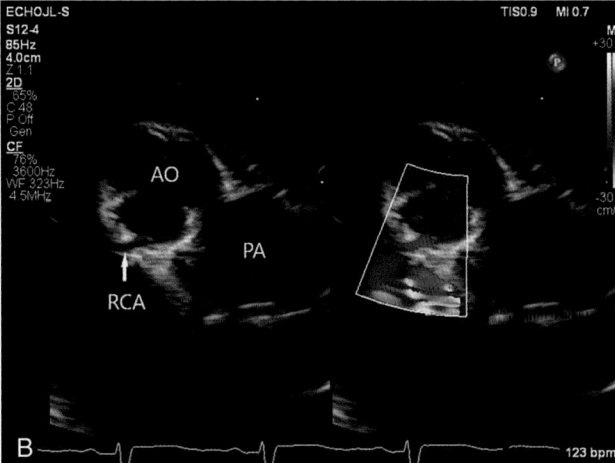

• **Fig. 29.11** Parasternal short-axis views with color Doppler comparison showing the origin of the **(A)** left and **(B)** right coronary arteries from the aorta in a patient with D-loop transposition of the great arteries. *AO,* Aorta; *LCA,* left coronary artery; *PA,* pulmonary artery; *RCA,* right coronary artery.

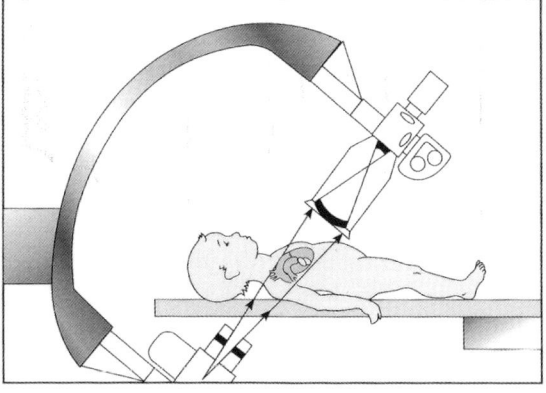

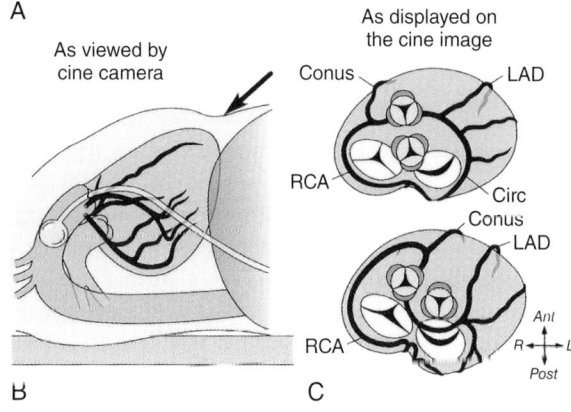

• **Fig. 29.12** The laid-back view to assess the coronary anatomy in transposition of the great arteries. **(A)** The anteroposterior position of the C-arm with maximal caudal angulation. **(B)** A lateral diagram to show the camera's view of the heart and, particularly, the great vessels and the coronary anatomy. **(C)** The cine image of anteroposterior great vessels *(upper diagram)* and side-by-side vessels *(lower diagram) Circ,* circumflex arter; *LAD,* left anterior descending; *RCA,* right coronary artery. (From Mandell VS, Lock JE, Mayer JE, Parness IA, Kulik TJ. The "laid-back" aortogram: An improved angiographic view for demonstration of coronary arteries in transposition of the great arteries. *Am J Cardiol.* 1990;65:1379–1383, with permission.)

coronary artery from the right coronary artery. Intramural coronary arteries, those with proximal segments within the wall of the aorta so that medial layers of the coronary and aorta are not separated by an adventitial layer, are surgically challenging. Careful echocardiographic analysis can detect the presence of intramural coronary arteries with acceptable precision. The variations of coronary anatomy in patients with D-transposition of the great vessels are discussed further in Chapter 42.

Cardiac Catheterization

Little information is needed beyond that furnished by echocardiography. The purpose of cardiac catheterization is to perform balloon atrial septostomy, when needed, and to confirm the coronary anatomy before an arterial switch procedure if the anatomy is incompletely defined by echocardiography. In most cases, the coronary course is well defined by echocardiography, obviating the need for coronary angiography, but when necessary, it is best visualized using the laid-back view (Fig. 29.12A–C).

Balloon atrial septostomy, introduced by Rashkind and Miller, remains the standard method of creating an atrial septal defect in cyanotic neonates with D-TGA.[8] Balloon atrial septostomy may be performed using biplane fluoroscopy or guided by bedside echocardiography (Fig. 29.9A–C). The duration of septal patency is often temporary and balloon septostomy is ineffective in most infants older than 2 months. In these circumstances, transseptal needle puncture with static balloon dilation and, occasionally, stent placement are widely employed to achieve septal patency.

Our approach to septostomy is to introduce a catheter through a 7-French sheath using an umbilical or percutaneous femoral venous entry site. Usually, the balloon is inflated with up to 3 mL of dilute contrast material and advanced into the left atrium guided often by bedside echocardiography and occasionally with fluoroscopy. Then the balloon is jerked rapidly across the septum and repeated at least once. The size of the defect is then measured by echocardiography and hemodynamic parameters are measured again.

Cardiac Computed Tomography

Cardiac computed tomography has a role in patients with D-TGA. Although rarely used in the neonatal period to diagnose coronary artery anomalies given technical challenges, routine coronary computed tomography angiography for long-term survivors following the arterial switch procedure has been described.[9] The rate of postoperative coronary abnormalities identified with coronary computed tomography is high; however, further investigation is needed to understand its impact on important long-term clinical outcomes.

Preoperative Management

In the case of known fetal diagnosis of D-TGA, optimal management includes delivery at a center where pediatric cardiologists are present to facilitate care of the neonate. At the very least, a neonatologist should be present at the delivery so that an early clinical assessment is possible. Low-dose prostaglandin E_1 infusion should be administered following vascular access securement. Anticipated side effects from prostaglandins include apnea that may lead to intubation and peripheral vasodilation that may lead to hypotension necessitating intravascular volume repletion. Following birth, the neonate should be transferred to a pediatric cardiovascular, general pediatric, or neonatal intensive care unit for further monitoring. Many neonates without prior *in utero* diagnosis are born in centers that not equipped to provide care and that may not possess prostaglandin infusions. These neonates can present with marked cyanosis and metabolic acidosis requiring prompt stabilization with prostaglandin infusion and transfer to a cardiac center by a specialized pediatric critical care transport team.

Echocardiography is performed to confirm anatomic impressions from previous fetal ultrasounds. Previously, balloon atrial septostomy was performed routinely in all neonates with TGA. However, with the introduction of the arterial switch procedure and the practice of performing surgical correction early in infancy, balloon atrial septostomy is now selectively applied to improve intra-atrial mixing in neonates with a restrictive or intact atrial septum or to facilitate an "arch watch" off of prostaglandins in the case of D-TGA with possible coarctation of the aorta. The shift away from universal balloon atrial septostomies is supported by its inability to eliminate the need for prostaglandins preoperatively and association with stroke.[10,11] When a sizable VSD is present, balloon atrial septostomy is less urgent and frequently can be avoided. Occasionally, neonates require anti-congestive therapy prior to definitive surgical repair to relieve increased work of breathing and tachypnea.

Surgery

Surgical creation of an atrial septal defect, by the Blalock-Hanlon technique, provided improved mixing of the pulmonary and systemic circuits prior to the introduction of the balloon atrial septostomy. It has been virtually abandoned as transcatheter creation of an atrial septal defect is favored in the neonate awaiting surgical repair.

Atrial switch procedures represented an important improvement in the management of the infant with D-TGA culminating in a physiologic repair of the underlying pathophysiology. In the Mustard procedure (Fig. 29.13),

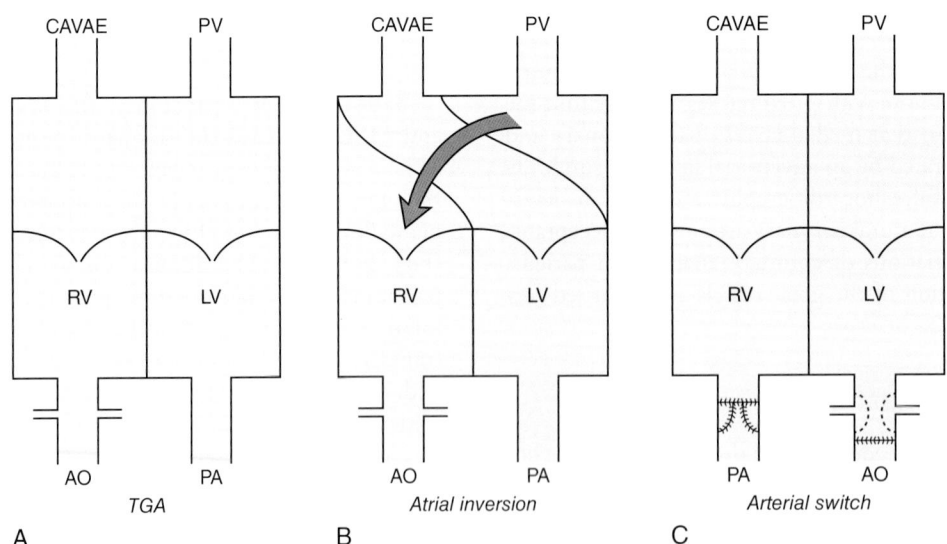

• **Fig. 29.13** Diagrammatic comparison of **(A)** unrepaired patient with transposition, **(B)** atrial inversion surgery in transposition of the great arteries, and **(C)** arterial switch surgery. Note that atrial inversion requires long atrial suture lines and results in the right ventricle being the systemic pump. Note the necessity to move the coronary arteries with arterial switching surgery; the left ventricle becomes the systemic pump. *AO*, aorta; *LV*, left ventricle; *PA*, pulmonary artery; *PV*, pulmonary vein; *RV*, right ventricle; *TGA*, transposition. (From Nadas AS, Fyler DC, eds. *Nadas' Pediatric Cardiology*. Philadelphia, PA: Hanley and Belfus; 1992.)

the pulmonary venous blood is baffled to the tricuspid valve and thus to the systemic arterial circuit, while the systemic venous blood is baffled to the mitral valve and thus to the pulmonary circuit using prosthetic material or fixed pericardium.[12] The Senning procedure accomplishes similar atrial baffling to the Mustard procedure; however, it utilizes native atrial septum and atrial free wall flaps.[13] There is little difference between the results of the two approaches with the mortality being less than 5%.[14] Timing of surgery was variable depending on institutional practice, but could be delayed for several months if necessary. Since the late 1980s, both the Mustard and Senning procedures are rarely used for management of D-TGA.

The first successful arterial switch procedure was reported by Jatene et al.[15] and involves transection and reanastomosis of the distal great arteries to the opposite proximal arterial roots as well as transposing the coronary arteries to the neoaortic root (Fig. 29.13). Lecompte et al.'s[16] modification of this technique is now widely utilized, transferring the distal pulmonary artery bifurcation anterior to the aorta (Fig. 29.14). Initially, the procedure was performed on older infants who had survived with a VSD and thus had systemic pressure in the left ventricle. Later, pulmonary artery banding was used to train the left ventricle to support the systemic circulation. Currently, neonates undergo the arterial switch procedure in the first 2 weeks of life, taking advantage of the fact that both right and left ventricles have faced similar afterload in the fetal circulation and the left ventricle is thus "prepared," obviating the need for pulmonary artery banding.[17] In the presence of large VSDs, the procedure may be delayed. However, delay in surgical repair

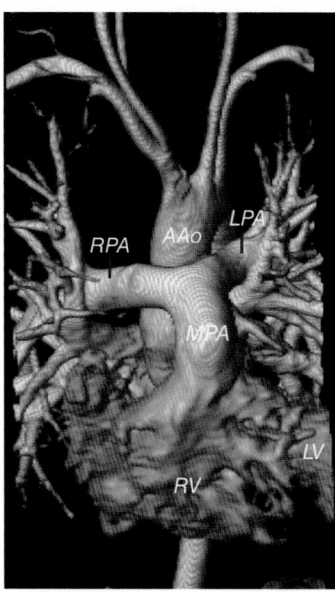

• **Fig. 12.14** Three-dimensional reconstruction from cardiac magnetic imaging dataset in patient with D-loop transposition after arterial switch operation. Note the branch pulmonary arteries which drape around the ascending aorta after Lecompte maneuver. *AAo,* Ascending aorta; *LPA,* left pulmonary artery; *LV,* left ventricle; *MPA,* main pulmonary artery; *RPA,* right pulmonary artery; *RV,* right ventricle. (Image courtesy of Dr. Tal Geva.)

can lead to the development of pulmonary vascular disease and with improvement in the management of cardiopulmonary bypass and perioperative critical care, neonates with D-TGA and VSDs are often repaired during the neonatal period. The results for either anatomic subset are excellent, although concomitant VSD closure carries a consistently higher risk. The major risk of the arterial switch procedure is inadequate myocardial perfusion related to anatomic obstruction to coronary blood flow, stenosis at the anastomotic sites of the great arteries, and neoaortic regurgitation or left ventricular failure in the case of later repairs.[17] In the initial experience with the arterial switch approach, certain variants of the coronary artery origins and distributions were associated with higher risk, but these effects have been mitigated with increasing experience.[18]

VSDs are closed by placing sutures or patches on the right side of the septum. In the era of atrial baffle repairs, VSD closure was through the tricuspid valve to avoid a ventriculotomy in the systemic right ventricle. Similarly, avoidance of damage to the tricuspid valve was critical. The poorer long-term outcomes of atrial switch procedures in D-TGA, particularly with associated VSD, provided significant motivation for the adoption of the arterial switch procedure, where tricuspid valve competence is less critical.

Relief of LVOT obstruction remains a challenge in neonates with D-TGA. Dynamic subpulmonic obstruction is the most common form due to leftward deviation of the ventricular septum in the setting of higher pressure in the right ventricular chamber relative to the left ventricle in those with intact ventricular septum. Following the arterial switch procedure, the pressure differential is reversed (left ventricle is greater than the right ventricle) and the obstruction generally resolves. After atrial baffle procedures, the obstruction may persist but is generally insignificant and rarely requires additional surgery. In neonates with fixed obstruction, the approach is dependent upon the anatomic cause. With discrete subpulmonic, fibromuscular obstruction or obstruction due to accessory AV valve tissue, resection may be possible in some using a transpulmonary approach. In the case of fixed LVOT obstruction and a sizeable VSD, the Rastelli, réparation à l'ètage ventriculaire (REV), or Nikaidoh procedures may be necessary. The Rastelli procedure involves closing the VSD so that the left ventricular output passes through the ventricular defect and into the aorta and a conduit is placed between the right ventricle and the main pulmonary artery.[19] If a restrictive VSD is present, it may require enlargement to make the Rastelli procedure feasible. The REV and Nikaidoh procedures are other options (see below).

Among the anatomic variations in patients with D-TGA, the subset with the highest surgical risk are those with D-TGA, VSD, and aortic arch obstruction. The Boston Children's approach has generally been to address all three lesions at the initial operation using techniques described above and in the chapter on coarctation and aortic arch hypoplasia. It should be noted that the mortality rate for this repair is at least 10% both locally and nationally. The major anatomic risk factor for this patient group is hypoplasia of the tricuspid valve, which is typically associated with hypoplasia of the right ventricular infundibulum. Patch augmentation of this sub-neopulmonary area is frequently required.

Conversion from an atrial switch to an arterial switch procedure has been used to make the left ventricle the systemic ventricle in failing Mustard or Senning patients. Conversion requires banding of the main pulmonary artery initially to "prepare" the left ventricle for systemic afterload by inducing ventricular hypertrophy. Once sufficient left ventricular hypertrophy is observed, the patient can undergo an arterial switch procedure with coronary reimplantation and takedown of the atrial baffle. The duration of the induced increase in left ventricular afterload is variable, although as a general rule, as patients are older at the time of banding, the duration of pre-arterial switch LV "training" seems to take longer, and may extend from months to years.

Palliative atrial baffle procedures are occasionally used in patients with D-TGA and inoperable levels of pulmonary vascular obstructive disease due to either a large VSD or patent ductus arteriosus.[20] Baffling full saturated, pulmonary venous blood to the ascending aorta via the right ventricle increases systemic arterial Po2, even in those with a VSD due to streaming within the ventricles. In those with a patent ductus arteriosus, preoperative cyanosis was often more obvious in the upper rather than lower limbs as the ductus perfused the descending aorta with fully saturated blood (reverse differential cyanosis). Postoperatively, the more obvious improvement was in the upper extremities.

Finally, patients with D-TGA (with or without a VSD) who are either diagnosed or seek care late may suffer from elevated pulmonary arterial pressures as a result of pulmonary vascular obstructive disease in addition to left ventricular deconditioning. In this rare subset of patients, a two-stage surgical approach may be warranted. Placement of a pulmonary artery band both re-trains the left ventricle and also may promote vascular remodeling of the pulmonary arterial tree. If the pulmonary arterial pressures diminish to an acceptable level, a subsequent arterial switch procedure may be possible. Occasionally, re-tightening of the pulmonary artery band is required prior to achieving anatomic correction.

Course Following Atrial Switch Repair

The natural history of D-TGA is marked by limited survival without surgery. Those with an intact ventricular septum generally do not survive beyond the first year of life, with most succumbing early in infancy.[21] Patients with a large VSD or patent ductus arteriosus may survive if not operated upon, but pulmonary vascular obstructive disease nearly always develops. In rare cases of balanced physiology, patients with D-TGA, large VSD, and pulmonic stenosis have survived for a number of years. Even more unusual is late survival of patients with D-TGA and intact ventricular septum with a large atrial septal defect. For the population of those who have undergone physiologic correction with an atrial switch, a sizable number have survived into adulthood with greater mortality in those with large VSDs versus those with intact ventricular septum.[22]

Despite survival into adulthood for those who had an atrial switch procedure, a number of late morbidities have been identified, including loss of sinus rhythm, systemic RV dysfunction, and systemic tricuspid valve regurgitation, and supported the near universal application of the arterial switch approach to neonates with D-TGA. The following sections highlight these key late morbidities.

Rhythm Abnormalities

Brady- and tachyarrhythmias are late complications frequently experienced in patients following an atrial switch operation. Supraventricular rhythm disturbances, especially atrial fibrillation and intra-atrial reentrant tachycardia, are common. Atrial tachyarrhythmias are thought to be a result of long-standing atrial enlargement in the setting of systemic right ventricular failure or tricuspid regurgitation. Sinus node dysfunction, manifested by brady-tachyarrhythmias and in some cases overt syncope, is thought to result from injury related to extensive atrial incisions and suture lines with damage to the sinus node artery. Many require pacemaker implantation to minimize recurrent symptomatic episodes since antiarrhythmic therapy alone may aggravate bradycardia. Sudden death, presumably related to rhythm disorders, is a well-recognized phenomenon occurring in up to 1% of patients who undergo physiologic correction of D-TGA with an atrial switch procedure.[22]

Baffle Obstruction and Leak

Obstruction of the superior limb of the systemic venous baffle at the right atrial–superior vena cava junction is a well-known sequela of the Mustard procedure. The clinical presentation may include chylothorax, edema of the upper extremities, or hydrocephalus. Occasionally, decompression via the azygous vein may mask the presence of severe baffle obstruction. Catheter intervention or surgical revision of the baffle may be required. Inferior vena caval obstruction is uncommon. Pulmonary venous obstruction is a more frequent complication of the Senning procedure. Early manifestations may be pulmonary venous congestion on chest radiograph in the early postoperative period or symptoms of reactive airway disease unresponsive to bronchodilator therapy as a late complication. Baffle leaks are not common, but when present are generally noted at the superior aspect of the right atrium. If the predominant shunt is right to left, the patient may show cyanosis, though most often the degree of leak is too small to be clinically apparent. Left-to-right shunts are generally not hemodynamically significant.

Systemic Tricuspid Regurgitation

Tricuspid regurgitation was commonly found following surgical repairs that include closure of a membranous VSD by a transatrial approach. Although generally of minimal significance in the case of an arterial switch procedure, tricuspid regurgitation is more critical after atrial switch operations. As the tricuspid valve is the systemic AV valve in patients who have undergone an atrial switch procedure, preservation of the tricuspid valve's function is linked to superior long-term clinical outcomes.

Systemic Right Ventricular Dysfunction

Failure of the morphologic right (systemic) ventricle is widely reported following the Senning or Mustard procedure, although most patients are asymptomatic. However, echocardiographic and stress testing criteria show abnormal ventricular response to stress as well as decreased exercise tolerance that have both chronotropic and ventricular function components. Cardiac transplantation may be necessary in a small number of patients with severe decompensation of ventricular function.

Course Following Arterial Switch Procedure

In an effort to mitigate the late morbidities experienced in patients who have undergone physiologic correction of D-TGA (i.e., atrial switch procedures), anatomic surgical correction with an arterial switch procedure is the typical approach in neonates presently. The overall outcomes following the arterial switch operation have progressively improved since the 1980s, but there still remain a few classic complications. Although the impact of atypical coronary artery patterns has been mitigated, increased postoperative risk experienced with VSD closure and aortic arch repair remain.[23]

Coronary Insufficiency

Kinking or stretching of the coronary arteries can lead to coronary artery obstruction following the arterial switch procedure. Coronary artery obstruction is typically apparent in the operating room or early in the perioperative period. Presentation manifests with electrocardiographic changes of ischemia (i.e., ST segment depression or elevation), ventricular arrhythmias or profound low output with concurrent left ventricular systolic dysfunction. When suspected intraoperatively, inspection and reconfiguration of the proximal coronary segments is mandatory. In some cases, infants with important obstruction identified at a routine follow-up catheterization can be completely asymptomatic and have developed arterial collateralization over time. If coronary insufficiency is considered, diagnosis should be confirmed as soon as possible as time from sentinel event to diagnosis has been associated with survival.

Supravalvar Obstruction

An incidence of supravalvar pulmonary stenosis following the arterial switch procedure was soon noted after this surgical approach was introduced. The most frequent types of obstruction are discrete narrowing at the suture line of the anastomosis and long segment obstruction in the pulmonary arteries, especially the right, as they are draped across and anterior to the ascending aorta (due to the Lecompte maneuver). In early series, the frequency of stenosis was quite high, however in the more recent era, with emphasis on more extensive branch pulmonary artery mobilization to reduce anastomotic tension, the incidence has fallen considerably. Transcatheter resolution of discrete pulmonary artery stenoses either with balloon dilation or stent placement has been met with reasonable success in relieving the gradients. For long segment narrowing, balloon dilation is generally inadequate necessitating stent placement or surgical reintervention. Supravalvar aortic obstruction is far less frequent than supravalvar pulmonic obstruction.

Rhythm Abnormalities

In contrast to the atrial switch procedure, rhythm disturbances following the arterial switch procedure have been far less prevalent. AV conduction is rarely impaired, with less than 2% developing complete AV block all following VSD closure. Though supraventricular tachycardia and ventricular ectopic activity were noted commonly in the postoperative period, late ventricular tachycardia has been documented in fewer than 1%. Early postoperative ventricular tachyarrhythmias should always raise the concern of coronary artery obstruction and necessitate further investigation (i.e., troponin trend, serial electrocardiograms, and potentially echocardiography or angiography).

Left Ventricular Function

Preservation of left ventricular function after the arterial switch procedure is well documented.[23] Following an arterial switch procedure, including those with VSD closure, echocardiographic and catheterization quantitative analysis of ventricular function, cardiac index, left ventricular filling pressures, wall dimensions and thickness, systolic function, loading conditions, and contractility were normal greater than 3 years following the procedure.[23] Those undergoing a two-stage repair with initial pulmonary artery banding for LV "retraining" showed some mild derangement in function and contractility. Exercise testing in patients with D-TGA that is repaired with a primary arterial switch procedure show excellent preservation of cardiopulmonary function as compared with patients who underwent an atrial switch procedure.

Neoaortic Regurgitation

By reversing the great arteries in the arterial switch procedure, the native pulmonic valve serves as the neoaortic valve. Mild aortic regurgitation following surgery is present frequently, but progression to a moderate or severe requiring surgical intervention is rare. Employing the trap door technique for coronary artery reimplantation and undergoing an arterial switch beyond 1 year of age have been associated with increased frequency of neoaortic regurgitation.[24]

Additionally, reports have shown that the neoaortic annulus and root are larger compared with those of controls several years following surgery and that the size of the aortic root increases over the first several years postoperatively, which can result in progressive neoaortic regurgitation. Those with native bicuspid pulmonary (future neoaortic) valves have been demonstrated to have earlier occurrence of both root dilation and neoaortic regurgitation.

Variations

D-Transposition of the Great Arteries With Intact Ventricular Septum and Pulmonary Stenosis

LVOT obstruction with D-TGA and intact ventricular septum occurs in approximately 10%–30% of patients. As described above, the obstruction is often dynamic and related to leftward displacement of the ventricular septum which resolves after the arterial switch procedure. The remainder of cases results from fibrous tissue in the ventricular septum sometimes in association with abnormal mitral valve attachments or rarely valvar pulmonic stenosis. Though early results for surgical intervention were variable, more recent data following the arterial switch procedure indicates an almost uniformly good outcome for this group.

D-Transposition and Coarctation of the Aorta

The combination of coarctation or interruption of the aorta in combination with D-transposition of the aorta is rare and generally occurs in the setting of a VSD. Though survival was uncommon previously, results have improved using a single-stage repair including an arterial switch, VSD closure, and aortic arch repair. However, the mortality rate still remains higher when compared to patients with D-TGA and VSD without arch obstruction.

D-Transposition of the Great Arteries With Ventricular Septal Defect and Pulmonary Stenosis

D-TGA with VSD and pulmonary stenosis is present in approximately 10% of cases. The number, size, and location of VSDs vary as does the degree of LVOT obstruction, ranging from mild subvalvar involvement to pulmonary atresia (Fig. 29.15). The clinical presentation is related to the degree of LVOT obstruction and size of the VSD. Large VSDs with lesser degrees of LVOT obstruction present with a murmur or signs of heart failure, while those patients with smaller VSDs or increasing degrees of LVOT obstruction will show prominent cyanosis early in the neonatal period.

The surgical approach to this combination of lesions is not straightforward. In cases of severe cyanosis related to marked LVOT obstruction, many centers favor placement of a systemic to pulmonary shunt in the neonate (i.e., Blalock-Taussig-Thomas shunt). This palliative procedure is

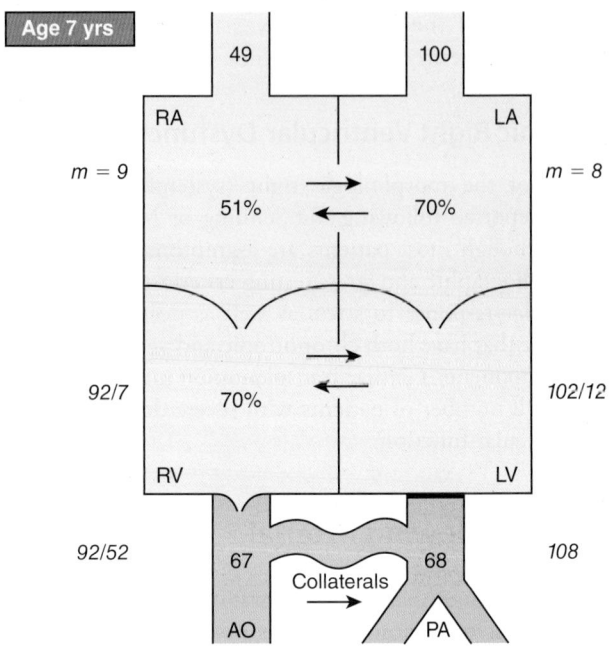

• Fig. 29.15 A hemodynamic diagram of a patient with transposition of the great arteries, ventricular defect, and pulmonary atresia. Note that the only blood supply to the lungs is via major collaterals arising from the descending aorta. Compare with a similar situation encountered in patients with tetralogy of Fallot and pulmonary atresia (see Chapter 26). *AO,* Aorta; italics, pressure in mm Hg; *LA,* left atrium; *LV,* left ventricle; *PA,* pulmonary artery; *RA,* right atrium; *RV,* right ventricle; %, percent oxygen saturation. (From Nadas AS, Fyler DC, eds. *Nadas' Pediatric Cardiology.* Philadelphia, PA: Hanley and Belfus; 1992.)

followed at a later date by a repair that achieves physiologic correction, most often a Rastelli procedure.[19] If the anatomic size and location of the VSD is acceptable, surgery involves closure of the defect with a baffle that directs left ventricular output to the aorta, in conjunction with placement of a right ventricular to pulmonary artery homograft. Alternatively, the Rastelli procedure can be performed in the neonatal period with anticipated conduit revision at a later time. An alternative approach was described by Lecompte et al.[16] and utilizes resection of the outlet septum via right ventriculotomy in order to facilitate left ventricular to aortic continuity. This approach requires transection of the pulmonary artery, closure of the native pulmonic valve, and anastomosis of the main pulmonary artery directly to the right ventricle in order to complete an anatomic and physiologic repair. This option is known as the REV procedure, which although similar to a Rastelli procedure is distinguished by resecting the infundibular septum to allow for a smaller VSD patch and thus less bulging of the patch into the right ventricle as well as creation of a direct connection from the right ventricle to the pulmonary artery, potentially obviating the need for an extracardiac conduit. Finally, in the Nikaidoh procedure, the native aortic root can be translocated into the native pulmonary root with native pulmonary (neoaortic) root enlargement using the same patch as used to close the VSD. This procedure is often used in younger patients as the incidence of late obstruction in the left ventricle to aorta pathway after the Rastelli procedure is significant. When comparing technical performance between a Rastelli, REV, and Nikaidoh procedure for patients with D-TGA with a VSD and LVOT obstruction, the Nikaidoh procedure is associated with minimal residual LVOT obstruction and normal left ventricular systolic function.[25] However, the Nikaidoh procedure is associated with increased resource utilization due to prolonged mechanical ventilation and length of stay.

Overriding Tricuspid Valve, Right Ventricular Hypoplasia, and Arch Obstruction With D-Transposition of the Great Arteries

When the tricuspid valve overrides the ventricular septum in D-TGA, the right ventricle may be small and arch hypoplasia or interruption may coexist (Fig. 29.16). In the case of a mildly hypoplastic right ventricle, an arterial switch procedure may be sufficient if the right ventricle and tricuspid valve can accept the systemic venous return at an acceptable filling pressure. In patients undergoing a complete primary repair of D-TGA with a VSD and aortic arch obstruction, the neonatal Z-score of the tricuspid valve is a predictor of mortality. Whereas, late development of right ventricular outflow tract obstruction is best predicted by the neonatal Z-score of the transverse aortic arch. If the right ventricle is diminutive, an arterial switch procedure can be performed in conjunction with an aortopulmonary shunt (i.e., Blalock-Taussig-Thomas shunt) to augment pulmonary blood flow. This initial approach is followed by a bidirectional Glenn and eventually a Fontan procedure. In some cases, the aortic arch may be so small as to require augmentation.

Summary

The management of D-TGA is a story of remarkable improvements. A uniformly lethal disease prior to surgical intervention, the care for these patients has seen exceptional improvements in quantity and quality of life with first the adoption of the atrial switch followed by the arterial switch procedures. The long-term outcomes of physiologic (atrial level) repair remain an issue for our adult congenital patients, but increased awareness and management have markedly improved their quality of life. With adoption of the arterial switch procedure, long-term morbidities appear minimal in comparison although still necessitate life-long follow-up. Finally, further investigation is warranted to determine the superior surgical procedure for patients with D-TGA, VSD, and LVOT obstruction.

References

1. Reller MD, Strickland MJ, Riehle-Colarusso T, et al. Prevalence of congenital heart defects in metropolitan Atlanta, 1998-2005. *J Pediatr.* 2008;153:807-813.
2. Pasquali SK, Hasselblad V, Li JS, et al. Coronary artery pattern and outcome of arterial switch operation for transposition of the great arteries: a meta-analysis. *Circulation.* 2002;106:2575-2580.
3. Lang P, Freed MD, Bierman FZ. Use of prostaglandin E1 in infants with d-transposition of the great arteries and intact ventricular septum. *Am J Cardiol.* 1979;44:76-81.
4. Anderson BR, Ciarleglio AJ, Hayes DA, et al. Earlier arterial switch operation improves outcomes and reduces costs for neonates with transposition of the great arteries. *J Am Coll Cardiol.* 2014;63:481-487.
5. Newfeld EA, Paul MM, Muster AJ, et al. Pulmonary vascular disease in complete transposition of the great arteries: a study of 200 patients. *Am J Cardiol.* 1974;34:75-82.
6. Escobar-Diaz MC, Freud LR, Bueno A, et al. Prenatal diagnosis of transposition of the great arteries over a 20-year period: improved but imperfect. *Ultrasound Obstet Gynecol.* 2015;45: 678-682.
7. Pasquini L, Sanders SP, Parness IA, et al. Coronary echocardiography in 406 patients with d-loop transposition of the great arteries. *J Am Coll Cardiol.* 1994;24:763-768.
8. Rashkind WJ, Miller WW. Creation of an atrial septal defect without thoracotomy. A palliative approach to complete transposition of the great arteries. *JAMA.* 1966;196:991-992.
9. Szymczyk K, Moll M, Sobczak-Budlewska K, et al. Usefulness of routine coronary CT angiography in patients with transposition of the great arteries after an arterial switch operation. *Pediatr Cardiol.* 2018;39:335-346.
10. Zaleski KL, McMullen CL, Staffa SJ, et al. Elective non-urgent balloon-atrial septostomy in infants with d-transposition of the great

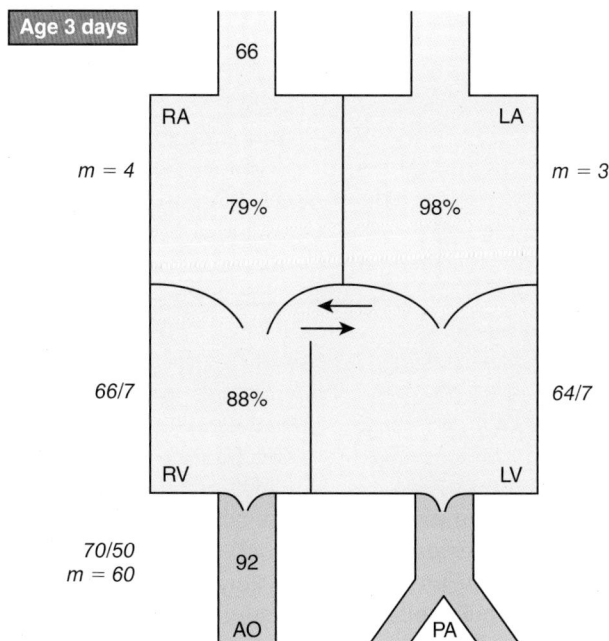

• **Fig. 29.16** Hemodynamic diagram of a patient with transposition of the great arteries, ventricular septal defect, and straddling tricuspid valve. The direct communication of the right atrium to the pulmonary ventricle (anatomic left ventricle) improves mixing of the pulmonary and systemic circulations. The arterial saturation is better than that in the usual patient with transposition of the great arteries despite an added major and surgically uncorrectable problem. *AO,* Aorta; italics, pressure in mm Hg; *LA,* left atrium; *LV,* left ventricle; *PA,* pulmonary artery; *RA,* right atrium; *RV,* right ventricle; *%,* percent oxygen saturation. (From Nadas AS, Fyler DC, eds. *Nadas' Pediatric Cardiology.* Philadelphia, PA: Hanley and Belfus; 1992.)

arteries does not eliminate the need for PGE1 therapy at the time of arterial switch operation. *Pediatr Cardiol.* 2021;42:597-605.

11. Hamzah M, Othman HF, Peluso AM, et al. Prevalence and outcomes of balloon atrial septostomy in neonates with transposition of great arteries. *Pediatr Crit Care Med.* 2020;21:324-331.

12. Mustard WT. Successful two-stage correction of transposition of the great vessels. *Surgery.* 1964;55:969-972.

13. Senning A. Surgical correction of transposition of the great vessels. *Surgery.* 1959;45:966-980.

14. Marx GR, Hougen TJ, Norwood WI, et al. Transposition of the great arteries with intact ventricular septum: results of Mustard and Senning operations in 123 consecutive patients. *J Am Coll Cardiol.* 1983;1:476-483.

15. Jatene AD, Fontes VF, Paulista PP, et al. Anatomic correction of transposition of the great vessels. *J Thorac Cardiovasc Surg.* 1976;72:364-370.

16. Lecompte Y, Zannini L, Hazan E, et al. Anatomic correction of transposition of the great arteries. *J Thorac Cardiovasc Surg.* 1981;82:629-631.

17. Wernovsky G, Hougen TJ, Walsh EP, et al. Midterm results after the arterial switch operation for transposition of the great arteries with intact ventricular septum: clinical, hemodynamic, echocardiographic, and electrophysiologic data. *Circulation.* 1988;77:1333-1344.

18. Blume ED, Altmann K, Mayer Jr JE, Colan SD, Gauvreau K, Geva T. Evolution of risk factors influencing early mortality of the arterial switch operation. *J Am Coll Cardiol.* 1999;33:1702-1709.

19. Villagra F, Quero-Jimenez M, Maitre-Azcarate MJ, et al. Transposition of the great arteries with ventricular septal defects: surgical considerations concerning the Rastelli operation. *J Thorac Cardiovasc Surg.* 1984;88:1004-1011.

20. Burkhart HM, Dearani JA, Williams WG, et al. Late results of palliative atrial switch for transposition, ventricular septal defect and pulmonary vascular obstructive disease. *Ann Thorac Surg.* 2004;77:464-469.

21. Liebman J, Cullum L, Belloc NB. Natural history of transposition of the great arteries: anatomy and birth and death characteristics. *Circulation.* 1969;40:237-262.

22. Williams WG, McCrindle BW, Ashburn DA, et al. Outcomes of 829 neonates with complete transposition of the great arteries 12-17 years after repair. *Eur J Cardiothorac Surg.* 2003;24:1.

23. Khairy P, Clair M, Fernandez SM, et al. Cardiovascular outcomes after the arterial switch operation for D-transposition of the great arteries. *Circulation.* 2013;127:331-339.

24. Formigari R, Toscano A, Giardini A, et al. Prevalence and predictors of neoaortic regurgitation after arterial switch operation for transposition of the great arteries. *J Thorac Cardiovasc Surg.* 2003;126:1753-1759.

25. Hu SS, Liu ZG, Li SJ, et al. Strategy for biventricular outflow tract reconstruction: Rastelli, REV, or Nikaidoh procedure? *J Thorac Cardiovasc Surg.* 2008;135:331-338.

30

Congenitally Corrected Transposition of the Great Arteries

KEVIN P. DALY AND JOHN E. MAYER JR.

KEY LEARNING POINTS

- Congenitally corrected transposition of the great arteries is the result of the combination of atrioventricular and ventriculoarterial discordance.
- Congenitally corrected transposition of the great arteries is frequently associated with other cardiac lesions, most commonly pulmonary (or subpulmonary) stenosis, ventricular septal defect, and Ebsteinoid-like tricuspid valve abnormalities.
- Complete heart block is a frequent complication with 5% having congenital complete heart block and there being

a relatively constant risk for the development of complete heart block over time (approximately 1% per year).
- Anatomic repair (frequently referred to as the "double switch operation") is the most common approach to surgical repair, especially if other cardiac lesions are present. Preparation of the morphologic left ventricle with a pulmonary artery band is frequently required.
- Long-term prognosis is determined by the development of complications, including heart failure with reduced ejection fraction, tricuspid regurgitation, and complete heart block.

Definition

Congenitally corrected transposition of the great arteries (ccTGA) is characterized by atrioventricular (AV) discordance and TGA (ventriculoarterial discordance). In such patients, systemic desaturated venous return passes from an atrium through a mitral valve into a morphologic left ventricle (mLV) and from there to the pulmonary artery (PA). The saturated pulmonary venous blood then traverses the opposite atrium to cross a tricuspid valve into a morphologic right ventricle (mRV) from which the aorta arises. Thus, because arterial oxygen saturation is normal in these patients in the rare case of complete absence of other cardiac lesions, the term "congenitally corrected" has been given to this entity based on the "correct" physiology. In this chapter, only patients with two ventricles are considered; those with a single ventricle or with one AV valve are discussed elsewhere (see Chapters 32, 35, 36, and 37).

Prevalence

TGA with two functionally adequate but inverted ventricles and levocardia (also called {S,L,L}; see Chapter 3) is a rare anomaly, with an incidence ranging from 0.03 to 0.07 per

1000 live births.[1-3] Familial clusters demonstrate that this is not always a sporadic defect and can be associated with other forms of transposition, laterality disorders, and primary ciliary dyskinesia.[4] At Boston Children's Hospital, 374 patients with this {S,L,L} anomaly have been evaluated since 1973 (Table 30.1). In addition, there were 50 others seen since 1973 with the next most common variety of congenitally corrected transposition, dextrocardia and a "mirror image" of the above, referred to as {I,D,D} (see Chapter 3).

Anatomy

The segmental anatomy (see Chapter 3) of this lesion is of two varieties: the more common is {S,L,L} and the next most common variant is its mirror image {I,D,D}. Dextrocardia or levocardia can exist with either segmental anatomy. In {S,L,L}, there is typically levocardia with situs solitus of the atria and viscera; the right-sided superior and inferior vena cavae drain into a right-sided atrium, which empties through a mitral valve with two papillary muscles into a finely trabeculated mLV (AV discordance), which in turn empties through a right-sided posterior pulmonary valve. The great vessel arrangement (ventriculoarterial [VA]

TABLE 30.1 Boston Children's Hospital experience, 1973–2022, with other cardiac problems associated with congenitally corrected transposition of the great arteries (*N* = 374). Each value represents the % of patients in a given column with each anomaly. Categories are not mutually exclusive. In total, 667 patients with single ventricle and {S,L,L} classification were excluded from the tables. The excluded patients included 459 with double inlet left ventricle, 54 with double-inlet ventricle of indeterminate morphology, 15 with double-inlet right ventricle, 43 with tricuspid atresia type IIIA–C, 20 with hypoplastic left heart syndrome, and 76 with other single-ventricle variants.

Year of Birth	1973–2022	1973–1987	1988–2002	2003–2022
Number (%)	*N* = 374 (100%)	*N* = 62 (17%)	*N* = 112 (30%)	*N* = 200 (53%)
Complete heart block	28	32	24	30
Present at birth	5	3	5	5
Pulmonary valve abnormality	54	61	55	51
Pulmonary stenosis	44	48	47	40
Subvalvar pulmonary stenosis	26	35	32	20
Pulmonary atresia	12	16	12	11
Ventricular septal defect	59	66	58	57
Atrioventricular canal type	9	6	11	10
Conal	3	0	1	4
Conoventricular	17	15	14	19
Membranous	17	19	15	18
Multiple	6	6	5	6
Muscular	12	6	5	18
Tricuspid valve anatomic problem	32	18	33	38
Ebstein anomaly	22	15	21	26
Tricuspid valve regurgitation (Moderate/severe)	39	34	43	38
Atrial septal defect	21	11	14	27
Aortic stenosis	11	3	15	11
Subaortic stenosis	7	2	12	7
Patent ductus arteriosus	12	8	7	17
Endocardial cushion defect	10	10	13	10
Coarctation of the aorta	8	3	8	10
Mitral valve disease	7	5	4	10

discordance) is also referred to as L-transposition. The left atrium empties through a tricuspid valve into a coarsely trabeculated mRV, which in turn empties through a left-sided anterior aortic valve. The two outflow tracts are parallel to one another, in contrast to their crossed positions in the normal heart, and the ventricular septum lies in a more anteroposterior position (Fig. 30.1). A mirror image form of this disease can also occur. This occurs when there is {I,D,D} segmental anatomy, usually associated with dextrocardia. The abdominal viscera are inverted, the superior and inferior vena cavae are left-sided and open into a morphologic right atrium, which empties through a mitral valve into mLV, which in turn connects to a left-sided posterior PA. Pulmonary venous return is to a right-sided morphologic left

atrium, which empties through a tricuspid valve into mRV (D-loop), which in turn connects to a right-sided anterior aorta (D-transposition).

Rarely, there are no associated cardiac defects. Survival of a 92-year-old woman who successfully carried 10 pregnancies and did not develop heart failure until 70 years old has been reported.[5] However, most patients have other cardiac anomalies (Table 30.1) that contribute to prognosis.[6] Tricuspid valve abnormalities are common, and regurgitation is frequent and, if left unrepaired, often progressive.[7,8] The tricuspid valve abnormality is frequently similar to Ebstein anomaly, and systolic dysfunction of the systemic right ventricle leading to heart failure is common with increasing age.[9]

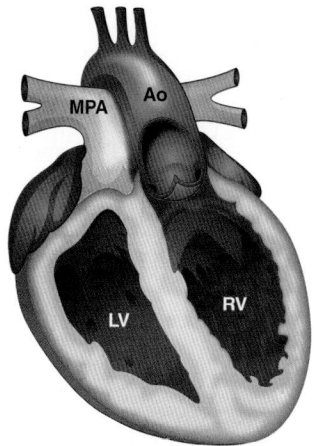

• **Fig. 30.1** Drawing of anteroposterior view of congenitally corrected transposition of the great arteries showing a trabeculated right-sided morphologic left ventricle *(mLV)* opening into posterior right-sided main pulmonary artery *(MPA)* and left-sided coarsely trabeculated morphologic right ventricle *(mRV)* opening into anterior left-sided aorta *(Ao)*. The mLV has a mitral valve with two papillary muscles originating from the free wall, whereas the mRV has a tricuspid valve, often "Ebstein-like" with at least one papillary muscle. (Adapted From Fyler DC, ed. *Nadas' Pediatric Cardiology.* Philadelphia: Hanley & Belfus; 1992.)

Pulmonary outflow obstruction is common and occurs most often in the subpulmonary area. It is usually due to impingement of the mitral valve apparatus or accessory valve–associated tissue into the outflow tract and rarely due to isolated valvar stenosis.[10] Pulmonary atresia does occur, although it is sometimes uncertain from which ventricle the pulmonary artery arises.

Ventricular septal defects (VSDs) may occur anywhere in the septum but are most commonly located in the membranous portion and adjacent areas. The pulmonary trunk may substantially override a membranous VSD and straddling of the tricuspid or mitral valve is associated with underdevelopment of either the mRV or mLV.

Conduction System

In {S,L,L} the sinus node is in the usual location. The atrial and ventricular septa are generally malaligned, unless the pulmonary trunk is underdeveloped.[11] The location of the AV node is variable. Anatomical studies have postulated the presence of two AV nodes, one in the normal location of the apex of the triangle of Koch and a second AV node located rightward and anterior of the first.[12] In our experience with intraoperative electroanatomic mapping, the presence of functional twin AV nodes is rare.[13] In most cases of {S,L,L}, the penetrating bundle of His arises from the right anterior AV node location. If a VSD is present, the His bundle and distal conduction system is often located on the superior margin. Anatomic studies have suggested that if there is pulmonary atresia or a small pulmonary trunk, then the atrial and ventricular septa are well aligned and the penetrating bundle can arise from the normally located inferoposterior AV node location.

AV block has been identified in the fetus and is present in about 5% of children; heart block spontaneously occurs over time with up to 40% of patients requiring pacemaker placement.[10,14] In contrast to {S,L,L}, children with {I,D,D} may have a normally located conduction system and spontaneous complete heart block is rare. However, recent intraoperative mapping studies have shown that there can be variations in AV node and His bundle anatomy in {I,D,D} hearts as well.[13]

Coronary Anatomy

Variations are frequent, but in general in those with {S,L,L}, the coronary artery origins are a mirror image of normal in that the right-sided vessel is morphologically similar to a normal left coronary with a circumflex and anterior descending, and the left-sided coronary resembles a right coronary artery.[15-17] In those with {I,D,D}, the coronaries are typically similar to usual coronary arteries in D-TGA.

Physiology

The physiologic problems presented by patients with ccTGA are directly related to the associated defects. Those without associated defects are fully saturated, and have outwardly normal physiology. Patients with pulmonary atresia are dependent on ductal patency at birth.

The systolic function of the mRV in the systemic position is a key determinant of prognosis. Right ventricular myofibers are primarily arranged longitudinally and right ventricular longitudinal strain has been demonstrated to decline over time and be an important marker of systemic right ventricular dysfunction and heart failure.[18] Maximal coronary flow reserve is decreased and correlates with ventricular function in both preoperative and postoperative patients.[19]

Clinical Manifestations

The clinical features are, similarly, a direct function of the associated cardiac anatomy. A relatively constant auscultatory finding, regardless of associated lesions, is the very loud (often palpable in the child) aortic valve closure component of the second heart sound (S2) at the upper left sternal border due to its proximity to the sternum. The infant may present with cyanosis, heart failure, or a heart murmur depending on the associated cardiac defects. An abnormal chest x-ray or ECG may also lead to cardiac referral.

Electrocardiography

In {S,L,L} an initial Q wave may be present in the right-sided chest leads and absent in the left due to depolarization of the ventricular septum from right to left (opposite of normal) (Fig. 30.2). Varying degrees of heart block, usually with a QRS complex of normal duration, are common—approximately

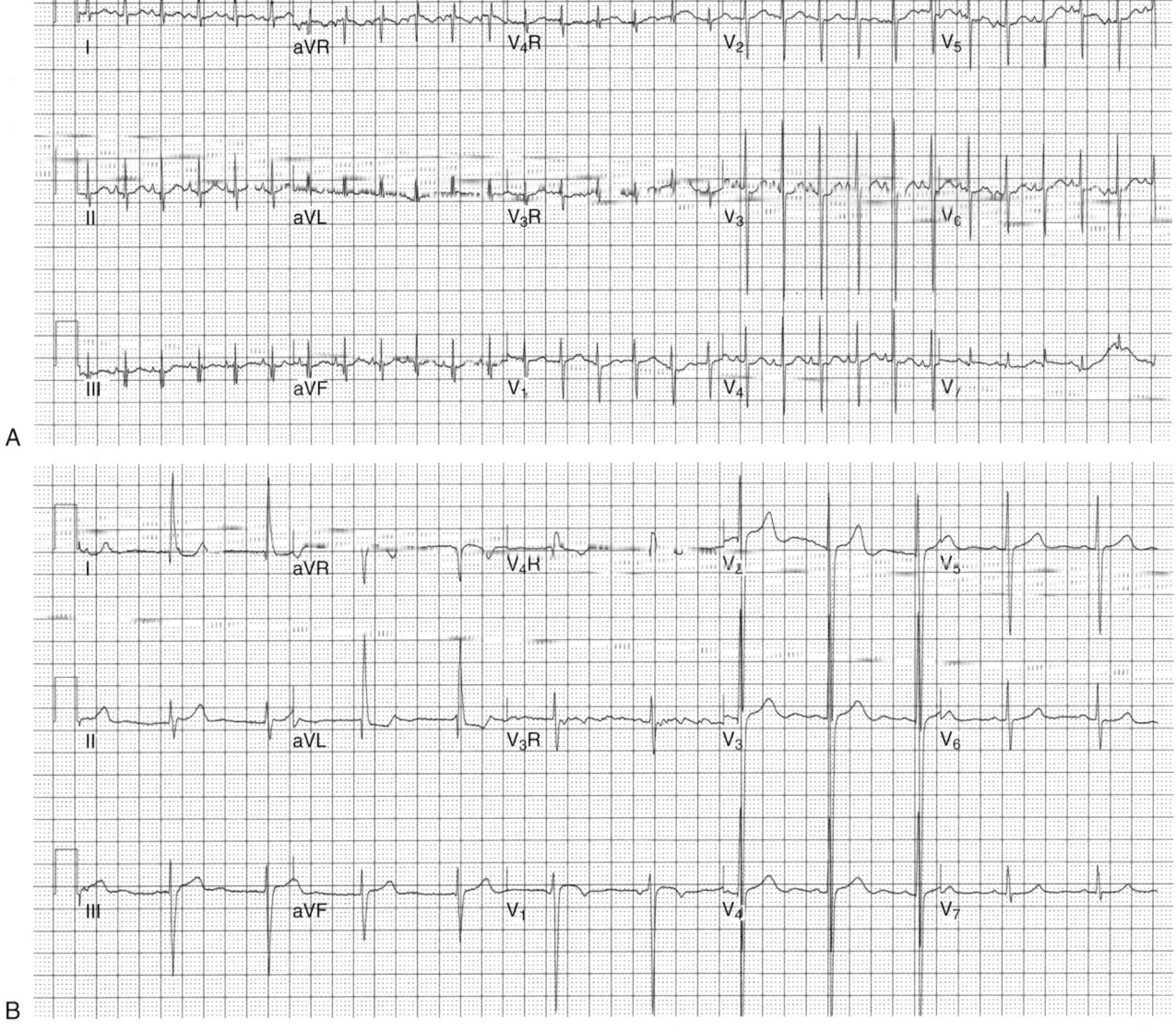

• **Fig. 30.2** Electrocardiograms of same patient with corrected transposition and coarctation of the aorta performed at: **(A)** 2-weeks-old showing reversed septal ventricular depolarization with a qR pattern in aVR, rsR pattern in aVL, small initial q wave in V_3R, V_1, and absent q wave in V_5, V_6; **(B)** 18-year-old, after neonatal end-to-end repair of coarctation of the aorta with pulmonary artery band placement and subsequent Mustard/arterial switch operation ("double switch"), showing absent r in aVR, qR pattern in aVL, small initial q wave in V_4R, and absent q wave in V_5, V_6.

5% of patients are born with complete heart block with approximately 40% developing AV block over time, spontaneous heart block occurs even in patients who have not undergone surgical intervention[10,14,20,21] (Table 30.1). In those with the {I,D,D} variety, the P wave is negative in lead 1 because the sinus node is left-sided. Since the ventricular septum depolarizes normally, the right chest leads usually have an initial R wave and the left chest leads an initial Q wave.

Chest X-Ray

The anterior and leftward ascending aorta can often be recognized on the plain chest x-ray (Fig. 30.3) as it extends and "smoothes" the left superior border of the cardiac silhouette.

Echocardiography

Echocardiography is a highly reliable means of identifying the anatomy. Inversion of the ventricles can be recognized by identification of the right-sided mitral valve and the left-sided tricuspid valve with {S,L,L} anatomy (Fig. 30.4). The papillary muscles of the bicuspid mitral valve attach only to the free wall of the mLV, whereas the tricuspid valve has chordal attachments to the septal surface of the mRV. The tricuspid valve annulus is more apically displaced than the

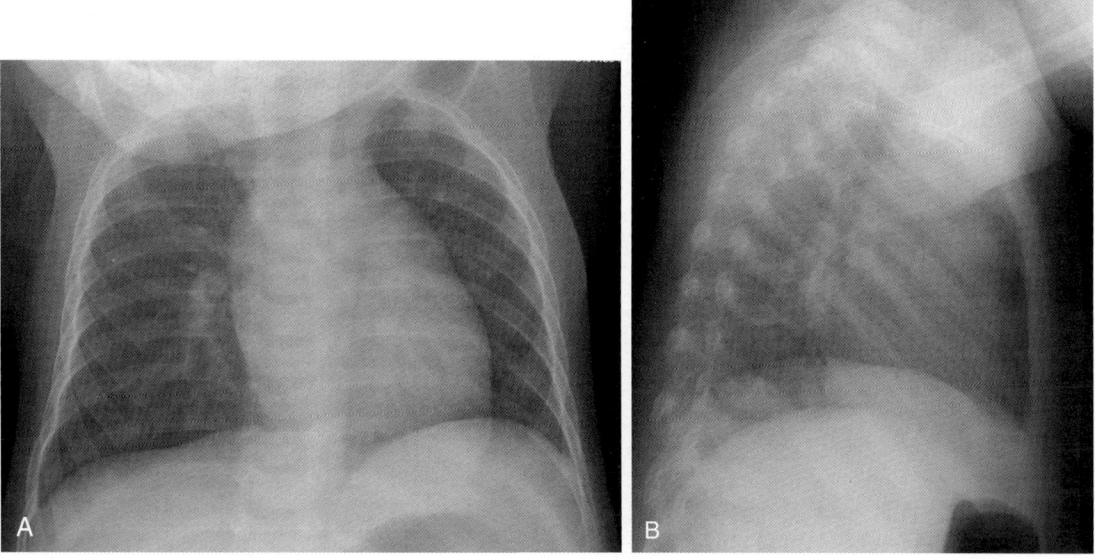

• **Fig. 30.3** (A) Anteroposterior and (B) lateral chest x-ray showing a prominent left-sided ascending aorta that extends and "smoothes" the left-superior border of the cardiac silhouette in an 8-month-old patient with congenitally corrected transposition of the great arteries.

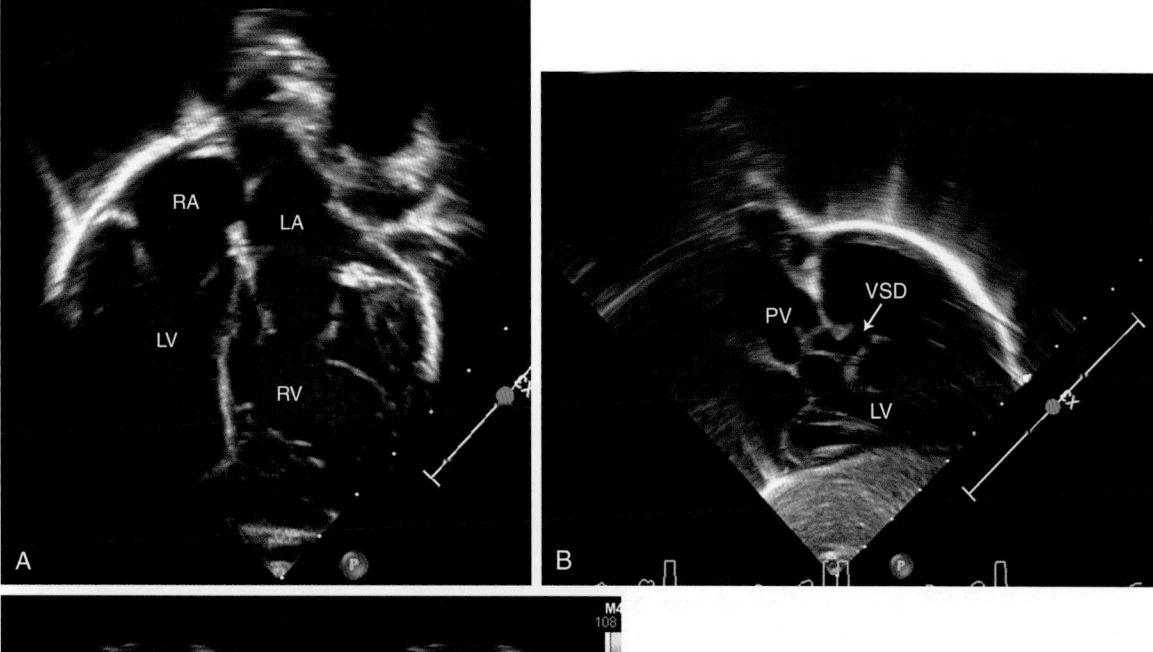

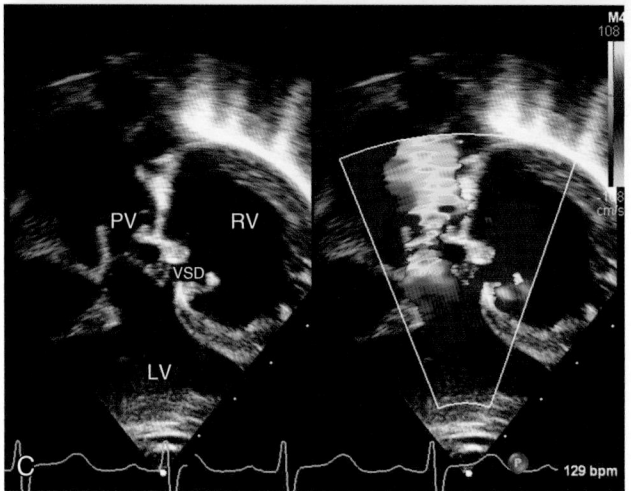

• **Fig. 30.4** Echocardiogram in {S,L,L} corrected transposition of the great arteries. (A) Apical four-chamber view. The ventricles are inverted, with the right atrium *(RA)* connecting to the right-sided left ventricle *(LV)*, and the left atrium *(LA)* connecting to the left-sided right ventricle *(RV)*. The RV can be identified by the more apical location of the tricuspid valve and the trabeculations on the septal surface compared with the LV with a smooth septal surface. (B) Subxiphoid long-axis view. There is an anterior LV from which the pulmonary valve *(PV)* arises. A membranous ventricular septal defect *(VSD)* is present and is restricted by accessory tissue. (C) Subxiphoid long-axis view in color compare mode. RV to LV flow through the membranous VSD which is restricted by accessory tissue. There is a low gradient across the VSD due to elevated LV pressure in the context of subpulmonary stenosis caused by protrusion of accessory tissue from the membranous septum.

mitral valve which can help identify the inverted ventricles. The fine trabeculations of the left ventricle may distinguish it from the coarse trabeculations of the right ventricle. Usually, the transposed aortic valve and main PA are readily recognized. The function of the tricuspid valve should be evaluated because regurgitation is common.[7,10]

The diagnosis is generally apparent from the initial subxiphoid long- and short-axis scans. In {S,L,L} with levocardia, the anterior and right-sided mLV is seen aligned with the PA.

There is frequently pulmonary or subpulmonary stenosis. Scanning more anteriorly displays the anterior and left-sided aorta aligned with the mRV. Because a VSD is common, the septum should be scanned in multiple views with and without color flow Doppler mapping. The tricuspid valve should be imaged using apical views to assess the location of the septal leaflet, and a Doppler examination should be performed to detect and grade regurgitation (Fig. 30.5). A careful Doppler examination of the pulmonary outflow tract

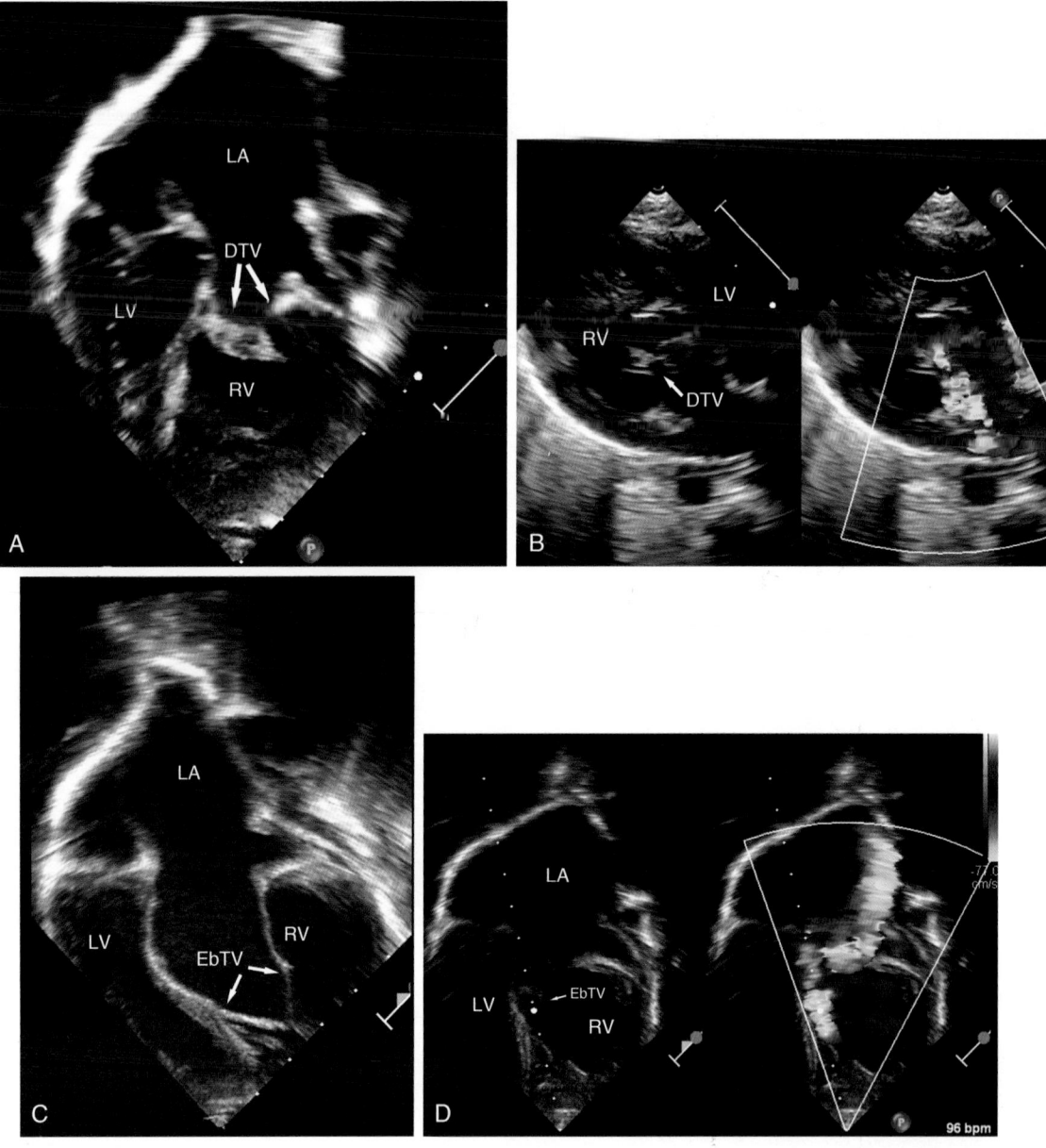

• **Fig. 30.5** Echocardiogram in patients with {S,L,L} corrected transposition of the great arteries demonstrating tricuspid valve anomalies. **(A)** Apical four-chamber view. Note the thickened and redundant leaflets of this dysplastic tricuspid valve *(DTV)*. The ventricles are inverted, with the right atrium connecting to the right-sided left ventricle *(LV)*, and the left atrium *(LA)* connecting to the left-sided right ventricle *(RV)*. **(B)** Parasternal long-axis view in color compare mode. The LV is anterior in this view with the trabeculated RV with DTV seen in the posterior part of the image. The color compare mode demonstrates regurgitation through the DTV. **(C)** Apical four-chamber view. Demonstrated is a dilated RV with an Ebstein malformation of the tricuspid valve *(EbTV)* during diastole. Note the tethering of the septal leaflet leading to apical displacement of the effective orifice. **(D)** Apical four-chamber view in color compare mode. With the EbTV closed, there is severe tricuspid regurgitation emanating along the RV septal surface.

should be performed from subxiphoid and apical transducer locations because subpulmonary obstruction is often present from mitral or accessory valve tissue.

Magnetic Resonance Imaging and Cardiac Computed Tomography

Magnetic resonance imaging (MRI) can help with quantification of morphologic right ventricular function, strain imaging, tricuspid regurgitation fraction, and evaluation for late gadolinium enhancement.[22] MRI or computed tomography (CT) can help assess mLV end-diastolic volume, mLV mass, and mLV mass/volume ratio. Cardiac CT can be utilized to create 3D models which can assist in planning for surgical procedures (Fig. 30.6). MRI may not be an option in patients with pacemakers, though many modern devices are MR conditional allowing for consideration of this imaging modality. In instances where MR is

contraindicated, quantitative cardiac CT angiography can be utilized.

Cardiac Catheterization

Because intracardiac anatomy and valve regurgitation can be delineated by echocardiography, catheterization is necessary only for specific indications, including: (1) PA pressure and resistance measurements along with anatomical delineation of PA architecture, particularly in those who have had prior aortopulmonary shunt procedures; (2) assessment of mLV systolic and end-diastolic pressure after PA banding; (3) interventional management (dilation or stent placement) of PA stenoses or previously placed obstructed LV–PA conduits; (4) device closure of surgically inaccessible VSDs; (5) delineating coronary artery anatomy or VSD locations; and (6) stenting of the ductus arteriosus in neonatal cases of pulmonary atresia. Newer catheter-based approaches such as

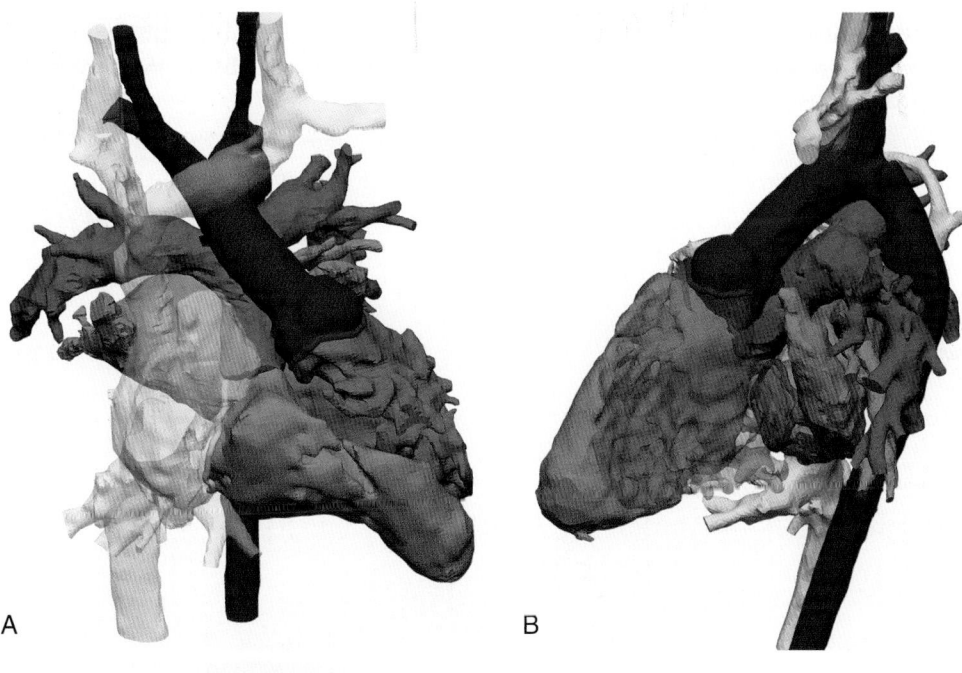

A   B

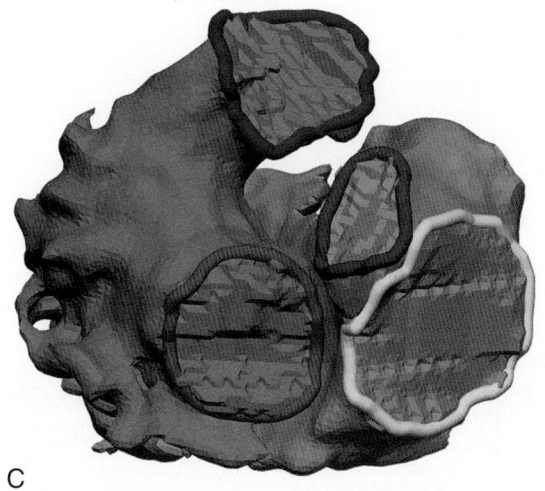

C

• **Fig. 30.6** Cardiac computed tomography imaging was utilized to create a three-dimensional model of a patient with {S,L,L} corrected transposition of the great arteries and a left aortic arch. The heart has been segmented with the systemic veins and right atrium represented by a light blue, the morphologic left ventricle with a sienna brown, the pulmonary veins and left atrium in pink, the morphologic right ventricle in purple, and the aorta in red. The annulus of the mitral valve is represented by a light blue ribbon, the tricuspid valve with pink, the pulmonary valve with blue, and the aortic valve in red. **(A)** A slightly rotated projection looking at the anterior-superior surface of the heart with the right atrium shown as a translucent structure helps demonstrate the relationship between the anterior aorta arising from the morphologic right ventricle and the posterior pulmonary artery arising from the morphologic left ventricle. **(B)** A projection of the heart seen from the patient's left with a translucent morphologic right ventricle helps demonstrate the presence of subaortic conus and separation of the tricuspid and aortic valve annulus. **(C)** A projection of the heart looking from the atria towards the ventricles demonstrates the relationships of all four valves. Again seen is subaortic conus with separation of the tricuspid and aortic valves. There is continuity between the mitral and pulmonary valves entering and exiting the morphologic left ventricle.

preoperative assessment of mLV function by measuring pressure-volume loops are worthy of further exploration.

Management

Because of the wide range of associated defects and the tendency of many of these to progress with time, no single management approach can be applied. In general, it is reasonable to follow medically (1) those with minor structural problems, (2) some asymptomatic patients with significant but balanced lesions, and (3) those with asymptomatic complete heart block because pacemaker placement alone is likely to result in increasing tricuspid regurgitation and right ventricular failure. The treatments that have been employed in patients followed at Boston Children's Hospital can be seen in Table 30.2.

Palliative operations such as a modified Blalock-Taussig-Thomas (BTT) aortopulmonary shunt were a common procedure in the past for severe pulmonary stenosis or atresia but had the potential for PA distortion in many if left alone for years. Currently, it is reasonable to stent the ductus arteriosus or place a BTT shunt for a short time in an infant with pulmonary atresia when conduit placement is not feasible or to allow for growth prior to definitive surgery. Patent ductus arteriosus stenting is a newer procedure, and our experience demonstrates that serial evaluation for PA and aortic distortion or obstruction must be performed.

The "physiologic repair" operations in which the AV and VA discordance was not addressed often included closure of a VSD and relief of pulmonary stenosis, with or without conduit placement from the mLV to PA. These operations were associated with significant early mortality rates and heart block, later conduit stenosis, tricuspid regurgitation, right ventricular failure, and unsatisfactory long-term survival.[14,22] Isolated tricuspid valve plasty or replacement has yielded

TABLE 30.2	Boston Children's Hospital experience, 1973–2022. Procedures required to treat congenitally corrected transposition of the great arteries {S,L,L} (N = 374). Numbers may be susceptible to incomplete ascertainment of procedures performed at outside institutions.				
Year of Birth	1973–2022 N (%)	1973–1987 N (%)	1988–2002 N (%)	2003–2022 N (%)
Patients	374 (100)	62 (17)	112 (30)	200 (53)
Male sex at birth	231 (62)	42 (68)	72 (64)	117 (59)
Underwent cardiac surgery	222 (59)	29 (47)	63 (56)	130 (65)
Double switch anatomic repair	118 (32)	1 (2)	31 (28)	86 (43)
Tricuspid valve replacement	13 (3)	5 (8)	8 (7)	0 (0)
Tricuspid valvuloplasty	27 (7)	0 (0)	6 (5)	21 (11)
Aortic arch repair	12 (3)	0 (0)	1 (1)	11 (6)
Aortic valve repair/replacement	12 (3)	0 (0)	7 (6)	5 (3)
Subaortic stenosis surgery	7 (2)	0 (0)	3 (3)	4 (2)
Palliative/preparatory				
Pulmonary artery band	113 (30)	6 (10)	19 (17)	88 (44)
BTT shunt	47 (13)	9 (15)	18 (16)	20 (10)
BDG shunt	10 (3)	0 (0)	2 (2)	8 (4)
1.5 Ventricle repair	5 (1)	0 (0)	0 (0)	5 (3)
Fontan	11 (3)	2 (3)	8 (7)	1 (1)
Transplant/MCS				
Heart transplant	6 (2)	1 (2)	2 (2)	3 (2)
Ventricular assist device	3 (1)	1 (2)	1 (1)	1 (1)
ECMO	13 (3)	0 (0)	5 (4)	8 (4)
Pacemaker	110 (29)	21 (34)	29 (26)	60 (30)
ICD	4 (1)	1 (2)	2 (2)	1 (1)
CRT	44 (12)	2 (3)	7 (6)	36 (18)

BDG, Bidirectional Glenn; *BTT,* Blalock-Taussig-Thomas; *CRT,* cardiac resynchronization therapy; *ECMO,* extracorporeal membrane oxygenation; *ICD,* implantable cardioverter defibrillator; *MCS,* mechanical circulatory support.

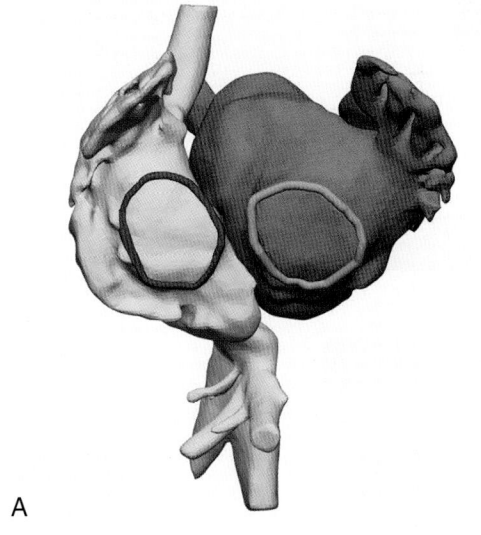

A

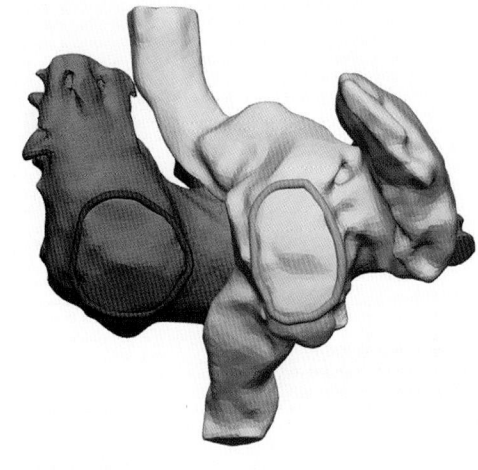

B

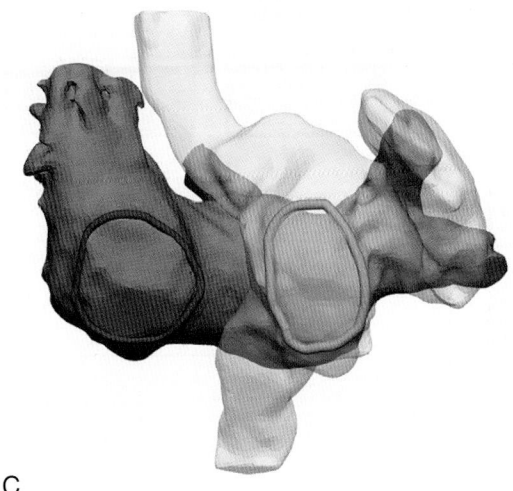

C

• **Fig. 30.7** Cardiac computed tomography imaging was utilized to create a smoothed three-dimensional model of a patient with {S,L,L} corrected transposition of the great arteries focused on the atrial anatomy. The systemic veins and right atrium are seen in light blue with the mitral valve annulus denoted by a purple ribbon. The pulmonary veins and left atrium are shown in purple with the tricuspid valve represented by a light blue ribbon. **(A)** The anatomy prior to atrial switch with the systemic veins draining to the mitral valve and pulmonary veins draining to the tricuspid valve. **(B)** After a Mustard type atrial switch, the systemic veins drain to the tricuspid valve with incorporation of the left atrial appendage and the pulmonary veins drain to the mitral valve with incorporation of the right atrial appendage. **(C)** The systemic venous pathway is made translucent to help visualize the relationships of the atrial pathways following a Mustard-type atrial switch.

acceptable intermediate-term outcomes, but patients with preoperative mRV dilation have unsatisfactory long-term outcomes.[23]

Because of complications with "physiologic repairs," the current surgical "anatomic repair" approach, which results in the mLV serving as the systemic ventricle providing blood flow to the aorta and the mRV serving as the subpulmonary ventricle, has been a preferred option. This "anatomic approach" requires an atrial-level switch operation for venous return (Mustard or Senning) in all (Fig. 30.7), together with either an arterial switch operation (frequently designated as a "double switch") in those with an intact ventricular septum or an isolated VSD, or a Rastelli procedure in which (1) the mLV is baffled to the aorta and (2) mRV to PA conduit is placed, in those patients with an outflow VSD +/− mLV outflow tract obstruction.

The Boston Children's Hospital surgical approach to patients with ccTGA has been recently described (Fig. 30.8).[21] Prior to considering the double switch operation, the mLV is assessed for its ability to function as the systemic ventricle. In the absence of a significant VSD or LV outflow

obstruction, placement of a PA band has been undertaken to "retrain" the mLV, which adversely remodels with decreased wall thickness when subjected to lower wall stress from subsystemic systolic pulmonary arterial pressures. The intraoperative goal of the PA band is to achieve a pressure that is two-thirds of the systemic pressure, which typically leads to ventricular septal shift and improvement in any tricuspid regurgitation without resulting in new-onset mitral regurgitation. The mLV is typically deemed prepared if the ejection fraction is > 60%, the end-diastolic volume is 40–100 mL/m², the indexed mass is > 50 g/m², the mass/volume ratio > 0.5, the pressure is > 90% of systemic, and the end-diastolic pressure is ≤ 10 mm Hg. It should be noted that these criteria are not perfect predictors of mLV preparedness to serve as a systemic ventricle. An additional physiologic consideration may be the development of the coronary microvasculature to provide nutrient flow to the hypertrophied LV myocytes,[24] although there are no currently available clinical methods to make this assessment. Others have advocated for creation of an atrial septal defect as well in order to increase both preload and afterload to the

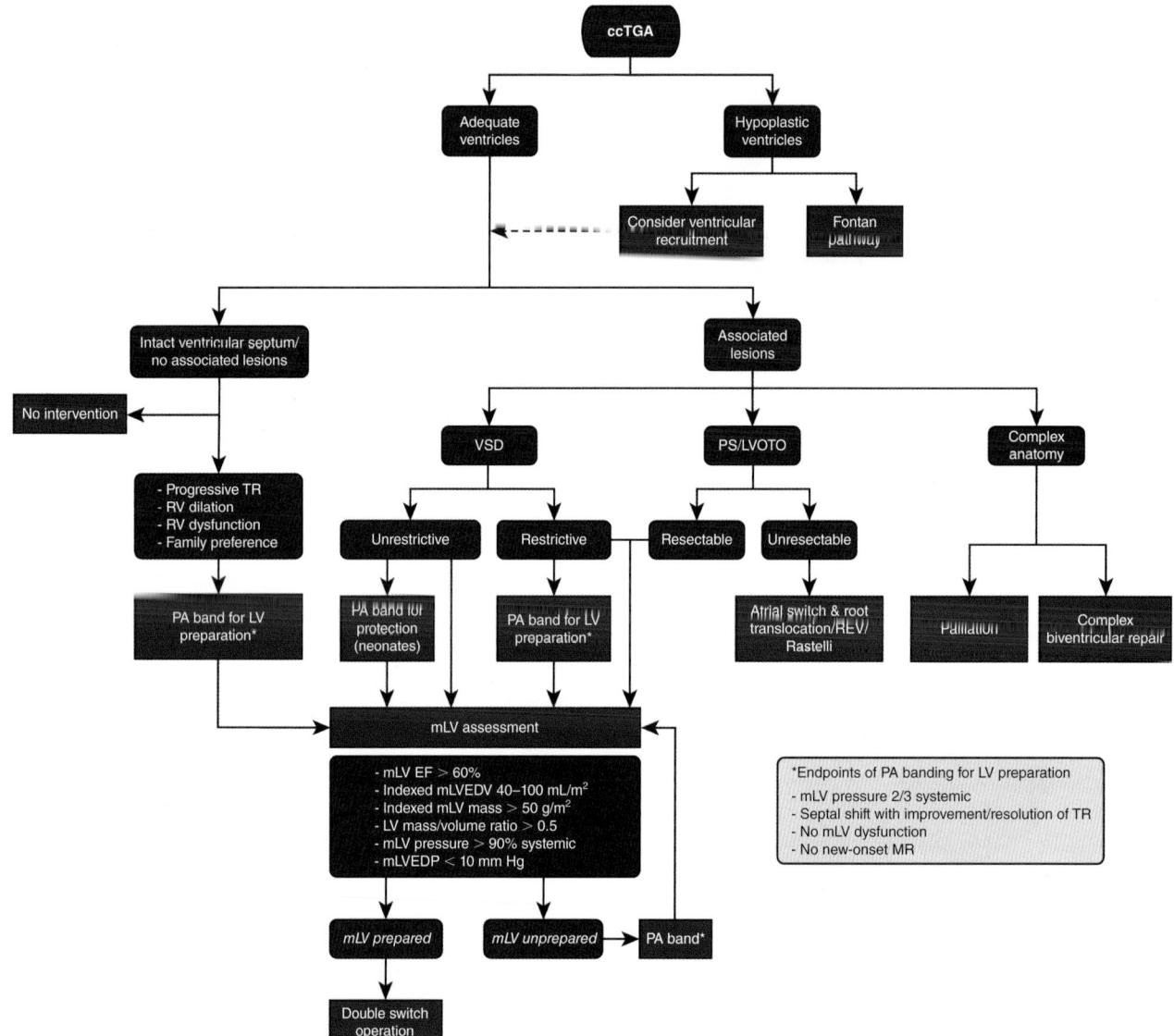

• **Fig. 30.8** Flow chart delineating the surgical approach to patients with congenitally corrected transposition of the great arteries *(ccTGA)* at Boston Children's Hospital. The criteria for morphologic left ventricle *(mLV)* preparedness are ideal measurements with decisions on individual patients made on case-by-case basis. *EF,* Ejection fraction; *LV,* left ventricle; *LVOTO,* left ventricular outflow tract obstruction; *mLV,* morphologic left ventricle; *mLVEDP,* morphologic left ventricle end-diastolic pressure; *mLVEDV,* morphologic left ventricle end-diastolic volume; *MR,* mitral regurgitation; *PA,* pulmonary artery; *PS,* pulmonary stenosis; *REV procedure,* Reparation a l'Etage Ventriculaire; *RV,* right ventricle; *TR,* tricuspid regurgitation; *VSD,* ventricular septal defect. (From Marathe SP, Chávez M, Schulz A, et al. Contemporary outcomes of the double switch operation for congenitally corrected transposition of the great arteries. *J Thorac Cardiovasc Surg.* 2022;164:1980–1990.)

mLV undergoing re-training and to serve as a "pop-off" mechanism to minimize the risk of mLV failure during retraining.[25] Timing of the double switch operation is of critical importance. In our experience younger children have superior outcomes and, where feasible, we prefer to perform the double switch operation prior to 5 years of age.

For the 103 patients who underwent double switch operation at Boston Children's Hospital between 1999 and 2019, 75% were alive without surgical reintervention at 5-year follow-up (excluding pacemakers); of the remaining 25% of patients, 3% had died, 3% had undergone heart transplant, 13% required reintervention on the neo-aortic valve, and 6% required other surgical reinterventions (Fig. 30.9).[21] Other large single-center series have reported 80% 15-year survival with the double switch operation.[26] Newer techniques for intraoperative mapping of the AV node and penetrating bundle should be considered to reduce the risk of surgical heart block. In our experience, the need for pacemaker was common; prior to double switch operation, 15% of patients had a pacemaker or cardiac resynchronization

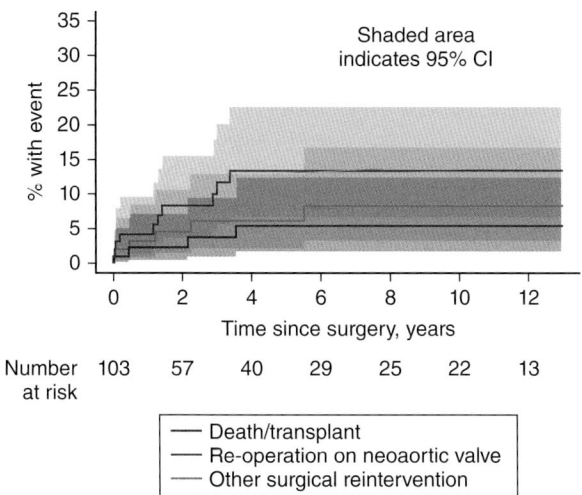

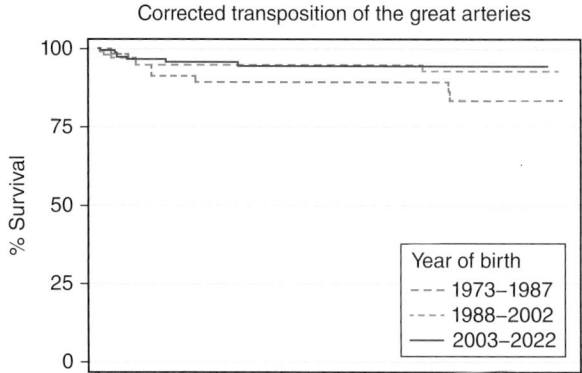

• **Fig. 30.9** Cumulative incidence of competing risk outcomes of death and transplant, neoaortic valve reintervention, and other surgical reintervention, excluding pacemaker placement, in 103 patients following double switch operation. *CI,* Confidence interval. (From Marathe SP, Chávez M, Schulz A, et al. Contemporary outcomes of the double switch operation for congenitally corrected transposition of the great arteries. *J Thorac Cardiovasc Surg.* 2022;164:1980–1990.)

therapy (CRT) system, 6% required pacemaker or CRT placement prior to discharge from the double switch operation, and 9% required pacemaker or CRT placement late after the double switch operation. When pacemaker placement is required, we prefer placement of a system capable of multisite pacing in order to provide CRT and optimize mLV systolic function.[27]

In patients who develop heart failure with reduced ejection fraction, referral to a congenital heart failure specialist should be made for optimization of medical management with guideline-directed medical therapy. In cases of refractory heart failure, support with pulsatile or continuous-flow ventricular assist devices has been successful and patients can be evaluated for cardiac transplantation. Patients who have had homografts used as mRV to PA conduits are at particular risk of anti-HLA allosensitization, which may increase the risk associated with heart transplant.[28] Use of decellularized homografts may help mitigate some of the risk of anti-HLA sensitization.[29]

Course

During follow-up, the natural history of unrepaired patients with some of the associated defects, particularly tricuspid regurgitation and AV conduction abnormalities, are well known to progress and are significant risk factors for survival. With regard to tricuspid regurgitation, increasing degrees of right ventricular systolic dysfunction commonly accompany this problem. Overall survival of patients treated at Boston Children's Hospital stratified by year of birth is presented in Fig. 30.10A. Spontaneous development of complete heart block is common, is present at birth in some, and progresses from first to second degree to complete

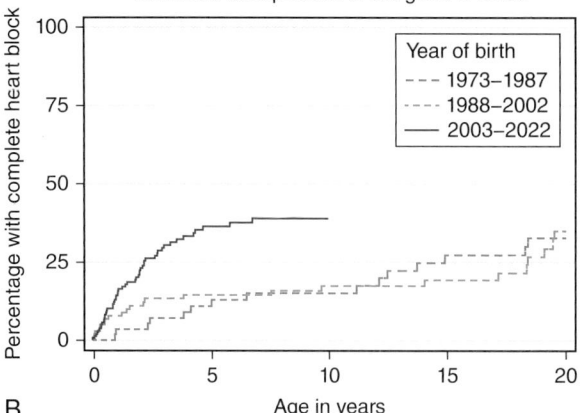

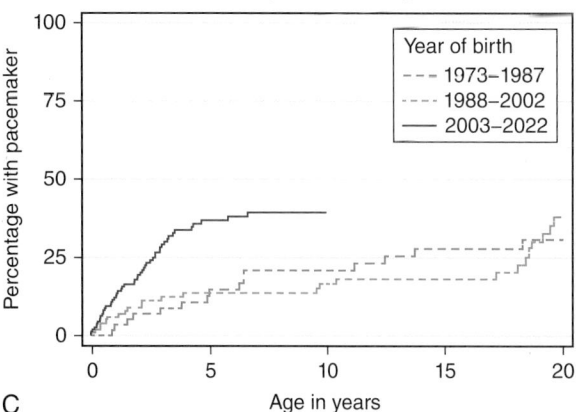

• **Fig. 30.10** **(A)** The modified natural history of patients with {S,L,L} corrected transposition of the great arteries is presented using Kaplan-Meier methodology stratified by year of birth (1973–1987; 1988–2002; 2003–2022). Censoring only takes place for loss-to-follow up. Percentage of {S,L,L} patients with **(B)** complete heart block and **(C)** implanted pacemakers (including cardiac resynchronization therapy devices), followed at Boston Children's Hospital stratified by year of birth is presented using Kaplan-Meier methodology. The most recent era is truncated at 10 years of follow-up due to the small number of patients remaining.

heart block in others, such that at least one-third of patients will acquire complete heart block during follow-up and require pacemaker placement (Table 30.2; Fig. 30.10B). In the earlier era of physiologic repair (with systemic mRV), and in the current era of anatomical repair with the double switch operation, development of mRV to PA conduit stenosis is common, and temporary relief by transcatheter stent placement is feasible in many patients. Development of heart failure with reduced ejection fraction was common in the era of physiologic repair (18% of patients developed severe subsystemic mRV systolic dysfunction, 7% patients were listed for heart transplant, and 5% of patients died).[14] In the current double switch operation era, the incidence of heart failure is reduced but not eliminated, and 8% of patients develop severe systemic mLV dysfunction, 5% are listed for heart transplant, and 3% of patients die. Time to development of the composite endpoint of death, heart transplant, moderate/severe subsystemic ventricular dysfunction, or moderate/severe subsystemic AV valve regurgitation was significantly longer in patients who have undergone double switch operation compared with physiologic repair.[14]

Anatomically Corrected Malposition of the Great Arteries

This rare entity has a {S,D,L} segmental arrangement consisting of AV and VA concordance but with the ascending aorta malpositioned to the left of the PA.[30,31] Associated lesions such as VSD, pulmonary stenosis, or subaortic stenosis are frequent and are amenable to surgical repair. Occasionally this segmental arrangement will be associated with complex defects and may only be amenable only to palliative procedures.[32]

References

1. Keane JF, Fyler DC. "Corrected" transposition of the great arteries. In: Keane JF, Lock JE, Fyler DC, eds. *Nadas' Pediatric Cardiology*. 2nd ed. Philadelphia: Elsevier; 2006:791-797.
2. Botto LD, Correa A, Erickson JD. Racial and temporal variations in the prevalence of heart defects. *Pediatrics*. 2001;107:E32.
3. Reller MD, Strickland MJ, Riehle-Colarusso T, et al. Prevalence of congenital heart defects in metropolitan Atlanta, 1998-2005. *J Pediatr*. 2008;153:807-813.
4. Tortigue M, Nield LE, Karakachoff M, et al. Familial recurrence patterns in congenitally corrected transposition of the great arteries: an international study. *Circ Genom Precis Med*. 2022;15:e003464.
5. Wissocque L, Mondésert B, Dubart AE. Late diagnosis of isolated congenitally corrected transposition of the great arteries in a 92-year old woman. *Eur J Cardiothorac Surg*. 2016;49:1524-1525.
6. Wallis GA, Debich-Spicer D, Anderson RH. Congenitally corrected transposition. *Orphanet J Rare Dis*. 2011;6:22.
7. Myers PO, Bautista-Hernandez V, Baird CW, et al. Tricuspid regurgitation or Ebsteinoid dysplasia of the tricuspid valve in congenitally corrected transposition: is valvuloplasty necessary at anatomic repair? *J Thorac Cardiovasc Surg*. 2014;147:576-580.
8. Furuya T, Hoashi T, Shimada M, et al. Serial changes of tricuspid regurgitation after anatomic repair for congenitally corrected transposition. *Eur J Cardiothorac Surg*. 2020;58:163-170.
9. Said SM, Burkhart HM, Schaff HV, et al. Congenitally corrected transposition of great arteries: surgical options for the failing right ventricle and/or severe tricuspid regurgitation. *World J Pediatr Congenit Heart Surg*. 2011;2:64-79.
10. Krummholz A, Gottschalk I, Geipel A, et al. Prenatal diagnosis, associated findings and postnatal outcome in fetuses with congenitally corrected transposition of the great arteries. *Arch Gynecol Obstet*. 2021;303:1469-1481.
11. Hosseinpour AR, McCarthy KP, Griselli M, et al. Congenitally corrected transposition: size of the pulmonary trunk and septal malalignment. *Ann Thorac Surg*. 2004;77:2163-2166.
12. Anderson RH. The conduction tissues in congenitally corrected transposition. *Ann Thorac Surg*. 2004;77:1881-1882.
13. Feins EN, O'Leary ET, Davee J, et al. Conduction mapping during complex congenital heart surgery: when to expect the unexpected. *J Thorac Cardiovasc Surg*. 2023;165:1618-1628.
14. Cui H, Hage A, Piekarski BL, et al. Management of congenitally corrected transposition of the great arteries with intact ventricular septum: anatomic repair or palliative treatment? *Circ Cardiovasc Interv*. 2021;14:e010154.
15. Dabizzi RP, Barletta GA, Caprioli G, et al. Coronary artery anatomy in corrected transposition of the great arteries. *J Am Coll Cardiol*. 1988;12:486-491.
16. Chiu IS, Wu SJ, Chen SJ, et al. Sequential diagnosis of coronary arterial anatomy in congenitally corrected transposition of the great arteries. *Ann Thorac Surg*. 2003;75:422-429; discussion 429.
17. Ismat FA, Baldwin HS, Karl TR, et al. Coronary anatomy in congenitally corrected transposition of the great arteries. *Int J Cardiol*. 2002;86:207-216.
18. Egbe AC, Miranda WR, Jain CC, et al. Prognostic implications of progressive systemic ventricular dysfunction in congenitally corrected transposition of great arteries. *JACC Cardiovasc Imaging*. 2022;15:566-574.
19. Hauser M, Meierhofer C, Schwaiger M, et al. Myocardial blood flow in patients with transposition of the great arteries – risk factor for dysfunction of the morphologic systemic right ventricle late after atrial repair. *Circ J*. 2015;79:425-431.
20. Simmons MA, Rollinson N, Fishberger S, et al. Modern Incidence of complete heart block in patients with L-looped ventricles: does univentricular status matter? *Congenit Heart Dis*. 2015;10:E237-E242.
21. Marathe SP, Chávez M, Schulz A, et al. Contemporary outcomes of the double switch operation for congenitally corrected transposition of the great arteries. *J Thorac Cardiovasc Surg*. 2022;164:1980-1990.
22. Wilson HC, Lu JC, Yu S, et al. Ventricular function in physiologically repaired and unrepaired congenitally corrected transposition of the great arteries. *Am J Cardiol*. 2022;165:95-100.
23. Deng L, Xu J, Tang Y, et al. Long-term outcomes of tricuspid valve surgery in patients with congenitally corrected transposition of the great arteries. *J Am Heart Assoc*. 2018;7:e008127.
24. Toba S, Sanders SP, Gauvreau K, et al. Histopathologic changes after pulmonary artery banding for retraining of subpulmonary left ventricle. *Ann Thorac Surg*. 2022;114:858-865.
25. Zartner PA, Schneider MB, Asfour B, et al. Enhanced left ventricular training in corrected transposition of the great arteries by increasing the preload. *Eur J Cardiothorac Surg*. 2016;49:1571-1576.
26. Barrios PA, Zia A, Pettersson G, et al. Outcomes of treatment pathways in 240 patients with congenitally corrected transposition of great arteries. *J Thorac Cardiovasc Surg*. 2021;161:1080-1093.e4.

27. Hofferberth SC, Alexander ME, Mah DY, et al. Impact of pacing on systemic ventricular function in L-transposition of the great arteries. *J Thorac Cardiovasc Surg.* 2016;151:131-138.
28. Shaddy RE, Hunter DD, Osborn KA, et al. Prospective analysis of HLA immunogenicity of cryopreserved valved allografts used in pediatric heart surgery. *Circulation.* 1996;94:1063-1067.
29. Coti I, Wenda S, Andreeva A, et al. Donor-specific HLA antibodies after fresh decellularized vs cryopreserved native allograft implantation. *HLA.* 2020;96:580-588.
30. Bernasconi A, Cavalle-Garrido T, Perrin DG, et al. What is anatomically corrected malposition? *Cardiol Young.* 2007;17:26-34.
31. Van Praagh R, Van Praagh S. Anatomically corrected transposition of the great arteries. *Br Heart J.* 1967;29:112-119.
32. Kari FA, Siddiqui S, Farooqi KM, et al. Staged surgical management of anatomically corrected malposition of great arteries. *World J Pediatr Congenit Heart Surg.* 2020;11:352-354.

31

Atrioventricular Canal Defects

SUNIL J. GHELANI, SARAH A. TEELE, AND JOHN E. MAYER JR.

KEY LEARNING POINTS

- There is a wide anatomical spectrum of atrioventricular canal defect (AVCD) with varying clinical presentations and surgical options.
- The pathophysiologic consequences of AVCD depend on the level and size of the septal defects and the function of the atrioventricular valves, ranging from development of heart failure in early infancy (complete AVCD) to a relatively asymptomatic state in the first several years (isolated primum atrial septal defect).
- Accurate anatomic diagnosis of AVCD is possible with echocardiography and may be supplemented with CT and

MRI studies in less common anatomies. All forms of AVCD present with a characteristic superior QRS axis on the ECG.
- AVCDs exhibit a strong association with Down syndrome.
- Surgical repair of complete AVCDs is required within the first months of life to relieve congestive heart failure and to prevent the development of pulmonary vascular disease. Repair of AVCDs without a ventricular septal defect component is optimally carried out in the pre-school age patient.
- Early results after surgical correction of AVCD are excellent; however, a significant proportion require later operations, most commonly for mitral valve regurgitation.

Definition

Atrioventricular canal defects (AVCDs) refer to a spectrum of abnormalities of the structures derived from the embryonic endocardial cushions. Other terms used to describe these anomalies include atrioventricular septal defects and endocardial cushion defects. The prototypical lesion in this spectrum is a complete AVCD, wherein there is a single (common) atrioventricular valve (AVV) and the portions of atrial and ventricular septa derived from the endocardial cushions are missing, resulting in large interatrial and interventricular level communications (Fig. 31.1).

Embryology and Genetics

Atrioventricular canal is the central common opening between the primitive atrium and future ventricular chamber and is the "normal" anatomy in the early stages of cardiac development. Endocardial cushions are four mesenchymal ingrowths that develop around the end of fourth embryonic week to ultimately septate the atrioventricular canal into two AVVs. The cushions contribute to the formation of mitral and tricuspid valves, the primum component of the septum between the atria and the inlet septum between the ventricles. AVCDs result when there is failure of normal development of the endocardial cushions. A significant role

for a second heart field origin structure, the dorsal mesenchymal protrusion, has also been identified in the formation of the atrial septum and AVCDs.[1,2]

AVCD is the ninth most common form of congenital heart disease with an incidence of 35 per 100,000 live births.[3] More than half of patients with complete AVCD have trisomy 21 (also referred to as Down syndrome), and about one in three patients with trisomy 21 has an AVCD.[4]

The superior bridging leaflet is commonly free of attachments in patients with AVCD and trisomy 21 (Rastelli type C, see below). AVCD is also seen frequently in association with asplenia (right atrial isomerism) heterotaxy syndrome. In polysplenia (left atrial isomerism) heterotaxy, a primum atrial septal defect (ASD) is more commonly found. Despite these known associations, no specific structural DNA variants have been identified. For patients with heterotaxy, many have primary ciliary dyskinesia which impacts normal right-left asymmetry, but the relationship to endocardial cushion development is unclear. Multiple candidate mechanisms have been proposed including Down syndrome cell adhesion molecule and epigenetic factors.[5,6] In animal experiments with induced genetic mutations, bone morphogenic protein 4, sonic hedgehog, and other cilia-related genes as well as the Wnt/β-catenin pathway, result in various forms of AVCD.[2] Numerous other genetic syndromes have been associated with mildly increased risk

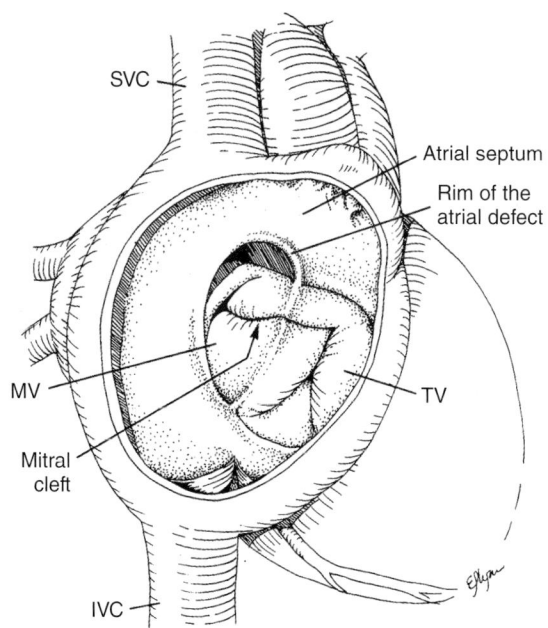

• **Fig. 31.1** Diagram depicting a complete atrioventricular canal defect as viewed from the right atrium. *IVC*, inferior vena cava; *MV*, mitral valve; *SVC*, superior vena cava; *TV*, tricuspid valve.

of AVCD, including Holt-Oram, Ellis-van Creveld, Noonan, Smith-Lemli-Opitz, DiGeorge, Bardet-Biedl, and CHARGE association.[7]

Anatomy And Classification

In a normal heart, the aorta is "wedged" between the mitral and tricuspid annuli. In AVCD, in the presence of a single large AVV, the aorta is displaced anteriorly and the plane of the common AVV is displaced apically (Fig. 31.2). This results in elongation of the left ventricular (LV) outflow tract and a longer distance from the ventricular apex to the aortic valve as compared with the AVV annulus. The outflow tract geometry is often referred to as "gooseneck deformity" due to its characteristic shape, and this anatomy is associated with a predisposition to development of LV outflow obstruction.

Variation in the development of the atrial and ventricular septa and leaflet tissue results in several anatomic AVCD variants (Fig. 31.3). In the complete form, a large primum ASD exists anteroinferior to the fossa ovalis, a large ventricular septal defect (VSD) exists posteriorly in the inlet

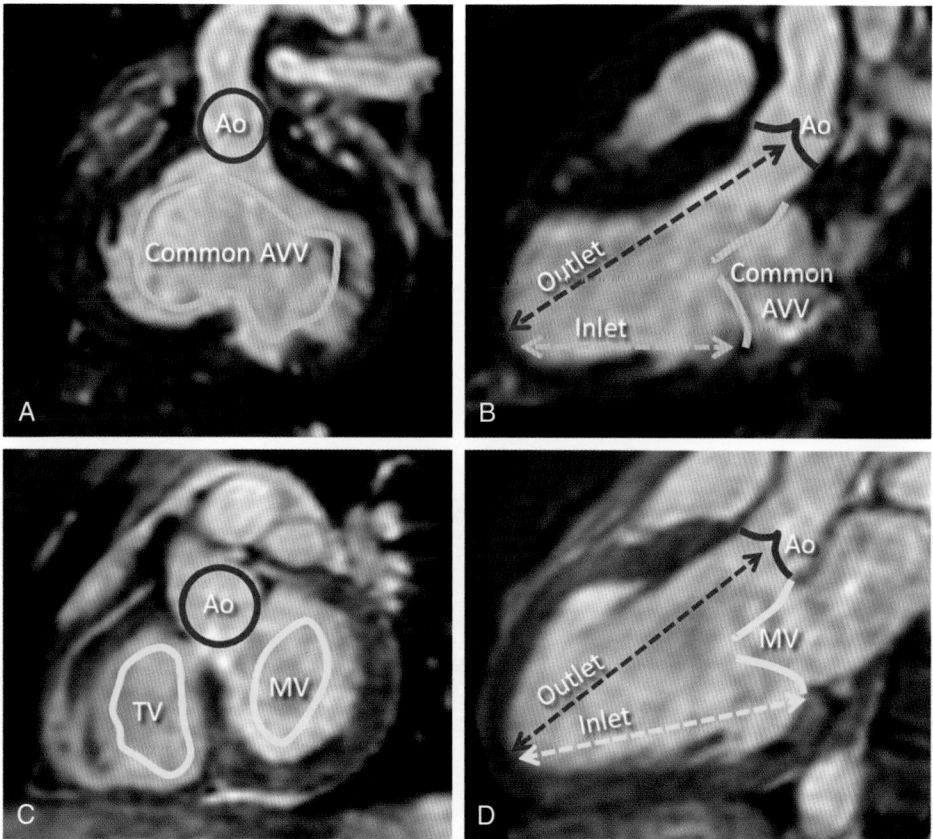

• **Fig. 31.2** **(A)** and **(B)** MRI images in short- and long-axis planes in a patient with atrioventricular canal defect depicting the anterior displacement of the aortic valve. The displacement results in increased length of the left ventricular outlet compared with its inlet **(B)**. This is in contrast to a normal heart in which the aorta *(Ao)* is "wedged" between the atrioventricular valve *(AVV)* annuli **(C)** with nearly equal lengths of the ventricular inlet and outlet **(D)** *MV*, mitral valve; *TV*, tricuspid valve.

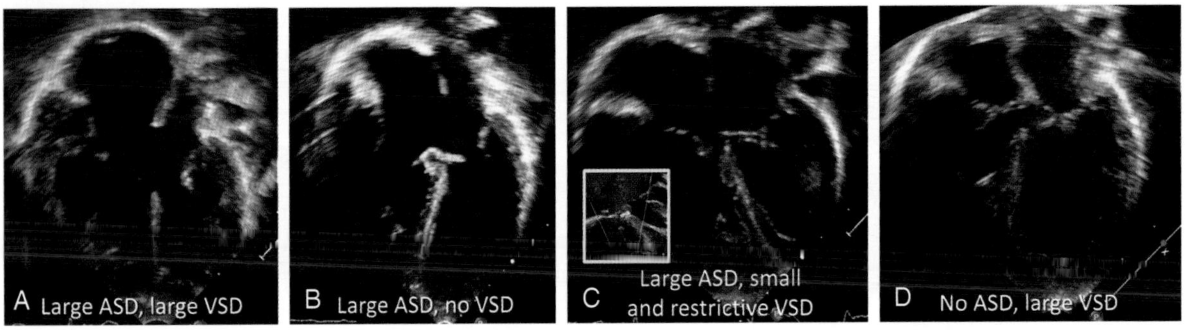

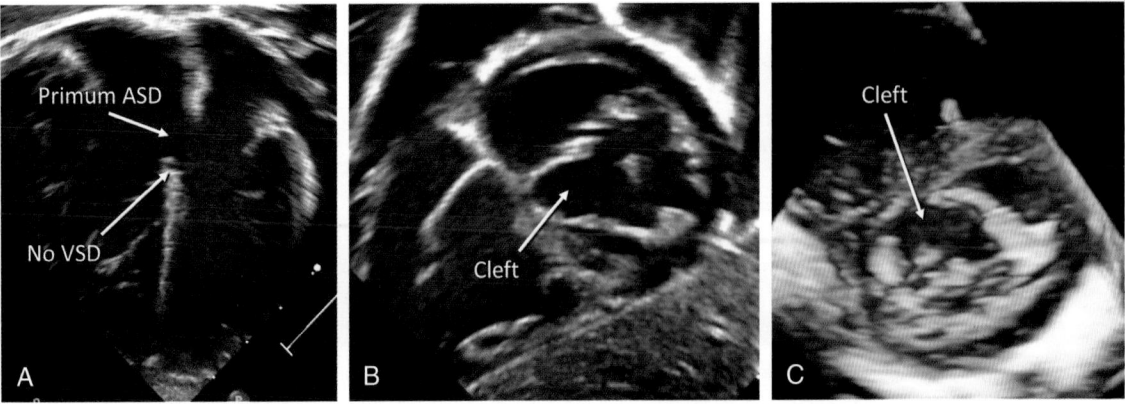

• **Fig. 31.3** Apical four-chamber echocardiographic views depicting **(A)** complete atrioventricular canal defect (AVCD), **(B)** partial AVCD with a primum atrial septal defect *(ASD)*, **(C)** transitional AVCD, and **(D)** isolated AVC-type ventricular septa defect *(VSD)*.

septum, and a single (common) AVV exists with a single annulus that spans over both ventricles (Fig. 31.3A). The VSD in AVCD commonly also involves the membranous septum which is often small or absent. Defects that lack one or more of these three features can be viewed as variants along a spectrum of AVCD. The most common variant is referred to as a "partial" or "incomplete" AVCD, and this occurs when the VSD component of the defect is completely closed by fibrous attachments from the valve leaflets to the crest of the ventricular septum resulting in a primum ASD and separate mitral and tricuspid valves (Fig. 31.4). When the VSD is only partially obliterated and allows for pressure restrictive shunting, the defect is referred to as "transitional" AVCD (Fig. 31.3C). Despite separate annuli, the valves do not have normal anatomy in this situation. The offset between the septal hinge points of the two valves is absent, and the mitral valve has a "cleft" representing the incomplete fusion of the superior and inferior bridging leaflets. Other varieties of AVCD such as those with small or absent primum ASDs or isolated AVC-type VSD are less common. A common anatomic feature of each of these variants is that the distance from the AVV annulus to the ventricular apex is reduced relative to the apex to aortic valve dimension, and thus all the variants will have a "gooseneck" deformity.

The common AVV leaflet anatomy has significant variability. Typically, there are five total leaflets and five commissures. The two leaflets that bridge the crest of the ventricular septum are called superior and inferior bridging leaflets. Leaflets along the lateral free walls of the LV and right ventricle (RV) are called lateral or mural leaflets. Typically, there is a single mural leaflet in the LV and two non-septal leaflets in the RV (Fig. 31.5).

The anatomy of the superior bridging leaflet forms the basis of the Rastelli classification (Fig. 31.6).[8] In Rastelli type A, the most common type, the superior bridging leaflet is divided, and each of the right and left components have attachments to the crest of the ventricular septum with no or minimal chordal bridging across the ventricular septum. In type B, the superior bridging leaflet has moderate chordal bridging over the crest of the septum and the leftward component of the anterior leaflet has attachments to a papillary muscle on the RV side of the septum. In type C, the superior bridging leaflet is undivided and has no septal chordal attachments and is thus "free floating." Rastelli type C may be viewed as the most primitive form of AVCD and is the most common variant found in patients with trisomy 21. The inferior bridging leaflet always has attachments to the ventricular septum.

AVCD may be associated with other cardiac lesions. Extension of the VSD anteriorly with anterior deviation of

• **Fig. 31.4** Partial atrioventricular canal defect with a primum atrial septal defect *(ASD)* and no ventricular septal defect *(VSD)* (seen well in apical four-chamber view, A) and a mitral valve cleft (by 2D short-axis view in B and 3D short-axis view in C).

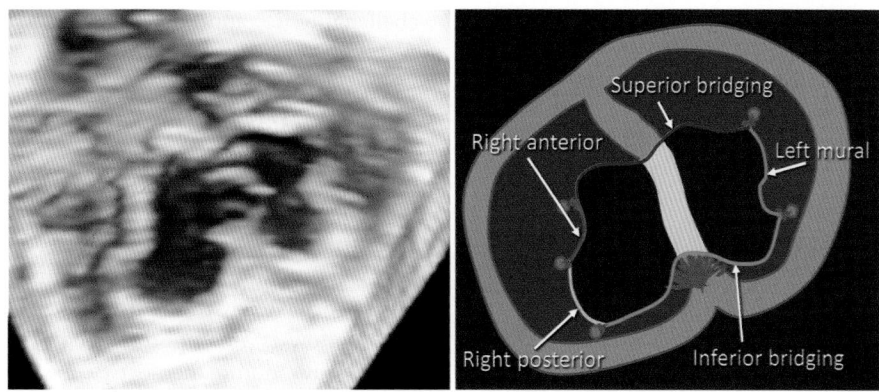

• **Fig. 31.5** Three-dimensional echocardiographic view of a common atrioventricular valve "en face" and a corresponding diagram showing the typical five leaflets of a balanced complete atrioventricular canal defect.

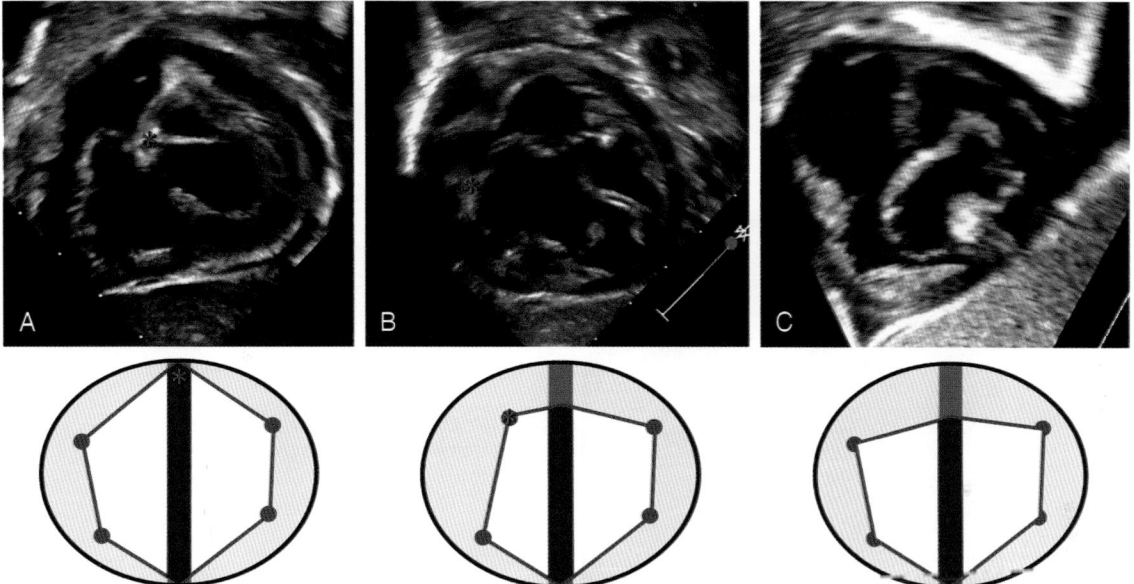

• **Fig. 31.6** "En face" views of the common atrioventricular valve from subxiphoid window and corresponding diagrams depicting the Rastelli classification. **(A)** Type A, the most common type, the superior bridging leaflet is divided by attachments to the crest of the ventricular septum (*) with no or minimal bridging. **(B)** Type B in which the superior bridging leaflet is divided and attached to a papillary muscle on the right ventricular septum (*). **(C)** Type C in which the superior bridging leaflet is undivided or "free floating." (Adapted from Pugnaloni F, Digilio MC, Putotto C, De Luca E, Marino B, Versacci P. Genetics of atrioventricular canal defects. *Ital J Pediatr*. 2020;46:61).

the infundibular septum (AVCD with tetralogy of Fallot) can be seen, especially with Rastelli type C AVCD (Fig. 31.7). This type is also rarely associated with other complex lesions such as double-outlet RV, D-loop transposition of the great arteries, and asplenia type of heterotaxy syndrome. Among the three types, Rastelli type A is most likely to be associated with LV outflow tract obstruction.

The LV papillary muscles are more closely spaced than in a normal heart and counterclockwise rotated as viewed from the apex. This brings the posteromedial papillary muscle away from the septum and the anterolateral papillary muscle closer to the septum. In approximately 5% of patients, the left AVV has additional abnormalities including parachute valve or double-orifice left AVV. In the parachute

variant, a single LV papillary muscle receives all the chordal attachments from the superior and inferior cushion components of the left AVV (Fig. 31.8). This results in absence of a mural leaflet and makes the surgical repair challenging, as complete cleft closure would occlude the left AVV and cause significant stenosis. A parachute left AVV is often associated with an imbalance in ventricular size and volume favoring the RV. A double-orifice left AVV results when there is a second opening in the leaflet that is separate from the main central opening between the leaflets (Fig. 31.9). The secondary orifice typically has its own separate chordal attachments to a papillary muscle. The combined opening of the two inlets for the left AVV is invariably smaller than if it were not a double-orifice valve. Double-orifice valves can be

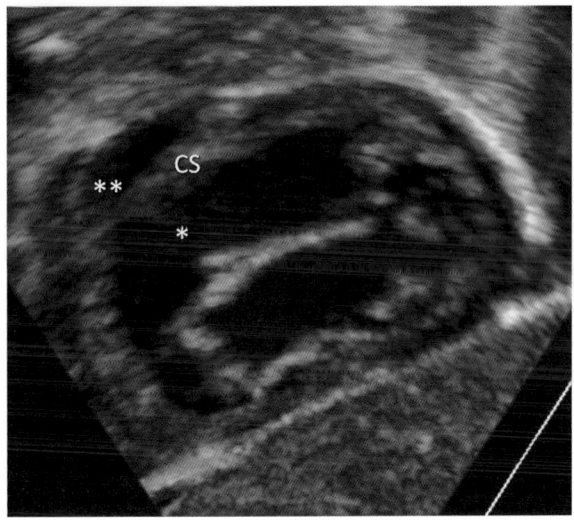

• **Fig. 31.7** Subxiphoid short-axis view showing tetralogy of Fallot with complete atrioventricular canal defect. Note the anterior and superior deviation of the conal septum *(CS)* resulting in a large conoventricular septal defect *(*)* and narrowing of the right ventricular outflow tract *(**)*.

challenging to appreciate in the setting of a complete AVCD.

Balanced Versus Unbalanced AVCD

In about 10% of AVCDs, the AVV favors one ventricle over the other, and when this occurs, the defect is referred to as an unbalanced AVCD. Unbalanced AVVD can either be LV or RV dominant. The relative commitment of the AVV is highly correlated with the size of the ventricles, and unequal AVV inflow is an important characteristic of unbalanced AVCDs. RV dominance is twice as common as LV dominance, and is associated with LV hypoplasia, parachute left AVV or closely spaced LV papillary muscles with a small or absent mural leaflet, bicuspid aortic valve, and coarctation of the aorta (Fig. 31.10). Conversely, LV dominant AVCD is associated with RV hypoplasia and outflow obstruction in the form of pulmonary valvar stenosis or atresia. Attempts have been made to quantify the degree of common AVV and ventricular imbalance to guide decision-making

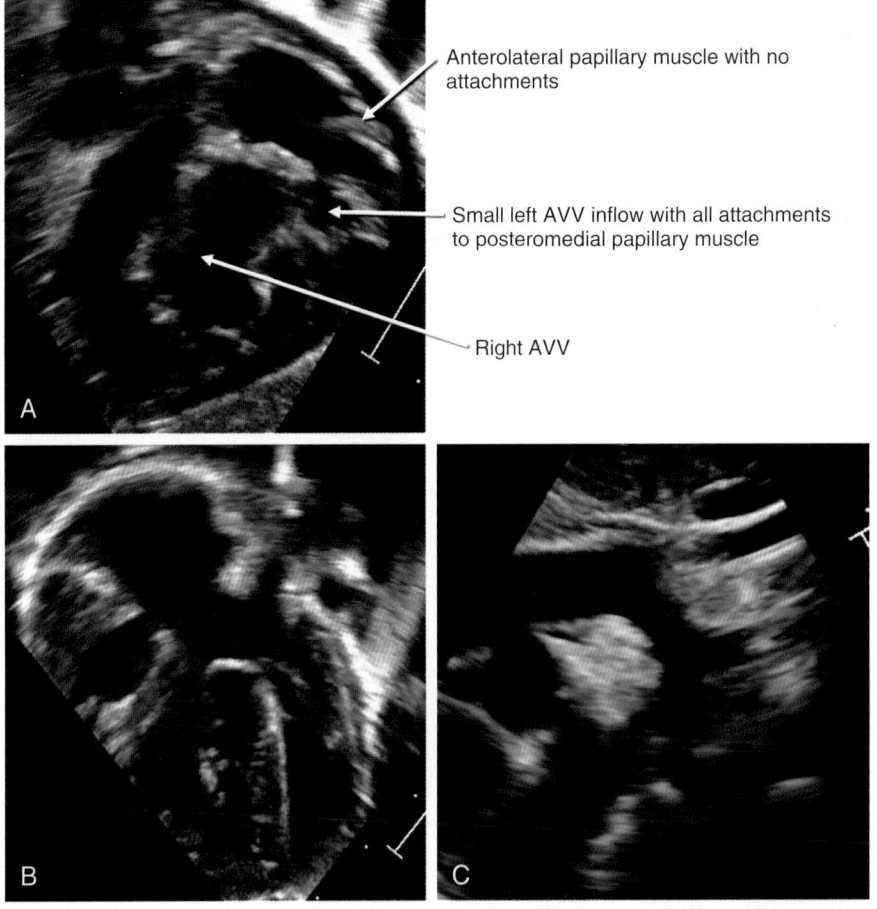

Anterolateral papillary muscle with no attachments

Small left AVV inflow with all attachments to posteromedial papillary muscle

Right AVV

• **Fig. 31.8** Parachute left atrioventricular valve *(AVV)*. **(A)** A subxiphoid short-axis view depicting a small inflow of the left AVV component overlying the posteromedial papillary muscle. A separate anterolateral papillary muscle exists but does not receive any chordal attachments. Parachute left AVV is associated with left heart hypoplasia (B and C). **(B)** A four-chamber view showing an apex-forming left ventricle with reduced lateral dimension and mildly reduced cavity size. **(C)** A long-axis view of the aortic arch and isthmic coarctation.

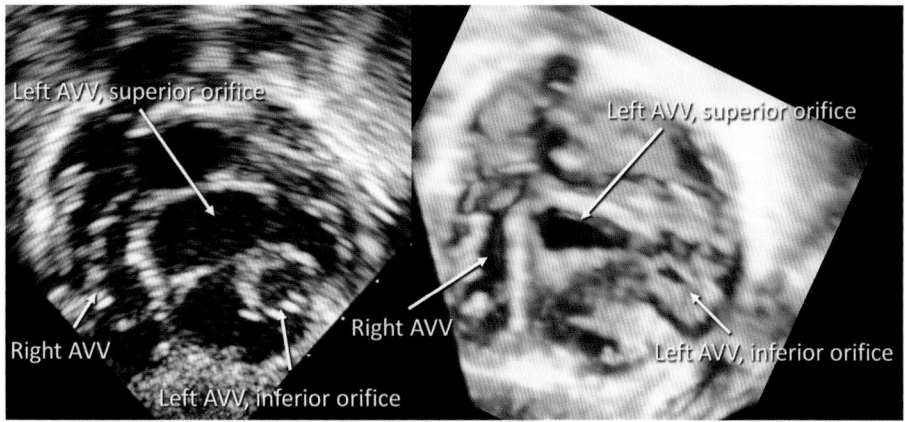

• **Fig. 31.9** Double-orifice left atrioventricular valve (AVV). Two- and three-dimensional echocardiographic views from a subxiphoid view showing the common AVV "en face." The left AVV has two orifices—a larger superior orifice and a smaller inferior orifice. The size discrepancy between the orifices is significant and is more readily apparent on the three-dimensional image.

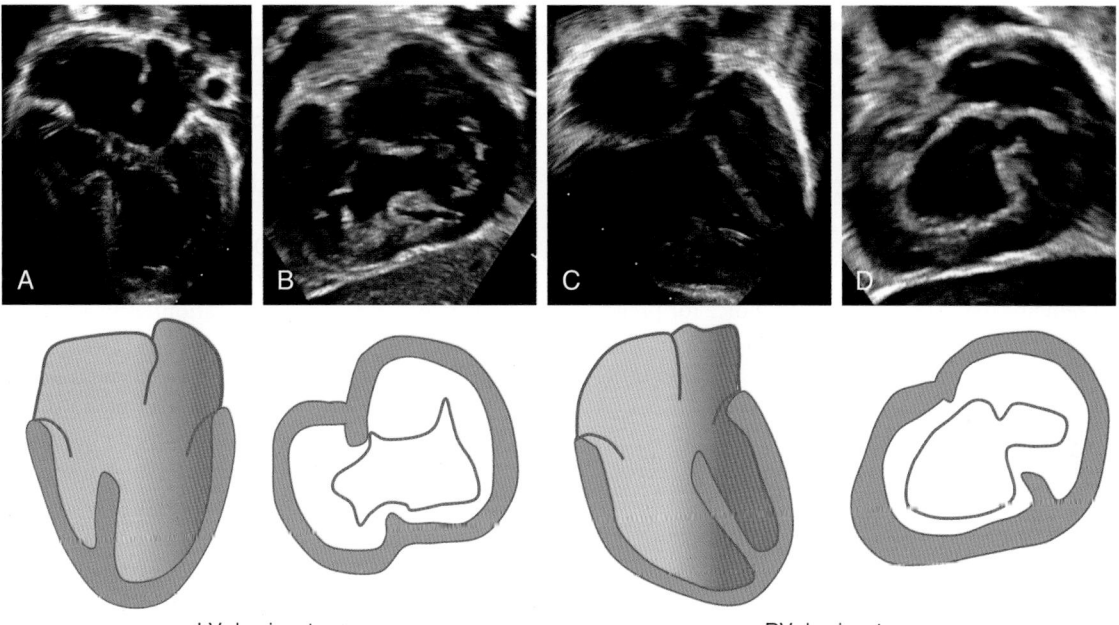

LV dominant   RV dominant

• **Fig. 31.10** Apical four-chamber view and subxiphoid short-axis views showing LV-dominant **(A and B)** and RV-dominant **(C and D)** atrioventricular canal defect (AVCD). In LV-dominant AVCD, the atrioventricular valve inflow predominantly overlies the left ventricle resulting in hypoplasia of the right ventricle, and vice versa.

regarding candidacy for full surgical repair. These include calculation of the ratio of relative AVV inflow overlying each of the ventricles using echocardiography (referred to as AVV index), relative angles of the AVV inflows, and metrics that use the size of the inflows relative to the size of the VSD.[9-11] These measurements are difficult to perform with a high degree of reproducibility and are not universally implemented. In recent years, cardiac magnetic resonance (CMR) and ECG-gated cine computed tomography (CT) scans have found an increasing role in visualization of the AVV and accurately quantifying ventricular volumes to guide surgical planning.[12]

Pathophysiology and Clinical Course

The pathophysiologic consequences of AVCDs vary among the anatomic subtypes; they depend upon the degree of shunting at the atrial and ventricular levels and presence of AVV regurgitation. In a balanced complete AVCD, there is typically a large left-to-right shunt in early infancy, beginning as the pulmonary vascular resistance drops over the initial several weeks of life. Left untreated, most infants develop progressive symptoms of congestive heart failure by the age of 6–8 weeks, including increased work of breathing, feeding difficulty, and failure to grow. In patients with primarily an atrial level shunt, such as transitional AVCDs with restrictive VSD or partial AVCD with no VSD (primum ASD), the presentation is like that of an isolated ASD. In these cases, the right heart volume load from the left-to-right shunt at the atrial level is typically well tolerated in early childhood. Some of these patients can become symptomatic earlier in life; in these uncommon cases, there are typically associated left-sided problems, including single LV papillary muscle, subaortic stenosis, and/or coarctation of the aorta. Ultimately, even isolated primum ASDs require surgery to eliminate increased pulmonary blood flow and chronic RV volume overload as these defects do not close spontaneously.

In all AVCD hearts with a large VSD component, the risk for development of pulmonary vascular disease is high without treatment. Irreversible pulmonary vascular disease can develop as early as the first year of life, similar to other patients with a large VSD. The risk of pulmonary vascular disease is higher in patients with trisomy 21 and seems to develop at an accelerated pace. The etiology of this phenomenon is multifactorial; reasons may include abnormal lung development, upper airway obstruction, and central hypoventilation.[13]

Diagnosis

Prenatal Diagnosis

Ultrasound remains the diagnostic tool of choice for prenatal diagnosis of AVCD. Despite inclusion of the four-chamber view in routine obstetric ultrasound protocols, the prenatal detection of AVCD is less than 50%.[14,15] Reasons for the relatively low prenatal detection rate are multifactorial; for example, lack of careful interrogation of the central "crux" of the heart may result in a missed diagnosis in the setting of generally preserved cardiac symmetry. A complete fetal echocardiogram, with careful assessment for associated lesions and balance of the AVV, allows for prognostication and comprehensive counseling. Genetic testing should be offered to all families given the higher prevalence of the above-mentioned conditions.

Postnatal Diagnosis

Newborns with complete AVCD may be diagnosed by a failed critical congenital heart disease screen due to mixing or bidirectional shunting at the atrial or ventricular levels. The screen is not infallible as at the time of the test, the intracardiac shunt may be all left to right, and oxygen saturations may be normal. Newborns with transitional AVCD may present with a holosystolic murmur arising as a result of the restrictive VSD, although this too is not dependable; the murmur may be soft or absent in the setting of a low transventricular pressure gradient in the early newborn period. ECG or echocardiogram performed for an unrelated reason may incidentally lead to the diagnosis of AVCD given the notable presence of a superior QRS axis in these patients. Physical examination in children presenting with congestive heart failure may include a hyperdynamic precordium, a crescendo-decrescendo ejection murmur over the upper left sternal border from increased flow across the pulmonary valve, and, in the presence of AVV regurgitation, a holosystolic murmur. These findings may be indistinguishable from those of a large VSD.

Echocardiography

When AVCD is among the considerations based on clinical symptoms in a child, echocardiography forms the basis of diagnosis and treatment planning. Echocardiographic protocol for initial evaluation of AVCD is summarized in Table 31.1.

In most children, the anatomy of the leaflets and subvalvar apparatus is best visualized from subxiphoid views. The so-called in-between view (also known as left anterior oblique view) shows the AVV "en face" allowing for assessment of its morphology, ventricular balance, and Rastelli classification (Fig. 31.6). Sweeping from the oblique view to a LV short axis view allows assessment of the subvalvar apparatus including the size, number, and spacing of the papillary muscles. The subxiphoid LV long-axis view demonstrates the anatomy of the LV outflow tract, highlighting the goose-neck deformity, and the presence of obstruction. Although the AVC VSD is difficult to assess in detail in subxiphoid views, atrial and ventricular septa are profiled very well for identification/exclusion of additional ASD and VSD.

In AVCD, the apical views are well suited for evaluation of the ASD and VSD. This is unlike most other septal defects in which apical views can be challenging to interpret. Apical four-chamber views aid in the assessment of AVV balance and relative lengths of two ventricles. Color Doppler imaging from apical and parasternal long-axis views is important in determining the degree of AVV regurgitation and LV outflow obstruction. Pulse and continuous wave Doppler can help quantify the degree of outflow obstruction when present.

Parasternal short-axis views can augment the subxiphoid short-axis views with respect to leaflet and subvalvar apparatus anatomy. Parasternal short-axis views are the mainstay for identification and localization of additional muscular VSDs when present. Parasternal short-axis views are also useful in localizing the site of regurgitation and understanding its mechanism; in most cases, AVV regurgitation is via the "cleft" between the superior and inferior bridging leaflets.

Three-dimensional (3D) echocardiography has the potential to augment the understanding of AVC anatomy obtained by two-dimensional (2D) imaging. It can provide a more complete picture in cases with double-orifice or parachute valves and can help localize the regurgitation when present (Fig. 31.8 and Fig. 31.9). While 2D and color Doppler imaging sweeps technically contain all the necessary information at a higher spatial and temporal resolution, 3D echo

TABLE 31.1	Echocardiography Protocol: A comprehensive anatomic and functional examination should be conducted including a complete cardiac anatomical survey. Elements listed in the Table should be evaluated in detail and given priority.

- Detailed long- and short-axis imaging of the atrial and ventricular components of the AV canal from the subcostal, apical, and parasternal windows.
- AVV morphology and attachments by sweeps in the subcostal (long-axis, short-axis, and in-between views), parasternal (long- and short-axis views), and in the apical 2C, 3C, and 4C views.
- Balance of AVV (commitment of AVV to underlying ventricle and size of ventricle) from apical four-chamber and subcostal and parasternal short-axis views.
- Subvalvar apparatus with special attention to papillary muscle anatomy, including oblique subcostal imaging in addition to standard views. Aim to exclude (or confirm when present) single LV papillary muscle or parachute deformity and double orifice left AVV by 2D, 3D, and color Doppler imaging.
- Evaluate for AVVR degree and mechanism by color Doppler (including color compare) in long- and short-axis views, including apical (2C, 3C, 4C) and parasternal windows.
- Detailed evaluation of the atrial and ventricular septa for additional septal defects. Adjust (lower) the Nyquist limit as needed to visualize low-velocity flow.
- Assess for LV outflow tract obstruction by 2D, color Doppler, and pulsed and continuous wave Doppler. Measure aortic annulus and root from the parasternal long-axis view.
- Rule out aortic arch obstruction by 2D, color Doppler, and pulsed and CW Doppler imaging, especially in RV-dominant AVC defects.
- Rule out RV outflow obstruction by 2D, color Doppler, pulsed and CW Doppler.

AVC, Atrioventricular canal; *AVV,* atrioventricular valve; *AVVR,* Atrioventricular valve regurgitation; *CW,* continuous wave; *LV,* left ventricular; *RV,* right ventricular.

allows demonstration of the anatomy in one look without the need to mentally reconstruct the structures from 2D.

Electrocardiography

The electrocardiogram in AVCD has a leftward, counterclockwise superior axis usually between −150 and −90 degrees in the frontal plane (Fig. 31.11). This ECG finding results from the abnormal ventricular activation as the conduction tissues courses along the inferior edge of the inlet VSD. The

ECG may also hint towards right heart dilation in the form of incomplete right bundle branch block, atrial enlargement, and ventricular hypertrophy when present.

Chest Radiography

Lung findings on chest radiograph depend on the size of the left-to-right shunt and pulmonary vascular resistance. In the presence of a significant left-to-right shunt, increased vascular markings, hyperinflation, and pulmonary

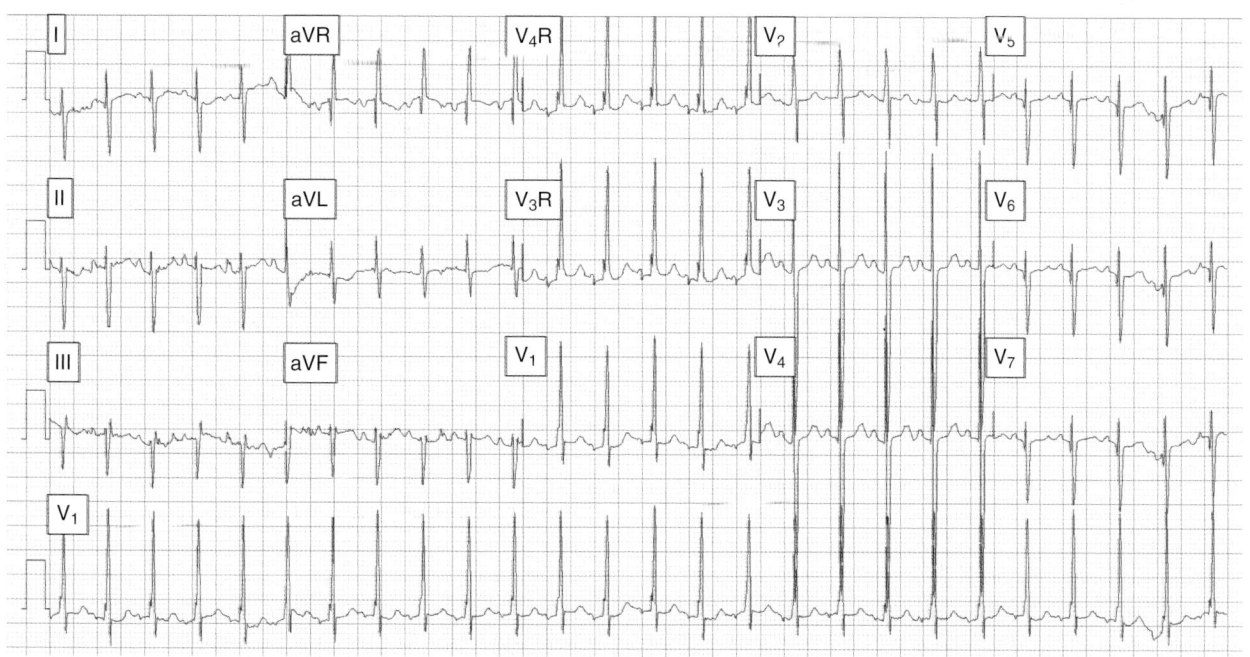

• **Fig. 31.11** ECG demonstrating the characteristic superior QRS axis in a patient with atrioventricular canal defect. Also note the presence of right ventricular hypertrophy on this ECG with prominent R waves in right precordial leads.

edema may be present. Cardiomegaly is common in uncorrected infants who are experiencing symptoms of heart failure. Additional abnormalities in the size and shape of the heart, symmetry of the lung fields, side of the aortic arch, thoracic and abdominal situs, and skeletal anomalies may provide clues with regards to the presence of associated conditions.

Cardiac Catheterization

Cardiac catheterization is not a part of routine diagnostic evaluation for patients with uncomplicated AVCDs undergoing surgical correction in early infancy. At older ages, cardiac catheterization may be considered to evaluate the pulmonary vascular resistance and perform vasodilator testing.

Computed Tomography Scan and Cardiac Magnetic Resonance

The majority of children with AVCD do not require imaging using CT scans or CMR, although they play an important role in specific subgroups of patients with AVCD. In presence of unbalanced defects, these imaging modalities can quantify ventricular volumes to guide surgical decision-making. In addition, CT has been found to have an important role in defining the vascular anatomy for initial palliation in patients with restrictive pulmonary blood flow being considered for transcatheter stenting of the ductus arteriosus. Patients with associated complex anatomy such as those with heterotaxy syndrome may benefit from detailed anatomical and functional assessment by CMR prior to interventions.

Management

Nearly all patients with AVCD ultimately require surgical correction. The median age at repair of a balanced complete AVCD at Boston Children's Hospital is 3.2 months.[16] Patients with transitional or partial canals typically undergo surgery at an older age. The role of medical therapy is limited to symptom control until surgery can be accomplished. Diuretic therapy is the mainstay of heart failure symptoms from left-to-right shunting and furosemide is the typical first-line agent. Angiotensin-converting enzyme inhibitors are occasionally used alongside diuretics.

Surgery

As noted above, AVCDs represent a spectrum ranging from an isolated primum ASD (typically with a "cleft" in the left AVV) to a complete AVCD with interatrial and ventricular septal communications and AVV abnormalities. The goals of surgical repair are to reconstitute the missing components of the interatrial and interventricular septa (typically with patch material) and to achieve separation and long-term competence of the AVV. The atrioventricular node and coronary sinus orifice are displaced inferiorly compared

with normal anatomy and are in close proximity to the posterior rim of the primum ASD component making the conduction system vulnerable to injury. Surgical techniques have improved such that the incidence of injury to the conduction system during repair of AVCDs is now < 5%.

Complete Atrioventricular Canal Defect

In the complete form of the AVCD, there is a large interventricular communication (inlet VSD), and a large interatrial communication (primum ASD), combined with a common AVV with a spectrum of anatomic variations (see Anatomy section). Because of the highly unfavorable natural history of the untreated complete AVCD, surgical intervention is generally undertaken between 3 and 6 months of age. Complete repair is favored over palliation with a pulmonary artery band unless there are significant associated medical or noncardiac abnormalities that make complete repair unacceptably risky. In general, patients will have much better outcomes with repaired lesions and normal, or nearly normal, physiology compared with palliated circulatory states.

Several variations of complete AVCD repair are commonly used, depending on surgeon preference. In almost all cases, except those with a single LV papillary muscle and absent or very hypoplastic mural leaflet of the left AVV, the "cleft" between the superior and inferior cushion leaflets must be completely closed to minimize the risk of acute or recurrent left AVV regurgitation. Assessment of left AVV competence can be made intraoperatively by injection of iced saline into the LV after valve repair, but this must be supplemented with echocardiographic assessment of the left AVV function by echocardiography. If residual moderate or greater left AVV regurgitation or stenosis is found, strong consideration should be given to re-repair. Supplemental techniques include commissuroplasty sutures at the commissures between the superior and/or inferior cushion leaflets and the mural leaflet, or the placement of an annuloplasty suture encompassing the (posterior) parts of the left AVV annulus not composed of patch material. Routine monitoring of left atrial pressure in the early period after surgery is frequently used to provide additional information about the adequacy of the left AVV repair. An additional consideration, regardless of the operative technique chosen, is to shorten the distance between the anterior and posterior aspects of the AV canal annulus (distance between the hinge points of the superior and inferior cushion elements) as a part of the repair. This technique provides an annuloplasty effect on the circumference of the right and left AVV orifices. In a complete AVCD, this is accomplished by making the VSD patch dimensions somewhat shorter in the anterior-posterior direction (front to back) than the dimensions of the VSD component of the defect. In addition, in any of the techniques, suture lines for the atrial and ventricular components should avoid the AV node and His bundle to prevent post-repair heart block. This can be accomplished by suturing the VSD patch to right side of the septum and suturing the ASD patch rightward along the right AVV annulus and then rightward of the coronary sinus orifice before reaching the posterior aspect of the primum ASD. In this approach, the coronary sinus will drain into the left side of the heart; although this is not a significant hemodynamic issue, it has implications for access during electrophysiologic mapping should that be necessary in the future. An alternative technique is to place this atrial patch suture line along the left AVV annulus and then on the leftward aspect of the atrial septal margin.

1. Single-patch technique: In this type of repair, one patch is used to close both the ventricular and atrial defects, and the right and left AVV components are separated. The right and left components of the separated AVV tissue components must be reattached to this new atrioventricular septum, and the cleft in the left AVV should be closed primarily. The patch material used at Boston Children's Hospital has generally been fresh autologous pericardium, and the level of the reattachment of the AVV tissue should favor proximity to the crest of the ventricular septum.
2. Two-patch technique: In this type of repair, the primum ASD and the inlet VSD components are closed with two separate patches. Dacron is commonly used for the VSD patch, and autologous pericardium is typically used for the atrial septal component. The cleft in the left AVV is closed in a similar fashion as for the single-patch technique. In addition to making the patch dimensions smaller than the VSD dimensions in the anterior-posterior dimension, the height of the patch should also be kept small to avoid displacement of the leaflet tissue into the atrium, as this seems to be associated with higher incidence of left AVV regurgitation.
3. Single-patch Australian technique: In this type of repair, the inlet VSD component is obliterated by suturing the common AVV tissue directly to the crest of the ventricular septum and then using a pericardial patch to close the remaining primum ASD component. Left AVV cleft closure is carried out in similar fashion as the other techniques.

Each of these techniques has been associated with high early success rates, but the risk for reoperation for residual or recurrent left AVV regurgitation has not been eliminated. The requirement for reoperation has been associated with more severe grades of preoperative AVV regurgitation, but all patients should be thoroughly evaluated with echocardiography prior to discharge and during extended follow-up after repair.

Transitional Atrioventricular Canal Defect

The transitional AVCD differs from the complete AVCD in that the ventricular component of the defect is small and therefore pressure restrictive. In a transitional AVCD, chordal attachments from the superior and inferior cushion leaflets to the ventricular septum (as in a Rastelli type A anatomy) fuse, partially obliterating the VSD component

of the AVCD, and leaving only the interchordal spaces as the interventricular communications. In the repair of this form of AV canal, the remaining interchordal spaces are closed with sutures in most cases, although small patches can also be used. The remainder of the repair consists of cleft closure and patch closure of the primum ASD component.

Partial Atrioventricular Canal Defect

The terms *partial AVCD* or *incomplete AVCD* refer to the situations in which the only communications between the right and left sides of the circulation occur at the level of the primum ASD. Repair then consists of patch closure of the primum ASD using similar techniques as used for the atrial component of the complete AVCD along with closure of the cleft in the left AVV.

Postoperative Management

Postoperative management of patients with AVCD should incorporate patient-specific considerations including preoperative anatomic details and physiology, indications for surgery and implications of timing, and noncardiac risk factors. Multi-organ comorbidities should be addressed in syndromic patients (e.g., thyroid function in patients with trisomy 21, splenic function in patients with heterotaxy syndrome). Which data are reassuring with regards to the technical success of the surgery and postoperative course? Which factors (patient specific and lesion specific) are concerning and require heightened awareness? For example, an 8-month-old patient with trisomy 21 and complete AVCD who demonstrates no symptoms of congestive heart failure in the preoperative period should be considered at risk for elevated pulmonary vascular resistance. Postoperative management could include more invasive monitoring than routine, pre-emptive use of inhaled or enteral pulmonary vasodilators, adjustments to sedation and fluid management strategies, and a modified approach to extubation.

Details of the surgical repair are critical for patient care in the immediate postoperative period, as they inform management and clinical thinking, especially when a patient's clinical course is not progressing as expected. The left AVV remains the Achille's heel in the repair of AVCD and its continuing competency should be questioned if a patient's cardiopulmonary status is, or becomes, vulnerable. Judicious use of fluid resuscitation, avoidance of abrupt shifts in intravascular volume, and thoughtful management of ventricular afterload may serve to protect the AVV repair as the patient recovers. In patients with unbalanced AVCD, factors associated with the nondominant chamber may impact medical strategies in order to optimize or mitigate physiologic implications. For example, in the patient with a parachute left AVV, left atrial hypertension and/or residual stenosis, and regurgitation might be expected. Strategies to optimize the circulation could include heart rate control in addition to the fluid and afterload management already noted. The presence of previously unappreciated additional VSD(s) as well as the potential for an LV to RA shunt should also be considered if a patient is struggling to progress. Although clinically significant LV outflow tract obstruction is uncommon in the immediate postoperative period, patients with small/dysmorphic left-sided structures (left AVV, LV cavity, aortic valve, and/or coarctation) are at increased risk.

Patients who are immediately status post-AVCD repair are at risk for dysrhythmias including complete heart block, accelerated junctional rhythm and junctional ectopic tachycardia, and atrial tachycardias. In patients with complete heart block, we typically wait 7 to 10 days postoperatively before placing a permanent pacemaker.[17]

The timing of extubation is variable as it considers all the patient factors previously discussed. Patients with known airway vulnerabilities, pulmonary hypertension, or left atrial hypertension may be transitioned off mechanical ventilation more smoothly with the use of noninvasive positive pressure ventilation.

Short- and Long-term Outcomes

Survival to discharge after surgical repair of complete AVCD is between 97% and 98%.[18,19] Risk factors for mortality include low birth weight and younger age at surgery. Some studies have found a lower risk of mortality and that of major complications for patients with trisomy 21 compared with those without.[18] Fewer than 3% develop complete heart block requiring a permanent pacemaker placement. Early outcomes for patients with partial or transitional AVCDs are better than those with complete forms.[20] About 15–20% of patients require reoperations after surgical correction of AVCD.[21-23] Common indications for reoperation include mitral valve dysfunction, tricuspid valve dysfunction, residual shunts, and LV outflow tract obstruction. Long-term survival after repair of tetralogy of Fallot associated with AVCD is excellent and the need for survival is affected by the choice of RV outflow reconstruction.[24]

Care of Adults With Repaired Atrioventricular Canal Defect

Patients with repaired AVCD need lifelong cardiac care. Depending on the physiologic state, clinical assessments including ECG and echocardiography are recommended at 1- to 3-year intervals.[25] Indications for surgical intervention on the mitral valve can be extrapolated from guidelines for mitral valve disease without history of AVCD. Surgical planning should consider differences in the annular geometry, scar and patch material from original surgery, and narrowness of the LV outflow tract. For example, struts of certain bioprosthetic valves may protrude more into the outflow increasing the risk of obstruction compared with mechanical valves. Similar to mitral valve disease, indications for reoperation for residual shunts or LV outflow tract obstruction may be extrapolated from their respective

isolated counterparts. Surgical repair of outflow obstruction can be more challenging in patients with AVCD when the mechanism of obstruction is not a discrete membrane.

Careful evaluation of hemodynamic burden of residual lesions should be undertaken in pregnant women or those planning a pregnancy. Residual left-to-right shunts and mitral regurgitation are generally well tolerated. Given the increased risk of congenital heart disease in the fetus of a woman with AVCD, a fetal echocardiogram is recommended during mid-second trimester. Women with Eisenmenger syndrome or severe pulmonary hypertension are at a high risk of major complications or mortality and should be advised against pregnancy.

References

1. Gittenberger-de Groot AC, Bartelings MM, Deruiter MC, et al. Basics of Cardiac development for the understanding of congenital heart malformations. *Pediatr Res.* 2005;57:169-176.
2. Burns T, Yang Y, Hiriart E, Wessels A. The dorsal mesenchymal protrusion and the pathogenesis of atrioventricular septal defects. *J Cardiovasc Dev Dis.* 2016;3:29. doi:10.3390/jcdd3040029.
3. Hoffman JIE, Kaplan S. The incidence of congenital heart disease. *J Am Coll Cardiol.* 2002;39:1890-1900.
4. Irving CA, Chaudhari MP. Cardiovascular abnormalities in Down's syndrome: spectrum, management and survival over 22 years. *Arch Dis Child.* 2012;97:326-330.
5. Barlow GM, Chen XN, Shi ZY, et al. Down syndrome congenital heart disease: a narrowed region and a candidate gene. *Genet Med.* 2001;3:91-101.
6. Dobosz A, Grabowska A, Bik-Multanowski M. Hypermethylation of NRG1 gene correlates with the presence of heart defects in Down's syndrome. *J Genet.* 2019;98:110.
7. Pugnaloni F, Digilio MC, Putotto C, De Luca E, Marino B, Versacci P. Genetics of atrioventricular canal defects. *Ital J Pediatr.* 2020;46:61.
8. Rastelli GC, Ongley PA, Kirklin JW, et al. Surgical repair of the complete form of persistent common atrioventricular canal. *J Thorac Cardiovasc Surg.* 1968;55:299-308.
9. Cohen MS, Jacobs ML, Weinberg PM, et al. Morphometric analysis of unbalanced common atrioventricular canal using two-dimensional echocardiography. *J Am Coll Cardiol.* 1996;28: 1017-1023.
10. Cohen MS, Jegatheeswaran A, Baffa JM, et al. Echocardiographic features defining right dominant unbalanced atrioventricular septal defect. *Circ Cardiovasc Imaging.* 2013;6:508-513.
11. van Son JA, Phoon CK, Silverman NH, et al. Predicting feasibility of biventricular repair of right-dominant unbalanced atrioventricular canal. *Ann Thorac Surg.* 1997;63:1657-1663.
12. Banka P, Schaetzle B, Komarlu R, et al. Cardiovascular magnetic resonance parameters associated with early transplant-free survival in children with small left hearts following conversion from a univentricular to biventricular circulation. *J Cardiovasc Magn Reson.* 2014;16:73.
13. Bush DS, Ivy DD. Pulmonary hypertension in the population with Down syndrome. *Cardiol Ther.* 2022;11:33-47.
14. Quartermain MD, Pasquali SK, Hill KD, et al. Variation in prenatal diagnosis of congenital heart disease in infants. *Pediatrics.* 2015;136:e378-e385.

15. ter Heide H, Thomson JDR, Wharton GA, et al. Poor sensitivity of routine fetal anomaly ultrasound screening for antenatal detection of atrioventricular septal defect. *Heart.* 2004;90:916-917.

16. IJsselhof R, Gauvreau K, Del Nido P, et al. Technical performance score: predictor of outcomes in complete atrioventricular septal defect repair. *Ann Thorac Surg.* 2017;104:1371-1377.

17. Romer AJ, Tabbutt S, Etheridge SP, et al. Atrioventricular block after congenital heart surgery: analysis from the Pediatric Cardiac Critical Care Consortium. *J Thorac Cardiovasc Surg.* 2019;157:1168-1177.e2.

18. St Louis JD, Jodhka U, Jacobs JP, et al. Contemporary outcomes of complete atrioventricular septal defect repair: analysis of the Society of Thoracic Surgeons Congenital Heart Surgery Database. *J Thorac Cardiovasc Surg.* 2014;148:2526-2531.

19. Atz AM, Hawkins JA, Lu M, et al. Surgical management of complete atrioventricular septal defect: associations with surgical technique, age, and trisomy 21. *J Thorac Cardiovasc Surg.* 2011;141:1371-1379.

20. Mery CM, Zea-Vera R, Chacon-Portillo MA, et al. Contemporary results after repair of partial and transitional atrioventricular septal defects. *J Thorac Cardiovasc Surg.* 2019;157:1117-1127.e4.

21. Stulak JM, Burkhart HM, Dearani JA, et al. Reoperations after repair of partial atrioventricular septal defect: a 45-year single-center experience. *Ann Thorac Surg.* 2010;89:1352-1359.

22. Fong LS, Betts K, Bell D, et al. Complete atrioventricular septal defect repair in Australia: Results over 25 years. *J Thorac Cardiovasc Surg.* 2020;159:1014-1025.e8.

23. Fong LS, Betts K, Ayer J, et al. Predictors of reoperation and mortality after complete atrioventricular septal defect repair. *Eur J Cardiothorac Surg.* 2021;61:45-53.

24. Shuhaiber JH, Robinson B, Gauvreau K, et al. Outcome after repair of atrioventricular septal defect with tetralogy of Fallot. *J Thorac Cardiovasc Surg.* 2012;143:338-343.

25. Stout KK, Daniels CJ, Aboulhosn JA, et al. 2018 AHA/ACC guideline for the management of adults with congenital heart disease: a report of the American College of Cardiology/American Heart Association Task Force on clinical practice guidelines. *Circulation.* 2019;139:e698-e800.

32

Heterotaxy Syndrome

DAVID SCHIDLOW, SITARAM M. EMANI, AND SARAH A. TEELE

KEY LEARNING POINTS

- Heterotaxy syndrome is a complex condition caused by abnormal establishment of left- or right-sidedness early in embryologic development. It affects the location and function of multiple organ systems throughout the body.
- Heterotaxy syndrome is classically divided into two subtypes: polysplenia (bilateral left-sidedness) and asplenia (bilateral right-sidedness). The subtypes have characteristic cardiac and noncardiac abnormalities, but there is substantial overlap.
- Screening for and treating noncardiac abnormalities in heterotaxy syndrome is important, as noncardiac disease

can contribute substantially to patient morbidity and mortality.
- Surgical repair or palliation of cardiac disease in heterotaxy syndrome presents unique challenges due to the underlying anatomic complexity. Detailed preoperative assessment and a thoughtful surgical approach are required to optimize outcomes
- Coordinated, data-driven, multidisciplinary care of heterotaxy syndrome is important and likely to improve outcomes in this challenging group of patients.

Introduction

Heterotaxy syndrome (HS) is a complex and multifaceted condition affecting the location and function of multiple organ systems throughout the body. The heart is often profoundly affected, resulting in some of the most complex and challenging congenital cardiovascular malformations encountered in pediatric cardiology. Cardiac disease may be exacerbated by abnormalities in other organ systems, and patients with HS remain a persistently challenging group with little change in prognosis over the last few decades.[1] Thankfully, care for HS is increasingly gravitating toward a data-driven multidisciplinary approach, and this along with innovations in medical and surgical therapies will hopefully improve outcomes in this complicated set of patients.

Human laterality begins early in embryonic development and is governed by complex molecular mechanisms underpinning ciliary motion. Usually the stomach, a single spleen, and a bi-lobed lung are left-sided, whereas the liver, gallbladder, and a tri-lobed lung are right-sided. The process of establishing laterality can be disrupted at any number of different stages, resulting in an abnormal distribution of organs within the thorax and abdomen.[2] In HS, organs within the thorax and abdomen assume a more symmetric arrangement, with two broad groups: those with tendencies toward bilateral right-sidedness and those with tendencies

toward bilateral left-sidedness. It should be noted, however, that perfect symmetry does not occur in HS.

The symmetry throughout the thorax and abdomen in HS is frequently accompanied by variable structural and/or functional abnormalities in the respiratory, immune, and gastrointestinal systems. The cardiovascular system is often but not always affected, with a seemingly limitless array of anatomic and physiologic aberrations, ranging from insignificant to life-threatening *in utero*. A substantial portion of morbidity and mortality associated with HS is due to cardiac disease. Nevertheless, non-cardiac disease can be severe and even life-threatening. At a minimum, the interplay between non-cardiac and cardiac disease is important and should not be dismissed.

The complexity of cardiac disease in HS patients may feel overwhelming, particularly for trainees new to congenital heart disease (CHD). Nevertheless, with the application of fundamental diagnostic principles and physiologic reasoning, the heart in HS can be readily understood. This chapter is intended as a practical guide for individuals caring for patients with HS. It begins with a review of commonly used definitions, nomenclature, and a brief discussion of the prevalence and etiology of HS. Following that are three sections pertaining to the cardiac manifestations, noncardiac manifestations, and cardiac surgical approaches. The chapter concludes with a discussion of the importance of a multidisciplinary approach to HS care.

Definitions and Nomenclature

A variety of terms is used to describe HS. Unfortunately for new learners, the language is inconsistently applied among institutions and authors. The following section reviews commonly encountered nomenclature and notes the authors' institutional preference where relevant.

The term "heterotaxy" is itself derived from a combination of two Greek words, *heteros* (ετερο) meaning "other" and *taxos* (ταξος) meaning "arrangement"; this "other arrangement" refers to the departure from normal human right-left asymmetry. Heterotaxy is typically divided into two broad categories based on the tendency toward bilateral left-sidedness or bilateral right-sidedness. For reasons that are poorly understood, HS is almost universally associated with abnormalities in the presence, location, number, and/or function of the spleen(s).

Patients with bilateral left-sidedness are typically referred to as having heterotaxy with polysplenia, the spleen being a left-sided organ. Another term frequently used is left atrial isomerism. Patients with polysplenia typically have multiple right- or left-sided spleens. Typically encountered in heterotaxy with polysplenia are lungs with bilateral left-sided bronchial morphology (bi-lobed lungs, see Fig. 32.6) with accompanying bilateral hyparterial bronchi. Hyparterial refers to anatomy in which branches of the bronchi originate below the point where the branch pulmonary artery crosses the bronchus. The liver is frequently midline, and gallbladder abnormalities, either gallbladder absence and/or associated biliary atresia, can be encountered. The stomach in polysplenia may be right-sided or left-sided, and malrotation may be present.

Patients with bilateral right-sidedness are typically referred to as having heterotaxy with asplenia. The term right atrial isomerism is sometimes employed to describe this group. On occasion, this patient population is referred to as having Ivemark syndrome, after the 1955 publication by Biörn Ivemark.[3] Typically encountered in heterotaxy with asplenia are lungs with bilateral right-sided bronchial morphology (tri-lobed lungs, see Fig. 32.6) with accompanying eparterial bronchi. Eparterial refers to the right superior lobe bronchus which originates above the level of the branch pulmonary artery. Abdominal findings may include abnormalities of liver position and absence of the spleen. Like its contralateral counterpart, the stomach may be right-sided or left-sided, and malrotation may be present.

Occasionally, bronchopulmonary and abdominal situs inversus totalis are accompanied by complex congenital heart disease. This group of patients strays from the tendency toward symmetry encountered in many with heterotaxy. Nevertheless, such patients are reasonably considered part of the heterotaxy spectrum based on contemporary criteria. It should also be noted that so-called "disharmonious" patterns of heterotaxy are increasingly recognized, wherein the tendency toward bilateral right- or left-sidedness is inconsistent among various involved organs.[4]

While the designations of polysplenia and asplenia are preferred at our institution, a brief discussion of term "isomerism" is useful. Among cardiac structures affected by HS, the atria, specifically the atrial appendages, tend to be the most symmetric, with bilateral finger-like appendages (left atrial appendage morphology) typical of polysplenia and bilateral broad-based atrial appendages (right atrial appendage morphology) typical of asplenia. It should be noted that the atria themselves do not assume a symmetric morphology. In fact, frequently the atria in HS lack enough features to reliably determine left or right morphology and by extension atrial situs; indeed many patients with HS have atrial situs ambiguus and a common atrium. Atrial appendage morphology might be informative in some instances, but many individuals with HS have indistinct or distorted atrial appendage morphology, limiting their utility in determining HS subtype.

Regardless of nomenclature used, neither the spleen (its number, location, or functional status) nor the anatomy of the atrial appendages should be used to derive firm conclusions about the cardiac or extra-cardiac anatomy, as there is substantial overlap between the two categories.[5] Conversely, cardiac (or non-cardiac) disease should not be used to make any inferences about the presence and function of the spleen or any other organ system. Despite their limitations, the terms asplenia and polysplenia provide some framework for the spectrum of potential abnormalities in a specific individual and will be used throughout the remainder of this chapter.

Two scenarios merit special attention: (1) situs inversus totalis (SIT) and (2) abnormalities of cardiac position in the absence of other visceral situs abnormalities. In situs inversus totalis, thoraco-abdominal asymmetry is maintained, albeit in the mirror image of usual. Organ anatomy and function are otherwise normal, and this group is usually not considered to have HS. This is also true of Kartagener syndrome, where SIT is accompanied by primary ciliary dyskinesia (PCD). It should be noted that, while ciliary abnormalities underpin them both, PCD and HS may or may not co-exist in any individual patient.

Another common temptation is to apply the label of HS to patients with abnormalities of cardiac position and/or with very complex anatomy. Dextrocardia (the majority of the cardiac mass in the right hemi-thorax) and mesocardia (the majority of the cardiac mass being midline) refer only to cardiac position and say nothing of the remaining viscera. Indeed, those with HS frequently have levocardia, whereas many with dextrocardia or mesocardia do not have HS. It can be particularly tempting to assign the label of heterotaxy to those with superior-inferior (upstairs/downstairs) ventricles. The ventricles in heterotaxy may occasionally assume such a relationship, but in most instances of superior-inferior ventricles, there is normal abdominal, thoracic, and atrial solitus.[6] These points are not purely academic, because diagnosing an individual with HS implies a potential array of noncardiac abnormalities requiring subspecialty testing and care.

At our institution, a standard set of criteria are applied to define HS (Table 32.1).[7–9] At least three criteria are required to meet the diagnosis of HS. Once the diagnostic criteria are met, patients can be broadly categorized into polysplenia and asplenia subtypes based upon specific anatomic features.

TABLE 32.1 **Heterotaxy Diagnostic Criteria from the National Birth Defects Prevention Study (Modified from Lin et al.[8] and Foerster et al.[9]) Classically, the Diagnosis of HTX Requires Three out of Eight Features**

1. Characteristic congenital heart defect
   a. Pulmonary venous anomalies (TAPVR, PAPVR)
   b. Atrial anomalies (atrial situs ambiguus or inversus, common atrium)
   c. Common atrioventricular canal (or septal) defects
   d. Ventricular abnormalities (hypoplastic or single left ventricle, hyoplastic or single right ventricle, ventricular malposition (e.g. L-loop, superior-inferior, criss-cross))
   e. Ventriculo arterial alignment abnormalities (double-outlet ventricle, D-loop TGA, L-loop TGA, truncus arteriosus, TOF (including TOF/PS, TOF/PA, and TOF/APV))
   f. Ventricular outflow abnormalities (subvalvar/valvar PS, PA with intact ventricular septum, PA with ventricular septal defect (not TOF-type), valvar or subvalvar aortic stenosis, coarctation of the aorta)

2. Biliary atresia

3. Abdominal situs abnormality
   a. Abdominal situs inversus
   b. Midline or transverse liver
   c. Midline aorta
   d. Ipsilateral aorta and IVC

4. Spleen abnormality
   a. Asplenia
   b. Polysplenia
   c. Single right-sided spleen

5. Isomerism of bronchi
   a. Bilateral left bronchial morphology (bilateral hyparterial bronchus)
   b. Bilateral right bronchial morphology (bilateral eparterial bronchus)

6. Isomerism of lungs
   a. Bilateral two lobes (left-sidedness)
   b. Bilateral three lobes (right-sidedness)

7. Similar morphology of atrial appendages ("atrial isomerism")

8. Two of the following
   a. A systemic venous anomaly
      1. Bilateral SVC
      2. Interrupted IVC
      3. Unroofed (absent) coronary sinus
   b. Intestinal malrotation (nonrotation, incomplete rotation, reverse rotation)
   c. Absent gallbladder

APV, absent pulmonary valve; *IVC,* inferior vena cava; *PAPVR,* partial anomalous pulmonary venous return; *PA,* pulmonic atresia; *PS,* pulmonic stenosis; *SVC,* superior vena cava; *TAPVR,* total anomalous pulmonary venous return; *TGS,* transposition of the great arteries; *TOF,* tetralogy of fallot

As stated above, however, additional cardiac and non-cardiac details require careful evaluation, and the dichotomous categories should not be used to derive any firm conclusions about the location and function of any organ system. As the genetic underpinnings of this syndrome are increasingly understood, more precise definitions across the HS spectrum are likely to emerge.

Prevalence and Etiology

The incidence of HS is thought to be approximately 1 in 5000–7000 of live births with CHD. Although HS is relatively rare, these complex patients are known for their challenging medical and surgical management. Heterotaxy may exhibit autosomal dominant, autosomal recessive, or X-linked patterns of inheritance. Most instances are sporadic, however, and in only about 40% of individuals is the responsible gene

identified. Even in the absence of diagnostic genetic testing, the recurrence in families is up to 25%.[10] Genetic counseling and prenatal screening for affected individuals and families are important.[11]

Cardiac Manifestations and Diagnostic Tools

Cardiac care for the patient with HS is often highly specialized and frequently requires contributions from numerous cardiac subspecialists, including those with expertise in imaging, electrophysiology, catheterization, intensive care, and advanced therapies including transplant. The following text is therefore intended as a general overview of cardiac disease in HS.

Despite their limitations, the terms polysplenia and asplenia permit a guide for the possible cardiac abnormalities in a given patient (Table 32.2). Frequently encountered in polysplenia HS are interruption of the inferior vena cava (IVC), normal or ipsilateral pulmonary venous connections, the presence of two ventricles, the presence of two separate atrioventricular valves, normally related great arteries, and systemic outflow obstruction (Fig. 32.1). In contrast, asplenia HS is frequently associated with an intact IVC, totally anomalous pulmonary venous connection (which may be obstructed), single-ventricle CHD, atrioventricular canal defects, transposition or malposition of the great arteries, and pulmonary stenosis or atresia (Fig. 32.2). Cardiac anomalies tend to be more complex in asplenia HS than in

TABLE 32.2 Commonly Encountered Cardiac Manifestations Among Heterotaxy Subtypes

	Polysplenia	Asplenia
Inferior vena cava	Interrupted	Intact
Pulmonary veins	Normal or ipsilateral	Totally anomalous, sometimes obstructed
Atrioventricular valves	Normal	Common (i.e., CAVC)
Ventricles	Two	Single
Great arteries	Normally related	Transposed or malposed (DORV)
Outflow obstruction	Systemic	Pulmonary
Rhythm	Sinus node dysfunction Heart block	Dual sinoatrial nodes Dual atrioventricular nodes

Cardiac manifestations of heterotaxy. Table displays cardiac abnormalities more likely to be encountered in polysplenia and asplenia as opposed to their contralateral counterparts. This is to be taken as a general guide, as there is substantial overlap between categories. *CAVC*, complete atrioventricular canal defect; *DORV*, double outlet right ventricle.

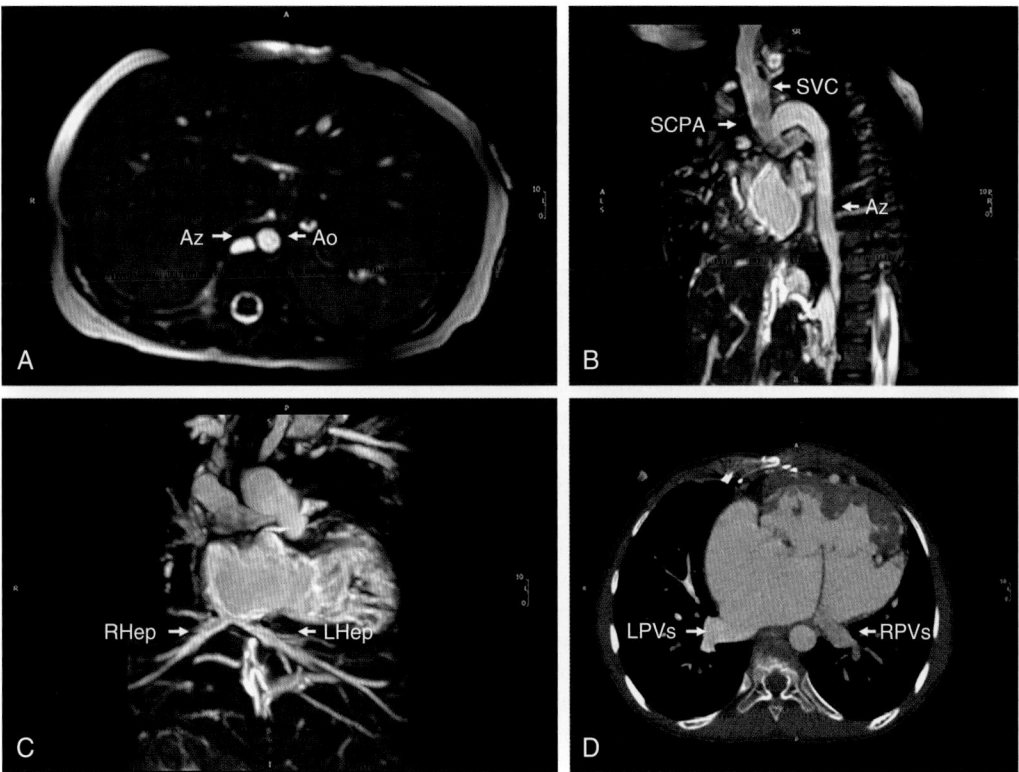

• **Fig. 32.1** Some of the cardiac findings commonly encountered in polysplenia syndrome. **(A)** Axial view of a dilated azygos vein consistent with interruption of the suprarenal inferior vena cava. **(B)** Sagittal view of a dilated azygos vein connecting to a right-sided superior vena cava in a patient with interrupted inferior vena cava; a Kawashima type superior cavopulmonary anastomosis is seen. **(C)** Coronal view of ipsilateral hepatic venous connections. **(D)** Axial view of ipsilateral pulmonary venous connections. *Ao*, Aorta; *Az*, azygos vein; *LHep*, left hepatic veins; *LPVs*, left pulmonary veins; *RHep*, right hepatic veins; *RPVs*, right pulmonary veins; *SCPA*, superior cavopulmonary anastomosis; *SVC*, superior vena cava.

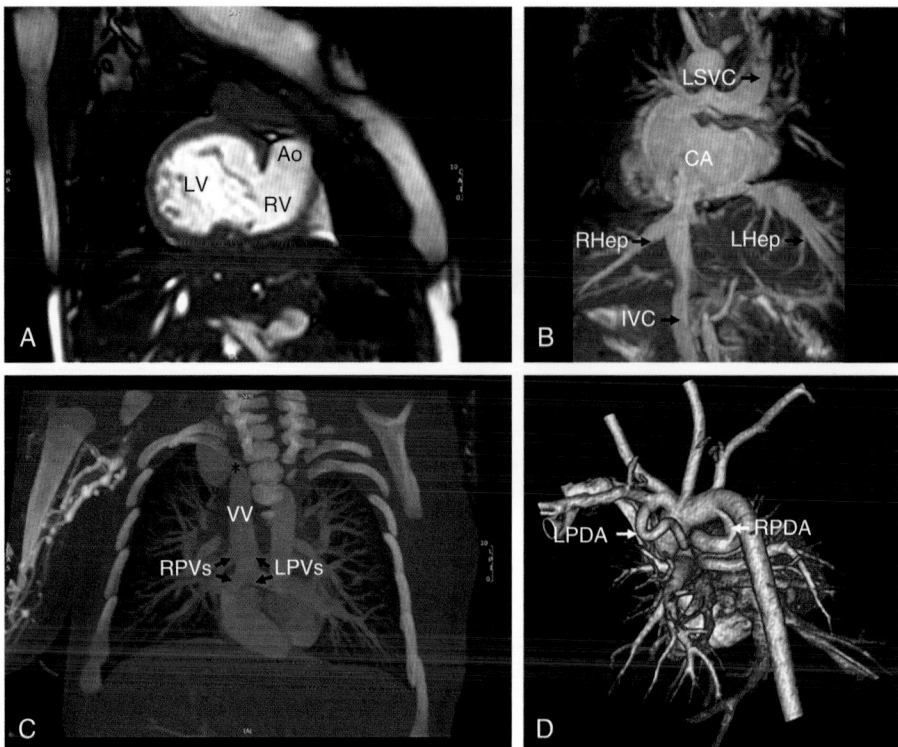

• **Fig. 32.2** Some of the cardiac findings commonly encountered in asplenia syndrome. **(A)** Modified coronal view of dextrocardia with L-loop ventricles, a left-dominant complete atrioventricular canal defect, and double-outlet right ventricle with pulmonary atresia. **(B)** Coronal view of venous anatomy in asplenia syndrome; a right-sided inferior vena cava, separate left hepatic veins, and a left superior vena cava status-post left bidirectional Glenn are seen. **(C)** coronal view of obstructed supracardiac totally anomalous pulmonary venous connection to the innominate vein-right superior vena cava junction. **(D)** Pulmonary atresia with confluent branch pulmonary arteries supplied by bilateral patent ductus arteriosi. *Ao,* Aorta; *CA,* common atrium; *IVC,* inferior vena cava; *LHep,* left hepatic veins; *LPDA,* left patent ductus arteriosus, *LPVs,* left pulmonary veins; *LSVC,* left superior vena cava; *LV,* left ventricle; *RHep,* right hepatic veins; *RPDA,* right patent ductus arteriosus; *RPV,* right pulmonary veins; *RV,* right ventricle; *VV,* vertical vein; *,* site of obstruction.

polysplenia HS, but both subtypes can have significant disease and substantial overlap exists (Table 32.3). From an electrophysiologic perspective, those with polysplenia HS frequently lack normal sinoatrial and atrioventricular nodes and may develop high-grade or complete atrioventricular block; this phenomenon may be lethal *in utero*.[12] Those with asplenia HS frequently have dual sinus and atrioventricular nodes, which can be appreciable on surface ECG as two p-wave and/or QRS axes. These patients have a greater likelihood of reentrant supraventricular tachycardia, with antegrade conduction through one AV node and retrograde conduction through the other.[13]

Given the limitations of the polysplenia and asplenia categories, a detailed anatomic evaluation is critical. Unusual portosystemic venous connections (Fig. 32.3), which functionally permit systemic venous-to-systemic venous collateralization, may occur in HS and must be diligently scrutinized, particularly among those undergoing single-ventricle palliation.[14] The myocardial architecture may be abnormal in HS, with the relatively frequent finding of ventricular non-compaction in polysplenia, a feature which may predispose to early or late cardiomyopathy.[15] Finally, a thorough understanding of the conduction system in any given patient is important.[13]

The appropriate diagnostic imaging modality in HS varies based upon patient age and the desired information. Given the severity of anatomic disease and readily appreciable situs abnormalities, HS is often identified in the prenatal period on screening obstetric ultrasound. A detailed fetal echocardiogram usually follows, allowing many aspects of cardiac anatomy, function, and physiology to be correctly delineated. This information can be used (1) to provide detailed prenatal counseling and support to families and (2) to permit the perinatal care team to appropriately prepare for the neonate's needs.[16] This might include initiation of a prostaglandin infusion after birth for those with ductus arteriosus-dependent blood flow, chronotropic or pacemaker therapy for those with heart block, and potentially emergency catheterization-based or surgical interventions for those with obstructed totally anomalous pulmonary venous connection or other life-threatening anomalies.[17] Timely fetal diagnosis is also important for those considering termination of the pregnancy or palliative induction.

Beyond the fetal period, the diagnostic assessment in HS varies considerably depending on the patient's age and the clinical scenario. A detailed discussion of imaging technique and technology is beyond the scope of this chapter. Some

TABLE 32.3	Incidence of Specific Cardiac Anomalies Among Heterotaxy Subtypes	
	Polysplenia (%)	Asplenia (%)
Dextrocardia	27–45	27–41
Interrupted IVC	65–92	0–3
Continuous IVC entering the RA	0–34	48–77
Continuous IVC entering the LA	0–16	20–52
Hepatic veins entering the atria directly	84–96	16–38
Unroofed coronary sinus	26–46	32–100
Bilateral superior venae cavae	33–50	38–71
TAPVC to a systemic vein	0–13	31–87
Pulmonary veins to RA (partial or total)	37–74	2–19
Common atrium	30–53	40–84
Atrial situs solitus	78	50
Atrial situs inversus	22	31
Atrial situs ambiguous	0	19
CAVC	16–66	69–92
Pulmonary stenosis/atresia	28–43	78–96
Systemic outflow obstruction	17–25	2–12
Single ventricle	26–43	29–73
TGA - D, -L/DORV	16–48	47–91
Abnormal coronary artery pattern	8–24	10–64
Left aortic arch	33	56
Right aortic arch	67	32–49

CAVC, Complete atrioventricular canal; *DORV,* double-outlet right ventricle; *IVC,* inferior vena cava; *LA,* left atrium; *RA,* right atrium; *TAPVC,* totally anomalous pulmonary venous connection; *TGA,* transposition of the great arteries. Reproduced with Permission from Lai WW, Mertens LL, Cohen MS, Geva T. *Echocardiography in Pediatric and Congenital Heart Disease: From Fetus to Adult,* 2nd edn. Wiley Blackwell; 2016.

general considerations follow, and consultation with a cardiac imaging specialist can be useful to help determine the best modality for a given patient.

Echocardiography is the mainstay of cardiac imaging in HS. In the neonatal period, echocardiography alone is often sufficient to provide the detailed anatomic and physiologic information needed to guide clinical decision-making. Transesophageal echocardiography is typically reserved for perioperative decision-making, although it may be useful in older patients if there are particularly nuanced questions pertaining to valvar anatomy and function not answerable by routine transthoracic assessment. As the patient ages, echocardiography remains the standard assessment tool for valvar function, ventricular function, and vascular assessment, and it is universally utilized in the outpatient setting.

Cardiovascular magnetic resonance (CMR) also has an important role in HS. The need for CMR is less common in infancy, but its clinical utility increases as the patient ages. General strengths of CMR include: (1) quantification of ventricular volumes and function, valvar regurgitation, and flow distributions; (2) detailed characterization of vascular anatomy and myocardial viability (e.g., presence of scar); and (3) the ability to readily reconstruct cardiac anatomy in three dimensions. CMR is particularly useful in HS when evaluating complex intracardiac anatomy prior to biventricular reconstruction (Fig. 32.4), to understand potential flow distribution in planning staged single-ventricle (Fontan) palliation,[18] and/or in older individuals in whom echocardiographic windows are poor. In contrast to echocardiography, the young patient (less than approximately 10 years) usually requires general anesthesia for a high-quality CMR, and there is a small risk of renal injury with gadolinium-containing contrast agents when utilized.[19] CMR typically cannot be performed in patients with a pacemaker, which is a common consideration given its relatively frequent occurrence in the HS population.

Cardiac computed tomography (CCT) is assuming an increasingly important role in HS.[20] Among infants and young children, a particular strength of CCT is excellent

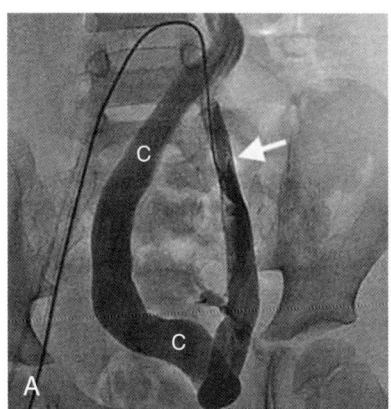
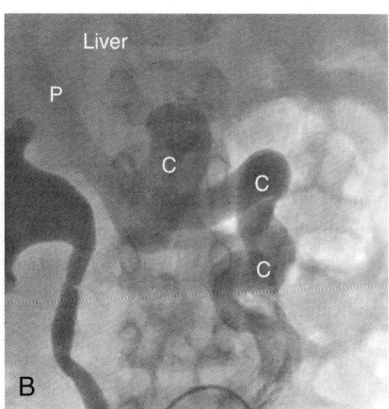
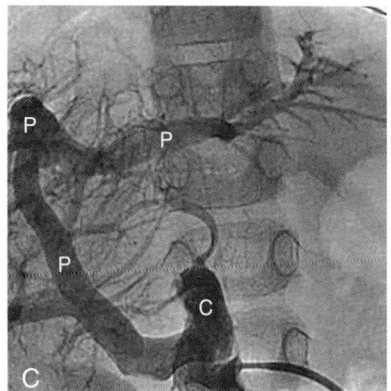

• **Fig. 32.3** (A–C) Pre-Fontan angiograms in a patient with heterotaxy and a portosystemic venous connection. A large collateral vein *(C)* from the left internal iliac vein *(arrow)* connects to the extrahepatic portal system *(P)*, which ultimately drains to the right atrium. This permits decompression of the superior cavopulmonary anastomosis and serves as a right-to-left shunt.

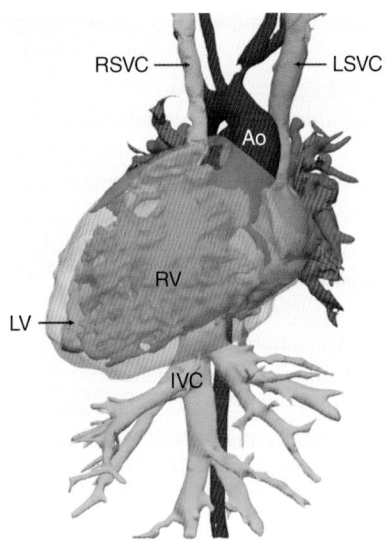

• **Fig. 32.4** Example of 3D modeling for pre-surgical planning in heterotaxy syndrome in a patient with heterotaxy, dextrocardia, rightward apex, {A,L,L} balanced complete atrioventricular canal defect, double outlet right ventricle, pulmonary atresia, bilateral superior venae cavae with no innominate ("bridging") vein, intact right-sided inferior vena cava, and a right aortic arch. *Ao,* Aorta; *IVC,* inferior vena cava; *LSVC,* left superior vena cava; *LV,* left ventricle; *RSVC,* right superior vena cava; *RV,* right ventricle. (Image courtesy of Emily Eickhoff.)

visualization of complex vascular anatomy frequently encountered in HS. These scans are typically performed without anesthesia and require very modest doses of radiation and contrast. Functional CCT is also possible if cine imaging is needed and there is a contraindication to CMR (e.g., pacemaker); however, these scans require a higher dose of radiation and should be utilized more judiciously. In addition, these studies require careful breath-holding and the ability to remain still. Therefore, in the pediatric population, general anesthesia may be required for functional CCT.

Finally, cardiac catheterization plays an integral role in assessment of HS. While non-invasive imaging modalities have supplanted the need for some invasive angiographic assessment, cardiac catheterization remains the mainstay for hemodynamic evaluation. This can be critically important for a complete physiologic understanding of a patient and is routinely utilized prior to many surgical interventions. Cardiac catheterization also has an important therapeutic role with the potential to address numerous hemodynamic lesions while avoiding the need for operative intervention.

From an electrophysiologic perspective, baseline assessment with electrocardiogram is a requisite, and strong consideration should be given to a period of prolonged electrophysiologic monitoring (e.g., 24-hour or longer Holter monitor) to identify any subtle abnormalities or predisposition to pathologic arrhythmia not detectable on a 10-second electrocardiogram. For patients with complex arrhythmias, catheterization-based electrophysiologic study and intervention can be required at any point in the care spectrum. Of note, intraoperative mapping of the conduction system at the time of complex intracardiac repair is increasingly utilized to avoid damage to the conduction system, which can be unusual in its course through the heart in HS (Fig. 32.5).[21]

As the phenotypic presentation of HS is highly variable, so too is the need for routine cardiac care. Patients with mild cardiovascular abnormalities (isolated interrupted IVC) may not suffer any obvious ill cardiac effects. Nevertheless, periodic follow-up is warranted, as late physiologic and electrical abnormalities are certainly known to occur. At the extreme other end of the spectrum, a patient could require numerous interventions in the neonatal period, require single-ventricle palliation, undergo complex biventricular reconstruction, or have significant arrhythmia burden requiring substantially more intensive outpatient follow-up. Outpatient care must be tailored to the individual patient, with a strong emphasis on a multidisciplinary approach among cardiac subspecialists, non-cardiac providers, the primary physician, and the patient's family.

Extra-Cardiac Manifestations

Background

In the most basic sense, HS is the sequela of abnormal signaling in early embryonic development. It is therefore not surprising that the incidence of extra-cardiac anomalies is high and CHD patients with HS can have substantial comorbidities requiring management in the acute care and outpatient settings. As previously noted, sophisticated prenatal imaging guides prenatal counseling and perinatal management and should consider extracardiac manifestations. Many of the associated anomalies exacerbate or are exacerbated by CHD medical and surgical management. Overall, these factors may contribute to the increased morbidity and mortality in HS patients independent of the complexity of the cardiac defects. It is therefore important to be aware of the more common extracardiac anomalies and proactively incorporate multidisciplinary expertise. This section focuses on three of the more clinically challenging organ systems that may be affected in these patients: respiratory, gastrointestinal, and immunologic (Table 32.4).

Respiratory

In addition to the aforementioned abnormalities of bronchial morphology (Fig. 32.6), the respiratory phenotype of atelectasis, recurrent respiratory infections, pneumothoraces, failed extubations, and chronic respiratory failure is familiar to clinicians caring for heterotaxy patients. Often it is difficult to determine whether the primary etiology is cardiac or pulmonary, as it can be both. The physiologic stressors of cardiopulmonary bypass, mechanical ventilation, and vulnerable cardiopulmonary interactions further compound this scenario. Perioperative and chronic respiratory complications in a subset of heterotaxy patients may reflect intrinsic pulmonary abnormalities genetically linked to the underlying CHD. There is considerable overlap between PCD, CHD with situs ambiguus, and CHD with situs solitus with regards to abnormal ciliary function and lower mean nasal nitric oxide (NO) levels.[22] A 2012 study found 18/43 (42%) patients with HS CHD had ciliary

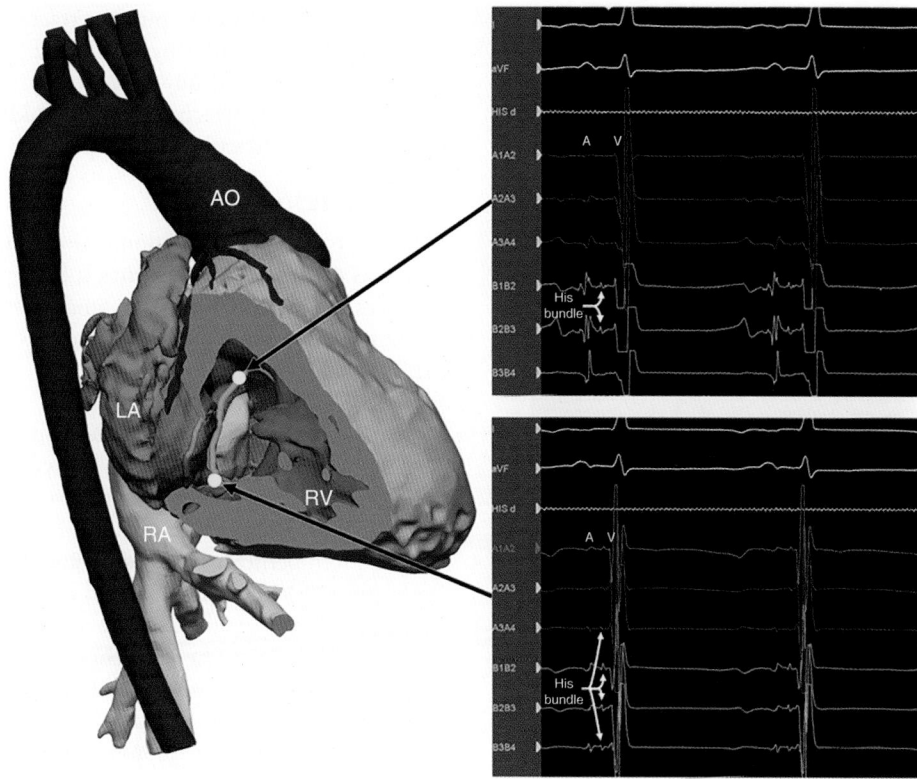

• **Fig. 32.5** Example of intraoperative conduction mapping a patient with heterotaxy, asplenia, {I,D,D} segmental anatomy, dextrocardia, left-dominant complete atrioventricular canal, and pulmonary atresia. Intraoperative conduction mapping was performed to localize His bundle electrograms (HBE) as a marker of the conduction axis location. Two discrete regions with HBE were identified consistent with twin atrioventricular nodes. In the top panel, an HBE was identified at the superior aspect of the ventricular septal defect (VSD). An additional HBE suggestive of a second node was noted at the inferior rim of the canaltype VSD. *AO,* Aorta; *LA,* left atrium; *RA,* right atrium; *RV,* right ventricle. (Image courtesy of Dr. Elizabeth DeWitt and Jocelyn Davee)

TABLE 32.4	Non-Cardiac Manifestations of Heterotaxy Syndrome	
	Polysplenia	**Asplenia**
Pulmonary	Bilateral bi-lobed lungs	Bilateral tri-lobed lungs
	Bilateral hyparterial bronchi	Bilateral eparterial bronchi
	Ciliary dyskinesia	Ciliary dyskinesia
Gastrointestinal	Malrotation	Malrotation
	Pancreatic anomalies	Hiatal or diaphragmatic hernia
	Biliary atresia and absence of gallbladder	
	Congenital absence of the portal vein	
	Abernethy malformation	
	Intestinal atresia	
Splenic function	May have functional asplenia	Likely absent

dyskinesia (CD). The risk of CD was higher in patients with both cardiac and pulmonary/abdominal laterality defects.[23] This group of patients has been shown to have a higher incidence of respiratory complications and need for tracheostomy than patients with HS without CD.[24]

Until more sophisticated therapies are developed, treatment of affected patients is limited. Many patients with HS have severe forms of CHD requiring staged palliation. Targeting surgical interventions that optimize cardiopulmonary physiology is important. Approaching respiratory insufficiency in these patients from a nuanced perspective that includes the support of pulmonologists is critical. A complete history and physical exam as well as consideration of pulmonary function testing, nasal NO measurement, and genetic testing, may inform acute and long-term management including the need for tracheostomy. Nasal epithelial biopsy for diagnostic ciliary electron microscopy (Fig. 32.7), which is minimally invasive, may be particularly useful for identifying structural abnormalities associated with CD.

Minimizing mechanical ventilation in the perioperative period is ideal, as spontaneous coughing is one of the best ways for patients to clear secretions. Intensive scheduled chest physiotherapy should be considered, even in the context of a reassuring chest radiograph. There is evidence that beta agonist treatment increases ciliary beat frequency and therefore empiric use of therapy may be helpful in some patients. Extended antibiotic therapy may be necessary to prevent overgrowth of respiratory tract organisms that normally would be cleared by unaffected epithelia or normal immune function. Ideally this therapy is informed by airway culture data. Tracheostomy should be considered in patients unable to wean from respiratory support.

Gastrointestinal

Although many of the abdominal organ anomalies follow patterns according to a patient's splenic phenotype, abnormalities in intestinal rotation and fixation appear to be common in both groups with a cited incidence of 33–90%. This is substantially higher than the normal population with a reported incidence of 0.5–4%.

Early in embryonic and fetal development, the small bowel develops outside the abdomen and goes through a predictable process of herniation, rotation, reduction, and fixation back inside the fetus. If this occurs normally, the duodenum lies in a retroperitoneal position behind the superior mesenteric artery (SMA) and anterior to the aorta, the duodenojejunal junction is anchored to the retroperitoneum in the left upper quadrant with the ligament of Treitz, and the cecum is anchored in the retroperitoneum in the right lower quadrant. From these two widely spaced retroperitoneal fixation points, a broad fan of mesentery supports the SMA and its branches. If, however, the duodenojejunal junction is malpositioned and/or the cecum is mobile or located in the upper abdomen, the mesentery between the two fixation points may be narrow. This creates risk for volvulus with interruption of SMA perfusion to the small bowel leading to small bowel ischemia and/or infarction. In addition, abnormal fixation points are frequently associated with Ladd's bands, abnormal fibrous bands that have the potential to cause bowel obstruction or to exacerbate the high-risk anatomic relationship for volvulus. Symptoms of volvulus can be subtle including feeding intolerance and failure to thrive or present as a surgical emergency with significant morbidity and mortality.

Imaging modalities for diagnosis of malrotation are discussed at length in the pediatric radiology literature. The spatial relationship of the SMA and superior mesenteric vein has been used as a marker of malrotation; however, abnormal positioning is not pathognomonic for malrotation,

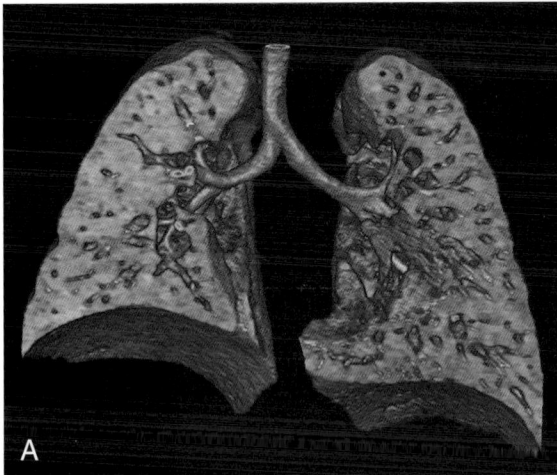
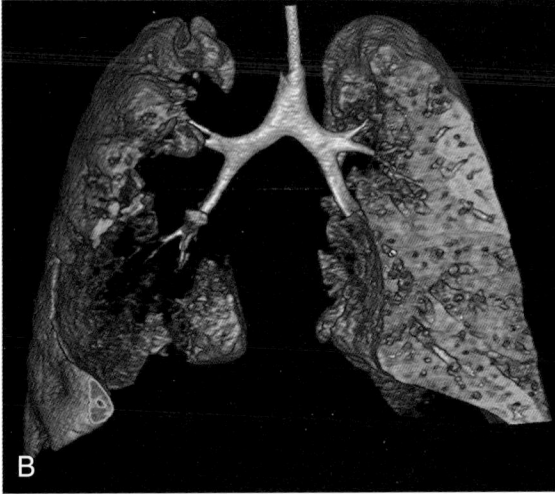

• **Fig. 32.6** Three-dimensional renderings of bronchial morphology in heterotaxy syndrome. **(A)** Bilateral left bronchial morphology in a patient with polysplenia. **(B)** Bilateral right bronchial morphology in a patient with asplenia.

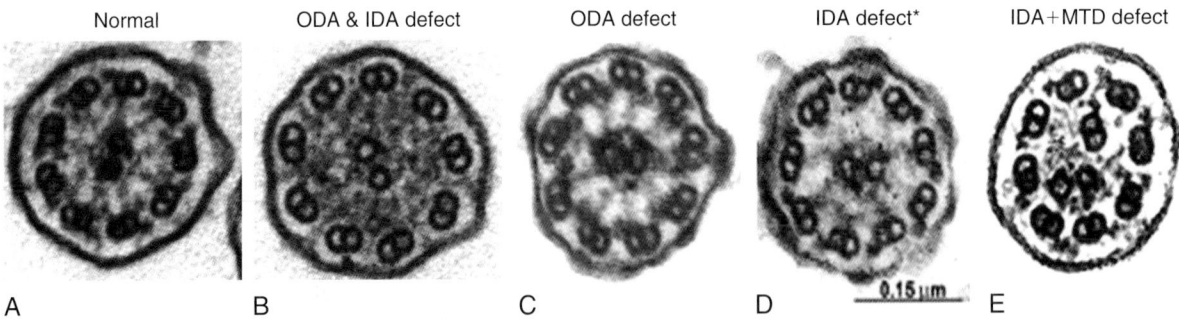

• **Fig. 32.7** Diagnostic ciliary electron microscopy findings in primary ciliary dyskinesia. (A) Normal ciliary ultrastructure. (B) Outer *(ODA)* and inner dynein arm *(IDA)* defect. (C) ODA defect. (D) IDA defect alone. (E) IDA defect with microtubule *(MTB)* disorganization. (From Shapiro AJ, Zariwala MA, Ferkol T, et al. Diagnosis, Monitoring, and Treatment of Primary Ciliary Dyskinesia: PCD Foundation consensus recommendations based on state of the art review. *Pediatr Pulmonol.* 2016;51:115–132.)

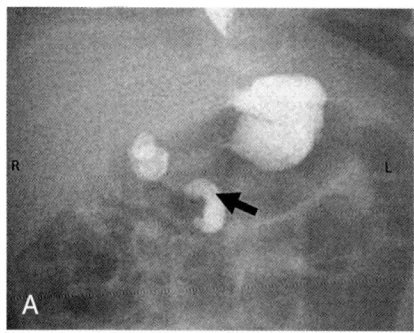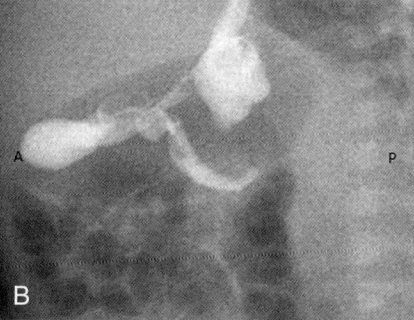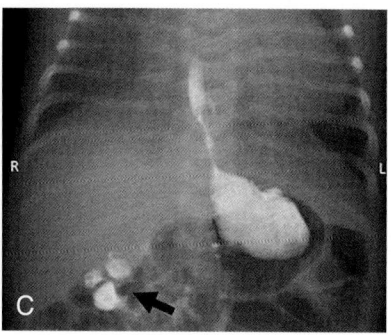

• **Fig. 32.8** Upper gastrointestinal series in a patient with malrotation. **(A)** Anteroposterior (AP) view: the duodenojejunal junction *(arrow)*, which is normally to the left of the vertebral pedicle, is to the right of the spine and low in position, below the level of the duodenal bulb; the duodenum does not cross the midline and ascend toward the ligament of Treitz, as would be expected in normal intestinal rotation. **(B)** Lateral view, the second portion of the duodenum, which normally courses posteriorly, is anteriorly positioned. **(C)** AP view: the proximal jejunum *(arrow)*, which is normally in the left upper quadrant, is in the right upper quadrant in this patient. (Images courtesy of Dr. Neha Kwatra.)

nor does a normal spatial relationship rule out disease. A truly normal small bowel study should document a retroperitoneal duodenum crossing the spine and ascending to the level of the gastric antrum, and a cecum in the opposite corner in the lower quadrant. Ultrasound can be diagnostic of malrotation and helpful with regard to screening for additional abdominal anomalies; however, its sensitivity and specificity are highly operator-dependent and patient-specific. An upper gastrointestinal series (UGI; Fig. 32.8) with small bowel follow through to the cecum and proximal colon remains the gold standard for diagnosis with high sensitivity in the 90s%. False negatives are possible if there is a mobile cecum.[25] Thoughtful evaluation is indicated in patients presenting with abdominal symptoms suggestive of intermittent or complete obstruction.

In the past, significant variability existed among subspecialists with regard to screening for malrotation and subsequent Ladd procedure in asymptomatic HS patients. Malrotation predisposes to volvulus, which is a life-threatening emergency. In broad epidemiologic studies, approximately 80% of cases of small bowel volvulus occur in the first month of life, and the vast majority occur within the first year.[26] Furthermore, many patients with HS and CHD have abnormal bowel perfusion at baseline. On the other hand, heterotaxy patients with unrepaired or palliated CHD are often high-risk surgical candidates, especially in the neonatal period. In addition, the Ladd procedure itself carries a non-trivial risk of postoperative complications including small bowel obstruction. Contemporary approaches balance risk and benefit, combining family and patient education, careful monitoring, and consideration for elective surgical intervention if other abdominal surgeries are required. Current data do not, however, support routine upper gastrointestinal screening or routine prophylactic Ladd procedure for the asymptomatic patient.[27,28]

Several additional gastrointestinal anomalies including esophageal hiatal hernia, diaphragmatic hernia, gastric volvulus, microgastria, pre-duodenal portal vein (can be associated with duodenal web or atresia, mechanical obstruction of the bile duct), congenital absence of the portal vein, biliary atresia, and pancreatic anomalies such as truncated or annular pancreas, have been described consistently in patients with HS. Pre-duodenal vein, congenital absence of the portal vein, biliary atresia, and pancreatic anomalies are more typically associated with polysplenia HS. Patients with more complex CHD requiring palliation to a circulation with abnormal hemodynamics (e.g., elevated central venous pressure) may be poor candidates for abdominal surgery such as the Kasai procedure.

Immunologic

Patients with either polysplenia- or asplenia-type HS (Fig. 32.9) may have functional asplenia. The spleen is important for bacterial clearance and the humoral immune response, especially to encapsulated organisms. In a systematic review assessing the risk of infection in patients with HS, affected patients were found to be at high risk for severe community-acquired bacterial infection with an associated high mortality, especially within the first 2 years of life.[29] This was true in patients with HS regardless of whether a spleen was present or not. Interestingly, patients with HS have not been found to be at increased risk for severe nosocomial bacterial infections when compared with non-HS CHD patients.[30]

Patients with polysplenia typically have two to six small spleens clustered alongside the greater curvature of the stomach which is on the right side of the patient in approximately 50% of cases.[31] The presence of one or multiple spleens, however, does not correspond to adequate splenic function in patients with HS. Objective measures of splenic function such as the presence of Howell-Jolly bodies on a peripheral blood smear or the pitted erythrocyte count using microscopy are indicated. Both studies are alternatives to scintigraphy which has been considered the gold standard but involves radiation exposure, is labor intensive, and expensive. Of note, there is a false-negative rate with Howell-Jolly body testing especially in patients prior to 2 years of age.

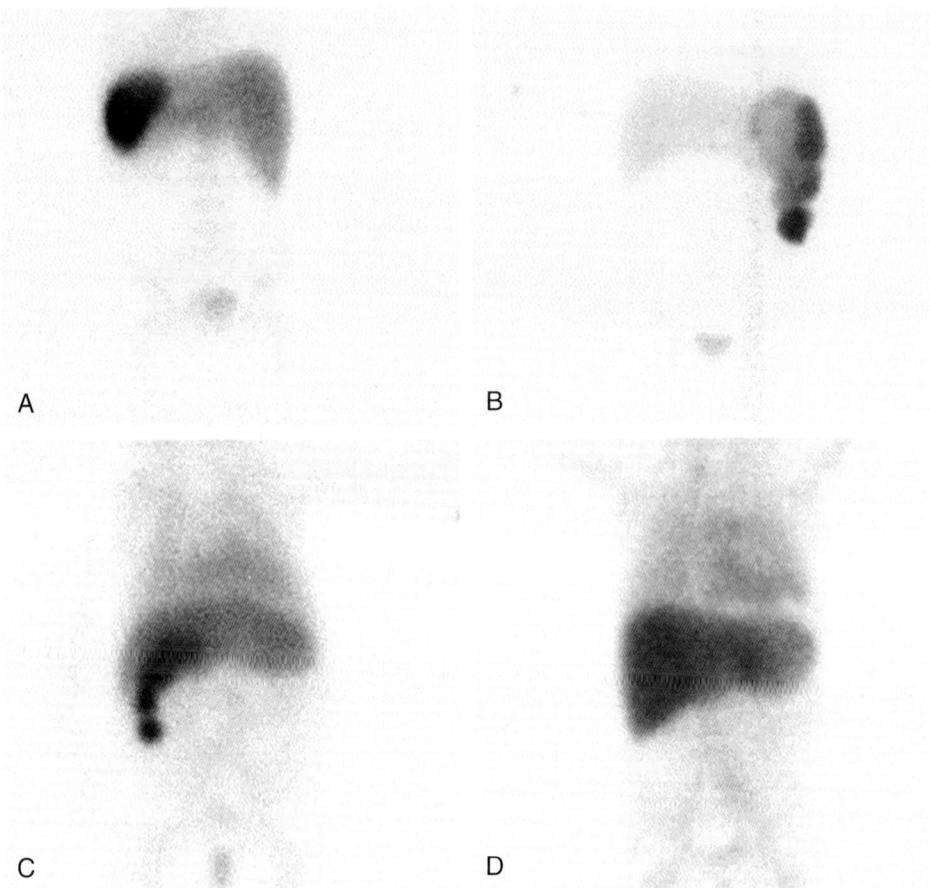

• **Fig. 32.9** Planar anterior images from heat-damaged ^{99m}Tc-RBC scintigraphy in patients with heterotaxy. **(A)** Single right-sided spleen. **(B)** Multiple left-sided spleens in a patient with polysplenia. **(C)** Multiple right-sided spleens in a patient with polysplenia. **(D)** Asplenia. (Images courtesy of Dr. Neha Kwatra.)

Rapid identification of at-risk patients and long-term effective prophylaxis is an area of research potential as most guidelines for management of the asplenic/hyposplenic HS patient are adopted from data in patients with sickle cell disease. The role of antibiotics remains regionally variable, but the literature typically advocates using prophylactic antibiotics with amoxicillin or penicillin starting in infancy and continuing through age 5 years or possibly longer. Management approaches to the asplenic/hyposplenic HS patient with a febrile illness also look to the sickle cell disease literature for support. Ill-appearing patients or those with a fever > 38.5°C should undergo evaluation including blood cultures, complete blood count with differential, and inflammatory markers.[29] Immunizations for encapsulated bacteria are an important part of preventative care. It is recommended that providers follow the guidelines set forth by the American Academy of Pediatrics with additional considerations as noted in the Red Book of adjustments for patients with asplenia.[32]

Surgical Approaches

Patients with HS have special surgical considerations. These can be divided into anatomic considerations, intraoperative management, and early postoperative care. A structured approach to perioperative evaluation is essential. Abnormalities of heart position such as dextrocardia or mesocardia may complicate intracardiac repair and alter the point of access to the intracardiac structures. Axial imaging with MRI or CT scan in such patients is advisable to assist with surgical planning.

Atrioventricular Canal Defect

In patients with atrioventricular canal defect, the most common morphology includes single superior bridging leaflet, inferior bridging leaflet, and right and left mural leaflets with two spaced papillary muscles on the left side subtending the superior and inferior bridging leaflets. In patients with HS, abnormal morphology of the atrioventricular valves can be noted. Particularly, there may be multiple scallops with deep recesses or fronds present on both the superior and inferior bridging leaflets, and regurgitation emanating between the scallops. Traditional operative techniques with closure of the cleft and annuloplasty may be insufficient to eliminate the atrioventricular valvular regurgitation, and closure of spacing between the fronds or scallops may be necessary. The presence of closely spaced papillary muscles or single fan-shaped papillary muscle may result in left-sided atrioventricular valvular stenosis following repair. Detailed preoperative evaluation and careful intraoperative inspection are necessary to achieve an acceptable physiologic result.

Systemic Venous Drainage

Careful assessment of systemic venous drainage is essential in the management of congenital heart defects in patients with HS. Bilateral superior vena cavae without a bridging innominate vein are a common feature of patients with asplenic HS. Patients with polysplenic HS often have an interrupted IVC with azygous continuation to the superior vena cava (SVC); the isolated hepatic veins flow directly into an atrium. Preoperative evaluation of the systemic venous circulation prior to surgical repair is essential to ensure that adequate systemic venous drainage is performed at the time of cardiopulmonary bypass. Separate cannulation of bilateral SVC as well as separate cannulation of ipsilateral hepatic veins may be necessary in certain circumstances.

Furthermore, the venous anatomy should be carefully delineated prior to single ventricle palliation, as it determines the timing and approach to superior cavopulmonary connections. In patients with interrupted IVC with azygous continuation, a cavopulmonary connection will result in Qp/Qs ratio of up to 0.8 which may lead to elevated SVC pressures in small infants. Delay of the superior cavopulmonary palliation (known as Kawashima procedure in patients with interrupted IVC and azygos continuation) may be advisable to avoid elevated SVC pressures. The azygos vein to SVC connection must be maintained to avoid obstruction of IVC flow. On the other hand, for patients with azygos drainage into a SVC and sizable intra-abdominal connections of the IVC to hepatic veins, ligation of the azygos vein is advisable. Maintenance of an azygos vein at the time of the bidirectional Glenn in these patients can lead to reversal of flow from the SVC into the IVC and result in severe cyanosis.

For patients with bilateral SVC, bilateral superior cavopulmonary anastomosis should be performed. In patients with an adequate bridging vein from the right to left SVC, however, ligation or banding of the non-dominant SVC may be appropriate. Another option in patients with bilateral SVC undergoing superior cavopulmonary anastomosis is creation of a neo-innominate vein; the nondominant SVC is anastomosed to the dominant SVC and thus creates a single source for cavopulmonary anastomosis. The advantage of this approach will be described below.

At time of the third stage of palliation (Fontan procedure), the IVC and hepatic veins are redirected into the pulmonary arteries. In patients with HS, abnormalities of hepatic venous drainage and IVC drainage should be considered. Separate drainage of hepatic veins into ipsilateral atria may be present, and these must be baffled together to avoid isolation of hepatic veins. A core principle that must be considered in patients with heterotaxy undergoing stage III palliation is even distribution of hepatic venous blood flow to both pulmonary arteries. Asymmetric flow into the branch pulmonary arteries may lead to arteriovenous malformations (AVMs) in the lung receiving less hepatic blood flow. These AVMs can lead to pulmonary venous desaturation and severe cyanosis. Several important cases should be considered.

1. Normal IVC and hepatic venous drainage into the right-sided atrium in a patient with normal heart position, and single right superior cavopulmonary anastomosis. A traditional Fontan procedure can be performed in which the IVC and hepatic veins are baffled into the pulmonary arteries at the site of entry of the right-sided SVC into the pulmonary arteries. This configuration usually results in adequate mixing of hepatic venous flow and normal distribution of hepatic venous drainage into both right and left pulmonary arteries.

2. Bilateral SVC with normal IVC drainage into the right atrium. In this scenario, insertion of inferior cavopulmonary connection into the right pulmonary artery may lead to maldistribution of hepatic venous flow to the right lung preferentially and predispose the patient to left AVMs. Several options exist for this patient including positioning of the inferior cavopulmonary anastomosis into the central pulmonary artery, thus deviating the anastomosis further leftward than usual, or takedown of the left SVC to create a neo-innominate vein followed by traditional insertion site of the inferior cavopulmonary anastomosis. Increasingly, use of computational flow dynamics (CFD) and 4D flow by MRI have been used to assist with surgical planning of the Fontan procedure in these patients to determine the ideal location of insertion point.[33]

3. Interrupted IVC with the azygos continuation. If a traditional Fontan is performed in which the hepatic veins are redirected into the right pulmonary artery, the superior cavopulmonary blood flow may lead to maldistribution of hepatic venous flow to one lung versus the other. This is markedly pronounced in patients with bilateral SVC with unilateral interrupted IVC with azygos continuation to the left SVC and leads to preferential hepatic drainage into the right lung and development of left AVM. Management of venous drainage in this subset of patients is extremely difficult. Options include redirection of the hepatic venous flow to the IVC/azygos vein posteriorly (by direct anastomosis or tube graft) to promote mixing of blood and even distribution to both lungs through the azygos vein. In patients with bilateral SVC, creation of a neo-innominate vein in conjunction with hepatic to azygos venous connection may be necessary. In this patient population, CFD analysis can be beneficial to assist with surgical planning (Fig. 32.10).

It is important to note that patients with HS undergoing total cavopulmonary anastomosis may be at higher risk for poor long-term outcomes. There have been conflicting reports regarding long-term outcomes in this patient population.[34,35]

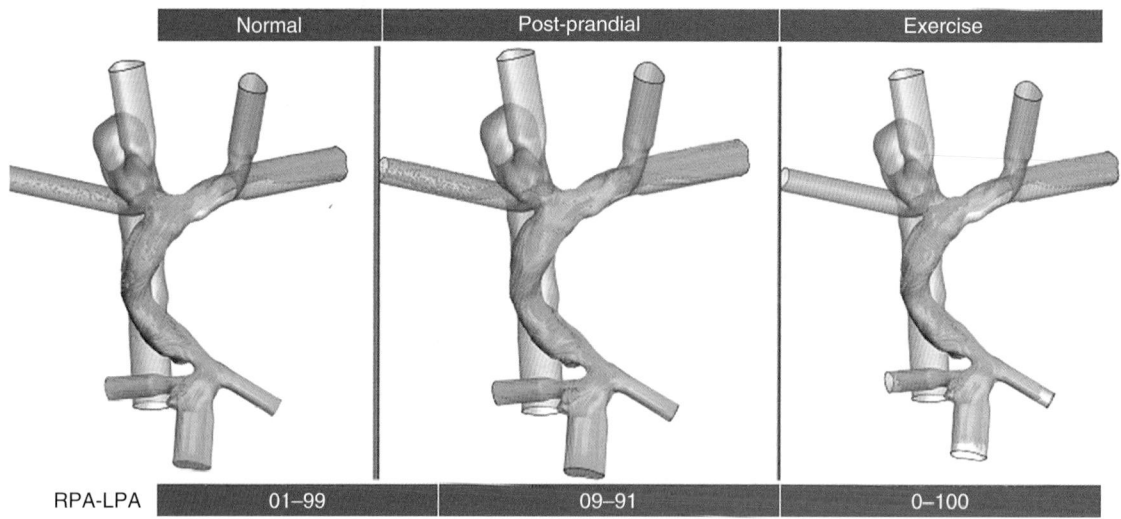

Normal	Post-prandial	Exercise

RPA-LPA	01–99	09–91	0–100

• **Fig. 32.10** Flow distribution modeling in a patient with heterotaxy who has undergone single-ventricle palliation with a Fontan operation. In normal, post-prandial, and exercise states, there is maldistribution of hepatic venous return to the left lung, consistent with this patient's known history of right-sided pulmonary arteriovenous malformations. *LPA,* Left pulmonary artery; *RPA,* right pulmonary artery.

Pulmonary Venous Drainage

Patients with HS may present with partial or total anomalous pulmonary venous connection. Compared with non-heterotaxy patients, they may have more unusual pulmonary venous drainage anatomy with vertical orientation of the pulmonary venous confluence, mixed drainage patterns (supracardiac versus intracardiac), and varying levels of obstruction. Patients with HS, total anomalous pulmonary venous connection, and single ventricle anatomy have amongst the highest mortality rates amongst neonates undergoing single ventricle palliation.

Management of Cardiopulmonary Bypass

Patients with HS have special considerations for intraoperative management. The presence of ciliary dysfunction affects various organ systems including the respiratory, intestinal, and hepatic systems. Intraoperative monitoring of lactate levels, near-infrared spectroscopy, and urine output reflect adequacy of perfusion and venous drainage of end organs during cardiopulmonary bypass. In patients with aortopulmonary collaterals, moderate hypothermia and higher flows may be advisable to adequately perfuse end organs. Evidence of inadequate venous drainage should be carefully assessed. Patients with ciliary dysmotility have a predisposition to pulmonary atelectasis following cardiopulmonary bypass, and maintenance of low-level positive pressure during the procedure may help prevent atelectasis. Suctioning of the airway to prior to separation from cardiopulmonary bypass is advisable to avoid mucus plugging.

A common challenge in the management of HS undergoing cardiac surgical repair is the potential for inadequate hepatic venous drainage due to anatomic abnormalities and difficulties associated with cannula position. If an IVC cannula is positioned within the branch hepatic vein and an IVC snare is applied during intracardiac repair, obstruction of hepatic venous and IVC flow may occur. Prolonged obstruction can lead to intraoperative hepatic and renal injury. Careful monitoring of markers of perfusion and abdominal girth are warranted in these patients. An alternative to traditional IVC cannulation may be open drainage with the use of cardiotomy suction into the hepatic veins and IVC during intracardiac repair.

Considerations Regarding Abdominal Situs

The presence of a right-sided stomach may be important in surgical decision-making. If a permanent pacemaker is necessary, placement of the generator contralateral to the side of the stomach may be advisable in case a patient requires subsequent G-tube placement.

Multidisciplinary Approach to Heterotaxy Care

As illustrated by the foregoing text, HS affect may significantly affect the function of multiple organ systems, yet non-cardiac care has historically been inconsistent. Despite the known association between PCD and postoperative respiratory complications, not all patients were screened and treated. Despite the risk for overwhelming sepsis, not all patients were assessed for splenic malfunction, prescribed prophylactic antibiotics, or received appropriate supplemental vaccinations. Despite many well-characterized genes that may cause HS, not all patients received genetic testing and counseling. Finally, approaches to malrotation were inconsistent. Consequently, at the authors' institution, a dedicated multidisciplinary team was formed to provide comprehensive HS evaluation and management with the hope of improving outcomes in this challenging group of patients. As of the writing of this textbook, our current institutional

TABLE 32.5	Multidisciplinary Approach to Heterotaxy Syndrome*

Cardiac
Holter monitor

Immunology
Complete blood count with differential
Peripheral smear for Howell-Jolly bodies
Pitted erythrocyte count
Immunoglobulin quantification
Flow cytometry for B-cell and T-cell subsets
Prophylactic amoxicillin

Pulmonary
Nasal brush biopsy for diagnostic ciliary electron microscopy
Nasal nitric oxide testing for patients > 5 years

Genetics
Chromosomal microarray
Heterotaxy/situs inversus gene panel

Gastrointestinal
Current data do not support routine upper gastrointestinal
    screening or routine prophylactic Ladd procedure for
    the asymptomatic patient
Direct bilirubin

*Usual approach for patients with heterotaxy syndrome. Note that the care for individual patients may vary. All testing is performed in conjunction with subspecialty consultation and follow-up as appropriate.

approach to HS screening, in consultations with individual specialists, is presented in Table 32.5.

Although individual patients with HS are unique and complex, certain predictable patterns of disease exist. Clinicians fluent with the cardiac anomalies, knowledgeable about the surgical considerations, and attuned to the presence of extracardiac manifestations may significantly improve patients' short and long-term outcomes.

Acknowledgments

The authors wish to acknowledge previous iterations of this chapter by Stella Van Praagh (1927–2006), whose chapter remains an outstanding and invaluable resource for those seeking greater depth of understanding of the embryologic and anatomic underpinnings of this disease.

References

1. Banka P, Adar A, Schaetzle B, et al. Changes in prognosis of heterotaxy syndrome over time. *Pediatrics*. 2020;146:e20193345.
2. Shiraishi I, Ichikawa H. Human heterotaxy syndrome. *Circ J*. 2012;76:2066-2075.
3. Ivemark B. Implications of agenesis of the spleen on the pathogenesis of conotruncus anomalies in childhood. *Acta Paediatr*. 1955; 44:590-592.
4. Yim D, Nagata H, Lam CZ, et al. Disharmonious Patterns of Heterotaxy and Isomerism: How Often Are the Classic Patterns Breached? *Circ Cardiovasc Imaging*. 2018;11(2):e006917. doi:10.1161/CIRCIMAGING.117.006917.
5. Jacobs JP, Anderson RH, Weinberg PM, et al. The nomenclature, definition and classification of cardiac structures in the setting of heterotaxy. *Cardiol Young*. 2007;17:1-28.
6. van Praagh S. Supero-inferior ventricles: anatomic and angiocardiographic findings in ten postmortem cases. In: van Praagh R, Takao A, eds. *Etiology and Morphogenesis of Congenital Heart Disease*. Mt Kisco, New York: Futura Publishing Company;1980:317-378.
7. Saba TG, Geddes GC, Ware SM, et al. A multi-disciplinary, comprehensive approach to management of children with heterotaxy. *Orphanet J Rare Dis*. 2022;17(1):351. doi:10.1186/s13023-022-02515-2.
8. Lin AE, Krikov S, Riehle-Colarusso T, et al. Laterality defects in the national birth defects prevention study (1998–2007): birth prevalence and descriptive epidemiology. *Am J Med Genet A*. 2014;164:2581-2591.
9. Foerster SR, Gauvreau K, McElhinney DB, Geva T. Importance of totally anomalous pulmonary venous connection and postoperative pulmonary vein stenosis in outcomes of heterotaxy syndrome. *Pediatr Cardiol*. 2008;29(3):536-544.
10. Shapiro AJ, Davis SD, Ferkol T, et al. Laterality defects other than situs inversus totalis in primary ciliary dyskinesia: Insights into situs ambiguus and heterotaxy. *Chest*. 2014;146:1176-1186.
11. Hu H, Chen W, Sheng W, Huang G. High familial recurrence of congenital heart defects in laterality defects patients: an evaluation of 184 families. *Pediatr Cardiol*. 2021;42:1722-1729.
12. Escobar-Diaz MC, Tworetzky W, Friedman K, et al. Perinatal outcome in fetuses with heterotaxy syndrome and atrioventricular block or bradycardia. *Pediatr Cardiol*. 2014;35:906-913.
13. Niu MC, Dickerson HA, Moore JA, et al. Heterotaxy syndrome and associated arrhythmias in pediatric patients. *Heart Rhythm*. 2018;15:548-554.
14. McElhinney DB, Marx GR, Newburger JW. Congenital portosystemic venous connections and other abdominal venous abnormalities in patients with polysplenia and functionally univentricular heart disease: a case series and literature review. *Congenit Heart Dis*. 2011;6:28-40.
15. Ramachandran P, Woo JG, Ryan TD, et al. The impact of concomitant left ventricular non-compaction with congenital heart disease on perioperative outcomes. *Pediatr Cardiol*. 2016;37:1307-1312.
16. Escobar-Diaz MC, Friedman K, Salem Y, et al. Perinatal and infant outcomes of prenatal diagnosis of heterotaxy syndrome (asplenia and polysplenia). *Am J Cardiol*. 2014;114:612-617.
17. Romanowicz J, Sinha P, Donofrio MT, et al. Predicting cardiac anatomy, physiology, and surgical management based on fetal echocardiography in heterotaxy syndrome. *Am J Perinatol*. 2021. doi:10.1055/s-0041-1732457.
18. Santoro G, Capozzi G, Caianiello G, et al. Pulmonary artery growth after palliation of congenital heart disease with duct-dependent pulmonary circulation: arterial duct stenting versus surgical shunt. *J Am Coll Cardiol*. 2009;54:2180-2186.
19. Lunyera J, Mohottige D, Alexopoulos AS, et al. Risk for nephrogenic systemic fibrosis after exposure to newer gadolinium agents: a systematic review. *Ann Intern Med*. 2020;173:110-119.
20. Sriharan M, Lazoura O, Pavitt CW, et al. Evaluation of high-pitch ungated pediatric cardiovascular computed tomography for the assessment of cardiac structures in neonates. *J Thorac Imaging*. 2016;31:177-182.
21. Feins EN, O'Leary ET, Hoganson DM, et al. Intraoperative conduction mapping in complex congenital heart surgery. *JTCVS Tech*. 2022;12:159-163.
22. Sherman F, Wodrich M, Zampi JD, Lee J, McCaffery H, Saba TG. Phenotypic features of ciliary dyskinesia among patients

with congenital cardiovascular malformations. *Pediatr Pulmonol.* 2020;55:2674-2682.

23. Nakhleh N, Francis R, Giese RA, et al. High prevalence of respiratory ciliary dysfunction in congenital heart disease patients with heterotaxy. *Circulation.* 2012;125:2232-2242.

24. Harden B, Tian X, Giese R, et al. Increased postoperative respiratory complications in heterotaxy congenital heart disease patients with respiratory ciliary dysfunction. *J Thorac Cardiovasc Surg.* 2014;147:1291-1298.

25. Sizemore AW, Rabbani KZ, Ladd A, et al. Diagnostic performance of the upper gastrointestinal series in the evaluation of children with clinically suspected malrotation. *Pediatr Radiol.* 2008;38:518-528.

26. Strouse PJ. Disorders of intestinal rotation and fixation ("malrotation"). *Pediatr Radiol.* 2004;34:837-851.

27. Collins Grant L, Hargis-Villanueva Angela E, Jayaraman Meghna S, et al. A prospective management strategy for heterotaxy syndrome with intestinal rotation abnormalities: Imaging does not predict need for surgery. *J Pediatr Surg.* 2023. 1531-5037. doi:10.1016/j.jpedsurg.2023.01.002. 36740478.

28. Huerta Carlos Theodore, Saberi Rebecca A, Lynn Royi, et al. Outcomes After Ladd Procedures for Intestinal Malrotation in Newborns with Heterotaxy Syndrome. *J Pediatr Surg.* 2023,58(6) 1095–1100. 1531-5037. doi:10.1016/j.jpedsurg.2023.02.013. 36941169.

29. Loomba RS, Geddes GC, Basel D, et al. Bacteremia in patients with heterotaxy: a review and implications for management. *Congenit Heart Dis.* 2016;11:537-547.

30. Shao PL, Chen MY, Wu MH, et al. Nosocomial severe bacterial infection after cardiac surgery for complex congenital heart disease in heterotaxy syndrome. *Pediatr Infect Dis J.* 2020;39:e163-e168.

31. Ticho BS, Goldstein AM, van Praagh R. Extracardiac anomalies in the heterotaxy syndromes with focus on anomalies of midline-associated structures. *Am J Cardiol.* 2000;85:729-734.

32. Kimberlin DW, Barnett ED, Lynfield R, et al., eds. *Red Book: 2021-2024 Report of the Committee on Infectious Diseases/ Committee on Infectious Diseases.* 32nd ed. American Academy of Pediatrics; 2021.

33. Tang E, Restrepo M, Haggerty CM, et al. Geometric characterization of patient-specific total cavopulmonary connections and its relationship to hemodynamics. *JACC Cardiovasc Imaging.* 2014;7:215-224.

34. Alsoufi B, McCracken C, Schlosser B, et al. Outcomes of multistage palliation of infants with functional single ventricle and heterotaxy syndrome. *J Thorac Cardiovasc Surg.* 2016;151:1369-1377.e2.

35. Marathe SP, Cao JY, Celermajer D, et al. Outcomes of the Fontan operation for patients with heterotaxy: a meta-analysis of 848 patients. *Ann Thorac Surg.* 2020;110:307-315.

33

Mitral Valve and Left Atrial Abnormalities

DIANA L. GEISSER AND MICHAEL N. SINGH

KEY LEARNING POINTS

- Mitral valve regurgitation is classified as primary (organic) or secondary (functional). Severe mitral regurgitation leads to progressive heart failure and the potential for atrial and/or ventricular arrhythmias. Medical and surgical management is based on the degree, mechanism, and etiology of regurgitation with engagement of a multidisciplinary team to determine the optimal approach.
- Mitral valve prolapse is one of the most common causes of chronic primary mitral regurgitation. Although typically benign, severe acute or chronic mitral regurgitation may occur, leading to heart failure symptoms. Medical and surgical management is based on mitral valve regurgitation guidelines with a multidisciplinary team.
- Congenital mitral valve stenosis is often multilevel (supravalvar, valvar, and subvalvar) and frequently occurs with

  other left-sided obstructive lesions. For patients who are symptomatic despite medical therapy, percutaneous transcatheter interventions or surgical mitral valvuloplasty are attempted prior to surgical mitral valve replacement when possible.
- There are two types of supravalvar mitral membrane: *supramitral* membranes for which surgical resection usually provides definitive treatment, and *intramitral* membranes that have a higher risk of requiring reintervention.
- Cor triatriatum is usually associated with other congenital cardiovascular anomalies. Severity of symptoms and timing of diagnosis are closely related to the size of the membrane opening and associated heart disease, with severe obstruction presenting earlier in life and mild obstruction sometimes going undiagnosed into adulthood.

Mitral Valve Disease

The mitral valve (MV) is an extremely complex connective tissue structure due to its cellular makeup, various components, and continuous movement within the heart. MV disease is classified as either congenital or acquired and further divided into stenotic, regurgitant, or mixed valve disease. Congenital MV abnormalities are rare, affecting ~0.4% with patients with congenital heart disease or ~0.005% of the general population. Most congenital MV lesions are associated with other congenital heart defects (~60%). Rheumatic mitral disease is a common acquired etiology worldwide, although it is rare in developed nations. Other acquired conditions include cardiomyopathy, infective endocarditis, and ischemic heart disease.[1]

Mitral Regurgitation

Definition

Mitral regurgitation (MR) is retrograde blood flow from the left ventricle to the left atrium during left ventricular

contraction due to an anatomical or functional impairment of a single abnormality or combination of abnormalities involving the MV apparatus, which includes the annulus, leaflets, chordae tendineae, and papillary muscles. The regurgitant volume from the left atrium causes volume overload of the left ventricle during diastole, leading to left ventricular dilation and eventual left ventricular dysfunction if not treated.[1]

Prevalence

The prevalence of mild to moderate MR in children with structurally normal hearts is ~1%. In a population-based cohort of older individuals, the prevalence of mild or more MR was ~19%. Isolated congenital MR is uncommon with an estimated incidence between 0.21% and 0.42% of total MR.

Pathology

MR is broadly classified as either primary or secondary. Primary (organic) MR is caused by abnormalities of the MV apparatus: leaflets (anterior or septal and posterior or mural), annulus, papillary muscles, and chordae tendineae. Secondary (functional) MR involves left ventricular and/or left atrial size, shape, or function abnormalities that result in papillary muscle displacement, leaflet tethering, and annular dilation with structurally normal or near normal leaflets.[2]

Primary developmental abnormalities involving the MV leaflets include isolated cleft of the anterior MV leaflet with an intact septum with the cleft directed toward the left ventricular outflow tract (LVOT) rather than the interventricular septum as in atrioventricular canal defects. Other leaflet abnormalities include underdevelopment of leaflets or redundancy of leaflets, as in mitral valve prolapse (MVP). Destruction of leaflets results from endocarditis, rheumatic heart disease, and autoimmune disorders such as systemic lupus erythematosus. Genetic conditions associated with leaflet abnormalities include Marfan syndrome, Loeys-Dietz syndrome, and osteogenesis imperfecta. Left atrial tumors can interfere with leaflet coaptation. Congenitally abnormal shortened (parachute MV) or elongated (Marfan syndrome) chordae, ruptured chordae (infection, trauma), or chordae displacement (congenital MR) are other etiologies of MR. Papillary muscle disorders include papillary muscle rupture (anomalous origin of left coronary artery from the pulmonary artery, myocardial infection, trauma) and abnormal position of the papillary muscles in the setting of endocardial fibroelastosis (papillary muscles originate high on the left ventricular wall). Mitral annular calcification, annular dilatation from connective tissue disorders, and destruction of the mitral annulus from infection can also lead to MR.[3]

Causes of secondary MR include dilated and ischemic cardiomyopathy, with the severity related to heart rhythm and conduction disturbances, and left ventricular loading conditions.[4]

Physiology

Left ventricular volume load imposed by MR leads to a cascading series of hemodynamic and structural cardiac change.[1] The left ventricle increases contractility in order to maintain antegrade stroke volume and cardiac output. Left ventricular dilation, left atrial enlargement, and eccentric ventricular hypertrophy can progress to ventricular remodeling and a chronic disease process. If untreated, failure of these compensatory adaptations develops and ventricular dysfunction and heart failure ensues. A normal ejection fraction in the setting of severe MR represents myocardial dysfunction.

Mitral regurgitant volume and the time period over which regurgitation developed determine the clinical effects of the disorder. Mitral regurgitant volume is in part determined by mitral orifice area, pressure gradient across the orifice, and duration of flow.[5] Indirect determinants include systemic vascular resistance, left ventricular afterload, and myocardial contractility.

The physiologic categories of MR are divided into three types: acute MR, chronic primary MR, and chronic

secondary MR. Acute MR results in abrupt volume overload of an unprepared left ventricle and left atrium leading to low cardiac output and pulmonary congestion secondary to pulmonary venous hypertension. If left untreated, severe and sustained volume overload in chronic primary and secondary MR leads to myocardial dysfunction, heart failure, pulmonary hypertension, arrhythmias, and death.

Etiologies of acute MR include infective endocarditis resulting in leaflet perforation, MVP with chordal rupture, and papillary muscle rupture. Other causes include carditis in the setting of acute rheumatic fever.

Chronic primary and secondary MR are divided into four stages of the disease process determined by valve anatomy, valve hemodynamics, hemodynamic consequences, and symptoms, which helps inform management in the adult population. The four stages consist of: at risk of MR (stage A), progressive MR (stage B), asymptomatic severe MR (stage C), and symptomatic severe MR (stage D).[2]

Clinical Manifestations

Symptoms

The clinical presentation of MR is variable and dependent on MR severity, progression from onset, and other associated valve abnormalities. Individuals with normal filling pressures and cardiac output are usually asymptomatic, particularly with mild or moderate MR. Acute MR presents with exertional dyspnea early in the course of the disorder due to the heart's inability to maintain normal filling pressures in the acute setting. Individuals with chronic MR initially develop fatigue and palpitation, with exertional dyspnea, orthopnea, and paroxysmal nocturnal dyspnea occurring late in the disease process and usually indicating elevated filling pressures and ventricular dysfunction. As the disease progresses and pulmonary hypertension develops, symptoms of right heart failure become evident with lower extremity edema and hepatic congestion. Symptoms of arrhythmia, such as atrial fibrillation, may also develop.[1]

Physical Examination

Ventricular enlargement and increased ventricular contractility lead to examination findings of an apically displaced and hyperdynamic impulse. S1 may be dampened. S3 is common with severe MR. There is an associated high-pitched, holosystolic, blowing murmur located at the left ventricular apex with radiation to the axilla and back with a posterolaterally directed regurgitant jet and radiation to the cardiac base with an anteromedially directed jet. Maneuvers that increase afterload or left ventricular volume cause an increase in the murmur (isometric exercise, sustained hand grip), whereas maneuvers that decrease left ventricular volume, such as Valsalva and standing, decrease the murmur. In the setting of acute MR, the murmur occurs in early systole and ends by mid-systole due to the rapid increase in left atrial pressure.[1]

Diagnostics

Electrocardiogram
Left atrial and left ventricular enlargement can be seen on electrocardiogram with moderate to severe MR. Right ventricular hypertrophy can be seen as pulmonary hypertension develops. Atrial flutter or atrial fibrillation can occur with severe MR.

Chest Radiography
Left atrial enlargement, left ventricular enlargement, and signs of congestive heart failure, including Kerley B lines and pulmonary edema are findings seen on chest radiography.

Noninvasive Imaging
Transthoracic echocardiogram (TTE) is the imaging modality of choice for the initial evaluation of MR as it provides structural, qualitative Doppler, semiquantitative, and quantitative parameters. For primary MR, information elucidated includes: MV apparatus anatomy, MR severity, atrial/ventricular size/function, mechanism of regurgitation with two-dimensional (2D) and three-dimensional (3D) imaging, continuous wave Doppler, color flow jet area, proximal isovelocity surface area, vena contracta width, mitral inflow, pulmonary vein flow profile, and effective regurgitant orifice (ERO) area. For secondary MR, additional information obtained includes: extent of regional/global left ventricular remodeling and degree of pulmonary hypertension.

If data from TTE is inadequate or discrepant with the clinical assessment, transesophageal echocardiogram (TEE) is indicated to assess MR severity, mechanism, and ventricular size/function. TEE is also beneficial for evaluation of vegetations in endocarditis or intraoperatively if surgical repair of the valve is required. Three-dimensional imaging of the MV from both the left ventricle and left atrial view is helpful when determining optimal surgical approach for repair based on the mechanism of disease.

If there is discordant information between echocardiography and clinical information, cardiac magnetic resonance (CMR) is indicated to objectively assess ventricular size/function and MR severity, including regurgitation fraction. Characteristics of severe MR include: moderate/severe left atrial enlargement, left ventricular enlargement, central mitral regurgitant jet of > 40% left atrium, holosystolic eccentric jet, vena contracta $\geq$ 0.7 cm, regurgitant volume $\geq$ 60 mL, regurgitant fraction $\geq$ 50%, and ERO $\geq$ 0.4 cm^2 in the adult.

Stress echocardiography is useful to assess the etiology of MR and assess myocardial viability, especially in secondary MR. Intracardiac echocardiography is an important complement to TEE for percutaneous transcatheter edge-to-edge MV repair in patients with anesthesia and intubation risks, as well as suboptimal imaging with other modalities due to post-surgical anatomy.[2]

Exercise Testing
Exercise testing using treadmill or bicycle ergometry with or without a metabolic cart (cardiopulmonary exercise test) is an objective modality to confirm the absence of symptoms in the presence of severe MR and define an individual's functional capacity. For individuals with less than severe regurgitation, it also helps distinguish between cardiac and pulmonary etiologies as the mechanism of exertional dyspnea.

Cardiac Catheterization
The accuracy of noninvasive imaging decreases the need for cardiac catheterization to diagnose or grade MR. If noninvasive testing and clinical assessment are conflicting or not conclusive, cardiac catheterization with hemodynamic measurements and left ventriculography is useful to grade MR severity, assess left ventricular function, and determine potential need for surgery.

Findings of elevated filling pressures with prominent "V" waves can support a cardiac etiology for dyspnea or demonstrate significantly abnormal pathophysiology in an asymptomatic patient. Normal hemodynamics in a symptomatic patient can point away from a cardiac etiology and allow focus on determining noncardiac sources of symptoms. Careful hemodynamic assessment can also differentiate between pre-capillary pulmonary hypertension (pulmonary vascular remodeling) with the finding of a high transpulmonary gradient and post capillary pulmonary hypertension (elevated pulmonary venous pressure) with the finding of elevated left atrial or pulmonary artery wedge pressure.

Evaluation of the density of contrast in the left atrium with left ventriculography can aid in determining the degree of MR. When the left atrium is opacified as intensely as the left ventricle and aorta there is angiographic grade 3+ MR. If the left atrium is more densely opacified than the left ventricle or aorta, the MR is angiographically grade 4+.

Exercise during hemodynamic assessment may be useful if resting hemodynamics are ambiguous. Coronary angiography may be necessary to establish the etiology in secondary MR and/or for individuals with coronary artery disease risk factors undergoing MV surgery.[2]

Management
Management of MR necessitates a precise evaluation to determine if it is primary MR (Fig. 33.1) versus secondary MR (Fig. 33.2) as well as the degree, the mechanism, and the etiology of regurgitation.

Acute Mitral Regurgitation

Vasodilator therapy may result in improved compensatory hemodynamics by decreasing aortic flow impedance to maintain cardiac output in the setting of acute severe primary MR but does not change the natural history. Nicardipine or sodium nitroprusside infusion is typically used, but limited by hypotension secondary to decrease in peripheral vascular resistance. Intra-aortic balloon pump can also be effective by decreasing left ventricular afterload. Expedited MV repair is required for symptomatic patients and improves mortality.[2]

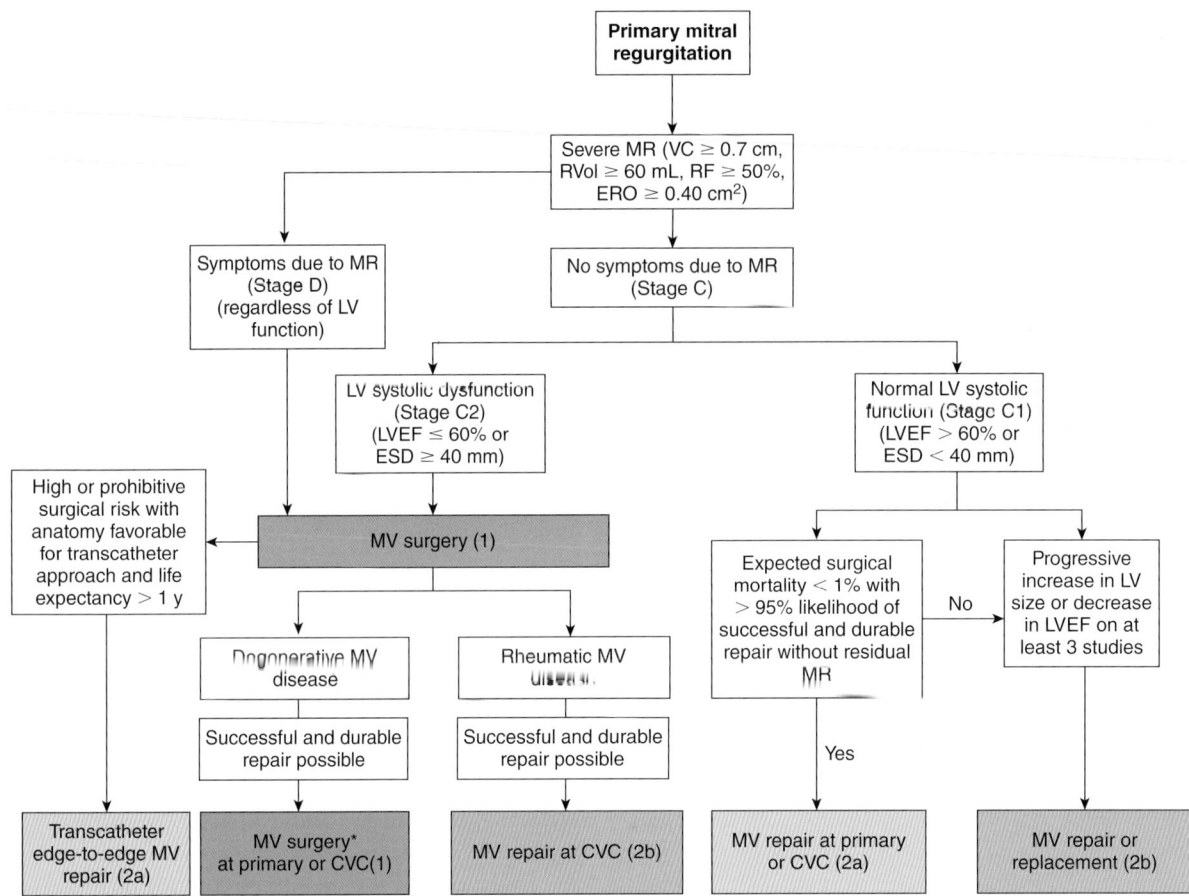

• **Fig. 33.1** Flowchart illustrating recommendations for the management of primary mitral regurgitation according to the 2020 ACC/AHA guideline for the management of patients with valvular heart disease. *CVC,* comprehensive valve center; *ERO,* effective regurgitant orifice; *ESD,* end-systolic dimension; *LV,* left ventricular; *LVEF,* left venticular ejection fraction; *MR,* mitral regurgitation; *MV,* mitral valve; *MVR,* mitral valve replacement; *RF,* regurgitant fraction; *RVol,* regurgitant volume; and *VC,* vena contracta. (2020 ACC/AHA Guideline for the Management of Patients With Valvular Heart Disease: A Report of the American College of Cardiology/American Heart Association Joint Committee on Clinical Practice Guidelines - Otto, Catherine M; Nishimura, Rick A; Bonow, Robert O; Carabello, Blase A; Erwin, 3rd, John P; Gentile, Federico; Jneid, Hani; Krieger, Eric V; Mack, Michael; McLeod, Christopher; O'Gara, Patrick T; Rigolin, Vera H; Sundt, 3rd, Thoralf M; Thompson, Annemarie; Toly, Christopher, Journal of the American College of Cardiology, 2021, Vol.77 (4), p.e25-e197 (Figure 8))

Chronic Primary Mitral Regurgitation

In the setting of asymptomatic chronic severe primary MR, periodic monitoring with TTE to evaluate ventricular size/function, ventricular longitudinal strain, and estimated pulmonary artery pressure, as well as biomarkers (brain natriuretic peptide levels) are important to determine appropriate timing for intervention. Surgical repair techniques include MV annuloplasty, cleft suture closure, leaflet patch augmentation, papillary muscle relocation, and artificial chordal implantation. Most of the data for surgical and medical management is based on adult studies and extrapolated to pediatric management as there are limited large-scale studies in the pediatric population.

Individuals with stage A or B chronic primary MR (at risk or progressive, respectively) can develop severe regurgitation slowly over time with no clinical manifestations or symptoms. Symptoms are an important prompt that an intervention is required and may be determined by a formal exercise stress test. Medical therapy with vasodilators is not indicated in asymptomatic, normotensive patients (stage B and C1) with primary MR and normal ventricular function. Once left ventricular dysfunction develops, intervention is indicated despite being asymptomatic.

If surgery is prohibitive or requires a delay due to other circumstances, medications with guideline-directed medical therapy, (GDMT) including angiotensin-converting enzyme inhibitors (ACE-I), angiotensin receptor blockers (ARBs), beta-adrenergic blocking agents, aldosterone antagonists, and/or diuretics, are used. Clinical trials with the use of vasodilator therapy have shown little or no clinical benefit in chronic asymptomatic MR with normal ventricular function.

MV intervention is indicated for severe primary MR with symptoms (stage D) or without symptoms and left ventricular ejection fraction ≤ 60% and/or left ventricular end systolic dimension ≥ 40 mm (stage C2). There are currently no left ventricular dimension criteria to consider surgical repair

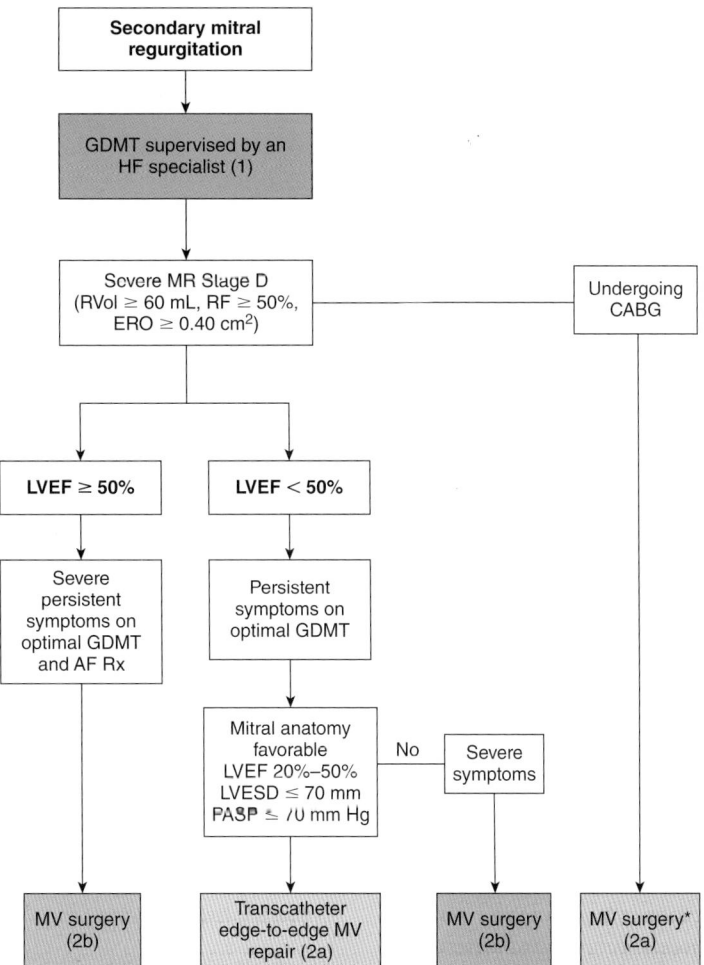

• **Fig. 33.2** Flowchart illustrating recommendations for the management of secondary mitral regurgitation according to the 2020 ACC/AHA guideline for the management of patients with valvular heart disease. *AF,* atrial fibrillation; *CABG,* coronary artery bypass graft; *ERO,* effective regurgitant orifice; *GDMT,* guideline-directed management and therapy; *HF,* heart failure; *LVEF,* left ventricular ejection fraction; *LVESD,* left ventricular end-systolic dimension; *MR,* mitral regurgitation; *MV,* mitral valve, *PASP,* pulmonary artery systolic pressure; *RF,* regurgitant fraction; *RVol,* regurgitant volume; *Rx,* medication. (2020 ACC/AHA Guideline for the Management of Patients With Valvular Heart Disease: A Report of the American College of Cardiology/American Heart Association Joint Committee on Clinical Practice Guidelines - Otto, Catherine M; Nishimura, Rick A; Bonow, Robert O; Carabello, Blase A; Erwin, 3rd, John P; Gentile, Federico; Jneid, Hani; Krieger, Eric V; Mack, Michael; McLeod, Christopher; O'Gara, Patrick T; Rigolin, Vera H; Sundt, 3rd, Thoralf M; Thompson, Annemarie; Toly, Christopher, Journal of the American College of Cardiology, 2021, Vol.77 (4), p.e25-e197 (Figure 8))

in the pediatric age group. The ideal time for MV surgery is when the left ventricle approaches but has not arrived at the parameters that indicate systolic dysfunction.

MV repair is the preferred method of surgery rather than MV replacement, especially if the etiology is degenerative in nature and there is a high chance of successful and long-lasting repair. Compared with MV replacement, MV repair permits a higher freedom from reoperation and recurrent moderate or severe MR. The durability of a simple posterior leaflet intervention and/or mitral annuloplasty is higher than an anterior and/or bileaflet repair, which tends to be more complex and extensive. It is preferred that MV repair be performed at a high-volume valve surgery center with a multidisciplinary team (non-invasive cardiologist with cardiac imaging expertise, cardiac surgeon, and interventional cardiologist) since successful

repair increases with surgeon-specific mitral surgery volume and expertise.

Overall, MV replacement is preferred to a substandard MV repair. Consideration of early MV repair prior to development of symptoms, left ventricular dysfunction, and/or pulmonary hypertension could be considered if there is a very high likelihood of a durable repair.

Transcatheter edge-to-edge MV repair is an option for symptomatic patients with primary MR and a high or prohibitive risk for surgery. A good result is gauged by a decrease in MR by two to three grades resulting in left ventricular reverse remodeling.

MV repair for rheumatic MR is not ideal given thickened/calcified leaflets, subvalvar disease, choral fusion/shortening, and progressive rheumatic disease compared with repair for complex degenerative disease. MV repair is considered standard of care for isolated severe primary MR with disease limited to less than half of the posterior leaflet with data showing improved long-term survival and reduction of symptoms. It is recommended that MV replacement not be performed unless there has been a failed attempt at repair at a comprehensive MV reference center.[1,2]

Chronic Secondary Mitral Regurgitation

Left ventricular systolic dysfunction and heart failure symptoms related to chronic secondary MR should be treated with GDMT including ACE-I, ARB, beta-blockers, aldosterone antagonist, and/or neprilysin inhibitors as they can decrease left ventricular volume and MR severity. Cardiac resynchronization therapy may be indicated in certain patients. GDMT should be maximized prior to consideration of a surgical or transcatheter intervention. MR that is proportionate to the degree of left ventricular dilation may have a better response to GDMT and devices that decrease left ventricular end diastolic volume. MR that is disproportionate to the degree of left ventricular dilation may have increased benefit from MV intervention.

Once optimized with GDMT, patients who remain symptomatic may be offered transcatheter edge-to-edge repair if their anatomy meets criteria. The mechanism of MR and MV anatomy need to be determined prior to consideration of transcatheter repair.

In patients undergoing coronary revascularization with coronary artery bypass graft surgery for myocardial ischemia, concomitant MV surgery would be reasonable for severe secondary MR with or without symptoms (stage C or D), since hibernating myocardium recruitment with revascularization alone may not improve the MR severity.

Gradual left atrial dilation may lead to mitral annular enlargement resulting in MV leaflet malcoaptation and MR with heart failure with preserved ejection fraction, restrictive cardiomyopathy, and non-obstructive hypertrophic cardiomyopathy. Patients who develop atrial fibrillation from these conditions can develop progressive left atrial dilation and mitral annular dilatation, which further increases the degree of MR. Successful pulmonary vein isolation for atrial fibrillation may decrease the MR severity.

It may be possible to treat isolated mitral annular dilation using a percutaneous transcatheter coronary sinus annuloplasty device. Since the coronary sinus runs almost parallel to the posterior mitral annulus, a coronary sinus device may be able to pull the posterior leaflet forward, allowing better coaptation with the anterior leaflet, thus reducing MR.

MV surgery for symptomatic chronic severe secondary MR may decrease cardiac chamber size, increase peak oxygen consumption, and improve symptoms/quality of life. Ischemic and dilated cardiomyopathy results in mitral annular dilatation and apical/lateral papillary muscle displacement as the mechanism of MR, which poses a challenge for surgical repair. Progression or improvement in ventricular dilation helps predict the repair longevity. MV replacement results in a lower recurrence rate of moderate to severe MR than MV repair, resulting in decreased symptoms of heart failure and rehospitalizations. The decision as to the preferred type of mitral prosthesis, mechanical versus bioprosthetic, should be based on the individual patient with a shared decision-making process. Factors to consider for the optimal prosthesis include age, life expectancy, risk of long-term anticoagulation, risk of reoperation, comorbidities, and quality of life. Percutaneous transcatheter MV replacement via a transapical or transseptal approach may be a viable option in the future for select patients.[2,6]

Mitral Valve Prolapse

MVP is a pathologic precursor to primary (organic) acute or chronic MR. Several descriptions are linked to the disease including myxomatous or degenerative MV disease, Barlow syndrome, and fibroelastic deficiency. The extent of leaflet thickening, redundancy, length, area, and matrix composition are used to distinguish the various types of pathology. Barlow syndrome is associated with leaflet myxoid infiltration and varying degrees of prolapse. Fibroelastic deficiency results from extracellular matrix protein deficiency with leaflet and chordae thinning, and increased risk of rupture. Variants span the spectrum from benign disease to death. Approximately 10% of individuals with MVP present with progressive severe MR, heart failure, and pulmonary hypertension.[7,8]

Definition

Abnormalities in the MV apparatus result in displacement of the anterior and/or posterior MV leaflets past the mitral annulus into the left atrium during systole (Fig. 33.3). Sudden tightening of the chordae tendineae and/or leaflets result in the mid-systolic click followed by malcoaptation of the leaflets during ventricular systole, producing the late systolic murmur of MR.[9]

Prevalence

MVP is one of the most common causes of chronic primary MR with a wear-and-tear phenomenon overlaying MV apparatus abnormalities, likely contributing to the increased prevalence with age. The estimated prevalence is approximately 2–5%.

Pathology

The pathology of MVP can involve aberration of a single component or multiple components of the MV apparatus. The laminated leaflet structure contains a collagenous ventricular surface layer, elastic atrial surface layer, and inner spongiosa layer. Excessive production of acid mucopolysaccharides and glycosaminoglycans containing spongiosa tissue leads to focal fibrosa interruption and myofibroblast cell differentiation into chondrocytes, leading to cartilaginous thickening resulting in primary MVP with varying degrees of MR. MVP can be congenital or syndromic in nature (Table 33.1) and associated with Marfan syndrome or other

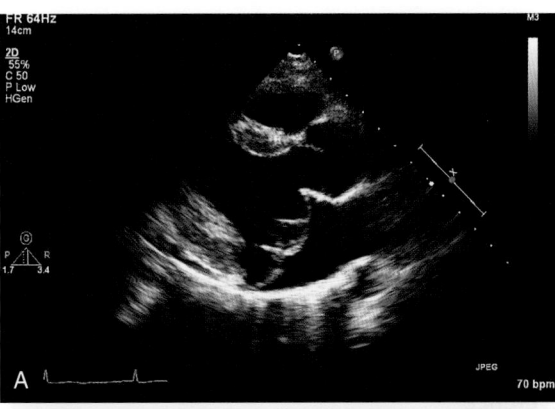

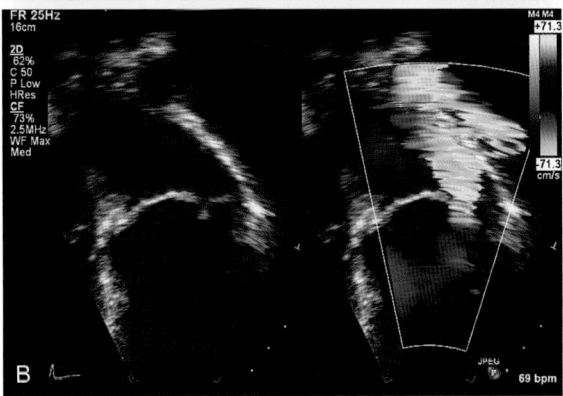

• **Fig. 33.3** Mitral valve prolapse from the parasternal long view **(A)** showing displacement of the anterior and posterior MV leaflets past the mitral annulus into the left atrium during systole, and from the apical four-chamber view **(B)** showing two-dimensional and color comparison images of mitral valve prolapse with associated mitral regurgitation.

TABLE 33.1	Classification of Mitral Valve Prolapse (MVP) as Syndromic Versus Non-Syndromic

Syndromic MVP
    Marfan syndrome/MASS phenotypes
    Loeys-Dietz
    Aneurysm osteoarthritis syndrome
    Ehlers-Danlos syndrome
    Juvenile polyposis syndrome
    Osteogenesis imperfecta
    Pseudoxanthoma elasticum
    BDCS or FTH syndromes
    Larsen-like syndrome
    Williams-Beuren syndrome
    Syndrome with sinus node dysfunction, arrhythmias,
        LVNC (HCN4)
    Trisomies 18, 13, 15
Non-syndromic MVP
    MMVP1 (16p11.2-p12.1 locus)
    MMVP2 (11p15.4 locus)
    MMVP3 (13q31.3e31.2 locus)
    Filamin A-MVP (FLNA)
    DCHS1
    Dilated cardiomyopathy (FLNC, LMNA)

Used with permission from Musella F, Azzu A, Antonopoulos AS, La Mura L, Mohiaddin RH. Comprehensive mitral valve prolapse assessment by cardiovascular MRI. *Clin Radiol.* 2022;77:e120–e129. Page e121, Table 1. *BDCS,* Borrone dermato-cardio-skeletal; *DCHS1,* Dachsous 1; *FLNA,* Filamin-A; *FLNC,* Filamin-C; *FTH,* Frank-Ter Haar; *HCN4,* hyperpolarisation-activated cyclic nucleotide channel 4; *LMNA,* Lamin-A; *LVNC,* left ventricular noncompaction; *MASS,* mitral valve, myopia, aorta, skin, and skeletal features; *MMVP,* myxomatous mitral valve prolapse; *MVP,* mitral valve prolapse.

related connective tissue disorders with a prevalence of approximately 57%. Secondary causes include acquired high flow states such as hyperthyroidism or pregnancy. It can also occur as a complication of chordal rupture or endocarditis.[2] Extracardiac manifestations are usually not present with non-syndromic (isolated or familial) MVP, which has an autosomal dominant or X-linked inheritance with varying degree of penetrance and phenotypic expression. Mitral annular disjunction (MAD) and myocardial fibrosis are associated with MVP. In MAD, portions of the posterior-lateral MV annulus hinge point at the ventricular myocardium are abnormally atrially displaced during ventricular systole. The mitral annulus slides and detaches from the myocardium from a few mm to > 10 mm.[9]

Physiology

The MV anatomy is used to classify MVP within the four stages of chronic primary MR. Mild MVP with normal leaflet coaptation is at risk of MR (stage A). Moderate to severe MVP with normal leaflet coaptation constitutes progressive MR (stage B). Severe MVP with loss of coaptation or flail leaflet defines stage C (asymptomatic severe MR) and stage D (symptomatic severe MR). Conditions resulting in the sudden onset of MVP with severe MR, such as chordal rupture, generate the same physiology of acute severe MR as discussed above.[2]

Clinical Manifestations

Symptoms

Most individuals with MVP are asymptomatic, but if present, common symptoms include fatigue, dizziness, palpitation, and chest pain. Children and adolescents have less frequent symptoms than adults do. Symptoms of transient ischemic attack or stroke may occur secondary to platelet or fibrin emboli from the MV or endocarditis. Sudden death may result from the rare occurrence of ventricular fibrillation. Palpitations and premature ventricular complexes are frequently seen with MAD with a propensity for sustained ventricular tachycardia and sudden cardiac death.[9]

Physical Examination

MVP is commonly associated with a mid-systolic click and late systolic murmur. Other manifestations include an isolated early- or mid-systolic click, isolated late systolic murmur, or holosystolic murmur. The click/murmur increases in intensity and occurs earlier in systole with isometric exercise (increases left ventricular afterload) or Valsalva maneuver/standing (decreases left ventricular end-diastolic volume). Conversely, increasing left ventricular preload (squatting or passive leg raising) decreases the intensity of the click/murmur and causes it to occur later in systole. Since MVP is a dynamic process, the click and/or murmur may be intermittently present. The physical appearance of individuals with MVP ranges from normal to an asthenic body habitus with other features suggestive of a connective tissue disorder (chest wall deformity, scoliosis, high arched palate, etc.).[9]

Diagnostics

Electrocardiogram

Electrocardiographic finds are dependent on the degree of cardiac chamber enlargement secondary to the severity of MR. Nonspecific abnormalities include T wave inversion and/or ST segment depression in the inferior or left precordial leads in some individuals with MVP. Premature atrial or ventricular complexes, atrial flutter, or atrial fibrillation may occur. Ambulatory cardiac monitoring may show episodes of non-sustained ventricular tachycardia.[9]

Chest Radiography

There are no specific findings on chest radiography related to isolated MVP without MR. Chest radiographic findings are similar to other etiologies of moderate or severe, acute or chronic MR.[9]

Noninvasive Imaging

TTE M-mode findings define MVP as posterior displacement of the anterior and/or posterior leaflet $\geq$ 2 mm during late systole or $\geq$ 3 mm holosystolic displacement. Other features include thickened and elongated myxomatous leaflets, varying degrees of MR, left atrial dilation, and MAD. Tissue Doppler with a high-velocity positive systolic wave at the lateral mitral annulus is suggestive of MAD. TEE is beneficial to evaluate the mechanism of MR and prolapsing leaflet components to inform optimal surgical approach to repair. CMR allows for evaluation of the MV leaflet components in multiple planes, MAD, and late gadolinium enhancement for myocardial fibrosis, which is associated with ventricular arrhythmias and sudden cardiac death.[7]

Exercise Testing

Exercise stress testing may be indicated to evaluate the etiology of nonspecific symptoms related to MVP. Stress echocardiogram may demonstrate transient moderate to severe MR that is not apparent at rest in individuals with exercise-induced symptoms and can provide prognostic and risk stratification information.

Cardiac Catheterization

Cardiac catheterization is not indicated for the diagnosis of MVP. Left ventricular angiography findings are nonspecific. Hemodynamic assessment and left ventriculography are useful to grade MR severity, left ventricular function, or potential need for surgery as documented above.[2]

Management

Vasodilator therapy decreases left ventricular size and mitral closing force. This may decrease the degree of MVP and severity of MR, except in the setting of systemic hypertension. Anti-platelet therapy is sometimes considered in individuals with severe leaflet redundancy or thickening. Anticoagulation with vitamin K antagonists or direct oral anticoagulants may be indicated with a history of stroke, atrial fibrillation, or recurrent transient ischemic attacks

despite anti-platelet therapy. Endocarditis prophylaxis is not indicated for MVP with or without MR, unless there is a previous history of endocarditis, prosthetic valve, or within 6 months after placement of prosthetic material by surgery or transcatheter intervention. Surgical indications for MVP are based on guidelines for primary acute or chronic MR with a preference for MR repair over MV replacement at a high-volume valve surgery center. Transcatheter edge-to-edge MV repair may be an option for select patients.[2]

Mitral Stenosis

Prevalence

Congenital MV stenosis is a rare condition that occurs in approximately 0.4% of patients with congenital heart disease.[10] While clinically significant MV lesions are very rare, with an estimated frequency in the general population of 5/100,000 people, advances in echocardiogram technology have allowed diagnosis of minor MV defects in up to 1% of healthy school-aged children.[10] Worldwide, most cases represent acquired disease from rheumatic fever, but in developed nations, congenital lesions are more common.[11] Congenital mitral stenosis often occurs with other left-sided obstructive lesions including supravalvar mitral membrane, subaortic obstruction, and variations of small left-sided structures including hypoplastic left heart syndrome and Shone's complex (supravalvar mitral membrane, parachute MV, subaortic obstruction, and coarctation of the aorta).[10,12]

Pathology

Various classification systems for congenital mitral stenosis have been developed—some based on anatomic features seen on postmortem exam and others based on surgical observation or associated repair techniques.[10] It has become widely recognized that most MV lesions are multilevel and do not fit into a single classification.[10,13] Abnormalities can be supravalvar (supravalvar mitral membrane), valvar (annular hypoplasia, abnormal leaflets or commissures), or subvalvar (abnormal chordae tendineae or papillary muscles).[10,13] Nevertheless, there is historical significance to older descriptive terms, and they are still commonly used to define MV lesions in conjunction with more precise descriptions of affected MV segmental anatomy.

In 1978, Ruckman and van Praagh proposed anatomic classifications of mitral stenosis. By their description, typical congenital mitral stenosis (Fig. 33.4) consisted of thickened and rolled leaflet margins, shortened and thickened chordae tendineae, interchordal spaces that are partially or completely obliterated by fibrous tissue, and underdeveloped papillary muscles with reduced interpapillary distance. In parachute MVs all the chordae tendineae, which are usually shortened and thickened, insert into a single papillary muscle group, and the anterolateral papillary muscle is often absent. A variation on this condition is parachute like asymmetric MV, in which there are two papillary muscles, one hypoplastic and the other more dominant and receiving the majority of tendinous chords.[10] In anomalous mitral arcade,

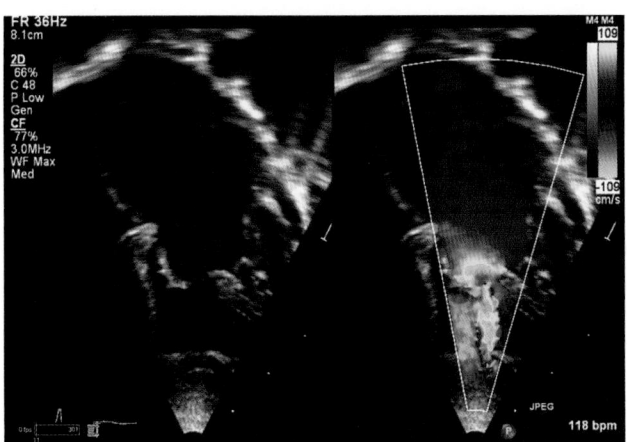

• **Fig. 33.4** Congenital mitral stenosis in an apical four-chamber view with two-dimensional and color comparison images. The mitral valve leaflets are thickened, with short chordae tendineae. Color comparison demonstrates flow acceleration beginning at the leaflet tips.

the left ventricular papillary muscle connects to the anterior mitral leaflet either directly or by unusually short chordae. A hammock MV refers to the appearance of the MV apparatus from the left atrial aspect when the valvar orifice is at least partially obstructed by tendinous chords attached to an abnormal papillary muscle implanted just below the posterior leaflet. Double-orifice MV occurs when there are two orifices with their own supporting apparatus or a bridge of valvar tissue dividing the MV inlet.[10] All components of the MV are small in hypoplastic mitral stenosis, which is commonly associated with LVOT anomalies and hypoplastic left heart syndrome.

Physiology

The degree of obstruction depends on the valve area, cardiac output, and heart rate. Cardiac output in turn is affected by coexisting shunts that may increase or decrease transmitral valve flow.[14] Post-tricuspid valve left-to-right shunts (i.e., ventricular septal defect, aortopulmonary window, or patent ductus arteriosus) will increase blood return to the left atrium, resulting in a larger cardiac output that needs to cross the MV and an increased gradient. Presence of an atrial septal defect with left-to-right shunt, in contrast, will result in less flow across the MV and a lower gradient. The gradient across the MV is also heart rate dependent. Since diastole is shortened with increased tachycardia, faster heart rates result in less diastolic filling time, elevated left atrial pressure, increased flow rate across the MV, and an increased transmitral gradient to maintain cardiac output.[15] Doppler velocity time integral of the MV inflow can be used to estimate a mean gradient that has fair correlation with direct measurements in the cardiac catheterization laboratory.[14] In pediatrics, widely accepted cut-offs to define mild, moderate, and severe mitral stenosis are as follows: valve area (cm²) >1.5, 1–1.5, and <1; mean gradient (mm Hg) <5, 5–10, and >10; and mean pulmonary artery pressure (mm Hg) <30, 30–50, and >50.[14]

Mitral stenosis is associated with elevated left atrial pressure, which is transmitted to the pulmonary circulation and can lead to pulmonary artery hypertension and pulmonary edema.[12,15] If pulmonary hypertension is severe, it can lead to right ventricular dysfunction and tricuspid regurgitation.[15] Following relief of mitral stenosis, left atrial pressure improves acutely, but pulmonary artery hypertension may not change immediately if morphologic changes have occurred in the pulmonary vasculature as a response to longstanding atrial hypertension.[12] Atrial fibrillation may worsen left atrial hypertension and decrease cardiac output since atrial contraction helps to augment transmitral flow in the presence of mitral stenosis.[15]

Clinical Manifestations

Symptoms

Mild mitral stenosis is not associated with symptoms. With moderate obstruction, patients develop dyspnea or exercise intolerance, and with severe obstruction, patients can be symptomatic at rest. For patients with moderate or severe obstruction, maintaining cardiac output can come at the expense of increased left atrial pressure, pulmonary venous congestion, pulmonary artery hypertension and resultant cough, wheeze, and occasionally hemoptysis. If cardiac output cannot be increased at rest or with exertion because of limitations to transmitral flow, patients experience fatigue, orthopnea, and exercise intolerance. In infants and young children, this can also manifest as poor oral intake, slow growth, diaphoresis, and recurrent pneumonia. Atrial fibrillation increases the risk of systemic embolic events.[15] Rarely, a markedly dilated left atrium can compress the recurrent laryngeal nerve and produce hoarseness, known as Ortner's syndrome.[16]

Physical Examination

The hallmark of the cardiac examination is an apical, low-pitched, rumbling diastolic murmur. The length of the murmur correlates with the severity of stenosis. There usually is presystolic accentuation. The murmur is easier to hear when the patient is in the left lateral decubitus position, during expiration, and after mild exercise to accentuate the effects of increased cardiac output. The intensity of the murmur is less in the setting of increased chest wall thickness, low cardiac output, or severe associated pulmonary disease.[15] An opening snap created by sudden tensing of the opened valve leaflets can be heard, and the intensity of S_1 depends on the excursion of the valve leaflets during closing; patients with mild or moderate obstruction have a loud S_1, whereas those with severe obstruction have a soft S_1. Patients with pulmonary hypertension have a prominent right ventricular heave, increased intensity of S_2, and occasionally a murmur of tricuspid regurgitation or pulmonary regurgitation (Graham Steele murmur).

Diagnostics

Electrocardiography

The electrocardiogram is normal in patients with mild stenosis. With advancing degrees of obstruction, P-mitrale develops with broad notched P waves in lead II and biphasic P waves in V_1. If pulmonary hypertension develops, right ventricular hypertrophy and right atrial enlargement can also be present. Chronic moderate or severe stenosis can produce atrial tachyarrhythmias, most notably atrial fibrillation.[15]

Chest Radiography

If mitral stenosis is severe enough, chest radiograph will show left atrial enlargement,[15] which can create a double density sign and splaying of the tracheal bifurcation due to superior displacement of the left mainstem bronchus. Signs of pulmonary arterial hypertension and pulmonary congestion can also be seen.[15]

Echocardiography

Echocardiography, including 2D images, continuous and pulse wave Doppler, and color echocardiography, is the primary mode of evaluating mitral stenosis in children. Since mitral stenosis is often complex and multilevel, assessment requires a detailed segmental approach with evaluation of the supravalvar region, MV annulus, leaflets, commissures, chordae tendineae, and papillary muscles in order to identify the anatomic contributions to MV obstruction (Table 33.2).[10,14] General assessment of the atria, ventricles, and outflow tracts is also necessary to identify associated cardiac disease and physiologic effects of mitral stenosis on the heart and pulmonary vasculature.[14] When possible, quantitative measurements should be obtained to define the degree of mitral stenosis and associated physiologic changes. Doppler velocity time integral of MV inflow is commonly used to estimate the mean gradient across the MV.[14] Assessment of early diastolic velocity (E wave) and late diastolic velocity (A wave) can also be performed, taking into consideration that the normal profiles change with age.[14] Although estimates of MV orifice area calculated using Doppler pressure half time and the Gorlin formula are poorly correlated in children, increasing use of 3D echo

may provide more accurate anatomic information about multilevel obstruction and the orifice size at the narrowest point.[14] Measurements of annulus size, left atrial size, and left ventricular size can be compared to established nomograms, and tricuspid regurgitation provides an indirect estimate of pulmonary pressures.[14]

Cardiac Catheterization

A thorough echocardiographic examination, in conjunction with the patient's history and physical examination, generally provide necessary information to determine patient management. Cardiac catheterization is performed if there is discrepancy between echocardiographic findings and clinical features, for catheter-based intervention, or prior to surgical intervention.[12] Simultaneous left atrial and left ventricular pressures permit direct measurement of transmitral pressure gradient, and pressure tracings can be used to calculate the effective orifice area using the Gorlin method.[12]

Management

Patients with mild mitral stenosis who are asymptomatic may only need close follow-up. For symptomatic patients, diuretics are used to treat pulmonary venous congestion and to limit intravascular volume that contributes to left atrial hypertension.[11] Beta-blockers and ivabradine can be used for heart rate control to increase diastolic filling time and decrease the transmitral gradient, but this is based on adult studies since evidence in pediatrics is lacking.[11] Also based on adult literature, patients with atrial fibrillation require antiarrhythmic mediation and anticoagulation to minimize risk of embolic events.[15]

Patients with poor growth, respiratory symptoms, hemoptysis, or severe pulmonary hypertension require intervention. Treatment options include percutaneous transcatheter balloon mitral valvuloplasty, surgical mitral valvuloplasty, and surgical MV replacement.[12,13] Balloon

TABLE 33.2	Segmental Approach to Echocardiography Evaluation of the Mitral Valve and Its Components	
Anatomic Region	**Evaluation**	
Supravalvar region	Atrial membrane	- Cor triatriatum: proximal to left atrial appendage
		- Supravalvar mitral membrane: distal to left atrial appendage
Annulus	Size	- Normal, hypoplastic, atretic, dilated
Leaflets and commissures	Anatomy	- Normal, dysplastic, thickened, deficient, underdeveloped, presence of accessory tissue, presence of a cleft, single versus multiple orifices
	Function	- Normal, restricted movement, valve prolapse
Chordae tendineae	Site of attachments	- 1 versus 2 papillary muscles, equal versus unequal distribution, septal attachments
	Morphology	- Fused, thickened, shortened
Papillary muscles	Number	- Normal, single papillary muscle, >2 papillary muscles
	Symmetry	- Symmetric versus asymmetric
	Position	- Normal, basal or apical displacement, closely spaced

valvuloplasty can decrease the mean transmitral gradient by up to 40%, but 28% of patients develop new moderate to severe MR due to a tear in the MV or disruption of chordal structures, and up to half of survivors will ultimately require reintervention.[12] Surgical intervention is favored for isolated supravalvar mitral membrane since resection provides definitive repair with less MR than balloon valvuloplasty. Surgery is also favored when there are associated cardiac lesions needing surgical correction or preexisting moderate or greater MR.[12] Surgical valvuloplasty techniques vary by the anatomy and include commissuroplasty, leaflet thinning, leaflet augmentation, chordal division or fenestration, and splitting of papillary muscles.[12,13] Surgical intervention can decrease the mean transmitral gradient by up to 70%, but rates of reintervention are still approximately 20–40%.[12,13] Risks of prosthetic valves include heart block necessitating permanent pacemaker placement, prosthesis thrombosis, and need for up-sizing to accommodate growth.[12,13] Supraannular implantation is often necessary due to small MV annular size, and is associated with decreased left atrial compliance and risk of obstructing pulmonary venous return.[12] More recently, implantation of the Melody valve in the mitral position has become an alternative to traditional prosthetic valves for younger and smaller patients. This technique has the benefits of allowing for future expansion in the catheterization laboratory after somatic growth and delaying or avoiding the need for reoperation.[17] Overall, survival after MV intervention for congenital mitral stenosis is favorable with 91–98% survival at 1 year and 87–96% survival at 5 years.[12,13] However, many patients will require reintervention at some point, and there is increased mortality in patients aged < 2 years and those requiring MV replacement at the time of initial intervention.[12,13]

Left Atrial Problems

Supravalvar Mitral Membrane

Definition

A supravalvar mitral membrane consists of a ring of connective tissue that is adherent to the atrial surface of the MV leaflets or slightly superior to the valve annulus. This fibrous tissue is distal to the left atrial appendage, which distinguishes it from the membrane of cor triatriatum.[18,19]

Prevalence

Supravalvar mitral membrane is an extremely rare congenital lesion with an estimated incidence of < 0.001% of congenital and acquired heart disease.[20]

Pathology

The supravalvar mitral membrane ranges from a thin membrane to a thick discrete fibrous ridge that partially or completely encircles the mitral orifice, and frequently adheres to the mitral leaflets.[18] Two types have been described; *supramitral* with a shelf-like membrane above the mitral annulus and normal MV leaflets and subvalvar apparatus and *intramitral* with the membrane adherent to the valve leaflets and resulting in impaired leaflet mobility (often associated with Shone's complex).[18] This condition can be an isolated finding but is associated with other congenital cardiac defects up to 89% of the time, including abnormalities of the MV apparatus, Shone's complex, bicuspid aortic valve, left ventricular hypoplasia, subvalvar and valvar aortic stenosis, coarctation, aortic arch hypoplasia, ventricular septal defect, or persistent left superior vena cava draining to the coronary sinus.[18,19]

Physiology and Clinical Manifestations

The clinical manifestations depend on the severity of obstruction and are the same symptoms seen with other forms of mitral stenosis, including secondary pulmonary edema and pulmonary hypertension. Cases are frequently found during evaluation of associated lesions.[13,18]

Diagnostics

Echocardiography

The membrane can be identified with the use of 2D echocardiography (Fig. 33.5). Multiple views, including parasternal long-axis, subxiphoid four-chamber, and apical four-chamber, are used for assessment, and measurements are typically made from the apical four-chamber view.[19,20] In one study, 25% of patients had lesions that could not be seen from the parasternal long-axis view, highlighting the importance of assessment from multiple views.[19] A multimodal approach using 2D, color flow, and 3D echocardiography and pulse wave and continuous wave doppler should be used to assess MV annular size, chordae length, number of papillary muscles, and measurement of the gradient across the MV.[13,19,20]

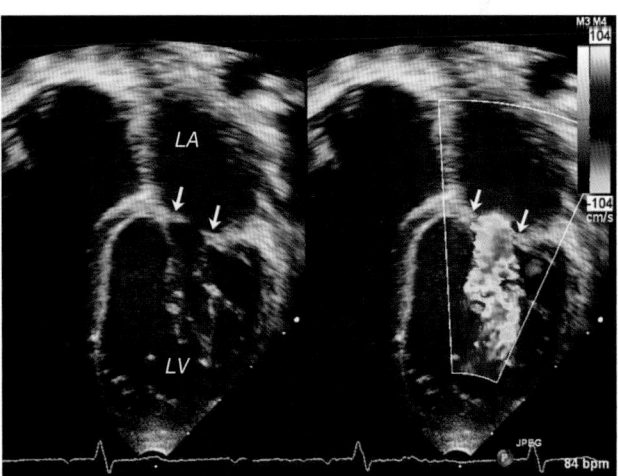

• **Fig. 33.5** Supravalvar mitral membrane as seen in the apical four-chamber view. In the two-dimensional image, the supravalvar mitral membrane *(arrows)* can be seen above the mitral annulus with extension onto the proximal leaflet tissue. Color comparison demonstrates flow acceleration beginning at the level of the membrane. *LA,* Left atrium; *LV,* left ventricle. (Used with permission from Schidlow DN, Zaidi A, Gauvreau K, Emani SM, Geva T. Echocardiographic characteristics of annulo-leaflet mitral ring. *J Am Soc Echocardiogr.* 2015; 28:541–548. Page 546, Figure 4.)

Cardiac Catheterization

Cardiac catheterization can be performed for diagnostic purposes and measurement of pulmonary artery pressure and transmembrane pressure gradient.[18,19] Intervention with balloon mitral valvuloplasty is performed in a minority of cases, and often does not eliminate the need for surgical intervention.[19]

Management

Surgical resection is the mainstay of treatment.[12] If the supravalvar mitral membrane is above the mitral annulus, it can be directly resected. If it is intramitral, surgical intervention may include removing adherent tissue from the MV leaflets and intervention on the chordae or papillary muscles.[13,18,19] Patients requiring surgical resection tend to be younger at the time of diagnosis, have a higher MV gradient at the time of diagnosis, have shortened chordae, and greater left atrial dilation.[19] The majority of patients undergo additional surgical procedures to repair associated defects at the same time.[18,19] Surgical resection usually provides definitive therapy with durable improvement in the mean gradient across the MV to < 5 mm Hg and insignificant MR.[18,19] Reintervention is often associated with intramitral rings, Shone's complex, MV annular hypoplasia, or abnormal subvalvar apparatus,[18] and rarely recurrence.[19] However, this highlights the importance of lifelong follow-up.

Cor Triatriatum

Definition

Cor triatriatum sinister is a rare cardiac anomaly in which a fibromuscular membrane divides the left atrium into a proximal posterior-superior chamber which typically receives the pulmonary veins, and a distal anterior-inferior chamber which communicates with the left atrial appendage and MV (Figs. 33.6 and 33.7).[21] Cor triatriatum dexter refers to the even more rare occurrence of a subdividing chamber in the right atrium, which will not be discussed here.

Prevalence

Cor triatriatum has an estimated prevalence of about 0.1% of congenital heart disease.[21]

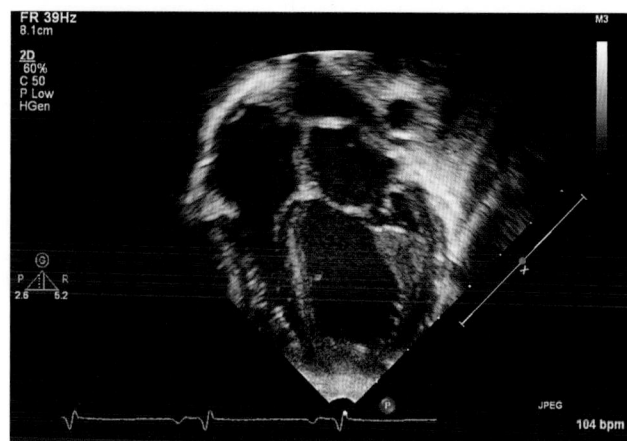

• **Fig. 33.7** Cor triatriatum as seen from the apical four-chamber view. There is a fibromuscular membrane dividing the left atrium into a proximal posterior-superior chamber, which typically receives the pulmonary veins, and a distal anterior-inferior chamber which communicates with the left atrial appendage (not seen on this image) and the mitral valve.

Pathology

Several developmental theories for cor triatriatum have been proposed with mal-incorporation (incomplete incorporation of the common pulmonary vein to the posterior portion of the primitive left atrium) being most accepted.[21] Pathologic examination of postmortem cases and human embryos has suggested that the membrane is composed of common pulmonary vein on the inferior/dorsal surface, septum primum and left atrial free wall on the superior/ventral surface, and a fibroelastic layer adjacent to the opening in the membrane.[21] There usually is a single opening in the membrane of variable size and an atrial communication or patent foramen ovale connecting the right atrium and distal chamber. Many variations have been described including no or multiple openings in the membrane.[21] Although cor triatriatum can be an isolated defect, the largest reviews found that 75–84% of cases are associated with other congenital cardiovascular anomalies, frequently including atrial septal defect, ventricular septal defect, partial or total anomalous pulmonary venous return, or left superior vena cava.[21-23] More complex congenital heart disease such as tetralogy of

• **Fig. 33.6** Typical example of cor triatriatum, as illustrated in 1969 by R. van Praagh. Diagram of left heart chambers and subdividing diaphragm. *CPVC,* Common pulmonary vein chamber; *LA,* left atrium; *LV,* left ventricle; *MV,* mitral valve. (Used with permission from Van Praagh R, Corsini I. Cor triatriatum: pathologic anatomy and a consideration of morphogenesis based on 13 postmortem cases and a study of normal development of the pulmonary vein and atrial septum in 83 human embryos. *Am Heart J.* 1969;78:379–405. Page 383, Figure 1D.)

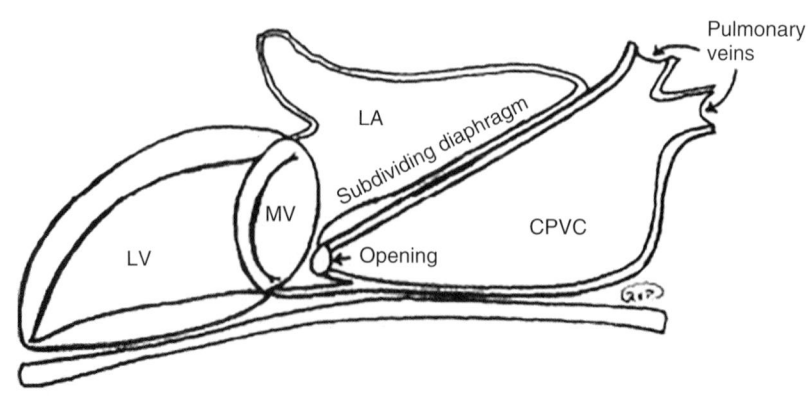

Fallot, D-transposition of the great arteries, atrioventricular canal defect, hypoplastic left heart syndrome, and others have also been reported in association with cor triatriatum, but with less frequency.[21-23]

Physiology

The effects on the cardiovascular system are similar to those seen in patients with mitral stenosis, being minimal or absent if the membrane opening is large, and associated with pulmonary venous obstruction, pulmonary edema, pulmonary hypertension, decreased cardiac output, or cardiogenic shock when the opening is small. The degree of obstruction is not expected to be progressive.[22] Symptoms of pulmonary venous obstruction are ameliorated not only by the presence of a large opening in the membrane but also by a large atrial communication between the proximal chamber and right atrium, other cardiac conditions that limit pulmonary blood flow, or partial anomalous pulmonary venous connection.[23]

Clinical Manifestations

Symptoms

Symptoms correlate directly with the diameter of the opening in the membrane as well as with the presence of associated cardiac defects.[22] With severe obstruction, patients can develop tachycardia, tachypnea, dyspnea, failure to thrive, feeding difficulties, recurrent pneumonia, neonatal cyanosis, heart failure, and arrhythmias.[22] With minimal or mild obstruction, diagnosis and repair may occur when patients are > 70 years old.[23] Cor triatriatum should be suspected in patients with unexplained pulmonary edema.[23]

Physical Examination

The physical examination differs from patients with mitral stenosis in having no apical diastolic murmur. Patients with pulmonary hypertension have a parasternal right ventricular lift and loud second heart sound. Symptomatic patients frequently have pulmonary rales.

Diagnostics

Electrocardiography

Electrocardiogram often shows right axis deviation and right ventricular hypertrophy, with right and left atrial hypertrophy being more variable.

Chest Radiography

Severe obstruction produces pulmonary venous obstruction, pulmonary edema, and Kerley B lines. In patients with pulmonary hypertension, the main pulmonary artery and right ventricle are dilated.

Echocardiography

Two-dimensional echocardiography is effective for diagnosis of cor triatriatum.[14] Multiple views, including parasternal, subxiphoid, and apical, are useful for detecting the left atrial membrane that often curves anteroinferiorly, the number of openings in the membrane, the location of atrial communications, and the presence of other congenital cardiac defects. The left atrial appendage is distal to the membrane, a characteristic that distinguishes this condition from supravalvar mitral membrane. The entry site of each pulmonary vein should be determined since total and partial anomalous pulmonary venous connection are known to be found in association with cor triatriatum.[22,23] Color and Doppler echocardiography are useful in assessing the degree of obstruction created by the membrane, estimating pulmonary artery pressure, and assessing valve function. In patients with limited transthoracic imaging or for intraoperative assessment, transesophageal echocardiography provides diagnostic imaging.[14]

Advanced Imaging

CMR imaging and computed tomography are additional modalities that can effectively detect the presence of a left atrial membrane.[24]

Cardiac Catheterization

Cardiac catheterization is generally not needed for management of patients with cor triatriatum. Patients with severe obstruction typically have pulmonary artery hypertension, elevated pulmonary capillary wedge pressure, normal pressure in the distal left atrial chamber, and normal left ventricular end-diastolic pressure. While catheter-based balloon dilation of the membrane has been reported both as a primary management strategy and as part of a staged treatment with later surgical intervention, surgery remains the mainstay of management.[25]

Management

The left atrial membrane is resected surgically for patients who are symptomatic, have pulmonary hypertension, or are undergoing repair of other cardiac defects. In two large review studies, 72–80% of patients had additional cardiac procedures performed at the same time as cor triatriatum repair. There is wide variability in patients' age at time of repair, ranging from a few days to 73 years.[22,23] In one review, patients undergoing surgical repair had a median age of 7 months, with 57% of patients being < 12 months and 25% being > 5 years.[22] In contrast, a second review reported a median age of 19 years, with 60% being > 5 years.[23] In all cases, surgical repair was definitive with no residual obstruction in the atrium at follow-up, although subsequent catheter or surgical interventions may have been performed for coexisting cardiac disease.

References

1. Iddawela S, Joseph PJS, Ganeshan R, et al. Paediatric mitral valve disease: from presentation to management. *Eur J Pediatr.* 2022;181:35-44.
2. Otto CM, Nishimura RA, Bonow RO, et al. 2020 ACC/AHA guideline for the management of patients with valvular heart disease: a report of the American College of Cardiology/American Heart Association Joint Committee on Clinical Practice Guidelines. *Circulation.* 2021;143:e72-e227.

3. Apostolidou E, Maslow AD, Poppas A. Primary mitral valve regurgitation: update and review. *Glob Cardiol Sci Pract*. 2017; 2017:e201703.

4. O'Gara PT, Mack MJ. Secondary mitral regurgitation. *N Engl J Med*. 2020;383:1458-1467.

5. Gaasch WH, Meyer TE. Left ventricular response to mitral regurgitation: implications for management. *Circulation*. 2008; 118:2298-2303.

6. Weiner MM, Hofer I, Lin HM, et al. Relationship among surgical volume, repair quality, and perioperative outcomes for repair of mitral insufficiency in a mitral valve reference center. *J Thorac Cardiovasc Surg*. 2014;148:2021-2026.

7. Musella F, Azzu A, Antonopoulos AS, et al. Comprehensive mitral valve prolapse assessment by cardiovascular MRI. *Clin Radiol*. 2022;77:e120-e129.

8. Guicciardi NA, De Bonis M, Di Resta C, et al. Genetic background of mitral valve prolapse. *Rev Cardiovasc Med*. 2022;23:96.

9. Jeresaty RM. Mitral valve prolapse: definition and implications in athletes. *J Am Coll Cardiol*. 1986;7:231-236.

10. Remenyi B, Gentles TL. Congenital mitral valve lesions: correlation between morphology and imaging. *Ann Pediatr Cardiol*. 2012;5:3-12.

11. Vahanian A, Beyersdorf F, Praz F, et al. 2021 ESC/EACTS Guidelines for the management of valvular heart disease. *Eur J Cardiothorac Surg*. 2021;60:727-800.

12. McElhinney DB, Sherwood MC, Keane JF, del Nido PJ, Almond CS, Lock JE. Current management of severe congenital mitral stenosis: outcomes of transcatheter and surgical therapy in 108 infants and children. *Circulation*. 2005;112:707-714.

13. Baird CW, Marx GR, Borisuk M, et al. Review of congenital mitral valve stenosis: analysis, repair techniques and outcomes. *Cardiovasc Eng Technol*. 2015;6:167-173.

14. Cantinotti M, Giordano R, Koestenberger M, et al. Echocardiographic examination of mitral valve abnormalities in the paediatric population: current practices. *Cardiol Young*. 2020; 30:1-11.

15. Chandrashekhar Y, Westaby S, Narula J. Mitral stenosis. *Lancet*. 2009;374:1271-1283.

16. Zaki SA, Banur D. Ortner's syndrome as a presenting feature of congenital heart disease in infants. *Heart Views*. 2020;21:118-120.

17. Pluchinotta FR, Piekarski BL, Milani V, et al. Surgical atrioventricular valve replacement with Melody valve in infants and children. *Circ Cardiovasc Interv*. 2018;11:e007145.

18. Toscano A, Pasquini L, Iacobelli R, et al. Congenital supravalvar mitral ring: an underestimated anomaly. *J Thorac Cardiovasc Surg*. 2009;137:538-542.

19. Schidlow DN, Zaidi A, Gauvreau K, et al. Echocardiographic characteristics of annulo-leaflet mitral ring. *J Am Soc Echocardiogr*. 2015;28:541-548.

20. Silverman NH. Echocardiography of congenital mitral valve disorders: echocardiographic-morphological comparisons. *Cardiol Young*. 2014;24:1030-1048.

21. Van Praagh R, Corsini I. Cor triatriatum: pathologic anatomy and a consideration of morphogenesis based on 13 postmortem cases and a study of normal development of the pulmonary vein and atrial septum in 83 human embryos. *Am Heart J*. 1969; 78:379-405.

22. Yaroglu Kazanci S, Emani S, McElhinney DB. Outcome after repair of cor triatriatum. *Am J Cardiol*. 2012;109:412-416.

23. Saxena P, Burkhart HM, Schaff HV, et al. Surgical repair of cor triatriatum sinister: the Mayo Clinic 50-year experience. *Ann Thorac Surg*. 2014;97:1659-1663.

24. Fuchs MM, Connolly HM, Said SM, et al. Outcomes in patients with cor triatriatum sinister. *Congenit Heart Dis*. 2018;13:628-632.

25. Li WW, Koolbergen DR, Bouma BJ, et al. Catheter-based interventional strategies for cor triatriatum in the adult: feasibility study through a hybrid approach. *BMC Cardiovasc Disord*. 2015;15:68.

34

Ebstein Anomaly and Other Tricuspid Valve Problems

EDWARD P. WALSH, GERALD R. MARX, AND PEDRO J. DEL NIDO

KEY LEARNING POINTS

- Ebstein anomaly involves adherence of the septal and inferior leaflets of the tricuspid valve (TV) to the underlying right ventricular myocardium. The anterior leaflet is mobile but is typically elongated and tethered.
- The degree of TV dysfunction varies widely. Some patients are critically ill at birth, while others remain asymptomatic for decades.
- Arrhythmias are common and sometimes fatal. Ebstein anomaly is the only congenital heart defect with an

incidence of accessory pathways (10%–38%) that far exceeds that of the general population.
- Critically ill neonates will require aggressive support, but may improve over days to weeks as pulmonary resistance falls.
- Surgical options for Ebstein anomaly have improved in recent years with the introduction of the cone operation.

Tricuspid valve (TV) dysfunction may be anatomic or physiologic, primary or secondary, regurgitant or stenotic, alone or in various combinations. The most important anatomic abnormality is Ebstein anomaly, which will be the central topic of this chapter. Other important subgroups include regurgitation from TV dysplasia (most commonly seen in patients with pulmonary atresia and intact septum) and tricuspid regurgitation secondary to annular dilatation in a variety of postoperative lesions (e.g., hypoplastic left heart syndrome [HLHS]). Isolated tricuspid stenosis is uncommon but may accompany repair of certain difficult atrioventricular (AV) canal defects.

Ebstein Anomaly

Anatomy

Ebstein anomaly is a relatively rare congenital cardiac malformation (0.012–0.06/1000 live births) that can pose serious management challenges from both a hemodynamic and electrophysiologic perspective. The primary anatomic derangement involves a distinctive malformation of the TV with adherence of the septal and inferior leaflets to the underlying right ventricular (RV) myocardium due to failure of embryologic delamination.[1] The anterior leaflet retains

mobility but is typically elongated, fenestrated, and tethered. Consequently, the functional TV orifice becomes displaced toward the RV apex with inflow oriented toward the RV outflow tract, resulting in variable degrees of regurgitation and occasionally stenosis. This in turn causes right atrial (RA) enlargement with expansion of the true right AV annulus, along with dilation of the *atrialized* portion of the RV above the functional TV orifice (but below the true AV annulus) where the tissue is remarkably thin-walled (Fig. 34.1). The majority of patients will have an interatrial communication (patent foramen ovale or atrial septal defect) with potential right-to-left shunting. The volume of the functional RV chamber varies but is usually smaller than the left ventricle. However, when combined with atrialized RV, total RV volume is increased, sometimes massively so. At a certain point, severe right heart dilation can negatively impact left ventricular function through ventricular-ventricular interaction, which can be an ominous development in this disease.[2] Roughly 30% of patients with Ebstein anomaly have significant secondary lesions that can include pulmonary stenosis, pulmonary atresia, or ventricular septal defect.

An Ebstein-like malformation of the left-sided TV can also occur in patients with L-loop transposition of the great arteries ("congenitally corrected" transposition). The free edge of

447

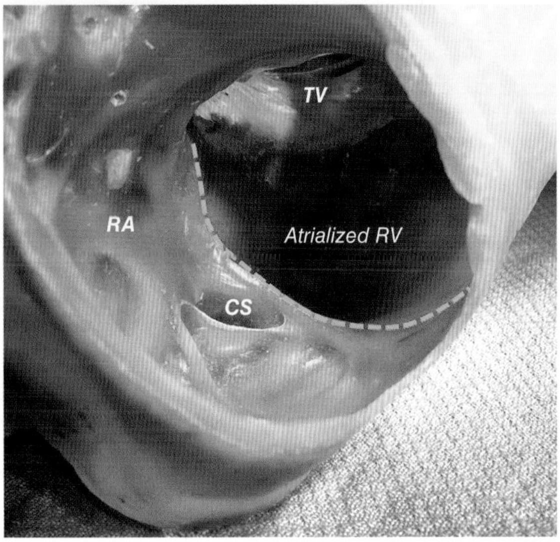

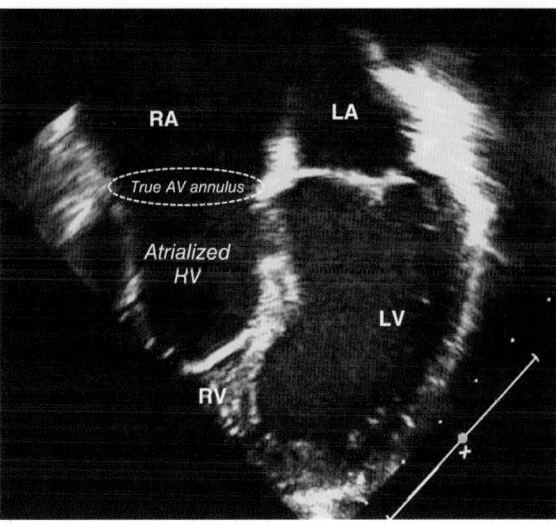

• **Fig. 34.1** Pathology specimen of severe Ebstein anomaly looking toward the right ventricular apex from the right atrium. The *blue line* marks the true atrioventricular annulus. The *red line* marks the mobile edge of the tricuspid valve loaflet. Atrialized right ventricle is the large area between lines. *CS,* Coronary sinus; *RA,* right atrium; *RV,* right ventricle; *TV,* tricuspid valve.

• **Fig. 34.2** Echocardiogram (apical four-chamber view) of severe Ebstein anomaly. Note the adherence of septal tricuspid leaflet to right ventricular muscle, and the large separation between the true atrioventricular annulus and the mobile edge of the leaflet. The functional right ventricular cavity is small in comparison with the volume of the atrialized right ventricle. *AV,* Atrioventricular; *LA,* left atrium; *LV,* left ventricle; *RA,* right atrium; *RV,* right ventricle.

the septal and inferior TV leaflets is displaced toward the RV apex, but the anterior leaflet will usually not display the elongated sail-like deformity seen in classic Ebstein anomaly, nor is the extent of atrialized RV ever as dramatic. Nonetheless, the resulting TV dysfunction can be significant, which is especially problematic, since it must function as the systemic AV valve in this anatomy (see Chapter 30).

Diagnosis

In the current era, moderate-severe forms of Ebstein anomaly are usually first suspected on screening fetal ultrasound and confirmed by fetal echocardiogram or by transthoracic echocardiogram shortly after delivery (Fig. 34.2). Milder forms might escape early detection. The degree of TV leaflet tethering, and hence TV and RV dysfunction, varies widely from patient to patient, so that some are critically ill at birth while others may remain asymptomatic for decades.[3]

Physical exam finding will vary according to severity of the TV defect and age. The degree of cyanosis ranges from none to profound. Recognition of tricuspid incompetence depends on the presence of a pansystolic (usually high frequency) murmur audible at the lower sternal border that varies with respiration. Tricuspid stenosis is suggested by the presence of a diastolic rumbling murmur at the lower sternal border, seeming to occur somewhat earlier in diastole than a mitral diastolic murmur. The cardiac impulse may be undulating. Both first and second heart sounds may be widely split. An S3 and/or S4 gallop is an auscultatory hallmark of this condition.[4]

Chest x-ray findings are similarly variable, but in all except mild forms there is some degree of cardiomegaly, with wall-to-wall heart possible in severe cases.

Echocardiographic data are usually unambiguous. Two-dimensional and three-dimensional imaging can provide detailed analysis of the size and mobility of the valve leaflets, as well as regurgitant orifice area. Cardiac MRI allows measurement of the atrialized and functional RV and percent tricuspid regurgitation (Fig. 34.3).[5] Catheterization may be required in select cases for: (1) electrophysiologic study and arrhythmia ablation; (2) coronary artery angiography; and (3) detailed hemodynamics (including measurements during balloon occlusion of an atrial septal defect) to assist in surgical planning, especially when partial diversion of systemic venous return by a superior cava-pulmonary artery anastomosis (bidirectional Glenn procedure) is contemplated.

Electrocardiogram and Arrhythmias

The electrocardiogram for the vast majority of patients with Ebstein anomaly (71%–94%) exhibits a pattern of complete right bundle branch block in the absence of preexcitation from an accessory atrioventricular pathway (AP). When preexcitation is present, it can fuse with the right bundle branch block pattern, and the resultant QRS complex can become pseudo-normalized to some degree (Fig. 34.4). A relatively normal appearing QRS in a patient with Ebstein anomaly should make one suspicious of a cryptic AP. Many patients with Ebstein anomaly will also have first-degree AV block in the absence of preexcitation, which is usually a consequence of RA enlargement with long interatrial conduction time rather than true delay at the AV node.

Patients with Ebstein anomaly must contend with a high incidence of tachyarrhythmias, some of which can be life-threatening.[6] The most important of these relate to APs

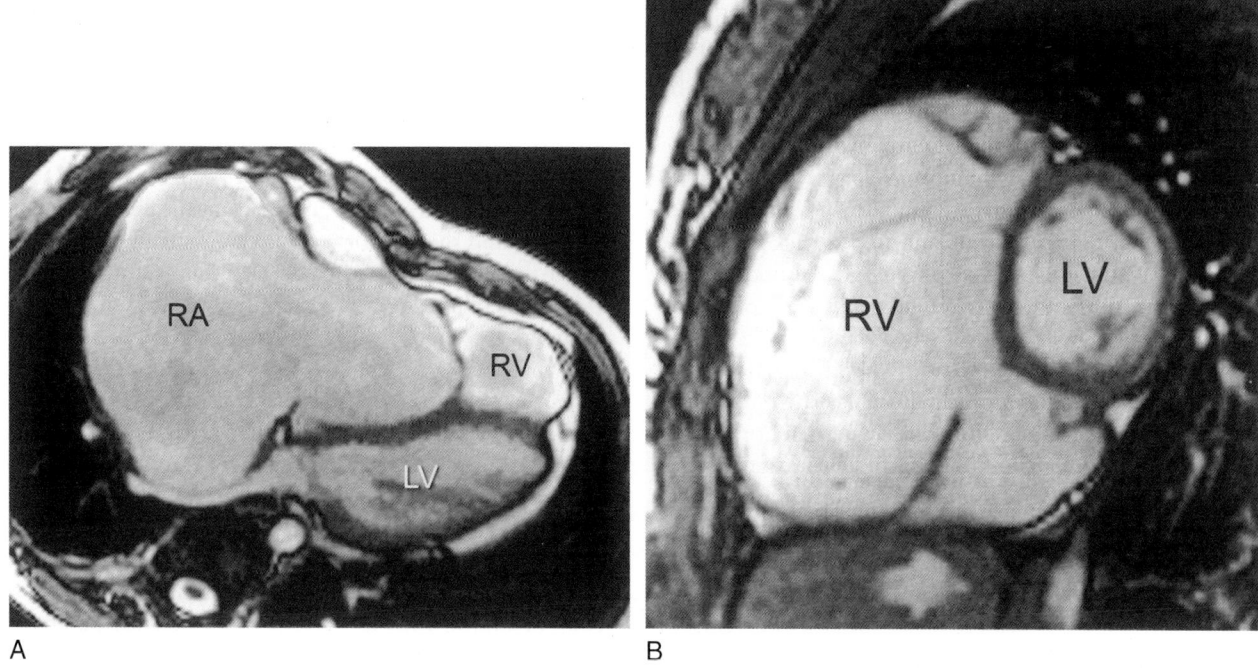

• **Fig. 34.3** Magnetic resonance images from a patient with Ebstein anomaly showing: **(A)** four-chamber view with dilated right atrium and apically displaced tricuspid valve; **(B)** short-axis view with enlarged right ventricle. *LV,* Left ventricle; *RA,* right atrium; *RV,* right ventricle.

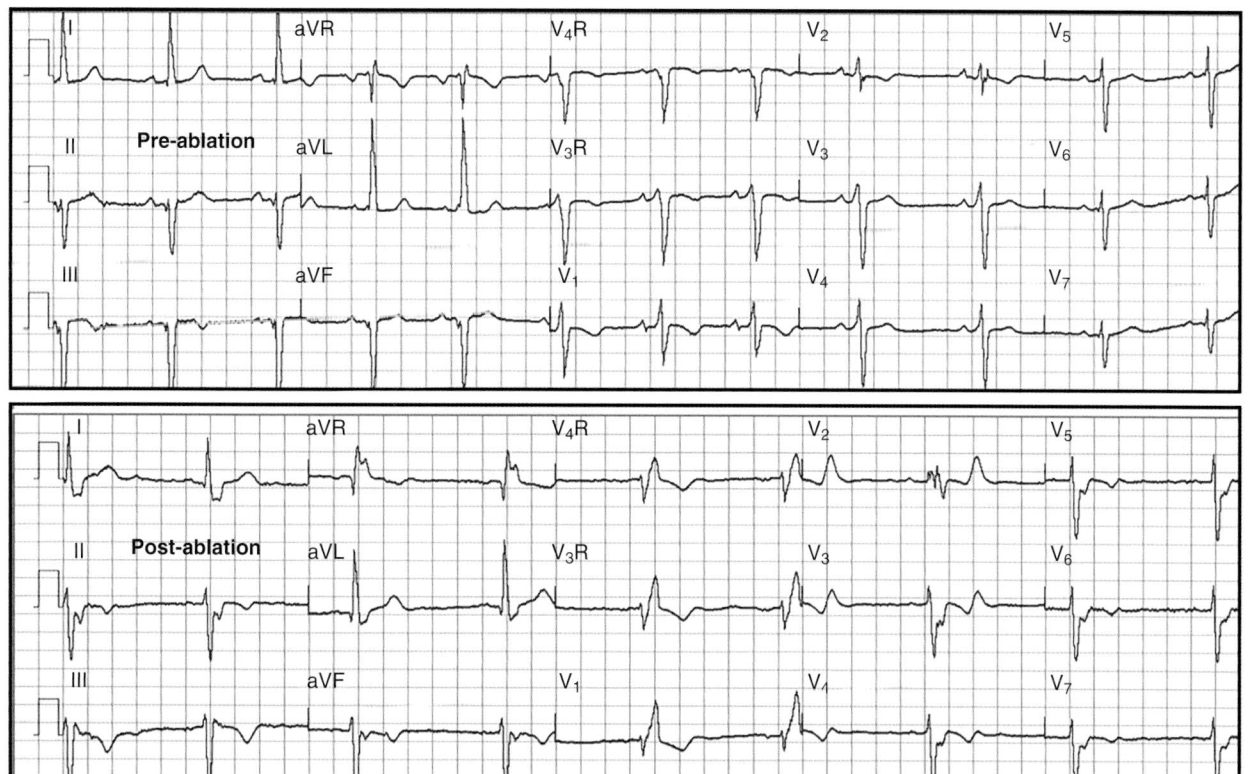

• **Fig. 34.4** Electrocardiograms from a patient with Ebstein anomaly, before and after catheter ablation for Wolff-Parkinson-White syndrome. Note that the pre-ablation QRS is relatively narrow (see leads I, aVR, aVL, and V1) due to fusion of preexcited activation over a right-sided accessory pathway with underlying complete right bundle branch block. Once the preexcitation was eliminated, the right bundle branch block pattern was exposed.

that tend to cluster along the septal and inferior aspects of the AV ring where the leaflet tissue is most abnormal. These APs can be either manifest (i.e., Wolff-Parkinson-White syndrome) or concealed (retrograde-only). Ebstein anomaly is the only form of congenital heart disease with an incidence of APs (10%–38%) that far exceeds that of the general population. As many as 50% of patients with Ebstein anomaly who undergo formal AP mapping will be found to have multiple separate pathways and/or complex AP insertion patterns. Atriofascicular pathways and AV nodal reentrant tachycardia are also quite common in this condition (see Chapter 17). Other notable arrhythmias include monomorphic ventricular tachycardia circuits arising from the congenitally abnormal muscle in the atrialized portion of the RV,[7] as well as acquired atrial flutter or atrial fibrillation that develop in response to abnormal hemodynamics and degenerative atrial remodeling. Catheter ablation of the various arrhythmia substrates in patients with Ebstein anomaly has become a standard approach to the issue. Many centers, including our own, have adopted a policy of routine electrophysiologic study prior to major surgical intervention to detect and eliminate arrhythmia substrates that could be difficult to address postoperatively.[8] Ablation procedures tend to be more challenging than in normal hearts, but improved imaging of fine anatomic details with intracardiac echo has improved ablation outcomes.[9]

Management

For newborns with critical cyanosis, aggressive efforts are needed to support the infant through the period of transitional circulation, including prostaglandins and/or nitric oxide to increase pulmonary blood flow. Many will improve over days and weeks as pulmonary resistance falls.[10] Support with extracorporeal membrane oxygenation may be necessary in severe cases to bridge the period of high pulmonary resistance or stabilize the patient through emergency procedures.[11] Complex surgical interventions, such as closure of the TV orifice using a fenestrated patch with a systemic-to-pulmonary shunt (the *Starnes procedure*), can be considered in extreme cases.[12]

Patients who do well through the neonatal period can be followed medically for some time. Very mild cases can be expected to have a nearly normal life expectancy unless complicated by arrhythmias. Indeed, survival to age 87 years has been reported.[13] Nevertheless, moderate or severe cases who survive infancy are likely to develop difficulties at some point without surgical or electrophysiologic intervention. Natural history data suggest poorer outcome in patients who had significant cyanosis at birth, those who develop heart failure, and those who experience arrhythmias.[14-16] Brain abscess, cerebral emboli, and endocarditis also remain a threat.

Until recently, the surgical options for this disease were somewhat limited, consisting primarily of TV plasty or replacement along with RA and RV wall plication, atrial septal closure, and sometimes a bidirectional Glenn shunt

to unload the right heart. The survival rate was roughly 80% at 20 years using these older techniques.[17,18] Surgery was usually reserved for those with significant symptoms. The introduction of the *cone procedure* by da Silva and colleagues in 2007[19] has had a major impact on the surgical approach to Ebstein anomaly. The goal of this operation is to utilize native TV tissue to create a competent cone-shaped valve with cordal support from the apex of the right ventricle and the base of the cone positioned at the level of the true AV annulus. To accomplish this, the adherent inferior and septal leaflets are carefully separated from the underlying RV endocardium and reshaped into a configuration that restores coaptation (Fig. 34.5). Reduction of the atrialized portion of the right ventricle in conjunction with reduction of the circumference of the TV annulus reduces the effective orifice of the TV closer to an appropriate size for the patient. A Glenn shunt may still be considered in select cases where the effective RV is felt to be too thin walled and dysfunctional to support the entire systemic venous return. Functional outcomes and durability of the cone operation thus far have been quite encouraging,[20-22] even for severe forms of this disease. Operation mortality of less than 1% and medium-term (6-year) survival rates of 98% have now been reported with the cone technique.[23] The threshold for recommending surgery has lowered considerably as a result.

Other Tricuspid Valve Problems

Tricuspid Valve Dysplasia

A dysplastic TV resulting in severe regurgitation is sometimes seen in association with pulmonary atresia and intact ventricular septum (see Chapter 37), and occasionally with critical congenital pulmonary stenosis. It should not be confused with Ebstein anomaly (Fig. 34.6). The distinguishing feature of dysplastic TV is that all three leaflets attach at the level of the true AV annulus. However, abnormal tethering of the valve leaflets by accessory cords restricts leaflet movement in systole resulting in central regurgitation, which often progresses rapidly causing RV and TV annulus dilation.

Functional Tricuspid Regurgitation

Functional tricuspid regurgitation refers to the presence of regurgitation in an otherwise well-formed TV. It is most commonly seen when the right ventricle is subjected to increased workload, such as when it is the systemic ventricle or when there is pulmonary hypertension, either secondary to elevated left atrial pressures or from primary pulmonary hypertension. In children the most common scenario is when the TV is the systemic AV valve as in HLHS. While there is no consistent structural defect in the valve leaflets or subvalve apparatus, the two mechanisms of regurgitation most commonly seen are splaying of the anteroseptal commissure and anterior leaflet prolapse, both associated with

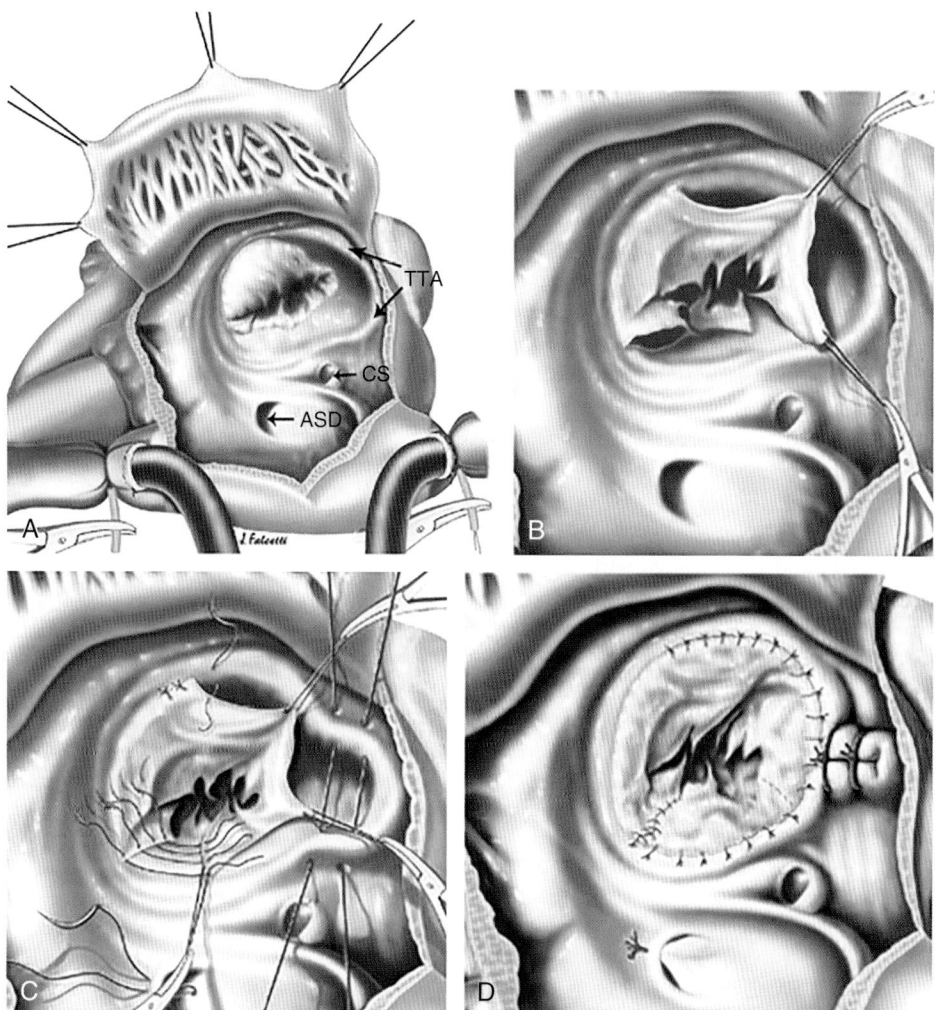

• **Fig. 34.5** The cone operation. **(A)** Opened right atrium showing displaced tricuspid valve. **(B)** Detached part of the anterior and inferior leaflet forming a single piece. **(C)** Clockwise rotation of the inferior leaflet to be sutured to the anterior leaflet septal edge and plication of the true tricuspid annulus. **(D)** Complete valve attachment to the true annulus and closure of the atrial septal defect. *ASD,* Atrial septal defect; *CS,* coronary sinus; *TTA,* true tricuspid annulus. (From da Silva JP, Baumgratz JF, da Fonseca L, et al. The cone reconstruction of the tricuspid valve in Ebstein's anomaly. The operation: early and midterm results. *J Thorac Cardiovas Surg.* 2007;133:215–223. Reproduced with permission).

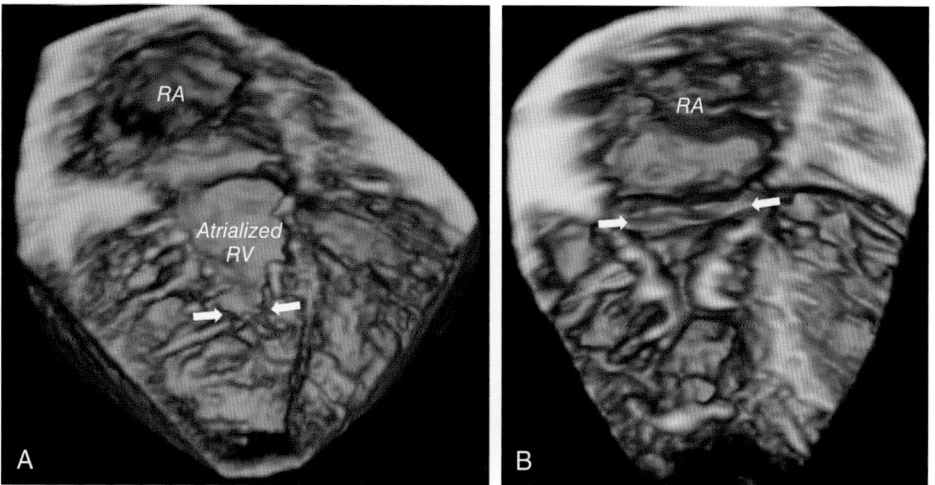

• **Fig. 34.6** Three-dimensional echocardiograms showing the contrast in tricuspid valve anatomy between **(A)** true Ebstein anomaly and **(B)** dysplastic tricuspid valve. The *arrows* mark the level of functional tricuspid valve orifice in the two conditions. *RA,* Right atrium; *RV,* right ventricle.

annular dilation.[24] The higher severity of the TV regurgitation as well as the presence of anterior leaflet prolapse are associated with higher risk of mortality and need for reoperation.

Surgical repair of the TV is indicated for moderate or greater regurgitation, either as a stand-alone procedure or in conjunction with staged palliation for HLHS (see Chapter 35). Surgical techniques include closure of the anteroseptal commissure when a large portion of the regurgitant jet is located in this region, along with annulus reduction. In young infants, suture annuloplasty is most commonly performed, although there is a significant risk of recurrent TV regurgitation, often from re-dilation of the annulus. In older children and adults, insertion of an annuloplasty reinforcing ring has been shown to be superior to simple suture annuloplasty, with the former having a substantially lower risk of need for reintervention. Valve replacement is rarely necessary and is associated with a lower long-term survival than valve repair.

References

1. Schreiber C, Cook A, Ho SY, Augustin N, Anderson RH. Morphologic spectrum of Ebstein's malformation: revisitation relative to surgical repair. *J Thorac Cardiovasc Surg.* 1999;117:148-155.
2. Fujioka T, Kühn A, Sanchez-Martinez S, et al. Impact of interventricular interactions on left ventricular function, stroke volume, and exercise capacity in children and adults with Ebstein's anomaly. *JACC Cardiovasc Imaging.* 2019;12:925-927.
3. Jaiswal PK, Balakrishnan KG, Saha A, Venkitachalam CG, Tharakan J, Titus T. Clinical profile and natural history of Ebstein's anomaly of tricuspid valve. *Int J Cardiol.* 1994;46:113-119.
4. Kumar AE, Fyler DC, Miettinen OS, Nadas AS. Ebstein's anomaly: clinical profile and natural history. *Am J Cardiol.* 1971;28:84-95.
5. Qureshi MY, O'Leary PW, Connolly HM. Cardiac imaging in Ebstein anomaly. *Trends Cardiovasc Med.* 2018;28:403-409.
6. Walsh EP. Ebstein's anomaly of the tricuspid valve: a natural laboratory for reentrant tachycardias. *JACC Clin Electrophysiol.* 2018;4:1271-1288.
7. Moore JP, Shannon KM, Gallotti RG, et al. Catheter ablation of ventricular arrhythmia for Ebstein's anomaly in unoperated and post-surgical patients. *JACC Clin Electrophysiol.* 2018;4:1300-1307.
8. Shivapour JKL, Sherwin ED, Alexander ME, et al. Utility of preoperative electrophysiology studies in patients with Ebstein's anomaly undergoing the cone procedure. *Heart Rhythm.* 2014:11;182-186.
9. El-Assaad I, DeWitt ES, Mah DY, et al. Accessory pathway ablation in Ebstein anomaly: a challenging substrate. *Heart Rhythm.* 2021;18:1844-1851.
10. Freud LR, McElhinney DB, Kalish BT, et al. Risk factors for mortality and circulatory outcome among neonates prenatally diagnosed with Ebstein anomaly or tricuspid valve dysplasia: a multicenter study. *J Am Heart Assoc.* 2020;9:e016684.
11. Carmichael TB, Walsh EP, Roth SJ. Anticipatory use of venoarterial extracorporeal membrane oxygenation for a high-risk interventional cardiac procedure. *Respir Care.* 2002;47:1002-1006.
12. Starnes VA, Pitlick PT, Bernstein D, Griffin ML, Choy M, Shumway NE. Ebstein's anomaly appearing in the neonate: a new surgical approach. *J Thorac Cardiovasc Surg.* 1991;101:1082-1087.
13. Hennebry TA, Calkins HG, Chandra-Strobos N. Successful interventional treatment of an octogenarian presenting with syncope and Ebstein's anomaly of the tricuspid valve. *J Invasive Cardiol.* 2002;14:44-47.
14. Attenhofer Jost CH, Tan NY, Hassan A, et al. Sudden death in patients with Ebstein anomaly. *Eur Heart J.* 2018;39:1970-1977.
15. Celermajer DS, Bull C, Till JA, et al. Ebstein's anomaly: presentation and outcome from fetus to adult. *J Am Coll Cardiol.* 1994;23:170-176.
16. Geerdink LM, Kapusta L. Dealing with Ebstein's anomaly. *Cardiol Young.* 2014;24:191-200.
17. Renfu Z, Zengwei W, Hongyu Z, et al. Experience in corrective surgery for Ebstein's anomaly in 139 patients. *J Heart Valve Dis.* 2001;10:396-398.
18. Chauvaud S, Berrebi A, d'Attellis N, Mousseaux E, Hernigou A, Carpentier A. Ebstein's anomaly: repair based on functional analysis. *Eur J Cardiothorac Surg.* 2003;23:525-531.
19. da Silva JP, Baumgratz JF, da Fonseca L, et al. The cone reconstruction of the tricuspid valve in Ebstein's anomaly. The operation: early and midterm results. *J Thorac Cardiovasc Surg.* 2007;133:215-223.
20. Vogel M, Marx GR, Tworetzky W, et al. Ebstein's malformation of the tricuspid valve: short-term outcomes of the "cone procedure" versus conventional surgery. *Congenit Heart Dis.* 2012;7:50-58.
21. Sainathan S, da Fonseca da Silva L, da Silva JP. Ebstein's anomaly: contemporary management strategies. *J Thorac Dis.* 2020;12:1161-1173.
22. Del Nido PJ. Commentary: cone reconstruction for Ebstein's anomaly is here to stay. *J Thorac Cardiovasc Surg.* 2021;161:1110-1111.
23. Schulz A, Marathe SP, Chávez M, et al. The association of age and repair modification with outcome after cone repair for Ebstein's malformation. *Semin Thorac Cardiovasc Surg.* 2022;34:205-212.
24. Bautista-Hernandez V, Brown DW, Loyola H, et al. Mechanisms of tricuspid regurgitation in patients with hypoplastic left heart syndrome undergoing tricuspid valvuloplasty. *J Thorac Cardiovasc Surg.* 2014;148:832-840.

35

Hypoplastic Left Heart Syndrome

JOSHUA W. SALVIN AND PETER LANG

KEY LEARNING POINTS

- Hypoplastic left heart syndrome (HLHS) is a rare congenital heart defect responsible for significant morbidity and mortality in the neonatal period.
- At birth, survival is dependent on both a patent ductus arteriosus to allow systemic perfusion from the right ventricle to the aorta and a nonrestrictive atrial-level communication to allow adequate mixing.
- The goals of palliation include establishment of an unobstructed pathway from the right ventricle to the aorta, limiting pulmonary blood flow with preservation of pulmonary artery architecture, and relief of pulmonary venous obstruction.
- The Single Ventricle Reconstruction Trial compared clinical outcomes in patients undergoing stage 1 palliation with a

Sano shunt versus the traditional Blalock-Thomas-Taussig shunt. It demonstrated some benefit in 12-month transplant-free survival in the Sano group.[1] At 6-year follow-up, however, there was no survival benefit, and the Sano group required more catheter interventions.[2]
- Overall survival in HLHS has improved due to the use of prostaglandin, prenatal diagnosis and diagnostic technologies, innovations in surgical and catheter-based interventions, advancements in postoperative management, and enhanced interstage follow-up. With improved survival, focus is now on optimizing neurodevelopmental outcomes, functional outcomes, and quality of life.

Definition

The term *hypoplastic left heart syndrome* (HLHS) describes a syndrome in which there is a diminutive left ventricle (LV) with underdevelopment of the mitral and aortic valves.[3] Because of its small size, the LV is incapable of supporting the systemic circulation.

Some patients have mitral and/or aortic stenosis, but most have aortic or mitral atresia. A rare subtype includes aortic atresia with a nearly normal-sized LV. These cases are not proper examples of HLHS. Similarly, cases of mitral atresia with a double-outlet right ventricle (DORV) are not examples of HLHS, nor are those rare instances of mitral atresia with L-malpositioned ventricles.

Prevalence and Genetics

HLHS is the most common form of functional univentricular heart disease, with an incidence of approximately 2–3 cases per 10,000 live births, and accounts for 2–3% of all congenital heart diseases. A male predominance (male-to-female ratio approximately 1.5:1) is observed in most population-based and clinical studies.[4,5] Despite a low prevalence, HLHS is responsible for 25–40% of all neonatal cardiac deaths. There may be genetic factors linked to the development of HLHS, with a recurrence risk in

subsequent siblings reported at 8%.[6,7] The majority of cases, however, are non-syndromic. The incidence of prematurity and associated extracardiac anomalies is low.

Anatomy

There are several important classifications of HLHS.[8] In each type, the LV is underdeveloped and the aortic valve is often atretic and hypoplastic, although some neonates have severe stenosis. Similarly, the mitral valve may be hypoplastic, severely stenotic, or atretic. The ascending aorta is hypoplastic. Above an atretic aortic valve, the diameter of the aorta may be 2 mm or less but sufficient to supply adequate coronary circulation in a retrograde fashion. The left atrium is small, reflecting the limited blood flow *in utero*. The atrial septum is thickened; the foramen ovale may be small and, occasionally, may be closed. A patent ductus arteriosus (PDA) is required for survival (Fig. 35.1). Anomalies of the brain have associated with HLHS.[9]

Physiology

Fetal Circulation

In HLHS, as in most forms of congenital heart disease, the intrauterine circulation is adequate to meet many of the

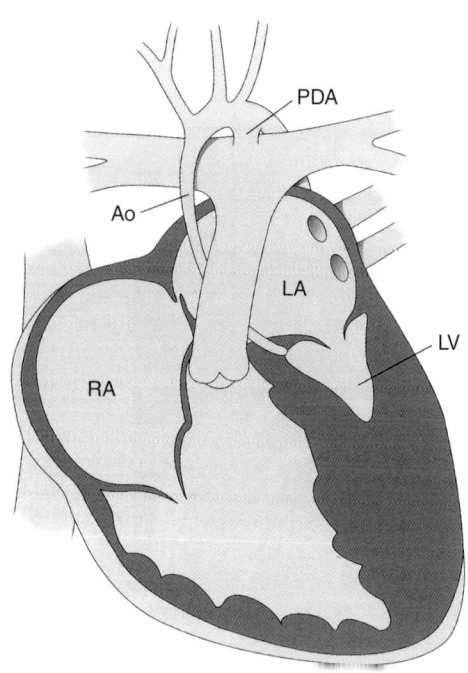

• **Fig. 35.1** Drawing of the anatomy of the hypoplastic left heart syndrome. Note the tiny ascending aorta *(Ao)* that supplies the coronary circulation in a retrograde direction. No blood passes through the diminutive left ventricle *(LV)*. The left atrium *(LA)* empties through an incompetent foramen ovale into the right atrium *(RA)*, where all systemic and pulmonary venous blood becomes mixed. The ductus arteriosus *(PDA)* supplies the entire circulation to the body. (From Nadas AS, Fyler DC, eds. *Nadas' Pediatric Cardiology*. Philadelphia: Hanley & Belfus, 1992.)

needs of the developing fetus. *In utero*, all circulation, with the exception of the small amount of pulmonary venous return, passes through the right side of the heart. Streams of superior and inferior vena cava blood return to the right atrium and join the pulmonary venous return (5% to 10% of the cardiac output). The complete admixture of all venous return (that from the placenta as well as the fetus) results in blood flow with identical oxygen saturation to all parts of the fetus. The right atrial return then crosses the tricuspid valve (TV) to the right ventricle (RV). The lack of LV contribution to cardiac output results in modest RV volume overload.

At this point in the fetal circulation, certain physiological questions emerge, even *in utero*. The relative flow to the pulmonary or systemic circulation is largely dependent on the relative resistance of the pulmonary and systemic vascular beds. Of equal importance is the status of the pulmonary venous return. In the face of mitral valve atresia, or even severe mitral valve stenosis, an obstructive interatrial septum can result in left atrial hypertension. Even though pulmonary blood flow is low *in utero*, altered intrauterine pulmonary venous pressure might be the best explanation for the abnormal muscularization of the pulmonary veins and lymphatic congestion seen in these patients. Similarly, the abnormal atrial septal thickness may be caused by fetal left atrial hypertension.

There is less speculation about the fetal circulation beyond the ductus arteriosus (DA). It is common to see a posterior aortic ridge of tissue opposite the insertion site of the DA; systemic blood flow bifurcates at this point. In cases of aortic valve atresia, in which the sole source of systemic blood flow is from the DA, the aortic arch becomes progressively smaller between ductal insertion and the coronary arteries. Sometimes the origin of the left subclavian artery is intercalated with ductal tissue, and it may become stenotic with time. The ascending aorta, carrying retrograde flow, is an end artery (a common coronary artery) and is frequently 2 mm or less in diameter. This small size is appropriate for the coronary flow required by the newborn heart. It must be remembered, however, that coronary blood flow is dependent on a long unobstructed path from the RV to the ascending aorta via the DA.

Novel therapies have evolved for fetuses with HLHS. In patients with severe aortic stenosis, fetal aortic balloon valvuloplasty aims to decrease the LV pressure load *in utero*; this may promote left heart growth and prevent formation of endocardial fibrosis. Patient selection is limited to those likely to have evolving sequalae of LV outflow tract obstruction (i.e., moderate LV dysfunction, retrograde arch flow, altered patent foramen ovale (PFO) flow, and monophasic mitral valve inflow). Patients considered for fetal aortic valvuloplasty must also demonstrate a capacity for LV recovery following the procedure. Technically successful fetal aortic balloon valvuloplasty may result in biventricular circulation in a subset of cases. Another subset of fetuses with HLHS in which fetal intervention has been attempted are those with an intact atrial septum or restrictive atrial septal defect (ASD). The rationale for fetal intervention in these patients is to prevent neonatal hypoxia and/or circulatory collapse, and to prevent worsening of the lung disease that occurs as a result of *in utero* pulmonary venous hypertension. Current data suggest that survival to hospital discharge is similar in patients who undergo fetal intervention on the atrial septum *in utero* compared with high-risk patients who undergo only postnatal intervention. Additional work in this novel area of fetal intervention is necessary.[10]

Transitional Circulation

With an atretic aortic valve, survival beyond birth is dependent on the RV supplying both the pulmonary and the systemic circulations via a PDA. The coronary arteries and brachiocephalic vessels are supplied in retrograde fashion. The relative flow to the pulmonary and systemic circuits depends on the relative resistances of the two vascular beds. One of the major influences on total pulmonary resistance is the size of the interatrial communication. A restrictive ASD tends to raise left atrial pressure and total pulmonary resistance which limits pulmonary blood flow, whereas a nonrestrictive atrial communication does not.

There is a nearly direct relationship between the amount of pulmonary blood flow and the systemic arterial oxygen saturation. The greater the pulmonary blood flow, the greater

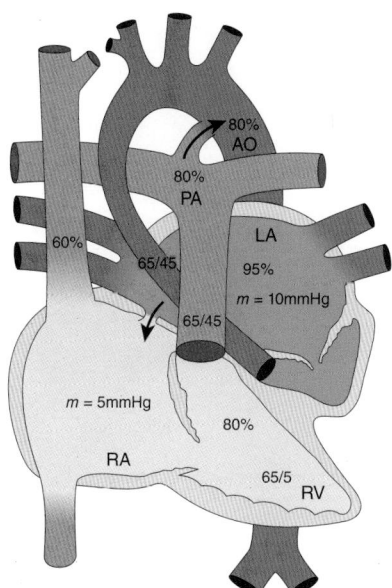

• **Fig. 35.2** Diagram showing ideal preoperative physiology. Low systemic vascular resistance and high pulmonary vascular resistance result in a Q_p/Q_s of approximately 1. (From Nadas AS, Fyler DC, eds. *Nadas' Pediatric Cardiology*. Philadelphia: Hanley & Belfus, 1992.)

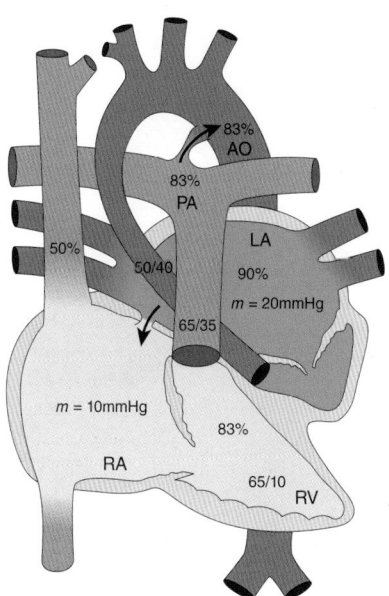

• **Fig. 35.3** Diagram showing closing ductus physiology: decreased systemic blood flow, poor coronary perfusion, increased pulmonary blood flow, and the Q_p/Q_s is approximately 3. There is an increase in right ventricular volume overloading, right ventricular end-diastolic pressure, and left atrial pressure. There is right ventricular dysfunction. (From Nadas AS, Fyler DC, eds. *Nadas' Pediatric Cardiology*. Philadelphia: Hanley & Belfus, 1992.)

the quantity of oxygenated pulmonary venous blood that will return to the heart and mix with the systemic venous return (Fig. 35.2). Neonates with completely unrestrictive pulmonary blood flow are likely to have to severe congestive heart failure secondary to RV volume overload, whereas those individuals with some resistance to pulmonary blood flow will have preserved systemic perfusion.

At birth, if the DA is widely patent and the pulmonary arteriolar resistance is relatively high, a brief honeymoon period may exist. A large PDA does not restrict systemic blood flow at a normal RV systolic pressure. In the absence of ductal constriction, it is unusual to have narrowing of the aortic arch, ensuring good coronary and renal perfusion. A modestly restrictive foramen ovale limits pulmonary blood flow to some extent. More importantly, the elevation in pulmonary arteriolar resistance typically seen in the newborn period maintains pulmonary blood flow at manageable levels. The moderate limitation in pulmonary blood flow caused by the relatively high resistance is not enough to produce dangerously low systemic arterial oxygen saturation (Fig. 35.2).

Unfortunately, this ideal state of physiologic palliation is short-lived. Although infants diagnosed *in utero* receive medical care during this period, neonates without a prenatal diagnosis of HLHS often pass through this honeymoon period without recognition. They behave normally and, unless their duskiness is questioned or captured on pre-discharge screening for congenital heart disease, are often thought to be well.

Two normal physiologic events conspire to bring neonates with a postnatal diagnosis of hypoplastic left heart to medical attention: the PDA begins to close and pulmonary vascular resistance decreases. Partial closure of the DA has several profound effects. The first, and the most obvious, is

the alteration in the relative resistances of blood flow to the systemic and pulmonary circulation. A decrease in systemic output in a newborn has many manifestations; the child's color may be poor despite a rise in the systemic oxygen saturation, the peripheral pulses are weak with a narrow pulse pressure and clinical evidence of poor end-organ perfusion, and the child may become lethargic. Concomitant with these changes is an absolute and relative increase in pulmonary blood flow. The major manifestation of this change is tachypnea, with an inability to breathe and eat at the same time. The force feeding of the pulmonary circulation by the closure of the DA is abetted by the normal fall in pulmonary resistance. The relaxation of the pulmonary bed, which may be seen even in the first day of life,[11] may be tempered by the development of acidosis secondary to poor cardiac output.

Usually the end result of progressive DA closure and decreasing pulmonary vascular resistance is profound cardiogenic shock. The decreased systemic blood flow is accompanied by poor coronary perfusion. Thus, the RV may have an increased pressure load (secondary to ductal constriction), an increased volume load (secondary to increased pulmonary blood flow), and jeopardized myocardial oxygen delivery. RV dysfunction and dilation results in tricuspid regurgitation (TR) which exacerbates volume overload. Finally, the increased pulmonary blood flow, with restricted egress from the left atrium, increases pulmonary venous pressure, contributing to the progression of cardiogenic shock and respiratory collapse (Fig. 35.3). Children with postnatal diagnosis of HLHS have high rates of morbidity and mortality.[12]

Before the introduction of prostaglandin E_1 (PGE1), a child in profound cardiogenic shock secondary to HLHS

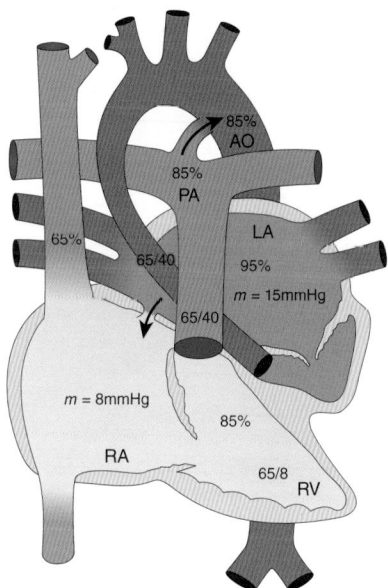

• **Fig. 35.4** Diagram showing acceptable physiology. The Q_p/Q_s is approximately 2. There is mild right ventricular volume overloading (approximately three times that of normal), a mild increase in right ventricular end-diastolic pressure, and a mild increase in left atrial pressure. (From Nadas AS, Fyler DC, eds. *Nadas' Pediatric Cardiology*. Philadelphia: Hanley & Belfus, 1992.)

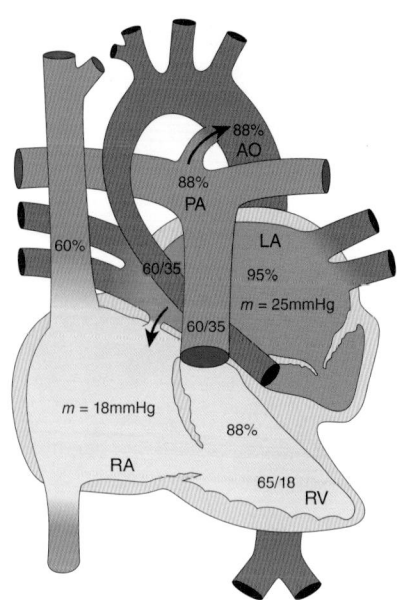

• **Fig. 35.5** Diagram of the low pulmonary resistance physiology. The Q_p/Q_s is approximately 4. There is severe right ventricular volume overloading (approximately five times that of normal), an increase in right ventricular end-diastolic pressure, an increase in left atrial pressure, poor systemic perfusion, low urine output, acidosis, poor right ventricular performance, right ventricular dilation, and tricuspid regurgitation. (From Nadas AS, Fyler DC, eds. *Nadas' Pediatric Cardiology*. Philadelphia: Hanley & Belfus, 1992.)

died quickly, often before surgical intervention could be mobilized. Although some children did survive to undergo palliative surgery, they were a select few whose systemic circulation was maintained by a persistent PDA. With the use of PGE1, the DA almost invariably reopens. Once an unobstructed pathway from the RV to the aortic arch has been secured, support for the RV is needed. Usually, the ventricle has suffered from a period of relative ischemia secondary to poor coronary perfusion; indeed, RV infarctions have been seen occasionally. In addition, the ventricle has had both a pressure and a volume overload and may have been deprived of adequate metabolic substrate because of hypoglycemia and hypocalcemia. Renal failure may result in an additional fluid overload and hyperkalemia. Finally, hepatic insufficiency, a frequent finding in the setting of low systemic output, may exacerbate the problems of hypoglycemia and acidosis. Inotropic support of the RV must be dosed thoughtfully so as to maintain optimal balance of systemic and pulmonary vascular resistance, support end-organ recovery, and minimize drug toxicity.

The physiologic state following resuscitation is never quite as ideal as that seen shortly after birth (Fig. 35.4). The relative resistance of the pulmonary and systemic circuits will have changed over the first days of life and that change may be influenced by the systemic and pulmonary vasodilatory properties of PGE1, the patient's clinical state, and medical management strategies. The overall pulmonary-to-systemic flow ratio is likely to be at least 2, with resulting systemic arterial oxygen saturation in the range of 85%. Consequently, the RV needs to pump three times the normal volume in order to maintain an adequate systemic cardiac output. An increase in RV end-diastolic pressure is a

usual finding. Excessive pulmonary blood flow results in a volume load to the left atrium. Obstruction to atrial outflow results in pulmonary venous hypertension.

All of this is relatively acceptable, but this transitional circulation is not stable. With the passage of hours and improvement in metabolic derangements, there is a continued decrease in pulmonary vascular resistance. Because the relative resistance of the pulmonary and systemic circulations determines the relative flows to the two circuits, when the maximum volume capacity of the RV is reached, there is a decrease in systemic output. This time, the low output state is not a function of ductal obstruction, but simply a product of the inability of the RV to meet the ever increasing volume demand caused by a decreasing pulmonary vascular resistance. The result of all of this is a continuation of the earlier evolution of the transitional circulatory changes. There is severe RV volume overloading, the RV end-diastolic pressure rises, and ventricular dilation results in TR, further worsening the volume load. Once again, poor systolic perfusion may result in acidosis and end-organ injury. Left atrial hypertension will impair gas exchange and, in all probability, necessitate intubation and assisted ventilation (Fig. 35.5).

Diagnosis and Clinical Manifestations

The diagnosis of HLHS is made by echocardiogram in the prenatal period in 50–75% of the cases during routine screening ultrasound between 18 and 24 weeks' gestation. Prenatal diagnosis allows for counseling, planning delivery at a cardiac center, or termination of pregnancy.[13]

The timing and severity of presentation in neonates who are not diagnosed prenatally is dependent upon the presence of a PDA and an ASD. Due to right-to-left flow across the PDA and mixing of oxygenated and deoxygenated blood, most neonates with HLHS will have an abnormal postductal saturation on pulse oximetry. For neonates not diagnosed prenatally, pulse oximetry screening may be more sensitive for detecting HLHS than physical examination alone.[14] Frequently, no murmur is heard. If there is an adequate ASD, the baby may present with cyanosis or tachypnea. As the DA closes, or in the case of an inadequate ASD, the infant suffers circulatory collapse, becoming gray and dusky. There are no palpable pulses. The infant is resuscitated, infusion of PGE1 is begun, and the baby is transferred immediately to the nearest pediatric cardiac center.

Electrocardiography

Although, statistically, the electrocardiogram (ECG) in infants with HLHS tends to show less than the usual LV voltages for a newborn infant, this feature is not helpful because many normal newborns also have this pattern. The ECG of an infant with HLHS usually shows slightly more RV hypertrophy than normal. Other nonspecific findings on ECG include a longer PR interval, wider QRS complex, and absent Q waves in the lateral precordial leads. Approximately 20% of neonates with HLHS, however, present with normal ECG findings.

Chest Radiography

There is little about the chest radiograph that is specific to this disease. The size of the heart and the amount of pulmonary vasculature are variable; the heart may be very large and the pulmonary vasculature increased.

Echocardiography

HLHS is diagnosed in detail by echocardiography (Fig. 35.6). The abnormal mitral and aortic valves, the diminutive LV, and the hypoplastic ascending aorta, as well as the flow of blood from the left atrium to the right, are readily identified and confirm the diagnosis. The coronary arteries are supplied from a tiny ascending aorta, often only a few millimeters in diameter. Doppler imaging may reveal retrograde flow in the ascending aorta. The left atrium is small and the atrial septum typically bulges toward the right. An absent or hypoplastic mitral valve is recognized and the diminutive LV is often visualized. The DA is large and carries blood from the pulmonary artery to the aorta.

The atretic or hypoplastic mitral valve and the hypoplastic LV can be seen in subxiphoid or apical views. Doppler examination of the mitral valve is useful to determine if it is atretic. A potential pitfall in evaluating LV size results from the tendency for the LV long-axis dimension to be reduced before the short-axis dimension. If the LV is evaluated using two-dimensional echocardiography in short-axis projection only, the severity of hypoplasia can be underestimated.

Parasternal and suprasternal views are best for imaging the hypoplastic ascending aorta and aortic arch. The point of juncture of the DA and the arch is often narrow, with a discrete coarctation being present.

The atrial septum can be imaged using subxiphoid views. The TV function should be evaluated with Doppler technique

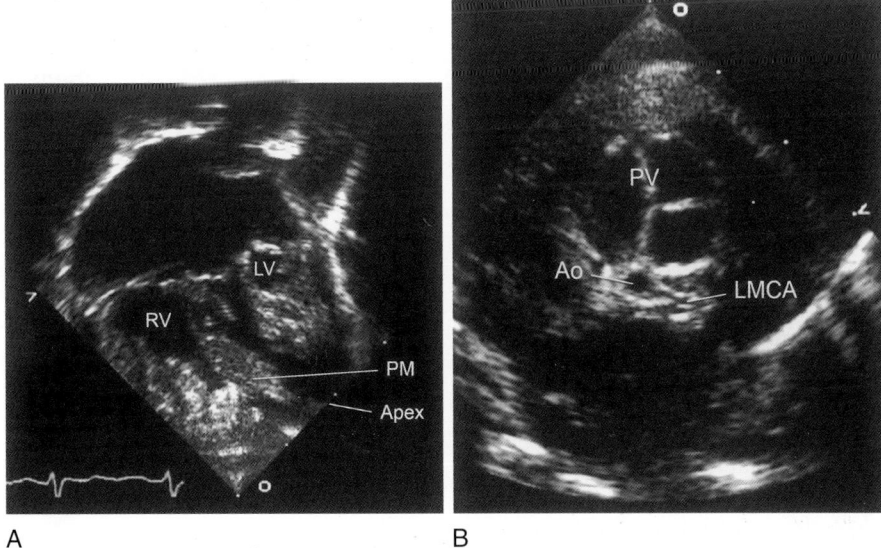

• **Fig. 35.6** Echocardiographic images in newborn with hypoplastic left heart syndrome. (A) The apical four-chamber view shows the large, apex-forming right ventricle (RV) containing hypertrophied papillary muscles (PM). The diminutive chamber of the left ventricle (LV) extends only a fraction of the heart length. (B) In parasternal short-axis views, the tiny ascending aorta (Ao) giving rise to the left main coronary artery (LMCA) is seen to lie directly posterior to the very large pulmonary valve (PV).

from apical and parasternal views, noting that TR occurs in a significant proportion of patients. RV function can be evaluated using subxiphoid views.

Cardiac Catheterization

Cardiac catheterization is rarely necessary in the newborn period, except in those with a virtually intact atrial septum. In those cases, it is undertaken to create a septal defect to relieve left atrial hypertension and pulmonary edema before the stage I surgical procedure.[15] Although patients typically undergo catheterization at age 4–6 months prior to the bidirectional Glenn or hemi-Fontan operations, long-term outcomes of low-risk patients undergoing MRI in lieu of catheterization are favorable and catheterization may be deferred.[16] Catheterization remains a standard procedure before the Fontan operation. Goals of pre-Fontan catheterization include a careful assessment of Glenn pressure, RV end-diastolic pressure, and calculation of pulmonary vascular resistance. The architecture of the branch pulmonary arteries and aorta are investigated angiographically, and abnormalities may be addressed in the lab or planned for the time of surgery. Coil occlusion of aortico-pulmonary collaterals may be performed. Pulmonary angiography may reveal arteriovenous malformations which guides post-Fontan expectations.

Management

Most infants with an adequate ASD and PDA arrive at a cardiac center receiving PGE1. The goal of therapy is to ensure a balance of oxygen demand to oxygen delivery. When this balance is not met, the use of inotropic agents, controlled mechanical ventilation, and anesthetics is necessary. Inotropic agents at low doses, such as an epinephrine infusion, aid in RV contractility. Controlled mechanical ventilation may modulate pulmonary vascular resistance. The Fio_2 should be reduced to as close to 0.21 as possible to maintain an arterial Po_2 of 35–40 mm Hg. The Pco_2 should be allowed to rise to 40 mm Hg in an attempt to maintain a pH of 7.35 to 7.40. Positive end-expiratory pressure may also be beneficial in increasing total pulmonary resistance. Narcotics and chemical paralysis may be used to limit oxygen demand. The desired result of these maneuvers is improved RV contractility, appropriate balance of pulmonary-to-systemic blood flow (Qp/Qs), mitigation of RV volume load, decreased metabolic demand, and thus improved oxygen delivery to end-organs.

A small subgroup of patients requires separate consideration. Rarely, the interatrial communication can be so obstructive that left atrial hypertension limits pulmonary blood flow to levels which do not permit adequate oxygenation despite the medical maneuvers described above. In this case, the Po_2 may be below 20 mm Hg. In this setting, rapid relief of the pulmonary venous obstruction by an emergency atrial septostomy with or without stent placement at catheterization is indicated.[15]

Surgical Palliation

Most patients with HLHS undergo a series of three-staged palliative procedures which include stage 1 (Norwood or Sano modification), bidirectional Glenn or hemi-Fontan, and the Fontan operation. Based on the initial attempts to manage HLHS, the following goals for successful palliation were established. First is the need to establish a permanent unobstructed communication between the RV and the aorta with preservation of RV function. Second is the necessity of limiting pulmonary blood flow with preservation of pulmonary artery architecture. The third goal is to relieve pulmonary venous obstruction (Fig. 35.7).

The stage 1 procedure developed by Norwood satisfies the goals for initial palliation and subsequent repair of children with HLHS.[17] Minimal prosthetic material is used in both the systemic and pulmonary circulations, allowing for maximal potential growth. The prosthetic aortopulmonary shunt placed at the time of initial palliation is removed at the time of subsequent palliative shunts. The first-stage operation consists of transection of the distal main pulmonary artery. The aorta, from the takeoff of the left subclavian artery to the ascending aorta, is incised, and an anastomosis is established between the proximal main pulmonary artery and the ascending aorta and the aortic arch. This connection is almost always augmented with homograft tissue in order to avoid arch obstruction. Pulmonary blood flow can be established by a modified Blalock-Thomas-Taussig shunt (mBTTS), a central shunt, or RV to distal main pulmonary artery shunt (Fig. 35.8). The latter modification, popularized

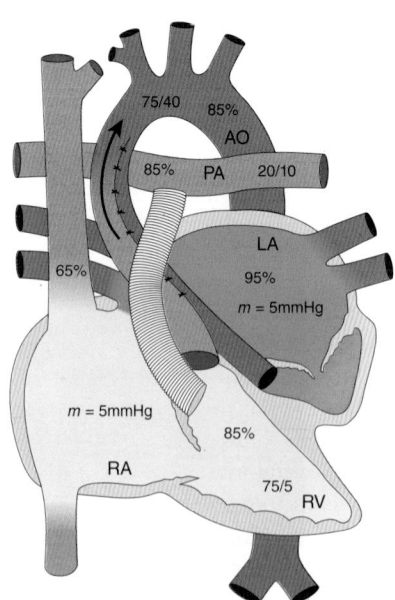

• **Fig. 35.7** Diagram showing ideal postoperative physiology. Widely patent pathway from the right ventricle to the aorta, limitation of pulmonary blood flow without distortion to the pulmonary arteries, unrestricted pulmonary venous return, normal-sized right ventricle, and normal tricuspid valve. (From Nadas AS, Fyler DC, eds. *Nadas' Pediatric Cardiology*. Philadelphia: Hanley & Belfus, 1992.)

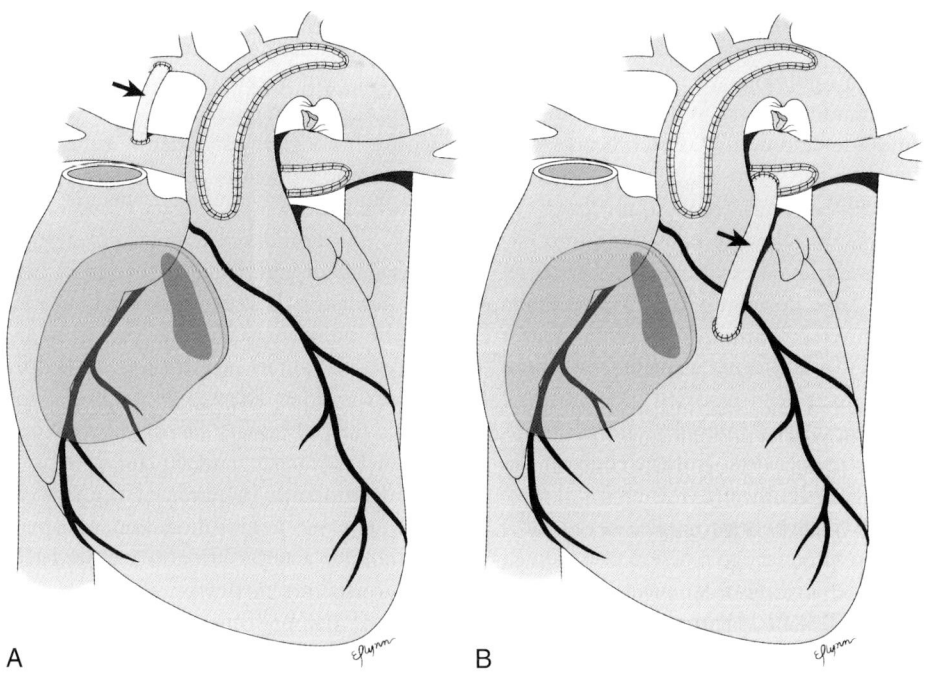

• **Fig. 35.8** Drawing showing pulmonary blood supplied by (A) modified Blalock-Taussig shunt *(arrow)* and (B) right ventricle-to-pulmonary artery shunt *(arrow)*.

by Sano, has the disadvantage of a small systemic ventriculotomy, but the advantage of avoiding diastolic pulmonary artery run-off which can compete with flow to the small ascending aorta and the coronary arteries.[18] This stage of the operation is completed by ligating the DA and opening the atrial septum.

The first randomized controlled trial in congenital heart surgery was designed to compare outcomes for the stage 1 Norwood approach versus the stage 1 with Sano modification. Transplant-free survival was higher at 12 months following a Sano shunt than mBTTS; however, there were more complications in the Sano group.[1] By 6 years, there was no difference in transplant-free survival between the Sano versus mBTTS groups.[2]

Surgical Complications

There are numerous potential challenges after stage 1 palliation. Some relate primarily to the underlying anatomic defect, some to the physiologic derangements associated with the circulatory collapse that first signaled the presence of heart disease, and some to the surgery.

The atrial septum is thicker and more leftward in orientation than it is in healthy individuals. It is not readily amenable to balloon septostomy. If obstructive, catheter-directed septostomy, often stabilized with a stent, is performed preoperatively to achieve left atrial decompression for stabilization before surgery.[15] At surgery, septectomy is an integral part of the initial palliative operation in all. Even with purported wide excision of atrial septal tissue, obstruction to flow has developed (Fig. 35.9). Because pulmonary venous hypertension can adversely affect the development of the pulmonary vascular bed, a restrictive ASD should be treated aggressively.

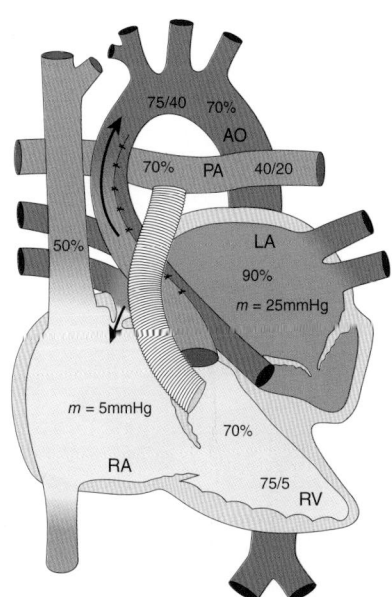

• **Fig. 35.9** Diagram showing restrictive atrial septal defect physiology. The Q_p/Q_s is approximately 1. There is pulmonary artery hypertension due to high left atrial pressure and decreased oxygen saturation caused by low Q_p/Q_s and pulmonary venous desaturation. (From Nadas AS, Fyler DC, eds. *Nadas' Pediatric Cardiology*. Philadelphia: Hanley & Belfus, 1992.)

Postoperative development of obstruction to flow across the interatrial septum may be subtle. Increasing cyanosis before the time when the child should be outgrowing the systemic-to-pulmonary shunt might be the first indication that there is a problem. The intensity of the shunt murmur may decrease as pulmonary artery pressure increases subsequent to pulmonary venous hypertension. Two-dimensional echocardiography may provide a definitive diagnosis of the problem; however, cardiac catheterization may be required.

Progressive stenosis of the pulmonary veins may be associated with extreme left atrial hypoplasia. Whether this occurs because of ongoing underdevelopment of the left heart structures, progressive mediastinal fibrosis, or inflammatory difficulties based on the initial surgery remains unclear.

The next level of concern following palliative surgery is the status of the TV. As mentioned earlier, the RV carries an excess volume and may have been subjected to metabolic and ischemic injury prior to palliation. Thus, some degree of TR may be expected. In addition, intrinsic/congenital abnormalities of the TV have been reported in a subset of patients which may require surgical intervention. A regurgitant TV often requires reintervention, and the effect of TR on early and late mortality is significant.

The RV myocardium may fare poorly regardless of the status of the TV. RV dysfunction secondary to a period of ischemia, acidosis, or severe volume loading may preclude normal (or even adequate) functional status. Ventriculocoronary connections may play a role in poor RV function in HLHS. Thick-walled coronary arteries and myocardial fibrillar disarray have been demonstrated in a subset of these patients, particularly those with a patent LV inflow and obstructed LV outflow tract (i.e., patients with mitral stenosis and aortic atresia). The potentially deleterious effect of the ventriculotomy if the RV to pulmonary artery shunt is used to supply pulmonary blood flow is an important consideration.

The development of recoarctation following stage 1 palliation for HLHS is a known complication (Fig. 35.10). The etiology of postoperative arch obstruction is likely multifactorial and includes constriction of ductal tissue in the arch, patch material, and surgical manipulation. Current practice is to perform an augmented aortic arch reconstruction with an extensive homograft patch at the time of initial palliation.[11] If recoarctation develops, the resulting increase in RV pressure and the increased pulmonary blood flow will produce symptoms; the diminished femoral pulses may provide diagnosis. Management with balloon dilation in the cardiac catheterization laboratory has been successful.

The pulmonary vascular bed must evolve normally if a successful Fontan operation is to be performed when the patient is older. The excess of blood volume and pressure to which the pulmonary vasculature is exposed must be kept in mind. Pulmonary vascular disease may be as devastating as RV dysfunction in terms of the subsequent suitability of a patient for a modified Fontan operation. Undistorted pulmonary arteries are also required (Fig. 35.11). Central pulmonary artery deformity may result when a long segment of the proximal main pulmonary artery is used in reconstructing the ascending aorta. Residual constricting ductal tissue may produce obstruction at the point of insertion of the DA into the origin of the left pulmonary artery. Severe narrowing at the takeoff of the proximal left pulmonary artery may be seen in those cases. Finally the point of insertion of the aortopulmonary shunt may cause distortion of the pulmonary artery. These potential complications must be considered at the time of initial palliation.

While a right mBTTS may provide a favorable regulation of overall pulmonary blood flow, the distribution to

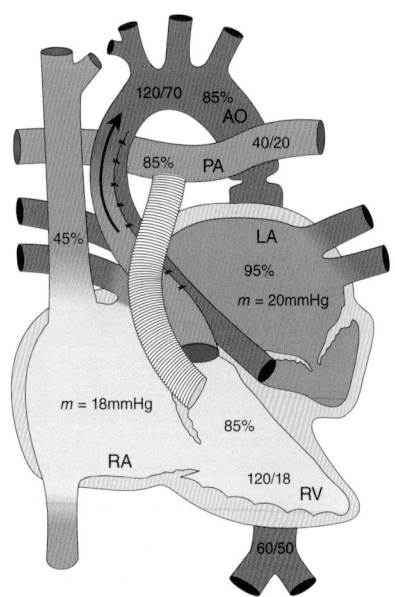

• **Fig. 35.10** Diagram showing coarctation physiology. The Q_p/Q_s is approximately 4. There is increased right ventricular end-diastolic pressure because of decreased ventricular function and tricuspid regurgitation, pulmonary artery hypertension due to increased pulmonary flow, and increased left atrial pressure. (From Nadas AS, Fyler DC, eds. *Nadas' Pediatric Cardiology*. Philadelphia: Hanley & Belfus, 1992.)

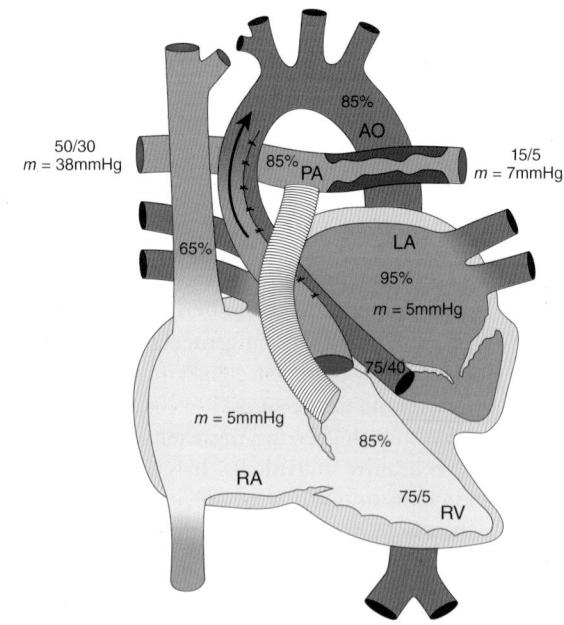

• **Fig. 35.11** Diagram showing distorted pulmonary artery physiology. The Q_p/Q_s is approximately 2. There is right pulmonary artery hypertension and left pulmonary artery hypoplasia because of low flow. (From Nadas AS, Fyler DC, eds. *Nadas' Pediatric Cardiology*. Philadelphia: Hanley & Belfus, 1992.)

right and left lungs is not symmetric. The usual 2:1 (ipsilateral: contralateral) distribution of blood flow that occurs following a mBTTS is exaggerated by whatever degree of proximal left pulmonary artery obstruction is present. This combination of factors can lead to potential right pulmonary artery hypertension and left pulmonary artery hypoplasia. Once again, the adverse effects on a subsequent Fontan operation are substantial. A potential benefit of the RV-to-pulmonary artery shunt as a source of pulmonary blood flow is the more central location of the distal anastomosis; a more symmetric distribution of pulmonary blood flow is often seen.

Hybrid Strategies

An alternative strategy to the stage 1 palliation in the neonatal period is a hybrid approach in which the atrial septum is stented, the branch pulmonary arteries are banded, and a PDA is maintained with PGE1 or a stent. In some institutions, this approach is more often undertaken in neonates with significant comorbidities such as prematurity or cerebral hemorrhage that would put them at greater risk for cardiopulmonary bypass. Recent data suggest that this approach has comparable outcomes to the traditional stage 1 palliation.[19,20] The hybrid approach can be followed by a surgical stage 1 palliation, or a comprehensive bidirectional Glenn shunt.

Management After Initial Palliation

The initial surgical palliation must allow the patient to accommodate to the changes in pulmonary arteriolar resistance that occur during the first weeks of life, as well as support the infant's doubling or tripling of body size in the first few months. Indeed, cardiopulmonary bypass (with or without a period of circulatory arrest), general anesthesia, and neuromuscular blockade, followed by a period of intensive pharmacological support and mechanical ventilation, all have profound effects on the pulmonary vasculature. It is not unusual to have an anatomically large shunt appear to be physiologically small immediately following cardiopulmonary bypass. Within hours, there may be a profound lowering of the pulmonary arteriolar resistance that alters the physiology again. The RV often requires a significant degree of inotropic support in the days following surgery. Following hospital discharge, the use of digoxin, ACE inhibitors, and diuretics is thought to be beneficial.

The status of the interatrial septum, RV and TV function, aortic arch reconstruction, and the pulmonary artery architecture should be monitored using oximetry and two-dimensional echocardiography. Cardiac catheterization or cardiac MRI is performed some time before the child is 6 months old. Assuming an adequate atrial septectomy, good RV and TV function, an unobstructed pathway from the RV around the aortic arch, and normal growth of the pulmonary arterial bed with a normal pulmonary arteriolar resistance, it is safe to proceed to a bidirectional Glenn shunt (or a hemi-Fontan). If preoperative

evaluation demonstrates a restrictive ASD, significant aortic arch obstruction, or hemodynamically significant aortic to pulmonary artery collaterals, these are usually addressed in the cardiac catheterization laboratory. Major pulmonary artery distortion or TR can be repaired at the time of the second stage procedure.

Fontan Operation

Despite the initial success of the Fontan operation,[17] a number of problems have been recognized during longer-term follow-up. In part, these are a consequence of poor patient selection. Many of the problems that adversely affect the outcome of Fontan operation are the result of the preoperative physiology and the complicated surgical manipulation required for survival. Today, with an eventual Fontan procedure in mind, every effort is made to avoid RV injury, to support normal pulmonary vascular bed growth and resistance, and to avoid distortion of the pulmonary arteries. Current practice calls for aggressive catheter-directed treatment of residual structural defects following the initial stage I procedure, a Glenn operation at 4 to 6 months to relieve the volume load on the single RV, and a Fontan procedure, often with a fenestration in the intra-atrial lateral tunnel wall, at 2 years of age.

Cardiac Transplantation

Cardiac transplantation is an alternative form of therapy for infants born with HLHS. The technical feasibility of such a procedure has never been seriously questioned. Issues include the availability of donors and the problems of organ rejection. Cardiac transplantation will remain as an alternative form of treatment.[21-23]

Ethical Issues

The management of children with HLHS, whether by palliation leading to a Fontan procedure or by transplantation, has provoked vigorous ethical discussion.[24] The discussion is complicated by many factors. First, untreated HLHS is rapidly and virtually 100% fatal. Postoperative care following surgical palliation has not only improved mortality but also long-term functional outcome. Heart transplantation may reduce the risk for early mortality provided a donor heart is found, but the long-term outcomes are still potentially problematic. It is clear that not all physicians would recommend either route and not all parents would choose to risk their child's suboptimal quality of life as well as the emotional and financial sacrifices associated with either form of treatment. The present standard of practice does not require that either form of treatment be recommended by the cardiologist or that the parents should agree. A responsible physician may recommend against either approach, but no responsible physician would withhold his or her opinion or deny full disclosure of information to anyone.

Other Anatomic Variants of HLHS

Mitral Atresia With Normal Aortic Root

Patients with mitral atresia and a normal aortic outflow are not properly classified under HLHS[25]; yet, by convention, this lesion complex appears in the hypoplastic LV file of Boston Children's Hospital.

Pathophysiology

Mitral atresia with a good-sized LV is associated with a ventricular septal defect if the aorta arises from the LV. Sometimes the TV is straddling. There may be a DORV with the LV being a blind pouch, or the ventricles may be L-malposed, with the physiology being that of tricuspid atresia. The great vessels may be transposed, the aorta arising from the RV. A PFO is usually present, although egress from the left atrium may take other routes (i.e., via a sinoseptal defect). Often the orifice of the foramen ovale is small enough to raise left atrial pressure, and the atrial septum is thickened. Most patients are classified as having a DORV, the aorta arising from the RV. Sometimes the aorta arises from the LV, in which case the size of the ventricular septal defect may have important hemodynamic consequences. Roughly half of these patients have pulmonary stenosis, and occasionally one sees a patient who has pulmonary valve atresia. Coarctation of the aorta has been noted in about 10% of patients with this anatomic variant.

Clinical manifestations

All of these patients are cyanotic, although among those with excessive pulmonary blood flow this may not be apparent at first. Tachypnea is common because left atrial pressures are often high, causing pulmonary edema, or there is excessive pulmonary blood flow. When there is limited pulmonary blood flow because of pulmonary stenosis or atresia, cyanosis may be the chief complaint. Most are symptomatic in the first weeks of life.

Electrocardiography

In most cases, the ECG shows RV hypertrophy.

Chest Radiography

Chest radiograph demonstrates variably enlarged heart size depending on the amount of pulmonary blood flow, and the pulmonary vasculature may be prominent because of excess flow or diminished because of pulmonary stenosis. There may be evidence of pulmonary edema. Pulmonary edema is possible in the presence of pulmonary stenosis because the size of the PFO determines left atrial pressure, and it may be restrictive even in the presence of normal or reduced amounts of pulmonary flow.

Echocardiography

The detailed anatomy can be documented by two-dimensional echocardiography using previously described techniques.

Cardiac Catheterization

Cardiac catheterization may be important to the successful management. If pulmonary artery flow, pressure, and resistance cannot be assessed by noninvasive imaging, then catheterization can measure these parameters. In addition, relief of an obstructive interatrial septum, likely critical for the development of the pulmonary vasculature, can be accomplished.

Management

With excessive pulmonary blood flow, pulmonary artery banding may be needed. In cases where there is inadequate pulmonary blood flow, an arterial-to-pulmonary shunt may be helpful. Enlargement of the ASD should be considered in all patients, particularly if a shunt procedure is being considered.

Aortic Atresia With Normal Left Ventricle

Aortic atresia with RV and LV of functionally normal capacity is an extremely rare anomaly; repair has been reported.

References

1. Ohye RG, Sleeper LA, Mahony L, et al. Comparison of shunt types in the Norwood procedure for single-ventricle lesions. *N Engl J Med*. 2010;362:1980-1992.
2. Newburger JW, Sleeper LA, Gaynor JW, et al. Transplant-free survival and interventions at 6 years in the SVR trial. *Circulation*. 2018;137:2246-2253.
3. Noonan JA, Nadas AS. The hypoplastic left heart syndrome: an analysis of 101 cases. *Pediatr Clin North Am*. 1958;5:1029-1056.
4. Gordon BM, Rodriguez S, Lee M, Chang RK. Decreasing number of deaths of infants with hypoplastic left heart syndrome. *J Pediatr*. 2008;153:354-358.
5. Reller MD, Strickland MJ, Riehle-Colarusso T, et al. Prevalence of congenital heart defects in metropolitan Atlanta, 1998-2005. *J Pediatr*. 2008;153:807-813.
6. Benson DW, Martin LJ, Lo CW. Genetics of hypoplastic left heart syndrome. *J Pediatr*. 2016;173:25-31.
7. Hinton Jr RB, Martin LJ, Tabangin ME, et al. Hypoplastic left heart syndrome is heritable. *J Am Coll Cardiol*. 2007;50:1590-1595.
8. Tchervenkov CI, Jacobs ML, Tahta SA. Congenital Heart Surgery Nomenclature and Database Project: hypoplastic left heart syndrome. *Ann Thorac Surg*. 2000;69:S170-S179.
9. Rollins CK, Ortinau CM, Stopp C, et al. Regional brain growth trajectories in fetuses with congenital heart disease. *Ann Neurol*. 2021;89:143-157.
10. Friedman KG, Tworetzky W. Fetal cardiac interventions: where do we stand. *Arch Cardiovasc Dis*. 2020;113:121-128.
11. Jonas RA, Lang P, Hansen D, et al. First-stage palliation of hypoplastic left heart syndrome: the importance of coarctation and shunt size. *J Thorac Cardiovasc Surg*. 1986;92:6-13.
12. Brown DW, Cohen KE, O'Brien P, et al. Impact of prenatal diagnosis in survivors of initial palliation of single ventricle heart disease: analysis of the National Pediatric Cardiology Quality Improvement Collaborative database. *Pediatr Cardiol*. 2015;36:314-321.

13. Morris SA, Ethen MK, Penny DJ, et al. Prenatal diagnosis, birth location, surgical center, and neonatal mortality in infants with hypoplastic left heart syndrome. *Circulation*. 2014;129:285-292.

14. de-Wahl Granelli A, Wennergren M, Sandberg K, et al. Impact of pulse oximetry screening on the detection of duct dependent congenital heart disease: a Swedish prospective screening study in 39,821 newborns. *BMJ*. 2009;338:a3037.

15. Vlahos AP, Lock JE, McElhinney DB, et al. Hypoplastic left heart syndrome with intact or highly restrictive atrial septum: outcome after neonatal transcatheter atrial septostomy. *Circulation*. 2004; 109:2326-2330.

16. Brown DW, Gauvreau K, Powell AJ, et al. Cardiac magnetic resonance versus routine cardiac catheterization before bidirectional Glenn anastomosis: long-term follow-up of a prospective randomized trial. *J Thorac Cardiovasc Surg*. 2013;146:1172-1178.

17. Norwood WI, Lang P, Hansen DD. Physiologic repair of aortic atresia-hypoplastic left heart syndrome. *N Engl J Med*. 1983;308:23-26.

18. Sano S, Ishino K, Kado H, et al. Outcome of right ventricle-to-pulmonary artery shunt in first-stage palliation of hypoplastic left heart syndrome: a multi-institutional study. *Ann Thorac Surg*. 2004;78:1951-1957; discussion 1957-1958.

19. Ho AB, Hribernik I, Shillaker D, et al. Hybrid palliation for hypoplastic left heart syndrome: association with contemporary outcomes. *Circulation*. 2021;144:1189-1191.

20. Ceneri NM, Desai MH, Tongut A, et al. Hybrid strategy in neonates with ductal-dependent systemic circulation and multiple risk factors. *J Thorac Cardiovasc Surg*. 2022;164:1291-1303.

21. Bailey LL, Nehlsen-Cannarella SL, Doroshow RW, et al. Cardiac allotransplantation in newborns as therapy for hypoplastic left heart syndrome. *N Engl J Med*. 1986;315:949-951.

22. Alsoufi B, Mahle WT, Manlhiot C, et al. Outcomes of heart transplantation in children with hypoplastic left heart syndrome previously palliated with the Norwood procedure. *J Thorac Cardiovasc Surg*. 2016;151:167–174, 175.e1-2.

23. Mahle WT, Hu C, Trachtenberg F, et al. Heart failure after the Norwood procedure: an analysis of the Single Ventricle Reconstruction Trial. *J Heart Lung Transplant*. 2018;37:879-885.

24. Spike JP. The ethics of treatment for hypoplastic left heart syndrome (HLHS). *Am J Bioeth*. 2017;17:65-66.

25. Moreno F, Quero M, Diaz LP. Mitral atresia with normal aortic valve: a study of eighteen cases and a review of the literature. *Circulation*. 1976;53:1004-1010.

36

Tricuspid Atresia

PETA M.A. ALEXANDER AND JOHN E. MAYER JR.

KEY LEARNING POINTS

- Tricuspid atresia is defined as absence of the tricuspid valve tissue and is commonly associated with hypoplasia of the right ventricle.
- Classification of tricuspid atresia subgroups depends on the degree of obstruction to pulmonary blood flow and the relationship of the great arteries.
- Management of neonates and infants should be focused on measures to protect the pulmonary vasculature from excessive blood pressures and flows and to protect the single left ventricle from excessive pressure and volume loading.
- The treatment goal is a Fontan-type circulation, which is dependent on low pulmonary vascular resistance and good function of the single left ventricle.
- Patients with tricuspid atresia have among the most favorable long-term outcomes after Fontan procedures.

Definition

Tricuspid atresia is characterized by absence of the tricuspid valve and hypoplasia of the right ventricle. By convention, patients are divided into groups, namely type I: those with normally related great arteries; type II: those with transposition of the great arteries (TGA); and type III: those with other complex anomalies. Tricuspid atresia is further classified into subtypes A–C based on the presence of a ventricular septal defect (VSD) and the degree of obstruction to pulmonary blood flow (PBF). This chapter is confined to those with type I and type II lesions, some of which are depicted in Fig. 36.1.

Prevalence

Tricuspid atresia occurred in 2.6% of infants hospitalized for congenital heart disease in New England, with a frequency of 0.057/1000 live births, comparable with other reports.[1,2]

Anatomy

In tricuspid atresia, there is no valvar orifice or valve tissue in the position of the tricuspid valve, and in most of these children there is no suggestion that a valve ever existed or that the right atrium was ever aligned toward the right ventricle.[3] In addition, there is absence of the inlet component of the right ventricular chamber. Systemic venous return blood passes from the right atrium through an atrial septal defect (ASD) or, more often, a patent foramen ovale to the left atrium and from there to left ventricle (LV). In patients with normally related great arteries (type I: about 80%; Table 36.1), entry to the pulmonary circulation occurs through a VSD (bulboventricular foramen), a hypoplastic right ventricular infundibular chamber, and then across the pulmonary valve into the pulmonary circulation (Fig. 36.2). When the great arteries are transposed (type II), the aorta arises from the infundibular chamber and the VSD carries blood from the LV to the aorta. In these cases, restriction at the VSD level results in functional subaortic stenosis (Figs. 36.1 and 36.2).

Tricuspid Atresia With Normally Related Great Arteries (Type I)

In a subset of type I patients, there may be infundibular or pulmonary valvar atresia. The patent ductus arteriosus initially contributes to PBF, and may be the only source of pulmonary blood in the uncommon patient with an intact ventricular septum or pulmonary valvar atresia. The VSD is usually perimembranous, less frequently muscular (single or multiple) in location. The right ventricle is variably small and typically represents only the infundibular portion of a normal right ventricle; in some patients, it consists of no more than a channel from the LV to the pulmonary artery. The passage through the VSD to the pulmonary artery is typically pressure-restrictive, and there may be additional

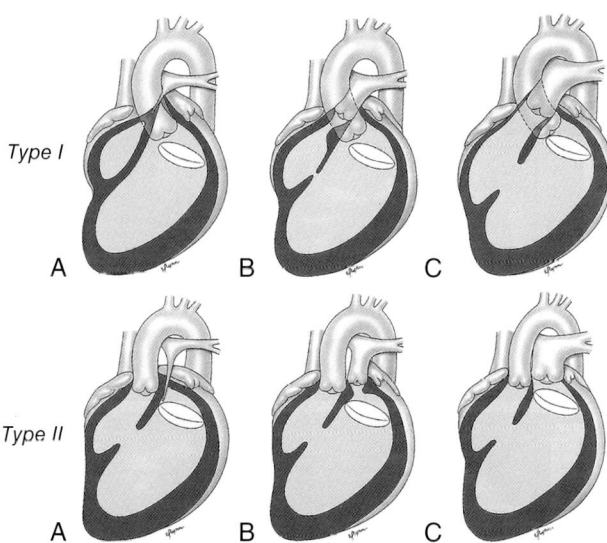

• **Fig. 36.1** Type 1: normally related great arteries without a ventricular septal defect (VSD), with pulmonary atresia (PA) **(A)**; small VSD and pulmonary stenosis (PS) **(B)**; and large VSD, no PS **(C)**. Type II: transposed great arteries with a VSD and PA/PS **(A)**; VSD and PS **(B)**; and VSD and no PS **(C)**. The VSD varies considerably in size and over time tends to get smaller. It may provide obstruction to pulmonary flow (type IB) or, in the presence of transposition, obstruct outflow to the aorta (functional subaortic stenosis). (From Nadas AS, Fyler DC, eds. *Nadas' Pediatric Cardiology.* Philadelphia, PA: Hanley and Belfus; 1992.)

TABLE 36.1	**Boston Children's Hospital (BCH) Experience**	

Anatomy	1988–2002 N = 233	2003–2022 N = 255
Type 1 – normally related great arteries	N = 161	N = 143
1A – no VSD, PA	18%	22%
1B – small VSD, PS	68%	51%
1C – large VSD, no PS	14%	26%
Type 2 – D-transposed great arteries	N = 49	N = 67
2A – VSD, PA	12%	9%
2B – VSD, PS	37%	42%
2C – VSD, no PS	51%	50%
Type 3 – complex	N = 23	N = 15
Intervention	1988–2002	2003–2022
Neonatal surgery at BCH	59	65
Fontan circulation	154	180
Outcome	1988–2002	2003–2022
Known dead[a]	20	23

PA, pulmonary atresia; *PS,* pulmonary stenosis; *VSD,* ventricular septal defect.

[a]With incomplete follow-up, these patients were documented as deceased.

pulmonary valvar stenosis, subvalvar obstruction, or pulmonary valvar atresia. Usually, the ventricular defect is small, tends to get smaller with time, and may ultimately close. The ductus arteriosus typically has a small diameter and without intervention, usually closes in the first days of life. In a few individuals (13%) with type IC tricuspid atresia, the passage of blood from the LV to the main pulmonary artery is completely unobstructed.

Tricuspid Atresia With Transposition of the Great Arteries (Type II)

When the great arteries are transposed (type II), the aorta arises from the infundibular chamber and the VSD carries blood to the aorta. In these cases, restriction at the VSD level results in functional subaortic stenosis (Fig. 36.2). Aortic coarctation is more common in this group (about 33%), often in patients with functional subaortic stenosis. The pulmonary artery is directly connected to the LV, and excessive pulmonary blood is more likely in these patients than in those with normally related great arteries (type I).

Tricuspid Atresia Variations

Some additional cardiac anatomic variations such as right aortic arch, left juxtaposition of the atrial appendages, and persistent left superior vena cava occur in patients with either type I or II tricuspid atresia.[3,4] Patients with L-looped ventricles may have left-sided (tricuspid) atrioventricular valve atresia and a diminutive, left-sided right ventricle and have circulatory physiology comparable to mitral atresia.

Physiology

The entire systemic venous return must pass through the foramen ovale throughout fetal life and after birth; less than 6% of our patients with untouched foramina ovale have had pressure gradients of more than a few millimeters of mercury (mm Hg) between the two atria. The pulmonary venous return and systemic venous return join in the left atrium and pass into the morphologic LV, which functions as a single ventricle. Cyanosis results from the systemic venous return entering the systemic arterial blood without passing through the lungs, typically referred to as a right-to-left shunt. The degree of arterial desaturation depends on the relative amounts of systemic and pulmonary venous return and on the oxygen saturations in the systemic and pulmonary venous returns. In those with normally related great vessels (type I), blood passes directly from the LV to the aorta and, some part of the left ventricular output passes through the VSD to the diminutive right ventricle and pulmonary artery (Fig. 36.2). The amount of PBF depends on the relative resistances of these two outlets from the single LV. Anatomic contributions to the total resistance to PBF include obstructions at the ventricular defect, right ventricular outflow tract, and the pulmonary valve, which are additive to the pulmonary arteriolar resistance, which in

Tricuspid atresia

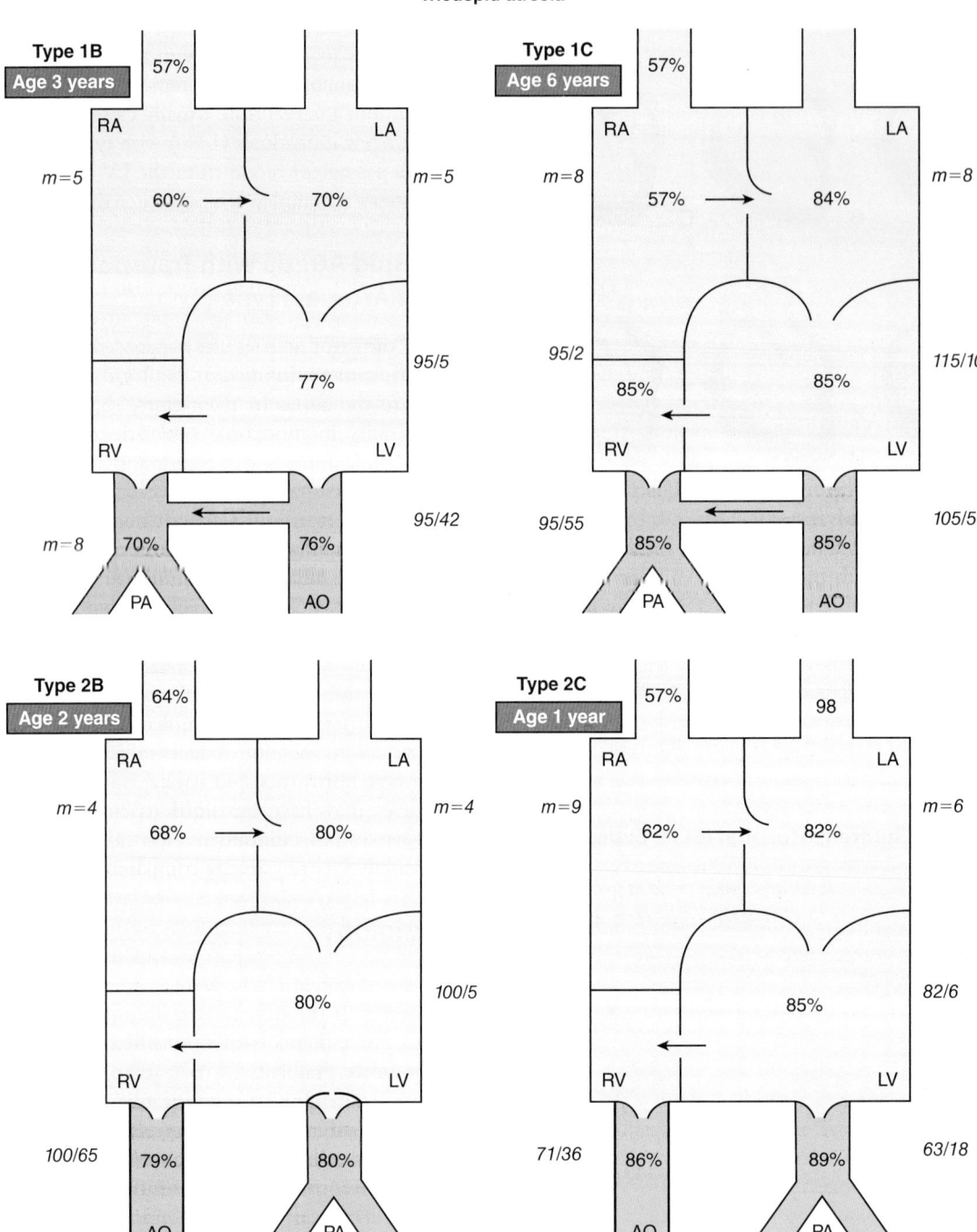

• **Fig. 36.2** Physiologic diagrams of patients with tricuspid atresia. Type 1B: tricuspid atresia with normally related great arteries is usually associated with low pulmonary artery pressure either because of a small ventricular defect, or, less often, because of pulmonary stenosis. Type 1C: tricuspid atresia with normally related great arteries and a pulmonary artery pressure that approaches the systemic level is unusual. Type 2B: tricuspid atresia and transposition of the great arteries may be associated with pulmonary stenosis or type 2C without pulmonary stenosis. *AO*, Aorta; *Italics*, mm Hg; *LA*, left atrium; *LV*, left ventricle; *PA*, pulmonary artery; *RA*, right atrium; *RV*, right ventricle; %, oxygen saturation. (From Nadas AS, Fyler DC, eds. *Nadas' Pediatric Cardiology*. Philadelphia, PA: Hanley and Belfus; 1992.)

early infancy can reflect persistent elevation of fetal pulmonary resistance. In general, the course of these patients is characterized by increasing cyanosis because of progressively diminishing PBF, most often because the ventricular defect becomes smaller relative to the size of the infant.

Uncommonly in type I, there may be relatively little obstruction PBF, which can be sufficiently high to result in congestive failure. The ductus arteriosus provides some blood flow to the pulmonary circulation after birth, but most often it closes in the first days of life.

In those with TGA (type II), subaortic stenosis frequently occurs because of an obstructive and closing VSD (Fig. 36.2). As the ventricular defect gets smaller, there is increasing obstruction to outflow to the aorta. To provide adequate cardiac output, left ventricular pressure must rise. With no change in pulmonary arteriolar resistance, this increased left ventricular pressure increases PBF, ultimately resulting in congestive heart failure. When the pulmonary artery has been banded, the ventricular defect becomes more obstructive, likely due to the pressure induced ventricular hypertrophy.[5]

Clinical Manifestations

Advanced prenatal screening including fetal echocardiogram programs in the New England region result in most patients receiving this diagnosis before birth.[6] Genetic testing could be considered as tricuspid atresia has been associated with trisomies and other clinical syndromes.[7]

Cyanosis

Virtually all patients with tricuspid atresia have cyanosis due to the obligate right-to-left shunt at atrial level, and most have a murmur. The diagnosis is typically made by echocardiography in early infancy. Cyanosis is the most common presenting clinical sign, particularly in those patients with restricted PBF. Those with severe obstruction to PBF, typically due to associated pulmonary valvar atresia, are dependent on a patent ductus for PBF and may become deeply cyanotic when the ductus closes in the first week of life. Others with less severe PBF restriction gradually become more cyanotic as the months go by. When the cyanosis

becomes intense, cyanotic spells may occur. Hepatomegaly is rarely observed in the more cyanotic children, although may occasionally result from an obstructed foramen ovale.

Congestive Heart Failure

Patients with unrestricted PBF (typically those with type II or type IC) develop signs of congestive failure, with minimal cyanosis, tachypnea, congested lungs, and hepatomegaly. There is usually, but not invariably, a moderate systolic murmur and the second heart sound is single and quite accentuated in those with transposed vessels.

Electrocardiography

Right atrial enlargement may be present, especially in older patients (Fig. 36.3). The QRS axis is usually leftward and superior, right ventricular anterior forces are diminished, and left ventricular dominance is frequent. Some patients with transposition (type II) have a leftward inferior QRS axis, and some may have left-sided S-T and T-wave abnormalities. The frequent findings of left superior axis and diminished anterior right ventricular forces are clinically useful in distinguishing this lesion from pulmonary atresia with intact ventricular septum (left inferior axis and diminished right anterior ventricular forces) and pulmonary atresia with VSD (right axis deviation and right ventricular hypertrophy).

Chest Radiography

The heart size is proportionate to the PBF. Because the most common forms of tricuspid atresia have relatively limited

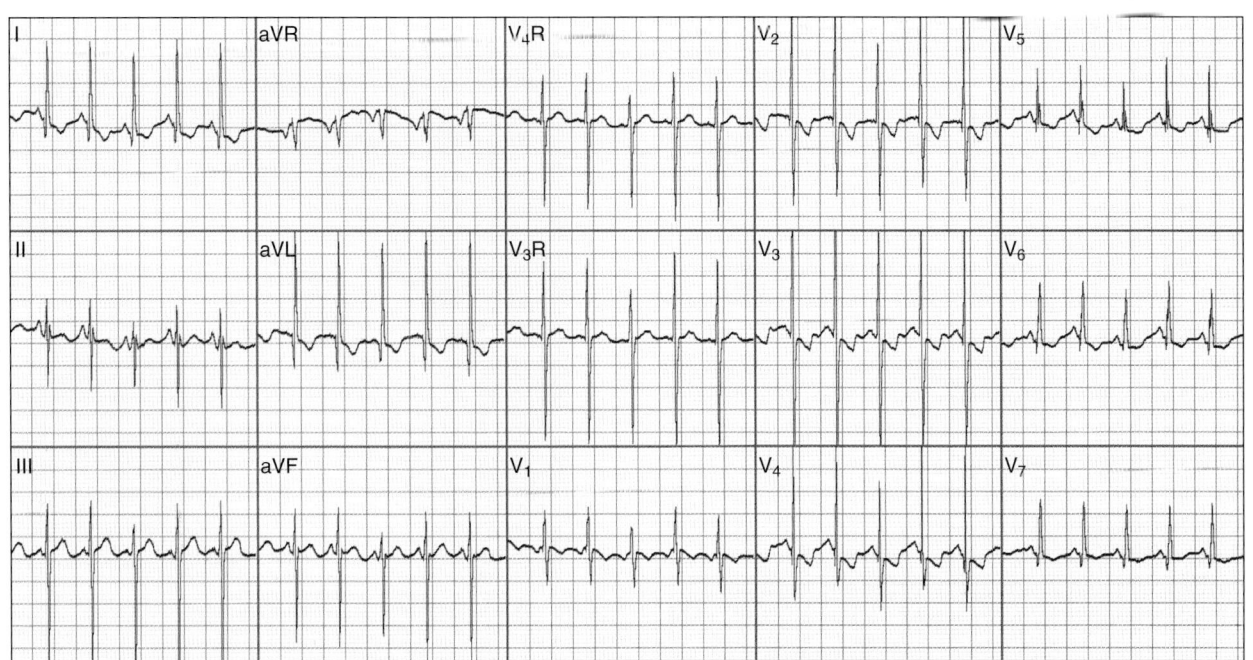

• **Fig. 36.3** Electrocardiogram demonstrating features of right atrial enlargement, leftward and superior QRS axis, and diminished right ventricular anterior forces.

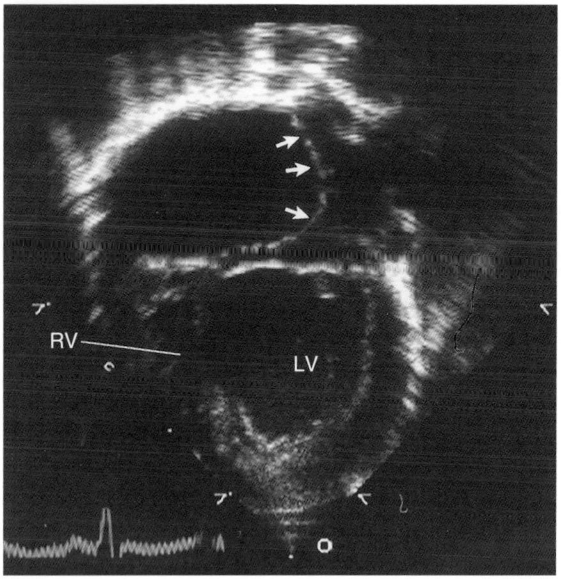

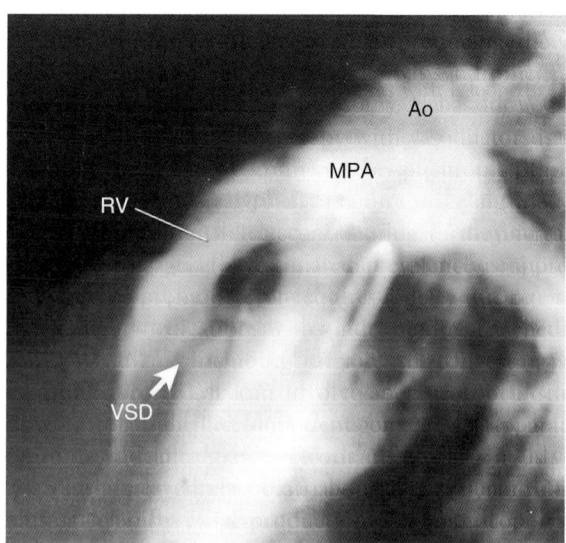

• **Fig. 36.4** Apical echocardiogram in a patient with tricuspid atresia. Note the small right ventricle *(RV)* with absence of a right atrioventricular connection. There is a muscular ventricular septal defect allowing the left ventricle *(LV)* to supply pulmonary blood flow. The atrial septum bows strikingly into the left atrium *(arrows)*.

blood flow, the heart size tends to be small or minimally enlarged; the resemblance to patients with tetralogy of Fallot is often striking. With increased PBF, the heart becomes proportionately enlarged and pulmonary vascular markings are increased.

Echocardiography

The anatomic features (Fig. 36.4) are readily demonstrable by echocardiography. These include the absence of a tricuspid valve, the presence and dimensions of ASD and VSD, the diminutive right ventricle, the great vessel relationships to the LV and right ventricular infundibulum, patency status of the ductus arteriosus, and the status of the outflow tracts and semilunar valves. Doppler echocardiography quantitates the degrees of obstruction at atrial, ventricular septal, and pulmonary levels.

Usually the right atrioventricular junction is filled with fibrous tissue. Occasionally there is tricuspid valve tissue present, but the valve is imperforate because of leaflet fusion. In such cases, the valve leaflets may move with the cardiac cycle, but Doppler examination determines if the valve is patent. An uncommon cause of tricuspid atresia is complete malalignment of a common atrioventricular valve over the LV so that the tricuspid portion of the valve is atretic. The clue to this diagnosis is the presence of a defect in the location of a primum ASD.

Pulmonary valvar stenosis is common in infants with normally related great arteries (type I), and is usually due to subvalvar muscular hypertrophy and/or a small VSD. The pulmonary valve can be well formed and nearly normal in size. In patients with TGA (type II), a small VSD or mid-cavity obstruction of the outflow chamber can produce

subaortic stenosis. If subaortic obstruction is seen on Doppler examination or if the VSD and outflow chamber appear small by imaging, then coarctation should be suspected. If the ductus arteriosus is widely patent, coarctation may not be completely excluded: right-to-left shunting in the ductus suggests proximal restriction of systemic blood flow in the proximal aorta, due to intracardiac or proximal arch obstruction, resulting in a ductus-dependent systemic circulation.

Cardiac Catheterization

While catheterization in earlier years was required to precisely define the anatomic details (Fig. 36.5), it is no longer necessary in the unoperated newborn as both anatomy and physiology are very well demonstrated by echocardiography. In the older patient who has not undergone surgical correction, and in those with prior surgical or catheterization procedures, cardiac catheterization is necessary, particularly to visualize pulmonary arteries, measure pressures to calculate arteriolar resistance, outline systemic venous return anatomy, and identify and coil occlude any unwanted channels such as a small left superior vena cava to coronary sinus or systemic–pulmonary venous collaterals.

Management

The ultimate goal for management for patients with tricuspid atresia is to achieve a successful Fontan circulation, which allows the patient to have nearly normal systemic arterial saturation.[8] To maximize the likelihood of a successful Fontan operation, there should be (1) no significant pulmonary arterial distortion from prior surgery (a potential problem resulting from prior shunting or banding

• **Fig. 36.5** Left ventricular angiogram, four-chambered view, in a 2-month-old baby with tricuspid atresia (type 1B) with contrast passing via a small *(arrow)* ventricular septal defect *(VSD)* to a hypoplastic right ventricle *(RV)* and then to main pulmonary artery *(MPA)*. The aorta *(Ao)* is normally located and fills directly from the left ventricle.

operations); (2) normal pulmonary arteriolar vascular resistance (a potential problem resulting from excess pulmonary artery pressures and flows due to prior shunting procedures or inadequate pulmonary artery bands [PABs]); (c) preserved left ventricular systolic and diastolic function (a potential problem resulting from concentric hypertrophy due to ventricular outlet obstruction or ventricular dilation due to volume load by excess pulmonary blood flow); and (4) a well-functioning mitral valve.[9-11] Multivariate analysis has shown that elevated pulmonary resistance, distorted pulmonary arteries, and left ventricular dysfunction and hypertrophy are risk factors for an unsuccessful Fontan operation.[10-12]

Neonatal Management

The neonatal management of the tricuspid atresia patient is therefore focused on achieving adequate oxygenation without creating these adverse outcomes which would add to the risk of the Fontan procedure.

Tricuspid Atresia with Pulmonary Obstruction

In patients with restrictions to PBF, most commonly seen in tricuspid atresia type I, the initial management frequently involves administration of PGE1 to maintain ductal patency followed by establishment of a reliable but controlled additional source of PBF. This is accomplished by creating a systemic-to-pulmonary artery shunt, generally a modified Blalock-Thomas-Taussig shunt with a prosthetic graft interposed between the innominate or subclavian artery and the pulmonary artery or by stenting the ductus arteriosus.

Tricuspid Atresia With Unrestricted Pulmonary Blood Flow

In patients with unrestricted PBF, typically occurring in patients with tricuspid atresia type II (and the rare type IC), a PAB is placed to limit PBF and pulmonary artery pressures and to manage congestive heart failure. Placement of a PAB alone should be carried out only after confirmation that the VSD is large (cross-sectional area > 2 cm^2/m^2) and aortic arch obstruction has been ruled out.

Tricuspid Atresia with D-Transposition of the Great Arteries and Subaortic Obstruction

In a significant number of cases with tricuspid atresia type II, there is associated subaortic stenosis at the VSD level and aortic arch hypoplasia or coarctation.[13] In these cases, the therapeutic choice is between a PAB plus aortic arch reconstruction and a Norwood stage 1 procedure, as would be carried out for hypoplastic left heart syndrome. The risk with the PAB plus arch reconstruction approach is that subaortic obstruction will develop due to narrowing at the VSD level, with the result that there will be obstruction to LV emptying to both the pulmonary and systemic circulations from the

single LV, and that progressive ventricular hypertrophy with systolic and diastolic dysfunction will result. For this reason, the Boston Children's approach to such patients with tricuspid atresia type II and aortic arch obstruction has been to carry out a stage 1 procedure similar to the approach for the analogous (physiologically) hypoplastic left heart syndrome.

Bidirectional Cavopulmonary Shunt

The routine use of an interim bidirectional cavopulmonary shunt in the first 6 months of life provides adequate oxygenation and reduction of potentially excess pulmonary artery pressures and flows that could raise pulmonary arteriolar resistance, as well as reducing the volume load on the single LV with its potential negative effects on ventricular function.[14] All patients are catheterized within the first 6 months of age primarily to determine pulmonary artery anatomy, pressure, and resistance. Also, catheterization can identify and treat any accessory venous channels such as a small left superior vena cava to coronary sinus, which, because of the higher upper body venous pressures following a bidirectional Glenn procedure and small veno-venous connections, will enlarge and cause cyanosis from significant right-to-left shunting. Most patients undergo a bidirectional Glenn shunt after 3–4 months of age, which is better tolerated than before age 2 months.[15] The exceptions to this approach are the unusual patients who have a restrictive VSD with normally related great vessels (type IB) with normal pulmonary artery anatomy, pressures, and resistances, and an adequate arterial saturation who may be able to have a primary Fontan procedure at 2–3 years of life. Although this interim bidirectional cavopulmonary shunt procedure represents an additional operative procedure, it allows additional time for patient growth and continued maturation of the pulmonary vascular bed and is generally accepted practice for most patients with single ventricle.

Fontan Procedure

Conceptually the Fontan operation would be accomplished as early in life as possible to minimize the morbidities associated with the palliated single-ventricle state, but Fontan procedures are less well tolerated in early infancy.[12] The explanation for this observation is thought to be related to the normal ongoing decline in pulmonary arteriolar resistance during infancy as well as concerns about growth of the systemic venous pathways and pulmonary artery structures post-Fontan. Problems with recurrent pleural effusion are more common in the younger age group. The observed difficulties with Fontan surgery in infants decreases with age, and it is current institutional practice to carry out the Fontan procedure after age 2 years, following the interim step of creation of a bidirectional cavopulmonary shunt. Prior to the Fontan procedure, all patients are again catheterized for delineation of pulmonary artery anatomy, pulmonary pressure and resistance, detection of any pulmonary arteriovenous malformations, and coil occlusion of any systemic venous to pulmonary–venous collaterals, which may result following the bidirectional Glenn shunt with its higher systemic venous pressures.[16] These collaterals may produce significant right-to-left shunting and increased cyanosis.

A fenestrated lateral tunnel modified Fontan operation or a fenestrated extracardiac Fontan is then performed (see Chapter 59 for further discussion of Fontan procedures and its complications).

Course

Without treatment, patient survival to age 1 year is only 10% to 20%.[17,18] Our management plan, comparable with that at other institutions with similar patient populations, has been in effect for more than 30 years. Since the Fontan procedure for tricuspid atresia was first published in 1971, iterative modifications have resulted in the current era lateral tunnel or extracardiac Fontan operations.[10,11,19] The lateral tunnel or extracardiac modifications performed for most patients appear hemodynamically more satisfactory, and the addition of a fenestration has proven quite beneficial in reducing postoperative effusions and length of stay.[11,20] (see Chapter 59 for further discussion of Fontan procedures and complications.) In general, however, Fontan surgery has greatly helped these patients: many have a nearly normal life, and most are gainfully employed. Although some participate in sports, most are somewhat limited by the restricted ability to increase cardiac output associated with this type of circulation.[21,22] It is remarkable that despite living with the equivalent of mild, chronic, right-sided congestive heart failure, patients with Fontan circulation report health-related quality of life that which approaches the general population norms.[23]

References

1. Fyler DC, Buckley LP, Hellenbrand WE, et al. Report of the New England Regional Infant Cardiac Program. *Pediatrics.* 1980;65 (suppl):375-461.
2. Langlois PH, Marengo L, Lupo PJ, et al. Evaluating the proportion of isolated cases among a spectrum of birth defects in a population-based registry. *Birth Defects Res.* 2023;115:21-25.
3. Van Praagh R, Ando M, Dungan WT. Anatomic types of tricuspid atresia: clinical and developmental implications. *Circulation.* 1971;44:115.
4. Melhuish BP, Van Praagh R. Juxtaposition of the atrial appendages: a sign of severe cyanotic heart disease. *Br Heart J.* 1968;30:269.
5. Freedom RM, Benson LN, Smallhorn JF, Williams WG, Trusler GA, Rowe RD. Subaortic stenosis, the univentricular heart, and banding of the pulmonary artery: an analysis of the courses of 43 patients with univentricular heart palliated by pulmonary artery banding. *Circulation.* 1986;73:758-764.
6. Donofrio MT, Moon-Grady AJ, Hornberger LK, et al. Diagnosis and treatment of fetal cardiac disease: a scientific statement from the American Heart Association. *Circulation.* 2014;129:2183-2242.
7. Berg C, Lachmann R, Kaiser C, et al. Prenatal diagnosis of tricuspid atresia: intrauterine course and outcome. *Ultrasound Obstet Gynecol.* 2010;35:183-190.
8. Fontan F, Baudet E. Surgical repair of tricuspid atresia. *Thorax.* 1971;26:240-248.
9. Juaneda E, Haworth SG. Pulmonary vascular structure in patients dying after a Fontan procedure. The lung as a risk factor. *Br Heart J.* 1984;52:575-580.
10. Khairy P, Fernandes SM, Mayer Jr JE, et al. Long-term survival, modes of death, and predictors of mortality in patients with Fontan surgery. *Circulation.* 2008;117:85-92.
11. d'Udekem Y, Iyengar AJ, Galati JC, et al. Redefining expectations of long-term survival after the Fontan procedure: twenty-five years of follow-up from the entire population of Australia and New Zealand. *Circulation.* 2014;130:S32-S38.
12. Gentles TL, Mayer Jr JE, Gauvreau K, et al. Fontan operation in five hundred consecutive patients: factors influencing early and late outcome. *J Thorac Cardiovasc Surg.* 1997;114:376-391.
13. Franken LC, Admiraal M, Verrall CE, et al. Improved long-term outcomes in double-inlet left ventricle and tricuspid atresia with transposed great arteries: systemic outflow tract obstruction present at birth defines long-term outcome. *Eur J Cardiothorac Surg.* 2017;51:1051-1057.
14. Rychik J, Jacobs ML, Norwood Jr WI. Acute changes in left ventricular geometry after volume reduction operation. *Ann Thorac Surg.* 1995;60:1267-1273; discussion 1274.
15. Reddy VM, McElhinney DB, Moore P, Haas GS, Hanley FL. Outcomes after bidirectional cavopulmonary shunt in infants less than 6 months old. *J Am Coll Cardiol.* 1997;29:1365-1370.
16. Banka P, Sleeper LA, Atz AM, et al. Practice variability and outcomes of coil embolization of aortopulmonary collaterals before Fontan completion: a report from the Pediatric Heart Network Fontan Cross-Sectional Study. *Am Heart J.* 2011;162:125-130.
17. Dick M, Fyler DC, Nadas AS. Tricuspid atresia: clinical course in 101 patients. *Am J Cardiol.* 1975;36:327-337.
18. Keating P, Van der M, Shipton. Tricuspid atresia—profile and outcome. *Cardiovasc J S Afr.* 2001;12:202-205.
19. Kreutzer J, Keane JF, Lock JE, et al. Conversion of modified Fontan procedure to lateral atrial tunnel cavopulmonary anastomosis. *J Thorac Cardiovasc Surg.* 1996;111:1169-1176.
20. Bridges ND, Lock JE, Castaneda AR. Baffle fenestration with subsequent transcatheter closure. Modification of the Fontan operation for patients at increased risk. *Circulation.* 1990;82:1681-1689.
21. Diller GP, Giardini A, Dimopoulos K, et al. Predictors of morbidity and mortality in contemporary Fontan patients: results from a multicenter study including cardiopulmonary exercise testing in 321 patients. *Eur Heart J.* 2010;31:3073-3083.
22. Cunningham JW, Nathan AS, Rhodes J, Shafer K, Landzberg MJ, Opotowsky AR. Decline in peak oxygen consumption over time predicts death or transplantation in adults with a Fontan circulation. *Am Heart J.* 2017;189:184-192.
23. Marshall KH, D'Udekem Y, Sholler GF, et al. Health-related quality of life in children, adolescents, and adults with a Fontan circulation: a meta-analysis. *J Am Heart Assoc.* 2020;9:e014172.

37

Pulmonary Atresia with Intact Ventricular Septum

JAMI LEVINE AND JOHN E. MAYER JR.

KEY LEARNING POINTS

- There is a wide spectrum of tricuspid valve, pulmonary valve, coronary artery, and right ventricular (RV) pathology in pulmonary valve atresia. Most have at least mild RV hypoplasia and elevated RV pressure.
- A small percentage with pulmonary atresia have RV dilation, low RV pressure, and severe tricuspid valve disease. There are fewer therapeutic options for those with this variant and a higher risk for poor outcome.
- Those with right heart hypoplasia are at risk for coronary artery abnormalities that can significantly impact prognosis and result in fewer therapeutic options.

- Diagnostic evaluation starts with transthoracic echocardiography but often includes cardiac catheterization for evaluation of the coronary artery anatomy.
- Surgical strategies may include surgical and catheter-based interventions and depending on anatomic details, may result in single-ventricle, 1.5-ventricle, or biventricular circulation. In some high-risk patients, heart transplant may be pursued. In particular, two groups of patients should not undergo pulmonary valve interventions in the newborn period: those with severe tricuspid regurgitation and low RV pressures, and those with RV-dependent coronary circulations.

Definition

Pulmonary atresia with intact ventricular septum (PA/IVS) is a condition in which there is either an absent or imperforate pulmonary valve and no ventricular septal defect.

Prevelance

In the New England Regional Infant Cardiac Program, PA/IVS was the 10th most common defect encountered among sick cardiac infants. The incidence rate in population studies varies from 0.069 to 0.074/1000 live births.[1,2] In the current era, the prevalence is slightly lower, likely secondary to pregnancy termination following prenatal diagnosis.

Prenatal Development

No clear genetic etiology has been described, though some familial cases have been reported. The wide variation in size of the right heart structures at birth as well as the anatomic variation in right heart anatomy suggest that valvar atresia can develop at any time during gestation and that its etiology is variable.[3] Our general understanding is that

decreased flow through any cardiac structure will lead to decreased growth. In PA/IVS, causes of decreased flow through the right heart may include primary abnormalities of the pulmonary valve, tricuspid valve (TV), and/or right ventricle (RV). As antegrade flow through the right heart is reduced, growth of the right heart structures slows and may completely stop. If an atretic pulmonary valve is not the primary insult, the lack of antegrade flow can lead to "acquired" valve atresia. Fetal cardiologists have observed that those that develop atresia earlier in gestation tend to have severe hypoplasia of the RV, whereas those that progress to atresia late in pregnancy can have nearly normal RV size.

Morphology

A number of classification systems have been proposed, but none are universally in use. Most agree that there are two main groups of patients; those with associated RV dilation (5%–10%) and those with associated right heart hypoplasia (90%–95%).[4,5]

Newborns with *PA/IVS and right heart dilation* have distinctly different anatomic and physiologic features from those with hypoplasia, often with concomitant severe tricuspid regurgitation, severe dilation of the RV and right atrium, and low RV pressure (Fig. 37.1). TV anomalies include Ebstein malformation or other severely dysplastic features. It appears that the to-and-fro flow across the TV contributes to better RV growth during gestation but can lead to depressed RV function, fetal arrhythmias, and hydrops fetalis. The physiology and the interventional options are very different from the group with right heart hypoplasia.

Among those with *right heart hypoplasia*, there is a wide spectrum of right heart pathology. At one end of the spectrum are patients with tiny RV cavities and a diminutive, poorly

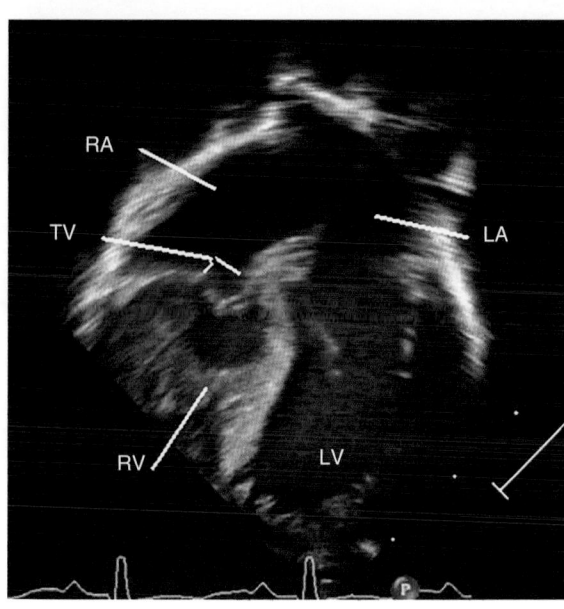

• **Fig. 37.2** Pulmonary atresia with intact ventricular septum and right ventricular hypoplasia. Apical view highlights a moderately hypoplastic tricuspid valve annulus (marked) and right ventricle. Note the size discrepancy between the two ventricles and the two atrioventricular valves. *LA,* Left atrium; *LV,* left ventricle; *RA,* right atrium; *RV,* right ventricle; *TV,* tricuspid valve.

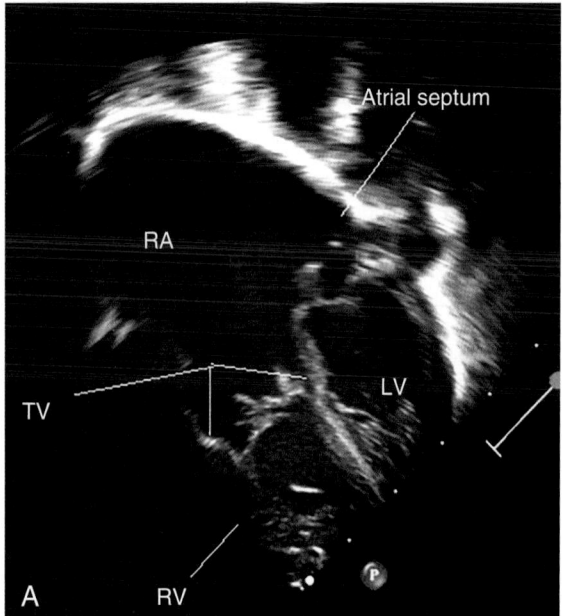

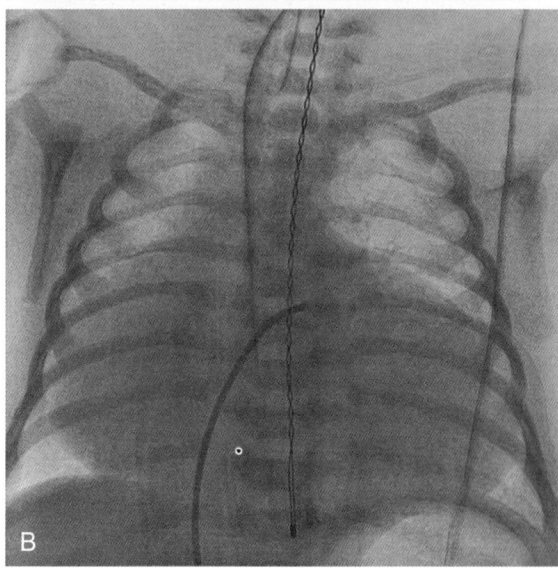

• **Fig. 37.1** Pulmonary atresia with intact ventricular septum and right heart dilation. **(A)** Apical view of the heart illustrating severe dilation of the right atrium and tricuspid valve annulus (marked). Note the "ragged" appearance of the tricuspid valve tissue. The atrial septum bows leftward due to high right atrial pressure, compressing the left atrium. **(B)** Fluoroscopic image of the same patient showing severe cardiomegaly due to right heart dilation. *LV,* Left ventricle; *RA,* right atrium; *RV,* right ventricle; *TV,* tricuspid valve.

developed TV. At the other end are those with a nearly normal-sized RV and TV annulus. TV annulus and RV cavity size are usually concordant (Figs. 37.2 and 37.3).

Ventricular anatomy: In most patients, the RV is at least mildly hypoplastic, is often hypertrophied, and may be anatomically abnormal.[4] A small subset have infundibular muscular atresia and no identifiable pulmonary valve tissue. This group has a high risk for coronary artery anomalies, including coronary ostial atresia.[6]

TV anatomy: In addition to annular hypoplasia, valves are often anatomically abnormal, including thickened or abnormally positioned valve leaflets, absent or thickened chordal apparatus, fused commissures, and absent or fused papillary muscles.

Pulmonary valve anatomy: Most patients have an identifiable pulmonary valve with morphology ranging from thickened, fused leaflets with annular hypoplasia to relatively normal leaflets, fused commissures, and a nearly normal annular diameter.

Pulmonary artery anatomy: The main and branch pulmonary arteries are typically normal in caliber. When hypoplasia is present, it is usually mild. Absent main pulmonary artery is uncommon. When present, it is often associated with ventricular infundibular atresia. Diminutive branch pulmonary arteries are rare.

Coronary artery anatomy: Coronary artery abnormalities are common.[6,7] RV sinusoids are the most common abnormality. These are persistent embryonic connections between the RV and the coronary arteries. These are of variable significance, but for patients who also have coronary obstructions or coronary ostial atresia, the sinusoids can represent a significant source of blood flow to the ventricular

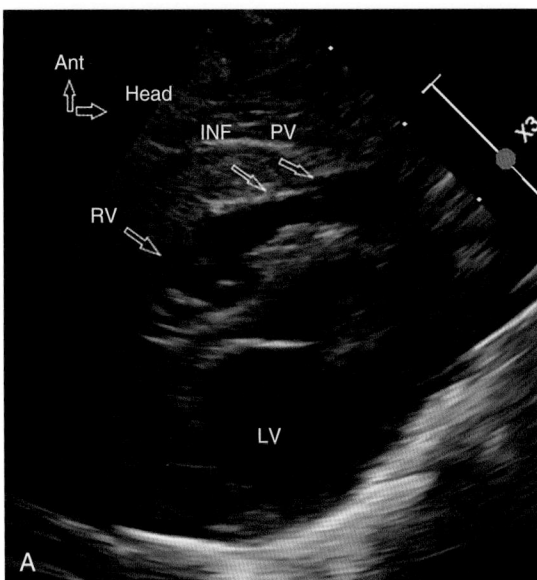

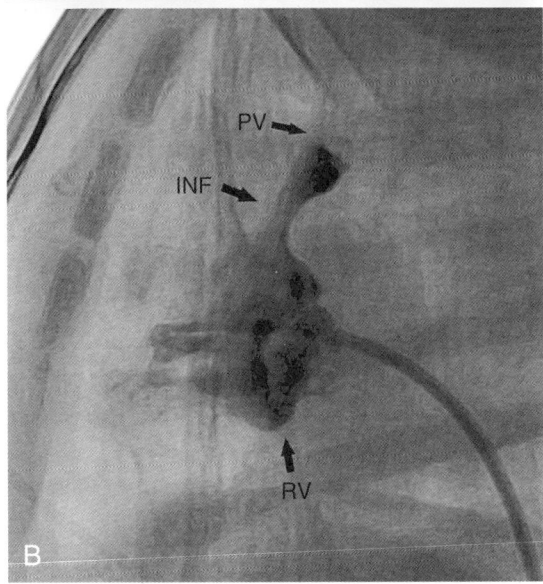

• **Fig. 37.3** Right ventricular outflow tract in membranous pulmonary atresia. **(A)** Parasternal short-axis view of the right ventricular outflow tract. The right ventricular cavity is moderately small and the infundibular segment is narrow. Thin pulmonary valve tissue is visible. **(B)** Angiogram from the same patient, confirming a small right ventricular cavity and a narrowed infundibulum. The pulmonary valve annulus looks nearly normal in size with no antegrade flow. *INF,* Infundibulum; *LV,* left ventricle; *PV,* pulmonary valve; *RV,* right ventricle.

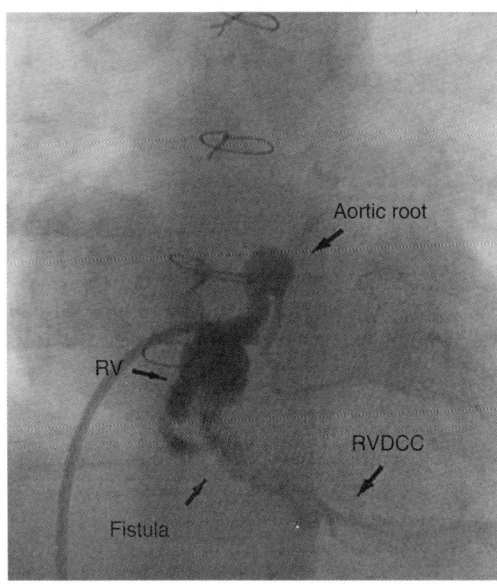

• **Fig. 37.4** Right ventricular-dependent coronary artery. Angiogram after injection of dye into a severely hypoplastic right ventricle. A prominent fistula (marked) comes from the apical region, giving rise to a coronary artery that courses along the surface of the left ventricle. This was the only blood supply to this region of the heart. The aortic root also fills revealing an abnormal connection superiorly between the aortic root and the right ventricle. *RV,* Right ventricle; *RVDCC,* right ventricular-dependent coronary circulation.

Physiology

Normally, deoxygenated blood returns to the RA and traverses the TV, RV, and pulmonary valve en route to the lungs. Oxygenated blood returns from the lungs to the left atrium, traverses the mitral valve, left ventricle, and aortic valve to deliver oxygenated blood to the systemic circulation (Fig. 37.5A). In PA/IVS, the obstruction to antegrade flow through the right heart forces the deoxygenated and oxygenated blood to mix (Fig. 37.5B). The deoxygenated blood crosses from right to left atrium through the patent foramen ovale, to mix with the pulmonary venous blood, resulting in arterial desaturation.

Two major adaptations must occur when there is no antegrade flow across the pulmonary valve *in utero*. First, blood entering the RV must be able to exit the RV. Right ventricular egress is typically via TV regurgitation, but may also occur via ventricular sinusoids to the coronary arteries. Second, an alternative mechanism to provide blood flow to the branch pulmonary arteries and developing lungs must exist.

In fetal life, blood flow to the pulmonary arteries occurs via the ductus arteriosus (DA), which is always patent in the fetus. Normal ductal flow *in utero* is from the pulmonary artery to the descending aorta and placenta. When the pulmonary valve is atretic, ductal blood flow is instead retrograde from the aorta to the pulmonary artery. The DA normally closes in the first hours to days after birth. If pulmonary valve atresia is present, this will cause cessation of perfusion to the lungs, leading to hypoxemia and death within hours.

myocardium, a situation referred to as RV-dependent coronary circulation (Fig. 37.4). When both coronary ostia are atretic, the RV becomes the only source of coronary flow. Varying amounts of LV myocardium can be at risk if the RV pressure is lowered. The smaller the RV and tricuspid annulus, the more likely there are to be coronary artery abnormalities. In those with coronary stenoses, there can be progressive changes over time, including narrowing/atresia of the distal coronary vessels and formation of coronary artery aneurysms, both of which can negatively impact long term outcome. In some, the degree of RV dependence can decrease, perhaps improving the long-term outcome.[8]

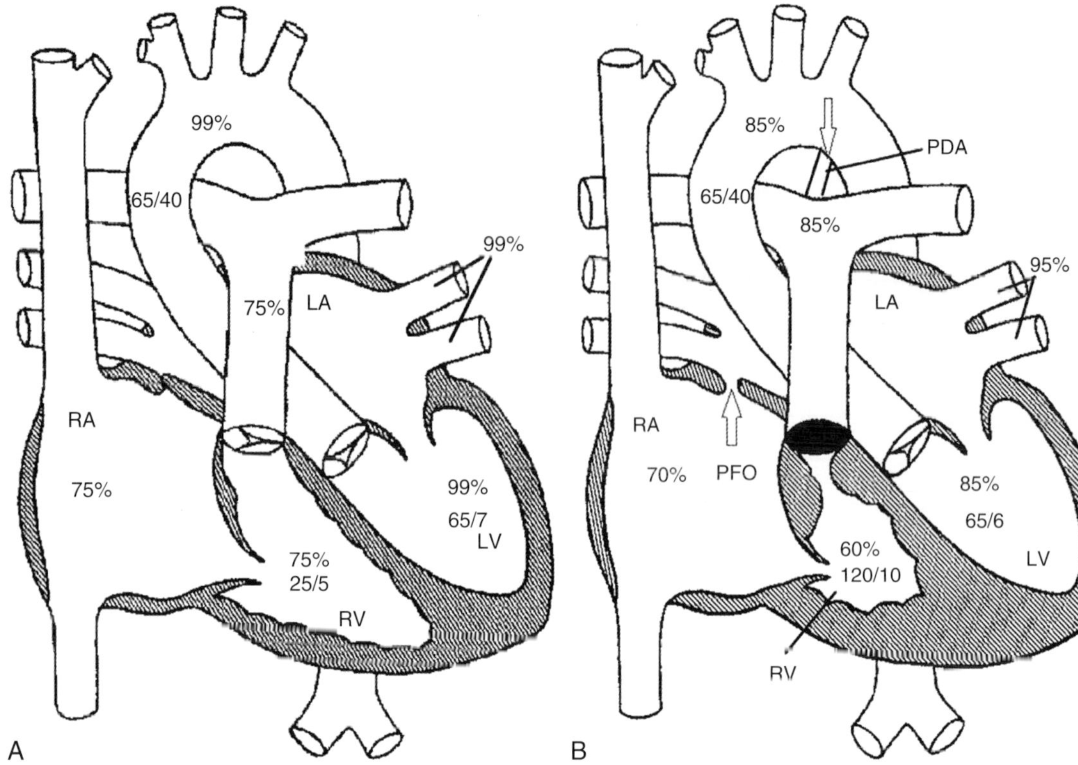

• **Fig. 37.5** Hemodynamics. **(A)** Newborn with normal valve function and no ductus arteriosus. The pressure in the right ventricle *(RV)* is well below the pressure in the left ventricle *(LV)*. The left heart is fully saturated, and the saturation in the pulmonary artery equals the saturation in the RV. **(B)** Newborn with pulmonary atresia and a patent ductus arteriosus *(PDA)*. The pressure in the RV is suprasystemic and the left heart saturations are reduced due to mixing of the pulmonary and systemic venous return. Saturations in the pulmonary artery equal those in the aorta. *LA*, Left atrium; *PFO*, patent foramen ovale; *RA*, right atrium.

The remedy is to maintain DA patency while assessment and decision-making proceed.

Postnatally, the RV pressure is usually elevated and may be higher than in the left ventricle, though a small subset will have unusually low RV pressure. In those with RV-dependent coronary arteries, the elevated pressures are needed to perfuse the sinusoidal connections between the RV and the coronary arteries, thus are important for survival. In this group, a fall in RV pressure typically results in decreased coronary perfusion and myocardial ischemia.[8-10] However, elevated RV pressure can also have negative effects. In some it can cause changes in ventricular septal geometry that impact left ventricular function. In addition, some have proposed that it can promote regional myocardial ischemia by limiting the ability of normal coronary flow to reach the ventricular septal segments of the myocardium.[11]

Clinical Presentation

In the current era, most newborns with PA/IVS are prenatally diagnosed. With prenatal diagnosis, life-threatening hypoxemia at birth is averted by initiating prostaglandin therapy to maintain DA patency. When there is no prenatal diagnosis, newborns are typically identified prior to nursery discharge due to cyanosis and/or decreased oxygen saturations on pulse oximetry. Less commonly, newborns may be

referred for evaluation of a heart murmur; resulting from either tricuspid regurgitation or a patent DA. If no signs or symptoms are detected prior to DA closure, presentation may instead be that of a critically ill newborn.

Diagnostic Evaluation

Electrocardiography

The electrocardiogram typically shows a QRS axis between 0 and 120 degrees with decreased anterior right ventricular forces.

Chest Radiography

Heart size can be quite variable, with normal or decreased pulmonary vascularity, depending on DA patency and size. In the dilated right heart variant, the cardiac silhouette can be severely enlarged with lung hypoplasia.

Echocardiography

Postnatal evaluation begins with a transthoracic echocardiogram. Though associated heart disease is uncommon, initial study should be a complete anatomic survey as well as additional images from multiple imaging planes of those anatomic details that are closely associated with prognosis and surgical outcome. These include TV annulus dimensions, RV size, estimated RV pressure, and abnormalities of the coronary arteries.[12-17] TV z scores have been an excellent predictor of both RV-dependent coronary circulation and of a successful biventricular repair. While echocardiography can confirm the presence of ventricular sinusoids, it cannot confirm or exclude RV-dependent coronary circulation. Echocardiography is also used at regular intervals throughout childhood to evaluate biventricular function and growth of right heart structures.

Cardiac Catheterization

In the current era, cardiac catheterization can be both diagnostic and therapeutic. Angiography is the gold standard for diagnosing coronary artery abnormalities and for confirming or excluding RV-dependent coronary circulation. Catheterization also provides an opportunity for therapeutic interventions in some.[13,18-20] For those without RV-dependent coronary circulation, it is desirable to create pulmonary valve patency. This may be done by creating an opening in the pulmonary valve with a radiofrequency ablation catheter and then dilating the valve to allow antegrade flow.

For those who cannot have a valve dilation or for whom valve dilation does not provide adequate antegrade flow, a stent may be placed across the DA to prevent duct closure when prostaglandins are withdrawn and delay the need for surgical intervention. In older patients, catheterization may be undertaken for additional interventions, including device closure of the foramen ovale, further dilation of the pulmonary valve, pulmonary valve replacement, and rarely coronary artery intervention.

Computed Tomography and Magnetic Resonance Imaging

There is rarely a role for MRI in the newborn, but it may be used as patients age to define pulmonary artery growth, ventricular growth, and ventricular function. The role of ultrafast CT for this condition is in evolution. In this institution, we often consider a pre-catheterization CT in newborns to delineate DA shape/size and pulmonary artery anatomy to allow for better procedural planning in newborns. CT is also used to image the coronary arteries, though in newborns with high heart rates, proximal coronary artery imaging is sufficiently variable to limit its reliability for decision-making. In older children, however, visualization is excellent, and this provides a less invasive method to follow those with concerning coronary artery pathology. This technology is progressing rapidly and is likely to have expanded utility in the future.

Management

Management is usually based on the size of the RV and TV, the RV pressure, and the anatomy of the coronary circulation. The goal is achievement of a two-ventricle circulation in as many children as possible. At the core of the treatment strategy is the expectation that improving antegrade flow through the right heart can lead to improved right heart growth.[12,13,19-21]

When the TV and RV are well developed, simply perforating and dilating the pulmonary valve may be all that is needed. In some, this provides sufficient antegrade pulmonary flow that the DA can safely close. The smaller the right heart structures, the more likely it is that this will not be adequate, and a staged approach will be required, involving opening the valve while assuring a second source of pulmonary flow by surgically placing a systemic-pulmonary shunt or stenting the DA. When pulmonary annular dimensions are small and/or there is muscular obstruction below the valve annulus, it is likely that the RV outflow tract will also require surgical enlargement. In the first years of life, additional interventions may include closure of the atrial level communication, surgical TV repair, and less commonly, procedures to improve branch pulmonary artery geometry or size. All interventions have the goal of improving antegrade flow early in life to maximize the opportunity for right heart growth and remodeling.

For those with RV hypoplasia, if ventricular growth is adequate, ultimately there will be a plan for closure of the foramen ovale and removal of any accessory sources of pulmonary blood flow (surgically or in the cath lab). If growth is inadequate, a single-ventricle strategy (Fontan operation) or a hybrid strategy (sometimes termed a 1.5-ventricle repair) may be pursued. The single-ventricle strategy is designed to separate the systemic (deoxygenated) and pulmonary venous (oxygenated) returns by only having the oxygenated blood enter the functional single ventricle (detailed discussion in Chapter 59). This typically involves ligation of the pulmonary artery so that there is no longer ejection from the RV into the lungs and then creation of a superior cavopulmonary anastomosis which redirects the upper body venous return directly to the lungs. The palliation is completed with redirection of the venous return from the lower body to the lungs (typically by age 2–4 years). In the 1.5-ventricle repair, a superior cavopulmonary anastomosis is created and the foramen ovale is closed so that upper body venous blood goes directly to the lungs.[10] The venous return from the lower body continues to enter the right heart with ejection from RV to the pulmonary arteries. This strategy allows for separation of the pulmonary and systemic circulations while decreasing the volume load on the small RV. In this scenario the RV is contributing to pulmonary blood flow, but only needs to be responsible for a fraction of the cardiac output to the lungs.

In those with RV-dependent coronary circulation, the pulmonary valve cannot be opened because the induced reduction in intracavitary pressure can cause significant myocardial ischemia. Treatment options involve a single-ventricle strategy or heart transplant.

Patients with low RV pressure and severe tricuspid regurgitation are at increased risk for a poor outcome with the strategy described above. In this group, opening the pulmonary valve and adding a systemic to pulmonary shunt creates a "circular shunt" which leads to inadequate systemic perfusion (Fig. 37.6). There may also be associated lung

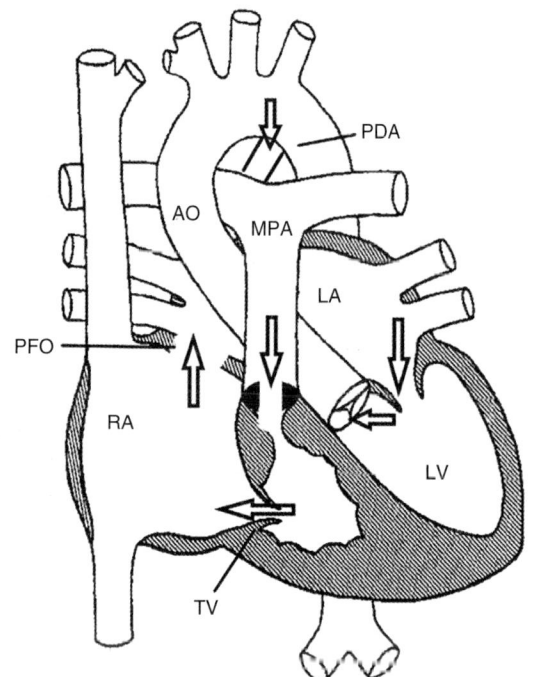

• **Fig. 37.6** Hemodynamics in pulmonary atresia with intact ventricular septum and a circular shunt. This physiology may occur after pulmonary valve dilation in patients with significant tricuspid regurgitation. Deoxygenated blood in the right atrium *(RA)* continues to cross into the left heart due to increased right ventricular compliance. It mixes with the pulmonary venous return before being ejected into the aorta. Some of this output crosses the ductus arteriosus to the pulmonary artery. After valve dilation, pulmonary regurgitation enables some ductal flow to return to the right ventricle *(RV)*, bypassing the lungs and ultimately returning to the RA via tricuspid regurgitation. This creates an ineffective circuit where a percentage of the cardiac output never picks up or delivers any oxygen, leading to hypoxia and low cardiac output. *AO,* Aorta; *LA,* left atrium; *LV,* left ventricle; *MPA,* main pulmonary artery; *PDA,* patent ductus arteriosus; *PFA,* patent foramen ovale; *TV,* tricuspid valve.

hypoplasia secondary to the severe cardiomegaly. For this group, therapeutic strategies will require case-by-case decision-making, depending on the anatomic details of the heart. Options have included surgical reduction of the RA and RV with TV repair, patch closure of the TV to surgically exclude the RV, followed by single-ventricle management, and heart transplant.

The small group with coronary ostial atresia typically do poorly with any interventions, and our current strategy is to maintain ductal patency while evaluating for a heart transplant.

An algorithm for neonatal assessment and management is diagrammed in Fig. 37.7.

Prognosis

As experience with this multipronged approach has increased, survival has improved, in part related to increased understanding of which patients benefit from which treatment strategies.[12,18,21,22] In the current era, all three strategies have good survival in short- and medium-term follow-up. Overall, survival has been over 80% in most series for biventricular, 1.5- and single-ventricle groups. The reported long-term outcomes suggest lower overall survival, but frequently include infants from the earlier eras of intervention. Because treatment has evolved significantly, those treated in the current era may have fewer late events. The subset of patients with coronary ostial atresia have the lowest survival rate in all series due in part to a high risk for death in infancy. Survival is also reduced for those with severe right heart dilation, severe tricuspid regurgitation, and low RV pressure. Outcomes mirror those described for neonates with severe tricuspid regurgitation and cardiomegaly due to Ebstein anomaly of the TV.

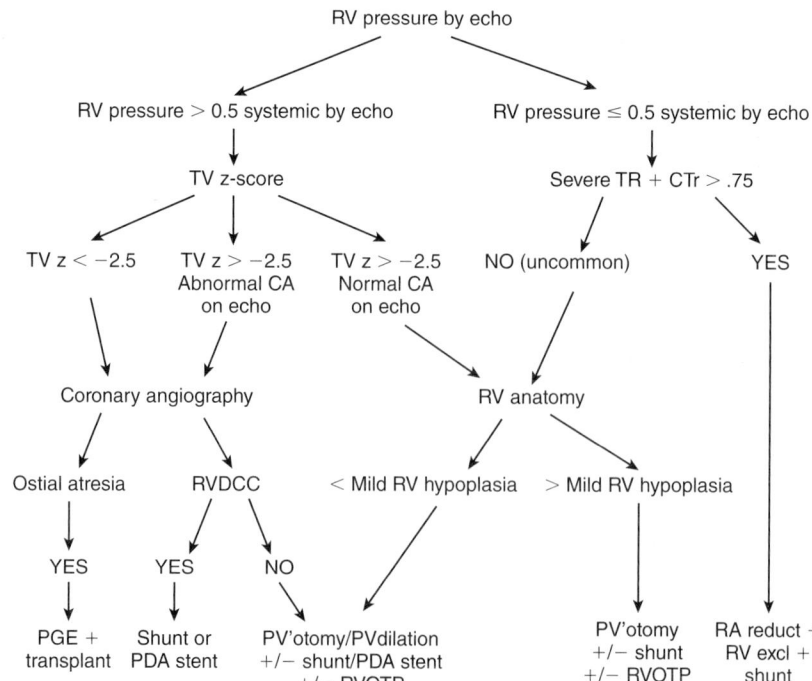

• **Fig. 37.7** Schematic outlining newborn management. *CA,* Coronary artery; *CTr,* cardiothoracic ratio; *PDA,* patent ductus arteriosus; *PGE,* prostaglandin; *PV,* pulmonary valve; *RV,* right ventricle, *RVDCC,* right ventricular-dependent coronary circulation; *RVOTP,* right ventricular outflow tract patch; *TR,* tricuspid regurgitation; *TV z,* tricuspid valve z score.

Late complications have been described and may include tricuspid and pulmonary valve dysfunction, sometimes requiring reintervention, liver disease from elevated right atrial pressures, and arrhythmias.[23-28]

References

1. Fyler DC, Buckley LP, Hellenbrand WE, et al. Report of the New England Regional Infant Cardiac Program. *Pediatrics.* 1980;65:375-461.

2. Mitchell SC, Korones SB, Berends HW. Congenital heart disease in 56,109 births. *Circulation.* 1971;43:323-332.

3. Erikson NL, Buttino LJ, Juberg RC. Congenital pulmonary atresia and patent ductus arteriosus in two sibs. *Am J Med Genet.* 1989;32:187-188.

4. Daubeny PE, Delaney DJ, Anderson RH, et al. Pulmonary atresia with intact ventricular septum. Range of morphology in a population–based study. *J Am Coll Cardiol.* 2002;39:1670-1679.

5. Zuberbuhler JR, Anderson RH. Morphological variations in pulmonary atresia with intact ventricular septum. *Br Heart J.* 1979;41:281-288.

6. Kipps AK, Powell AJ, Levine JC. Muscular infundibular atresia is associated with coronary ostial atresia in pulmonary atresia with intact ventricular septum. *Congenit Heart Dis.* 2011;6:444-450.

7. Freedom R, Anderson R, Perrin D. The significance of ventriculo-coronary arterial connections in the setting of pulmonary atresia with an intact ventricular septum. *Cardiol Young.* 2005; 15:447-468.

8. Guleserian KJ, Armsby LB, Thiagarajan RR, et al. Natural history of pulmonary atresia with intact ventricular septum and right ventricle-dependent coronary circulation managed by the single-ventricle approach. *Ann Thorac Surg.* 2006;6:2250-2257.

9. Giglia TM, Mandell VS, Connor AR, et al. Diagnosis and management of right ventricular dependent coronary circulation in pulmonary atresia with intact ventricular septum. *Circulation.* 1992;86:1516-1528.

10. Gentles TL, Colan SD, Giglia TG, et al. Right ventricular decompression and left ventricular function in pulmonary atresia with intact ventricular septum. The influence of less extensive coronary anomalies. *Circulation.* 1993;88:183-188.

11. Sholler GF, Colan SD, Sanders SP. Effect of isolated right ventricular outflow obstruction on left ventricular function in infants. *Am J Cardiol.* 1988;62:778-784.

12. Mainwaring RD, Lamberti JJ. Pulmonary atresia with intact ventricular septum. Surgical approach based on ventricular size and coronary anatomy. *J Thorac Cardiovasc Surg.* 1993;106: 733-738.

13. Jahangiri M, Zurakowski D, Bichell D, et al. Improved results with selective management in pulmonary atresia with intact ventricular septum. *J Thorac Cardiovasc Surg.* 1999;118:1046-1055.

14. Giglia TM, Jenkins KJ, Matitiau A, et al. Influence of right heart size on outcome in pulmonary atresia with intact ventricular septum. *Circulation.* 1993;88:2248-2256.

15. Peterson RE, Levi DS, Williams RJ, et al. Echocardiographic predictors of outcome in fetuses with pulmonary atresia with intact ventricular septum. *J Am Soc Echocardiogr.* 2006;19:1393-1400.

16. Salvin J, Colan SD, McElhinney DB, et al. Fetal tricuspid valve annulus as a predictor of single vs. biventricular outcome in pulmonary atresia with intact ventricular septum. *Pediatrics.* 2006;118:415-420.

17. Satou GM, Perry SB, Gauvreau K, Geva T. Echocardiographic predictors of coronary artery pathology in pulmonary atresia with intact ventricular septum. *Am J Cardiol.* 2000;85: 1319-1324.

18. Humpl T, Soderberg B, McCrindle B, et al. Percutaneous balloon valvotomy in pulmonary atresia with intact ventricular septum: impact on patient care. *Circulation.* 2003;108:826-832.

19. Chubb H, Pesonen E, Sivasubramanian S, et al. Long–term outcome following catheter valvotomy for pulmonary atresia with intact ventricular septum. *J Am Coll Cardiol.* 2010;59: 1468-1476.

20. Hoashi T, Kagisaki K, Kitano M, et al. Late clinical features of patients with pulmonary atresia or critical pulmonary stenosis with intact ventricular septum after biventricular repair. *Ann Thorac Surg.* 2012;94:833-841.

21. Cleuziou J, Schreiber C, Eicken A, et al. Predictors for biventricular repair in pulmonary atresia with intact ventricular septum. *Thorac Cardiovasc Surg.* 2010;58:339-344.

22. Montanaro C, Merola A, Kempny A, et al. The outcome of adults born with pulmonary atresia: high morbidity and mortality irrespective of repair. *Int J Cardiol.* 2019;280:61-66.

23. Zheng, J, Gao B, Zhu A, et al. Surgical results for pulmonary atresia with intact ventricular septum: a single center 15 year experience and medium term follow up. *Eur J Cardiothorac Surg.* 2016;50:1083-1088.

24. Wright LK, Knight JH, Thomas AS, et al. Long-term outcomes after intervention for pulmonary atresia with intact ventricular septum. *Heart.* 2019;105:1007-1013.

25. Muneuchi J, Watanabe M, Sugitani Y, et al. Long-term outcomes after an individualized strategy in patients with pulmonary atresia and intact ventricular septum. *Pediatr Cardiol.* 2022;43: 435-442.

26. Sukhavasi A, McHugh-Grant S, Glatz AC, et al. Pulmonary atresia with intact ventricular septum: intended strategies. *J Thorac Cardiovasc Surg.* 2022;16:325-327.

27. Schneider AW, Blom NA, Bruggemans EF, et al. More than 25 years of experience in managing pulmonary atresia with intact ventricular septum. *Ann Thorac Surg.* 2014;98:1680-1686.

28. Shi JZ, Chow PC, Li W, et al. Fifty-Five years follow-up of 111 adult survivors after biventricular repair of PAIVS and PS. *Pediatr Cardiol.* 2019;40:374-383.

38

Truncus Arteriosus and Hemitruncus

LAURA GELLIS AND DAVID W. BROWN

KEY LEARNING POINTS

- Truncus arteriosus is defined as a single arterial vessel that arises from the heart, and gives rise to the coronary arteries, aorta, and pulmonary arteries. The majority of patients with truncus arteriosus also have a conoventricular septal defect.
- DiGeorge syndrome (22q11 deletion syndrome) is present in 30%–35% of patients with truncus arteriosus.
- Babies who are not prenatally diagnosed are symptomatic within the first weeks of life, and often in the neonatal period. Evidence of congestive heart failure is the common presenting symptom with tachypnea and increased work of breathing.
- Survival after neonatal repair has improved, but a significant burden of morbidity and mortality remains both in the neonatal period and over follow-up. In the contemporary era (1995 onward), early mortality rates, defined as within 30 days of surgery or prior to hospital discharge, have fallen from previously ~20% to ~8%–11%. Among those who survived to discharge, survival at 1, 10, and 20 years is ~93%, ~80%–87%, and ~75%–81%, respectively.

- These patients require life-long follow-up. Catheter and surgical re-interventions are an expected part of a patient's clinic course. In particular, the right ventricular pulmonary homograft will require dilation and stenting of the via cardiac catheterization and ultimately surgical upsizing to accommodate for somatic growth. Additionally, the need for truncal valve repair and replacements remains a frequent component of long-term care with ~25% of patients requiring truncal valve intervention by 20 years.
- Hemitruncus or origin of a branch pulmonary artery from the ascending aorta is defined when a pulmonary valve and main pulmonary artery are present but one of the pulmonary artery branches comes off the ascending aorta and the other arises from the main pulmonary artery. Previously and in literature, this has also been referred to as "hemitruncus" despite no known direct embryologic or morphological relationship with truncus arteriosus.

Truncus Arteriosus

Definition

Truncus arteriosus is defined as a single arterial vessel that arises from the heart, and gives rise to the coronary arteries, aorta, and pulmonary arteries. The majority of patients with truncus arteriosus also have a conoventricular septal defect. Only one semilunar valve is present in truncus arteriosus and typically overrides the VSD. Unlike in tetralogy of Fallot with pulmonary atresia in which the pulmonary circulation is supplied by aortopulmonary collaterals or a ductus arteriosus, in truncus arteriosus, the main pulmonary artery or at least one pulmonary artery arises directly from the arterial trunk.

Prevalence

Truncus arteriosus is a rare lesion and is reported to occur in ~2%–4% of patients with congenital heart disease.[1] DiGeorge syndrome, also known as 22q11 deletion syndrome, results

from a chromosomal microdeletion at 22q11 and is present in 30%–35% of patients with truncus arteriosus.[2,3] Genetics of conotruncal heart disease together with recurrence risk data are discussed in detail in Chapter 5.

Embryology

In the normal embryo, septation of the single truncus arteriosus into aorta and main pulmonary artery together with aortic and pulmonary valve formation occurs by the end of the 5th week. Ectomesenchymal cells derived from the cardiac neural crest are involved in septation. Shortly thereafter, conal septum formation is completed. It is thought that disturbances during these weeks result in conotruncal abnormalities including truncus arteriosus.[4,5]

Anatomy

Typically, the single arterial trunk is positioned above a conoventricular VSD with the single semilunar valve (truncal valve) typically overriding the VSD. Rarely the ventricular septum is intact.[6]

Truncal valve morphology is tricommissural in ~55%–70%, bicuspid in ~10%–16%, and quadricuspid in 30%–33%. Even when tricommissural, the truncal valve cusps are often thickened and dysplastic. Neonatal truncal valve dysfunction is frequent with ~45%–52% of patients having at least mild truncal regurgitation at birth (14%–16% greater than mild) and ~10%–34% having at least mild degree of truncal stenosis (4%–9% greater than mild).[7-10] Additionally, the truncal root is typically dilated and larger truncal root z-scores both at birth and over follow-up have been shown to be associated with progressive truncal regurgitation.[9]

Truncus arteriosus classification is based primarily on the origin of pulmonary blood flow. The Van Praagh and Van Praagh classification is outlined in Fig. 38.1. In type I, the branch pulmonary arteries arise from a short main pulmonary artery off the arterial trunk (45%–68% of cases). In type II, the branch pulmonary arteries arise from separate, usually closely spaced origins off the arterial trunk (29%–48% of cases). Type III is characterized by having one branch pulmonary artery arising from the ascending portion of the arterial trunk and collateral vessel(s) supply

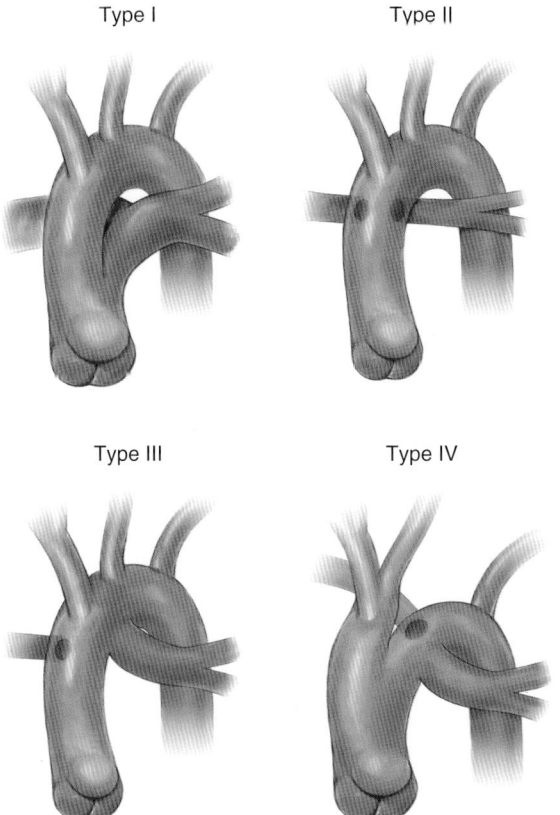

• **Fig. 38.1** Van Praagh and Van Praagh classification of truncus arteriosus. Type I: the branch pulmonary arteries arise from a short main pulmonary artery off the arterial trunk. Type II: the branch pulmonary arteries arise from separate origins off the arterial trunk. Type III: one branch pulmonary artery arising from the ascending portion of the arterial trunk and collateral vessel(s) supply the contralateral lung. Type IV: aortic coarctation or interruption and both branch pulmonary arteries arise from the arterial trunk.

the contralateral lung (6%–10% of cases). In type IV, there is aortic coarctation or interruption (interruption occurring in 11%–19% of cases) and both branch pulmonary arteries arise from the arterial trunk. The modification of "A" is used if a VSD is present and "B" if there is no VSD. The branch pulmonary arteries typically arise from the posterior-lateral aspect of the arterial trunk. A right aortic arch occurs in ~25%–36% of patients, and in the majority of cases a patent ductus arteriosus (PDA) is absent, except from type IV in which a ductus is necessary to supply lower body blood flow.[1,11,12]

Coronary artery anomalies are frequent and can include a prominent right conal artery, and ostial anomalies such as single coronary artery, as well as high or low origins or narrowing of the vessels.[7,9,13]

Additional frequent associations with truncus arteriosus include atrial septal defects, aberrant subclavian artery, persistent left superior vena cava, retro-aortic left innominate vein, and partial anomalous pulmonary venous return (Table 38.1).

Physiology

The single outflow tract receives the output of both ventricles and, within a short distance, the blood destined for pulmonary circulation is diverted to the lungs (Fig. 38.2). The amount of pulmonary blood flow is determined by the presence of pulmonary stenosis (which is uncommon) and by the balance between systemic vascular and pulmonary arteriolar resistance. In the absence of pulmonary stenosis, the expected reduction in pulmonary resistance in the first days of life leads to pulmonary overcirculation that is often not well tolerated. Systemic arterial saturation is determined by the amount of pulmonary blood flow, which is typically excessive and saturations remain high. Truncal regurgitation of some degree is present in many patients, and when severe, the added burden of the diastolic regurgitant flow may be more than can be tolerated and can lead to early congestive heart failure and low diastolic coronary perfusion pressure with the risk of ischemia. Because of the excessive pulmonary blood flow, development of pulmonary vascular obstructive disease is common among survivors who have not undergone surgery and it can occur as early as 6 months of age.

Clinical Manifestations

Truncus arteriosus is readily identified on fetal echocardiogram, which shows an abnormal four-chamber view and single outflow tract with the majority of cases diagnosed prenatally in the contemporary era. Babies who are not prenatally diagnosed are symptomatic within the first weeks of life, and often in the neonatal period. Evidence of congestive heart failure is the common presenting symptom with tachypnea and increased work of breathing. The peripheral pulses are bounding and there is a widened pulse pressure due to the run off to the pulmonary arteries during

TABLE 38.1	Boston Children's Hospital Experience 1985–2020	
	Overall (N = 170)	
Male	87 (51.2%)	
Median age at surgery, days	10.5 (5.0–35.0)	
Age at Surgery		
≤ 7 days	69 (40.6%)	
8–30 days	55 (32.4%)	
31–90 days	22 (12.9%)	
> 90 days	24 (14.1%)	
TA Classification		
A1	76 (45.0%)	
A2	51 (30.2%)	
A3	13 (7.7%)	
A4	29 (17.2%)	
Truncal Valve Morphology		
Tricuspid	87 (56.5%)	
Bicuspid	16 (10.4%)	
Quadricuspid	51 (33.1%)	
Associate Anomalies		
DiGeorge syndrome	31 (18.2%)	
Right aortic arch	47 (27.6%)	
Patent ductus arteriosus	40 (23.5%)	
Anomalous vein	15 (8.8%)	
Mitral valve anomaly	11 (6.5%)	
Coronary anomalies	50 (29.4%)	
Extracardiac anomaly	25 (14.7%)	
At the Time of Initial Surgery		
Concomitant truncal valve repair	14 (8.2%)	
Concomitant arch repair	25 (14.7%)	
Non-biventricular repair	4 (2.4%)	
Mortality		
Early (≤30 days postoperative or prior to discharge)	22 (31%)	
Late (>30 days post repair or after hospital discharge)	28 (16%)	

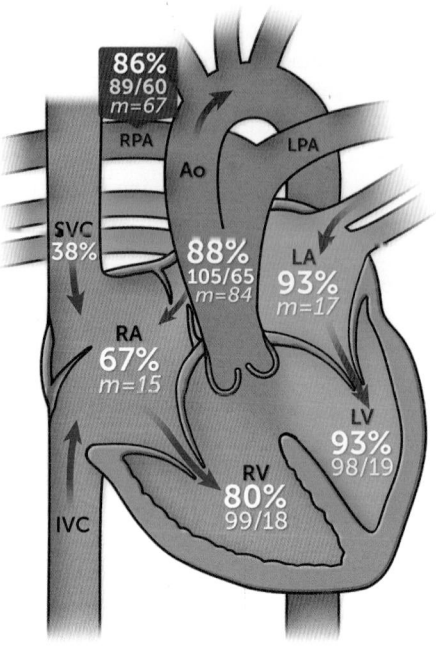

• **Fig. 38.2** Diagram of the hemodynamics in a patient with truncus arteriosus. Equilibration of systemic and pulmonary pressures; the complete mixing of systemic and pulmonary blood as evidenced by similar systemic and pulmonary oxygen concentrations. *Ao*, Aorta; *IVC*, inferior vena cava; *LA*, left atrium; *LPA*, left pulmonary artery; *LV*, left ventricle; *RA*, right atrium; *RPA*, right pulmonary artery; *RV*, right ventricle; *SVC*, superior vena cava.

diastolic flow rumble due to relative mitral stenosis and a huge pulmonary blood flow is common. Some infants can be visibly cyanotic in the rare situation of pulmonary artery stenosis or persistently elevated pulmonary vascular resistance. In older infants and children who are not repaired, pulmonary vascular obstructive disease may develop with associated cyanosis and other clinical features that reflect the elevated pulmonary vascular resistance.

Electrocardiography

The electrocardiogram may show left or right ventricular hypertrophy, with left or combined ventricular hypertrophy being more common.

Chest Radiography

Chest radiographs show cardiomegaly and increased pulmonary vasculature. There may be a right aortic arch.

Echocardiography

From a subcostal long-axis view, the echocardiogram shows the overriding truncal root and its leftward posterior originating pulmonary artery is visualized atop a large conoventricular septal defect together with truncal valve thickness and mobility (Fig. 38.3) The atrial and ventricular septa, atrioventricular valves, and truncal valve commissural

diastole and if truncal regurgitation is present. There is generally an easily palpable and often visible right ventricular impulse. There is usually a systolic murmur at the left sternal border, sometimes associated with the diastolic murmur of truncal regurgitation. There is frequently a prominent ejection click audible at the apex or the left sternal border, and the second heart sound is usually single although this may be difficult to detect in a small sick infant. An apical

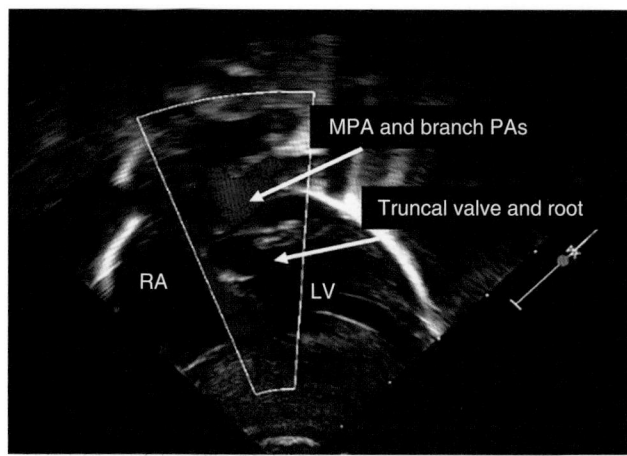

• **Fig. 38.3** Echocardiogram subcostal long axis. Subcostal echocardiographic image showing overriding truncal valve with the main pulmonary artery *(MPA)* arising from the single arterial root. *LV,* Left ventricle; *PAs,* pulmonary arteries; *RA,* right atrium.

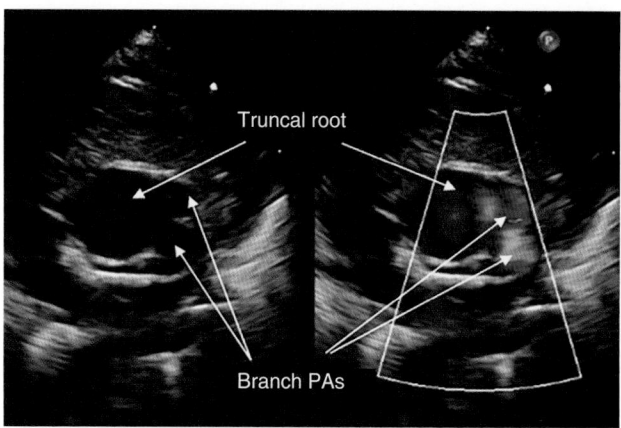

• **Fig. 38.5** Echocardiogram parasternal short-axis imaging of branch pulmonary artery *(PA)* origins. Two-dimensional imaging on the left and color Doppler interrogation on the right from the parasternal short-axis imaging plane demonstrating unobstructed flow into the separate pulmonary artery branches as they originate from the truncal root (truncus arteriosus type II).

details may be evaluated using a short-axis subcostal view. Truncal valve stenosis may be quantitated using Doppler from apical, suprasternal, or right sternal border views, and regurgitation from parasternal or apical transducer locations. Truncal valve morphology, coronary artery origins, and branching details, including ostial to pulmonary artery origin measurements, are available from parasternal long- and short-axis views (Fig. 38.4).

The proximal pulmonary artery anatomy and the truncus type (Fig. 38.5) are displayed using parasternal short-axis and suprasternal notch views.

The ascending and transverse aortic arch, brachiocephalic arterial, and ductal origin anatomy can be outlined on a suprasternal notch short-axis view.

Cardiac Computed Tomography and Magnetic Resonance Imaging

Cardiac computed tomography can provide additional anatomic clarification of branch pulmonary arteries, arch, and

occasionally coronary arteries in the neonatal period without sedation and with using low radiation doses (Fig. 38.6). In older children and repaired adults, magnetic resonance imaging can also serve as an alternative to echocardiography for comprehensive anatomic and functional assessments.

Cardiac Catheterization

Catheterization is rarely needed prior to repair as echocardiogram, supplemented with cardiac computed tomography

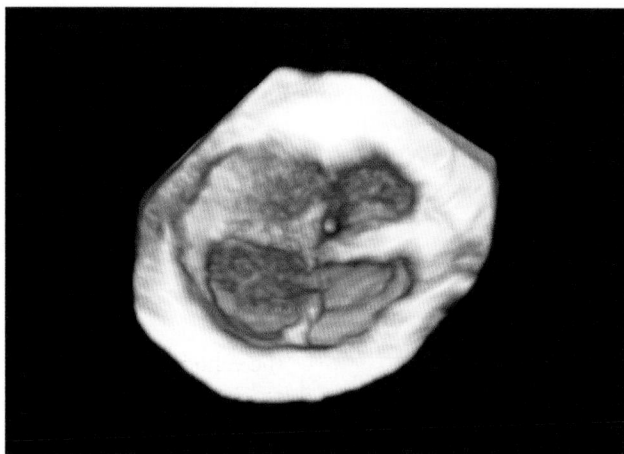

• **Fig. 38.4** Three-dimensional echocardiogram reconstruction of a quadricuspid truncal valve in diastole as viewed from above.

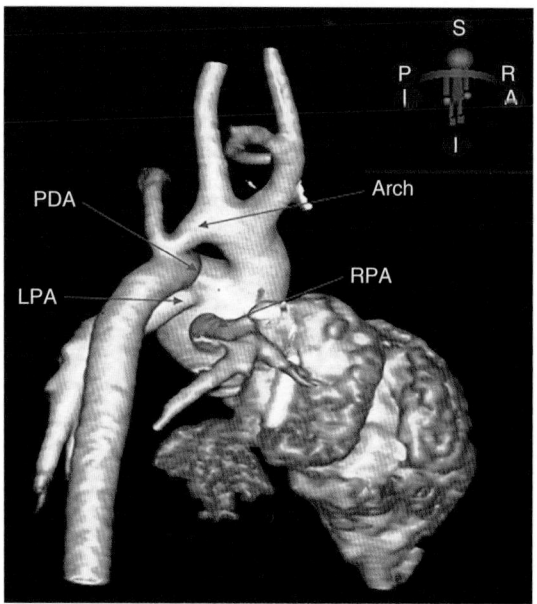

• **Fig. 38.6** Cardiac computed tomography (CT) of truncus type IV with coarctation of the aorta. Three-dimensional reconstruction of cardiac CT viewed posteriorly demonstrating separate origins of the right and left pulmonary arteries off the single arterial trunk. There is coarctation of the aortic arch and a patent ductus arteriosus *(PDA)* is present consistent with type IV truncus arteriosus. *LPA,* Left pulmonary artery; *RPA,* right pulmonary artery.

in some cases, provides precise anatomic details as well as characterizing ventricular function, truncal, and atrioventricular valve function. The only preoperative indications for such a study would include uncertainty about anatomic information or suspicion of pulmonary vascular obstructive disease, which does occur even in infants with this lesion. The purpose of the study in the latter is to evaluate pulmonary resistance response to vasodilators such as oxygen and nitric oxide.

Management

Since most of these patients will develop heart failure in the neonatal period, since the mid-1980s, the management strategy has focused on complete neonatal repair. Repair consists of VSD closure, removal of the branch pulmonary arteries from the common trunk with patch closure of the defect in the trunk, and placement of a valved homograft from the right ventricle to the detached pulmonary arteries, and aortic arch interruption or coarctation repair if present (type IV). Concomitant truncal valve repair in patients with significant truncal valve dysfunction continues to evolve.

Survival after neonatal repair has improved, but a significant burden of morbidity and mortality remains both in the neonatal period and over follow-up. In the contemporary era (1995 onward), early mortality rates, defined as within 30 days of surgery or prior to hospital discharge, have fallen from previously ~20% to ~8%–11%. Among those who survived to discharge, survival at 1, 10, and 20 years is ~93%, ~80%–87%, and ~75%–81%, respectively.[7-9,14] (Fig. 38.7).

These patients require life-long follow-up. Catheter and surgical re-interventions are an expected part of a patient's clinic course. In particular the right ventricular pulmonary homograft will require dilation and stenting of the via cardiac catheterization and ultimately surgical upsizing to accommodate for somatic growth. Additionally, the need for truncal valve repair and replacements remains a frequent component of long-term care with ~25% of patients requiring truncal

valve intervention by 20 years.[9,10] The majority of patients who survive into adulthood have no or mild limitation in functional status (New York Heart Association functional class I or II), though reduced objective measures of exercise capacity and neurodevelopmental delays are common.[15] Subacute bacterial endocarditis prophylaxis is only needed in the initial 6 months after surgical repair when prosthetic material is used, in patients who have undergone surgical repair and have residual defects at the site or adjacent to the site of the prosthetic material, if there is a history of endocarditis, or in patients who are cyanotic.[16]

Hemitruncus (Origin of Branch Pulmonary Artery From the Ascending Aorta)

Definition

Origin of a branch pulmonary artery from the ascending aorta is defined when a pulmonary valve and main pulmonary artery are present but one of the pulmonary artery branches comes off the ascending aorta and the other arises from the main pulmonary artery. Previously and in literature, this has also been referred to as "hemitruncus" despite no known direct embryologic or morphological relationship with truncus arteriosus.

Prevalence

Hemitruncus is a rare disease that is reported to account for ~0.12% of all congenital heart defects. It is often associated with other cardiac malformations such as tetralogy of Fallot and pulmonary atresia and chromosome 22q11 microdeletion for genetic syndromes.[17-20] At Boston Children's Hospital over the most recent 20-year period (2003–2022), there were 14 cases of hemitruncus, 3 of which were associated with tetralogy of Fallot with pulmonary atresia. Right hemitruncus was present in 12 (86%), with a left aortic arch in all of those cases. Of two patients with left hemitruncus,

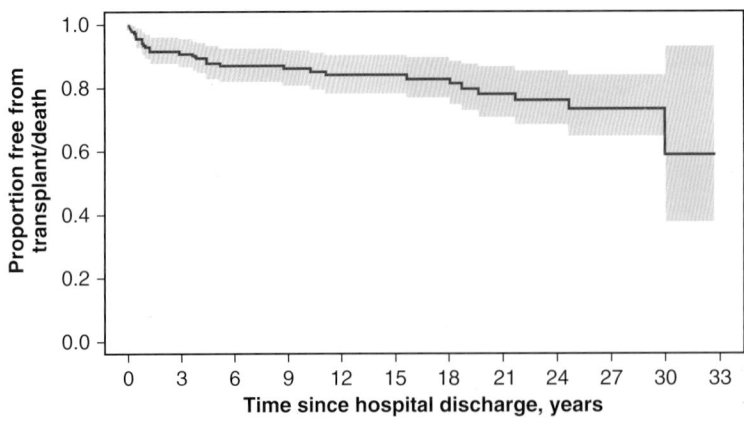

at risk 148 124 107 91 79 67 57 43 30 16 4 0

• **Fig. 38.7** Freedom from death or transplant for those who survive to hospitalization. Kaplan-Meier curve for long-term survival at Boston Children's Hospital among patients undergoing full repair since 1985.

one had a right aortic arch. Associated congenital heart defects other than tetralogy of Fallot included interrupted aortic arch (1), VSD (1), and atrial septal defect (1).

Embryology

Unlike truncus arteriosus, origin of a branch pulmonary artery from the ascending aorta occurs in the setting of normal separation of the aortic and pulmonary valves. Overall, the embryological development remains not clearly defined. Theories include incomplete migration of branch pulmonary arteries versus failure of the sixth arch to fuse correctly with the main pulmonary artery.[17]

Pathology

The anomalous branch pulmonary artery typically arises from the posterolateral wall of the ascending aorta just above the sinotubular junction or more distally just proximal to the innominate artery. Anomalous origin of the right pulmonary artery is more common than the left and is associated with a left aortic arch and left-sided PDA. Alternatively, anomalous origin of the left pulmonary artery is typically associated with a right aortic arch and right-sided PDA.

Physiology

After birth, due to the falling pulmonary resistance there is increased pulmonary blood flow into the lung supplied by the aorta. Blood flow to the opposite lung (supplied by normal origin of pulmonary artery) is also increased in that it receives the entire venous return (cardiac output). The pulmonary artery pressure in both lungs is elevated (Fig. 38.8) Congestive heart failure (a nearly universal phenomenon) occurs within the first weeks of life and is often severe if not repaired.

Clinical Manifestations

A systolic murmur is heard at birth. Within days or a week or so after birth, tachypnea, dyspnea, and the clinical syndrome of congestive heart failure become evident if left unrepaired. The infant has the clinical picture of a large left-to-right shunt without cyanosis. Pulses may be bounding due to diastolic runoff from the aorta into the anomalously arising pulmonary artery.

Electrocardiography

The electrocardiogram shows right ventricular hypertrophy.

Chest X-Ray

The heart is large, and the pulmonary vasculature is increased bilaterally. Sometimes the difference in vascularity between right and left lung is distinguishable, especially if tetralogy of Fallot is also present, but usually only in retrospect.

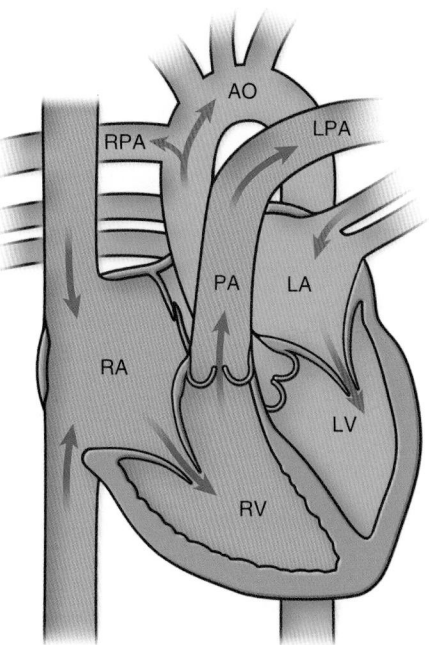

• **Fig. 38.8** Diagram of origin of the right pulmonary artery from the ascending aorta. Depiction of the right pulmonary artery (RPA) arising from the ascending aorta in the presence of a separate pulmonary valve and main pulmonary artery giving rise to the left pulmonary artery (LPA). RPA from the ascending aorta is more common than LPA arising from the ascending aorta. RPA can arise proximally by the aortic sinotubular junction or more distally by the origin of the innominate artery (shown here). *AO,* aorta; *LA,* left atrium; *LV,* left ventricle; *PA,* pulmonary artery; *RA,* right atrium; *RV,* right ventricle.

Echocardiography

The pulmonary artery arising from the aorta (usually the right) is well seen in a parasternal long- or short-axis view. Color flow Doppler mapping or the pulsed Doppler examination demonstrates continuous flow into the pulmonary artery from the aorta. The other pulmonary artery (usually the left) connects normally with the main pulmonary trunk. A persistent ductus arteriosus is commonly associated. If the ductus is large, the pulmonary trunk may appear erroneously to bifurcate normally.

Cardiac Catheterization

This is no longer necessary in the neonate because echocardiography provides all anatomic details. If considered necessary at a later age, the evaluation of right pulmonary resistance response to dilators may be necessary, at which time angiography in the left ventricle or ascending aorta may be done to confirm the diagnosis (Fig. 38.9).

Management

As soon as the diagnosis is established, the infant is stabilized on anti-congestive medications, and cardiac surgery is carried out by anastomosis (typically directly) of the pulmonary artery arising from the aorta to the contralateral

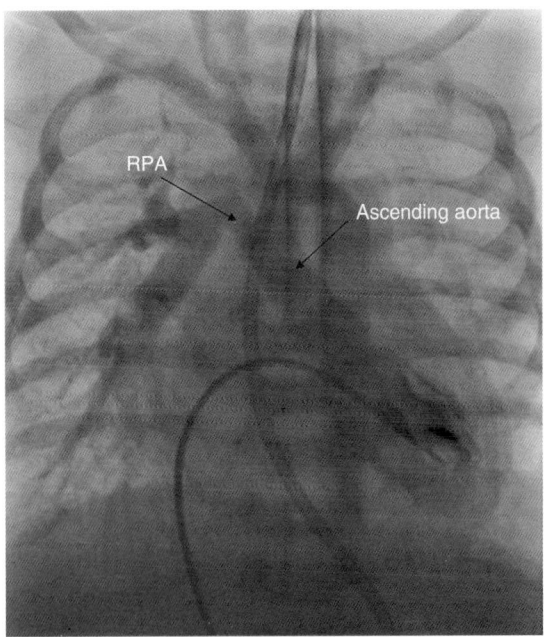

• **Fig. 38.9** Catheterization with injection into the left ventricle showing contrast filling the ascending aorta, aortic arch, and the right pulmonary artery *(RPA)* off the ascending aorta.

pulmonary artery. Due to the rarity of this lesion, there are few long-term outcome studies; during follow-up, the patient should be monitored for hypoplasia or stenosis of the pulmonary artery and management with balloon dilation or stenting may be necessary.[20-22]

Acknowledgment

The authors would like to thank and acknowledge Drs. John F. Keane and Donald C. Fyler for their contributions to a previous version of this chapter.

References

1. Van Praagh R, Van Praagh S. The anatomy of common aorticopulmonary trunk (truncus arteriosus communis) and its embryologic implications. A study of 57 necropsy cases. *Am J Cardiol.* 1965;16:406-425.
2. Goldmuntz E, Clark BJ, Mitchell LE, et al. Frequency of 22q11 deletions in patients with conotruncal defects. *J Am Coll Cardiol.* 1998;32:492-498.
3. Hamzah M, Othman HF, Daphtary K, et al. Outcomes of truncus arteriosus repair and predictors of mortality. *J Card Surg.* 2020; 35:1856-1864.
4. de la Cruz MV, da Rocha JP. An ontogenetic theory for the explanation of congenital malformations involving the truncus and conus. *Am Heart J.* 1956;51:782-805.
5. Kirby ML. Cellular and molecular contributions of the cardiac neural crest to cardiovascular development. *Trends Cardiovasc Med.* 1993;3:18-23.
6. Carr I, Bharati S, Kusnoor VS, Lev M. Truncus arteriosus communis with intact ventricular septum. *Heart.* 1979;42: 97-102.
7. Naimo PS, Bell D, Fricke TA, et al. Truncus arteriosus repair: a 40-year multicenter perspective. *J Thorac Cardiovasc Surg.* 2021; 161:230-240.
8. Naimo PS, Fricke TA, Yong MS, et al. Outcomes of truncus arteriosus repair in children: 35 years of experience from a single institution. *Semin Thorac Cardiovasc Surg.* 2016;28: 500-511.
9. Gellis L, Binney G, Alshawabkeh L, et al. Long-term fate of the truncal valve. *J Am Heart Assoc.* 2020;9:e019104.
10. Guariento A, Doulamis IP, Staffa SJ, et al. Long-term outcomes of truncus arteriosus repair: a modulated renewal competing risks analysis. *J Thorac Cardiovasc Surg.* 2022;163:224-236.e6.
11. Bharati S, McAllister HA, Rosenquist GC, et al. The surgical anatomy of truncus arteriosus communis. *J Thorac Cardiovasc Surg.* 1974;67:501-510.
12. Calder L, Praagh R Van, Praagh S Van, et al. Clinical, angiocardiographic, and pathologic findings in 100 patients. *Am Heart J.* 1976;92:23-38.
13. de la Cruz M V, Cayre R, Angelini P, et al. Coronary arteries in truncus arteriosus. *Am J Cardiol.* 1990;66:1482-1486.
14. Russell HM, Pasquali SK, Jacobs JP, et al. Outcomes of repair of common arterial trunk with truncal valve surgery: a review of the society of thoracic surgeons congenital heart surgery database. *Ann Thorac Surg.* 2012;93:164-169.
15. Marino BS, Lipkin PH, Newburger JW, et al. Neurodevelopmental outcomes in children with congenital heart disease: evaluation and management. *Circulation.* 2012;126:1143-1172.
16. Wilson W, Taubert KA, Gewitz M, et al. Prevention of infective endocarditis. *Circulation.* 2007;116:1736-1754.
17. Aru GM, English WP, Gaymes CH, et al. Origin of the left pulmonary artery from the aorta: embryologic considerations. *Ann Thorac Surg.* 2001;71:1008-1010.
18. Peng E, Shanmugam G, Macarthur K, et al. Ascending aortic origin of a branch pulmonary artery? Surgical management and long-term outcome. *Eur J Cardiothorac Surg.* 2004;26: 762-766.
19. Fong L V, Anderson RH, Siewers RD, et al. Anomalous origin of one pulmonary artery from the ascending aorta: a review of echocardiographic, catheter, and morphological features. *Heart.* 1989;62:389-395.
20. Dong S, Yan J, Xu H, et al. The surgical treatment of anomalous origin of one pulmonary artery from the ascending aorta. *J Cardiothorac Surg.* 2019;14:82.
21. Prifti E, Bonacchi M, Murzi B, et al. Anomalous origin of the right pulmonary artery from the ascending aorta. *J Card Surg.* 2004;19:103-112.
22. Goldstein BH, Bergersen L, Powell AJ, et al. Long-term outcome of surgically repaired unilateral anomalous pulmonary artery origin. *Pediatr Cardiol.* 2010;31:944-951.

39

Total Anomalous Pulmonary Venous Connection

CHRISTINA RONAI AND DAVID W. BROWN

KEY LEARNING POINTS

- In total anomalous pulmonary venous connection (TAPVC), all pulmonary venous blood returns to the right atrium. Some form of interatrial communication between the right and left sides of the heart is essential for survival.
- Clinical presentation depends on whether or not there is some degree of pulmonary venous obstruction.
- Supracardiac connection, or connection of the pulmonary venous confluence via a vertical vein to the innominate vein or superior vena cava, is the most common form of TAPVC.

- Early mortality has improved dramatically over the years, even as the age at surgery has decreased. Among series of patients operated on in the past two decades, early mortality rates have ranged from 2% to 10%.
- The most important problem survivors encounter is pulmonary venous obstruction (stenosis), either in individual veins or at the anastomotic connection to the left atrium. It occurs in about 10% of patients (more common in those with infradiaphragmatic or mixed types), is often progressive, and is associated with high mortality rates, from 25% to 46%.

Definition

Drainage of the entire pulmonary venous circulation into systemic venous channels characterizes total anomalous pulmonary venous connection (TAPVC).

Incidence

TAPVC has been described in 9 in 100,000 of the population.[1,2] TAPVC has syndromic associations with cat-eye, Holt-Oram, and the asplenia syndromes.

Embryology

Normally, by the end of the first month of human development, lung buds and the tracheobronchial tree have developed from derivatives of the foregut, with vascular supply from the splanchnic plexus. Portions of the splanchnic plexus become the pulmonary vascular bed, which has numerous connections with the cardinal and omphalovitelline systems. Shortly thereafter, a common pulmonary vein appears, connecting the pulmonary venous plexus and the sinoatrial portion of the heart, and later becomes incorporated into the left atrial wall, by which time the pulmonary–splanchnic venous connections have regressed. When failure of the common pulmonary vein to unite with the left atrium occurs, some of the pulmonary–splanchnic venous connections may persist, allowing pulmonary venous connections at various systemic venous–right atrial levels, such as the left innominate vein, portal vein, and coronary sinus levels.

Anatomy

Any pulmonary vein, or combination of pulmonary veins, may drain anomalously into the systemic venous or right heart circulation, producing a left-to-right shunt. When all pulmonary veins drain to the systemic venous circulation, the patient is said to have TAPVC (drainage, return). There are several anatomic variations (Fig. 39.1; Table 39.1). Common to all types, other than mixed, is the presence of a common horizontal pulmonary vein, usually large and draining both lungs immediately posterior to the left atrium. This structure is more vertically oriented in infradiaphragmatic

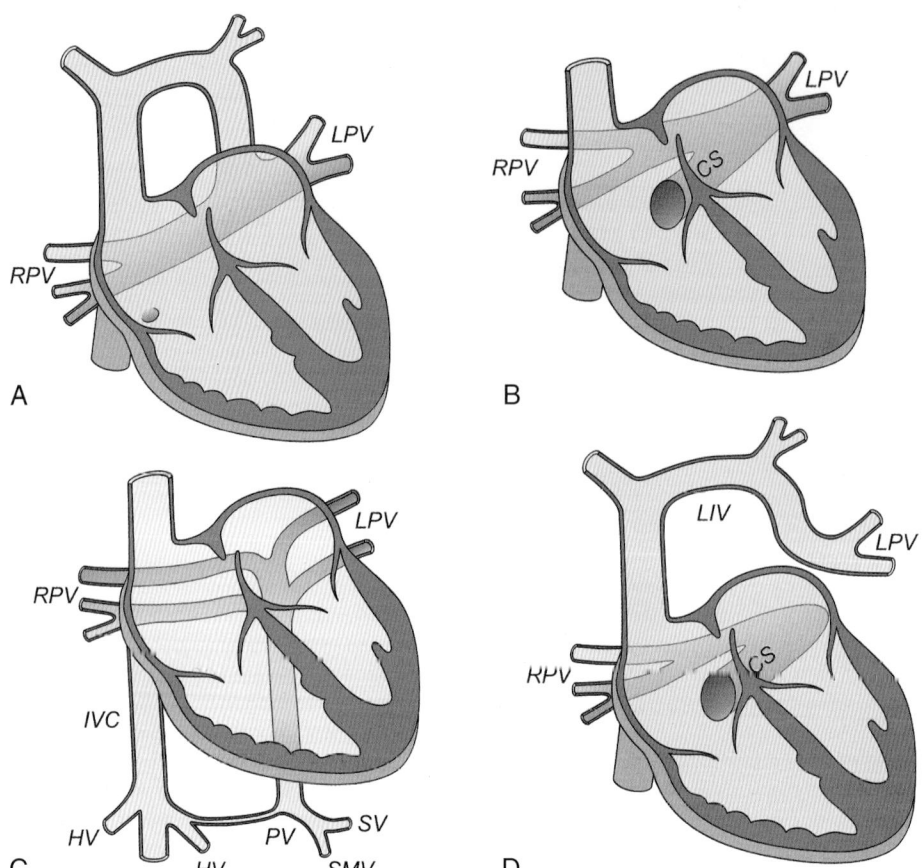

• **Fig. 39.1** Variants of total anomalous pulmonary venous connection. **(A)** Supracardiac: both right *(RPV)* and left *(LPV)* pulmonary veins join a common pulmonary venous confluence behind the heart, which drains via a vertical vein to the undersurface of the left innominate vein and then to the right atrium. **(B)** Cardiac: the pulmonary venous confluence connects to the coronary sinus *(CS)*, and then to the right atrium via the coronary sinus ostium. **(C)** Infradiaphragmatic: the pulmonary venous confluence drains inferiorly via a vertical vein to the portal vein *(PV)* or hepatic veins *(HV)* and then to the right atrium. **(D)** Mixed connections: the left pulmonary veins *(LPV)* drain to the left innominate vein *(LIV)*, and the RPV drain to the CS in this example. *IVC,* Inferior vena cava; *SMV,* superior mesenteric vein; *SV,* splanchnic vein. (Brown DW, Pulmonary Venous Anomalies. From: Lai WW, Mertens LL, Cohen MS, Geva T, eds. *Echocardiography in Pediatric and Congenital Heart Disease*, 3rd edition. Hoboken NJ: Wiley-Blackwell, 2022. Figure 10.4, page 193, with permission).

TABLE 39.1	Boston Children's Hospital Experience

Between January 2002 and January 2022, 275 patients under 1 year of age with total anomalous pulmonary venous connection (TAPVC) were seen and operated on.

Type of TAPVC	Number (%)
Total Cases TAPVC	275
Supracardiac TAPVC	123 (45)
Infracardiac TAPVC	72 (26)
Mixed TAPVC	38 (14)
TAPVC to coronary sinus	31 (11)
TAPVC to right atrium	11 (4)

total veins and may vary somewhat in anomalous connection to the coronary sinus, but it is this vein that allows the surgeon to repair this lesion by anastomosing it to the back of the left atrium.

1. **Supracardiac**. This is the most common type of TAPVC. All the pulmonary veins connect to a confluence posterior to the left atrium and then a left-sided ascending "vertical" vein typically connects to the innominate vein. This vertical vein usually passes anterior to the left pulmonary artery and mainstem bronchus, but occasionally can pass between these two structures, leading to obstruction. Sometimes there can be right-sided supracardiac connections to other cardinal system derivatives, wherein the right-sided vertical vein drains directly into the superior vena cava and occasionally into the azygous system.

2. **Cardiac**. All pulmonary veins drain into a common pulmonary vein, which then drains into the coronary sinus, which then drains normally into the right atrium; the coronary sinus septum is usually intact.

3. **Infradiaphragmatic**. This occurs when the pulmonary venous confluence has connection with the umbilicovitelline system below the diaphragm. A descending vertical vein originates from the confluence and descends through the diaphragm to the portal vein (most commonly), ductus venosus, or hepatic vein, reentering the heart through the inferior vena cava.

4. **Mixed**. This is the least common form of TAPVC. Any combination of anatomic entry of the pulmonary veins into the venous circulation is possible. For example, the right-sided veins may enter the right atrium, whereas the left veins travel upward to the left innominate.

Among large surgical series with available information, the averages of the connection sites were supracardiac, 47%; cardiac, 16%; infradiaphragmatic, 13%–23%; and mixed, 7%–10%.[3-7] The pulmonary venous system may be variably, absolutely, or relatively obstructed.[8,9] The point of obstruction may be caused by compression by adjacent structures; for example, the vertical vein to the left innominate vein may be compressed if it passes between the left bronchus and left pulmonary artery. Veins draining below the diaphragm are almost always obstructed at the diaphragm, within the liver, or with constriction of the ductus venosus. Those entering the coronary sinus are less often obstructed, whereas all other types may be obstructed in variable locations.[10] Often, increased pulmonary flow accentuates the obstruction. When there is obstruction, there is pulmonary venous hypertension and reflex pulmonary arterial hypertension, often at suprasystemic pressure levels.

Rarely, other isolated, simple cardiac anomalies, such as ventricular septal defect, are associated with total anomalous veins; however, other major cardiac abnormalities are more likely to be present in heterotaxy syndromes when there is asplenia and polysplenia (see Chapter 32).

Physiology

All venous blood returns to the right atrium. Some form of communication between the right and left sides of the heart is essential for survival in TAPVC. The entire pulmonary venous blood flow is returned to the systemic venous circulation, where there is mixing of the two venous returns. Characteristically, mixing is virtually complete, each chamber of the heart receiving blood of similar oxygen content. The level of arterial oxygen saturation is dependent on the amount of pulmonary blood flow. When there is increased pulmonary blood flow, the percentage of arterial oxygen saturation may reach the high 80s, but with limited pulmonary blood flow, it may be much lower.

The amount of pulmonary blood flow is governed by the pulmonary arteriolar resistance and by the degree of obstruction of the pulmonary veins. When the obstruction is severe, the amount of pulmonary blood flow is small; when this is mixed with the systemic venous return, the result is a low arterial oxygen saturation. Pulmonary arterial pressure may be suprasystemic with severe obstruction, and because of this, in the first days of life, the ductus arteriosus may shunt right to left. Detection of the ductal right-to-left shunt is not possible by comparing the arterial oxygen saturation above and below the ductus because all oxygen saturations in the heart are identical, negating the value of this otherwise useful test.

TAPVC below the diaphragm is characterized by severe obstruction. Less often, there is obstruction in the tortuous pulmonary venous channels of the supracardiac types. Asymmetric obstructions in some pulmonary veins and not in others, in certain mixed varieties, forces increased blood flow to the least obstructed area of lung, thereby stimulating persistence of fetal pulmonary arteriolar vasculature, which may help the patient survive. With minimal obstruction, the amount of pulmonary blood flow can be enormous; the patient may be pink and in congestive heart failure.

Generally, the left atrium, left ventricle, mitral, and aortic valves may be relatively small compared with the very dilated right ventricle and other right-sided heart structures.[11,12] If the ductus arteriosus is patent, some of the cardiac output may bypass the left heart, further contributing to the impression of a small left ventricle.

Clinical Manifestations

Patients with totally anomalous pulmonary venous connection range from those with maximally obstructed pulmonary venous connection to those with completely unrestricted pulmonary blood flow. Although the extremes will be described in some detail, it must be recognized that most cases fall some place between them.

Obstructed Pulmonary Veins

When there is severe obstruction of the pulmonary venous connection, the infant is discovered to be acutely ill within days after birth. As described, this is usual when the venous connection is to the umbilicovitelline system (infradiaphragmatic), and occurs in about 50% of connections to the supracardiac structures.[13] Usually, there is rapid onset of tachypnea, gasping, and retractions indicative of pulmonary edema. The more severe the obstruction, the earlier the infant is symptomatic and discovered to have heart disease. Because the infradiaphragmatic connection variety is invariably severely obstructed, it is not surprising that, although uncommon overall, it is the type most frequently found at autopsy among babies with TAPVC, many undiagnosed.[9]

Physical Examination

On physical examination, the infant often appears very ill. There is cyanosis, tachypnea, and hepatomegaly. Often there is no murmur, the only abnormality being a loud second heart sound.

Electrocardiography

The electrocardiogram shows right ventricular hypertrophy, but because these patients are usually neonates, it is difficult to be certain that this is abnormal. There is usually right atrial enlargement (tall peaked P wave in lead II) and right axis deviation in older infants, although in neonates this finding may not be present.

Chest X-Ray

On chest x-ray, the heart is of normal size or slightly enlarged. There is evidence of pulmonary edema, sometimes marked (Fig. 39.2).

Echocardiography

Typically the first clue to the diagnosis is an exclusive right-to-left shunt at the atrial level. This is never a normal physiologic finding and, when present, should always be further investigated. The common vein receiving all pulmonary veins is often seen behind the heart, as is the connection to the systemic venous circulation,[14] and this may be well seen from the subxiphoid view in infants. Right ventricular and pulmonary hypertension are usually present, and if the ductus is open, right-to-left shunting may be visible. Each pulmonary vein is visualized, and Doppler techniques are used to assess the presence or absence of pulsatile pulmonary venous blood flow; absence of pulsatility suggests obstruction. The confluence and individual pulmonary veins are best seen from the suprasternal notch or high left sternal border. If the venous channel is obstructed, the confluence is usually dilated, and the velocity of blood flow is low. If at least four pulmonary veins are not identified, multiple drainage sites should be suspected.

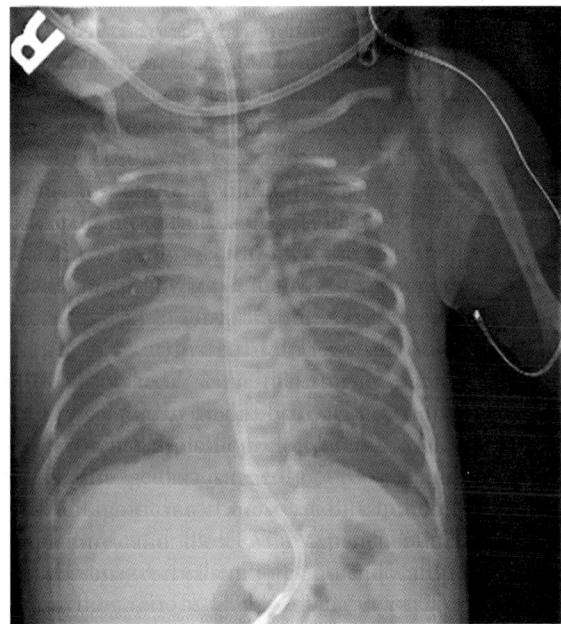

AP-port-supine

• **Fig. 39.2** This infant with obstructed infradiaphragmatic total anomalous pulmonary venous connection has gross pulmonary edema with poorly visible pulmonary structures on chest x-ray.

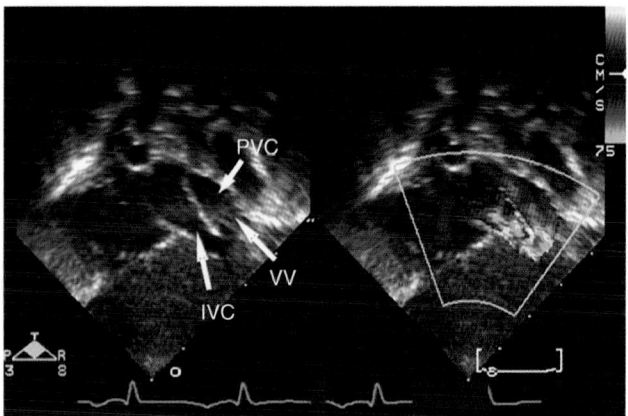

• **Fig. 39.3** Infradiaphragmatic total anomalous pulmonary venous connection (TAPVC): subxiphoid short-axis view. The subxiphoid short-axis view in this patient with infradiaphragmatic TAPVC with 2D and color Doppler flow mapping shows the vertical vein *(VV)* descending just below the level of the diaphragm, and then coursing anteriorly to drain directly into the inferior vena cava *(IVC)*. Note the color flow acceleration at the connection to the IVC. *PVC,* Pulmonary venous confluence. (Brown DW, Pulmonary Venous Anomalies. From: Lai WW, Mertens LL, Cohen MS, Geva T, eds. *Echocardiography in Pediatric and Congenital Heart Disease*, 3rd edition. Hoboken NJ: Wiley-Blackwell, 2022. Figure 10.29, page 208, with permission).

Once the pulmonary venous confluence and individual pulmonary veins have been identified, the sites of communication with the systemic venous circuit are identified. The most common drainage site for obstructed anomalous venous connection is the portal-hepatic system. The descending vertical vein can be seen in a subxiphoid transverse view as a third vascular channel crossing the diaphragm between the inferior vena cava and the descending aorta (Fig. 39.3) and, using color-flow Doppler mapping, can be traced into the liver. Pulmonary venous flow returns to the right atrium through a dilated inferior vena cava.

Less commonly, obstruction occurs in supracardiac total anomalous pulmonary venous drainage (Fig. 39.4). One cause of obstruction in this type of drainage is compression of the vertical vein if it passes between the left pulmonary artery and the left main bronchus (usually the vertical vein passes anterior to the left pulmonary artery and left main bronchus). The innominate vein and superior vena cava are usually dilated in relation to the severity of obstruction of pulmonary venous flow.

Rarely, TAPVC to the coronary sinus is obstructed,[10] either at the junction of the common pulmonary vein with the coronary sinus or within the coronary sinus. Other sites of obstruction include the azygous vein and the right superior vena cava. Pulsed and continuous-wave Doppler echocardiography identifies non-pulsatile points of obstruction. The flow pattern should also be sampled in the individual veins, as well as in the venous confluence, because obstruction may occur at multiple sites.

Other echocardiographic findings with TAPVC include a small left atrium, and an enlarged and hypertensive right ventricle. With severe obstruction, the right ventricular

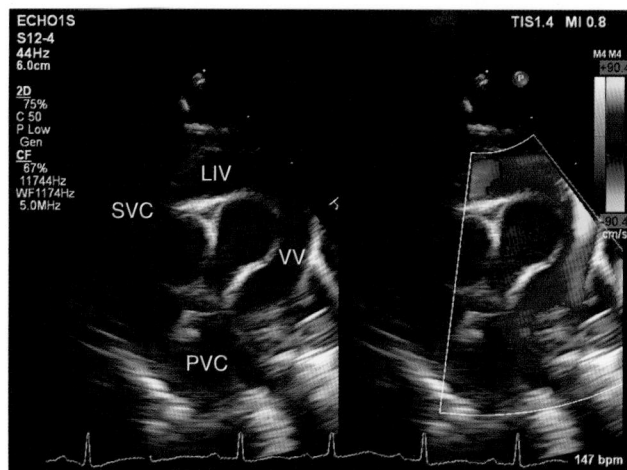

• **Fig. 39.4** Supracardiac total anomalous pulmonary venous connection (TAPVC). Parasternal short-axis view with color Doppler flow mapping in this patient with supracardiac TAPVC to the left innominate vein (*LIV*) shows the pulmonary venous confluence (*PVC*) that drains via the vertical vein (*VV*) toward the leftward aspect of the innominate vein. *SVC*, Superior vena cava. (Brown DW, Pulmonary Venous Anomalies. From: Lai WW, Mertens LL, Cohen MS, Geva T, eds. *Echocardiography in Pediatric and Congenital Heart Disease*, 3rd edition. Hoboken NJ: Wiley-Blackwell, 2022. Figure 10.20, page 202, with permission).

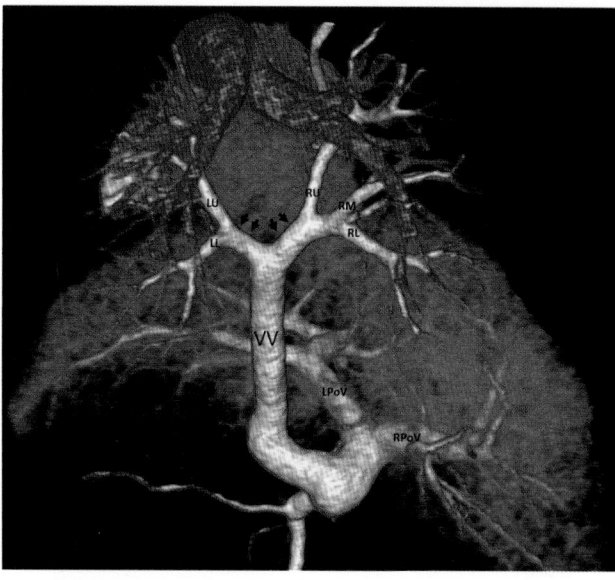

• **Fig. 39.5** Computed tomography showing infradiaphragmatic total anomalous pulmonary venous connection with all five pulmonary veins joining a confluence (*arrows*) and the vertical vein (*VV*) connection to the portal venous system. *LL*, Left lower pulmonary vein; *LPoV*, left portal vein; *LU*, left upper pulmonary vein; *RL*, right lower pulmonary vein; *RM*, right middle pulmonary vein; *RPoV*, right portal vein; *RU*, right upper pulmonary vein. (Image courtesy of Dr. David N. Schidlow).

pressure is often suprasystemic, with posterior bowing of the ventricular septum. Tricuspid regurgitation, if present, allows estimation of the right ventricular pressure.

Magnetic Resonance Imaging and Computed Tomography

Cardiac MRI or CT, if needed, provides high-quality imaging data with a fast acquisition time, but CT does require exposure to ionizing radiation (Fig. 39.5). Such axial imaging may be helpful to guide surgical planning, particularly if acoustic interference by lung tissue hinders the complete demonstration of pulmonary venous connections by echocardiography.

Cardiac Catheterization

Cardiac catheterization has been unnecessary in this lesion for many years, as noninvasive imaging techniques can typically provide all of the necessary information for the surgical team. Transcatheter intervention may be helpful in special situations, such as balloon dilation/stenting of obstructed vertical veins, in those patients who have immediate contraindications to surgical repair.

Unrestricted Pulmonary Blood Flow

The neonate with unrestricted pulmonary blood flow is generally not very ill. In the current era, the diagnosis is frequently made within days as the detection of a heart murmur or mild cyanosis leads to echocardiography. Infants with unrestrictive pulmonary blood flow and high pulmonary flow ratios could often have an oxygen saturation level in the 90s, which for most would mean no

apparent cyanosis and often a delayed diagnosis. However, following the recommendation for universal newborn oximetry screening in the United States in 2011, infants with TAPVC are more frequently diagnosed in the first 2 days of life even if not obviously cyanotic. However, occasionally the diagnosis may be made after some years—we evaluated and surgically repaired unobstructed TAPVC to the azygous vein in a 16-year-old virtually asymptomatic patient.

Physical Examination

On physical examination, the infant may be thin, is often tachypneic, and has minimal or no visible cyanosis. Often there is hepatomegaly. There may be a prominence of the left side of the chest with a palpable right ventricular impulse (prominent right ventricular heave), a gallop rhythm, and an accentuated pulmonary component of a widely split fixed second heart sound. A systolic ejection murmur, rarely more than grade 3, is audible at the left upper sternal border, followed by an early diastolic rumble at the lower sternal border. In the uncomplicated situation, the physical findings are similar to those of a large atrial septal defect. A loud systolic murmur suggests some additional cardiac anomaly.

Electrocardiography

The electrocardiogram shows abnormal right ventricular hypertrophy for age when the infant is more than a few weeks old. Right atrial enlargement as demonstrated by a tall peaked P wave in lead II is often present as is right axis deviation.

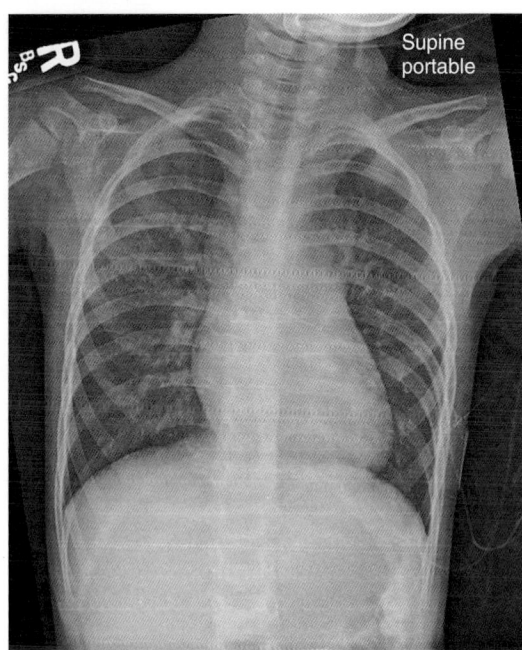

• **Fig. 39.6** Chest x-ray in a 5-year-old with unrepaired supracardiac total anomalous pulmonary venous connection depicting the typical "snowman" appearance caused by the dilated innominate vein in.

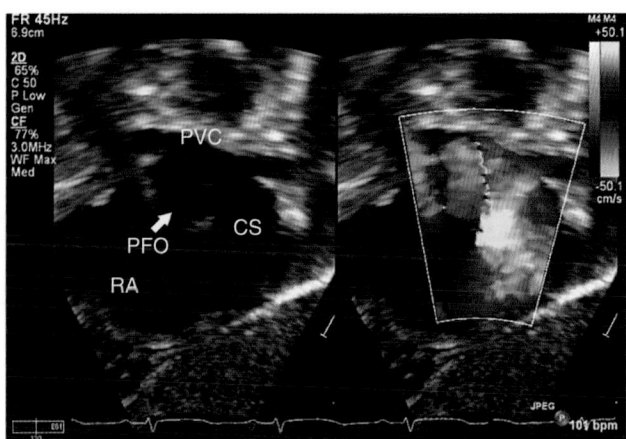

• **Fig. 39.7** Subcostal oblique view with color Doppler of total anomalous pulmonary venous connection to the coronary sinus (CS), which is markedly dilated. The image depicts the typical "whale's tail" appearance of the pulmonary venous confluence (PVC) and connection of the vertical vein to the CS. Note the obligate right-to-left shunt across the patent foramen ovale (PFO). RA, Right atrium.

Chest X-Ray

On chest x-ray, the heart is enlarged, and there is pulmonary vascular engorgement. Compared with the obstructive type, there is excessive pulmonary blood flow, often marked, but usually without pulmonary edema. Supracardiac TAPVC to the innominate vein is often noted to have a "snowman appearance" if the patient is older (Fig. 39.6).

Laboratory Data

The level of oxygen saturation by skin oximetry is often only minimally reduced, at about 90%, a degree of desaturation often unappreciated by the naked eye. With the advent of universal oximetry screening in the newborn period, this is less of a clinical problem than in prior eras.

Echocardiography

On echocardiographic examination, the common pulmonary vein is visible behind the left atrium, and each pulmonary vein can be identified. Often TAPVC to the coronary sinus is unrestricted and the pulmonary venous confluence appears to be a "whale tail" (Fig. 39.7). Pulmonary artery and right ventricular pressure can be determined when tricuspid regurgitation is present. If transthoracic imaging is unsatisfactory, transesophageal echocardiography can provide much better anatomic information.

Magnetic Resonance Imaging and Computed Tomography

Because precise anatomic details are outlined by echocardiography in the very young, there is little need for MRI in

this age group, whether or not pulmonary venous obstruction is present. In the older, larger patients with poor windows, MRI or CT can provide exquisite anatomic information.

Cardiac Catheterization

In these patients with uncomplicated total anomalous unrestricted pulmonary venous connection, cardiac catheterization for anatomic reasons has not been necessary for many years. However, beyond infancy, it would be indicated when significant pulmonary hypertension or vascular obstruction was suspected, to quantitate pulmonary vascular resistance and study responses to vasodilators.

Management

Most patients with uncomplicated TAPVC have neither maximally obstructed nor completely unrestricted pulmonary blood flow and present clinical problems somewhere between those two extremes. It is important to emphasize, however, that most patients with infradiaphragmatic connection have severe obstruction and are very likely to become extremely ill rapidly within days after birth, particularly when the patent ductus arteriosus constricts.

Once the diagnosis is made, surgical repair is undertaken. Almost all patients have a large pulmonary venous confluence behind the left atrium. This structure is horizontal or oblique in those with supracardiac and cardiac anomalous connection sites, and vertical in those with the infradiaphragmatic variety. The surgical procedure essentially consists of making as large an anastomosis as possible between this pulmonary venous confluence and the posterior wall of the left atrium. Perhaps the one exception to this management plan is in the group with mixed total anomalous connection in whom the single large posterior pulmonary venous confluence is absent. In this group, if stable and without significant pulmonary hypertension or pulmonary venous obstruction, it is not unreasonable to follow these patients medically until such time when the individual anomalous veins are large enough to anastomose directly to the left atrium.

Early mortality has improved dramatically over the years, even as the age at surgery has decreased.[15] Among series of patients operated on in the past two decades, early mortality rates have ranged from 2% to 10% (median, 10%).

Clinical Course

Most often, late follow-up shows an excellent result. Late postoperative arrhythmias, mostly supraventricular, have been reported in some patients.[16] The major problem that survivors have encountered is pulmonary venous obstruction (stenosis), either at the anastomosis site or in individual pulmonary veins. Anastomotic site obstruction can be simply due to scar tissue at the anastomosis of the pulmonary venous confluence to the back wall of the left atrium, and thus may respond well to reoperation. Stenosis of the individual pulmonary veins is a more feared complication; it occurs in about 11%–17% of patients, is often progressive, requires frequent surgical and interventional catheterization procedures, and is associated with high mortality rates, from 25% to 46%.[17-20] This has been reported by some to be more common after repair of infradiaphragmatic or mixed types.[20,21] In patients with associated single-ventricle heart disease, mortality is significantly higher. Pathologic studies have demonstrated proliferation of myofibroblasts that narrow the lumen of the veins. Currently a multimodality approach to therapy including "sutureless" surgical techniques,[22] transcatheter balloon dilation and/or stent placement, and medical therapy with targeted biologic inhibition agents such as tyrosine kinase inhibitors for aggressive pulmonary vein stenosis have demonstrated some promise in halting disease progression and prolonging survival.[23-25]

TAPVC is either an isolated phenomenon or is associated with the complex cardiac abnormalities found in the asplenia-polysplenia syndromes. The physiologic effect of the anomalous connection may be negligible in this situation, in that these syndromes usually include other cardiac defects that allow common mixing, such as single ventricle, common atrium, and common atrioventricular canal. It is very common in patients with asplenia, much less so in the polysplenia group (see Chapter 32). It is customary to repair the total veins at the initial surgery, whether it be shunt placement for pulmonary atresia or stenosis or a stage one procedure as a prelude to a later Fontan procedure. In the asplenia group, pulmonary vein stenosis is unfortunately a common complication, occurring in 38% in our patients.

References

1. Ferencz C, Rubin JD, McCarter RJ, et al. Congenital heart disease: prevalence at livebirth. The Baltimore-Washington Infant Study. *Am J Epidemiol.* 1985;121:31-36.
2. Hoffman JI, Kaplan S. The incidence of congenital heart disease. *J Am Coll Cardiol.* 2002;39:1890-1900.
3. Burroughs JT, Edwards JE. Total anomalous pulmonary venous connection. *Am Heart J.* 1960;59:913-931.
4. Michielon G, Di Donato RM, Pasquini L, et al. Total anomalous pulmonary venous connection: long-term appraisal with evolving technical solutions. *Eur J Cardiothorac Surg.* 2002;22:184-191.
5. Hyde JA, Stumper O, Barth MJ, et al. Total anomalous pulmonary venous connection: outcome of surgical correction and management of recurrent venous obstruction. *Eur J Cardiothorac Surg.* 1999;15:735-740; discussion 740-741.
6. Sinzobahamvya N, Arenz C, Brecher AM, Blaschczok HC, Urban AE. Early and long-term results for correction of total anomalous pulmonary venous drainage (TAPVD) in neonates and infants. *Eur J Cardiothorac Surg.* 1996;10:433-438.
7. Lupinetti FM, Kulik TJ, Beekman RH III, Crowley DC, Bove EL. Correction of total anomalous pulmonary venous connection in infancy. *J Thorac Cardiovasc Surg.* 1993;106:880-885.
8. Lucas Jr RV, Lock JE, Tandon R, Edwards JE. Gross and histologic anatomy of total anomalous pulmonary venous connections. *Am J Cardiol.* 1988;62:292-300.
9. James CL, Keeling JW, Smith NM, Byard RW. Total anomalous pulmonary venous drainage associated with fatal outcome in infancy and early childhood: an autopsy study of 52 cases. *Pediatr Pathol.* 1994;14:665-678.
10. Jonas RA, Smolinsky A, Mayer JE, Castaneda AR. Obstructed pulmonary venous drainage with total anomalous pulmonary venous connection to the coronary sinus. *Am J Cardiol.* 1987;59:431-435.
11. Lima CO, Valdes-Cruz LM, Allen HD, et al. Prognostic value of left ventricular size measured by echocardiography in infants with total anomalous pulmonary venous drainage. *Am J Cardiol.* 1983;51:1155-1159.
12. Rosenquist GC, Kelly JL, Chandra R, et al. Small left atrium and change in contour of the ventricular septum in total anomalous pulmonary venous connection: a morphometric analysis of 22 infant hearts. *Am J Cardiol.* 1985;55:777-782.
13. Norwood WI, Hougen TJ, Castaneda AR. Total anomalous pulmonary venous connection: surgical considerations. *Cardiovasc Clin.* 1981;11:353-364.
14. Chin AJ, Sanders SP, Sherman F, Lang P, Norwood WI, Castaneda AR. Accuracy of subcostal two-dimensional echocardiography in prospective diagnosis of total anomalous pulmonary venous connection. *Am Heart J.* 1987;113:1153-1159.
15. Bando K, Turrentine MW, Ensing GJ, et al. Surgical management of total anomalous pulmonary venous connection. Thirty-year trends. *Circulation.* 1996;94:II12-II16.
16. Korbmacher B, Buttgen S, Schulte HD, et al. Long-term results after repair of total anomalous pulmonary venous connection. *Thorac Cardiovasc Surg.* 2001;49:101-106.
17. Ricci M, Elliott M, Cohen GA, et al. Management of pulmonary venous obstruction after correction of TAPVC: risk factors for adverse outcome. *Eur J Cardiothorac Surg.* 2003;24:28-36; discussion 36.
18. Lacour-Gayet F, Zoghbi J, Serraf AE, et al. Surgical management of progressive pulmonary venous obstruction after repair of total anomalous pulmonary venous connection. *J Thorac Cardiovasc Surg.* 1999;117:679-687.

19. Hancock Friesen CL, Zurakowski D, Thiagarajan RR, et al. Total anomalous pulmonary venous connection: an analysis of current management strategies in a single institution. *Ann Thorac Surg.* 2005;79:596-606.

20. Seale AN, Uemura H, Webber SA, et al. Total anomalous pulmonary venous connection: outcome of postoperative pulmonary venous obstruction. *J Thorac Cardiovasc Surg.* 2013;145:1255-1262.

21. Seale AN, Uemura H, Webber SA, et al. Total anomalous pulmonary venous connection: morphology and outcome from an international population-based study. *Circulation.* 2010;122:2718-2726.

22. Kalfa D, Belli E, Bacha E, et al. Outcomes and prognostic factors for postsurgical pulmonary vein stenosis in the current era. *J Thorac Cardiovasc Surg.* 2018;156:278-286.

23. Callahan R, Kieran MW, Baird CW, et al. Adjunct targeted biologic inhibition agents to treat aggressive multivessel intraluminal pediatric pulmonary vein stenosis. *J Pediatr.* 2018;198:29-35.e5.

24. Feins EN, Ireland C, Gauvreau K, et al. Pulmonary vein stenosis: anatomic considerations, surgical management, and outcomes. *J Thorac Cardiovasc Surg.* 2022;163:2198-2207.e3.

25. Feins EN, Callahan R, Baird CW. Pulmonary vein stenosis-evolving surgical management of a challenging disease. *Children (Basel).* 2021;8:631.

40

Pulmonary Vein Stenosis

RYAN CALLAHAN, CHRISTOPHER W. BAIRD, ERIC N. FEINS, AND KATHY JENKINS

KEY LEARNING POINTS

- Intraluminal pulmonary vein stenosis results from neoproliferation of myofibroblast-type cells in the subendothelium, potentially as a response to increased wall shear stress. Anatomic locations resulting in turbulence are especially vulnerable. Both recurrence and progression can occur as wall shear stress changes with flow redistribution as the disease advances.
- Outcomes for anatomically focused surgical repair with a goal to remove areas of turbulence have been demonstrated to be superior to sutureless repair.
- Serial catheter-based intervention is used as primary therapy or to treat recurrence and allows for interval vessel growth.

- Stenting can be used for refractory lesions and as anatomically focused therapy. Intravascular ultrasound can be used diagnostically to evaluate the extent and mechanism of obstruction.
- Reducing inciting factors and utilizing targeted antineoproliferative treatment to suppress myofibroblasts can reduce the likelihood and rate of recurrence.
- A multidisciplinary team centered around the needs of patients and families with shared decision-making is necessary to care for this complex, medically fragile, and high-risk population.

Clinical Description

Pulmonary vein stenosis (PVS) is a rare and poorly understood condition characterized by intraluminal obstruction of individual pulmonary veins occurring with an estimated prevalence of 1.7 cases per 100,000 children under 2 years of age.[1] PVS results from neoproliferation of myofibroblast-like cells within the subendothelium,[2,3] causing luminal obliteration, flow redistribution with V/Q mismatch, pulmonary edema, pulmonary hypertension, and secondary ventricular dysfunction, and, if untreated, death from respiratory failure, pulmonary hypertensive crisis, and/or low cardiac output (Fig. 40.1). PVS occurs in association with congenital heart disease (CHD), developmental or acquired lung disease, or in isolation, and in both normally connected and anomalous pulmonary veins. A hallmark feature of the disease, in contrast to CHD from abnormal cardiac development, is recurrent obstruction after successful surgical or transcatheter intervention; the disease progresses to previously uninvolved vessels or longitudinally to new areas within the involved veins. The rate of recurrence or progression varies considerably among patients, with the most aggressive forms of the disease recurring within 3–4 weeks after surgery or transcatheter intervention.

In many cases, initial PVS diagnosis occurs during surveillance testing in infants with CHD, prematurity, or as part of an evaluation for respiratory symptoms. Characteristic chest radiograph findings include increased interstitial, reticular, and ground-glass opacity with distributional heterogeneity (Fig. 40.2). PVS is commonly diagnosed using echocardiography, with examination of individual pulmonary veins and Doppler flow patterns demonstrating typical findings of reduced luminal contour with accelerated and dampened flow patterns with loss of phasic variation (Fig. 40.3A–C). Delineation of pulmonary veins and identification of areas of obstruction can also be seen using computerized tomography (CT) angiography[4] with three-dimensional reconstruction most accurately correlating with invasive angiographic findings. Other secondary abnormalities demonstrated by CT includes: pleural thickening, interlobar pulmonary vein collateral formation, mediastinal and perihilar induration, interlobular septal thickening, ground glass opacity, cyst formation, and lobar or lung hypoplasia.[4] Left atrial wall thickening has also been described (Fig. 40.4).

Risk Factors and Prognosis

While the etiology of PVS in individual patients remains uncertain, well-known risk factors include prematurity with bronchopulmonary dysplasia and CHD with both normally connected and anomalous pulmonary venous

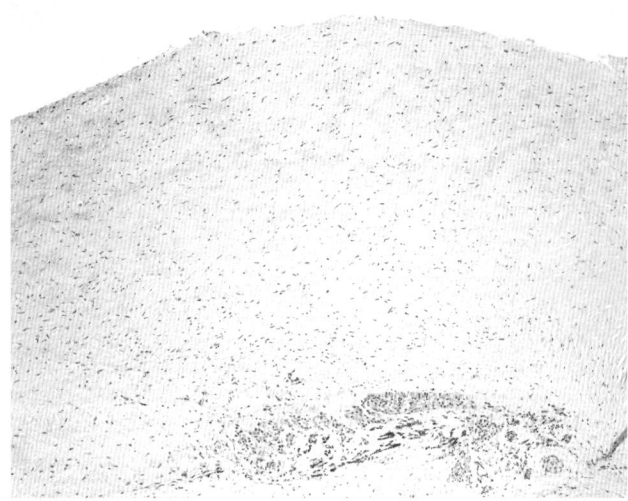

• **Fig. 40.1** A 2-month-old girl who developed bilateral pulmonary vein stenosis after neonatal repair of supracardiac total anomalous pulmonary venous connection. Biopsy specimen from the common pulmonary vein orifice shows mural thickening composed of (myo)fibroblastic proliferation and an abundant myxoid extracellular matrix (hematoxylin and eosin, original magnification; 100x).

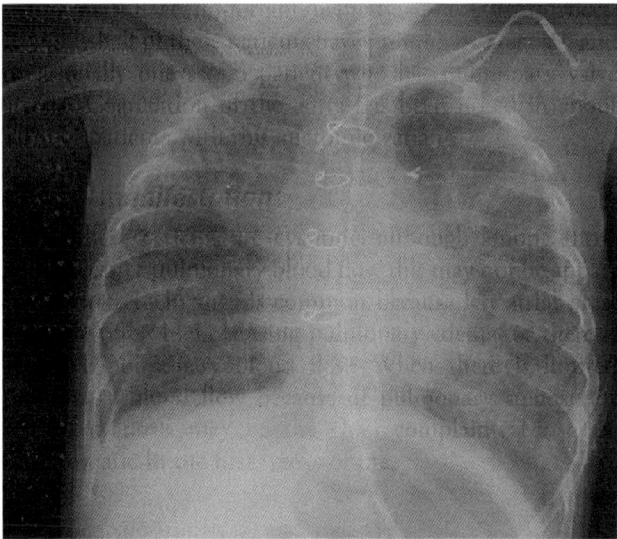

• **Fig. 40.2** A typical chest radiograph for an infant with severe pulmonary vein stenosis is shown; interstitial, reticular, and ground-glass opacities in a heterogeneous distribution are demonstrated.

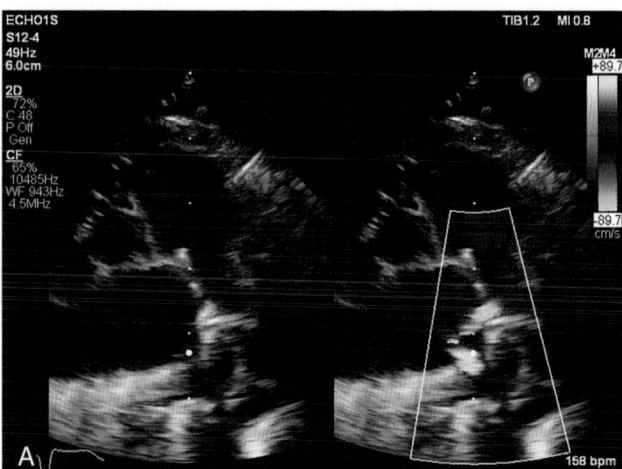

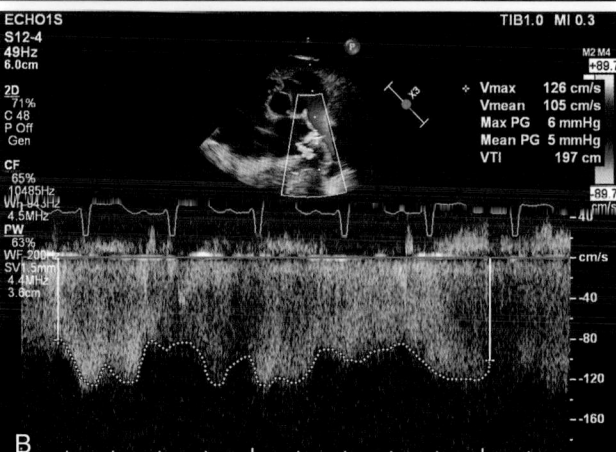

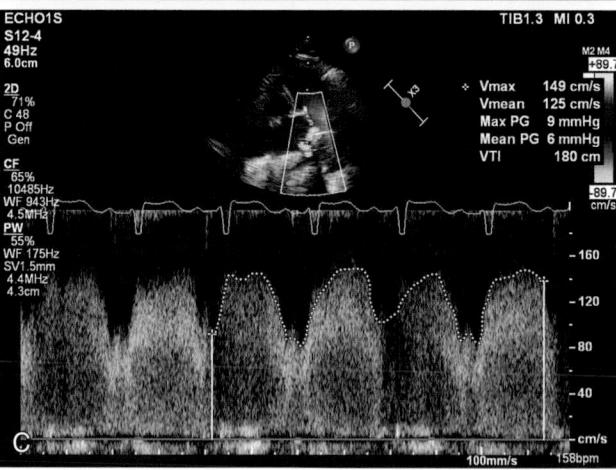

• **Fig. 40.3** Two-dimensional echocardiogram with color flow Doppler depicting abnormal flow velocity in both the upper and lower left pulmonary veins **(A)** and pulsed wave Doppler signals with increased velocity and loss of phasic variation in the left upper **(B)** and left lower **(C)** pulmonary vein.

return. A summary of the literature is shown in Table 40.1. Early age at presentation, bilateral disease, and involvement of distal (or upstream) vasculature are well-known risk factors for poor outcome. More recently, longer exposure to left-to-right shunts has been associated with the development of PVS in patients with trisomy 21[5] and aspiration has been associated with poor response to therapy[6]; these conditions are likely inciting factors. In addition, obstruction often occurs at sites where anatomic structures cause turbulent flow.[4] Genetic factors may also play a role as PVS has occurred in patients with known genetic defects, though the issue is complex, and no single genetic cause has been identified.

A new unifying hypothesis about what may stimulate subendothelial neoproliferation is increased wall shear stress.[18] Wall shear stress is the frictional drag on the endothelium caused by the moving blood. It is increased at areas of turbulence, is flow-dependent, and is known to cause vascular obstruction in other diseases, such as sickle cell

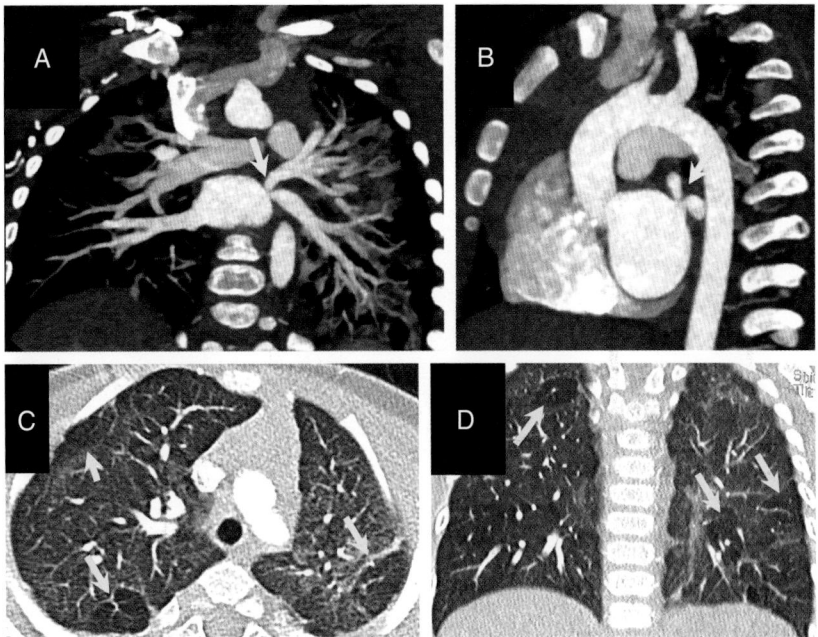

• **Fig. 40.4** Computerized tomography angiography in an infant with chronic lung disease of prematurity and left-sided pulmonary vein stenosis. Severe proximal stenosis of the left upper and lower pulmonary veins that insert obliquely into the superior aspect of the left atrium (*yellow arrows*, **A** and **B**) with associated mosaic attenuation of both lungs with hyperlucent lobules from air trapping (*yellow arrows*, **C** and **D**).

| TABLE 40.1 | Risk Factors Associated with Pulmonary Vein Stenosis Mortality, Re-Intervention, and Re-Stenosis |

Risk Factor	N	Outcome	Predictor	Statistical Value	Reference
Age	82	Mortality	Age < 5 months at PVS diagnosis	HR 3.4 [95% CI 1.6–7.6], P = .002	Balasubramanian et al. 2012*[7]
	49	Mortality	Age < 6 months at operation	Log-rank test, P = .004	Quinonez et al. 2015*[8]
	39	Mortality	Age < 6 months at PVS diagnosis	Log-rank test, P < .01	Mahgoub et al. 2017[9]
	93	Mortality	Age < 6 months at PVS diagnosis	HR 3.4 [95% CI 1.5–7.5], P = .003	DiLorenzo et al. 2019[10]
Weight	49	Mortality	< 3 kg at operation	Log-rank test, P < .001	Quinonez et al. 2015*[8]
	39	Mortality	Small for gestational age	Log-rank test, P < .046	Mahgoub et al. 2017[9]
Unilateral versus bilateral disease at diagnosis	82	Mortality	Bilateral disease	HR 3.9 [95% CI 1.7–9.2], P = .002	Balasubramanian et al. 2012*[7]
	39	Mortality	Bilateral disease	Log-rank test, P < .01	Mahgoub et al. 2017[9]
	34	Re-intervention Mortality	Bilateral disease	HR 5.64 [95% CI 1.07–29.77], P = .041 HR 6.26 [95% CI 1.14–34.4], P = .035	Rosenblum et al. 2020[11]
Number of veins involved at diagnosis	31	Mortality	Greater number of stenotic veins	Parameter estimate = 1.5, SE 0.56, P = .007, Reliability 50%	Lo Rito et al. 2016[12]

Continued

TABLE 40.1	Risk Factors Associated with Pulmonary Vein Stenosis Mortality, Re-Intervention, and Re-Stenosis—cont'd				
Risk Factor	**N**	**Outcome**	**Predictor**	**Statistical Value**	**Reference**
	39	Mortality	>/= 3 veins	Log-rank test, P < .01	Mahgoub et al. 2017[9]
	93	Mortality	> 1 vein	HR 2.1 per additional vein affected [95% CI 1.3–3.4], P = .004	DiLorenzo et al. 2019[10]
PVS disease severity	31	Mortality	Smaller upstream vessels	Parameter estimate = –0.008, SE 0.004, P = .03, Reliability 53%	Lo Rito et al. 2016[12]
	30	Re-stenosis Mortality	High postoperative severity score at 1 month	HR 1.34 [95% CI 1.17–1.50], P = .002 HR 1.33 [95% CI 1.14–1.55] P < .001	Kalfa et al. 2017[13]
	34	Mortality	Severity score > 6	HR 7.21 [95% CI 1.01–51.3], P = .049	Rosenblum et al. 2020[11]
Systolic PA:Ao pressure ratio	54	Mortality	Increasing PA:Ao ratio	Log-rank test, P < .001	Sykes et al. 2018*[14]
Right ventricular function	68	Mortality	Worsening right ventricular function	Log-rank test, P < .001	Sykes et al, 2018*[14]
Surgical approach	174	Mortality	Anatomically focused surgery (vs. conventional)	HR 0.19 [95% CI 0.05–0.72], P = .014 (survival benefit)	Feins et al. 2022*[15]
Medical therapy	48	Stabilization (no re-stenosis × 6 months)	Higher drug intensity of Adjunct Imatinib	90% (54–99) vs. 83% (55–99), P = .03	Callahan et al. 2018*[16]
	174	Mortality	Adjunct imatinib +/- bevacizumab	HR 0.47 [95% CI 0.25–0.92], P = .026 (survival benefit)	Feins et al. 2022*[15]
	67	Survival	Adjunct sirolimus	Log-rank test, P = .027	Patel et al. 2021[17]

Ao, Aorta; *CI*, Confidence interval; *HR*, hazards ratio; *PA*, pulmonary artery; *PVS*, pulmonary vein stenosis.
*Boston Children's Hospital.

anemia. Importantly, increased wall shear stress as the inciting cause of neoproliferation also can explain the progression of disease to uninvolved vessels. When PVS occurs in one vessel, there is vascular obstruction and subsequent flow redistribution to other vessels; the increased flow in these vessels increases wall shear stress, which may trigger neoproliferation. Measuring wall shear stress directly is challenging, but it can be estimated using computational fluid dynamics.

Prognosis for specific patients must be individualized given the disease heterogeneity. Prognosis is based on the ability to arrest the intraluminal neoproliferation and achieve disease stabilization with a sufficiently intact pulmonary bed to provide adequate gas exchange and respiratory function. The therapeutic window is narrow for single-ventricle physiology compared to patients with a biventricular circulation. Prognosis is based on the

effectiveness of surgery and interventional catheterization to relieve anatomic obstruction, maintain vessel patency, and reduce areas with high wall shear stress ***and*** the response of the neoproliferation to removal of potential inciting factors (e.g., aspiration) and the use of antineoproliferative therapy. Prognosis is also determined by variable preservation of right ventricular function and the presence or absence of reactive pulmonary hypertension. Survivors with PVS have limitations in pulmonary reserve due to loss of portions of the pulmonary vascular bed and scarring within areas where there was previous neoproliferation. Survival for a recent cohort of patients treated at our institution with multivessel PVS stratified by the presence of prematurity or CHD, and for those treated with antiproliferative therapy stratified by the number of affected vessels at onset of therapy, is shown in Table 40.2 and Fig. 40.5.

TABLE 40.2	Description of Pulmonary Vein Stenosis Population (1998–2020)	
Patient Demographics	**Median (Q1–Q3) or n (%)**	
Total number of patients	242	
Age at diagnosis (months)	5 (3–10)	
PVS diagnosis		
CHD (excluding PDA/PFO/small ASD)	196 (81)	
TAPVC	71 (36.2)	
PAPVC	20 (10.2)	
Isolated prematurity (<37 weeks)	32 (13.2)	
Primary (full term/structurally normal heart)	14 (5.8)	
Ventricular physiology		
Single ventricle	43 (17.8)	
Biventricular conversion	16 (6.6)	
Two ventricles	183 (75.6)	
Number of veins affected at initial diagnosis		
1	7 (2.9)	
2	72 (29.8)	
3	65 (26.9)	
4	87 (35.9)	
5	11 (4.5)	
Disease presence at diagnosis		
Unilateral	69 (28.5)	
Bilateral	173 (71.5)	
Tracheostomy +/– ventilator dependent	20 (8.3)	
Treated with imatinib mesylate	114 (47.1)	
Treated with bevacizumab	23 (9.5)	
Lung transplant	7 (2.89)	

ASD, Atrial septal defect; *CHD*, congenital heart disease; *PAPVC*, partial anomalous pulmonary venous connection; *PDA*, patent ductus arteriosus; *PFO*, patent foramen ovale; *PVS*, pulmonary vein stenosis; *TAPVC*, total anomalous pulmonary venous connection.

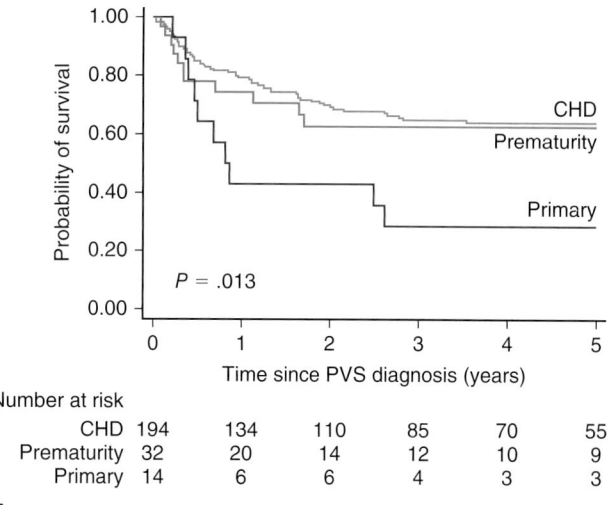

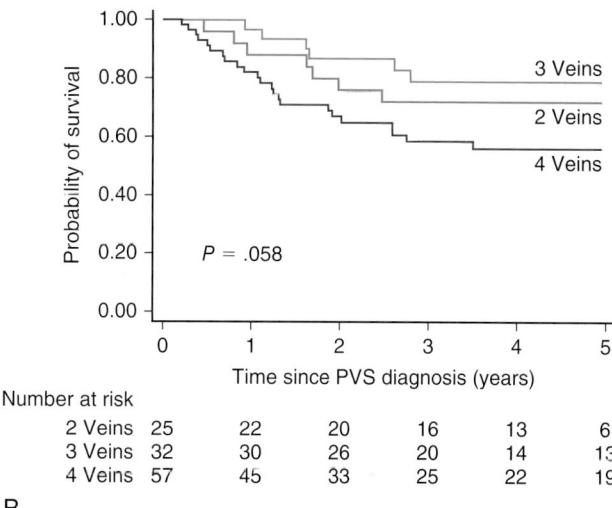

• **Fig. 40.5** Kaplan-Meier curves of patients with multi vessel pulmonary vein stenosis *(PVS)* from 1998 to 2020. **(A)** Five-year survival of all patients by diagnosis. **(B)** Five-year survival of all patients treated with imatinib +/– bevacizumab by number of affected veins at diagnosis. *CHD*, Congenital heart disease.

Management

Cardiac Catheterization

Indication

Cardiac catheterization is considered the gold-standard imaging study for the diagnosis of PVS and is the most common invasive treatment modality for PVS (initial presentation and recurrence). An initial catheterization is performed when there is suspicion for PVS based on the clinical presentation and noninvasive imaging. For patients with known PVS, new or worsening symptoms (e.g., respiratory failure, feeding intolerance, irritability, low cardiac output), right ventricular dysfunction, right ventricular hypertension and/or pulmonary vein gradients, or decrease in lobar perfusion by nuclear lung perfusion scan, a catheterization to evaluate for restenosis is warranted.

Goals

A complete right and left heart catheterization with angiography is performed in order to evaluate the hemodynamics, specifically the degree of right heart failure and severity of pulmonary hypertension. The pulmonary venous anatomy is delineated using a combination of balloon wedge pulmonary artery angiography and selective retrograde pulmonary venography (Fig. 40.6). Next, the mechanism of pulmonary venous obstruction and the overall severity (number of

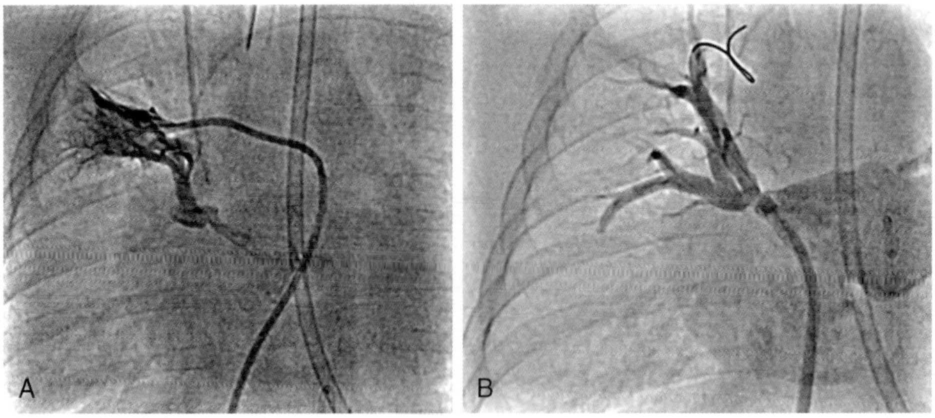

• **Fig. 40.6** Cardiac angiography of the right upper pulmonary vein (RUPV). **(A)** Right upper pulmonary artery wedge angiography suggestive of RUPV ostial stenosis. **(B)** RUPV retrograde venography via long sheath injection demonstrating ostial stenosis.

veins involved, extent of disease within each vein) is defined using a combination of angiography, pulmonary vein pressure assessment, and intravascular ultrasound (IVUS). Transcatheter interventions are then performed to relieve stenosis either as a primary therapy or as a palliation prior to surgical repair. With rare exceptions, vascular access below the diaphragm in either the femoral vein or the hepatic vein is required in order to enter the pulmonary veins.

Angiography

Pulmonary artery wedge angiography and retrograde venography determine the pulmonary venous connections and the severity of luminal narrowing of PVS, if present. Mechanisms of obstruction from non-opacified structures such as obstructive atrial tissue can be challenging to diagnose by cardiac angiography alone. In the case of PVS, early luminal narrowing occurs focally, either at the veno-atrial junction or at a location just distally that is unique to each vein (i.e., the left upper pulmonary vein at the level of the left bronchus). The vein distal or upstream to the stenosis initially dilates as the vein wall characteristics in this area remain normal and compliant (Fig. 40.7A). As the disease progresses, there is extension of the disease toward the lung as well as flow redistribution away from the affected lobe, both of which cause long segment luminal narrowing (Fig. 40.7B). The final stage is vein atresia with or without collateral formation to a non-atretic ipsilateral pulmonary vein (Fig. 40.7C and D).

Pressure Assessment

The pulmonary vein pressure is assessed directly with a catheter cannulating the vein or indirectly via a pulmonary artery wedge pressure. Of note, the indirect pressure measurement can significantly underestimate the actual pulmonary vein pressure and is paired with other techniques when attempting to confidently rule out PVS. A gradient of 4 mm Hg in the absence of significantly elevated pulmonary blood flow confirms the presence of a pulmonary venous obstruction. A pressure assessment while slowly

pulling a catheter from the vein to the left atrium is important when localizing the area of pulmonary venous obstruction, particularly in a surgically repaired total anomalous pulmonary venous connection (TAPVC; i.e., within the individual vein, at the surgical anastomosis, or both).

Intravascular Ultrasound

IVUS can not only demonstrate the lumen of the pulmonary vein but also characterize the wall architecture. IVUS can assist in determining the mechanism of obstruction such as vein distortion, obstructive atrial tissue, or luminal narrowing with or without wall thickening. The intravascular ultrasonographic features of PVS have been defined using *in vivo* and *ex vivo* models, and the presence of luminal narrowing is associated with future restenosis.[19,20] Lastly, IVUS can assist in accurately measuring lumen diameter for guided interventions such as stent implantation.

Interventional Tools

The goals of transcatheter intervention are to relieve the stenosis and minimize or eliminate the veno-atrial gradient. Conventional balloon venoplasty is the first-line therapy and requires low to ultra-high pressure for an effective dilation depending on the mechanism and chronicity of the stenosis. Cutting balloons are required for resistant lesions, noncompliant veins from severe disease, and for the treatment of in-stent restenosis in the case of a failed previously placed stent.[21] Stent implantation is reserved for a severe residual obstruction/gradient despite effective balloon venoplasty, recurrent PVS despite effective balloon venoplasty, following recanalization of vein atresia, and dilation of large veins of at least 8 mm in diameter where the incidence of in-stent restenosis is low.[22] Drug-eluting stents have a lower in-stent restenosis growth rate than bare metal stents and are considered if a stent is placed in a vein less than 6 mm (max diameter = 5 mm).[23] It is noteworthy that stent implantation requires re-intervention for stent re-dilation until the vein is adult size. There are evolving recanalization techniques using chronic total occlusion and radiofrequency

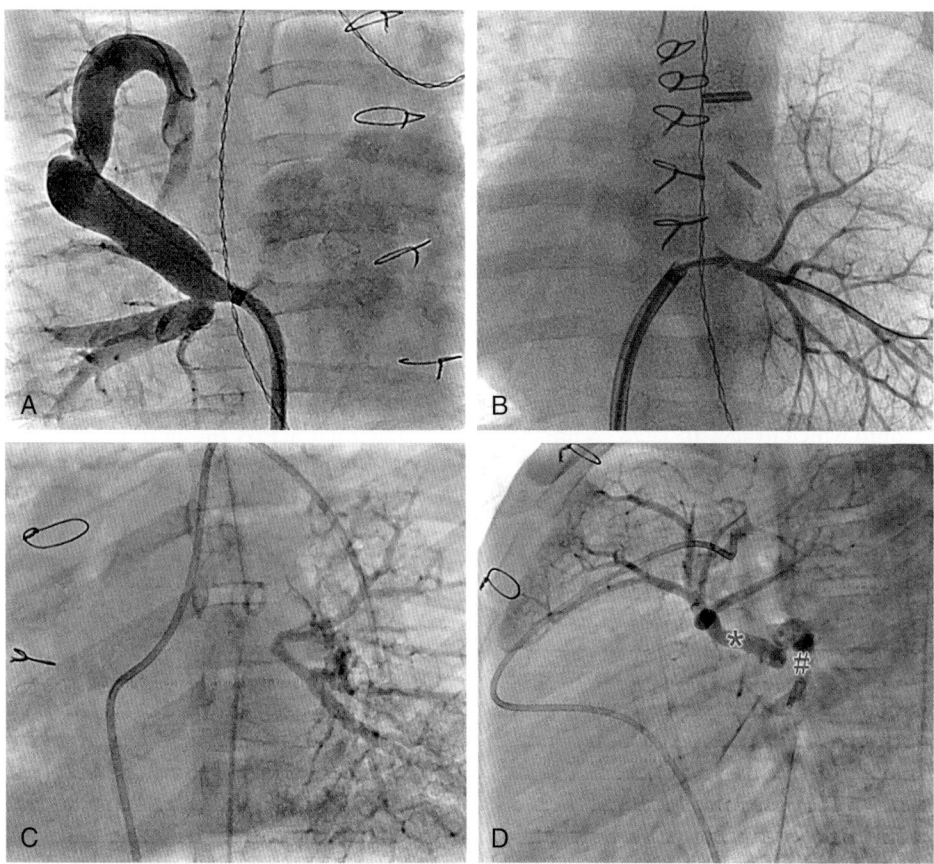

• **Fig. 40.7** Cardiac angiography of pulmonary vein stenosis (PVS). **(A)** Right common pulmonary vein ostial stenosis extending into the right lower pulmonary vein (RLPV) and dilation of the right upper pulmonary vein. **(B)** Diffuse PVS of the left lower pulmonary vein with hypoplasia of the distal vasculature. **(C)** Atresia of the RLPV without collateralization. **(D)** Atresia of the right upper pulmonary vein *(*)* with collaterals to the superior segment of the right lower pulmonary vein *(#)*.

ablation wires for the treatment of vein atresia. Other tools such as drug-coated balloons and bioresorbable stents are currently under investigation.

Peri-Catheterization Care

Cardiac catheterizations for patients with PVS are time-intensive, technically demanding procedures requiring multidisciplinary expertise. While most patients recover on the cardiology ward overnight and are discharged the following day, patients with more severe disease and secondary hemodynamic burdens may require admission to the intensive care unit. Higher-risk patients include those who are younger, have severe respiratory failure, low cardiac output, bilateral disease, secondary pulmonary hypertension, and/or right ventricular dysfunction. Serious adverse events such as hemodynamic instability, pulmonary hemorrhage, or embolic cerebral vascular accidents can occur.[24] Further, transcatheter interventions can result in pulmonary edema, which in high-risk patients can cause challenges with oxygenation, ventilation, and low cardiac output. Diuretics with or without short-term positive pressure are the mainstays of therapy in the post-catheterization period. Twenty-four hours of systemic anticoagulation followed by antiplatelet therapy is usually given to prevent clot

propagation in veins following venoplasty and for femoral vessel preservation.

Surgery

Kawashima was one of the first to describe the repair of PVS in 1971 in a 15-year-old boy with an atrial septal defect and presumed ventricular septal defect. Pulmonary vein disease was unexpectedly discovered upon opening the atrium where membranes were excised from bilateral pulmonary vein ostia.[25] More complex repair techniques were subsequently developed to address more extensive disease and in younger patients.[26] These operations included excision of the stenotic regions with direct reimplantation of the healthy pulmonary veins into the left atrium, venoplasty, use of prosthetic material to widen the vein-atrial junction, and the use of autologous atrial tissue to patch-enlarge the venous pathway.[27] Unfortunately, early outcomes were quite poor, particularly when surgical repair was required in infancy.

Given the overall poor outcomes of primary PVS repair, as well as the significant problem of post-TAPVC repair pulmonary vein obstruction, surgical techniques evolved. "Sutureless" repair techniques were developed in the 1990s by multiple groups. In 1996, Lacour-Gayet et al.[18] in Paris first described the sutureless repair to specifically address post-TAPVC repair pulmonary vein obstruction. Inspired by the Senning operation, the sutureless technique involved the use of a pedicle of *in-situ* vascularized pericardial flap which was sewn directly to the atrial wall thereby avoiding suturing directly to the pulmonary vein tissue (Fig. 40.8). The virtue of this technique was based upon the concern that manipulation/suturing onto vein tissue served as a nidus for inflammation, scar formation, and recurrent stenosis. Moreover, suturing the atrium to the pericardium was felt to allow for a more aggressive resection of diseased vein tissue since the surgeon would not have to rely on unresected vein tissue onto which to sew. In 1998, Najm et al.[29] in Toronto reported a similar approach. When compared with older PVS repair techniques, outcomes utilizing the sutureless technique for the treatment of post-TAPVC repair PVS were generally favorable.[30,31]

Calderone and colleagues then described extending the sutureless repair to primary PVS, including primary repair of TAPVC.[32] In addition to avoiding direct suturing to pulmonary vein tissue, the sutureless repair was thought to simplify the anastomosis. Since the suture lines are atrio-pericardial, the anastomosis was felt to be less prone to distortion in the way that direct vein-atrium connections might be. Unfortunately, mixed outcomes have been reported without significant benefit over direct primary repair of TAPVC.[13,33–35] These variable outcomes largely speak to the complex, multifactorial pathophysiology underlying PVS. While sutureless repair techniques aim to avoid direct manipulation and suturing on the pulmonary veins, there are other significant factors that drive the overactivity of myofibroblast-like cells in the pulmonary vein subendothelium leading to PVS recurrence.[36]

While much of the focus on PVS has been on the pulmonary veins themselves, little attention has been given to the surrounding intrathoracic structures that impact pulmonary vein course. We have increasingly recognized, through preoperative imaging and intraoperative assessment, a fulcrum effect on the pulmonary veins of PVS patients. We have observed that as the pulmonary veins pass from the lung parenchyma, they must pivot over and pass neighboring mediastinal structures and across the pericardial reflection before reaching the back of the more medial left atrium. This creates a long, angulated, and tortuous pulmonary vein course from the lung parenchyma to the heart. It is well known that vessel angulation leads to variations in wall shear stress,[37] which contribute to vascular remodeling, intimal hyperplasia, and stenosis.[38]

The specific mediastinal structures that impact pulmonary vein course vary with location. The left upper pulmonary vein passes anterior to the left mainstem bronchus and then across the pericardial reflection before entering the left atrium medially and posteriorly. Enlargement of the bronchus in the setting of chronic lung disease with elevated airway pressures can exacerbate pulmonary vein angulation. The left lower pulmonary vein passes anteriorly to the descending thoracic aorta and then crosses the pericardial reflection before reaching the left atrium medially. The right upper pulmonary vein angulates over the right pulmonary artery and then passes across the pericardial reflection before entering the left atrium medially. Importantly, when pulmonary hypertension exists, a common condition with PVS, the pulmonary arteries are enlarged and hypertensive, which accentuates their impact on the pulmonary vein course. The right lower pulmonary vein is the least commonly involved vessel in PVS, a finding noted in an analysis by Callahan et al.[39] of the disease patterns and outcomes for the specific pulmonary veins. When right lower PVS does occur, there is angulation as the vein passes across the pericardial reflection and into the left atrium. This is typically seen with a more posteriorly directed right lower pulmonary vein, in contrast to the more typical orientation that has a straight pathway to the left atrium.

Given the recognition of the long, angulated course that the pulmonary veins can take as they pass from the lung parenchyma to the left atrium, we now place greater emphasis

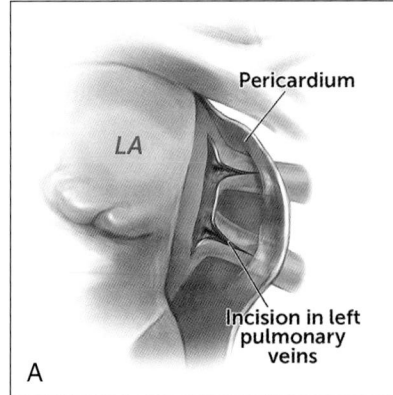 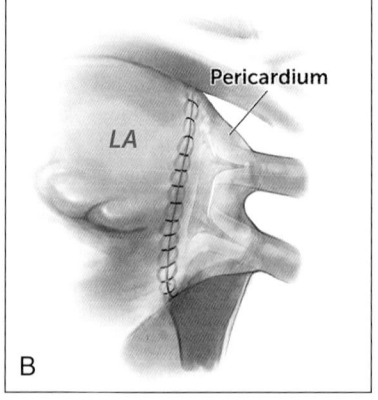

• **Fig. 40.8** Illustration representing "sutureless" repair of left pulmonary vein stenosis. **(A)** The pericardium has been opened, an incision made extending from the left atrium *(LA)* into the left upper and lower pulmonary veins across the ostial stenosis. **(B)** Completed repair showing the pericardium sutured to LA. Termed "sutureless" as no sutures are placed directly into the pulmonary veins.

on the extrinsic anatomy when repairing PVS of all forms. The goal of the anatomic-based PVS repair strategy is to remove the fulcrum effect that adjacent mediastinal structures and the pericardial reflection can have on the pulmonary veins, creating a shorter straighter course of the veins into the left atrium.[40]

Preoperatively, this involves having a clear understanding of both the location and extent of the pulmonary vein disease as well as the actual course of the veins in the mediastinum. Cardiac catheterization remains the gold standard for assessing pulmonary vein disease severity and includes hemodynamics, angiography, pressure assessment, IVUS, and balloon compliance testing. In addition, we are increasingly using preoperative CT for surgical planning to get a more global sense of the pulmonary veins, the adjacent mediastinal structures, and the degree of vessel angulation/tortuosity.

There are three primary components of the anatomic-based PVS repair strategy. First, takedown of the pericardial reflection and aggressive mobilization of the pulmonary veins as they enter the pericardial space to eliminate any angulation as the veins cross the pericardium. Second, resection of any stenotic or thickened pulmonary vein tissue. Third, lateralizing and enlarging the pulmonary vein–left atrial junction such that the course of the pulmonary veins into the left atrium is shorter, less angulated, and therefore less prone to disturbed flow. On the right side, we now prefer using autologous atrial flaps to augment the pulmonary vein-left atrial pathway, thereby using only native tissue on the pulmonary veins themselves. Alternatively, a decellularized homograft patch may be required. On the left side, the venotomy is extended into the base of the left atrial appendage and the vein-atrial connection is patch augmented to lateralize the vein-atrial confluence (Fig. 40.9). In select cases with severely hypoplastic or atretic pulmonary veins (i.e., less than 2 mm in luminal diameter), we have opted to place a short stent intraoperatively at the pulmonary vein-left atrial connection to prevent any potential for anastomotic recoil. This is typically reserved for cases where there is concern about the pulmonary vein-left atrial connection getting compressed and narrowing down despite patch enlargement.

This newer anatomic-focused approach has yielded encouraging results to date. While only implemented in the last several years, we have observed an improvement in mortality when compared with more conventional PVS repair techniques, with a 2-year survival of 82.1% versus 61.8% for conventional repair ($p = 0.03$).[30] Importantly, this mortality benefit was observed after controlling for potential confounding factors including age, number of vessels involved, surgical era, and use of adjuvant chemotherapy. Nonetheless, ongoing surveillance is crucial to better understand the longer-term durability of this repair strategy. We have not observed a significant change in re-intervention rate; however, re-intervention, especially transcatheter, should not be considered a "failure." PVS is a challenging and chronic disease, and the expectations should be that despite evolving surgical techniques, re-intervention is a likely and even expected management strategy.

Medical Therapy

Patients with intraluminal myofibroblastic neoproliferation remain at risk for recurrent obstruction or progression after successful anatomic intervention. Antineoproliferative treatment should be considered whenever ongoing neoproliferation is present. Pulmonary vein biopsies obtained at surgery can be useful in cases where the etiology of obstruction is uncertain, such as reoperations with potential anastomotic obstruction. Current therapeutic regimens at our institution are based on the identification of tyrosine kinase receptors on the surface of myofibroblasts in a series of patients with PVS[11] and the results of a prospective investigator-sponsored Investigational New Drug trial in 48 patients.[16] In most cases, an oral agent, imatinib

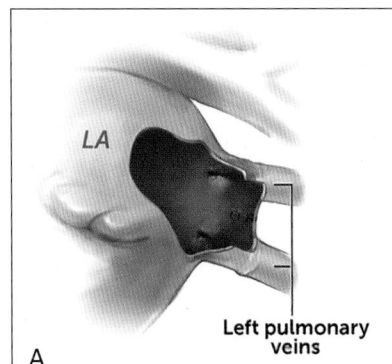 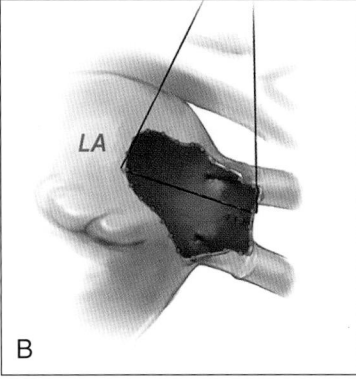 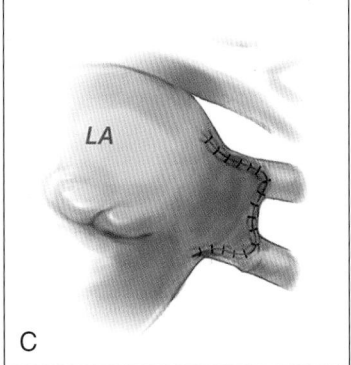

• **Fig. 40.9** Illustration representing anatomic-focused repair of left pulmonary vein stenosis. **(A)** A portion of the lateral aspect of the base of the left atrial appendage has been resected, with incisions extending across the upper and lower left pulmonary vein ostia. The left atrium *(LA)* has been lateralized by suturing the posterior-medial aspect of the pulmonary veins. **(B)** The LA-pulmonary vein connection is lateralized by suturing the left atrial appendage *(blue dots)* to the pulmonary vein confluence *(orange dots)*. **(C)** Completed repair with lateralized left atrial-pulmonary vein confluence.

mesylate, targeting platelet-derived growth factor receptor, is started when the patient is identified or 7–10 days after PVS surgery. During the treatment period, the rate of recurrence is monitored closely and interventional catheterization to relieve pulmonary vein obstruction is performed if needed. If the PVS progresses to involve new areas of the vasculature, a biweekly intravenous agent, bevacizumab, targeting vascular endothelial growth factor, is added to the regimen. Therapy is continued until disease stabilization, defined as 6 months without evidence of neoproliferative recurrence, typically 1–2 years. Once the antineoproliferative therapy is withdrawn, the disease is monitored closely, and treatment is reinitiated if there is recurrence. Patients on imatinib mesylate and/or bevacizumab are monitored for potential effects on the bone marrow, kidneys, and liver, and are at increased risk for infection.

In addition to tyrosine kinase blockade, other medications are used to prevent recurrence or progression. Our catheterization laboratory routinely uses short courses of sirolimus as a mechanistic target of rapamycin (mTOR) to reduce occurrence of in-stent restenosis after various types of stent-based therapy, including PVS; we have demonstrated the effectiveness of this regimen.[42] Sirolimus has also been used as a primary antineoproliferative therapy and a retrospective analysis showed improved survival.[7,17] Studies of losartan targeting transforming growth factor (TGF) beta have also been attempted, but evidence of effectiveness thus far is limited. Targeted medical agents are promising adjuncts to anatomically focused therapy to arrest neoproliferation, but current understanding of the underlying biology, intrinsic differences between patients, or over time, is limited.

Surveillance and Involvement of Subspecialists

One of the most important components of management of PVS is active surveillance to identify disease recurrence or progression during times when the rate of neoproliferation is high or unknown. Recurrence or progression can occur rapidly in just 3–4 weeks after surgery or transcatheter intervention, especially if antineoproliferative therapy is not used, resulting in rapid clinical deterioration or insidious development of vessel atresia. High-quality echocardiograms with sedation if needed, together with lung perfusion scans (using pediatric protocols to reduce radiation exposure) performed monthly, can usually detect changes in PVS obstruction (Fig. 40.10).

Limitations in each of these two testing modalities (i.e., imaging, Doppler interrogation, and low flow states for individual veins by echocardiography and measures of relative flow only or the presence of collaterals for lung perfusion scan) can be overcome by performing the two simultaneously. CT angiography can also be used to visualize anatomic changes, but the importance of anatomic narrowings can be difficult to interpret which limits the use of the test for clinical decision-making during treatment. Surveillance is typically done monthly at times of high risk and at longer intervals as the rate of neoproliferation slows and the disease stabilizes. It is important to repeat testing after intervention to establish a non-invasive baseline to detect future changes. The overall disease trajectory and rate of recurrences as indicative of the degree of neoproliferation should be monitored closely, with additional antineoproliferation or consideration for lung transplant if there is lack of treatment response.

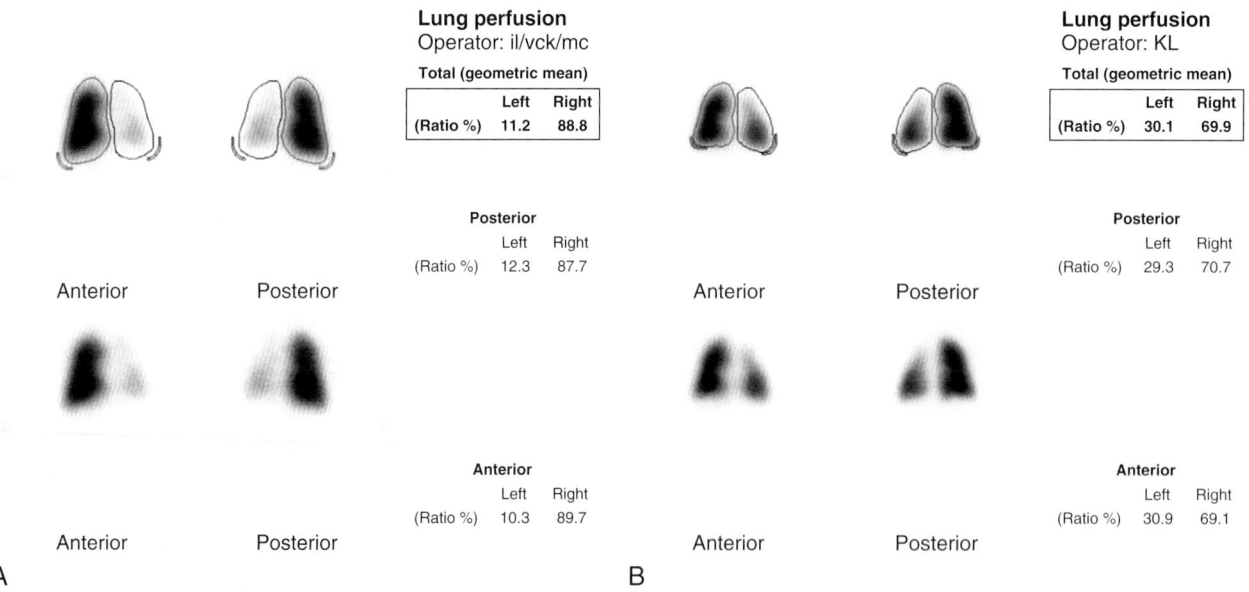

• **Fig. 40.10** Perfusion scans are shown for a patient with severe left-sided pulmonary vein stenosis before **(A)** and after **(B)** interventional catheterization and balloon dilation of the left pulmonary veins, resulting in increased flow the left lung.

Care for patients with PVS requires a multidisciplinary team of pediatric professionals. Pediatric cardiologists, cardiac interventionalists, surgeons, transplant specialists, intensivists, and anesthesiologists are all required to support the care of this high-risk population. Certain patients also require expertise in the management of pulmonary hypertension and anticoagulation. Treatment with antineoproliferative agents can require co-management by a pediatric oncologist given the unfamiliarity of use of chemotherapeutic agents by most pediatric cardiologists and the known drug toxicities. PVS patients also commonly have coexisting pulmonary diseases or gastrointestinal disorders, both of which can be complicated to diagnose and manage, requiring input from additional subspecialists.

Beyond the need for medical expertise, the high-risk nature of the disease, inherent uncertainty, requirement for frequent testing and intervention, use of antineoproliferative agents with inherent toxicity and side effects, and difficult decisions such as whether to seek treatment a distance from home or list for transplant put enormous burden and stress on families. Dedicated nurse practitioners, social workers, nutrition and other multidisciplinary team members, and palliative care teams can augment the primary cardiology teams and level of family support. This comprehensive care approach is needed to provide for the well-being of parents and other family members as they navigate this difficult disease.

References

1. McLennan DI, Solano EC, Handler SS, et al. Pulmonary vein stenosis: moving from past pessimism to future optimism. *Front Pediatr.* 2021;9:747812.
2. Sadr IM, Tan PE, Kieran MW, et al. Mechanism of pulmonary vein stenosis in infants with normally connected veins. *Am J Cardiol.* 2000;86:577-579, A10.
3. Pogoriler JE, Kulik TJ, Casey AM, et al. Lung pathology in pediatric pulmonary vein stenosis. *Pediatr Dev Pathol.* 2016;19:219-229.
4. Sena L, Callahan R, Sleeper LA, Beroukhim RS. Prognostic significance of computed tomography findings in pulmonary vein stenosis. *Children.* 2021;8:402.
5. Choi C, Gauvreau K, Levy P, et al. Longer exposure to left-to-right shunts is a risk factor for pulmonary vein stenosis in patients with trisomy 21. *Children.* 2021;8:19.
6. Niccum M, Callahan R, Gauvreau K, et al. Aspiration is associated with poor treatment response in pediatric pulmonary vein stenosis. *Children.* 2021;8:783.
7. Balasubramanian S, Rehman M, Gauvreau K, et al. Bilateral disease and early age at presentation are associated with shorter survival in patients with congenital heart disease and intraluminal pulmonary vein stenosis. *Congenit Heart Dis.* 2012;7:378-386.
8. Quinonez LG, Gauvreau K, Borisuk M, et al. Outcomes of surgery for young children with multivessel pulmonary vein stenosis. *J Thorac Cardiovasc Surg.* 2015;150:911-917.
9. Mahgoub L, Kaddoura T, Kameny AR, et al. Pulmonary vein stenosis of ex-premature infants with pulmonary hypertension and bronchopulmonary dysplasia, epidemiology, and survival from a multicenter cohort. *Pediatr Pulmonol.* 2017;52:1063-1070.
10. DiLorenzo MP, Santo A, Rome JJ, et al. Pulmonary vein stenosis: outcomes in children with congenital heart disease and prematurity. *Semin Thorac Cardiovasc Surg.* 2019;31:266-273.
11. Rosenblum JM, Altin HF, Gillespie SE, et al. Management outcomes of primary pulmonary vein stenosis. *J Thorac Cardiovasc Surg.* 2020;159:1029-1036.e1.
12. Lo Rito M, Gazzaz T, Wilder TJ, et al. Pulmonary vein stenosis: severity and location predict survival after surgical repair. *J Thorac Cardiovasc Surg.* 2016;151:657-666.e2.
13. Kalfa D, Belli E, Bacha E, et al. Primary pulmonary vein stenosis: outcomes, risk factors, and severity score in a multicentric study. *Ann Thorac Surg.* 2017;104:182-189.
14. Sykes MC, Ireland C, McSweeney JE, et al. The impact of right ventricular pressure and function on survival in patients with pulmonary vein stenosis. *Pulm Circ.* 2018;8:2045894018776894.
15. Feins EN, Ireland C, Gauvreau K, et al. Pulmonary vein stenosis: anatomic considerations, surgical management, and outcomes. *J Thorac Cardiovasc Surg.* 2022;163:2198-2207.e3.
16. Callahan R, Kieran MW, Baird CW, et al. Adjunct targeted biologic inhibition agents to treat aggressive multivessel intraluminal pediatric pulmonary vein stenosis. *J Pediatr.* 2018;198:29-35.e5.
17. Patel JD, Briones M, Mandhani M, et al. Systemic sirolimus therapy for infants and children with pulmonary vein stenosis. *J Am Coll Cardiol.* 2021;77:2807-2818.
18. Hammer PE, McEnaney K, Callahan R, et al. The role of elevated wall shear stress in progression of pulmonary vein stenosis: evidence from two case studies. *Children.* 2021;8:729.
19. Callahan R, Jenkins KJ, Gauthier Z, et al. Preliminary findings on the use of intravascular ultrasound in the assessment of pediatric pulmonary vein stenosis. *Catheter Cardiovasc Interv.* 2021;97:E362-E370.
20. Callahan R, Gauthier Z, Toba S, et al. Correlation of intravascular ultrasound with histology in pediatric pulmonary vein stenosis. *Children.* 2021;8:193.
21. Peng LF, Lock JE, Nugent AW, et al. Comparison of conventional and cutting balloon angioplasty for congenital and postoperative pulmonary vein stenosis in infants and young children. *Catheter Cardiovasc Interv.* 2010;75:1084-1090.
22. Suntharos P, Prieto LR. Treatment of congenital and acquired pulmonary vein stenosis. *Curr Cardiol Rep.* 2020;22:153.
23. Khan A, Qureshi AM, Justino H. Comparison of drug eluting versus bare metal stents for pulmonary vein stenosis in childhood. *Catheter Cardiovasc Interv.* 2019;94:233-242.
24. Esch JJ, Porras D, Bergersen L, et al. Systemic embolic complications of pulmonary vein angioplasty in children. *Pediatr Cardiol.* 2015;36:1357-1362.
25. Kawashima Y, Ueda T, Naito Y, et al. Stenosis of pulmonary veins: report of a patient corrected surgically. *Ann Thorac Surg.* 1971;12:196-202.
26. Bini RM, Cleveland DC, Ceballos R, et al. Congenital pulmonary vein stenosis. *Am J Cardiol.* 1984;54:369-375.
27. Pacifico AD, Mandke NV, McGrath LB, et al. Repair of congenital pulmonary venous stenosis with living autologous atrial tissue. *J Thorac Cardiovasc Surg.* 1985;89:604-609.
28. Lacour-Gayet F, Rey C, Planche C. Pulmonary vein stenosis. Description of a sutureless surgical procedure using the pericardium in situ. *Arch Mal Coeur Vaiss.* 1996;89:633-636.
29. Najm HK, Caldarone CA, Smallhorn J, et al. A sutureless technique for the relief of pulmonary vein stenosis with the use of in situ pericardium. *J Thorac Cardiovasc Surg.* 1998;115:468-470.
30. Lacour-Gayet F. Surgery for Pulmonary venous obstruction after repair of total anomalous pulmonary venous return. *Semin Thorac Cardiovasc Surg Pediatr Card Surg Annu.* 2006;9:45-50.

31. Devaney EJ, Ohye RG, Bove EL. Pulmonary vein stenosis following repair of total anomalous pulmonary venous connection. *Semin Thorac Cardiovasc Surg Pediatr Card Surg Annu.* 2006;9:51-55.

32. Honjo O, Atlin CR, Hamilton BC, et al. Primary sutureless repair for infants with mixed total anomalous pulmonary venous drainage. *Ann Thorac Surg.* 2010;90:862-868.

33. Kanter KR, Kirshbom PM, Kogon BE. Surgical repair of pulmonary venous stenosis: a word of caution. *Ann Thorac Surg.* 2014;98:1687-1692.

34. Shi G, Zhu Z, Chen H, et al. Surgical repair for primary pulmonary vein stenosis: single-institution, midterm follow-up. *J Thorac Cardiovasc Surg.* 2015;150:181-188.

35. Viola N, Alghamdi AA, Perrin DG, et al. Primary pulmonary vein stenosis: the impact of sutureless repair on survival. *J Thorac Cardiovasc Surg.* 2011;142:344-350.

36. Kovach AE, Magcalas PM, Ireland C, et al. Paucicellular fibrointimal proliferation characterizes pediatric pulmonary vein stenosis. *Am J Surg Pathol.* 2017;41:1198-1204.

37. Han HC. Twisted blood vessels: symptoms, etiology and biomechanical mechanisms. *J Vasc Res.* 2012;49:185-197.

38. Cunningham KS, Gotlieb AI. The role of shear stress in the pathogenesis of atherosclerosis. *Lab Invest.* 2004;85:9-23.

39. Callahan R, Gauvreau K, Marshall AC, et al. Outcomes in establishing individual vessel patency for pediatric pulmonary vein stenosis. *Children.* 2021;8:210.

40. Feins EN, Callahan R, Baird CW. Pulmonary veins stenosis: evolving surgical management of a challenging disease. *Children.* 2021;8:631.

41. Riedlinger WF, Juraszek AL, Jenkins KJ, et al. Pulmonary vein stenosis: expression of receptor tyrosine kinases by lesional cells. *Cardiovasc Pathol.* 2006;15:91-99.

42. Callahan R, Esch JJ, Wang G, et al. Systemic sirolimus to prevent in-stent stenosis in pediatric pulmonary vein stenosis. *Pediatr Cardiol.* 2020;41:282-289.

41

Aortopulmonary Window

SARAH W. GOLDBERG AND MUHAMMAD BAKR GHBEIS

KEY LEARNING POINTS

- An aortopulmonary (AP) window is a communication between the ascending aorta and the pulmonary trunk, occurring above two distinct and separate semilunar valves.
- AP window is associated with other cardiac defects in up to two-third of patients, most commonly aortic arch abnormalities such as interrupted aortic arch and coarctation of the aorta.
- Isolated AP window is not typically associated with genetic abnormalities.

- As opposed to other septal defects, AP windows do not close spontaneously or get smaller with somatic growth over time; due to a high incidence of pulmonary vascular disease in unrepaired patients, surgical management is indicated as soon as possible after diagnosis.
- A two-patch surgical repair technique is used in most cases with excellent long-term outcomes.
- Other associated cardiac lesions are typically addressed at the time of AP window repair.

Definition

An aortopulmonary (AP) window is a communication between the ascending aorta and the pulmonary trunk, occurring above two distinct and separate semilunar valves.[1-3] The presence of the two separate semilunar valves distinguishes an AP window from truncus arteriosus.[2]

Prevalence

AP window is a rare congenital heart defect accounting for 0.1–0.2% of all congenital heart disease.[1,4-7] AP window is not associated with any genetic abnormalities. Despite being an abnormality of the conotruncus, AP window is not associated with 22q11 deletion syndrome.[8] AP window occurs equally between the males and females and has not been associated with any *in utero* exposures.[1,3,6]

Embryology

The AP septum forms during the 9th week of embryonic development.[9] AP window results from a failure of the two opposing conotruncal ridges of the truncus arteriosus to fuse, producing a deficiency in the AP septum.[3,4] A large AP window defect may result in abnormal incorporation of the right sixth aortic arch, which gives rise to the right pulmonary artery. This can result in the right pulmonary artery arising abnormally from the rightward aspect of the ascending aorta.[9]

AP window is associated with other cardiac defects in 50–75% of patients,[1,5,6,8,10] most commonly aortic arch abnormalities such as interrupted aortic arch (IAA) and coarctation of the aorta (Table 41.1).[7,11] In a study of 42 patients, IAA occurred in 50% of patients with an AP window.[1] Conversely, AP window occurs in approximately 4% of patients with IAA.[8] Other commonly associated congenital heart defects include ventricular septal defect, D-transposition of the great arteries, tetralogy of Fallot, and other variations of the pulmonary arteries, head and neck vessels, and coronary arteries.[4] Berry syndrome is a combination of a distal AP window, an abnormal origin of the right pulmonary artery from the aorta, and IAA or coarctation of the aorta with an intact ventricular septum.[12,13]

Anatomy

The defect of an AP window can vary in size and position in the wall between the ascending aorta and the main pulmonary artery (MPA).[14,15] Defects are classified into four types based on their position related to the MPA (Fig. 41.1)[2]:
- Type I: Proximal defect, located above the sinus of Valsalva on the posteromedial wall of the ascending aorta. This defect has a superior rim of tissue but little inferior rim separating the defect from the semilunar valves.
- Type II: Distal defect, located adjacent to the origin of the right pulmonary artery with possible extension into the origin.

TABLE 41.1	Children's Hospital Boston 20 Years' Experience: Aortopulmonary (AP) Window 2002–2022	
Total number of patients		49
Isolated AP window		12 (24%)
Other CHD		37 (76%)
VSD		6
ASD		6
IAA		4
TOF		3
ARCAPA		3
Other		12
Age at surgical repair (days, median)		34 (range 2–589)
Surgical mortality		0

ARCAPA, Anomalous right coronary artery originating from the pulmonary artery; *ASD,* atrial septal defect; *CHD,* congenital heart disease; *IAA,* interrupted aortic arch; *TOF,* tetralogy of Fallot; *VSD,* ventricular septal defect.

- Type III: Large or total defect, involving the entire AP septum.
- Type IV: Intermediate defect, involving portions of the proximal and distal AP septum. This defect often has adequate superior and inferior tissue rims that may be amenable to transcatheter device closure.[11]

As opposed to other septal defects, AP windows do not close spontaneously or get smaller with somatic growth over time.[1]

Physiology

The physiological effects of an AP window are those of a left-to-right shunt lesion, such as a ventricular septal defect or patent ductus arteriosus. The degree of shunting depends on the size of the defect and the ratio of the systemic and pulmonary vascular resistances.[1] As the pulmonary vascular resistance declines in the days and weeks after birth, the left-to-right shunt will increase, resulting in excess pulmonary blood flow. If aortic arch obstruction is present,

left-to-right shunting will be increased. As the ductus arteriosus starts to close in IAA, systemic perfusion will decline and pulmonary blood flow will increase further, potentially resulting in cardiogenic shock. The presence of any associated severe congenital heart defect may mask the presence of an AP window.[1]

Clinical Manifestations

AP window is rarely diagnosed in the antenatal period.[4,10] Although the severity of clinical symptoms will vary with the size of the defect, due to the timing of normalization of the pulmonary vascular resistance, and associated cardiac lesions, most patients will present within the first several weeks of life, particularly if the lesion is unrestrictive.[1,11] The clinical features of AP window are often indistinguishable from those of a large left-to-right shunt lesions such as a patent ductus arteriosus or ventricular septal defect.[4] The most common symptoms on presentation include increased work of breathing, tachypnea, diaphoresis, poor feeding, and difficulty with weight gain.[4] Patients with smaller, restrictive AP windows may be asymptomatic on presentation.[1] Cyanosis is not usually a prominent feature of AP windows but bidirectional shunting across large defects can produce systemic desaturation in early infancy, when the pulmonary vascular resistance is still elevated, or later on after pulmonary vascular disease has developed.[17]

Because AP window defects are typically large and unrestrictive, the pulmonary vasculature is exposed to systemic hypertension. Without repair, chronic left-to-right shunting may result in the development of pulmonary vascular disease within the first several years of life. If left surgically uncorrected, 40% of patients with AP window will die within the 1st year of life with the major cause of mortality in older children being pulmonary vascular disease.[10,18] Therefore, it is important that these lesions are recognized and treated early to prevent irreversible pulmonary vascular changes.

On physical exam, patients may have tachypnea with accessory muscle use, a displaced apical impulse suggestive of

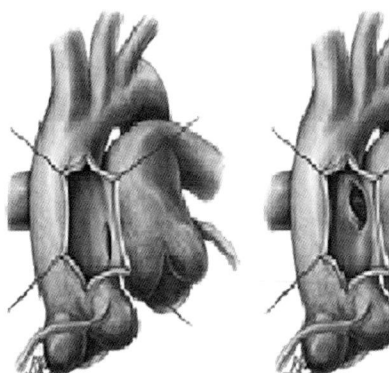 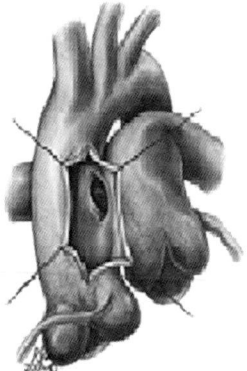 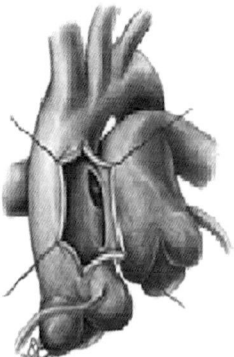 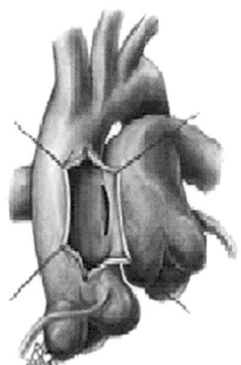

Type I - Proximal defect   Type II - Distal defect   Type III - Total defect   Type IV - Intermediate defect

• **Fig. 41.1** Anatomic classification of the types of aortopulmonary window by the Society of Thoracic Surgeons. (Reprinted from Backer CL, Mavroudis C. Surgical management of aortopulmonary window: a 40-year experience. *Eur J Cardiothorac Surg.* 2002;21:773–779, with permission from Elsevier.)

cardiomegaly, bounding pulses due to diastolic run-off, and failure to thrive.[4] A systolic murmur can often be heard along the left sternal border but, in contrast to a patent ductus arteriosus, a diastolic component to the murmur is uncommon with large lesions. Smaller AP windows will have continuous murmurs similar to a patent ductus arteriosus. A mid-diastolic rumble may be present due to left ventricular volume overload.

Patients with associated congenital heart defects may present differently. In particular, patients with IAA or severe coarctation can present in cardiogenic shock coinciding with ductal closure.[1,17] Preceding symptoms may include poor feeding, mottling, lethargy, and decreased urine output while, on exam, patients may have evidence of decreased systemic perfusion including diminished pulses and decreased capillary refill in addition to findings consistent with congestive heart failure.

Although rare, there are some patients who have been diagnosed with AP windows in adolescence and adulthood.[19,20] These patients usually present with significant pulmonary arterial hypertension progressing to Eisenmenger syndrome, making them inoperable.[21,22] Patients may have a history of symptoms consistent with congestive heart failure. On presentation, symptoms are consistent with pulmonary arterial hypertension, including tachypnea and increased work of breathing, exertional intolerance, and cyanosis. Findings on exam may include a pansystolic murmur, loud P2, and pulmonary ejection click consistent with elevated pulmonary vascular resistance.[21] Rarely, patients with smaller, restrictive defects may present with limited symptoms and a continuous murmur on exam in the setting of less pulmonary vascular disease.[19]

Electrocardiography

The electrocardiographic patterns are the same as those seen in patients with significant systemic-to-pulmonary circulation, or left-to-right shunt indicative of increased myocardial demand with increased pulmonary overcirculation. This can include sinus tachycardia and increased right- and left-sided voltages, as well as deep Q wave in lateral precordial leads.

Chest X-Ray

The chest x-ray shows evidence of left-to-right shunting with increased pulmonary vascular markings and mild to moderate cardiomegaly. Other possible findings can include absence of the aortic knuckle and prominence of the main pulmonary segment.

Echocardiography

The hyperdynamic function and the enlarged chambers provide useful clues to the presence and location of a left-to-right shunt. The defect itself can be easily visualized and the shunting documented by Doppler examination,

although the defect may be missed without careful evaluation of the ascending aorta and pulmonary artery. The diagnosis is made by scanning the AP septum in multiple views (including subxiphoid, parasternal, and suprasternal notch). Imaging the defect in multiple views and detecting the flow through it by color flow Doppler mapping allows confirmation of the true defect rather than false dropout. At the level of the defect, the joined vessels are elliptical in cross-section, whereas in contrast, false dropout is characterized by persistence of the normal circular contour of each vessel (Fig. 41.2). The distinguishing feature between AP window and truncus arteriosus is the presence of two separate semilunar valves in the former. The AP window is proximal to, or at the level of, the pulmonary artery branches, whereas a persistent ductus arteriosus is more distal and usually has some length.

Surgically important information that is readily derived from the echocardiogram includes the distance between the proximal border of the defect and the semilunar valves and coronary arteries, as well as the distance between the distal border and the pulmonary arteries. Although the incidence of additional defects is frequent, these are all now readily identifiable by careful echocardiography. In select patients with acoustic limitations, other imaging modalities such as cardiac magnetic resonance imaging or cardiac computed tomography may provide similar anatomic information (Fig. 41.3).

Cardiac Catheterization

From an anatomic or hemodynamic standpoint, catheterization is not typically necessary, particularly in neonatal and early infancy presentation. One indication at this age is if device closure is planned. There are few case reports of management with device closure with success in small

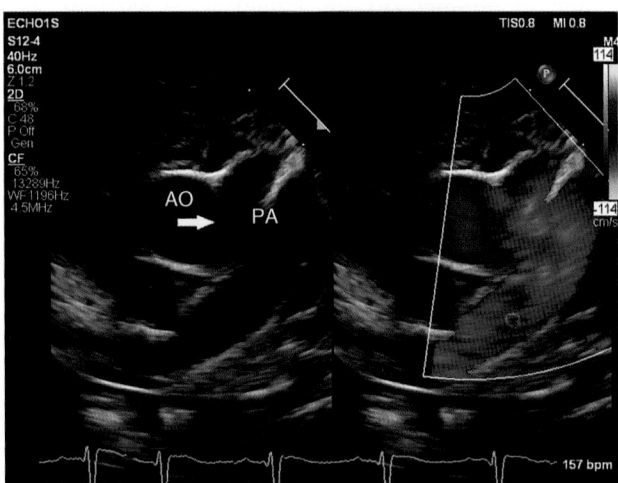

• **Fig. 41.2** Aortopulmonary window by echocardiography. Parasternal short-axis view with color Doppler comparison demonstrates the large window defect *(arrow)* between the ascending aorta *(AO)* and the adjacent main pulmonary artery *(PA)*. Note the loss of the circular two-dimensional contour of the ascending aorta which is a diagnostic hallmark.

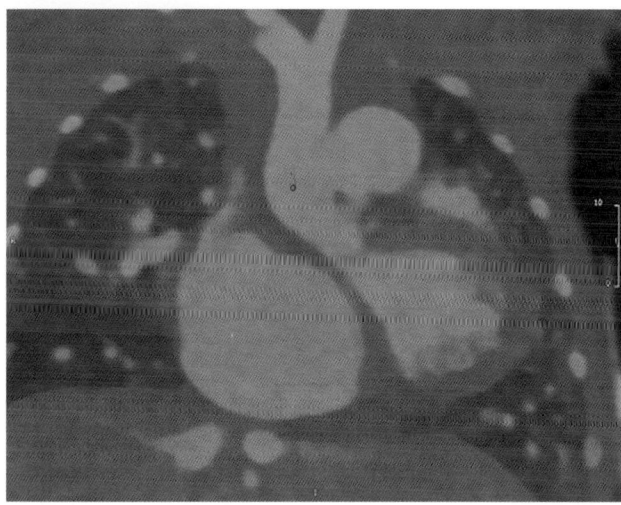

• **Fig. 41.3** Aortopulmonary window by computed tomography (CT). CT in this infant with an aortopulmonary window in a coronal plane demonstrates the large communication between the ascending aorta and the main pulmonary artery.

defects without other lesions, and if technically favorable with adequate superior and inferior rims of the defect.[23,24]

Other indications for cardiac catheterization is with late presentations where the assessment of pulmonary vascular resistance becomes vital in determining the surgical candidacy.

Management

The management of AP window is almost always surgical, whether with early or later presentation. If the AP window defect is large and unrestrictive, the clinical presentation may be profound, and indeed may lead to shock with inadequate systemic perfusion. Acute medical management may include inotropic support, measures to improve systemic output by limiting excessive pulmonary blood flow, and measures to decrease metabolic demands including intubation and mechanical ventilation, sedation, and sometimes neuromuscular blockade.

As noted previously, some select patients with small, uncomplicated lesions (type IV) may be candidates for catheter-delivered device closure, but this is uncommon. The vast majority of patients require surgical repair. Surgical closure, including repair of any other lesions, should be undertaken with minimal delay after diagnosis in infants. A brief period of intensive anticongestive therapy is probably useful perioperatively to improve physiologic readiness for surgery. For those with late presentations, pulmonary vasoreactivity testing should take place to assess surgical candidacy. Surgical outcomes are generally excellent, including presentations beyond infancy.[19]

In terms of operative technique, the two-patch repair is often used, as it requires minimal additional time and permits separate mobilization of the aorta and MPA in any future reoperation.[4] The two-patch technique also appears to result in less subsequent aorta or pulmonary artery stenoses

than a single-patch repair. Early morbidity includes pulmonary artery stenosis and residual AP septal defects. Long-term follow-up is indicated to look for recurrent lesions such as the development of branch pulmonary artery stenosis and arch obstruction.[6]

In a report from our hospital covering a 20-year period, among 49 patients operated on at median age of 5 weeks, there was no mortality. Two-patch repair following the AP window division was performed in 60% of the patients, while 30% underwent AP window division with primary aortotomy closure and patch closure of the pulmonary artery.

References

1. Bagtharia R, Trivedi KR, Burkhart HM, et al. Outcomes for patients with an aortopulmonary window, and the impact of associated cardiovascular lesions. *Cardiol Young.* 2004;14: 473-480.
2. Jacobs JP, Quintessenza JA, Gaynor JW, et al. Congenital Heart Surgery Nomenclature and Database Project: aortopulmonary window. *Ann Thorac Surg.* 2000;69:44-49.
3. Erez E, Dagan O, Georghiou GP, et al. Surgical management of aortopulmonary window and associated lesions. *Ann Thorac Surg.* 2004;77:484-487.
4. Barnes ME, Mitchell ME, Tweddell JS. Aortopulmonary window. *Semin Thorac Cardiovasc Surg Pediatr Card Surg Annu.* 2011;14:67-74.
5. Kutsche LM, van Mierop LHS. Anatomy and pathogenesis of aorticopulmonary septal defect. *Am J Cardiol.* 1987;59: 443-447.
6. Hew CC, Bacha EA, Zurakowski D, et al. Optimal surgical approach for repair of aortopulmonary window. *Cardiol Young.* 2001;11:385-390.
7. Šamánek M, Voříšková M. Congenital heart disease among 815,569 children born between 1980 and 1990 and their 15-year survival: a prospective bohemia survival study. *Pediatr Cardiol.* 1999;20:411-417.
8. Konstantinov IE, Karamlou T, Williams WG, et al. Surgical management of aortopulmonary window associated with interrupted aortic arch: A Congenital Heart Surgeons Society study. *J Thorac Cardiovasc Surg.* 2006;131:1136-1141.e2.
9. Anderson RH, Cook A, Brown NA, et al. Development of the outflow tracts with reference to aortopulmonary windows and aortoventricular tunnels. *Cardiol Young.* 2010;20:92-99.
10. van Son JAM, Puga FJ, Danielson G, et al. Aortopulmonary window: factors associated with early and late success after surgical treatment. *Mayo Clin Proc.* 1993;68:128-133.
11. Backer CL, Mavroudis C. Surgical management of aortopulmonary window: a 40-year experience. *Eur J Cardiothorac Surg.* 2002;21:773-779.
12. Berry TE, Bharati S, Muster AJ, et al. Distal aortopulmonary septal defect, aortic origin of the right pulmonary artery, intact ventricular septum, patent ductus arteriosus and hypoplasia of the aortic isthmus: a newly recognized syndrome. *Am J Cardiol.* 1982;49:108-116.
13. Binsalamah ZM, Greenleaf CE, Heinle JS. Type A interrupted aortic arch and type III aortopulmonary window with anomalous origin of the right pulmonary artery from the aorta. *J Card Surg.* 2018;33:344-347.

14. Mori K, Ando M, Takao A, et al. Distal type of aortopulmonary window. Report of 4 cases. *Heart*. 1978;40:681-689.

15. Richardson JV, Doty DB, Rossi NP, et al. The spectrum of anomalies of aortopulmonary septation. *J Thorac Cardiovasc Surg*. 1979;78:21-27.

16. Collinet P, Chatelet-Cheront C, Houze de l'Aulnoit D, et al. Prenatal diagnosis of an aorto-pulmonary window by fetal echocardiography. *Fetal Diagn Ther*. 2002;17:302-307.

17. Tweddell J. Aortopulmonary window. In: Kaiser LK, Spray T, eds. *Mastery of Cardiothoracic Surgery*. 2nd ed. Philadelphia: Lippincott, Williams and Williams; 2006.

18. Bertolini A, Dalmonte P, Bava GL, et al. Aortopulmonary septal defects. A review of the literature and report of ten cases. *J Cardiovasc Surg (Torino)*. 1994;35:207-213.

19. Talwar S, Siddharth B, Gupta SK, et al. Aortopulmonary window: results of repair beyond infancy. *Interact Cardiovasc Thorac Surg*. 2017;25:740-744.

20. Kumar V, Singh RS, Thingnam SKS, et al. Surgical outcome in aortopulmonary window beyond the neonatal period. *J Card Surg*. 2019;34:300-304.

21. Aggarwal SK, Mishra J, Sai V, et al. Aortopulmonary window in adults: diagnosis and treatment of late-presenting patients. *Congenit Heart Dis*. 2008;3:341-346.

22. El Dick J, El-Rassi I, Tayeh C, et al. Aortopulmonary window in adults: a rare entity leading to Eisenmenger syndrome. *Echocardiography*. 2019;36:1173-1178.

23. Guzeltas A, Ugan Atik S, Tanidir IC. Transcatheter closure of aortopulmonary window in infants with Amplatzer Duct Occluder-I. *Acta Cardiol Sin*. 2021;37:305-308.

24. Yıldırım A, Erdem A, Türkmen Karaağaç A. Transcatheter closure of the aortopulmonary window in a three-month-old infant with a symmetric membranous ventricular septal defect occluder device. *Turk Gogus Kalp Damar Cerrahisi Derg*. 2021;29:101-104.

42

Coronary Artery Anomalies

JANE W. NEWBURGER, REBECCA BEROUKHIM, AND LUIS QUINONEZ

KEY LEARNING POINTS

- Anomalous origin of a coronary artery from the pulmonary artery causes myocardial ischemia secondary to coronary steal; with timely surgical repair, the outlook is excellent in the majority of affected children.
- Anomalous origin of the left coronary artery with interarterial and intramural course carries a substantial risk of sudden cardiac death with exercise and should be repaired in the early school years.
- Anomalous origin of the right coronary artery in patients with symptoms or signs of ischemia should undergo surgical repair; for asymptomatic patients, choice of observation

without exercise restriction versus surgical repair requires consideration of individual patient circumstances and shared decision-making.
- Intraseptal left coronary artery usually has a benign clinical course; rare patients with inducible ischemia are treated with beta-blockers, non-dihydropyridine calcium channel inhibitors, or surgery.
- Management of coronary artery fistulae depends upon their size and hemodynamic burden, as well as technical considerations related to patient age and size.

Introduction

Most coronary artery anomalies, such as minor degrees of origin eccentricity or anomalous origin coronary arteries that do not run between the great arteries (interarterial) or in the wall of the aorta (intramural), are of no clinical significance. In this chapter, we will discuss a subset of coronary anomalies that present to the pediatric cardiologist and may impact patient well-being. These include: (1) anomalous origin of a coronary artery from the pulmonary artery, (2) anomalous aortic origin of a coronary artery (AAOCA) with an intramural course, and (3) coronary arterial venous fistulae. Coronary artery abnormalities that are associated with particular forms of congenital and acquired heart disease, such as tetralogy of Fallot, transposition of the great arteries, Williams syndrome, Kawasaki disease, or hyperlipidemia, are described in the relevant chapters.

Anomalous Origin of the Left Coronary Artery From a Pulmonary Artery

Pathology

Anomalous origin of a coronary artery from the pulmonary artery occurs in 1 in 300,000 births. In the vast majority of such cases, an anomalous left main coronary artery arises from

the pulmonary artery (ALCAPA, Fig. 42.1),[1] with only rare origin of the right coronary artery from the pulmonary artery (ARCAPA, Fig. 42.2). The other high-pressure coronary artery arising from the aorta provides perfusion for the myocardium, is bigger and, in most cases, provides retrograde flow through collaterals to the anomalous coronary and the pulmonary artery. An isolated left anterior descending or circumflex coronary artery may also arise from the pulmonary artery.[2] Extremely rarely, both coronary arteries may arise from the pulmonary artery, a condition that is fatal unless recognized very early. Patients who come to postmortem examination generally have evidence of myocardial infarction.

Physiology

Before birth, the pulmonary artery pressure is at systemic levels, allowing for satisfactory antegrade myocardial perfusion from the pulmonary artery through the anomalous coronary. With birth and falling pulmonary artery pressure, the antegrade perfusion of the anomalous coronary gradually decreases, and the normal coronary artery from the aorta takes over the circulation through collateral vessels. In most patients, the flow in the anomalous coronary artery reverses, and a coronary artery steal develops from the myocardium to the pulmonary artery. The size of this left-to-right shunt is rarely large enough to be a significant hemodynamic

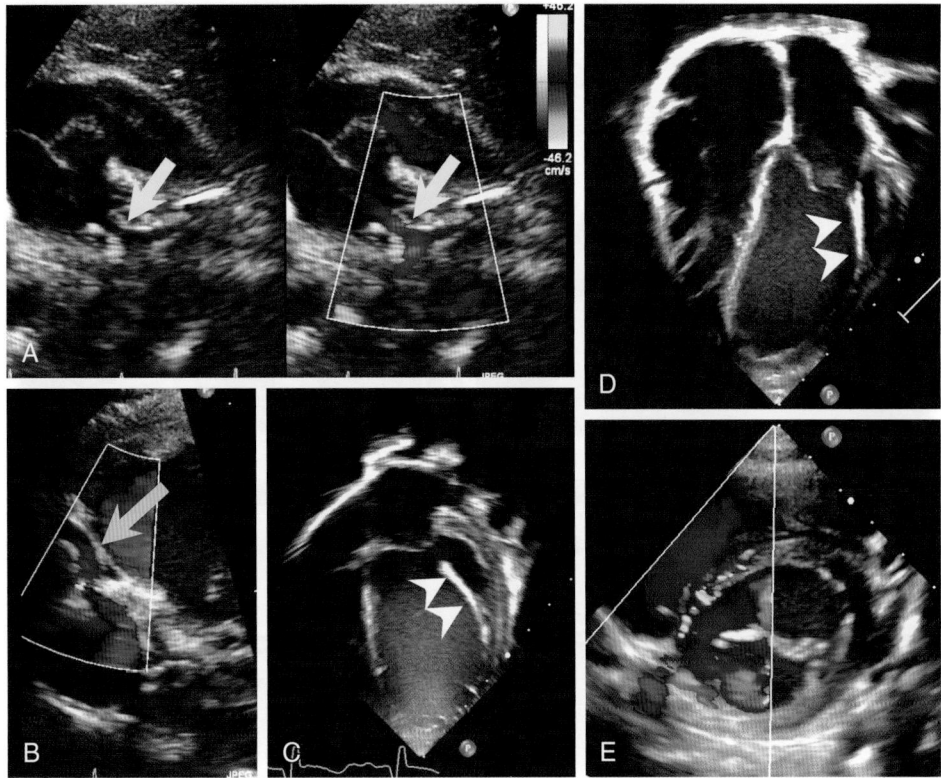

• **Fig. 42.1** Two patients with anomalous origin of the left coronary artery from the pulmonary artery. Retrograde flow is seen from an anomalous left coronary artery into the pulmonary artery in a 2-month-old infant (*yellow arrow*, **A**). The right coronary artery is mildly dilated with antegrade flow (*orange arrow*, **B**), and the left ventricle is severely dilated with echogenic, ischemic papillary muscles (*white arrowheads*, **C**). A 6-year-old with unrepaired anomalous left coronary artery from the pulmonary artery has a similar appearance of echogenic papillary muscles (*white arrowheads*, **D**), and has developed characteristic robust collateral flow in the interventricular septum (**E**).

burden, but it deprives the myocardium of perfusion. Sometime in the first week of reversed coronary flow, myocardial ischemia becomes sufficient to be recognizable on an electrocardiogram. The heart enlarges, congestive heart failure becomes manifest, and with ischemic damage to the left papillary muscles, mitral regurgitation often compounds an already deteriorating situation. Fibrosis secondary to hypoperfusion and subendocardial ischemia increase the risk of high-grade ventricular ectopy and sudden cardiac death.

If, for any reason, the patient maintains systemic pressure in the pulmonary arteries, this sequence of events will not occur, and the anomalous coronary will be perfused by blood originating from the pulmonary artery. Although this blood has substantially lower oxygen saturation than that of the other coronary, evidence of myocardial ischemia is not seen. Some patients with uncorrected anomalous coronary origin from the main pulmonary artery have enough coronary collateral circulation to survive to childhood, adolescence, and adulthood, when they may present with ischemic cardiomyopathy or sudden cardiac arrest.[3]

Diagnosis

Although patients with ALCAPA appear normal at birth, most have developed signs and symptoms of congestive heart failure by 1–2 months, with tachycardia, tachypnea, diaphoresis, irritability, and poor weight gain. Physical examination can reveal a gallop, mitral regurgitation from ischemia of papillary muscles, and hepatomegaly. Older patients sometimes are asymptomatic,[4] discovered via a murmur of mitral regurgitation or presence of cardiomegaly, or they may present with heart failure, myocardial ischemia, or sudden cardiac death. The electrocardiogram almost always shows evidence of an anterolateral myocardial infarction (Fig. 42.3), even in the asymptomatic patient. A chest radiograph typically reveals cardiomegaly, sometimes severe.

In diagnostic testing, the origin of the coronary arteries should be identified in any patient with unexplained myocardial disease. An enlarged, poorly functioning left ventricle is characteristic, as is mitral regurgitation. The anomalous origin of this coronary artery from the pulmonary artery is associated with inequality of coronary artery size.[5]

The parasternal short-axis view usually identifies the origins of the coronary arteries from the aorta. Scanning in a parasternal short- or long-axis view may identify clearly the orifice of the coronary artery in the pulmonary root. Color flow Doppler mapping is extremely valuable in demonstrating the direction of flow in the coronary, particularly into

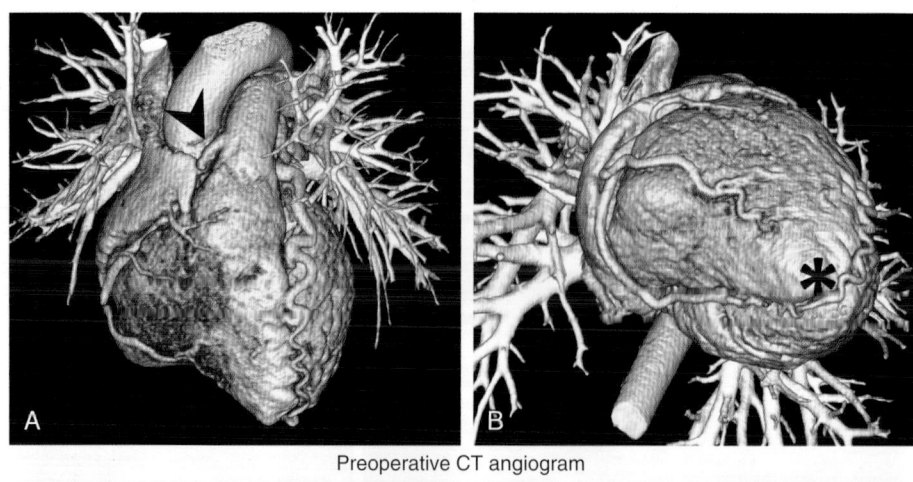

Preoperative CT angiogram

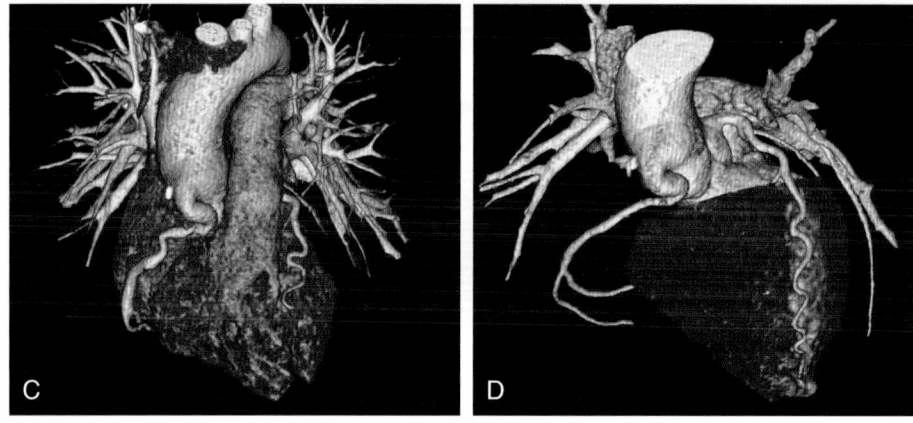

6 months after surgery   18 months after surgery

• **Fig. 42.2** A 6-year-old asymptomatic child with an incidental diagnosis of anomalous right coronary artery from the pulmonary artery. The right coronary artery is markedly dilated (*black arrow*, **A**) with large collateral vessels. The posterior descending coronary artery connects to the distal left anterior descending (*asterisk*, **B**). At follow-up computed tomography *(CT)* 6 months and 18 months after surgery, the distal right coronary artery is progressively smaller in size with persistent tortuosity of the proximal vessel (**C, D**).

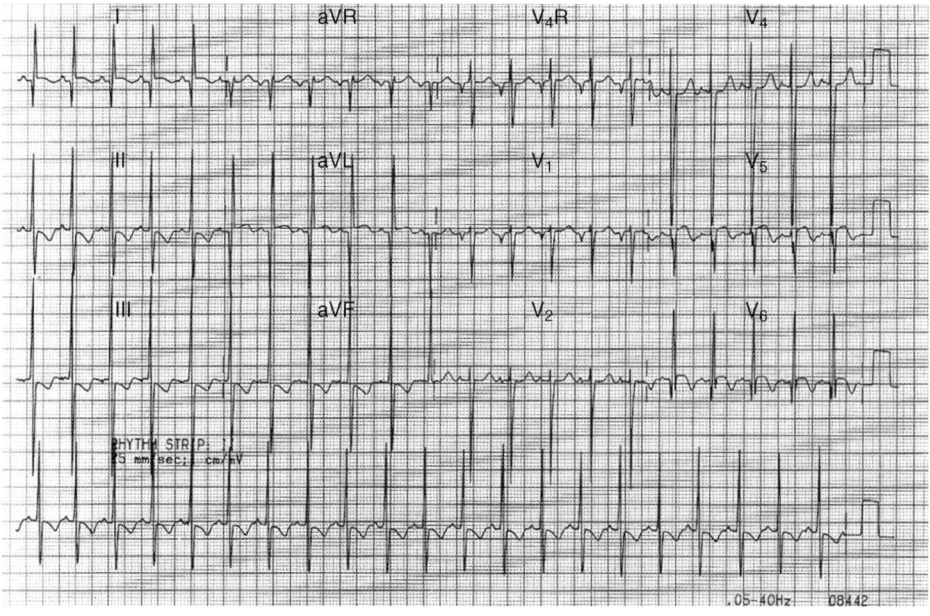

• **Fig. 42.3** Electrocardiogram from a 3-month-old infant with anomalous origin of the left coronary artery from the pulmonary artery showing evidence of extensive anterolateral infarction (deep Q waves in leads 1, aVL, V6); diminished anterior forces V1–V4; and left atrial enlargement V1).

the pulmonary root when the pulmonary resistance is low. Demonstration of antegrade flow in the coronary artery and branches by color flow Doppler mapping excludes anomalous origin of that vessel. Careful imaging and color flow Doppler mapping allow accurate diagnosis in the majority, such that surgery without cardiac catheterization can be undertaken.

When the diagnosis is uncertain by noninvasive imaging, cardiac catheterization with selective angiography confirms the diagnosis. With contrast injection, the normal coronary artery arising from the aorta is seen to be large and often tortuous and, through collaterals, fills the left coronary artery (LCA), which in turn is seen to drain into the pulmonary artery. In addition, findings of left ventricular systolic dysfunction, elevated left ventricular end-diastolic pressure secondary to ischemia, and associated elevated left atrial pressure are usually demonstrable.

Management

After the diagnosis has been recognized and the infant stabilized, surgery is undertaken as soon as possible to provide a normal two-coronary circulation. Years ago, ligation of the anomalous artery was used to eliminate the left-to-right shunt to prevent a steal from the myocardium; this approach had some success but also significant early and late mortality. In the past few decades, a number of surgical techniques have been used to connect the anomalous artery to the aorta with excellent outcomes. These include direct aortic reimplantation, or, if not possible, the Takeuchi procedure, which involves creation of an intrapulmonary baffle.[5] Some children with moderate or severe mitral regurgitation also undergo mitral valve repair. In a recent multicenter series of the Pediatric Cardiac Care Consortium, early mortality was 12.4%; among survivors to discharge with available follow-up, 30-year transplant-free survival was greater than 95%.[6] Interestingly neither the severity of left ventricular dysfunction nor mitral regurgitation at the time of initial surgery was predictive of short- or long-term outcomes. Following surgery, most patients become asymptomatic, and left ventricular function and mitral regurgitation improve on echocardiogram over time.[7-12]

Course

The improvement in symptoms and left ventricular function after successful repair is remarkable. However, abnormal global longitudinal and circumferential myocardial strain,[13] and abnormal exercise capacity[7] may be evident after repair even in patients with normal left ventricular ejection fraction and no symptoms. Moreover, long-term survivors with good LCA patency have reduced myocardial flow reserve in left coronary territory, possibly related to impaired vasodilation and/or residual patchy interstitial fibrosis or infarcts from the period of hypoperfusion.[8] Some patients have persistent mitral regurgitation, long-term left ventricular dysfunction and congestive heart failure, and/or proximal coronary artery stenosis or hemodynamically significant mitral regurgitation necessitating coronary artery reoperation or mitral valve repair or replacement. Those who have had a Takeuchi operation may have complications including pulmonary stenosis secondary to the baffle and baffle leaks. Cardiac transplantation is rarely needed except in patients with end-stage ischemic cardiomyopathy. Although long-term survival is excellent even in those who present to medical attention with severe congestive heart failure, the occurrence of late sequelae in some patients highlights the need for life-long cardiac surveillance.

Anomalous Aortic Origin of the Coronary Artery

Pathology

With increasing use and accuracy of non-invasive imaging techniques such as coronary computed tomography angiography (CTA), AAOCA, arising at or above the inappropriate sinus of Valsalva, is now recognized to be relatively common. Altogether, the incidence of such anomalies, including interarterial, subpulmonic, prepulmonic, retroaortic, and retrocardiac is ~0.7% in the general population (Fig. 42.4).[9] Among these, AAOCA with interarterial and intramural course have the highest risk of sudden cardiac death, generally related to vigorous aerobic exercise.

Physiology

Anatomic features associated with myocardial ischemia (e.g., exertional syncope, sudden cardiac arrest, inducible ischemia on stress testing, or angina) include anomalous left coronary artery (ALCA), intramural course, longer intramural length, and high and/or slit-like orifice.[10] Of note, the occurrence of ischemia and risk for arrhythmia in patients with AAOCA is indicated by myocardial fibrosis found on autopsy of patients who died suddenly with AAOCA as well as ischemic events or myocardial infarction in patients with AAOCA but no other risk factors.[11] Importantly, however, a normal stress test does not preclude sudden cardiac death events. Most patients die during or in close temporal association to exercise. Sudden death related to AAOCA is rare in patients over age 35 years, but this is thought to be related to the lower rate of participation in competitive or highly aerobic activities in older individuals. There is no age beyond which the presence of AAOCA is irrelevant; assessment may become more challenging in adult patients who have atherosclerotic coronary artery disease or other conditions.[11]

The mechanism of ischemia and sudden cardiac arrest in patients with AAOCA may be multifactorial.[12] For example, ischemia or myocardial scar from past ischemia may promote symptomatic or fatal arrhythmia. An increase in diameter and interarterial pressure in the great arteries with exercise, accompanied by tachycardia and

Surgical view

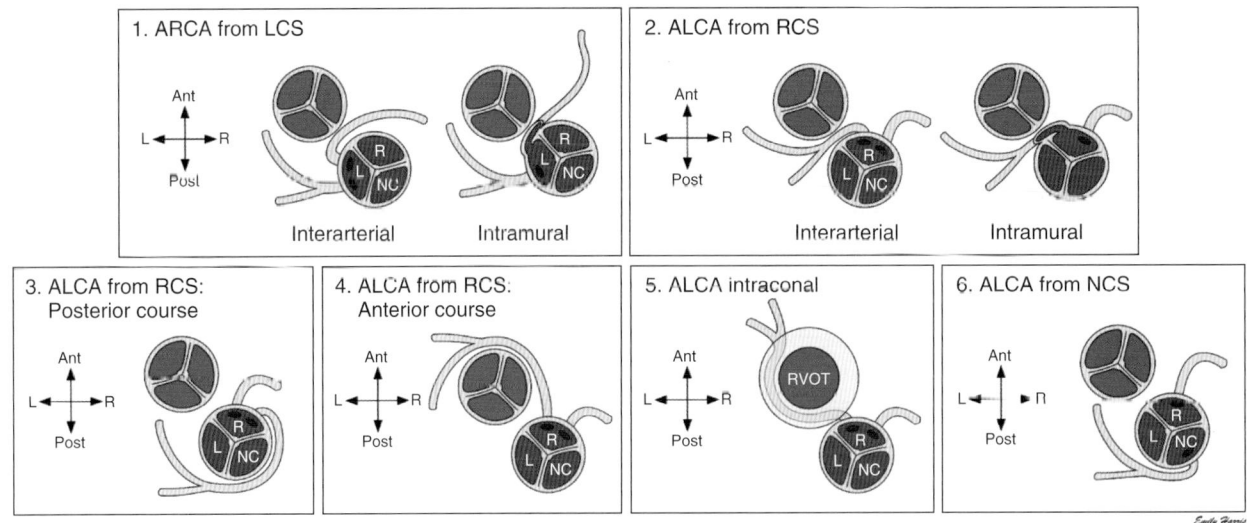

• **Fig. 42.4** Types of anomalous aortic origin of the coronary artery from the viewpoint of the surgeon. *ALCA,* Anomalous left coronary artery; *ARCA,* anomalous right coronary artery; *L,* left; *LCS,* left coronary sinus; *NC,* non coronary; *NCS,* non-coronary sinus; *R,* right; *RCS,* right coronary sinus; *RVOT,* right ventricular outflow tract. (Courtesy of Fabozzo A, DiOrio M, Newburger JW, et al. Anomalous aortic origin of coronary arteries: a single-center experience. *Semin Thorac Cardiovasc Surg.* 2016;28:791–800.)

lower diastolic filling time, may obstruct forward flow in a coronary artery with a slit-like orifice or compress arterial segments with tangential interarterial and intramural course. Some have hypothesized that the intercoronary commissure itself may restrict coronary flow in some patients with AAOCA.

Diagnosis

Patients with a suspected or definite diagnosis of AAOCA by echocardiography should undergo CTA (or CMR) to confirm the diagnosis and high-risk features (slit-like or stenotic orifice, high take-off, intramural course).

With respect to assessing ischemia, there are no data on the diagnostic test characteristics of stress tests in patients with AAOCA, so the choice of stress test is based on adult experience, institutional availability, and first principles. Because ischemia occurs with exercise, non-invasive tests for inducible ischemia should use exercise rather than pharmacologic stress. Among stress tests, exercise ECG has the lowest sensitivity (68%) and specificity (77%). Use of stress echocardiography increases the sensitivity to 76% and specificity to 88%, is practical for children, and avoids radiation exposure. Stress testing with Single Photon Emission Computed Tomography radionuclide Myocardial Perfusion Imaging (SPECT rMPI). increases the sensitivity to 88%, with some loss in specificity (77%), and positron emission tomography (PET) scanning is the most sensitive (91%) of all, with reasonable specificity (82%).[14,15] The type of stress imaging chosen should be tailored to coronary artery anatomy. For example, most stress imaging modalities only detect left ventricular ischemia, so a stress MRI is the best modality for assessing inducible ischemia in a patient with an interarterial/intramural non-dominant right coronary artery.

Management of AAOCA

Guidelines for management of AAOCA have been issued by national societies and individual experts.[11,16,17] There is broad agreement that patients with AAOCA and ischemia—manifested by angina, syncope with exercise suspected to be related to ventricular arrhythmia, or history of aborted sudden cardiac death—should be restricted from exercise and undergo surgical intervention. If surgery is felt to be prohibitively high risk, catheter-based therapy may be reasonable. For asymptomatic patients, recommendations diverge regarding those with anomalous aortic origin of the left (L AAOCA) and right (R AAOCA) coronary arteries with interarterial/intramural course.

Anomalous Aortic Origin of the Left Coronary Artery

The incidence of L AAOCA by CTA is ~0.05% and across imaging modalities is 0.03% (Figs. 42.5 and 42.6).[9] The risk of sudden cardiac death with vigorous exercise in patients with L AAOCA exceeds that of surgery in risk-benefit analyses.[18] For this reason, all individuals with L AAOCA with interarterial/intramural course should be restricted from competitive sports and undergo surgical repair. Because the risk of sudden cardiac death is extremely low in very young children and technical aspects of surgery may be facilitated by larger patient size, elective surgery in asymptomatic patients is generally deferred to school age. Patients may participate in competitive sports after surgical repair assuming there are no signs, symptoms, or diagnostic tests that suggest inducible ischemia. An exception exists for patients who present after aborted sudden cardiac death; in this group, exercise restrictions are recommended for at

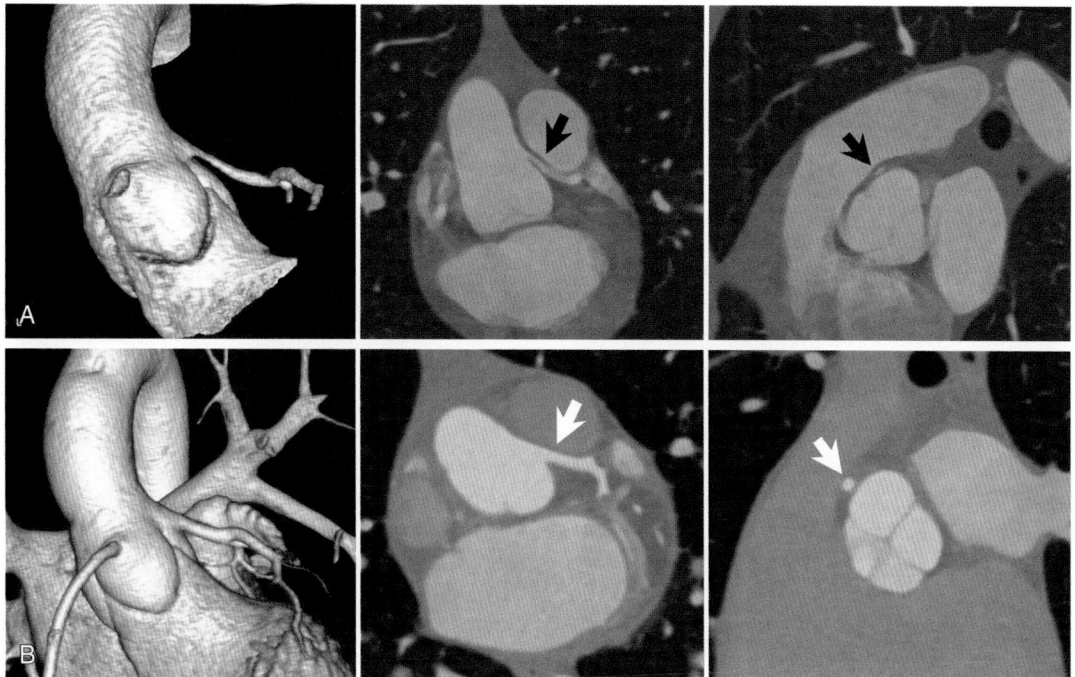

• **Fig. 42.5** Anomalous origin of the left main coronary artery from the aorta, above the sinotubular junction in a 14-year-old asymptomatic girl. **(A)** Preoperatively, the coronary artery arises high above the sinotubular junction with a slit-like ostium, and takes an interarterial course *(black arrows)*. **(B)** Following surgical unroofing of the left main coronary artery, the ostium is unobstructed with a normal takeoff angle and no residual interarterial course *(white arrows)*.

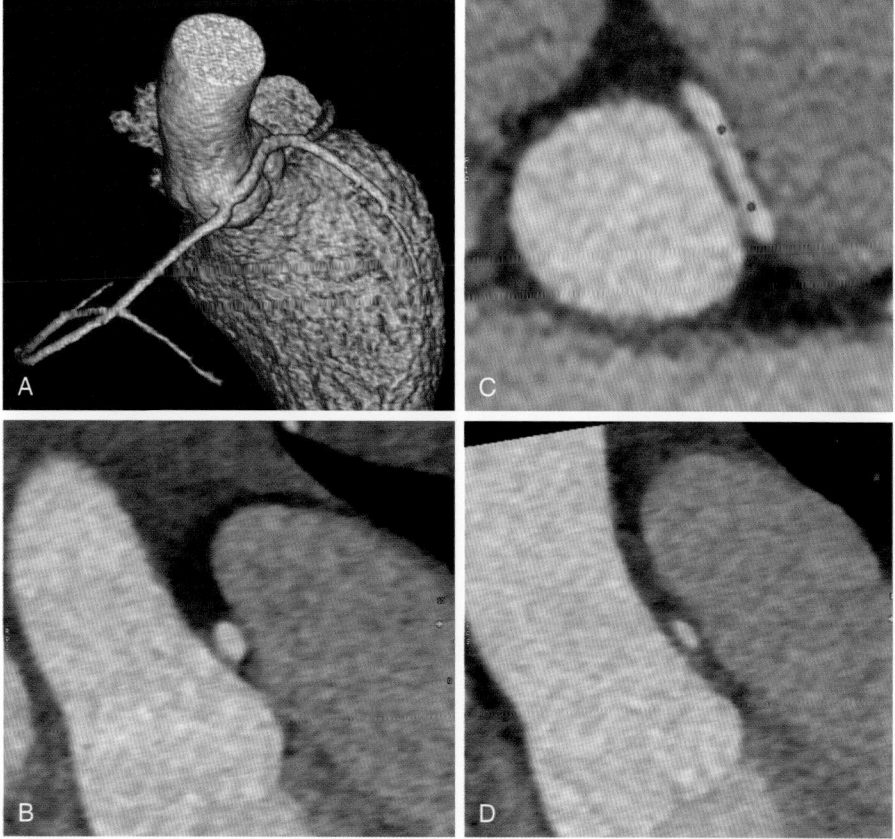

• **Fig. 42.6** Single coronary artery with intramural course of the left coronary artery. **(A)** Single coronary artery arises from the right aortic sinus, giving rise to the right and left main coronary arteries. **(B)** The orifice of the left coronary artery is normal in caliber. **(C)** and **(D)** A few millimeters into the left main coronary artery, the vessel becomes intramural with a slit-like vessel shape and intramural distance of 8.6 mm *(red dots)*.

least 1 year following surgical repair. These patients need to be monitored carefully as they may have areas of myocardial scar that promote lethal arrhythmias even after the risk of exercise-induced ischemia has been eliminated by surgery.

Anomalous Aortic Origin of the Right Coronary Artery

The diagnosis of R AAOCA with interarterial/intramural course is about 10-fold higher than L AAOCA; its incidence is 0.2–0.3% across imaging modalities (Fig. 42.7).[9] Until recently, it was regarded as a minor anomaly without clinical significance. The absolute risk of sudden death is exceedingly low, estimated to be about 0.02% per year (range between 0.0035% and 0.06% per year), and almost always in the context of vigorous exertion, with some variation according to age, with peak risk in adolescence and young adulthood.[18] In a series of 1049 sudden death events during competitive athletics, 16 patients had an anomalous right coronary artery.[19] Reasoning from the incidence of R AAOCA in the general population, the relative risk of sudden death with competitive sports among individuals with R AAOCA with intramural course is five to eight times greater than that in the general population.

In the asymptomatic patient with R AAOCA in whom observational management is elected, full participation in competitive athletics is allowed as long as there is always an automatic external defibrillator (AED) on the field.[16] For patients with ischemia, as indicated by angina, exertional syncope, sudden cardiac arrest, or diagnostic testing that shows inducible ischemia, coronary surgery is recommended. For the asymptomatic patient, a decision analysis was attempted to calculate the most favorable risk-benefit ratio of management strategies.[18] The strategy of exercise restriction was unequivocally inferior to observation without exercise restriction or surgical repair. However, the latter two strategies were more closely matched, with a slight benefit to observation without exercise restriction. The decision might be tipped toward surgical repair by patient or medical factors such as a very high-risk anatomic variant, lifestyle, and sports participation (for example, a patient with an unwavering commitment to a sport that does not lend itself to AED rescue, such as competitive swimming, cross-country running), or patient/family preference. The low absolute increase in risk of sudden cardiac death in asymptomatic patients with R AAOCA, and the uncertain relative risks of observation versus surgical repair, have led to considerable controversy regarding risk stratification and practice variation in management. The choice of management strategy thus involves shared decision-making between providers and families in light of individual circumstances.

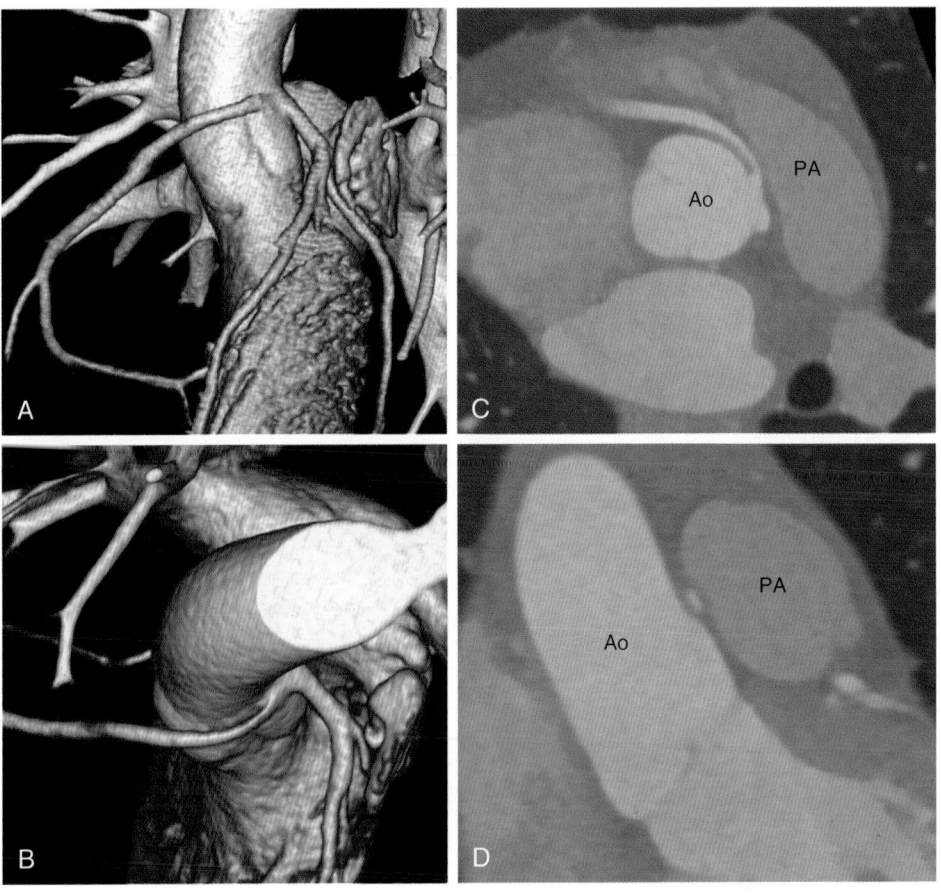

• **Fig. 42.7** Anomalous origin of the right coronary artery from the left aortic sinus. **(A)** The right coronary artery originates from the left aortic sinus at the sinotubular junction, adjacent to the origin of the left coronary artery. **(B–D)** The proximal vessel has a narrow, slit-like intramural course for 4 mm as it courses between the aorta *(Ao)* and pulmonary artery *(PA)*.

Risks of surgical repair of an anomalous coronary artery, although rare, include death, stroke, aortic regurgitation, perioperative myocardial infarction, persistent pleural effusions, post-pericardiotomy syndrome, and postoperative infections. In the Congenital Heart Surgeons' Society registry documenting 395 primary repairs, complications included coronary-related reoperations (3%), new mild (8%) or moderate (2%) aortic regurgitation associated with commissural manipulation, new low ejection fraction (2%), new positive postoperative ischemia test at any time (4%) or at the last test (2%), and death within 30 days (1%).[20] Risk factors included preoperative ischemia, surgery for L AAOCA, repair strategies other than unroofing, and unroofing with commissural manipulation. The long-term outcome of coronary ostial patency after coronary unroofing is unknown. Although unroofing is the most common surgical technique, other surgical repairs include re-implantation of the anomalous coronary to the appropriate sinus, and creation of a neo-ostium or an aortocoronary window. Coronary artery bypass with proximal ligation is also an option, but is not the preferred approach in children or young adults.

For asymptomatic individuals with anomalous right coronary artery who have no immediate plans for surgery, a practical plan is to follow the child every 3 years or so at the discretion of the cardiologist. All patients with AAOCA should have a fasting lipid profile to optimize preventive cardiology management, particularly because visual inspection at the time of surgery has revealed accelerated atherosclerosis in the intramural segments in some patients.

Intraseptal or Intraconal Left Coronary Artery

Pathology

Intraseptal or intraconal LCA arises from the right coronary cusp and follows a subpulmonic course below the pulmonary valve, running through the conal ventricular septum (Fig. 42.8). It occurs in 0.09% of the population in a pooled estimate of coronary CT angiograms.[9] Thus, it is twice as common as L AAOCA and one-third as common as R AAOCA. The left main coronary artery may emerge and become epicardial at the bifurcation, but in rare patients, extensive segments of the left coronary system, including the left anterior descending coronary artery, may be intramyocardial. The risk of sudden cardiac death with this anomaly appears to be exceedingly low.[19]

Physiology

The intraseptal anomalous LCA is a type of myocardial bridge, which may be associated with inducible myocardial ischemia even in the absence of atherosclerosis.[21] Coronary obstruction during systole should not significantly reduce total myocardial perfusion because two-thirds of blood flow in left coronary system occurs in diastole. However, there can be a "spillover" effect, in which narrowing persists in early diastole. The more severe the systolic narrowing, the more likely spill over. With tachycardia, one has more systolic compression, and systole occupies a greater percentage of the cardiac cycle because of shortening of the diastolic filling period. Assessment of dynamic obstruction in the symptomatic patient thus requires a fast heart rate.

Diagnosis

Diagnosis of intraseptal LCA is often suspected from echocardiography and confirmed with a coronary CTA or MRI. Testing for inducible ischemia may include exercise stress testing, advanced stress imaging tests (e.g., dobutamine stress MRI, exercise N[13]–ammonia PET scan), or cardiac catheterization, sometimes with intravascular ultrasound or dobutamine stress diastolic fractional flow reserve, when noninvasive data are insufficient to make a management decision.

Course

The vast majority of patients with intraseptal LCA are asymptomatic, with the diagnosis discovered incidentally. Rarely, patients can have symptoms of angina or exercise-induced arrhythmia reflecting inducible myocardial ischemia.

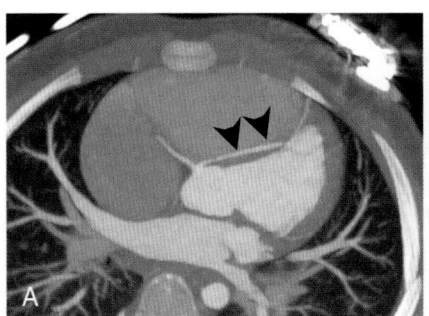 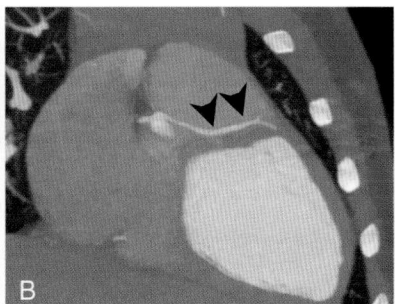 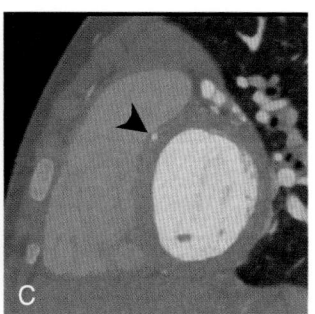

• **Fig. 42.8** Intraseptal course of the left main coronary artery *(black arrowheads)*. The left main coronary artery arises from the right aortic sinus, adjacent to the right coronary artery **(A)**, and courses through the infundibular septum before bifurcating into the left anterior descending and circumflex coronary arteries **(B** and **C)**.

Management

Management is based upon first principles and on successful strategies used in the more common clinical problem of myocardial bridges.[21] In symptomatic patients with inducible ischemia, beta-blocker therapy, which decreases heart rate and contractility and therefore coronary compression, is generally the first line of therapy. Non-dihydropyridine calcium channel blockers (verapamil, diltiazem) reduce heart rate and improve endothelial function. Patients with significant ischemia should be restricted from competitive sports. Surgery to unroof an intraseptal LCA may require infundibulotomy and intracavitary unroofing. As a consequence of this technical complexity combined with uncertain impact on long-term outcomes, surgical management of intraseptal LCA is generally reserved for patients in whom medical therapy has failed and who have persistent symptoms with proven ischemia or life-threatening ventricular arrhythmias.

Asymptomatic patients with intraseptal LCA do not need exercise restriction or medications.

Coronary Arterial Fistulae

Pathology

Coronary artery fistulae refer to connections between a coronary artery and another lower-resistance circuit, bypassing the capillaries. Coronary artery fistulae affect between 0.1% to 0.2% of the population.[22,23] When a coronary artery connects to a vein, it is called a coronary arteriovenous fistula, and when it connects to a cardiac chamber, it is called a coronary-cameral fistula. Coronary cameral fistulae most commonly arise from the right coronary artery or left anterior descending coronary artery and connect to the right atrium or right ventricle. Coronary artery fistulae can also connect to arteries and veins outside the heart itself, for example to the pulmonary arteries. Although usually congenital, coronary fistulae can also be acquired, for example, after trauma (e.g., cardiac biopsy, coronary angioplasty, radiofrequency ablation) or in the setting of chronic inflammation (e.g., endocarditis). The majority of coronary artery fistulae are too small to cause hemodynamic burden, with ~75% being noted incidentally during imaging tests. More than 80% of coronary artery fistulae are single, but some patients have multiple fistulae. Fistulae occasionally involve multiple arteries converging on one drainage site, or multiple drainage sites arising from a single arterial origin.

Physiology

The hemodynamic burden posed by a coronary artery fistula depends upon the resistance to flow through it, as determined by the structure into which it is draining, its size, span, and tortuosity. Flow through a coronary artery fistula may be continuous through the cardiac cycle, for example, as in a coronary-cameral fistula to the right atrium. More than 90% of coronary fistulae have a left-to-right shunt, and when the fistula is large, one may see both right and left ventricular enlargement. In the less common circumstance of a coronary-cameral fistula to left-sided cardiac structures (i.e., a left-to-left shunt), volume overload may be confined to the left atrium and/or left ventricle. Coronary artery fistulae can enlarge over time and can be immense, and some are associated with coronary artery aneurysm formation; aneurysm rupture is catastrophic. The largest fistulae can manifest with myocardial hypoperfusion and ischemia from a coronary steal in diastole, resulting in congestive heart failure, angina, and arrhythmias, as well as mitral regurgitation from papillary muscle ischemia. Rarely, thrombosis in a fistula can cause myocardial infarction or arrhythmia.

Diagnosis

The tiniest coronary fistulae occur in asymptomatic children with normal cardiac auscultation. Larger fistulae are associated with a continuous murmur that is louder in diastole than systole, and loudest at the point of drainage. The differential diagnosis includes patent ductus arteriosus, ruptured sinus of Valsalva aneurysm, and aorta-to-left ventricular tunnel. The diagnosis of coronary artery fistula is most often confirmed using two-dimensional echocardiography and color Doppler imaging, with advanced imaging by coronary CTA providing superior resolution of anatomy (Fig. 42.9).[24] Invasive coronary artery angiography remains the gold standard for anatomic and hemodynamic information, as well as for transcatheter device closure of fistulae (Video 42.1, video of angiogram). Exercise or pharmacologic stress testing with myocardial imaging may be performed to assess inducible ischemia in patients with possible angina.

Course

Small coronary artery fistulae sometimes regress. As a general rule, however, fistulae enlarge over time and occasionally become immense and/or associated with coronary artery aneurysm formation. The largest fistulae can lead to myocardial hypoperfusion and ischemia from coronary steal in diastole, resulting in congestive heart failure, angina, and arrhythmias, as well as mitral regurgitation from papillary muscle ischemia. Rarely, progressive stenosis due to myointimal hyperplasia or thrombosis in a fistula can cause myocardial infarction or arrhythmia. Fistulae arising from a proximal coronary artery have a propensity to become aneurysmal. Management of risk factors for later atherosclerotic coronary artery disease is key because of the propensity of fistulous connections to develop early atherosclerotic changes.

Management

Management of coronary artery fistulae depends upon their size and hemodynamic burden, as well as technical

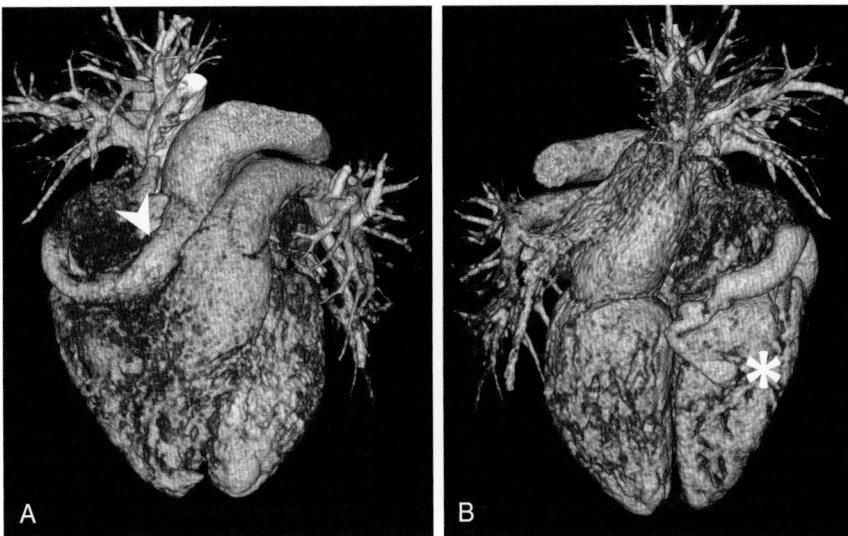

• **Fig. 42.9** A 14-year-old asymptomatic girl with a heart murmur was discovered to have a large fistula from the right coronary artery to the base of the right ventricle. The right coronary artery is severely dilated (*white arrowhead*, **A**), and connects to the base of the right ventricle (*white asterisk*, **B**).

considerations related to fistula anatomy and patient age and size.[22,23,25] Small fistulae in asymptomatic patients without cardiac chamber enlargement can be followed clinically by serial echocardiography and may regress over time. Large-sized fistulae and, some would argue, those that arise from proximal coronary artery segments should generally be closed. Intervention by percutaneous or surgical techniques is undertaken in patients with symptoms of heart failure or with significant left-to-right shunt causing volume overload and risk for coronary steal with myocardial ischemia. Transcatheter closure with coils or other closure devices is preferred over surgical ligation for single fistulae or when technically feasible; surgery may be needed for closure of large proximal fistulae, those with aneurysms, or complex fistulae not amenable to catheter closure. The optimal method of closure should be determined by interventional cardiologists and cardiac surgeons on the basis of the individual patient's fistula anatomy and technical factors involved in its closure. Regardless of the closure technique, patients should be followed with post-closure coronary anatomy surveillance, including evidence of recanalization and/or thrombus formation. Thromboprophylaxis should be used to avoid myocardial infarction from thrombus propagation in ectatic coronary vessels. Infants undergoing closure of a severely dilated proximal fistula segment or distal medium and large coronary artery fistulae appear to be at particularly high risk for adverse coronary events following fistula closure; experts recommend anticoagulation post closure until coronary re-evaluation in 3–6 months, followed by antiplatelet therapy.[25] The choice of long-term thromboprophylaxis with anticoagulants, antiplatelet agents, or both should be based upon the anatomy of the proximal coronary artery fistula and estimated likelihood of thrombosis.

References

1. Wesselhoeft H, Fawcett JS, Johnson AL. Anomalous origin of the left coronary artery from the pulmonary trunk. *Circulation.* 1968;38:403-425.
2. Guenther TM, Sherazee EA, Gustafson JD, et al. Anomalous origin of the circumflex or left anterior descending artery from the pulmonary artery. *World J Pediatr Congenit Heart Surg.* 2020;11:765-775.
3. Kwiatkowski DM, Mastropietro CW, Cashen K, et al. Characteristics and surgical outcomes of patients with late presentation of anomalous left coronary artery from the pulmonary artery: a multicenter study. *Semin Thorac Cardiovasc Surg.* 2021;33: 141-150.
4. Hegde S, Bell J, Zachariah B, Sitaram E, Maysky M. Echocardiographic diagnosis of Bland-White-Garland Syndrome in an asymptomatic adult. *JACC Case Rep.* 2020;2:1021-1024.
5. Takeuchi S, Imamura H, Katsumoto K, et al. New surgical method for repair of anomalous left coronary artery from pulmonary artery. *J Thorac Cardiovasc Surg.* 1979;78:7-11.
6. Thomas AS, Chan A, Alsoufi B, et al. Long-term outcomes of children operated on for anomalous left coronary artery from the pulmonary artery. *Ann Thorac Surg.* 2022;113:1223-1230.
7. Paridon SM, Farooki ZQ, Kuhns LR, Arciniegas E, Pinsky WW. Exercise performance after repair of anomalous origin of the left coronary artery from the pulmonary artery. *Circulation.* 1990; 81:1287-1292.
8. Singh TP, Di Carli MF, Sullivan NM, Leonen MF, Morrow WR. Myocardial flow reserve in long-term survivors of repair of anomalous left coronary artery from pulmonary artery. *J Am Coll Cardiol.* 1998;31:437-443.
9. Cheezum MK, Liberthson RR, Shah NR, et al. Anomalous aortic origin of a coronary artery from the inappropriate sinus of Valsalva. *J Am Coll Cardiol.* 2017;69:1592-1608.
10. Jegatheeswaran A, Devlin PJ, McCrindle BW, et al. Features associated with myocardial ischemia in anomalous aortic origin of a coronary artery: a Congenital Heart Surgeons' Society study. *J Thorac Cardiovasc Surg.* 2019;158:822-834.e3.

11. Stout KK, Daniels CJ, Aboulhosn JA, et al. 2018 AHA/ACC guideline for the management of adults with congenital heart disease: a report of the American College of Cardiology/American Heart Association task force on clinical practice guidelines. *J Am Coll Cardiol.* 2019;73:e81-e192.

12. Gräni C, Buechel RR, Kaufmann PA, Kwong RY. Multimodality imaging in individuals with anomalous coronary arteries. *JACC Cardiovasc Imaging.* 2017;10:471-481.

13. Cabrera AG, Chen DW, Pignatelli RH, et al. Outcomes of anomalous left coronary artery from pulmonary artery repair: beyond normal function. *Ann Thorac Surg.* 2015;99:1342-1347.

14. Garber AM, Solomon NA. Tests for coronary artery disease. *Ann Intern Med.* 1999;131:980.

15. Fleischmann KE, Hunink MGM, Kuntz KM, et al. Exercise echocardiography or exercise SPECT imaging? *JAMA.* 1998;280:913.

16. Brothers JA, Frommelt MA, Jaquiss RDB, Myerburg RJ, Fraser Jr CD, Tweddell JS. Expert consensus guidelines: anomalous aortic origin of a coronary artery. *J Thorac Cardiovasc Surg.* 2017;153:1440-1457.

17. Jegatheeswaran A, Brothers JA. Anomalous aortic origin of a coronary artery: learning from the past to make advances in the future. *Curr Opin Pediatr.* 2021;33:482-488.

18. Mery CM, Lopez KN, Molossi S, et al. Decision analysis to define the optimal management of athletes with anomalous aortic origin of a coronary artery. *J Thorac Cardiovasc Surg.* 2016;152:1366-1375.e7.

19. Maron BJ, Doerer JJ, Haas TS, Tierney DM, Mueller FO. Sudden deaths in young competitive athletes: analysis of 1866 deaths in the United States, 1980-2006. *Circulation.* 2009;119:1085-1092.

20. Jegatheeswaran A, Devlin PJ, Williams WG, et al. Outcomes after anomalous aortic origin of a coronary artery repair: a Congenital Heart Surgeons' Society Study. *J Thorac Cardiovasc Surg.* 2020;160:757-771.e5.

21. Matta A, Roncalli J, Carrié D. Update review on myocardial bridging: new insights. *Trends Cardiovasc Med.* 2022. doi:10.1016/j.tcm.2022.06.002.

22. Buccheri D, Chirco PR, Geraci S, Caramanno G, Cortese B. Coronary artery fistulae: anatomy, diagnosis and management strategies. *Heart Lung Circ.* 2018;27:940-951.

23. Al-Hijji M, El Sabbagh A, El Hajj S, et al. Coronary artery fistulas: indications, techniques, outcomes, and complications of transcatheter fistula closure. *JACC Cardiovasc Interv.* 2021;14:1393-1406.

24. Kalisz K, Sanders AE, Avery R, Allen BD. Coronary artery fistulas: a review of the current and future roles of imaging. *J Thorac Imaging.* 2021;36:333-344.

25. Gowda ST, Latson L, Sivakumar K, et al. Anatomical classification and posttreatment remodeling characteristics to guide management and follow-up of neonates and infants with coronary artery fistula: a multicenter study from the Coronary Artery Fistula Registry. *Circ Cardiovasc Interv.* 2021;14:e009750.

43

Vascular Rings, Slings, and Related Anomalies

ANDREW J. POWELL, STEPHEN P. SANDERS, AND CHRISTOPHER W. BAIRD

KEY LEARNING POINTS

- Knowledge of the development of the aortic arch and pulmonary arteries provides a framework for understanding and classifying vascular rings and related anomalies.
- A vascular ring results in complete encirclement of the trachea and the esophagus by vascular structures, some components of which may not be patent but rather consist of fibrous vessel remnants such as the ligamentum arteriosum.

- The two most common types of vascular rings are a double aortic arch and a right aortic arch with an aberrant left subclavian artery and a left ligamentum arteriosum.
- Vascular rings that cause significant symptoms are treated by surgical division of the ring.
- Left pulmonary artery sling is frequently associated with intrinsic airway abnormalities and is treated by surgical reimplantation of the left pulmonary artery and, in some cases, tracheal surgery.

This chapter reviews some of the more common developmental anomalies of the aortic arch and pulmonary arteries. The normal development of the aortic arch and pulmonary arteries is presented in Chapter 2. We will use the hypothetical double arch model originated by Edwards[1] and modified by Weinberg[2] to explain the development of these anomalies (Fig. 43.1).

Normal Left Aortic Arch

The normal left aortic arch results from involution of the segment of the right dorsal aorta between the right 7th segmental artery and the descending aorta[3] (Fig. 43.2). This results in an arch branching order, proximal to distal, of a right brachiocephalic artery giving rise to the right common carotid and right subclavian arteries, a left common carotid artery, and a left subclavian artery. The ligamentum arteriosum (ductus ligament) is a remnant of the 6th embryonic pharyngeal arch artery and courses between the proximal left pulmonary artery or distal pulmonary trunk and the aorta just distal to the left subclavian artery. A common arch branching variant has the left vertebral artery arising directly from the arch instead of the left subclavian artery.

Aortic Arch Variants

Left aortic arch with an aberrant right subclavian artery results from involution of the right 4th pharyngeal arch artery instead of the right dorsal aorta (Fig. 43.3).[1,2] The right subclavian artery is the last brachiocephalic artery arising from the arch and passes behind the esophagus to reach the right shoulder and arm. Most patients are asymptomatic, but in some dysphagia can result from compression of the esophagus which can be treated by relocation of the subclavian artery anteriorly by anastomosing it to the right common carotid artery. In symptomatic patients, this condition has been referred to as dysphagia lusoria (from the Latin, *lusus naturae*, "prank of nature"). Aneurysmal dilation with dissection or rupture of the proximal part of the aberrant artery (right dorsal aorta) has also been reported.[4]

Right aortic arch results from involution of the left (instead of the right) dorsal aorta distal to the left 7th segmental artery (Fig. 43.4).[2] Most cases have a mirror image branching pattern (proximal to distal: left brachiocephalic artery, right common carotid artery, and right subclavian artery) and are associated with congenital heart defects such as tetralogy of Fallot, truncus arteriosus, or transposition of

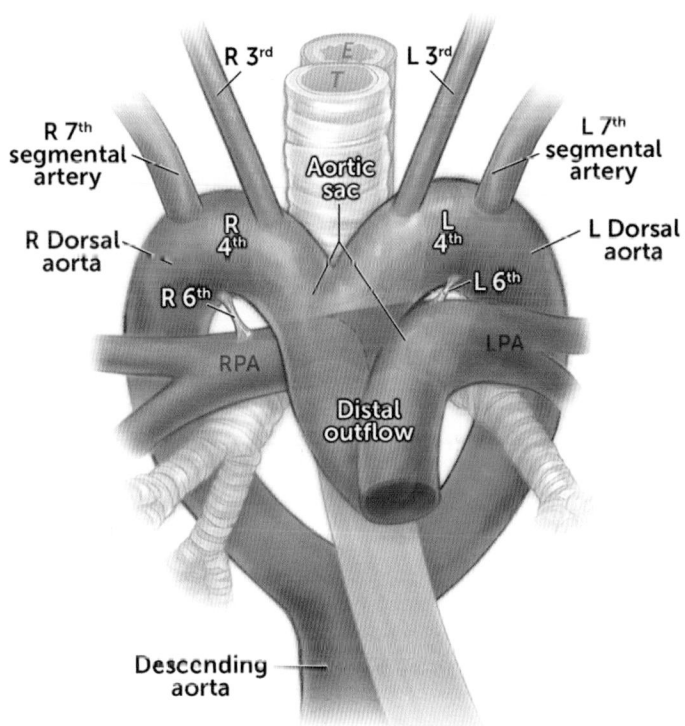

• **Fig. 43.1** Double aortic arch model used to explain the development of various arch anomalies. The pulmonary trunk and ascending aorta develop from the distal outflow of the embryonic heart which connects to the aortic sac at the dorsal pericardial wall. The pulmonary bifurcation and the extrapericardial ascending aorta are derived from the aortic sac. The right *(RPA)* and left *(LPA)* branch pulmonary arteries arise directly from the caudal aspect of the aortic sac and segregate with the pulmonary bifurcation and 6th pharyngeal arch arteries (R6th, L6th), which appear to arise after and from the branch pulmonary arteries. The aortic component of the aortic sac divides into a right and left horn from which the 3rd and 4th pharyngeal arch arteries arise. The segment of dorsal aorta between the insertion of the 3rd and 4th pharyngeal arch arteries (carotid duct, not shown) involutes leaving the 3rd arch as the common carotid artery and the 4th and 6th arches the only connections between the aortic sac and the caudal dorsal aorta. The 4th arch artery becomes the definitive aortic arch and the 6th becomes the ductus arteriosus. The 7th segmental branches of the dorsal aorta form part or all of the subclavian artery. *E,* Esophagus; *T,* trachea.

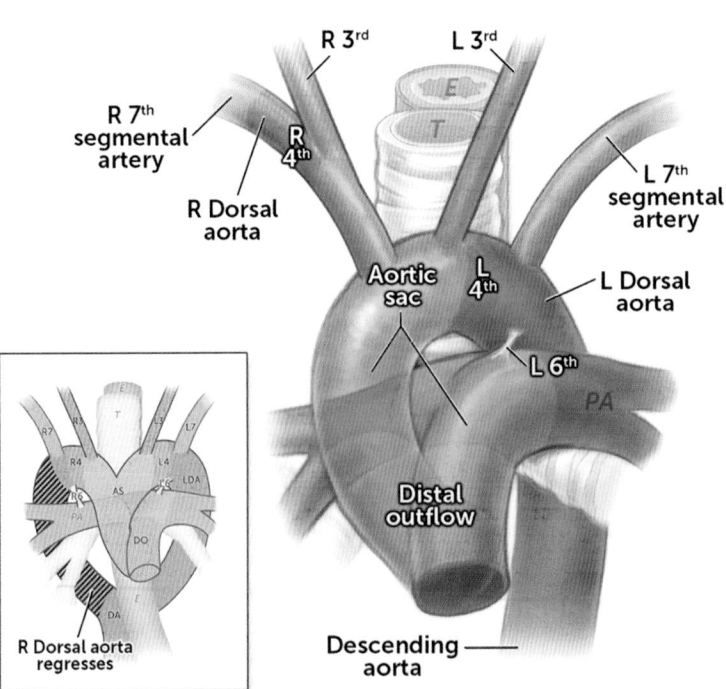

• **Fig. 43.2** Development and components of the normal left aortic arch. A left aortic arch forms by involution of the right dorsal aorta distal to the right 7th segmental artery (shown on inset double arch model). The components of the mature left aortic arch and pulmonary artery system are shown. *L,* Left; *R,* right.

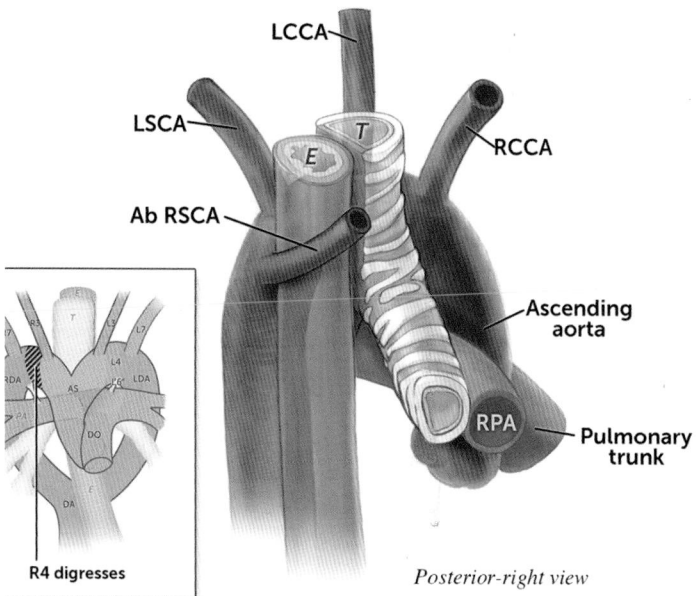

Posterior-right view

• **Fig. 43.3** Left aortic arch with aberrant right subclavian artery (Ab RSCA). This results from involution of the right 4th pharyngeal arch artery instead of the distal segment of the right dorsal aorta (shown on inset double arch model). The proximal part of the Ab RSCA derives from the right dorsal aorta. *LCCA,* Left common carotid artery; *LSCA,* left subclavian artery; *RCCA,* right common carotid artery; *RPA,* right pulmonary artery.

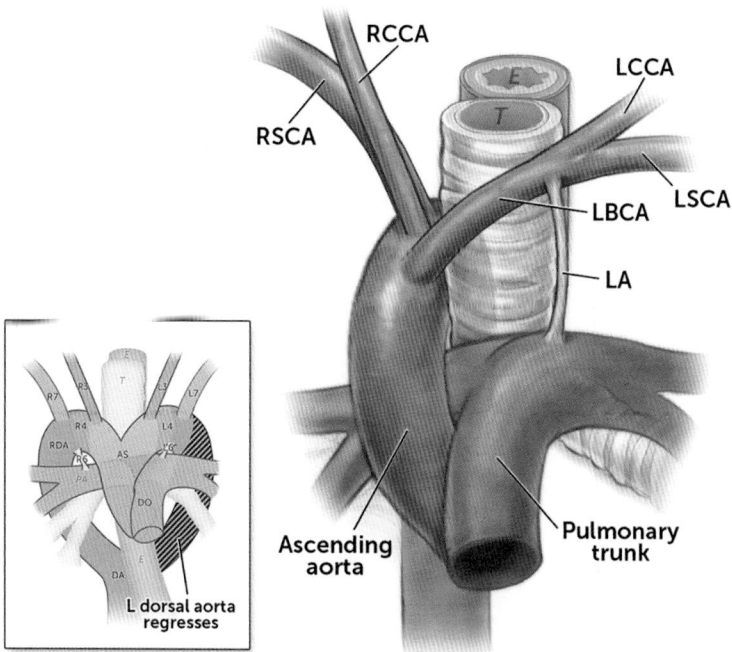

• **Fig. 43.4** Right aortic arch with mirror image branching. This results from involution of the left dorsal aorta distal to the left 7th segmental branch instead of the right (shown on the inset double arch model). Even with a right aortic arch, the right 6th pharyngeal arch artery usually involutes leaving the left 6th arch artery as the ductus arteriosus. It typically courses between the base of the left pulmonary artery and the left innominate artery near the origin of the left subclavian artery because that is the only remaining part of the left dorsal aorta. *E,* Esophagus; *LA,* ligamentum arteriosum or ductal ligament; *LBCA,* left brachiocephalic artery; *LCCA,* left common carotid artery; *LSCA,* left subclavian artery; *RCCA,* right common carotid artery; *RSCA,* right subclavian artery; *T,* trachea.

the great arteries. The ductus arteriosus is most commonly on the left arising from the left brachiocephalic artery.

Cervical aortic arch implies that the aortic arch extends superiorly through the thoracic inlet above the ipsilateral clavicle and can occur on either side (Fig. 43.5).[5] There are two main types of cervical arch: (1) associated with separate origins of the ipsilateral internal and external carotid arteries from the arch (thought to be due to involution of the 4th pharyngeal arch artery, persistence of the carotid duct, and the 3rd pharyngeal arch artery as the definitive aortic arch); and (2) associated with an ipsilateral common carotid artery (thought to be due to failure of descent of the aortic arch [4th pharyngeal arch artery] into the mediastinum). Most are asymptomatic but can cause a pulsatile neck mass. Arch branching anomalies are common. Associated congenital heart defects include coarctation, tetralogy of Fallot, ventricular septal defect, and double-outlet right ventricle. Treatment is rarely indicated in the absence of arch obstruction.

Isolated subclavian artery is one that is disconnected from the aortic arch and has a connection to the ipsilateral pulmonary artery via a persistent ductus arteriosus or ligamentum arteriosum. It usually occurs on the side opposite the arch, most often a right aortic arch, and is often associated with a congenital heart defect such as tetralogy of Fallot or interrupted aortic arch (Fig. 43.6).[6] The subclavian artery is separated from the arch by involution at two points, the ipsilateral dorsal aorta distal to the 7th segmental artery and the ipsilateral 4th pharyngeal arch artery.[2] The subclavian artery is supplied by the ipsilateral ductus arteriosus, the ipsilateral vertebral artery, and/or a collateral artery. The ductus arteriosus may close early in life. Persistent patency of the ductus arteriosus usually results in a left-to-right shunt and reversal of blood flow in the subclavian and vertebral arteries. Symptoms can include arm claudication or subclavian steal syndrome. The pulse in the involved arm is often diminished or absent. Repair involves establishing communication between the isolated subclavian artery and the aortic arch.

Vascular Rings

Definition

A vascular ring results in complete encirclement of the trachea and the esophagus by vascular structures, some components of which may not be patent but rather consist of fibrous vessel remnants such as the ligamentum arteriosum.[2]

Prevalence

The overall prevalence of vascular rings is difficult to ascertain because many are asymptomatic but appears to be approximately 1–3% of congenital cardiovascular

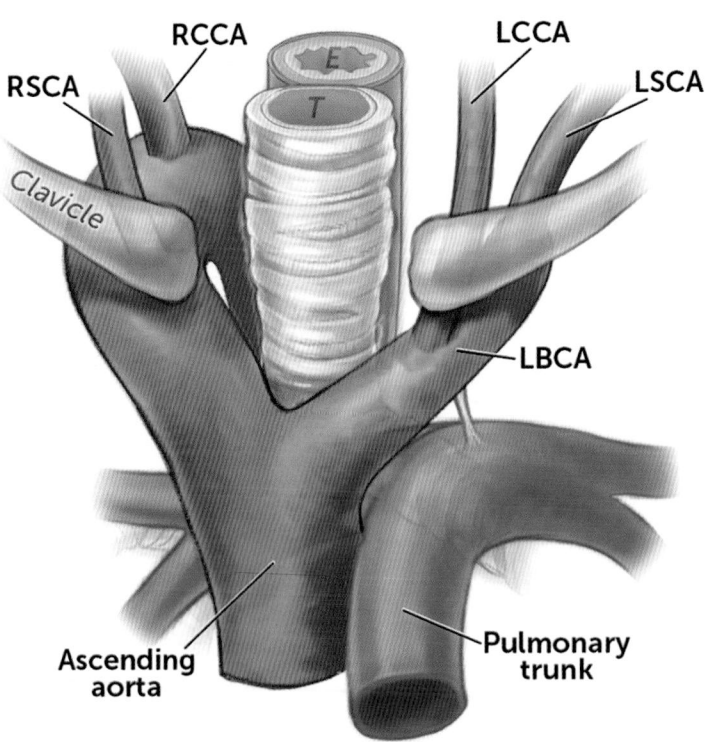

• **Fig. 43.5** Right cervical aortic arch. The aortic arch extends above the ipsilateral clavicle. The abnormal superior location of the definitive aortic arch is because either it is formed by the 3rd pharyngeal arch artery if there are separate origins of internal and external carotid arteries, or failure of descent of the aortic arch formed by the 4th arch artery if a common carotid artery is present.[5] *E,* Esophagus; *LBCA,* left brachiocephalic artery; *LCCA,* left common carotid artery; *LSCA,* left subclavian artery; *RCCA,* right common carotid artery; *RSCA,* right subclavian artery; *T,* trachea.

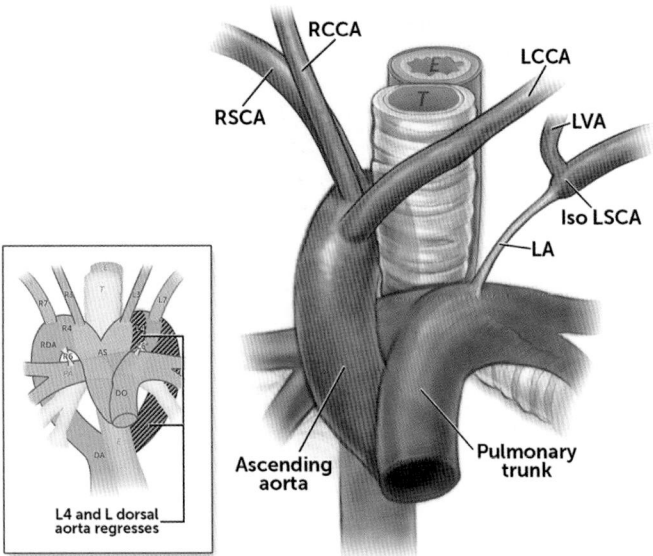

• **Fig. 43.6** Isolation of a subclavian artery. This usually occurs on the side opposite the aortic arch and is due to involution of both the ipsilateral distal dorsal aorta segment and the ipsilateral 4th pharyngeal arch artery (shown on the inset double arch model). The ipsilateral 6th arch artery (ductus arteriosus) joins the short dorsal aorta segment from which the subclavian artery (7th segmental artery) arises. The left vertebral artery *(LVA)* often supplies flow to the isolated subclavian artery. *E,* Esophagus; *Iso LSCA,* isolated left subclavian artery; *LA,* ligamentum arteriosum or ductal ligament; *LBCA,* left brachiocephalic artery; *LCCA,* left common carotid artery; *RCCA,* right common carotid artery; *RSCA,* right subclavian artery; *T,* trachea.

anomalies.[7] A right aortic arch with diverticulum of Kommerell, aberrant left subclavian artery, and left ligamentum (ductus) is most common followed by double aortic arch.[8] These two anomalies comprise more than 90% of vascular rings and will be the focus of this discussion.

Usually, double aortic arch and right aortic arch with an aberrant left subclavian artery and left ligamentum are isolated anomalies, although they may occur with other congenital heart defects, most commonly ventricular septal defect and tetralogy of Fallot.[7,9] The 22q11 microdeletions are associated with isolated aortic arch anomalies including vascular ring, as well as with conotruncal cardiac defects and non-cardiac abnormalities.[10] Because this mutation is often sporadic and clinical manifestations may be subtle, genetic testing of any patient with a vascular ring should be considered.

Embryology and Anatomy

Double Aortic Arch

Both of the embryonic distal dorsal aorta segments between the 7th segmental branch and the descending aorta persist resulting in complete aortic arches on both sides of the trachea and esophagus, joining posteriorly to form the descending aorta, thereby completely encircling the trachea and esophagus (Fig. 43.7).[1,2] A left ligamentum arteriosum is usually present as well. The common carotid and subclavian arteries arise separately from each arch and are usually symmetrically positioned around the trachea. The right arch is larger than the left in about 75% of cases and typically higher as well.[1,2] Occasionally, a segment of

an arch (usually the left) is atretic with a fibrous cord either distal to the left subclavian artery or between the carotid and subclavian arteries.

Right Aortic Arch With Diverticulum of Kommerell, Aberrant Left Subclavian Artery, and Left Posterior Ligamentum Arteriosum

A right aortic arch with an aberrant left subclavian artery is caused by regression of the left 4th pharyngeal arch artery (Fig. 43.8).[2] As a result, the left subclavian artery originates as the last branch from the aortic arch, at a relatively posterior location, coursing behind the esophagus to the left arm. A left ligamentum arteriosum originates from a bulbous dilation at the base of the left subclavian artery (the left dorsal aorta segment known as the diverticulum of Kommerell) and attaches to the left pulmonary artery, effectively pulling the aorta and the diverticulum forward, compressing the esophagus and trachea, and forming a ring. The diverticulum of Kommerell is the result of normal *in utero* pulmonary-to-aorta ductus arteriosus blood flow that must travel through the proximal left subclavian artery to reach the descending aorta. In rare cases that are associated with right ventricular outflow obstruction (e.g., tetralogy of Fallot), there is no diverticulum because of reduced or absent pulmonary-to-aorta ductal flow *in utero* resulting in uniform caliber of the aberrant left subclavian artery despite the presence of a ligamentum arteriosum completing a vascular ring.[11] Rarely, the ductus arteriosus is right-sided and connects the right pulmonary artery to the right-sided aortic arch, and thus no vascular ring is formed (Fig. 43.9). In such cases, there is no diverticulum

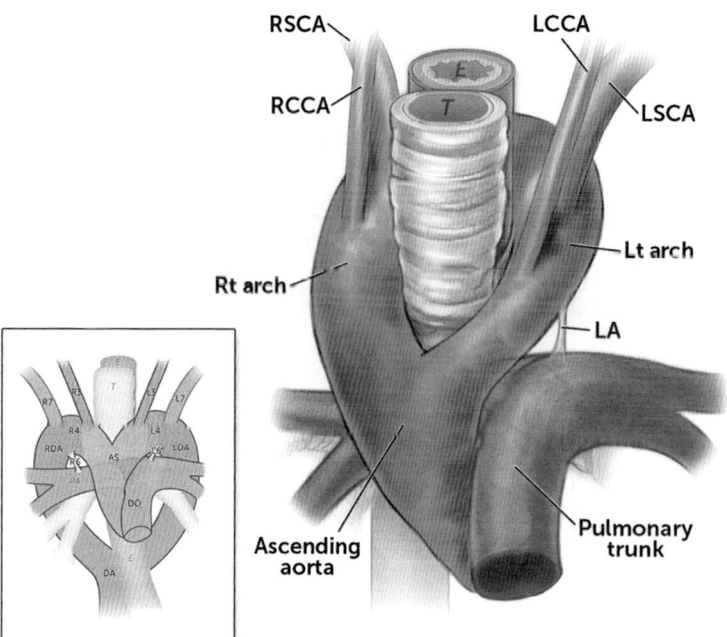

• **Fig. 43.7** Double aortic arch. This is due to failure of involution of either distal dorsal aorta segment. Each arch is formed by the aortic sac horn, the 4th pharyngeal arch artery, and the dorsal aorta. Common carotid (3rd pharyngeal arch artery) and subclavian (7th segmental artery) arteries arise from each arch. A left ligamentum arteriosum *(LA)* (or occasionally a ductus arteriosus) is usually present as well. *E*, Esophagus; *LA*, ligamentum arteriosum or ductal ligament; *LCCA*, left common carotid artery; *LSCA*, left subclavian artery; *Lt arch*, left aortic arch; *RCCA*, right common carotid artery; *RSCA*, right subclavian artery; *Rt arch*, right aortic arch; *T*, trachea.

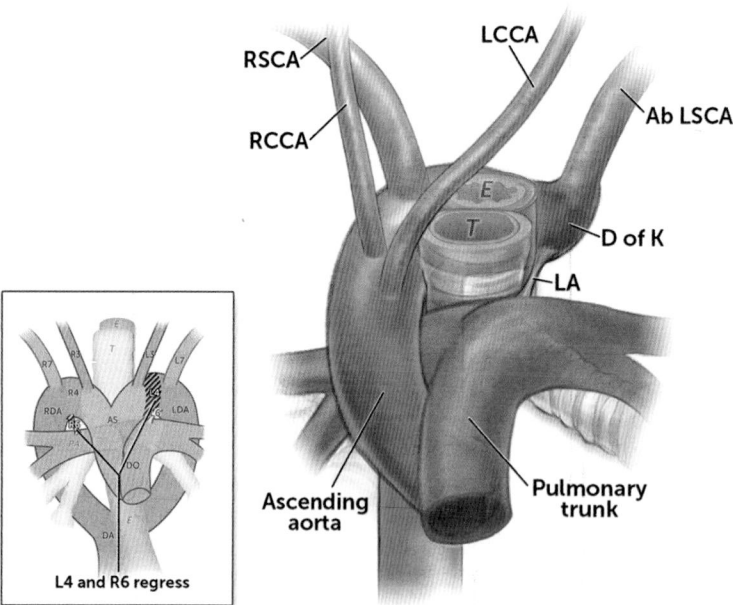

• **Fig. 43.8** Right aortic arch with aberrant left subclavian artery *(Ab LSCA)* and left ligamentum arteriosum *(LA)* from a diverticulum of Kommerell *(D of K)*. Involution of the left 4th pharyngeal arch artery results in the left subclavian artery being the last branch of the right aortic arch (shown on the inset double arch model). The left 6th arch artery (ductus arteriosus that becomes the ligamentum arteriosum on closure) persisted, attached to the left dorsal aorta (D of K) which also gives rise to the aberrant subclavian artery. The diverticulum is dilated because it carried the flow from the left ductus arteriosus *in utero*. *E*, Esophagus; *LCCA*, left common carotid artery; *RCCA*, right common carotid artery; *RSCA*, right subclavian artery; *T*, trachea.

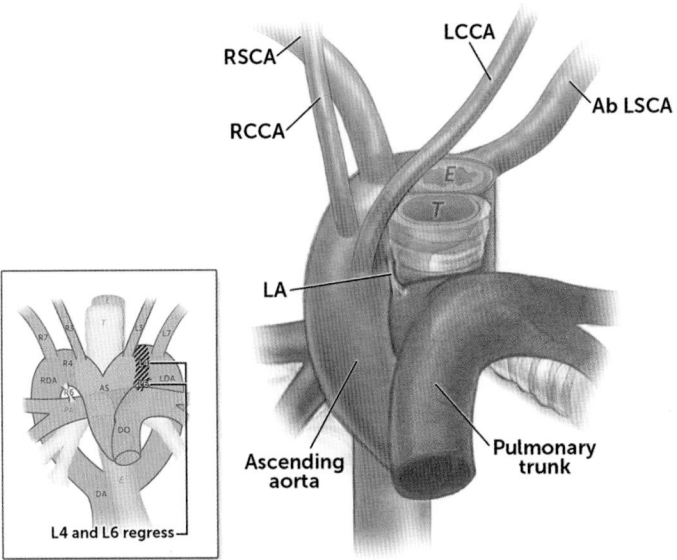

• **Fig. 43.9** Right aortic arch with aberrant left subclavian artery (*Ab LSCA*) and right ligamentum arteriosum (*LA*). Here the right 6th pharyngeal arch artery (right ductus arteriosus) persisted instead of the left (shown on the inset double arch model). In contrast to the situation in Fig. 43.8, the left dorsal aorta (origin of the aberrant left subclavian artery) did not dilate because it carried only flow to the subclavian artery *in utero E*, Esophagus; *LCCA*, left common carotid artery; *RCCA*, right common carotid artery; *RSCA*, right subclavian artery; *T*, trachea.

of Kommerell, and the caliber of the left subclavian artery is uniform throughout.

Symptoms

The symptoms of a vascular ring are due to tracheal compression and, less commonly, to esophageal compression.[7] Patients with double aortic arch usually present in early infancy with symptoms and signs that include stridor, dyspnea, and a barking cough, all of which are worse during feeding or exertion.[7,9] "Reflex apnea" lasting seconds or even minutes may be triggered by feeding. Older children may have a history of chronic cough or wheezing misdiagnosed as asthma. Recurrent respiratory infections may be a result of aspiration or inadequate clearing of secretions. Symptoms related to esophageal compression include vomiting, choking, and non-specific feeding difficulties in infants, and dysphagia and slow eating in older children.

In many patients with a right aortic arch, an aberrant left subclavian artery, and a left ligamentum, the ring is loose and causes no symptoms. The diagnosis is often discovered when imaging studies are performed for other reasons. However, in some cases, when the ligamentum arteriosum is short or the diverticulum of Kommerell is especially large, the ring may be tight. These patients have symptoms similar to those of patients with a double aortic arch. Occasionally, an older individual may complain of mild dysphagia as the aorta and left subclavian artery become larger and more tortuous over time and impinge on the posterior aspect of the esophagus because of tethering by the ligamentum.

Physical Examination

Symptomatic infants show signs of increased respiratory work such as intercostal retractions and nasal flaring. Sometimes they lie with their back arched and neck extended, which probably minimizes tracheal narrowing. Auscultation may reveal coarse upper airway sounds and wheezing. Mild intermittent cyanosis may be present. In patients with a right arch, an aberrant left subclavian, and a left ligamentum in whom the ring is loose, the physical examination may be completely normal.

Diagnostic Imaging

The diagnosis of a vascular ring requires a high index of suspicion because of the relative infrequency of this entity compared with other conditions that cause respiratory distress in children, such as asthma, respiratory infection, and reflux. Once suspected, diagnostic imaging studies should be obtained with the goals of (1) identifying the cause of a patient's symptoms by demonstrating the relevant vascular and airway anatomy, and (2) preoperative planning, in part to determine whether a right, left, or midline approach is most appropriate.

Development of a single universal diagnostic imaging algorithm is complicated by varying ages and modes of presentation and the numerous specialties involved in such cases. There are no reported studies that rigorously compare different imaging strategies with respect to accuracy, patient safety, and cost-effectiveness. In practice, a center's diagnostic testing algorithm is tailored to fit local expertise, experience, costs, and available technology. The approach is then individualized to the patient, taking into account severity of symptoms, previous findings, age, and other medical conditions. It is important to note that no imaging modality except direct visualization can reliably show ligamentous or atretic structures. Their presence is typically inferred based on anatomic patterns, the position of vessels, and the presence of a diverticulum.

A plain chest radiograph is useful to exclude other pathology but is of limited value for detecting vascular ring. A barium contrast esophagogram usually reveals a posterior indentation on the esophagus caused by prominent arch segments (Fig. 43.10).[7,9] This procedure is usually sufficient to determine whether a vascular ring is the likely cause of symptoms. However, it provides no direct information about the vascular anatomy. Bronchoscopy provides excellent visualization of the airway as well as respiratory dynamics and is especially valuable before and during surgery.[7,12] X-ray angiography can provide excellent visualization of the aortic vasculature, but care must be taken to avoid misdiagnosis from overlapping structures. Airway and vascular relationships, as well as the degree of airway compression, can be difficult to determine. Given its invasive nature and relatively high expense, x-ray angiography has been supplanted by noninvasive techniques. Echocardiography, including fetal echocardiography,[8,13] can provide good depiction of the relevant vasculature and in many cases is sufficient for diagnosis and surgical planning (Fig. 43.11).[7,14] It has the additional advantage of being able to define associated cardiovascular anomalies. Its principal weakness is poor visualization of the airway. In addition, some patients may have poor acoustic windows, and portions of the aortic arch system may be obscured by the trachea. In contrast, both magnetic resonance imaging (MRI) and computed tomography (CT) clearly define the vasculature, the airway, and their three-dimensional relationship with high reliability and accuracy (Fig. 43.12).[7] The most recent generation of dual-source, multi-row detector CT scanners can image the infant thorax with a very low dose of radiation in under 1 second, obviating the need for sedation and breath holding. For echocardiography and MRI, younger patients typically require sedation to reliably obtain high-quality studies.

Management and Course

Surgical division of a vascular ring is the only definitive treatment. This was first performed in a patient with a double aortic arch by Dr. Robert Gross at Boston Children's Hospital in 1945.[15] Surgical risk in the current era is low, so prompt surgery is indicated for patients with airway or esophageal symptoms. Asymptomatic patients, typically those with a relatively loose right aortic arch with an aberrant left subclavian artery, may be observed.

For surgical treatment of a double aortic arch, the smaller of the two arches and any contributing ligamentum arteriosum are divided, typically via a posterolateral thoracotomy on the side of the arch to be divided. For treatment of a right arch, aberrant left subclavian artery, and left ductal ligamentum, the ligamentum is divided via a left posterolateral

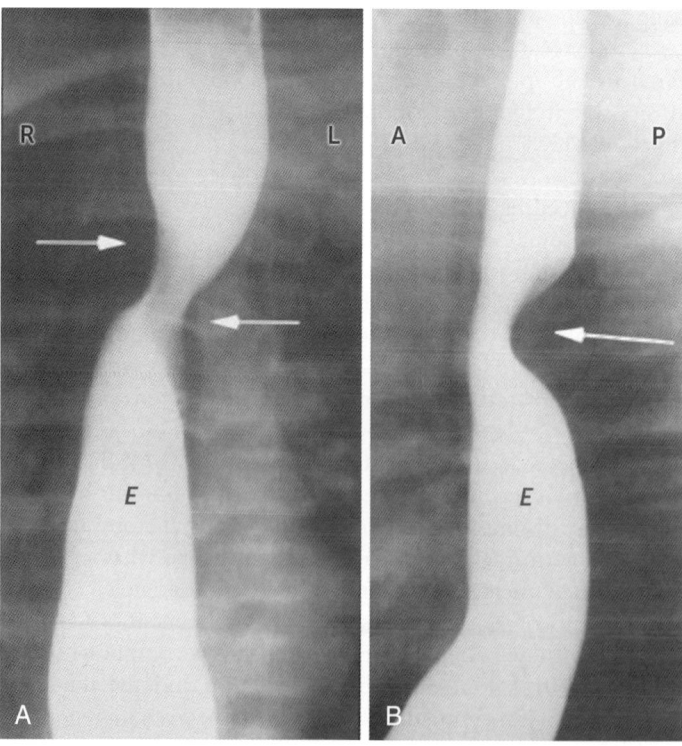

• **Fig. 43.10** Barium esophagram of a double aortic arch. (A) Anteroposterior projection showing indentations on both right and left sides of the esophagus (E) *(arrows)* from the two aortic arches. The right-sided arch is more superior, typical for double aortic arch. (B) Lateral projection showing the large posterior indentation *(arrow)* on the esophagus. *A,* Anterior; *L,* left; *P,* posterior; *R,* right.

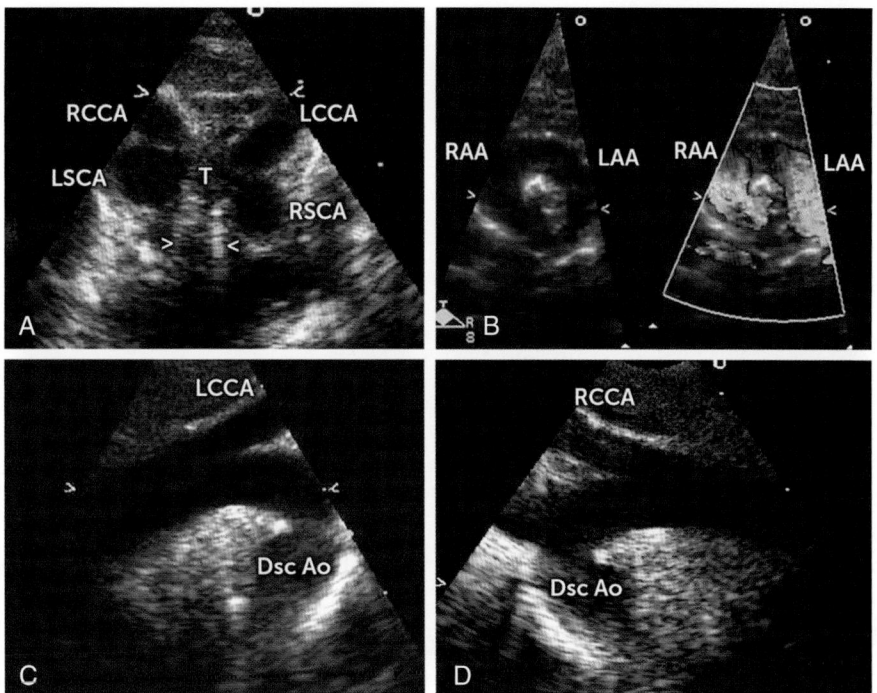

• **Fig. 43.11** Double aortic arch. Echocardiogram using a suprasternal notch window. **(A)** Transverse view superior to the arch level illustrating the symmetric origins of the right *(RCCA)* and left *(LCCA)* common carotid arteries and right *(RSCA)* and left *(LSCA)* subclavian arteries from their respective arches. The trachea *(T)* can be recognized by the characteristic acoustic shadow *(arrowheads)* it casts. **(B)** Transverse view demonstrating the right *(RAA)* and left *(LAA)* aortic arches with two-dimensional and color Doppler imaging. **(C)** Long-axis view of the unobstructed left aortic arch. **(D)** Long-axis view of the unobstructed right aortic arch. Note that by convention right aortic arches are displayed with the right-left screen orientation inverted so that superior structures are positioned to the left on the screen. *Dsc Ao,* Descending aorta. (From Powell AJ. Chapter 32: Vascular Rings and Slings (Fig. 32.4). In: Lai WW, Mertens LL, Cohen MS, Geva T, eds. *Echocardiography in Pediatric and Congenital Heart Disease: From Fetus to Adult*, 3rd edn. Wiley Blackwell; 2022. pp. 685–699.)

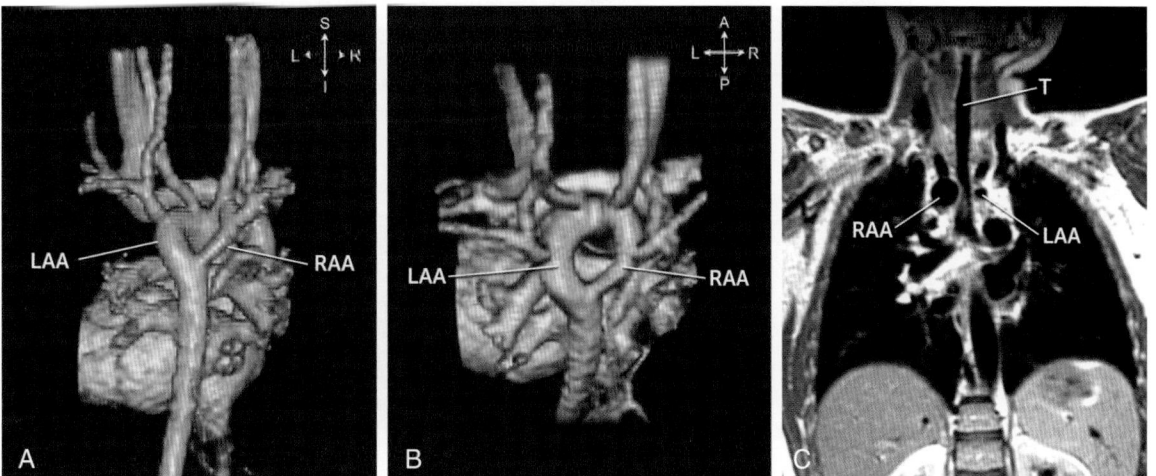

• **Fig. 43.12** Double aortic arch with both arches patent. Volume-rendered three-dimensional magnetic resonance angiogram viewed from posterior **(A)** and superior **(B)** vantage points. In this case, the left aortic arch *(LAA)* is larger than the right *(RAA)*. Note the symmetrical origins of the common carotid and subclavian arteries from each arch, as shown in Fig. 43.7. **(C)** Magnetic resonance imaging using fast spin echo imaging and blood signal suppression (black blood) in an oblique coronal plane from a different patient illustrating tracheal compression by RAA and LAA which are seen in cross-section. The right arch is larger than the left as is usually the case. *T,* Trachea.

thoracotomy, thereby severing the ring and freeing the trachea and esophagus. An important additional component with ring division is lysis of residual fibrotic tissue overlying the adventitia of the esophagus and trachea. Some centers have also recommended resection of the diverticulum of Kommerell with anterior relocation of the aberrant subclavian artery to the left carotid artery to avoid residual airway or esophageal obstruction.[12] Patients with a circumflex aortic arch and descending aorta on the opposite side of the arch (Fig. 43.13) often require more extensive arch surgery such as an aortic uncrossing procedure to avoid recurrent symptoms.[16] Operative mortality for ring division is reported to be less than 3%, with most of the complications occurring either in earlier eras or in patients with additional intracardiac abnormalities.[17] Video-assisted thoracoscopic surgery is favored at some institutions to divide rings with ligamentous or patent segments of small diameter.[18] Advantages of thoracoscopic surgery compared with open thoracotomy may include smaller incisions, improved visualization, reduced postoperative pain, lower risk for chest wall deformity, and earlier hospital discharge. However, complications such as bleeding, recurrent laryngeal nerve injury, and residual symptoms related to poor tissue mobilization can occur.

Frequently after vascular ring division, the postoperative course is uncomplicated with immediate improvement of airway symptoms. However, if there is significant associated tracheomalacia, complete resolution of noisy respirations may take months or even years.[7,17] Recurrent or persistent symptoms in the short term, mostly airway symptoms, occur in up to 50% of patients but only 2–3% undergo reoperation.[12,19] Recently, techniques to address tracheomalacia directly (e.g., tracheopexy) have been developed.[20] Longer-term follow-up studies indicate that most patients are asymptomatic, although abnormalities on airway imaging and pulmonary function tests may persist.[7,19]

Pulmonary Artery Sling

Definition

Left pulmonary artery sling, also known as anomalous origin of the left pulmonary artery from the right pulmonary artery, is a vascular anomaly in which the left pulmonary artery arises aberrantly from the proximal right pulmonary artery and courses posterior to the trachea and anterior to the esophagus to reach the left hilum (Fig. 43.14).[21] This arrangement creates a vascular "sling" around the trachea but not the esophagus. The ligamentum arteriosum is positioned to the left of the trachea and connects the descending aorta to the distal main pulmonary artery.

Embryology and Anatomy

The embryology of pulmonary artery sling is not understood. No normal vessel passes between the trachea and esophagus at any stage of development. The branch pulmonary arteries develop from the vascular plexus arising from the posterior aspect of the aortic sac.[3] It is possible that part of the plexus on the dorsal-caudal aspect of the tracheal bud persists, connecting the right and left branch pulmonary

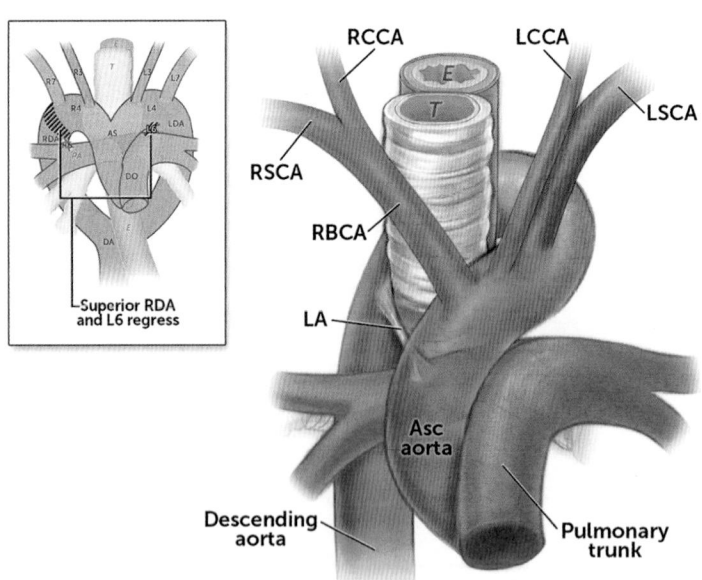

• **Fig. 43.13** Left circumflex aortic arch with right descending aorta and right posterior ligamentum arteriosum (*LA*). This anomaly appears to result from involution of the right dorsal aorta between the right 6th pharyngeal arch artery (right ductus arteriosus) and the right 7th segmental artery (shown on the inset double arch model). Persistence of part of the distal right dorsal aorta and flow-induced remodeling from the right ductus arteriosus might influence the position of the descending aorta. *Asc Aorta*, Ascending aorta; *E*, esophagus; *LCCA*, left common carotid artery; *LSCA*, left subclavian artery; *RBCA*, right brachiocephalic artery; *RCCA*, right common carotid artery; *RDA*, right dorsal aorta; *RSCA*, right subclavian artery; *T*, trachea.

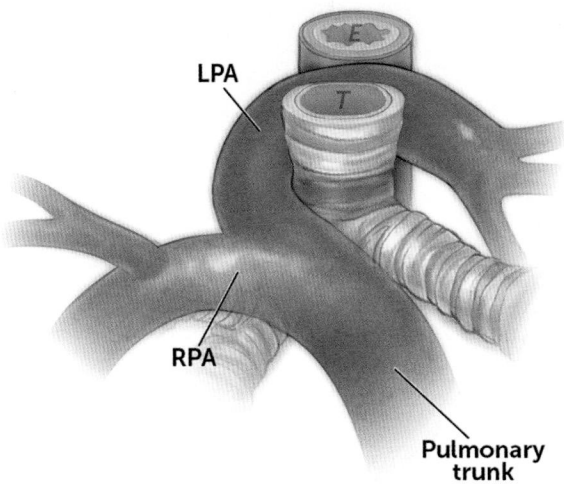

LPA

RPA

Pulmonary trunk

• **Fig. 43.14** Origin of the left pulmonary artery *(LPA)* from the right pulmonary artery *(RPA)* or LPA sling. The developmental origins of this anomaly are not understood, nor why only the left pulmonary artery is so affected. This is the only vascular anomaly in which a major vessel passes between the trachea *(T)* and esophagus *(E)*.

arteries with loss of the connection of the left branch to the aortic sac. A mechanism for this is unknown, especially one that explains why this anomaly only occurs on the left side.

A pulmonary artery sling can cause obstruction of the right main bronchus or trachea, or both. In at least half of the cases, there are associated complete cartilaginous tracheal rings in which the posterior membranous portion of the trachea and proximal bronchi is absent and the tracheal cartilage is circumferential, the so-called "ring-sling complex."[22] The complete rings may be localized to the area adjacent to the sling or extend throughout the trachea, suggesting a more extensive abnormality of airway development rather than just compression by the abnormal vessel. Complete rings are often but not always associated with significant airway narrowing and may be an important source of airway symptoms in addition to the sling itself. Other abnormalities associated with left pulmonary artery sling include a tracheal origin of the right upper lobe bronchus, agenesis or hypoplasia of the right lung,[23] hypoplastic left pulmonary artery, and other intracardiac defects.[7,21]

Symptoms

Usually, patients present in the first weeks of life with respiratory stridor and distress that is often severe. However, a few patients are asymptomatic and can be followed without surgery.[24]

Physical Examination

An affected infant may have stridor, dyspnea, tachypnea, wheezing, or intermittent cyanosis. The right lung may be either hyperinflated (and thus hyper-resonant), partly atelectatic, or hypoplastic. Peripheral breath sounds may be decreased, and there may be signs of a mediastinal shift, especially if the right lung is hypoplastic or absent.

Diagnostic Imaging

Chest radiograph findings are variable depending on the location and severity of airway obstruction and lung hypoplasia/agenesis or hyperinflation. Barium contrast esophagogram often demonstrates an anterior indentation on the esophagus in contrast to the posterior indentation seen in many vascular rings.[21,22] Usually, echocardiography can demonstrate the abnormal origin of the left pulmonary artery as well as associated intracardiac abnormalities, and is sufficient to establish the diagnosis.[25] Because of the high incidence of tracheal anomalies other than simple compression by the sling, bronchoscopy is also warranted in most cases.[26] This may be supplemented by CT or MRI as needed to ensure that the trachea, bronchi, and pulmonary arteries have been completely assessed (Fig. 43.15).[7,26] X-ray angiography and bronchography are rarely indicated.

Management and Course

For the symptomatic infant, morbidity and mortality without surgical repair are high; therefore, prompt surgical intervention is indicated. If there is extrinsic tracheal compression without fixed stenosis, the left pulmonary artery is transected from its right-sided origin and anastomosed to the main pulmonary artery, anterior to the trachea.[26] Commonly, however, there is significant fixed tracheal stenosis, and the affected segment must be resected or a tracheoplasty procedure performed with cardiopulmonary bypass.[26] In that case, the undivided left pulmonary artery may be translocated anteriorly through the divided trachea before the airway is reanastomosed. This technique avoids a vascular anastomosis and may decrease the incidence of left pulmonary artery stenosis. Surgical outcome is primarily related to the extent of intrinsic airway stenosis and the severity of any associated cardiovascular disease.[26] Cases with mild airway involvement have minimal operative mortality and a good long-term outlook. Those requiring extensive tracheal reconstruction have higher mortality, may require prolonged mechanical ventilation, and often have residual airway symptoms. All patients should be followed longitudinally for the development of left pulmonary artery stenosis.

Innominate Artery Compression Syndrome

Innominate artery compression syndrome refers to children with symptoms of airway obstruction who are found to have significant tracheal narrowing where the innominate artery passes anterior to it.[27] Typically, localized tracheomalacia with dynamic airway narrowing is found, but it remains controversial whether this is primarily due to compression or an intrinsic airway problem. Some reports have attributed the tracheal narrowing to a more distal, posterior, and leftward origin of the innominate artery from the aortic arch; however, careful studies have not found this to be a consistent

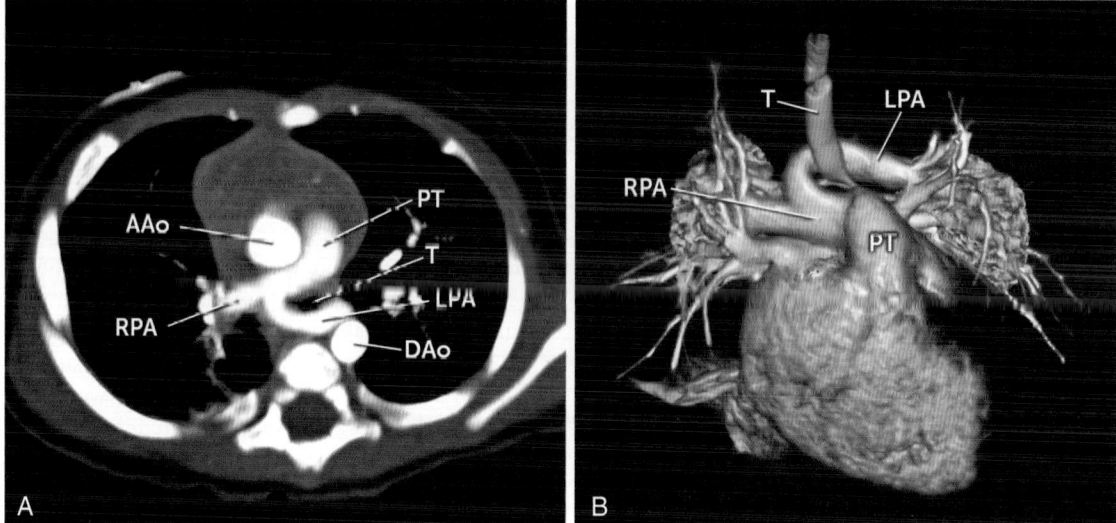

• **Fig. 43.15** Left pulmonary artery sling. Computed tomography with intravenous contrast. **(A)** Axial plane image illustrating the left pulmonary artery *(LPA)* arising from the right pulmonary artery *(RPA)* and coursing posterior to the narrowed trachea *(T)*. **(B)** Three-dimensional reconstruction viewed from an anterior perspective with the aorta removed. *AAo,* Ascending aorta; *DAo,* descending aorta; *PT,* pulmonary trunk. (From Crowell A.L. Chapter 02: Vascular Rings and Slings (Figure 32,13). In: Lai WW, Mertens LL, Cohen MS, Geva T, eds. *Echocardiography in Pediatric and Congenital Heart Disease. From Fetus to Adult,* 0⁰ edn. Wiley Blackwell; 2022. pp. 685–699.)

finding.[28] Others have proposed that mediastinal crowding and an enlarged thymus gland contribute to the pathology. Some degree of anterior tracheal compression on a lateral chest radiograph is commonly seen in asymptomatic children, and it is normal for the innominate artery to originate slightly to the left of the trachea and to course immediately anterior to it.[29] Innominate artery compression syndrome is rarely associated with congenital heart disease.

Presentation is in infancy with stridor, which may be sufficiently severe to cause apnea or syncope. Feeding difficulties (e.g., poor weight gain, gastroesophageal reflux), as well as a history of esophageal atresia and tracheoesophageal fistulae, are common. The diagnosis can be made by a combination of bronchoscopy and CT or MRI (Fig. 43.16).[28] On bronchoscopy, there is a characteristic anterior pulsatile indentation of the trachea 1 to 2 cm above the carina. The trachea should be narrowed at least 50% to 75% during spontaneous respiration to attribute symptoms to this diagnosis. Patients with mild symptoms should be managed conservatively because they usually improve over time.[28] Those with a history of apnea, severe stridor, or recurrent respiratory infections without an alternative explanation are candidates for surgery. Historically, the favored surgical technique consisted of an aortopexy procedure suturing the adventitia of the aorta to the posterior aspect of the sternum to lift both the aortic arch and the innominate artery in an anterior and leftward direction, as well as a partial thymectomy.[28] This low-risk procedure usually results in a dramatic decrease in stridor, although mild residual symptoms may remain because of persistent tracheomalacia. Some have advocated for reimplanting the innominate artery more proximally away from the trachea.[30] Most recently, a direct anterior tracheopexy guided by intraoperative bronchoscopy has been utilized as an adjunct to directly support the trachea.[31]

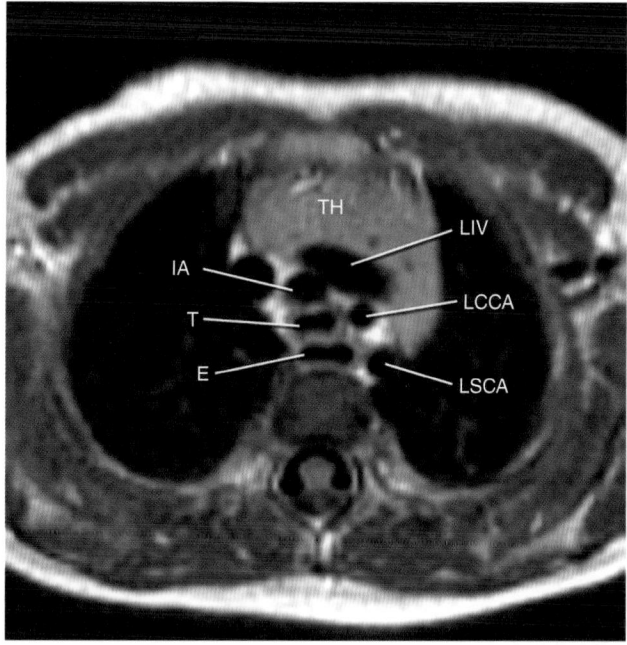

• **Fig. 43.16** Innominate artery compression syndrome. Magnetic resonance imaging using fast spin echo imaging and blood signal suppression (black blood) in an axial plane illustrating a narrow trachea *(T)* with the innominate artery *(IA)* located anteriorly. *E,* Esophagus; *LCCA,* left common carotid artery; *LIV,* left innominate vein; *LSCA,* left subclavian artery; *TH,* thymus.

Isolated Branch Pulmonary Artery

Isolated branch pulmonary artery occurs when the intrapulmonary portion of a branch pulmonary artery is not connected to the central pulmonary circulation but maintains connection to the ipsilateral ductus arteriosus

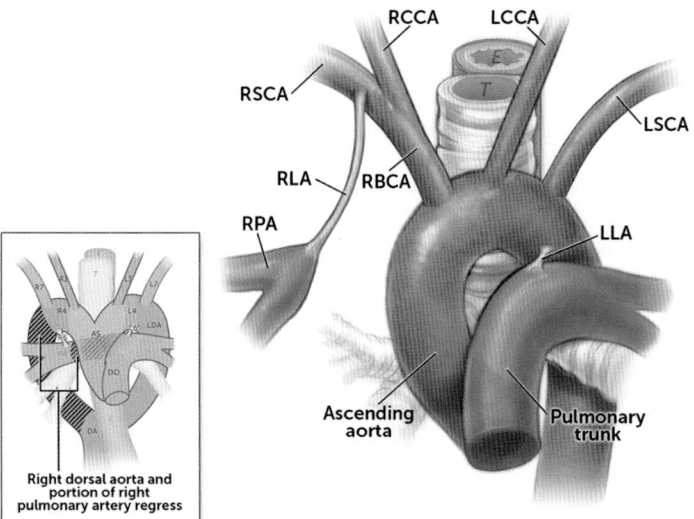

• **Fig. 43.17** Isolated right pulmonary artery *(RPA)* and a left aortic arch. The left aortic arch seems to form in the usual way, by involution of the right dorsal aorta distal to the right 7th segmental artery. Isolation of the RPA is due to involution of the RPA proximal to the insertion of the right 6th pharyngeal arch artery (right ductus arteriosus), with consequent loss of connection of the RPA to the pulmonary trunk (shown on the inset double arch model). The RPA is then supplied by the right ductus, which typically closes after birth forming the right ligamentum arteriosum *(RLA)* with loss of flow to the right lung. *E,* Esophagus; *LCCA,* left common carotid artery; *LLA,* left ligamentum arteriosum or ductal ligament; *LSCA,* left subclavian artery; *RBCA,* right brachiocephalic artery; *RCCA,* right common carotid artery; *RSCA,* right subclavian artery; *T,* trachea.

(Fig. 43.17).[32] The condition is also referred to as a "unilaterally absent pulmonary artery" and "isolated pulmonary artery of ductal origin." The affected pulmonary artery usually occurs on the side opposite the aortic arch. Isolated branch pulmonary artery may be part of more complex heart defects such as tetralogy of Fallot (with or without pulmonary valve atresia) and heterotaxy syndrome. Rarely, most often in heterotaxy syndrome, both branch pulmonary arteries are isolated. This anomaly appears to be due to involution of the branch pulmonary artery proximal to its junction with the ipsilateral ductus arteriosus. Ductal closure results in marked diminution of blood flow to the affected lung, with only collateral arterial supply. If not promptly treated, hypoplasia of the affected lung and underdevelopment of pulmonary vasculature ensue. Complications include heart failure early on, asymmetric chest and scoliosis, pulmonary hypertension, respiratory infections, and hemoptysis. However, many patients are asymptomatic for many years. Chest radiograph often shows asymmetry of the chest and reduced lung volume and vascular markings on the affected side. Imaging shows absence of the mediastinal portion of the affected pulmonary artery and often demonstrates the distal vessel in the lung hilum. Angiography at catheterization can usually demonstrate the intrapulmonary portion of the vessel, either by filling collateral arterial vessels or by pulmonary vein wedge angiography (Fig. 43.18). Unless treated as a neonate, a systemic-to-pulmonary shunt to the affected lung is usually necessary to induce growth and development of the vascular bed prior to establishing continuity between the affected pulmonary artery and the pulmonary

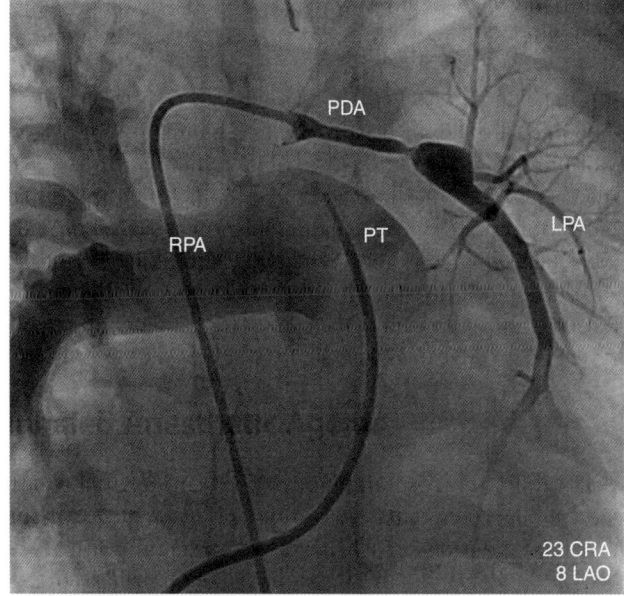

• **Fig. 43.18** Isolated left pulmonary artery *(LPA)* and a right aortic arch. Simultaneous injections into an isolated LPA and right pulmonary artery *(RPA)*. The RPA catheter courses antegrade through the right ventricle, whereas the isolated LPA is injected with a catheter ascending retrograde from the right-sided aorta into the left brachiocephalic artery and stenotic left persistent ductus arteriosus *(PDA)*. *PT,* Pulmonary trunk. (From Batlivala SP, McElhinney DB, Pigula FA, Marshall AC. Isolated pulmonary artery arising from a duct: a single-center review of diagnostic and therapeutic strategies. *J Thorac Cardiovasc Surg.* 2014;148:2245–2252.)

trunk.[32] Lung growth and pulmonary perfusion improve in most patients but often remain abnormal, especially in patients treated after infancy.

References

1. Edwards JE. Anomalies of the derivatives of the aortic arch system. *Med Clin North Am.* 1948;32:925-949.

2. Weinberg PM. Aortic arch anomalies. In: Allen HD, Gutgesell HP, Clark EB, Driscoll DJ, eds. *Moss and Adams' Heart Disease in Infants, Children, and Adolescents.* Philadelphia: Lippincott Williams & Wilkins; 2001:707-735.

3. Rana MS, Girard A, Christofolo VM, et al. Development of the human aortic arch system captured in an interactive three-dimensional reference model. *Am J Med Genet A.* 2014;164A: 1372-1383.

4. Fisher RG, Whigham CJ, Trinh C. Diverticula of Kommerell and aberrant subclavian arteries complicated by aneurysms. *Cardiovasc Intervent Radiol.* 2005;28:553-560.

5. Felson B, Strife JL. Cervical aortic arch: a commentary. *Semin Roentgenol.* 1989;24:114-120.

6. Zhu D, Zhou Y, Ji W, et al. Clinical and imaging characteristics of isolated subclavian artery in pediatric patients. *Clin Imaging.* 2021;77:224-229.

7. Yoshimura N, Fukahara K, Yamashita A, et al. Congenital vascular ring. *Surg Today.* 2020;50:1151-1158.

8. Yoo SJ, Min JY, Lee YH, et al. Fetal sonographic diagnosis of aortic arch anomalies. *Ultrasound Obstet Gynecol.* 2003;22:535-546.

9. Woods RK, Sharp RJ, Holcomb GW III, et al. Vascular anomalies and tracheoesophageal compression: a single institution's 25-year experience. *Ann Thorac Surg.* 2001;72:434-438.

10. McElhinney DB, Clark BJ III, Weinberg PM, et al. Association of chromosome 22q11 deletion with isolated anomalies of aortic arch laterality and branching. *J Am Coll Cardiol.* 2001;37:2114-2119.

11. Velasquez G, Nath PH, Castaneda-Zuniga WR, et al. Aberrant left subclavian artery in tetralogy of Fallot. *Am J Cardiol.* 1980; 45:811-818.

12. Labuz DF, Kamran A, Jennings RW, et al. Reoperation to correct unsuccessful vascular ring and vascular decompression surgery. *J Thorac Cardiovasc Surg.* 2022;164:199-207.

13. Young AA, Hornberger LK, Haberer K, et al. Prenatal detection, comorbidities, and management of vascular rings. *Am J Cardiol.* 2019;123:1703-1708.

14. Lillehei CW, Colan S. Echocardiography in the preoperative evaluation of vascular rings. *J Pediatr Surg.* 1992;27:1118-1120.

15. Gross RE. Surgical relief for tracheal obstruction from a vascular ring. *N Engl J Med.* 1945;233:586-590.

16. Kamran A, Friedman KG, Jennings RW, et al. Aortic uncrossing and tracheobronchopexy corrects tracheal compression and tracheobronchomalacia associated with circumflex aortic arch. *J Thorac Cardiovasc Surg.* 2020;160:796-804.

17. Amir G, Soffair N, Bruckheimer E, et al. Mid-term results of vascular ring surgery. *Cardiol Young.* 2022;32:1415-1420.

18. Herrin MA, Zurakowski D, Fynn-Thompson F, et al. Outcomes following thoracotomy or thoracoscopic vascular ring division in children and young adults. *J Thorac Cardiovasc Surg.* 2017;154:607-615.

19. ten Berge M, van der Laag J, van der Ent CK, et al. Clinical, radiological and functional follow-up after surgical decompression of double aortic arch. *Pediatr Radiol.* 2002;32:561-566.

20. Lawlor C, Smithers CJ, Hamilton T, et al. Innovative management of severe tracheobronchomalacia using anterior and posterior tracheobronchopexy. *Laryngoscope.* 2020;130:E65-E74.

21. Gikonyo BM, Jue KL, Edwards JE. Pulmonary vascular sling; report of seven cases and review of the literature. *Pediatr Cardiol.* 1989;10:81-89.

22. Berdon WE, Baker DH, Wung JT, et al. Complete cartilage-ring tracheal stenosis associated with anomalous left pulmonary artery: the ring-sling complex. *Radiology.* 1984;152:57-64.

23. Pu WT, Chung T, Hoffer FA, et al. Diagnosis and management of agenesis of the right lung and left pulmonary artery sling. *Am J Cardiol.* 1996;78:723-727.

24. Raj S, Chandra S. Left pulmonary artery sling without symptoms. *Ann Pediatr Cardiol.* 2017;10:98-99.

25. Yeager SB, Chin AJ, Sanders SP. Two-dimensional echocardiographic diagnosis of pulmonary artery sling in infancy. *J Am Coll Cardiol.* 1986;7:625-629.

26. Carlson L, Halder M, Liu H, et al. Left pulmonary artery sling: postoperative outcomes for patients at a single center. *World J Pediatr Congenit Heart Surg.* 2021;12:715-727.

27. Gross RE, Neuhauser EB. Compression of the trachea by an anomalous innominate artery. An operation for its relief. *Am J Dis Child.* 1948;75:570-574.

28. Gardella C, Girosi D, Rossi GA, et al. Tracheal compression by aberrant innominate artery: clinical presentations in infants and children, indications for surgical correction by aortopexy, and short- and long-term outcome. *J Pediatr Surg.* 2010;45:564-573.

29. Fawcett SL, Gomez AC, Hughes JA, et al. Anatomical variation in the position of the brachiocephalic trunk (innominate artery) with respect to the trachea: a computed tomography-based study and literature review of Innominate Artery Compression Syndrome. *Clin Anat.* 2010;23:61-69.

30. Grimmer JF, Herway S, Hawkins JA, et al. Long-term results of innominate artery reimplantation for tracheal compression. *Arch Otolaryngol Head Neck Surg.* 2009;135:80-84.

31. Bairdain S, Smithers CJ, Hamilton TE, et al. Direct tracheobronchopexy to correct airway collapse due to severe tracheobronchomalacia: Short-term outcomes in a series of 20 patients. *J Pediatr Surg.* 2015;50:972-977.

32. Batlivala SP, McElhinney DB, Pigula FA, et al. Isolated pulmonary artery arising from a duct: a single-center review of diagnostic and therapeutic strategies. *J Thorac Cardiovasc Surg.* 2014;148: 2245-2252.

Other Forms of Heart Disease

44

Preventive Cardiology

JACOB HARTZ, SHANNON LYON, AND SARAH D. DE FERRANTI

KEY LEARNING POINTS

- Cardiovascular disease (CVD) is a leading cause of morbidity and mortality in adulthood; risk factors for atherosclerotic heart disease can begin early in life.
- Hypertension affects approximately 2–4% of children and is a risk factor for renal insufficiency, left ventricular hypertrophy or dysfunction, and CVD later in life.
- Optimal nutrition and adequate physical activity may delay or prevent CVD in adulthood; lifestyle counseling is a cornerstone in the management of hypertension and dyslipidemia in youth.
- Familial hypercholesterolemia (FH) is inherited in an autosomal dominant fashion. The clinical form of heterozygous FH affects

- approximately 1 in 250 people and is characterized by high low-density lipoprotein (LDL) cholesterol, generally ≥ 190 mg/dL.
- For children who meet the LDL cholesterol threshold to begin a lipid-lowering medication, statins are the recommended agent as they are well tolerated with minimal adverse effects and can reduce LDL by 25–46%.
- Pharmacological treatment of hypertension is indicated in patients diagnosed with stage II hypertension and in patients with stage I hypertension who are at high risk for CVD, are symptomatic, or have evidence of end-organ damage.

Introduction

Cardiovascular disease (CVD) is the leading cause of death and disability. In 2019, there were 874,613 deaths attributed to CVD in the United States and over 18 million deaths occurred internationally (based on 2018 data). In the United States, CVD is responsible for more deaths each year than all forms of cancer and lower respiratory tract infections combined. The burden of CVD leads to $216 billion in direct costs and an additional $147 billion in indirect costs each year.[1]

The major risk factors for CVD, including hypertension, elevated low-density lipoprotein (LDL) cholesterol, and low high-density lipoprotein (HDL) cholesterol, have their antecedents in childhood. Pediatric cardiologists may be asked to evaluate and manage these conditions in youth with diseases associated with an increased CVD risk (e.g., type 2 diabetes mellitus or Turner syndrome) and during the usual care of their patients with congenital heart disease, particularly those who are at an increased risk for hypertension (e.g., patients who have undergone cardiac surgery or have left-sided obstructive lesions). For this reason, this chapter will focus on the identification, evaluation, and management of hypertension and dyslipidemia in youth.

Hypertension

Elevated blood pressure (previously called "prehypertension") and hypertension refer to a high systolic blood pressure, a high diastolic blood pressure, or both. In adults, thresholds for hypertension are based on levels associated with the risk for CVD. In childhood, cut points for abnormal blood pressure are based on population distributions and have been determined by consensus because there is limited data about the relationship between blood pressure and CVD endpoints. The most recent pediatric guidance, 2017 Clinical Practice Guideline for Screening and Management of High Blood Pressure in Children and Adolescents, proposes blood pressure cut points based on percentiles used for children less than 13 years old, while adult blood pressure thresholds are used for adolescents 13 years old and older (Table 44.1).[2] The blood pressure tables used to determine abnormal blood pressures are presented in Tables 44.2 and 44.3.

Elevated blood pressure readings are rather common in childhood, but diagnosed hypertension affects fewer youth. Studies generally report that 7–12% of girls and 15–19% of boys have blood pressure in the elevated range. A diagnosis of hypertension requires repeated high measurements, thus the prevalence of "clinically meaningful

TABLE 44.1 Categories of Blood Pressure by Age Group (mm Hg)

Category	< 13 Years Old	≥ 13 Years Old
Normal	< 90th percentile	< 120/< 80
Elevated*	≥ 90th to < 95th percentile *or* 120/80 to 129/80	120/< 80 to 129/< 80
Hypertension		
Stage 1	≥ 95th to < 95th percentile + 12 *or* 130/80 to 139/89	130/80 to 139/89
Stage 2	≥ 95th percentile + 12 *or* ≥ 140/90	≥ 140/90
Critical	>180/120 or ≥ stage 2 hypertension with symptoms	

*Use the lower of these two measurements to categorize the blood pressure for children < 13 years old.
Adapted from Flynn JT, Kaelber DC, Baker-Smith CM, et al. Clinical practice guideline for screening and management of high blood pressure in children and adolescents. *Pediatrics.* 2017;140:e20171904.

TABLE 44.2 Blood Pressure (BP) Levels for Boys by Age and Height Percentile

Age (y)	BP Percentile	SBP (mm Hg) Height Percentile or Measured Height							DBP (mm Hg) Height Percentile or Measured Height						
		5%	10%	25%	50%	75%	90%	95%	5%	10%	25%	50%	75%	90%	95%
1	Height (in)	30.4	30.8	31.6	32.4	33.3	34.1	34.6	30.4	30.8	31.6	32.4	33.3	34.1	34.6
	Height (cm)	77.2	78.3	80.2	82.4	84.6	86.7	87.9	77.2	78.3	80.2	82.4	84.6	86.7	87.9
	50th	85	85	86	86	87	88	88	40	40	40	41	41	42	42
	90th	98	99	99	100	100	101	101	52	52	53	53	54	54	54
	95th	102	102	103	103	104	105	105	54	54	55	55	56	57	57
	95th + 12 mm Hg	114	114	115	115	116	117	117	66	66	67	67	68	69	69
2	Height (in)	33.9	34.4	35.3	36.3	37.3	38.2	38.8	33.9	34.4	35.3	36.3	37.3	38.2	38.8
	Height (cm)	86.1	87.4	80.6	92.1	94.7	97.1	98.5	86.1	87.4	89.6	92.1	94.7	97.1	98.5
	50th	87	87	88	89	89	90	91	43	43	44	44	45	46	46
	90th	100	100	101	102	103	103	104	55	55	56	56	57	58	58
	95th	104	105	105	106	107	107	108	57	58	58	59	60	61	61
	95th + 12 mm Hg	116	117	117	118	119	119	120	69	70	70	71	72	73	73
3	Height (in)	36.4	37	37.9	39	40.1	41.1	41.7	36.4	37	37.9	39	40.1	41.1	41.7
	Height (cm)	92.5	93.9	96.3	99	101.8	104.3	105.8	92.5	93.9	96.3	99	101.8	104.3	105.8
	50th	88	89	89	90	91	92	92	45	46	46	47	48	49	49
	90th	101	102	102	103	104	105	105	58	58	59	59	60	61	61
	95th	106	106	107	107	108	109	109	60	61	61	62	63	64	64
	95th + 12mm Hg	118	118	119	119	120	121	121	72	73	73	74	75	76	76
4	Height (in)	38.8	39.4	40.5	41.7	42.9	43.9	44.5	38.8	39.4	40.5	41.7	42.9	43.9	44.5
	Height (cm)	98.5	100.2	102.9	105.9	108.9	111.5	113.2	98.5	100.2	102.9	105.9	108.9	111.5	113.2
	50th	90	90	91	92	93	94	94	48	49	49	50	51	52	52
	90th	102	103	104	105	105	106	107	60	61	62	62	63	64	64

Continued

TABLE 44.2   Blood Pressure (BP) Levels for Boys by Age and Height Percentile—cont'd

Age (y)	BP Percentile	SBP (mm Hg) Height Percentile or Measured Height							DBP (mm Hg) Height Percentile or Measured Height						
	90th	107	107	108	108	109	110	110	63	64	65	66	67	67	68
	95th + 12 mm Hg	119	119	120	120	121	122	122	75	76	77	78	79	79	80
5	Height (in)	41.1	41.8	43.0	44.3	45.5	46.7	47.4	41.1	41.8	43.0	44.3	45.5	46.7	47.4
	Height (cm)	104.4	106.2	109.1	112.4	115.7	118.6	120.3	104.4	106.2	109.1	112.4	115.7	118.6	120.3
	50th	91	92	93	94	95	96	96	51	51	52	53	54	55	55
	90th	103	104	105	106	107	108	108	63	64	65	65	66	67	67
	95th	107	108	109	109	110	111	112	66	67	68	69	70	70	71
	95th + 12 mm Hg	119	120	121	121	122	123	124	78	79	80	81	82	82	83
6	Height (in)	43.4	44.2	45.4	46.8	48.2	49.4	50.2	43.4	44.2	45.4	46.8	48.2	49.4	50.2
	Height (cm)	110.3	112.2	115.3	118.9	122.4	125.6	127.5	110.3	112.2	115.3	118.9	122.4	125.6	127.5
	50th	93	93	94	95	96	97	98	54	54	55	56	57	57	58
	90th	105	105	106	107	109	110	110	66	66	67	68	68	69	69
	95th	108	109	110	111	112	113	114	69	70	70	71	72	72	73
	95th + 12 mm Hg	120	121	122	123	124	125	126	81	82	82	83	84	84	85
7	Height (in)	45.7	46.5	47.8	49.3	50.8	52.1	52.9	45.7	46.5	47.8	49.3	50.8	52.1	52.9
	Height (cm)	116.1	118	121.4	125.1	128.9	132.4	134.5	116.1	118	121.4	125.1	128.9	132.4	134.5
	50th	94	94	95	97	98	98	99	56	56	57	58	58	59	59
	90th	106	107	108	109	110	111	111	68	68	69	70	70	71	71
	95th	110	110	111	112	114	115	116	71	71	72	73	73	74	74
	95th + 12 mm Hg	122	122	123	124	126	127	128	83	83	84	85	85	86	86
8	Height (in)	47.8	48.6	50	51.6	53.2	54.6	55.5	47.8	48.6	50	51.6	53.2	54.6	55.5
	Height (cm)	121.4	123.5	127	131	135.1	138.8	141	121.4	123.5	127	131	135.1	138.8	141
	50th	95	96	97	98	99	99	100	57	57	58	59	59	60	60
	90th	107	108	109	110	111	112	112	69	70	70	71	72	72	73
	95th	111	112	112	114	115	116	117	72	73	73	74	75	75	75
	95th + 12 mm Hg	123	124	124	126	127	128	129	84	85	85	86	87	87	87
9	Height (in)	49.6	50.5	52	53.7	55.4	56.9	57.9	49.6	50.5	52	53.7	55.4	56.9	57.9
	Height (cm)	126	128.3	132.1	136.3	140.7	144.7	147.1	126	128.3	132.1	136.3	140.7	144.7	147.1
	50th	96	97	98	99	100	101	101	57	58	59	60	61	62	62
	90th	107	108	109	110	112	113	114	70	71	72	73	74	74	74
	95th	112	112	113	115	116	118	119	74	74	75	76	76	77	77
	95th + 12 mm Hg	124	124	125	127	128	130	131	86	86	87	88	88	89	89
10	Height (in)	51.3	52.2	53.8	55.6	57.4	59.1	60.1	51.3	52.2	53.8	55.6	57.4	59.1	60.1
	Height (cm)	130.2	132.7	136.7	141.3	145.9	150.1	152.7	130.2	132.7	136.7	141.3	145.9	150.1	152.7

TABLE 44.2   Blood Pressure (BP) Levels for Boys by Age and Height Percentile—cont'd

Age (y)	BP Percentile	SBP (mm Hg) Height Percentile or Measured Height							DBP (mm Hg) Height Percentile or Measured Height						
	50th	97	98	99	100	101	102	103	59	60	61	62	63	63	64
	90th	108	109	111	112	113	115	116	72	73	74	74	75	75	76
	95th	112	113	114	116	118	120	121	76	76	77	77	78	78	78
	95th + 12 mm Hg	124	125	126	128	130	132	133	88	88	89	89	90	90	90
11	Height (in)	53	54	55.7	57.6	59.6	61.3	62.4	53	54	55.7	57.6	59.6	61.3	62.4
	Height (cm)	134.7	137.3	141.5	146.4	151.3	155.8	158.6	134.7	137.3	141.5	146.4	151.3	155.8	158.6
	50th	99	99	101	102	103	104	106	61	61	62	63	63	63	63
	90th	110	111	112	114	116	117	118	74	74	75	75	75	76	76
	95th	114	114	116	118	120	123	124	77	78	78	78	78	78	78
	95th + 12 mm Hg	126	126	128	130	132	135	136	89	90	90	90	90	90	90
12	Height (in)	55.2	56.3	58.1	60.1	62.2	64	65.2	55.2	56.3	58.1	60.1	62.2	64	65.2
	Height (cm)	140.3	143	147.5	152.7	157.9	162.6	165.5	140.3	143	147.5	152.7	157.9	162.6	165.5
	50th	101	101	102	104	106	108	109	61	62	62	62	62	63	63
	90th	113	114	115	117	119	121	122	75	75	75	75	75	76	76
	95th	116	117	118	121	124	126	128	78	78	78	78	78	79	79
	95th + 12 mm Hg	128	129	130	133	136	138	140	90	90	90	90	90	91	91
13	Height (in)	57.9	59.1	61	63.1	65.2	67.1	68.3	57.9	59.1	61	63.1	65.2	67.1	68.3
	Height (cm)	147	150	154.9	160.3	165.7	170.5	173.4	147	150	154.9	160.3	165.7	170.5	173.4
	50th	103	104	105	108	110	111	112	61	60	61	62	63	64	65
	90th	115	116	118	121	124	126	126	74	74	74	75	76	77	77
	95th	119	120	122	125	128	130	131	78	78	78	78	80	81	81
	95th + 12 mm Hg	131	132	134	137	140	142	143	90	90	90	90	92	93	93
14	Height (in)	60.6	61.8	63.8	65.9	68.0	69.8	70.9	60.6	61.8	63.8	65.9	68.0	69.8	70.9
	Height (cm)	153.8	156.9	162	167.5	172.7	177.4	180.1	153.8	156.9	162	167.5	172.7	177.4	180.1
	50th	105	106	109	111	112	113	113	60	60	62	64	65	66	67
	90th	119	120	123	126	127	128	129	74	74	75	77	78	79	80
	95th	123	125	127	130	132	133	134	77	78	79	81	82	83	84
	95th + 12 mm Hg	135	137	139	142	144	145	146	89	90	91	93	94	95	96
15	Height (in)	62.6	63.8	65.7	67.8	69.8	71.5	72.5	62.6	63.8	65.7	67.8	69.8	71.5	72.5
	Height (cm)	159	162	166.9	172.2	177.2	181.6	184.2	159	162	166.9	172.2	177.2	181.6	184.2
	50th	108	110	112	113	114	114	114	61	62	64	65	66	67	68
	90th	123	124	126	128	129	130	130	75	76	78	79	80	81	81
	95th	127	129	131	132	134	135	135	78	79	81	83	84	85	85
	95th + 12 mm Hg	139	141	143	144	146	147	147	90	91	93	95	96	97	97

Continued

TABLE
44.2 **Blood Pressure (BP) Levels for Boys by Age and Height Percentile—cont'd**

Age (y)	BP Percentile	SBP (mm Hg) Height Percentile or Measured Height							DBP (mm Hg) Height Percentile or Measured Height						
16	Height (in)	63.8	64.9	66.8	68.8	70.7	72.4	73.4	63.8	64.9	66.8	68.8	70.7	72.4	73.4
	Height (cm)	162.1	165	169.6	174.6	179.5	183.8	186.4	162.1	165	169.6	174.6	179.5	183.8	186.4
	50th	111	112	114	115	115	116	116	63	64	66	67	68	69	69
	90th	126	127	128	129	131	131	132	77	78	79	80	81	82	82
	95th	130	131	133	134	135	136	137	80	81	83	84	85	86	86
	95th + 12 mm Hg	142	143	145	146	147	148	149	92	93	95	96	97	98	98
17	Height (in)	64.5	65.5	67.3	69.2	71.1	72.8	73.8	64.5	65.5	67.3	69.2	71.1	72.8	73.8
	Height (cm)	163.8	166.5	170.9	175.8	180.7	184.9	187.5	163.8	166.5	170.9	175.8	180.7	184.9	187.5
	50th	114	115	116	117	117	118	118	65	66	67	68	69	70	70
	90th	128	129	130	131	132	133	134	78	79	80	81	82	82	83
	95th	132	133	134	135	137	138	138	81	82	84	85	86	86	87
	95th + 12 mm Hg	144	145	146	147	149	150	150	93	94	96	97	98	98	99

DBP, Diastolic blood pressure; *SBP,* systolic blood pressure.

TABLE
44.3 **Blood Pressure (BP) Levels for Girls by Age and Height Percentile**

Age (y)	BP Percentile	SBP (mm Hg) Height Percentile or Measured Height							DBP (mm Hg) Height Percentile or Measured Height						
		5%	10%	25%	50%	75%	90%	95%	5%	10%	25%	50%	75%	90%	95%
1	Height (in)	29.7	30.2	30.9	31.8	32.7	33.4	33.9	29.7	30.2	30.9	31.8	32.7	33.4	33.9
	Height (cm)	75.4	76.6	78.6	80.8	83	84.9	86.1	75.4	76.6	78.6	80.8	83	84.9	86.1
	50th	84	85	86	86	87	88	88	41	42	42	43	44	45	46
	90th	98	99	99	100	101	102	102	54	55	56	56	57	58	58
	95th	101	102	102	103	104	105	105	59	59	60	60	61	62	62
	95th + 12 mm Hg	113	114	114	115	116	117	117	71	71	72	72	73	74	74
2	Height (in)	33.4	34	34.9	35.9	36.9	37.8	38.4	33.4	34	34.9	35.9	36.9	37.8	38.4
	Height (cm)	84.9	86.3	88.6	91.1	93.7	96	97.4	84.9	86.3	88.6	91.1	93.7	96	97.4
	50th	87	87	88	89	90	91	91	45	46	47	48	49	50	51
	90th	101	101	102	103	104	105	106	58	58	59	60	61	62	62
	95th	104	105	106	106	107	108	109	62	63	63	64	65	66	66
	95th + 12 mm Hg	116	117	118	118	119	120	121	74	75	75	76	77	78	78
3	Height (in)	35.8	36.4	37.3	38.4	39.6	40.6	41.2	35.8	36.4	37.3	38.4	39.6	40.6	41.2
	Height (cm)	91	92.4	94.9	97.6	100.5	103.1	104.6	91	92.4	94.9	97.6	100.5	103.1	104.6
	50th	88	89	89	90	91	92	93	48	48	49	50	51	53	53
	90th	102	103	104	104	105	106	107	60	61	61	62	63	64	65

TABLE 44.3 Blood Pressure (BP) Levels for Girls by Age and Height Percentile—cont'd

Age (y)	BP Percentile	SBP (mm Hg) Height Percentile or Measured Height							DBP (mm Hg) Height Percentile or Measured Height						
	95th	106	106	107	108	109	110	110	64	65	65	66	67	68	69
	95th + 12 mm Hg	118	118	119	120	121	122	122	76	77	77	78	79	80	81
4	Height (in)	38.3	38.9	39.9	41.1	42.4	43.5	44.2	38.3	38.9	39.9	41.1	42.4	43.5	44.2
	Height (cm)	97.2	98.8	101.4	104.5	107.6	110.5	112.2	97.2	98.8	101.4	104.5	107.6	110.5	112.2
	50th	89	90	91	92	93	94	94	50	51	51	53	54	55	55
	90th	103	104	105	106	107	108	108	62	63	64	65	66	67	67
	95th	107	108	109	109	110	111	112	66	67	68	69	70	70	71
	95th + 12 mm Hg	119	120	121	121	122	123	124	78	79	80	81	82	82	83
5	Height (in)	40.8	41.5	42.6	43.9	45.2	46.5	47.3	40.8	41.5	42.6	43.9	45.2	46.5	47.3
	Height (cm)	103.6	105.3	108.2	111.5	114.9	118.1	120	103.6	105.3	108.2	111.5	114.9	118.1	120
	50th	90	91	92	93	94	95	96	52	52	53	55	56	57	57
	90th	104	105	106	107	108	109	110	64	65	66	67	68	69	70
	95th	108	109	109	110	111	112	113	68	69	70	71	72	73	73
	95th + 12 mm Hg	120	121	121	122	123	124	125	80	81	82	83	84	85	85
6	Height (in)	43.3	44	45.2	46.6	48.1	49.4	50.3	43.3	44	45.2	46.6	48.1	49.4	50.3
	Height (cm)	110	111.8	114.9	118.4	122.1	125.6	127.7	110	111.8	114.9	118.4	122.1	125.6	127.7
	50th	92	92	93	94	96	97	97	54	54	55	56	57	58	59
	90th	105	106	107	108	109	110	111	67	67	68	69	70	71	71
	95th	109	109	110	111	112	113	114	70	71	72	72	73	74	74
	95th + 12 mm Hg	121	121	122	123	124	125	126	82	83	84	84	85	86	86
7	Height (in)	45.6	46.4	47.7	49.2	50.7	52.1	53	45.6	46.4	47.7	49.2	50.7	52.1	53
	Height (cm)	115.9	117.8	121.1	124.9	128.8	132.5	134.7	115.9	117.8	121.1	124.9	128.8	132.5	134.7
	50th	92	93	94	95	97	98	99	55	55	56	57	58	59	60
	90th	106	106	107	109	110	111	112	68	68	69	70	71	72	72
	95th	109	110	111	112	113	114	115	72	72	73	73	74	74	75
	95th + 12 mm Hg	121	122	123	124	125	126	127	84	84	85	85	86	86	87
8	Height (in)	47.6	48.4	49.8	51.4	53	54.5	55.5	47.6	48.4	49.8	51.4	53	54.5	55.5
	Height (cm)	121	123	126.5	130.6	134.7	138.5	140.9	121	123	126.5	130.6	134.7	138.5	140.9
	50th	93	94	95	97	98	99	100	56	56	57	59	60	61	61
	90th	107	107	108	110	111	112	113	69	70	71	72	72	73	73
	95th	110	111	112	113	115	116	117	72	73	74	74	75	75	75
	95th + 12 mm Hg	122	123	124	125	127	128	129	84	85	86	86	87	87	87
9	Height (in)	49.3	50.2	51.7	53.4	55.1	56.7	57.7	49.3	50.2	51.7	53.4	55.1	56.7	57.7
	Height (cm)	125.3	127.6	131.3	135.6	140.1	144.1	146.6	125.3	127.6	131.3	135.6	140.1	144.1	146.6

Continued

TABLE 44.3 Blood Pressure (BP) Levels for Girls by Age and Height Percentile—cont'd

Age (y)	BP Percentile	SBP (mm Hg) Height Percentile or Measured Height							DBP (mm Hg) Height Percentile or Measured Height						
	50th	95	96	97	98	99	100	101	57	58	59	60	60	61	61
	90th	108	108	109	111	112	113	114	71	71	72	73	73	73	73
	95th	112	112	113	114	116	117	118	74	74	75	75	75	75	75
	95th + 12 mm Hg	124	124	125	126	128	129	130	86	86	87	87	87	87	87
10	Height (in)	51.1	52	53.7	55.5	57.4	59.1	60.2	51.1	52	53.7	55.5	57.4	59.1	60.2
	Height (cm)	129.7	132.2	136.3	141	145.8	150.2	152.8	129.7	132.2	136.3	141	145.8	150.2	152.8
	50th	96	97	98	99	101	102	103	58	59	59	60	61	61	62
	90th	109	110	111	112	113	115	116	72	73	73	73	73	73	73
	95th	113	114	114	116	117	119	120	75	75	76	76	76	76	76
	95th + 12 mm Hg	125	126	126	128	129	131	132	87	87	88	88	88	88	88
11	Height (in)	53.4	54.5	56.2	58.2	60.2	61.9	63	53.4	54.5	56.2	58.2	60.2	61.9	63
	Height (cm)	135.6	138.3	142.8	147.8	152.8	157.3	160	135.6	138.3	142.8	147.8	152.8	157.3	160
	50th	98	99	101	102	104	105	106	60	60	60	61	62	63	64
	90th	111	112	113	114	116	118	120	74	74	74	74	74	75	75
	95th	115	116	117	118	120	123	124	76	77	77	77	77	77	77
	95th + 12 mm Hg	127	128	129	130	132	135	136	88	89	89	89	89	89	89
12	Height (in)	56.2	57.3	59	60.9	62.8	64.5	65.5	56.2	57.3	59	60.9	62.8	64.5	65.5
	Height (cm)	142.8	145.5	149.9	154.8	159.6	163.8	166.4	142.8	145.5	149.9	154.8	159.6	163.8	166.4
	50th	102	102	104	105	107	108	108	61	61	61	62	64	65	65
	90th	114	115	116	118	120	122	122	75	75	75	75	76	76	76
	95th	118	119	120	122	124	125	126	78	78	78	78	79	79	79
	95th + 12 mm Hg	130	131	132	134	136	137	138	90	90	90	90	91	91	91
13	Height (in)	58.3	59.3	60.9	62.7	64.5	66.1	67	58.3	59.3	60.9	62.7	64.5	66.1	67
	Height (cm)	148.1	150.6	154.7	159.2	163.7	167.8	170.2	148.1	150.6	154.7	159.2	163.7	167.8	170.2
	50th	104	105	106	107	108	108	109	62	62	63	64	65	65	66
	90th	116	117	119	121	122	123	123	75	75	75	76	76	76	76
	95th	121	122	123	124	126	126	127	79	79	79	79	80	80	81
	95th + 12 mm Hg	133	134	135	136	138	138	139	91	91	91	91	92	92	93
14	Height (in)	59.3	60.2	61.8	63.5	65.2	66.8	67.7	59.3	60.2	61.8	63.5	65.2	66.8	67.7
	Height (cm)	150.6	153	156.9	161.3	165.7	169.7	172.1	150.6	153	156.9	161.3	165.7	169.7	172.1
	50th	105	106	107	108	109	109	109	63	63	64	65	66	66	66
	90th	118	118	120	122	123	123	123	76	76	76	76	77	77	77
	95th	123	123	124	125	126	127	127	80	80	80	80	81	81	82
	95th + 12 mm Hg	135	135	136	137	138	139	139	92	92	92	92	93	93	94

TABLE 44.3	Blood Pressure (BP) Levels for Girls by Age and Height Percentile—cont'd													
		SBP (mm Hg)							DBP (mm Hg)						
Age (y)	BP Percentile	Height Percentile or Measured Height							Height Percentile or Measured Height						
15	Height (in)	59.7	60.6	62.2	63.9	65.6	67.2	68.1	59.7	60.6	62.2	63.9	65.6	67.2	68.1
	Height (cm)	151.7	154	157.9	162.3	166.7	170.6	173	151.7	154	157.9	162.3	166.7	170.6	173
	50th	105	106	107	108	109	109	109	64	64	64	65	66	67	67
	90th	118	119	121	122	123	123	124	76	76	76	77	77	78	78
	95th	124	124	125	126	127	127	128	80	80	80	81	82	82	82
	95th + 12 mm Hg	136	136	137	138	139	139	140	92	92	92	93	94	94	94
16	Height (in)	59.9	60.8	62.4	64.1	65.8	67.3	68.3	59.9	60.8	62.4	64.1	65.8	67.3	68.3
	Height (cm)	152.1	154.5	158.4	162.8	167.1	171.1	173.4	152.1	154.5	158.4	162.8	167.1	171.1	173.4
	50th	106	107	108	109	109	110	110	64	64	65	66	66	67	67
	90th	119	120	122	123	124	124	124	76	76	76	77	78	78	78
	95th	124	125	125	127	127	128	128	80	80	80	81	82	82	82
	95th + 12 mm Hg	136	137	137	139	139	140	140	92	92	92	93	94	94	94
17	Height (in)	60.0	60.9	62.5	64.2	65.9	67.4	68.4	60.0	60.9	62.5	64.2	65.9	67.4	68.4
	Height (cm)	152.4	154.7	158.7	163.0	167.4	171.3	173.7	152.4	154.7	158.7	163.0	167.4	171.3	173.7
	50th	107	108	109	110	110	110	111	64	64	65	66	66	66	67
	90th	120	121	123	124	124	125	125	76	76	77	77	78	78	78
	95th	125	125	126	127	128	128	128	80	80	80	81	82	82	82
	95th + 12 mm Hg	137	137	138	139	140	140	140	92	92	92	93	94	94	94

DBP, Diastolic blood pressure; *SBP,* systolic blood pressure.

The 50th, 90th, and 95th percentiles were derived by using quantile regression on the basis of normal-weight children (BMI < 85th percentile). Adapted from Flynn JT, Kaelber DC, Baker-Smith CM, et al. Clinical practice guideline for screening and management of high blood pressure in children and adolescents. *Pediatrics.* 2017;140:e20171904.

hypertension" has been estimated to be lower, around 3.5%.[2] Even with the most recent guidelines lowering the threshold for diagnosing hypertension for adolescents, recent estimates suggest that the prevalence of stage 1 hypertension remains between 2% and 4%.[3,4]

Etiology

Blood pressure is determined by the product of cardiac output and systemic vascular resistance. Therefore, anything that increases either cardiac output (stroke volume × heart rate) or systemic vascular resistance will increase blood pressure. The systemic vascular resistance, determined primarily by the smaller arterioles, is the primary driver of blood pressure at rest. Causes of increased cardiac output or increased systemic vascular resistance include coarctation of the aorta, renovascular disease, renal insufficiency, obstructive sleep apnea, or more rarely Cushing syndrome, pheochromocytoma, neoplasms, tuberous sclerosis, and others.[5]

Prematurity is associated with a relative paucity of nephrons, which can result in renal insufficiency and hypertension. Further, *in utero* exposure to hypertension or gestational diabetes increases the risk of CVD later in life.[6] A history of an umbilical catheter in the neonatal period can be associated with renal artery or vein thrombosis or can be a marker for exposure to nephrotoxic agents. Coarctation, even if well repaired, is associated with abnormalities in vascular response and as many as 75% of patients with coarctation develop hypertension.[6] Primary hypertension, the most common etiology in older children and adolescents, can occur in the setting of poor nutrition, inadequate physical activity, an elevated body mass index (BMI), or a family history of CVD.[5]

Screening, Diagnosis, and Evaluation

The recommendation to routinely screen youth for elevated blood pressure and hypertension is based on the findings that hypertension may be a sign of an underlying disorder, can lead to end-organ damage, and is associated with having hypertension during adulthood, and therefore the risk of CVD. For the general pediatric population, blood pressure screening should be performed annually beginning at age 3 years during routine clinic visits. For patients with certain risk factors, such as obesity, prematurity, coarctation of the aorta, diabetes mellitus, renal disease, or those taking medications that increase blood pressure, blood pressure should be measured at each encounter.[2]

In the evaluation of patients with elevated blood pressure or suspected hypertension, an accurate measurement is essential. The diagnosis of hypertension is based on auscultatory blood pressure measurements in a clinic setting over three clinic visits. To obtain a clinic blood pressure, the patient should be seated in a quiet room for several minutes, with feet on the floor and arm resting at the level of the heart. The blood pressure should be taken using a cuff size appropriate for the patient's arm circumference (bladder length should be 80–100% of the circumference of the arm and the width should be at least 40%). Further, it is recommended that the blood pressure be obtained in the right arm if at all possible for consistency and because the left arm may lead to a falsely low reading in the setting of coarctation. However, in patients with a right aortic arch and coarctation, an isolated aberrant right subclavian artery, or known obstruction or injury to the right arm arterial bed, measurements should be taken on the left arm to avoid falsely low blood pressure measurements.

If the initial blood pressure is above the 90th percentile in patients aged < 13 years, or ≥ 120 mm Hg systolic or 70 mm Hg diastolic in patients aged ≥ 13 years, two additional blood pressures should be obtained during the clinic visit.[2] To obtain a blood pressure in the leg (to assess for coarctation of the aorta), the patient should be in the supine position. The systolic blood pressure in the legs is normally 10–20% higher than the upper extremity blood pressure.[2]

To confirm a diagnosis of hypertension, obtaining a 24-hour ambulatory blood pressure monitor (ABPM) is recommended to assess the blood pressure in a nonclinical setting. The ABPM measures blood pressure several times an hour during waking hours and at least once an hour during sleep hours. An ABPM can identify patients with reactive ("white coat") hypertension (elevated clinic blood pressure with normal ambulatory blood pressure) as well as those with masked hypertension (normal clinic blood pressure, but elevated ambulatory blood pressure). It is the best test for understanding the patient's blood pressure response to sleep. The diurnal variation ("dipping") refers to the percent change in the mean blood pressure during the wake and sleep periods. An abnormal diurnal variation (i.e., blunted) is defined as having less than a 10% difference between the wake and sleep periods. A blunted diurnal variation can be evidence of coarctation of the aorta[7] or renal disease.[8]

In patients with confirmed hypertension, the initial evaluation should assess for secondary causes of hypertension (Table 44.4), evidence of end-organ damage, and comorbidities associated with hypertension (e.g., dyslipidemia and

TABLE 44.4 Secondary Causes of Hypertension and Preferred Blood Pressure-Lowering Agent

Condition	Agent of Choice
Renovascular hypertension	ACE-I ARB Diuretic Vasodilator
Chronic kidney disease	ACE-I ARB
Acute nephritis	Diuretic Vasodilator
Proteinuria	ACE-I ARB
Plasma renin-activity abnormalities	
Non-suppressed (normal-high)	ACE-I ARB
Suppressed (low)	Vasodilator Diuretic
Diabetes mellitus	ACE-I ARB
Obesity-related hypertension	ACE-I ARB
Athlete with hypertension	ACE-I ARB CCB
Coarctation of aorta	Beta-blocker
Apparent mineralocorticoid excess	Spironolactone or eplerenone
Glucocorticoid remedial aldosteronism	Amiloride or triamterene Glucocorticoid
Congenital adrenal hyperplasia	Spironolactone or eplerenone
Liddle syndrome	Amiloride or triamterene
Gordon syndrome	Thiazide

ACE-I, Angiotensin converting enzyme inhibitor; *ARB,* angiotensin II receptor blocker; *CCB,* calcium channel blocker.

insulin resistance). Initial studies for those with confirmed elevated blood pressure or hypertension should include a chemistry panel with creatinine and blood urea nitrogen, and urinalysis. A lipid panel (non-fasting total cholesterol [TC] and HDL cholesterol is appropriate) should also be considered to assess for additional CVD risk factors and in those with obesity, obtaining a glycated hemoglobin and serum alanine transaminase is recommended. Due to the increased incidence of renal disease in hypertensive patients aged less than 6 years, a renal ultrasound with Doppler should be obtained; a renal ultrasound with Doppler should be obtained regardless of age if renovascular disease is suspected. If there is a high degree of suspicion for renal artery stenosis based on ultrasound (renal size discrepancy, concern on ultrasound, hypokalemia), computed tomographic angiography can be considered, as it has a higher sensitivity for detecting renal artery stenosis than a renal ultrasound, but does expose the patient to radiation.[2] Consultation with a nephrologist or radiologist helps determine the appropriate imaging modality in this setting.

Echocardiography is useful to assess for cardiac etiologies of hypertension, primarily coarctation, and to look for evidence of end-organ damage in the form of left ventricular hypertrophy or left ventricular dysfunction. An echocardiogram is typically obtained only after a patient is diagnosed with hypertension. Follow-up echocardiograms can be useful to monitor for changes in the ventricular mass in response to treatment; typically, the change in left ventricular mass is relatively slow, over the course of 6–12 months. Electrocardiograms are not helpful for patients with suspected or confirmed hypertension, as the positive predictive value in identifying left ventricular hypertrophy by electrocardiograph is low.

Treatment of Hypertension

While the benefits of reducing blood pressure in youth have been difficult to demonstrate in longitudinal studies, there is evidence that it reduces surrogate markers of CVD. Litwin et al.[9] demonstrated that left ventricular hypertrophy, a marker of increased CVD risk in adults, regresses with adequate blood pressure control. Further, youth with hypertension have been found to be more likely to have hypertension as adults,[10] pointing toward long-term benefits of blood pressure reduction during childhood.

Lifestyle Modifications

For children with stage 1 hypertension without evidence of end-organ damage, a structured intervention to improve health behaviors is the first step. All patients should be counseled to avoid tobacco; eat a diet rich in fruits and vegetables, whole grains, and lean proteins with a limited intake of foods with added sugar and sugar-sweetened beverages; obtain sufficient physical activity (i.e., ≥ 60 minutes of moderate-to-vigorous physical activity per day on most days); limit recreational screen time (i.e., less than 2 hours per day); and obtain sufficient sleep. Patients may also need to avoid medications that raise blood pressure, if possible. One important aspect of the diet is to recommend that the patient limit their sodium intake to less than 2300 mg per day.[2]

Pharmacotherapy

For patients with stage 1 hypertension with symptoms or evidence of end-organ damage or with stage 2 hypertension, pharmacotherapy is indicated. More urgent attention is indicated for those with neurologic symptoms or hypertensive urgency/emergency. The treatment goal for those under 13 years old is a systolic and diastolic blood pressure less than 90th percentile and for those 13 years and older, the goal is a systolic and diastolic blood pressure less than 130 mm Hg and 80 mm Hg, respectively.

The most commonly used medications have all been shown to reduce blood pressure effectively in youth (Table 44.5). While specific medications are indicated in certain circumstances, for most patients the best medications are the ones that sufficiently lower the blood pressure. Blood pressure medications are generally well tolerated with fewer adverse effects than are experienced by adults. However, there are certain contraindications for each of the medications. It should be remembered that it is not uncommon for patients to require more than one medication to adequately control their blood pressure, particularly those with secondary hypertension (e.g., coarctation, chronic renal insufficiency).

For the pediatric cardiologist, coarctation of the aorta is a common etiology of hypertension. The pathophysiology of hypertension in coarctation of the aorta is discussed elsewhere. It is estimated that over one-third of patients with coarctation will develop hypertension. While earlier age of repair appears to reduce the risk of hypertension,[11] other risk factors do not appear to be different from the general population. The recommendations for measuring blood pressure in patients with coarctation generally include obtaining blood pressure in all four extremities or at least in one upper and one lower extremity. However, the indications for assessing the severity of the blood pressure and subsequent treatment are not different than in the general population. One exception may be the inclusion of blood pressure measurement during exercise, although there are no clear-cut points for peak exercise blood pressure.

Dyslipidemia

Dyslipidemia refers to an abnormality in the cholesterol or triglyceride content of the lipoproteins including one or more of the following: (1) an elevated triglyceride level (i.e., hypertriglyceridemia); (2) a low HDL cholesterol level; (3) an elevated LDL cholesterol; or (4) a combination of these abnormalities. Two common lipid disorders in clinical practice are hypertriglyceridemia in the setting of insulin resistance and an elevated LDL cholesterol secondary to familial hypercholesterolemia (FH).

Population screening has identified that one in five school-aged children in the United States has an abnormal lipid level[12]; 7.1% of children and adolescents have an elevated TC and 6.4% have an elevated LDL cholesterol.[12,13] Obesity is an important driver of dyslipidemia; over 40% of children who are obese (i.e., BMI ≥ 95th percentile for sex, age, and height) have at least one lipid abnormality. However, an important proportion of children with dyslipidemia are of normal weight.[14] Severe dyslipidemias track into adulthood and are a risk factor for subclinical atherosclerosis and atherosclerotic cardiovascular disease (ASCVD),

TABLE 44.5   Commonly Used Blood Pressure-Lowering Medications

Drug	Age	Initial Dose	Maximal Dose	Dosing Interval	Formulations

ACE inhibitors - Contraindications: pregnancy, angioedema. Common adverse effects: cough, headache, dizziness, asthenia. Severe adverse effects: hyperkalemia, acute kidney injury, angioedema, fetal toxicity.

Drug	Age	Initial Dose	Maximal Dose	Dosing Interval	Formulations
Benazepril	≥6 y[a]	0.2 mg/kg per day (up to 10 mg per day)	0.6 mg/kg per day (up to 40 mg per day)	Daily	Tablet: 5, 10, 20, 40 mg (generic) Extemporaneous liquid: 2 mg/mL
Captopril	Infants Children	0.05 mg/kg per dose 0.5 mg/kg per dose	6 mg/kg per day 6 mg/kg per day	Daily to 4 times a day Three times a day	Tablet: 12.5, 25, 50, 100 mg (generic) Extemporaneous liquid: 1 mg/mL
Enalapril	≥1 mo[a]	0.08 mg/kg per day (up to 5 mg per day)	0.6 mg/kg per day (up to 40 mg per day)	Daily to twice a day	Tablet: 2.5, 5, 10, 20 mg (generic) Solution: 1 mg/mL
Fosinopril	≥6 y <50 kg ≥50 kg[a]	0.1 mg/kg per day (up to 5 mg per day) 5 mg per day	40 mg per day 40 mg per day	Daily	Tablet: 10, 20, 40 mg (generic)
Lisinopril	≥6 y[a]	0.07 mg/kg per day (up to 5 mg per day)	0.6 mg/kg per day (up to 40 mg per day)	Daily	Tablet: 2.5, 5, 10, 20, 30, 40 mg (generic) Solution: 1 mg/mL
Ramipril	—	1.6 mg/m² per day	6 mg/m² per day	Daily	Capsule: 1.25, 2.5, 5 10 mg (generic)
Quinapril	—	5 mg per day	80 mg per day	Daily	Tablet: 5, 10, 20, 40 mg (generic)

ARBs - Check chem 7 levels at baseline, 1–2 weeks after starting therapy, and at least yearly thereafter. Contraindications: pregnancy. Common adverse effects: headache, dizziness. Severe adverse effects: hyperkalemia, acute kidney injury, fetal toxicity.

Drug	Age	Initial Dose	Maximal Dose	Dosing Interval	Formulations
Candesartan	1–5 y[a] ≥6 y[a] <50 kg ≥50 kg	0.2 mg/kg per day (up to 4 mg per day) 4 mg per day 8 mg per day	0.4 mg/kg per day (up to 16 mg per day) 16 mg per day 32 mg per day	Daily to twice a day	Tablet: 4, 8, 16, 32 mg Extemporaneous liquid: 1 mg/mL
Irbesartan	6–12 y ≥13	75 mg per day 150 mg per day	150 mg per day 300 mg per day	Daily	Tablet: 75, 150, 300 mg (generic)
Losartan	≥6 y[a]	0.7 mg/kg (up to 50 mg)	1.4 mg/kg (up to 100 mg)	Daily	Tablet: 25, 50 100 (generic) Extemporaneous liquid: 2.5 mg/mL
Olmesartan	≥6 y[a] <35 kg ≥35 kg	— 10 mg 20 mg	— 20 mg 40 mg	Daily	Tablet: 5, 20, 40 mg Extemporaneous liquid: 2 mg/mL
Valsartan	≥6 y[a]	1.3 mg/kg (up to 40 mg)	2.7 mg/kg (up to 160 mg)	Daily	Tablet: 40, 80, 160, 320 mg (generic) Extemporaneous liquid: 4 mg/mL

Thiazide diuretics - Check chem 7 levels at baseline, 1–2 weeks after starting therapy, and at least yearly thereafter. Contraindications: anuria and sulfa allergies. Common adverse effects: dizziness, hypokalemia. Severe adverse effects: cardiac dysrhythmias, cholestatic jaundice, new-onset diabetes mellitus, pancreatitis.

Drug	Age	Initial Dose	Maximal Dose	Dosing Interval	Formulations
Chlorthalidone	Child	0.3 mg/kg	2 mg/k per day (50 mg)	Daily	Tablet: 25, 50, 100 mg (generic)
Chlorothiazide	Child[a]	10 mg/kg per day	20 mg/kg per day (up to 375 mg per day)	Daily to twice a day	Tablet: 250, 500 mg (generic) Suspension: 250/5 mL Extemporaneous liquid: 1 mg/mL

TABLE 44.5 Commonly Used Blood Pressure-Lowering Medications—cont'd

Drug	Age	Initial Dose	Maximal Dose	Dosing Interval	Formulations
Hydrochloro-thiazide	Child[a]	1 mg/kg per day	2 mg/kg per day (up to 37.5 mg per day)	Daily to twice a day	Tablet: 12.5, 25, 50 mg
Calcium channel blockers - Contraindications: hypersensitivity to CCBs. Common adverse effects: flushing, peripheral edema, dizziness. Severe adverse effects: angioedema.					
Amlodipine	1–5 y ≥6 y[a]	0.1 mg/kg 2.5 mg	0.6 mg/kg (up to 5 mg per day) 10 mg	Daily	Tablet: 2.5, 5, 10 mg Extemporaneous liquid: 1 mg/mL
Felodipine	≥6 y	2.5 mg	10 mg	Daily	Tablet (extended release): 2.5, 5, 10 mg (generic)
Isradipine	Child	0.05–0.1 mg/kg	0.6 mg/kg (up to 10 mg per day)	Capsule: twice daily to thrice a day; extended-release tablet: daily	Capsule: 2.5, 5 mg Extended-release tablet: 5, 10 mg
Nifedipine extended release	Child	0.2–0.5 mg/kg per day	3 mg/kg/day (up to 120 mg per day)	Daily to twice a day	Tablet (extended release): 30, 60, 90 mg (generic)

[a]Food and Drug Administration labeling for pediatrics.
ACE-I, Angiotensin converting enzyme inhibitor; *ARB,* angiotensin II receptor blocker; *CCB,* calcium channel blocker.
Adopted and modified from Flynn JT, Kaelber DC, Baker-Smith CM, et al. Clinical practice guideline for screening and management of high blood pressure in children and adolescents. *Pediatrics.* 2017;140:e20171904.

making it important to identify and treat some lipid disorders in childhood.[13]

Etiology

The lipids found in humans include sterols (primarily cholesterol) and fatty acids. While dyslipidemia is associated with an increased risk of CVD, lipids are an important component of a number of physiologic processes. For instance, cholesterol plays a role in the fluidity of cell membranes, steroid hormones, and bile acids, while fatty acids are the primary energy store for humans, are a constituent of phospholipids, and play a role in cell signaling.[15] As lipids are hydrophobic, they need to be carried in the circulation packaged as lipoproteins. Lipoproteins are composed of cholesterol (free cholesterol and cholesterol esters), triglycerides, and apolipoproteins. Lipoproteins can be differentiated based on their content of triglycerides and cholesterol; size and density; electrophoretic properties; and composition of apolipoproteins. They are categorized as chylomicrons (and chylomicron remnants), very low-density lipoproteins (VLDL), intermediate-density lipoproteins, LDL, and HDL. The key to the physiology of the lipoprotein particle lies in its composition of apolipoproteins, which provide structure, act as ligands for receptors, and activate enzymes necessary for lipid metabolism.[16]

Screening, Diagnosis, and Evaluation

Identification of patients with dyslipidemia (Table 44.6) can be difficult as it is often asymptomatic, can occur in patients who appear otherwise healthy, and the family history often provides insufficient information to identify all patients. Therefore, both the American Academy of Pediatrics and an Expert Panel of the National Heart, Lung, and Blood Institute recommend screening all children once who are 9–11 years old and again between the ages of 17–19 years old. Children with a family history of premature ASCVD or very high cholesterol should be screened beginning at age 2 years. Screening can be performed by obtaining a non-fasting TC and HDL cholesterol level to calculate a non-HDL cholesterol (HDL cholesterol from TC and non-fasting lipid profiles are reasonably good screening tests). It is recommended that if the non-HDL cholesterol is higher than 145 mg/dL, a fasting lipid profile should be obtained on two separate occasions to assess risks and next steps.[17,18]

FH is the most common disease inherited in an autosomal dominant fashion, and the phenotype is seen in approximately 1 in 250 people. It is characterized by high LDL, generally ≥ 160 mg/dL in childhood in the heterozygous form and is most often caused by defects in the LDL receptor, but can also be a result of a gain-of-function mutation in the *PCSK9* gene or Apo B production. Without treatment, FH increases the risk of CVD by as much as 20-fold. Currently, patients with FH typically are classified as either having heterozygous or homozygous FH, but may be better classified based on the phenotypic severity of the disease. Patients with homozygous FH, which occurs in about 1 in 1 million individuals, have severely elevated LDL cholesterol levels, often above 800 mg/dL. Unlike those with heterozygous FH, patients with homozygous FH often present in childhood with xanthomas or a family history of

TABLE 44.6   **Lipid Disorders**

Disease	Causes/Variants	Lipids	Notes
Familial hypercho-lesterolemia (FH)	1) LDL receptor defect 2) APOB defect (familial defective Apo B-100) 3) PCSK9 4) LDLRAP1 (autosomal recessive hypercholesterolemia)	H ↑ LDL-C	• Heterozygous FH is the most common autosomal dominant inherited disease. • Defects in the LDL receptor are most common. • Patients with homozygous FH have LDL-C that is often above 000 mg/dL.
Familial chylomi-cronemia syndrome	1) LPL deficiency 2) APO-CII deficiency 3) LMF1 4) APO-A5 5) GP1HBP1 (structural support protein for lipoprotein lipase)	↑TG	• Severely elevated TG levels, often >1000 mg/dL, but varies widely. • Primary treatment goal is lowering TG to reduce risk of TG-induced pancreatitis.
Lysosomal acid lipase deficiency (Wolman disease and CESD)	Defect in *LIPA* gene	↑ TG ↓ HDL-C	• Wolman disease is a more severe phenotype than CESD and presents in infancy with cholestasis, liver disease, failure to thrive, malabsorption, and adrenal insufficiency. • CESD presents later with liver disease and dyslipidemia.
Familial dysbetali-poproteinemia	Apo E-2 defect	↑ LDL-C ↑ TG ↓ HDL-C	• Diagnosis is made when the TG to Apo B ratio is < 10.
Familial hypertri-glyceridemia	Polygenic with VLDL production	↑ TG	• Often associated with other comorbidities, particularly insulin resistance.
Sitosterolemia	ABCG5/ABCG8	↑ LDL	• Hemolytic anemia and joint pain. • Often responds poorly to statins, but well to diet modification. • Patients may present with xanthomas with LDL-C levels lower than would be expected.
Cerebrotendinous xanthomatosis	Defect in 27-hydroxylase (CYP27A1)	↑ LDL-C ↓ HDL-C	• Primarily a neurologic disease secondary to cholesterol and cholestanol in the brain. • Symptoms begin in the second decade of life, with a diagnosis made in the third or fourth decade of life. • Additional symptoms include elevated cholestanol levels, increased bile alcohols in urine, jaundice, early atherosclerotic events, cataracts, chronic diarrhea, and osteoporosis. • LDL-C levels are lower than would be expected in the presence of xanthomas.

CESD, Cholesterol ester storage disease; *HDL-C*, high-density lipoprotein cholesterol; *LDL-C*, low-density lipoprotein cholesterol; *TG*, triglycerides; *VLDL*, very low-density lipoprotein.
Adapted from Circulation.2019;139:e603-e634, ©2019 American Heart Association, Inc.

severe hypercholesteremia. Unfortunately, if missed, patients may present in childhood or early adolescence with coronary ischemia. Patients with homozygous FH also are unlikely to respond to conventional medical therapy and must be treated with novel therapies often combined with weekly or biweekly LDL apheresis, despite being on multiple standard lipid-lowering medications.

The development of hypertriglyceridemia, either in isolation or in combination with other lipid abnormalities, is often multifactorial and influenced by genetics, health behaviors, and medications. Triglycerides are primarily produced by the liver or the intestine and delivered to the periphery packaged in VLDL or in chylomicrons,

respectively. Dysfunctional metabolism of either VLDL or chylomicrons can therefore lead to hypertriglyceridemia. In patients with insulin resistance, lipolysis of triglycerides by lipoprotein lipase in adipocytes and myocytes is unchecked. This leads to an increased return of fatty acids to the liver, which stimulates increased VLDL production by the liver. Insulin resistance also leads to an overproduction of both VLDL, by failing to properly limit apolipoprotein B production in the liver, possibly through increased expression of apolipoprotein CIII. In patients with severe hypertriglyceridemia (i.e., >400 mg/dL), these processes are compounded by delayed clearance of chylomicrons and chylomicron remnants.[19]

Management of Dyslipidemia

Lifestyle Modifications

All children with dyslipidemia should be counseled on a diet that is rich in fiber (fruits, vegetables, whole grains), lean protein, and poly- and monounsaturated fat. For those with hypertriglyceridemia, a focus on limiting the intake of sugar and simple carbohydrates should be emphasized, whereas in those with hypercholesterolemia (elevated LDL cholesterol), limiting saturated fats to less than 10% of total energy intake may be beneficial. Moderate to vigorous physical activity for at least 1 hour a day is recommended for all. In youth with dyslipidemia, one study showed lifestyle modifications initiated in the clinical setting were associated with an LDL reduction of 8–15% and triglyceride reduction of 27% (4–47%) over a 6-month period.[20]

Pharmacology for Hypercholesterolemia (Elevated LDL Cholesterol)

The indications for treatment are an elevated LDL cholesterol with cut points for pharmacotherapy related to the underlying risk of CVD (Table 44.7). High LDL cholesterol responds best to a lower intake of saturated and hydrogenated oils. All patients should be counseled to increase their intake of fruits and vegetables. Some patients, particularly those with the genetic disorder FH, do not respond sufficiently to lifestyle changes and require pharmacotherapy.

For the majority of youth who require lipid-lowering therapy to reduce their CVD risk, a statin is the preferred first-line medication (Fig. 44.1). Statins inhibit the enzyme HMG-CoA reductase, the rate-limiting factor in cholesterol synthesis, thus decreasing intracellular cholesterol levels. The reduction in intracellular cholesterol levels leads to increased production of LDL receptors, leading to improved clearance of LDL cholesterol. Depending on the statin and its dose, statins decrease LDL cholesterol by 25–45%.[21] As a rule of thumb, doubling the dose of a statin will decrease LDL cholesterol by an additional 6% from the baseline change. Statins also lower triglycerides by 15–30%. While cardiovascular events are exceedingly rare in youth, surrogate markers of CVD risk, such as carotid intima-medial

---

TABLE 44.7 Classification of Cardiovascular Risk Conditions and Lipid Treatment Thresholds for Children and Adolescents*

Category	Condition	Screening interval	Consider medication (mg/dL)	Goal level (mg/dL)
High risk	• Type 1 diabetes mellitus • Type 2 diabetes mellitus • End-stage renal disease • Kawasaki disease with persistent aneurysms (Zmax ≥ 2.5) • Solid-organ transplant vasculopathy • Childhood cancer survivor (or stem cell recipient) *Or* • Moderate risk *plus* > 2 at-risk factors	Every year	LDL-C > 130 *or* Non-HDL > 145 *or* TG > 400	LDL < 100 Non-HDL < 130
Moderate risk	• Severe obesity (BMI > 1.2 × 95th percentile) • Heterozygous familial hypercholesterolemia • Hypertension • Coarctation • Aortic stenosis • Elevated lipoprotein(a)* • Chronic kidney disease not requiring dialysis • Childhood cancer survivor or received chest radiation *Or* • >3 at-risk factors	Every 2 years	LDL-C > 160 *or* Non-HDL > 160 or TG > 400	< 130 or Non-HDL <130
At risk	• Obesity (BMI ≥ 95th percentile) • Insulin resistance with comorbidities (NAFLD, PCOS) • White-coat hypertension • Cardiomyopathy • Pulmonary hypertension • Chronic inflammatory conditions • Previous coronary artery translocation for anomalous coronary artery or transposition of the great arteries • Childhood cancer (cardiotoxic chemotherapy only) • Kawasaki disease with regressed aneurysms	Every 3 years	≥ 160	< 130 or Non-HDL < 130

BMI, Body mass index; *HDL-C*, high-density lipoprotein; *LDL-C*, low-density lipoprotein; *NAFLD*, non-alcoholic fatty liver disease; *PCOS*, polycystic ovarian syndrome; *TG*, triglycerides.

*Adapted from de Ferranti SD, Steinberger J, Amedur R, et al. Cardiovascular risk reduction in high-risk pediatric patients: a scientific statement from the American Heart Association. *Circulation*. 2019;139:e603–e634.

**Normal levels vary by assay.

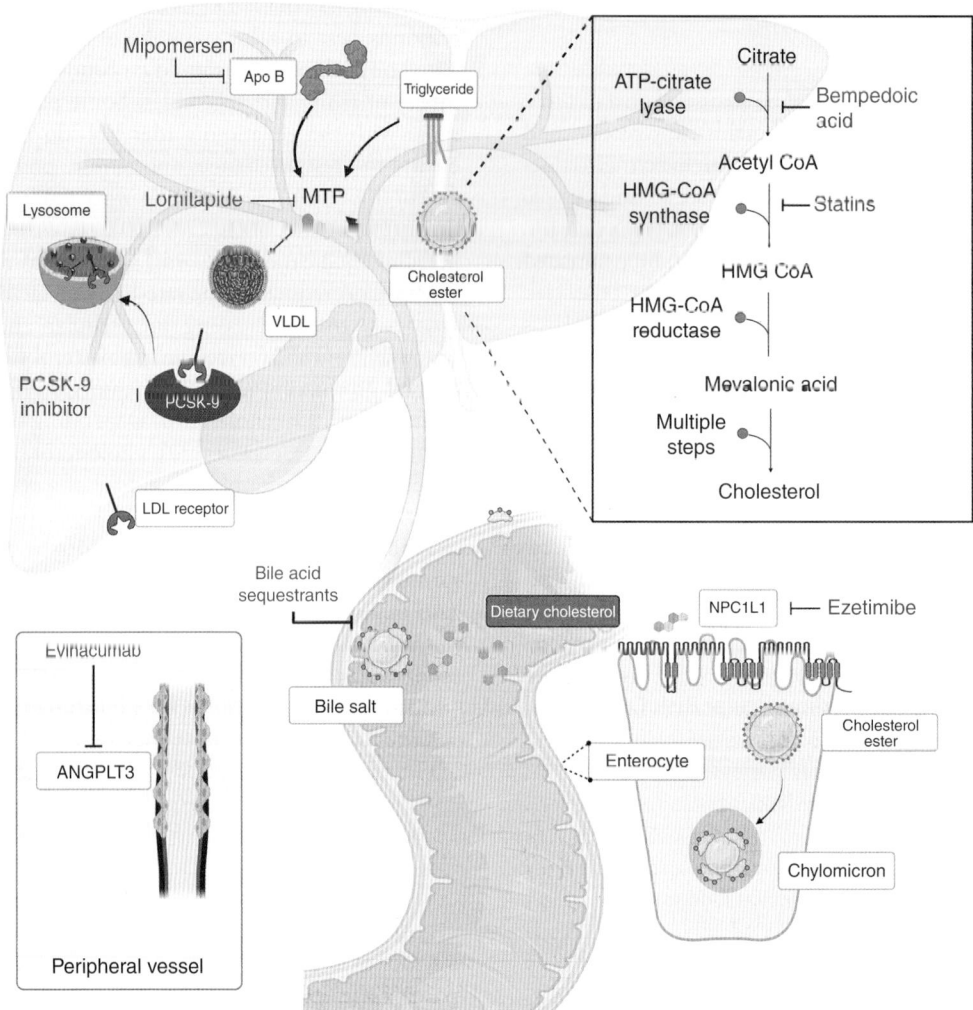

• **Fig. 44.1** Statins inhibit the production of HMG-CoA reductase which is the rate-limiting step in the mevalonate pathway, which produces cholesterol. Slightly upstream of HMG-CoA reductase is ATP citrate lyase, which is inhibited by bempedoic acid. Inhibitors of PCSK-9 reduce the breakdown of LDL receptors within the cell, leading to an increase in the availability of the receptor to uptake circulating LDL cholesterol. Bile acid sequestrates interrupt enterohepatic circulation, thus reducing cholesterol absorption from the small intestine. The mechanism of action of ezetimibe is not fully understood, but is currently thought to block NPC1 protein. This protein is important in the update of dietary and biliary cholesterol by the jejunum, which leads to an increased uptake of circulating LDL cholesterol. Mipomersen is an antisense oligonucleotide inhibitor of Apo B synthesis and reduces the production of Apo B. Lomitapide inhibits the action of microsomal triglyceride transfer protein *(MTP)*, which is critical to the assembly of the nascent Apo B and lipids into a lipoprotein. Evinacumab is a novel monoclonal antibody that inhibits angiopoietin-like protein 3. The role of angiopoietin-like protein 3 in lipid metabolism is still being understood. *ANGPLT3,* Angiopoietin-like protein 3; *Apo B,* apolipoprotein B; *ATP-citrate lyase,* adenosine triphosphate citrate lyase; *HMG-CoA synthase,* 3-hydroxy-3-methylglutaryl-CoA lyase; *LDL,* low-density lipoprotein; *NPC1L1,* Nieman Pick C1-like 1 protein; *PCSK-9,* proprotein convertase subtilisin/kexin type 9; *VLDL,* very-low-density lipoprotein.

thickness and flow-mediated dilation, improve in youth treated with statins.[22]

While a number of adverse effects are commonly attributed to statins, statins are generally well tolerated and adverse effects are rare. In randomized controlled trials in children with FH, rates of adverse effects do not differ between treatment and placebo groups. A small proportion of adult patients are not able to tolerate statins, but there was no significant difference in the rate of reported myalgias or discontinuation of statins as noted in a report by the American Heart Association.[22]

In patients who have a contraindication to statins or have not reached goal LDL cholesterol, **ezetimibe** is often recommended. Although initial trials showed mixed results regarding the efficacy of ezetimibe, the publication of the IMPROVE-IT study not only changed the perception of ezetimibe but also gave increased credence to the "LDL hypothesis."[23] When added to a statin, ezetimibe reduces LDL cholesterol by approximately 20% and triglycerides by 5–11%, and increases HDL cholesterol by 3–5%. Although adverse effects such as hepatotoxicity and myalgias have been reported, adverse reactions are rare.

Pharmacology for Hypertriglyceridemia

Hypertriglyceridemia is defined as a triglyceride level greater than 100 mg/dL for children less than 9 years old and greater than 130 mg/dL for youth over 9 years old. As triglycerides are typically much more responsive to lifestyle changes, treatment is primarily related to reducing the risk of pancreatitis. The goal of therapy is to reduce the presence of harmful apolipoproteins. Lifestyle counseling should be provided and physical activity is recommended for 60 minutes per day, most days of the week. Those with high triglyceride levels generally benefit from improving the quality and reducing the quantity of carbohydrates. Medications are indicated less frequently, except in the case of severe hypertriglyceridemia (i.e., >400 mg/dL) when the goal is to minimize the risk of acute pancreatitis. In patients with a normal LDL cholesterol, but a triglyceride level between 200 and 400 mg/dL, the decision to treat is based on the non-HDL cholesterol level or the apolipoprotein B level. For those patients, *statins* remain the first-line option as adult studies have demonstrated that they continue to have the strongest evidence for reducing CVD risk.[24]

The mechanism of action of *fibrates* likely includes increasing lipoprotein lipase activity, decreasing endogenous triglyceride production, and inhibiting peroxisome proliferator-activated receptor gamma. Fibrates are generally well tolerated but may lead to discomfort (e.g., diarrhea and gallstones), myalgias, and increased appetite. Fibrates also are generally contraindicated in patients with liver or kidney disease. However, when used to reduce severely elevated triglyceride levels, this risk should be weighed against the risk of triglyceride-induced pancreatitis. Gemfibrozil should not be used in combination with a statin because of an increased risk of myalgias. Fibrates have little-to-no role in the treatment of elevated LDL cholesterol.

The addition of polyunsaturated fats to the diet has a small, but statistically significant positive impact on CVD risk. Based on studies in adults, the use of one class of polyunsaturated fatty acids, *omega-3 polyunsaturated fatty acids*, has gained particular interest. Omega-3 fatty acids can be purchased as "fish oil," which is typically a combination of omega-6 fatty acids and omega-9 fatty acids. Although the formulation and dose ultimately determine the effects of omega-3 fatty acid supplements on the lipid profile, high doses (4 g/day) decrease triglycerides by approximately 30% while increasing LDL cholesterol by 6–8% and HDL cholesterol by 1–5%.[25] *Icosapent ethyl (Vascepa®)*, which is the purified form of the omega-3 fatty acid, eicosapentaenoic acid (EPA), was shown in the Reduction of Cardiovascular Events with Icosapent Ethyl–Intervention Trial (REDUCE-IT)[5] to reduce the risk of the CVD events by approximately 25%. However, the Long-Term Outcomes Study to Assess Statin Residual Risk with Epanova in High Cardiovascular Risk Patients with Hypertriglyceridemia (STRENGTH)[26] was recently halted because of futility. The results of the STRENGTH trial along with concerns about the placebo used in REDUCE-IT have raised concerns about the benefits of purified omega-3 supplements in preventing CVD. In addition, omega-3 supplements have adverse effects that limit adherence, including bad taste, belching, a small risk of bleeding mostly for those on antithrombotics or anticoagulants, and an increased risk of atrial fibrillation.

Nicotine, Physical Activity, and Cardiovascular Disease

Tobacco

In large part, CVD is preventable. It is estimated that lifestyle behaviors such as avoidance of tobacco, a healthy diet, and sufficient physical activity account for approximately 90% of the risk for CVD.[16,27] While tobacco use among youth is at its lowest levels in decades, electronic cigarettes (also known as vaping products) have been increasing. In 2021, 13.4% of high-school students reported using a tobacco product, nearly 80% of which was in the form of electronic cigarettes.[23] While a number of the carcinogens in tobacco cigarettes are missing from electronic cigarettes, electronic cigarettes still contain nicotine and their use increases the chances of using combustible tobacco.[28] Nicotine is the primary culprit for the increased risk of CVD related to smoking, causing endothelial injury, the initial step in the development of atherosclerosis. Further, through its effects on the sympathetic nervous system, abuse of nicotine leads to an increased heart rate, blood pressure, and myocardial oxygen demand. Of the modifiable risk factors, using tobacco products as a child or adolescent was shown to be the strongest predictor for fatal CVD events (odds ratio 1.61, confidence interval 1.21–2.13).[29]

Physical Activity

Physical activity also modifies CVD risk. For instance, increased amounts of moderate-to-vigorous physical activity led to improvements in mean waist circumference, systolic and diastolic blood pressure, fasting insulin, fasting glucose, and fasting triglycerides.[30] The Cardiovascular Risk in Young Finns found that low physical activity was associated with accelerated progression of carotid intima-media thickness (CIMT) over 27 years of follow-up.[31] Recommendations for physical activity for youth from the 2018 Physical Activity Guidelines for Americans[17] are based on age. In children aged less than 5 years, it is recommended that they are active throughout the day. For older children, it is recommended that children receive at least 60 minutes per day of moderate-to-vigorous physical activity along with 3 days of muscle- and bone-strengthening activities. Importantly, cardiovascular health tends to track into adulthood, emphasizing the importance of early identification and treatment.[32]

The role of the diet in reducing CVD risk is largely based on observational studies. Perhaps the best evidence in children and adolescents comes from the Diet Intervention Study in Children.[24] This randomized controlled trial provided dietary counseling and evaluated the safety and efficacy of a reduced-fat diet in youth with elevated LDL cholesterol. While the changes in LDL cholesterol were small, there were no adverse effects of the low-fat diet. For this reason, the most recent recommendations in the 2019 ACC/AHA Guideline on the Primary Prevention of Cardiovascular Disease[26] avoided specific amounts of fats and carbohydrates and focused on encouraging the intake of fruits and vegetables, whole grains, and lean meats.

Conclusion

While CVD events are rare in children, there is substantial evidence that the factors for CVD are present in children and track into adulthood. The pediatric cardiologist will likely be asked to manage patients with various severities of hypertension and dyslipidemia. There is growing literature on the importance of early identification and treatment of these conditions with a combination of lifestyle modifications and medications.

References

1. Virani SS, Alonso A, Aparicio HJ, et al. Heart disease and stroke statistics 2021 update: a report from the American Heart Association. *Circulation.* 2021;143:e254-e743.
2. Flynn JT, Kaelber DC, Baker-Smith CM, et al. Clinical practice guideline for screening and management of high blood pressure in children and adolescents. *Pediatrics.* 2017;140:e20171904.
3. Bell CS, Samuel JP, Samuels JA. Prevalence of hypertension in children. *Hypertension.* 2019;73:148-152.
4. Song P, Zhang Y, Yu J, et al. Global prevalence of hypertension in children: a systematic review and meta-analysis. *JAMA Pediatr.* 2019;173:1154-1163.
5. Flynn JT, Urbina EM, Brady TM, et al. Ambulatory blood pressure monitoring in children and adolescents: 2022 update: a scientific statement from the American Heart Association. *Hypertension.* 2022;79:e114-e124.
6. Bald M, Neudorf U. Arterial hypertension in children and adolescents after surgical repair of aortic coarctation defined by ambulatory blood pressure monitoring. *Blood Press Monit.* 2000;5:163-167.
7. Hauser M, Kuehn A, Wilson N. Abnormal responses for blood pressure in children and adults with surgically corrected aortic coarctation. *Cardiol Young.* 2000;10:353-357.
8. de la Sierra A, Segura J, Gorostidi M, et al. Diurnal blood pressure variation, risk categories and antihypertensive treatment. *Hypertens Res.* 2010;33:767-771.
9. Litwin M, Niemirska A, Sladowska J, et al. Left ventricular hypertrophy and arterial wall thickening in children with essential hypertension. *Pediatr Nephrol.* 2006;21:811.
10. Chen X, Wang Y. Tracking of blood pressure from childhood to adulthood: a systematic review and meta-regression analysis. *Circulation.* 2008;117:3171.
11. Canniffe C. Hypertension after repair of aortic coarctation—a systematic review. *Int J Cardiol.* 2013;167:2456-2461.
12. Kit BK. Prevalence of and trends in dyslipidemia and blood pressure among us children and adolescents, 1999-2012. *JAMA.* 2015;169:272-279.
13. Nicklas TA, Von Duvillard SP, Berenson GS. Tracking of serum lipids and lipoproteins from childhood to dyslipidemia in adults: the Bogalusa Heart Study. *Int J Sports Med.* 2002;23:39.
14. May AL, Kuklina EV, Yoon PW. Prevalence of cardiovascular disease risk factors among US adolescents, 1999–2008. *Pediatrics.* 2012;129:1035-1041.
15. Carmena R, Duriez P, Fruchart JC. Atherogenic lipoprotein particles in atherosclerosis. *Circulation.* 2019;109:III2-III7.
16. Jacobson TA, Ito MK, Maki KC, et al. National Lipid Association recommendations for patient-centered management of dyslipidemia: part 1 - executive summary. *J Clin Lipidol.* 2014;8:473-488.
17. U.S. Department of Health and Human Services. *Physical Activity Guidelines for Americans.* 2nd ed. Washington, DC: U.S. Department of Health and Human Services; 2018.
18. Expert Panel on Integrated Guidelines for Cardiovascular Health and Risk Reduction in Children and Adolescents. Expert panel on integrated guidelines for cardiovascular health and risk reduction in children and adolescents. *Pediatrics.* 2011;128:S213-S256.
19. Hartz JC, de Ferranti SD, Gidding SS. Hypertriglyceridemia in diabetes mellitus: implications for pediatric care. *J Endocr Soc.* 2018;2:297-512.
20. Zachariah JP, Chan J, Mendelson MM, et al. Adolescent dyslipidemia and standardized lifestyle modification: benchmarking real-world practice. *J Am Coll Cardiol.* 2016;68:2122-2123.
21. Feingold KR. *Cholesterol Lowering Drugs.* South Dartmouth, MA: MDText.com, Inc.; 2000.
22. Vuorio A, Kuoppala J, Kovanen PT, et al. Statins for children with familial hypercholesterolemia. *Cochrane Database Syst Rev.* 2019;2019.CD006401.
23. Gentzke AS, Wang TW, Cornelius M, et al. Tobacco product use and associated factors among middle and high school students – National Youth Tobacco Survey, United States, 2021. *Morb Mortal Wkly Rep.* 2022;71:1-29.
24. Grundy SM, Stone NJ, Bailey AL, et al. 2018 AHA/ACC/AACVPR/AAPA/ABC/ACPM/ADA/AGS/APhA/ASPC/NLA/PCNA guideline on the management of blood cholesterol. *J Am Coll Cardiol.* 2019;73:e285-e350.
25. Balk EM, Lichtenstein AH, Chung M, et al. Effects of omega-3 fatty acids on serum markers of cardiovascular disease risk: a systematic review. *Atherosclerosis.* 2006;189:19-30.
26. Arnett DK. 2019 ACC/AHA guideline on the primary prevention of cardiovascular disease: a report of the American College of Cardiology/American Heart Association Task Force on clinical practice guidelines. *Circulation.* 2019;140:e596.
27. Yusuf S, Hawken S, Ounpuu S, et al. Effect of potentially modifiable risk factors associated with myocardial infarction in 52 countries (the INTERHEART study): case-control study. *Lancet.* 2004;364:937-952.
28. Soneji S, Barrington-Trimis JL, Wills TA, et al. Association between initial use of e-cigarettes and subsequent cigarette smoking among adolescents and young adults: a systematic review and meta-analysis. *JAMA Pediatr.* 2017;171:788-797.
29. Jacobs D, Woo J, Sinaiko A, et al. Childhood cardiovascular risk factors and adult cardiovascular events. *N Engl J Med.* 2022;386:1877-1888.
30. Ekelund U. Independent associations of physical activity and cardiorespiratory fitness with metabolic risk factors in children: The European youth heart study. *Diabetologia.* 2007;50:1832-1840.
31. Juonala M, Viikari JS, Raitakari OT. Main findings from the prospective Cardiovascular Risk in Young Finns Study. *Curr Opin Lipidol.* 2013;24:57-64.
32. Telama R, Yang X, Leskinen E, et al. Tracking of physical activity from early childhood through youth into adulthood. *Med Sci Sports Exerc.* 2014;46:955-962.

45

Rheumatic Fever and Rheumatic Heart Disease

R. KRISHNA KUMAR

KEY LEARNING POINTS

- Rheumatic fever (RF) and rheumatic heart disease (RHD) have largely become confined to the poorest and marginalized populations across the globe; low- and middle-income countries have a substantial burden of disease.
- The entity of subclinical RHD is now well accepted, as a number of asymptomatic individuals can be identified through echocardiographic screening in endemic regions.

- The diagnostic criteria for RF are now context specific with different thresholds for high- and low-risk populations. Subclinical carditis is now included as a major criterion.
- Penicillin continues to be the cornerstone of primary and secondary prevention of RF and RHD.
- Public health initiatives to reduce burden of RF and RHD require strengthening of primary care services, maintenance of disease registries, and attention to the care continuum.

Introduction

Rheumatic fever (RF), although still without precise pathogenesis, is considered to be a delayed autoimmune reaction in predisposed individuals to group A, β-hemolytic, streptococcal infection. It is a self-limited disease that typically involves the joints, skin, brain, serous surfaces, and heart. Rheumatic heart disease (RHD) results from damage to the heart valves and the supporting tensor apparatus, which is perhaps the only long-term consequence of RF.

While it is traditionally believed that immune responses to streptococcal infections manifest as clinically overt episodes of acute rheumatic fever (ARF), it is now increasingly apparent that clinically silent smoldering inflammation of the valve may also contribute to the development of RHD. This covert phenomenon is demonstrable through echocardiographic screening of populations in endemic regions.[1]

Epidemiology

"In the 1920s RF was the leading cause of death in individuals between 5 and 20 years of age … in 1938 there were more than a thousand deaths in New York City alone ... In New England, childhood rheumatism accounted for nearly half of adult heart disease, and in Boston's crowded North End, hardly a family was spared"[2] (Fig. 45.1). In developed countries, RF and RHD had almost disappeared by the early 1980s. Some localized resurgences, peaking in 1985, then occurred.[3] The decline in RF incidence and RHD prevalence predated the introduction of penicillin and greatly accelerated thereafter.[4]

In stark contrast, RF and RHD remain a major problem in low- and middle-income countries that account for most of the global burden of 40 million patients with RHD.[5] It is increasingly apparent that the incidence of RF and prevalence of RHD mirrors human development and access to health care.[4] In the last three decades, RHD has become largely confined to the poorest and the marginalized populations across the globe where it is among the leading causes of death from heart disease in young adults.[4,5] The highest burden of disease is reported from many parts of Africa, the rural poor in South Asia, the aboriginal populations in Australia, and in select Polynesian nations.[5]

Echocardiographic screening has revealed the presence of clinically silent "latent rheumatic valve disease" that is largely confined to endemic regions.[1] Latent RHD has been shown to progress to clinically manifest disease and penicillin prophylaxis has been shown to prevent this progression.[6]

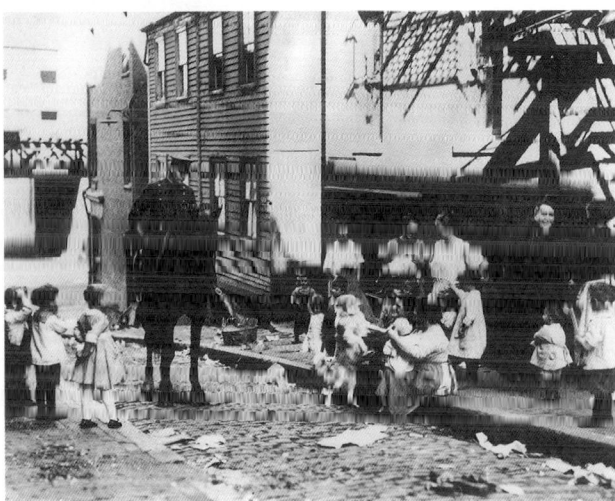

• **Fig. 45.1** Foster Street, North End, Boston, 1905. (Courtesy of Gates and Tripp.)

Pathogenesis

A "Social Disease"

RF is found mainly in poverty-stricken populations and marginalized communities. In the past, in the United States, it seemed to be predominantly a disease of the White ghettos and later a disease of Black populations. The complex interplay of factors relating to the agent, environmental, and host factors is depicted in Fig. 45.2. An understanding of these factors enables planning prevention at various stages of the RF-RHD continuum.

Group A Streptococcal Pharyngitis

Since Cheadle's[7] Harveian lectures first published in 1889, physicians have noted that pharyngitis often occurs a week or so before the onset of RF and that, at least in temperate climates, there is a seasonal incidence of RF. Throat cultures often grew β-hemolytic streptococci. Still, it was not generally accepted until the early 1960s that group A, β-hemolytic streptococcal infection invariably preceded an attack of ARF. The convincing evidence was the high rising levels of streptococcal antibodies (antistreptolysin O) in the sera of children with active RF. With the acceptance of group A, β-hemolytic streptococcal pharyngitis as being inextricably involved in the pathogenesis of RF, research focused sharply on the streptococcus as a causative agent. The following observations must be reconciled in any theory of the causation of RF:

1. The youngest age at which RF occurs is about 2 years, with the disease being rare in the third year. The age range at which a child has a first attack of RF is 5–15 years, the average being 8 years.
2. There is a latent period from the onset of streptococcal infection to the onset of RF (average, 18 days).
3. At most, during an epidemic of β-hemolytic streptococcal pharyngitis, RF occurs in 3% of untreated patients.
4. Chorea may manifest without evidence of preceding streptococcal infection, yet it may be followed some years later by mitral stenosis (MS).
5. The dramatic inflammatory suppression by adrenocorticotropic hormone or cortisone suggests that an immunologic mechanism is involved in the pathogenesis.
6. RF primarily damages the mitral valve, to a lesser extent the aortic valve, rarely the tricuspid valve, and extremely rarely the pulmonary valve.
7. Group A, β-hemolytic streptococcal pharyngitis in a child who has recovered from RF is likely to reactivate the disease; indeed, the second attack is likely to mimic the first in its manifestations.
8. Data from most regions of the world indicate that ARF occurs following pharyngeal infection with group A streptococcus (GAS). However, based on recent evidence from Aboriginal and Torres Strait Islander children who suffer the highest rates of ARF globally, GAS skin infections may also be responsible for ARF.[8] They have a low throat carriage rate of GAS but extremely high prevalence of impetigo from GAS.[8]

Genetic Factors

There is a tendency for clustering of ARF cases within families with a higher concordance among monozygotic twins than dizygotic twins (44% vs. 12%).[9] The exact basis of this genetic susceptibility is unclear and perhaps polygenic.

Several genes may confer susceptibility to ARF and RHD through alleles that code for proteins involved in both the innate and adaptive immune response to GAS infection.[9]

Pathogenetic Hypotheses

Despite extensive experience with and investigation of RF, questions remain about its exact pathogenesis. What is known is that of the streptococcal subgroups, group A is the most pathogenic to humans. In this group, the virulence of the organism appears to be related to its M-protein, of which there are at least 130 varieties. The exact basis of rheumatogenicity of the specific GAS strains is still elusive. It is postulated that the group A, β-hemolytic streptococcus with the appropriate M-protein with antigenic similarities with molecules found in the heart, synovium, basal ganglia, and subcutaneous tissues (molecular mimicry) adheres to the pharyngeal mucosa of the genetically susceptible host.[10] Antigens and superantigens are then produced that activate T-cell and B-cell lymphocytes, which produce cytokines and antibodies directed against these molecules (Fig. 45.3).

An alternative hypothesis, "neo-antigen" theory, postulates that a complex is formed between type IV collagen and the M-protein within the subendothelial collagen matrix that triggers the formation of anticollagen antibodies resulting in persistent inflammation of the heart valves.[11]

From a clinical standpoint, the following scenario seems reasonable. In a genetically susceptible individual, repeated,

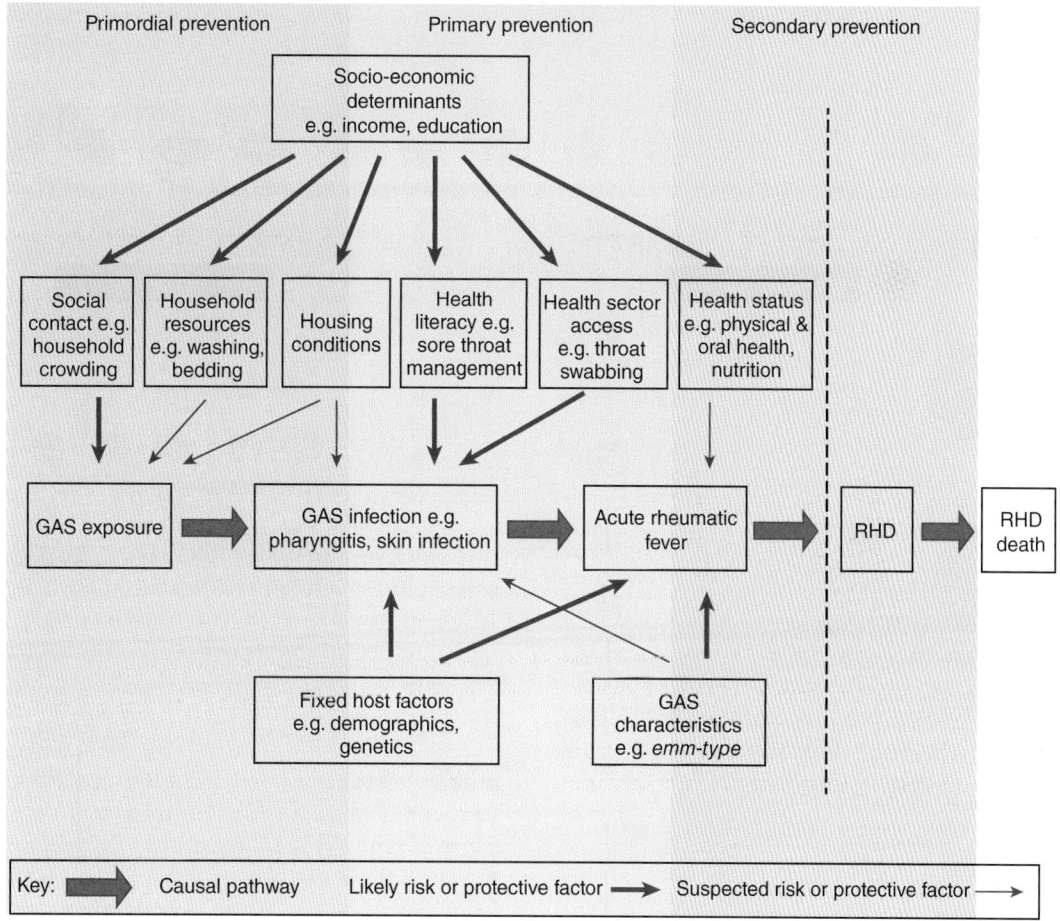

• **Fig. 45.2** Major hypothesized risk and protective factors along the causal pathway from group A streptococcal exposure to acute rheumatic fever and rheumatic heart disease. *ETS*, environmental tobacco smoke; *GAS*, group A streptococcus; *RHD*, rheumatic heart disease. (From Dougherty S, Okello E, Mwangi J, et al. Rheumatic heart disease. *J Am Coll Cardiol.* 2023;81: 81–94.)

untreated streptococcal infections in early life sensitize the child to the possibility of RF. Sometime after the age of 2 years, a group A, β-hemolytic streptococcal infection sets off an unusually high antibody response. After recovery from the infection, there is a 10-day latent period of relative well-being, following which an autoimmune response involving the excess streptococcal antibodies begins, lasts many weeks, and gradually damages the left heart valves. Later, a recurrent streptococcal infection may reactivate the disease. There is continuing valve damage after clinical evidence of rheumatic activity has subsided. The demonstration of subclinical valve affliction through echocardiographic screening supports the persistence of smoldering activity that is likely to scar the valves over time.[1]

Pathology

There are inflammatory lesions in the heart, blood vessels, brain, and serous surfaces of the joints and pleura. The pathologic picture is characterized by a distinctive and pathognomonic granuloma, consisting of perivascular infiltration of cells and fibrinoid protoplasm (Aschoff bodies).

Aschoff bodies (Fig. 45.4) are found in all patients with clinical rheumatic activity, in those who have died after RF, and in many with chronic rheumatic valvar abnormalities as well,[12] suggesting that many patients with this disease have subclinical, active, RF smoldering for years.

As many as half of patients with a first attack of RF have valve involvement.

The mitral valve is most commonly involved, being at first incompetent and, later, in some patients, becoming stenotic. Both stenosis and regurgitation are the result of extensive fibrosis or scarring of the valve leaflets and the tensor apparatus. MS results from a relatively uniform scarring with fusion of the leaflets at the commissures, while mitral regurgitation (MR) is the result of disproportionate restriction of motility of one of the leaflets (typically the posterior leaflet) with non-coaptation of the leaflets at the commissures. The resultant jet of MR is typically directed posteriorly and laterally. These features are readily demonstrable through conventional echocardiography (Fig. 45.5; Video 45.1).

When first involved, the aortic valve becomes incompetent, but unlike the mitral valve, almost never becomes stenotic. Aortic regurgitation (AR) does occur as a solitary

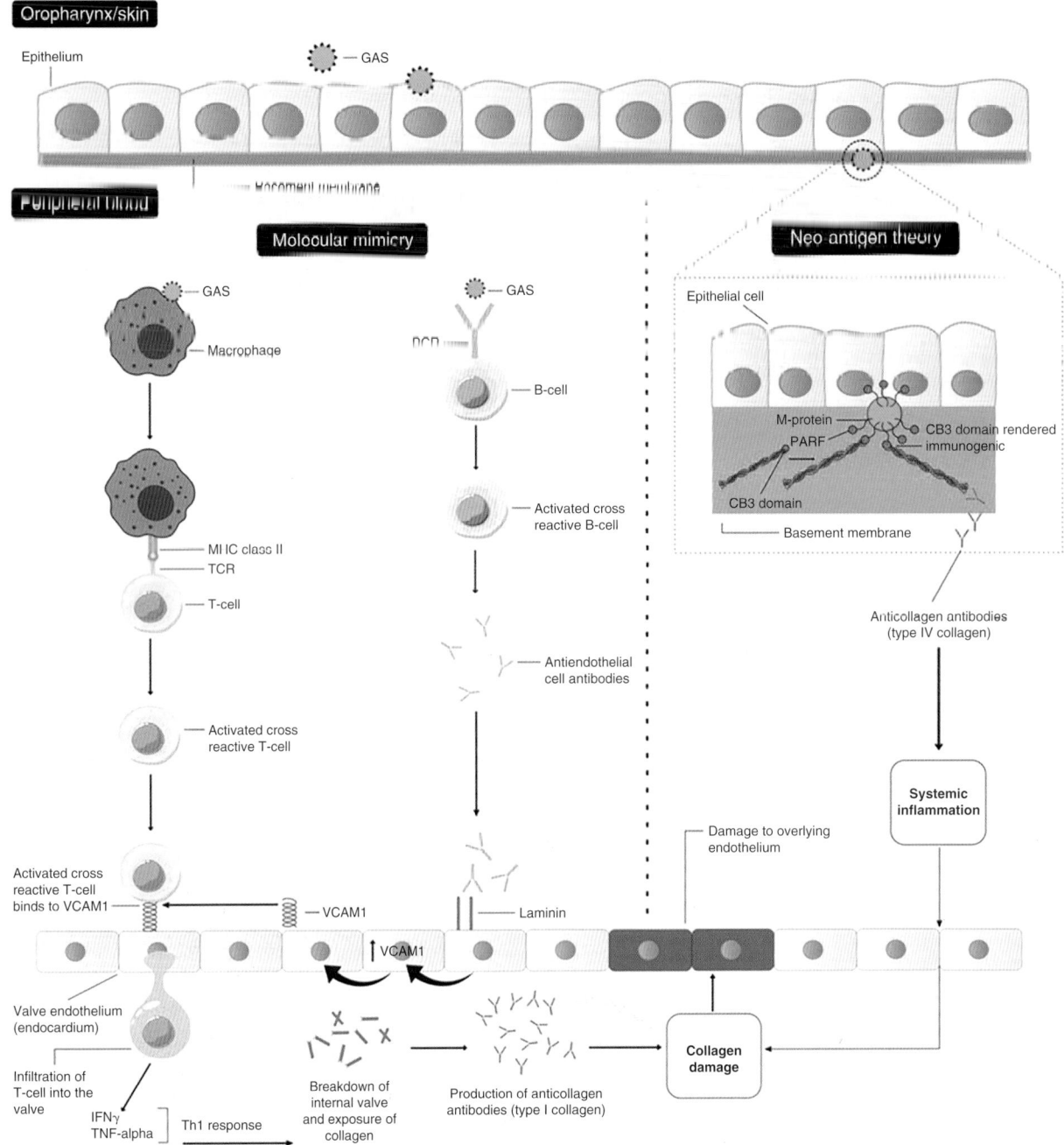

• **Fig. 45.3** Proposed pathogenesis of acute rheumatic fever in the heart tissues. Molecular mimicry theory (left-side): following infection, group A streptococcus (GAS) adheres to and invades the epithelial surface of the pharynx or skin, resulting in activation of both B- and T-cells in the peripheral blood. The activated B-cells generate antibodies (antiendothelial cell antibodies; AECAs) against the M-protein or GAS group A carbohydrate antigen (GlcNAc). AECAs bind to the endothelium that line the surface of heart valves (endocardium), upregulating (vascular cell adhesion molecule 1) (VCAM1). Upregulated VCAM1 allows activated T-cells (primarily CD4+ T-cells) to infiltrate into the avascular valve matrix, producing Aschoff bodies or granulomatous lesions underneath the endocardium and a Th1 response, all of which lead to valve breakdown, remodeling, and malformation. Breakdown of the valve also leads to exposure of type I collagen, resulting in further immune-mediated damage to the valve. Neo-antigen theory (right side): following infection, GAS enters the epithelial basement membrane in the pharynx or skin. An octapeptide motif on the GAS M-protein called peptide associated with rheumatic fever (PARF) binds to the CB3 region of type IV collagen (present in the basement membrane), which renders the CB3 domain immunogenic. Autoantibodies are then directed against type IV collagen resulting in systemic inflammation. Owing to the similarities between various forms of collagen, these antibodies may then target type I collagen in the valve, resulting in damage to the overlying valvular endothelium, leading to valve breakdown, remodeling, and malformation. *MHC*, major histocompatibility complex; *TCR*, T-cell receptor. (From Dougherty S, Okello E, Mwangi J, et al. Rheumatic heart disease. *J Am Coll Cardiol*. 2023;81: 81–94.)

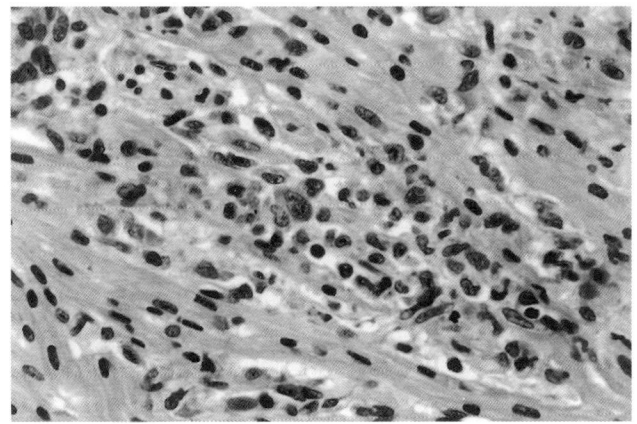

• **Fig. 45.4** Granulomatous stage of an Aschoff nodule showing central necrosis with fibrinoid degeneration and a mixed inflammatory infiltrate of lymphocytes, plasma cells, and large histiocytic cells (Anitschkow cells). (Courtesy of Antonio Perez-Atayde, MD PhD, Department of Pathology, Boston Children's Hospital.)

lesion (5% of patients) but is more often seen in combination with MR. MR alone or associated with AR is by far the most common lesion, so much so that the diagnosis of RHD without mitral disease is suspect. Incompetent and even stenotic tricuspid valves are seen, and rarely an incompetent pulmonary valve is reported.

Clinical Manifestations

A history of pharyngitis is reported by about half of patients with ARF. Pharyngitis ranges from typical symptoms of streptococcal pharyngeal infection to vague symptoms of upper respiratory illness. With spontaneous subsidence of the sore throat, there is a latent period when the child is afebrile and seems well. About 10 days later, the child becomes ill again. At this point, elevation of the antistreptolysin-O titer is demonstrable, and throat culture may yield β-hemolytic group A streptococci.

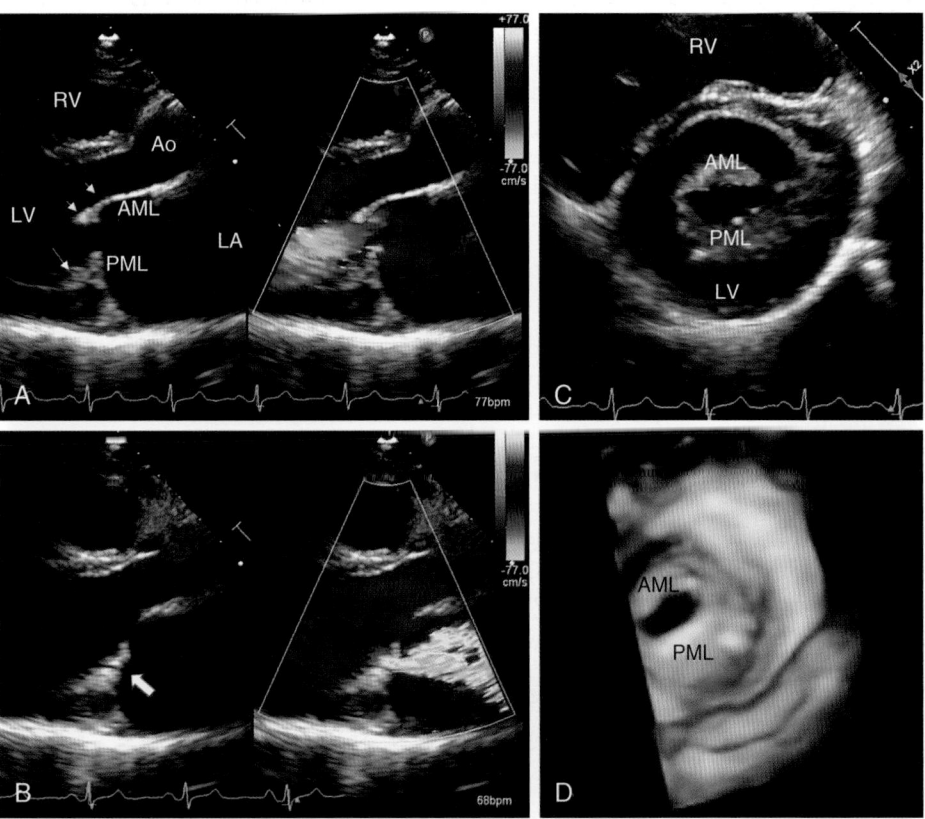

• **Fig. 45.5** Echocardiograms from a 18-year-old woman with rheumatic heart disease with mitral regurgitation and mitral stenosis. **(A)** and **(B)** Parasternal long- and short-axis views in diastole **(A)** and systole **(B)**. Note the thickened tip of the anterior mitral leaflet (*AML*, shown by *small yellow arrowheads*) together with the dog-leg or hockey stick appearance that results from relative fixity of the AML tip while the rest of the valve leaflet is mobile. Note also the thick posterior mitral leaflet *(PML)* together with the thickened chords *(white arrow)*. The mitral regurgitation seen in the systolic frame **(B)** results from reduced leaflet margin coaptation as a result of the relatively mobile free margin of AML. **(C)** A parasternal short-axis view of the mitral valve that demonstrates the stenotic orifice together with thickened AML and PML margins. **(D)** A frozen end-diastolic frame of a 3D echocardiogram with thickened leaflets and fused commissures. *Ao,* Aorta; *LA,* left Atrium; *LV,* left ventricle; *RV,* right ventricle.

The fever associated with ARF is not high, rarely over 103°F and sometimes recognized only with systematic recording on a temperature chart.

Polyarthritis

Most patients have some joint symptoms.[13] Several joints may be intermittently involved (polyarthritis), ranging from vague arthralgia to florid swelling, heat, redness, and demonstrable joint fluid. Occasionally, it is difficult to elicit objective evidence of arthritis; intermittent limping and other limitations of function to guard painful joints may be the only historical data. When there is active involvement (swollen, red, or tender joints), there is fever. The joints most involved are the knees, hips, ankles, elbows, wrists, and shoulders; characteristically the joint symptoms are migratory, rarely involving a single joint for more than 2 days. Unlike joint involvement in rheumatoid arthritis, the small joints of the hands and feet, the temporomandibular joints, and sternoclavicular joints are not commonly involved. The pain can be exquisite, the child reacting to any contact with the inflamed joint, including the weight of bed sheets. A swollen joint that is not tender results from some disease other than RF. The stage of acute arthritis associated with obvious fever is self-limited, commonly subsiding within a few days and rarely lasting longer than a month. It is a striking clinical observation that chorea and acute polyarthritis never occur together. This is readily believable because the combination of these two problems would produce memorable difficulties.

Carditis

Although roughly half of patients with RF have evidence of carditis on first examination, symptoms of congestive heart failure are relatively uncommon. When there is congestive failure, the patients are sometimes very ill with dyspnea, hepatomegaly, vomiting, tachycardia, and fever, as well as florid joint involvement.

When there is pericardial effusion, there may be cough and often precordial or left shoulder pain that varies with position.

Carditis is mainly manifested by the appearance of murmurs, of which the apical systolic murmur of MR is the commonest. It is characteristically blowing, of high frequency, and transmits to the axilla. It extends through most of systole, beginning with the first sound. Often, there is a short, apical, mid-diastolic rumble (Carey Coombs murmur) that does not signify MS. The presystolic crescendo of MS is not encountered in the first attack of ARF. A repeated, careful search for an early diastolic blowing murmur is required because there may be aortic insufficiency. Occasional rhythm irregularity can be documented with a variable 2:1 block. A friction rub indicates pericarditis. With pancarditis, there may be gross congestive heart failure, enlarged liver, visible pulsating neck veins when the patient is in the sitting position, shortness of breath, and pulmonary rales. It is increasingly recognized that carditis may not be apparent clinically but evident on echo as MR with morphologic changes.

Erythema Marginatum

In a small percentage of patients with active RF, a distinctive rash, erythema marginatum, may be observed. When present, it is virtually a certain sign of RF (Fig. 45.6). It is an irregular, geometric, circinate, marginate, red rash over the torso that is evanescent. This rash may be brought out by hot baths and does not itch.

Subcutaneous Nodules

Firm nodules over hard bony surfaces such as the elbows, wrists, shins, knees, ankles, vertebral column, and occiput are seen occasionally in patients with active RF. On microscopy, these structures resemble Aschoff nodules and almost invariably signify rheumatic activity. This phenomenon is uncommon in first attacks, generally being seen in patients who already have established RHD. Nodules are best detected under side-lighting when the skin is slowly moved over the bony surfaces such as the elbows or knees. Nodules are more often seen than palpated and are small, non-tender lumps attached to the underlying bone (Fig. 45.7).

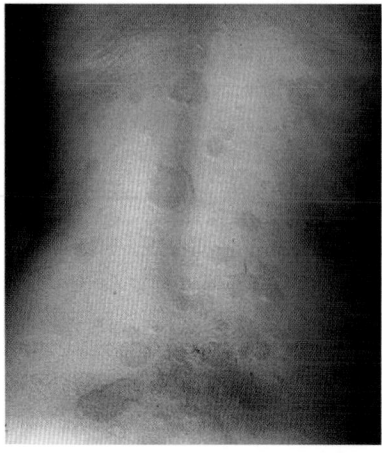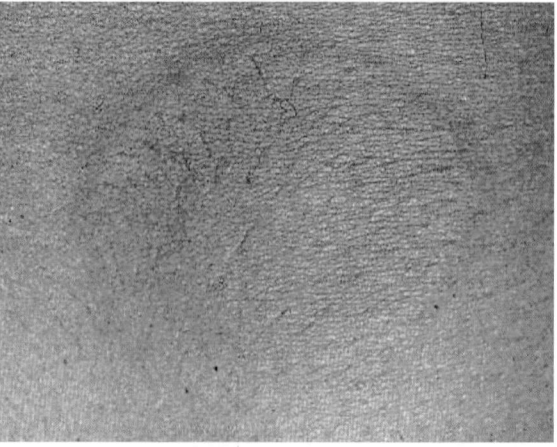

• **Fig. 45.6** Erythema marginatum of the thighs in an 8-year-old boy. (Courtesy of John K. Triedman, MD.)

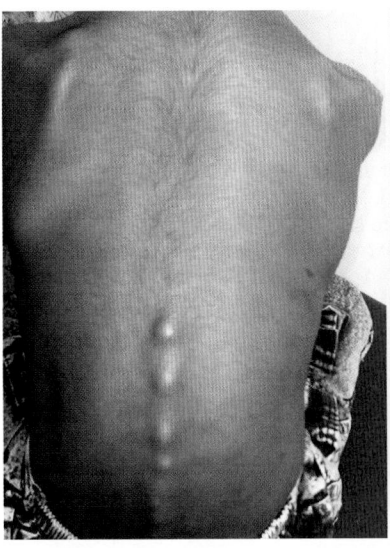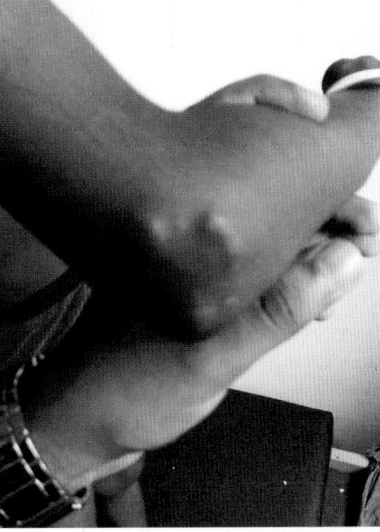

• **Fig. 45.7** Subcutaneous nodules in acute rheumatic fever. These are painless mobile nodules that are characteristically seen over bony prominences.

Chorea

Sydenham's chorea (St. Vitus' dance) is a distinctive clinical entity with virtually no differential diagnosis. There are purposeless, choreiform movements, aggravated by stress, in an emotionally labile child or young adolescent (usually female). Chorea is less common in older adolescents and is not seen in adults. There may be slurred speech, grotesque facial grimacing, and illegible penmanship. The outstretched hands assume a characteristic "spooning" position; asked to show the tongue, it flicks out and in like a snake's tongue; a fine tremor is palpable in the outstretched hands. In a severe attack, the child may be unable to feed, and the thrashing movements of the extremities may result in bruises. The more the parents chastise the child about spilling food, nervousness, and dropping things, the more the child's equanimity and coordination disintegrate. Often the onset of chorea is reported to have followed some major trauma such as a bad automobile accident.

Chorea may exist in two circumstances. It simply may be part of an otherwise active rheumatic process (almost never with simultaneous arthritis), in which case there is an elevated sedimentation rate, fever, and evidence of a preceding streptococcal infection; or it may be an isolated phenomenon (pure chorea) without evidence of rheumatic activity and no evidence of a preceding streptococcal infection.

Whether a child has chorea or not can usually be determined in the first minutes of the physical examination because the disease is readily recognized if it is has ever been seen before. If a question remains, the performance of the child should be observed under varying circumstances. The outstretched hands, the movements of the tongue, the ability to pronounce Methodist Episcopal or some other equally difficult phrase, the response to irritation (usually the examination alone is irritating enough), and the inability to write may resolve the question.

Abdominal Pain

At intervals in the past, children were hospitalized for abdominal pain with fever and ended up with abdominal exploration for appendicitis, after which it was discovered that the child had ARF. Whether this abdominal pain is a consequence of pericardial effusion or inflammation of the abdominal serous surfaces is not clear.

Clinical Manifestations of Established Rheumatic Heart Disease

The clinical features of RHD are largely dictated by the severity of individual valve lesions. MR and AR are often well tolerated over several years before decompensation can set in. Commonly reported symptoms include fatigue, palpitations, and dyspnea on exertion. Poor growth may be noticeable in younger children. As the disease advances, there is further limitation in the functional status. MS is typically associated with progressive dyspnea on effort as a result of pulmonary venous congestion.

Right heart failure often results from back pressure effects of severe left-sided valve lesions with pulmonary hypertension and "functional" tricuspid regurgitation (TR). Occasionally, the tricuspid valve is also involved by the rheumatic pathology with resultant stenosis or regurgitation and in these situations the right heart failure is often pronounced.

A careful physical examination often allows accurate assessment of the heart valves affected and their relative severity (Table 45.1).

Ancillary Studies

Laboratory Tests

A throat culture from an untreated patient often grows hemolytic streptococci. The antistreptolysin-O titer is elevated and may continue to rise, sometimes to remarkably high levels, as the period of observation continues. Other indirect tests of infection, such as rapid antigen diagnostic tests, may be positive but do not provide strain virulence information.[14]

The sedimentation rate is almost invariably elevated, as is the C-reactive protein. The possibility of finding a normal

TABLE 45.1	Physical Examination in Rheumatic Heart Valve Disease*
Valve Lesion	Physical Examination Findings
Mitral regurgitation (MR)	Moderate and severe MR is consistently associated with left ventricular enlargement and a hyperdynamic apex. The first heart sound may be normal or loud in the presence of associate mitral stenosis. The second heart sound is widely split and the pulmonary component is loud. MR is severe with associated PAH. An apical pan systolic murmur accompanies moderate or severe MR. Mild MR may be clinically silent. Severe MR is accompanied by a third heart sound or an apical mid diastolic flow murmur that may not have a pre-systolic accentuation.
Aortic regurgitation (AR)	Moderate or severe AR is accompanied by LV enlargement as in MR with a displaced hyperdynamic apex. The aortic component of the second heart sound may be attenuated. The early diastolic murmur of AR is characteristically a high frequency, blowing with a decreasing intensity (decrescendo). The "peripheral signs" of AR are seen in moderate or severe AR and result from diastolic steal from the aorta. They include a wide pulse pressure and bounding pulses.
Mitral stenosis (MS)	Rheumatic MS has a characteristic set of physical findings that are quite specific. The first heart sound in loud; the second heart sound is closely split with a loud pulmonary component in severe MS. The onset of diastolic filling is typically heralded by a sharp opening snap (not heard in congenital MS or in calcified valves) followed by a rumbling low-pitched mid-diastolic murmur with a presystolic accentuation. In mild MS, often only the presystolic component is audible.
Tricuspid regurgitation (TR)	Severe tricuspid regurgitation is typically identified through elevated jugular venous pulsations with prominent systolic waves of TR. This may be accompanied by liver enlargement with palpable systolic pulsations. The pansystolic murmur of TR is often heard in the left lower sternal border in moderate or severe TR.

*Aortic stenosis and tricuspid stenosis are not included in this table because they are quite uncommon. Multivalve involvement is common in rheumatic heart disease and physical examination has mixed findings of individual lesions. The relative severity of individual valve affliction determines the dominant manifestation.

sedimentation rate in a child with a severely congested liver should be kept in mind but is rarely seen in practice. The sedimentation rate must be corrected for anemia because anemia is common in these patients.

Electrocardiogram

Roughly 20% of patients have a prolonged PR interval, particularly if repeated electrocardiograms are taken. Atropine shortens the prolonged PR interval to normal. Occasionally, patients have intermittent 2:1 block, and rarely complete heart block has been reported.

Chest X-Ray

The heart size may be variably enlarged if there is carditis (Fig. 45.8). Pulmonary venous congestion accompanies severe acute MR and severe MS.

Echocardiogram

The commonest echocardiographic finding in patients with ARF is MR that could be clinically silent. Specific criteria that suggests a pathologic MR include a color Doppler jet that is clearly seen in two views and is ≥ 2 cm long in one of them with at least one complete spectral envelope and a peak gradient ≥ 3m/s. Accompanying morphologic changes may be subtle in the first episode of RF unlike in established RHD. They include leaflet thickening and excessive mobility with "prolapse" of the leaflet margin (Video 45.1).[15] Flail leaflet margins resulting from ruptured cords are well

described and often result in severe MR. The simultaneous presence of AR although relatively uncommon, points specifically towards the diagnosis of RF. Isolated AR, on the other hand, is exceptional in RF. Additional findings include pericardial effusion. Ventricular dysfunction is most unusual in RF and suggests an alternative diagnosis such as myocarditis.

The echocardiographic features of established RHD correlate well with pathological findings (Fig. 45.5). Echocardiography enables confirmation of RHD, quantification of the severity of regurgitation or stenosis, assessment of physiologic consequences in the form of chamber enlargement, and pulmonary hypertension, detection of complications (such as endocarditis, atrial thrombi), and planning of surgery or catheter intervention.

Diagnosis

There being no specific tests for RF, T. Duckett Jones, in 1944, published clinical criteria for the diagnosis of RF that have had widespread use with periodic modifications over the years. In Jones's scheme, two major or one major and two minor criteria are required to make the diagnosis of RF. The most recent update in 2015 has fundamental modifications.[16] The criteria are now context specific with liberal thresholds for endemic regions with "high-risk populations" and relatively stringent thresholds for non-endemic regions with low-risk population. This takes into account the pre-test probability of RF based on prevalence of RHD in the population. Additionally, subclinical carditis identified through echocardiography is now a major criterion.

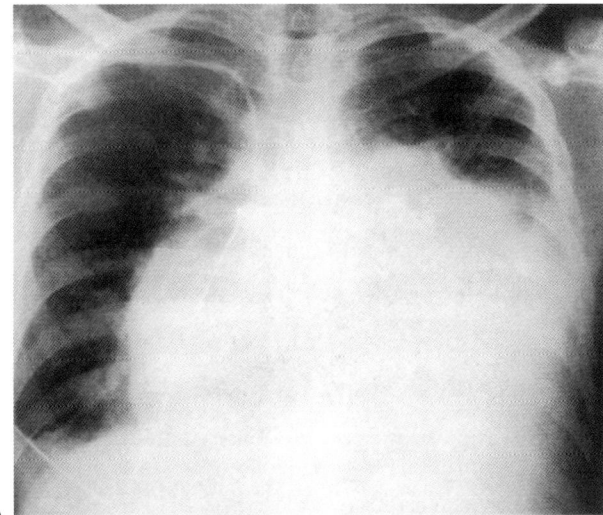

A

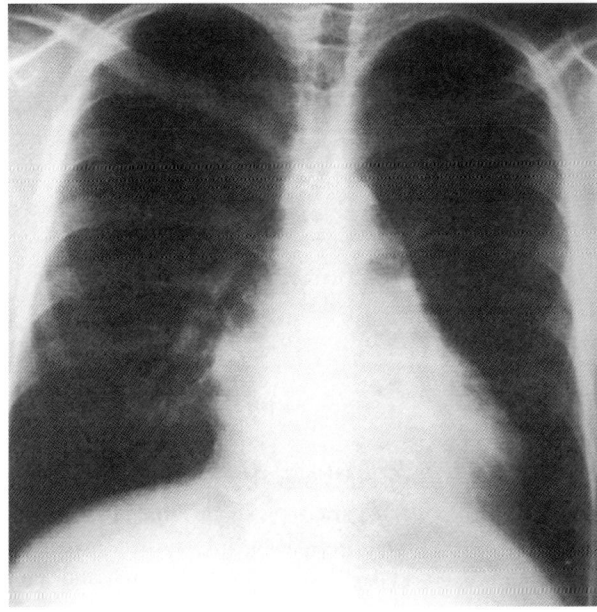

D

• **Fig. 45.8** Chest x-rays from a 14-year-old with active rheumatic fever for 8 months despite steroid and salicylate therapy. **(A)** Preoperative, without significant pericardial fluid. **(B)** Postoperative, following replacement of the mitral and aortic valves for gross congestive heart failure.

Finally, three minor criteria are sufficient for recurrences of RF. A summary of the revised criteria is presented in Table 45.2. While the revised Jones criteria should allow classification in the vast majority, the following situations merit specific consideration:

1. Chorea. For practical purposes, the presence of chorea alone proves the diagnosis of ARF. Confusion often arises when there is hemichorea or when the physician has not seen this disease. Usually, the diagnosis is self-evident.

2. Post streptococcal reactive arthritis. There is a sizeable group of patients who have arthritis, fever, and evidence of a preceding streptococcal infection. They are also labeled as having probable RF. For some of these patients, the diagnosis is ultimately shown to be erroneous, but

the group as whole tends to have a higher likelihood to develop valvar damage in significant numbers over the years.

For established RHD, there are now specific echocardiographic criteria developed by the World Heart Federation that are now used widely both to confirm diagnosis in individual cases and to screen populations.[15] These criteria include morphologic features of aortic and mitral valves as well as Doppler criteria for regurgitation of the mitral and aortic valves and stenosis of the mitral valve.[15]

Differential Diagnosis

The diagnosis of RF can sometimes be contested and needs to be distinguished from a few mimics.

Myocarditis

Apart from the clinical course, echocardiography, in a vast majority of circumstances, allows distinction between acute viral myocarditis and RF. Ventricular function is typically preserved in RF and MR is the dominant feature. Acute viral myocarditis is typically associated with varying degrees of ventricular dysfunction and MR is typically mild.

Rheumatoid Arthritis

Rheumatoid arthritis can be confused with ARF in two ways. With continued follow-up, the syndrome of arthritis, elevated antistreptolysin titer, and elevated sedimentation rate may turn out to be rheumatoid arthritis. One should be wary of this possibility, particularly if the joints involved are the small joints of the hands and feet. In any case, follow-up usually solves this problem.

A more pressing differential difficulty occurs when the patient has pericardial effusion, fever, evidence of a prior streptococcal infection, and an elevated sedimentation rate. Without murmurs typical of RHD, these patients have most often turned out to have rheumatoid arthritis or, rarely, lupus erythematosus.

Other Joint Diseases

Rarely, there may be more than one joint involved with septic arthritis. This differential resolves itself in days with observation. Trauma and aseptic forms of arthritis are almost invariably monoarticular and are usually readily recognized. For practical purposes, monoarticular arthritis is not RF.

Sickle Cell Disease

Sickle cell disease may mimic ARF in many respects, including cardiomegaly, systolic and diastolic murmurs, and joint pain. A family history may provide a clue, and a sickle cell preparation and electrophoresis of the hemoglobin will confirm the diagnosis.

Infective Endocarditis

Infective endocarditis may be the cause of fever in a child who has murmurs compatible with RHD. Differentiation

TABLE 45.2	Diagnosis of Rheumatic Fever, Revised Jones Criteria (2015) of American Heart Association and World Heart Federation
Low-Risk Population: Rheumatic fever incidence of < 2/100,000 in school going children; RHD prevalence < 1/1000)	**Moderate- or High-Risk Population:** Rheumatic fever incidence of ≥ 2/100,000 in school going children; RHD prevalence > 1/1000
Major Criteria	
Arthritis: polyarthritis only	Arthritis: polyarthritis or monoarthritis Polyarthralgia
Carditis, clinical or subclinical (identified through echocardiography)	
Chorea*	
Erythema marginatum	
Subcutaneous nodules	
Minor Criteria	
Polyarthralgia	Mono or polyarthralgia
Fever (>38.5°C)	Fever (>38.0°C)
ESR ≥ 60 mm in the first hour and/or CRP ≥3.0 mg/dL	ESR ≥ 30 mm in the first hour and/or CRP ≥ 3.0 mg/dL
Prolonged PR interval	

Minimum Requirements Common to all Populations:

- **Initial episodes of ARF:** two major or one major + two minor criteria
- **Recurrent episodes of ARF:** two major or one major + two minor or three minor
  Essential criteria: previous evidence of group A beta hemolytic streptococcal infection[#]

*The presence of characteristic rheumatic chorea in isolation is quite specific and does not require the simultaneous presence of other criteria or previous evidence of group A beta hemolytic streptococcal infection.
#Another possible exception for the essential criterion is in patients with longstanding or indolent rheumatic carditis.
ARF, Acute rheumatic fever; *CRP*, C-reactive protein; *ESR*, erythrocyte sedimentation rate; *RHD*, rheumatic heart disease.

between infective endocarditis and active RF may be difficult because both diseases cause murmurs and may be associated with elevated sedimentation rates and arthritis or arthralgia. Observation over a few days generally makes it possible to distinguish between the two possibilities. Any question of infective endocarditis is a mandatory indication for multiple blood cultures.

Management

Acute Rheumatic Fever (Table 45.3)

After throat cultures have been obtained, penicillin needs to be administered to eliminate the resident streptococcus. The doses used are therapeutic (600,000–900,000 U of benzathine penicillin intramuscularly for children, and 1,200,000 U for adolescents [or penicillin, 200,000 U orally, four times daily and continued until the patient has been treated for 10 days]). At that time, a preventive maintenance dose of penicillin is begun (200,000 U orally, twice daily, every day). Despite the absence of demonstrable streptococci or an elevated antistreptolysin titer, patients with chorea are given penicillin just like all others with ARF.

It is not necessary to limit physical activity in RF. Avoidance of vigorous activity is ordinarily left to the patient who, when sick, scarcely feels like moving around anyway.

Salicylates are used for control of pain and suppression of rheumatic activity in patients who do not have carditis or have only questionable evidence of cardiac involvement (Table 45.3). In those who cannot tolerate salicylates, a nonsteroidal anti-inflammatory drug such as naproxen (10–20 mg/kg/day) may be used. On the other end of the spectrum, it is mandatory that the child with pancarditis and congestive heart failure receives prednisone as a life-saving measure. There is room for debate about the use of prednisone for the child with valvulitis that is not life-threatening because unassailable evidence that further valve damage can be prevented is lacking.

Demonstrable response, often dramatic, occurs in 48–72 hours, and complete suppression in 7–10 days. The sedimentation rate returns to normal sooner when prednisone is used. After 2–3 weeks without clinical or laboratory evidence of activity, the dose of prednisone can be tapered and aspirin added while observing the response. Sometimes there is a reappearance of symptoms or laboratory findings (rebound phenomenon) despite this weaning process. The dose then should be increased until suppression is again attained. In any case, treatment is rarely needed beyond 12–16 weeks. Rheumatic pericardial effusion tends to accumulate slowly and rarely causes tamponade even with a large accumulation.

Management of congestive heart failure is usually best accomplished with diuretics. Digoxin is seldom needed. In

TABLE 45.3	Management of Acute Rheumatic Fever and Secondary Prophylaxis		
Goal	**Specific Treatment Modalities**	**Rationale**	**Recommendations**
Elimination of GAS skin or throat infection	Penicillin and alternatives	To limit the repetitive exposure to GAS antigens	A single intramuscular dose of benzathine penicillin injection (dose depends on weight; 1.2 MU for > 25 kg and 6 MU for < 25 kg) is ideal. Penicillin V 250 mg four times daily for 10 days can also be used. Azithromycin can be used for those with penicillin allergy.
Suppression of inflammation	NSAIDs (naproxen safer than aspirin) and steroids	Relief from symptoms of fever and arthritis. NSAIDs and steroids have not been shown to prevent the progression to RHD	Aspirin 50–100 mg/kg/day in four divided doses is the traditional recommendation; reduce dose by 25% after 1 week if good clinical response and continue for 6–8 weeks, tapering the dose in last 2 weeks. Naproxen is commonly preferred alternative: 10–20 mg/kg/day, divided every 12 hours (maximum 1000 mg/day), until pain is relieved, then taper the dose. Steroids are a useful alternative to NSAIDs in those who continue to worsen and develop heart failure. They enable rapid relief of symptoms and reduce the duration of hospitalization. Prednisone (1–2 mg/kg/day, maximum 80 mg/day) is generally preferred. It can be tapered after 2–3 weeks. Intravenous methylprednisolone can be used in life-threatening situations.
Prevention of recurrences	Secondary penicillin prophylaxis	Secondary prophylaxis prevents recurrences of ARF and progression of heart valve damage	3- to 4-weekly intramuscular BPG or daily oral penicillin V • **ARF without carditis:** until age 21 or for 5 years after last ARF (whichever is longer) • **ARF with carditis but no residual valve damage:** until age 21 or for 10 years after last ARF (whichever is longer) • **ARF with carditis and residual valve damage:** until age 40 or for 10 years after last ARF (whichever is longer); lifetime prophylaxis may be needed

ARF, Acute rheumatic fever; *BPG,* benzathine penicillin G; *BW,* body weight; *GAS,* group A streptococcus; *NSAID,* non-steroidal anti-inflammatory drug; *RHD,* rheumatic heart disease.

rare instances, heart failure may be severe and difficult to treat. This is usually the result of severe MR that results from inflammation of the leaflets and tensor apparatus together (Video 45.1). These patients will need intensive care and vasodilator therapy with milrinone. In refractory situations, it may be necessary to undertake emergent heart valve surgery. Most surgeons prefer to replace the acutely inflamed mitral valve.

Although chorea is a self-limited disease, the emotional distress can be alleviated with benzodiazepines. Haloperidol, carbamazepine, or pimozide are also useful alternatives. In severe cases, hospitalization may be needed, if for no other reason than to assist the child in eating and to prevent injury from flailing movements.

Management of Established Rheumatic Heart Disease

For isolated MS, there is a role for reducing heart rates using beta-blockers or ivabradine to improve diastolic filling.[17] This is often combined with diuretics until the stenosis is relieved through surgery or transcatheter balloon valvotomy (Fig. 45.9) Afterload reduction through

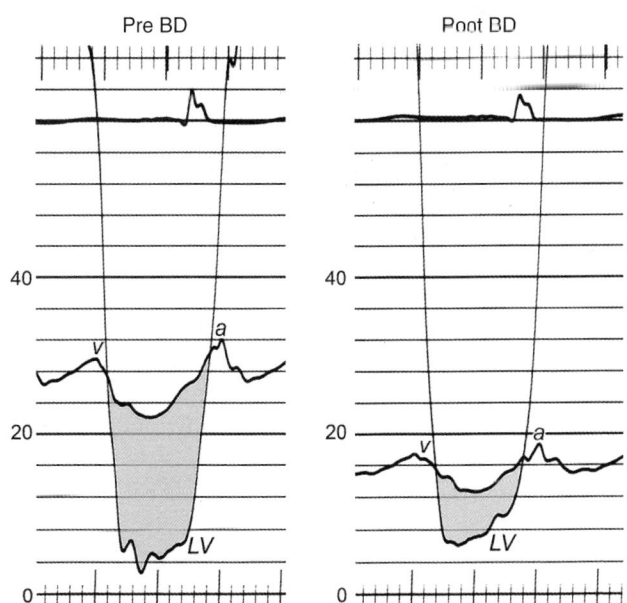

• **Fig. 45.9** Pressure tracings obtained at catheterization in a 14-year-old boy with severe mitral stenosis of rheumatic origin showing marked reduction of the gradient *(shaded area)* across the mitral valve following balloon dilation *(BD).*

angiotensin-converting enzyme inhibitors or angiotensin receptor blockers may have a possible role in severe regurgitation of the mitral or aortic valves to mitigate the physiological consequences to some degree. However, ultimately surgery is needed when symptoms develop or when there is unacceptable left ventricular (LV) enlargement with or without dysfunction. Unlike in adults, threshold LV dimensions for children with asymptomatic MR and AR are not clearly established (Table 45.4).

Most patients with rheumatic MR can undergo surgical mitral valve repair in expert hands. However, severe AR typically requires replacement. The tricuspid valve when affected can almost always be repaired. Following surgery, secondary penicillin prophylaxis must be continued. Oral anticoagulation is needed for those with prosthetic metallic valves and atrial fibrillation.

Patient and family education is of paramount importance. The specific areas that need focus include: the need for adherence to secondary penicillin prophylaxis, the potential risks of pregnancy in those with untreated RHD and those in need of oral anticoagulants, and the importance of dental hygiene to prevent endocarditis.

Clinical Course

Untreated active RF lasts from a few weeks to several months, averaging between 8 and 16 weeks for rheumatic activity as measured by the presence of an elevated sedimentation rate, congestive failure, nodules, erythema marginatum, or continued chorea. In those younger than age 5 years, carditis is more severe and chronic heart disease more common than in older patients.[18] Rheumatic activity persists longer in patients who have carditis.

At the time of initial presentation, as many as half of children with RF already have a significant murmur. As the days and weeks go by, under appropriate therapy, some children lose the murmur, whereas others develop murmurs for the first time. These changes are less frequent the longer the disease lasts, but the cardiac status perhaps never completely stabilizes; some individuals first develop new cardiac murmurs 20 years later.

When there is chorea with no other signs of rheumatic activity (pure chorea), ultimate heart damage is less frequent, appears late, and is most often pure MS without preceding MR.

Individuals with MR and/or AR may experience worsening of the existing valvar damage as the years go by.[17] Smoldering valve inflammation is the most likely basis for progression of valve damage and this is mitigated by adherence to penicillin prophylaxis. MS usually requires years to develop, sometimes as many as 20 years, although, in countries in which RF is common, MS develops more rapidly, being seen in small children. Biopsy specimens of the atrial appendages in patients undergoing mitral valve surgery show Aschoff nodules in high frequency the nearer the surgery is to the attack of active RF, but they are still present in some patients many years later. The presence of Aschoff

TABLE 45.4	Management of Established Rheumatic Heart Valve Disease: Indications for Intervention
Condition	**Specific Recommendations**
Mitral stenosis (MS)	Moderate to severe (≤ 1.5 cm^2) symptomatic MS requires relief and balloon mitral valvotomy (BMV) is generally preferred. Surgical valve repair or replacement is preferred for those with • Calcific MS with calcified commissures or extensive calcium deposits • Severe fusion of subvalvar apparatus precluding lasting relief with BMV • Associated mitral regurgitation: more than mild and/or at the commissures • Left atrial clot
Mitral regurgitation (MR)	Surgery (mitral valve repair or replacement) is indicated for • Severe symptomatic chronic MR • Acute MR resulting from chordal rupture during ARF that is unresponsive to therapy • Asymptomatic MR with LVEF $\leq 60\%$, LVESD ≥ 40 mm, LA volume ≥ 60 mL/m^2 or diameter ≥ 55 mm, systolic pulmonary arterial pressure > 50 mm Hg in adults; *atrial fibrillation
Aortic regurgitation (AR)	Surgery (typically aortic valve repair) is indicated Severe symptomatic chronic AR Asymptomatic AR with LVESD ≥ 50 mm or 25 mm/m^2 BSA, or LVEF $\leq 50\%$*
Tricuspid valve disease	Isolated tricuspid valve disease is rare in RHD. Any significant associated tricuspid valve disease must be addressed during valve repair or replacement of other valves. In general tricuspid valves can be repaired in the vast majority of patients.
Mixed heart valve disease	In general, symptomatic mixed or multivalve heart disease merits consideration for surgery. Approach should be individualized depending on the specifics of valve affliction.

*Left atrial and left ventricular (LV) dimension thresholds are not clearly established for children; however, Z scores of LV end-systolic dimensions of > 2 merit close follow-up and consideration for surgery after careful individualized attention.
ARF, Acute rheumatic fever; *LA,* left atrium; *LVEF,* left ventricular ejection fraction; *LVESD,* left ventricular end-systolic dimension; *RHD,* rheumatic heart disease.

nodules is taken as evidence of smoldering, low-grade rheumatic activity.

A second attack of RF represents either poor adherence to secondary prophylaxis or, less often, ineffectiveness of oral penicillin. A recurrent attack usually resembles the earlier attack, although valvar involvement may be extended.

The question of adequate prophylaxis must be examined. Perhaps a switch to intramuscular benzathine penicillin is needed for those on oral penicillin or shortening of intervals between doses to 3 weeks instead of 4 weeks for those receiving intramuscular injections.

The demonstration of morphological and Doppler features of rheumatic valve affliction in asymptomatic individuals with a normal cardiac examination is now a well-recognized entity that is particularly common in endemic regions with a high RHD prevalence.[1,6] This entity is known as subclinical RHD. The term "latent RHD" also includes patients with missed RHD that are incidentally identified through echocardiography screening. The progression of subclinical RHD to manifest RHD can be significantly mitigated by penicillin prophylaxis.[6]

Prevention

RHD prevention is traditionally classified as primordial, primary, and secondary prevention depending on the stage of intervention in the disease continuum (Fig. 45.2). Primordial prevention seeks to prevent streptococcal infection in the first place through improvement in living conditions and an effective vaccine. Primary prevention requires prompt treatment of streptococcal sore throat and skin infections. Secondary prevention seeks to halt the progression of heart valve damage in those with latent or manifest RHD or after the occurrence of RF. Secondary prevention is best accomplished using benzathine penicillin G intramuscularly every 4 weeks (every 3 weeks in high-prevalence regions).[17]

It is important to recognize that a life course approach needs to be adopted for those living with established RHD. This requires the maintenance of disease registers in those living in endemic regions. The disease runs a protracted course over many years and if often punctuated by destabilizing events such as pregnancy, intercurrent infections, and atrial fibrillation.[19]

It is essential to understand RHD prevention and control through a public health lens.[20] Much of the global decline in RHD burden has happened with improving access to health care and living standards and is not the result of specific RHD control strategies.[20] RHD control in affected populations has unique challenges because of absence of an effective vaccine, high dependence on penicillin, the long and protracted course of heart valve disease, and high dependence on expensive tertiary cardiac care to treat established disease.[21]

Much needs to be done to implement key elements of RHD prevention and control in vulnerable populations across the globe. These include creating robust and effective disease registries that are deeply integrated into primary health care, ensuring reliable availability and safe administration of penicillin, tailoring control strategies to regions with high disease burden, and improving access to affordable tertiary care that includes heart surgery and catheter interventions.[21]

Acknowledgment

The author and editors recognize Dr. Donald C. Fyler (1924–2011), a long-term member of the cardiology faculty at Boston Children's Hospital, who authored the chapters on this topic in earlier editions of the Nadas' textbook. Some of his excellent material has been retained in this new edition.

References

1. Marijon E, Ou P, Celermajer DS, et al. Prevalence of rheumatic heart disease detected by echocardiographic screening. *N Engl J Med*. 2007;357:470-476.
2. Bland EF. Rheumatic fever: the way it was. *Circulation*. 1987; 76:1190-1195.
3. Veasy LG, Wiedmeier SE, Orsmond GS, et al. Resurgence of acute rheumatic fever in the intermountain area of the United States. *N Engl J Med*. 1987;316:421-427.
4. Watkins DA, Baker M, Kumar RK, et al. Epidemiology, risk factors, burden and cost of ARF and RHD. In: Dougherty S, Carapetis J, Zühlke, Wilson N, eds. *ARF and RHD*. St Louis, MO: Elsevier; 2021:1-18.
5. Watkins DA, Johnson CO, Colquhoun SM, et al. Global, regional, and national burden of rheumatic heart disease, 1990-2015. *N Engl J Med*. 2017;377:713-722.
6. Beaton A, Okello E, Rwebembera J, et al. Secondary antibiotic prophylaxis for latent rheumatic heart disease. *N Engl J Med*. 2022;386:230-240.
7. Cheadle WB. Harveian lectures on the various manifestation of the rheumatic state as exemplified in childhood and early life. *Lancet*. 1889;821:871-921.
8. McDonald MI, Towers RJ, Andrews RM, et al. Low rates of streptococcal pharyngitis and high rates of pyoderma in Australian aboriginal communities where acute rheumatic fever is hyperendemic. *Clin Infect Dis*. 2006;43:683-689.
9. Engel ME, Stander R, Vogel J, et al. Genetic susceptibility to acute rheumatic fever: a systematic review and meta-analysis of twin studies. *PLoS One*. 2011;6:e2532.
10. Tandon R, Sharma M, Chandrashekhar Y, et al. Revisiting the pathogenesis of rheumatic fever and carditis. *Nat Rev Cardiol*. 2013;10:171-177.
11. Cunningham MW. Rheumatic fever revisited. *Nat Rev Cardiol*. 2014;11:123.
12. Thomas WA, Averill JH, Bland EF, et al. The significance of Aschoff bodies in the left atrial appendage: a comparison of 40 biopsies removed during mitral commissurotomy with autopsy material from 40 patients dying from rheumatic fever. *N Engl J Med*. 1953;249:761-765.
13. Lahiri K, Rane HS, Desai AG. Clinical profile of rheumatic fever: a study of 168 cases. *J Trop Pediatr*. 1985;31:273-275.
14. Stollerman GH. Rheumatic fever in the 21st century. *Clin Infect Dis*. 2001;33:806-814.

15. Remenyi B, Wilson N, Steer A, et al. World Heart Federation criteria for echocardiographic diagnosis of rheumatic heart disease: an evidence-based guideline. *Nat Rev Cardiol*. 2012;9:297-309.

16. Gewitz MH, Baltimore RS, Tani LY, et al. Revision of the Jones Criteria for the diagnosis of acute rheumatic fever in the era of Doppler echocardiography: a scientific statement from the American Heart Association. *Circulation*. 2015;131.1806 1818.

17. Kumar RK, Antunes MJ, Beaton A, et al. Contemporary diagnosis and management of rheumatic heart disease: implications for closing the gap: a scientific statement from the American Heart Association. *Circulation* 2020;142:e337-e357.

18. Tani LY, Veasy LG, Minich LL, et al. Rheumatic fever in children younger than 5 years: is the presentation different. *Pediatrics*. 2003;112:1065.

19. Zuhlke L, Engel ME, Karthikeyan G, et al. Characteristics, complications, and gaps in evidence-based interventions in rheumatic heart disease: the Global Rheumatic Heart Disease Registry (the REMEDY study). *Eur Heart J*. 2015;36:1115-1122.

20. Watkins DA, Hasan B, Mayosi B, et al. Structural Heart Diseases. In: Prabhakaran D, Anand S, Gaziano TA, Mbanya JC, Wu Y, Nugent R, eds. *Cardiovascular, Respiratory, and Related Disorders*. 3rd ed. Washington, DC: The International Bank for Reconstruction and Development/The World Bank; 2017.

21. Palafox B, Mocumbi AO, Kumar RK, et al. The WHF roadmap for reducing CV morbidity and mortality through prevention and control of rheumatic heart disease. *Glob Heart*. 2017;12. 47-62.

46

Kawasaki Disease

AUDREY DIONNE AND JANE W. NEWBURGER

KEY LEARNING POINTS

- Kawasaki disease is an acute, systemic vasculitis characterized by fever, bilateral non-exudative conjunctivitis, erythema of the lips and oral mucosa, changes in the extremities, rash, and cervical lymphadenopathy.
- Coronary artery aneurysms develop in up to 25% of cases and may lead to myocardial infarction, sudden death, or chronic coronary insufficiency.
- Timely treatment with high-dose intravenous immunoglobulin (IVIG) reduces the incidence of aneurysms fivefold, and

should ideally be administered within 7 days of fever onset. Those at highest risk should be treated with IVIG plus primary adjunctive immunomodulatory therapy.
- Long-term cardiovascular surveillance is tailored to initial severity of disease and current coronary status.
- Patients with large aneurysms have life-long risk of progressive coronary artery stenosis or occlusion and worsening ischemia.

Definition

Kawasaki disease (KD) is an acute, systemic vasculitis of uncertain etiology, occurring predominantly in infants and young children. It is characterized by fever, bilateral non-exudative conjunctivitis, erythema of the lips and oral mucosa, changes in the extremities, rash, and cervical lymphadenopathy. Coronary artery aneurysms or ectasia develop in 15% to 25% of cases and may lead to myocardial infarction, sudden death, or chronic coronary insufficiency.

Prevalence

Though noted initially in Japan in 1967 and most prevalent there, KD occurs worldwide in children of all races. The most recent Japanese statistics from a nationwide survey in 2017–2018 reported 32,528 patients with KD with annual incidence rate of 359 per 100,000 children aged 0–4 years; the highest incidence was in children 9–11 months old, at 572 and 398 per 100,000 boys and girls, respectively.[1] The steady increase in incidence over the decades since its first description may be related to an actual increase in disease incidence, increased awareness of the condition, or greater tendency to classify children with incomplete clinical features as having KD. For the first time, the incidence of KD was significantly lower during the COVID-19 pandemic, 40%–46% of the corresponding months of the previous 5 years.[2]

It is harder to estimate the prevalence of KD in the United States due to the lack of a mandatory national reporting system. Data from hospital discharge records by the Centers for Disease Control estimated an annual incidence of 20 per 100,000 children younger than 5 years in the United States, with rates that were highest in Asian and Pacific Islanders (30 per 100,000), followed by non-Hispanic African American (17 per 100,000) and Hispanics (16 per 100,000), and lowest among Caucasians (12 per 100,000).[3]

The pattern of involvement is generally endemic, with occasional epidemics among primarily younger children. Boys are affected as much as 50% more commonly than girls. Most cases occur in children younger than 5 years; however, the illness is being more commonly recognized in older children and adolescents. Outbreaks are more likely in the spring, suggesting an infectious trigger, but a steady background activity of cases is noted throughout the remainder of the year. In Japan, siblings have a 10-fold risk of developing KD. The disease recurs in approximately 3% in Japanese studies.

Etiology and Pathogenesis

The etiology of KD remains unknown, with infectious etiology, immunologic response, and environmental and genetic factors as possible contributors.[4]

An infectious cause or trigger to KD is supported by epidemiologic data. There is seasonal variation in the incidence of KD, and epidemics were previously described. The rates tend to follow those of other common viral infections in pediatrics. Cases may occur in clusters, and siblings are at increased risk of developing the disease within a week of onset of the index case. Interestingly, the number of cases of KD declined markedly during the COVID-19 pandemic, consistent with the decrease in infectious illnesses with universal masking and social isolation. The disease is also most common in children younger than 5 years but rare in those less than age 6 months; the rarity in infants may be explained by passive immunity to the relatively common infectious triggers by transplacentally acquired maternal antibodies. The signs and symptoms of KD overlap significantly with those of other febrile illnesses. In addition, the self-limiting illness with a low rate of recurrence supports an infectious etiology. Multiple candidate pathogens have been evaluated and excluded, most consistent with an exaggerated immune response to a common infectious trigger in a genetically predisposed individual.

Other hypotheses include a marked immune response to exposure of the host to a superantigen. A number of reports have implicated specific superantigens, including TSST-1–secreting strains of *Staphylococcus aureus* and streptococcal pyrogenic exotoxin B– and C–producing streptococci, as well as *Lactobacillus casei*, which induces coronary arteritis in mice. Other investigators have found support for a typical antigen immune response by demonstrating oligo-IgA plasma cells and IgA heavy-chain genes in vascular tissue of individuals with fatal KD.

Multiple environmental factors, including dust mites, rug shampoo, and pollen release, have been suggested, although more recent data have not supported those theories.

The potential trigger may be wind-born and carried by tropospheric wind, as suggested by analyses of epidemics and non-epidemic interannual fluctuation of cases consistent with large-scale winds originating in central Asia and traversing the north Pacific.

Regardless of the initiating event, KD is accompanied by significant derangements in the immunoregulatory system that lead to coronary inflammation and coronary artery abnormalities. Endothelial cell activation, CD68+ monocyte/macrophages, CD8 (cytotoxic) lymphocytes, and oligoclonal IgA plasma cells appear to be involved in coronary arteritis. Matrix metalloproteinase, vascular endothelial growth factor, monocyte chemotactic and activating factor, tumor necrosis factor-α (TNF-α), and various interleukins appear to have a role in the vasculitic process and aneurysmal dilatation.

Genome-wide association studies have identified polymorphisms associated with both disease susceptibility (e.g., FcγR2a, caspase 3, human leukocyte antigen class II, B-cell lymphoid kinase, inositol 1,4,5-triphosphate kinase C, and CD40) and coronary artery aneurysms (e.g., *TGFBR2*). Most studies on genetic risk factors have been performed in Asian populations, and to date, there are no studies on polygenic risk scores.

Pathology

KD may be accompanied by inflammation of systemic medium-sized extraparenchymal arteries,[5] but morbidity and mortality are largely related to coronary artery involvement. The proposed model for arteriopathy in KD includes three distinct processes.[6] The first is a necrotizing arteritis that destroys the arterial wall into the adventitia, causing aneurysms. This process occurs in the first 2 weeks of illness and involves a self-limited neutrophilic process. Next, a subacute/chronic vasculitis occurs, with infiltration of lymphocytes, plasma cells, and eosinophils; this process can continue for months in some patients. Lastly, there is luminal myofibroblastic proliferation with medial smooth muscle cell–derived myofibroblastic proliferation that can persist for years. This is the mechanism by which progressive stenosis occurs.

Myocardial inflammation with edema and cellular inflammatory infiltrate with neutrophils, monocytes, macrophages, and/or eosinophils is almost universal in KD and is the earliest cause of death. Giant aneurysms are also at risk of rupture in the first few weeks. The mortality from KD, although rare, peaks between 15 and 45 days after onset of fever due to a hypercoagulable state, thrombocytosis, and a disrupted vascular endothelium, which can lead to coronary thrombosis and myocardial infarction. The risk of mortality declines beyond the first year of illness, but progressive coronary stenosis and myocardial infarction remain a risk even into adulthood.[7]

Mildly dilated coronary arteries may be able to regress to normal during follow-up. However, in large aneurysms, the intima, media, and elastica were destroyed during the acute process. In such aneurysms, progressive thrombosis and myofibroblastic proliferation may decrease the internal lumen dimension to normal, but the coronary artery vasculature always remains abnormal (Fig. 46.1).[8]

Clinical Manifestations

Because no diagnostic test is available for KD, the diagnosis must be made on clinical grounds (Fig. 46.2; Table 46.1).[4] The diagnosis is based on the presence of fever with systemic and mucocutaneous inflammation. First described by Kawasaki in Japanese children, the classic criteria have continued to serve as the standard adopted by the American Heart Association for diagnosis and include fever for 4 days or more and at least four of the five following findings: (1) non-exudative, bilateral conjunctivitis; (2) oral changes with erythematous or dry fissured lips, strawberry tongue, or pharyngitis; (3) a rash involving the trunk, perineum, and extremities, often sparing the face; (4) erythema of the palmar and plantar surfaces, edema of the hands or feet, or periungual desquamation; and (5) unilateral anterior cervical lymphadenopathy of 1.5 cm or greater. It is important to note that these findings are often not present at the same time, making serial evaluation of the patient essential.

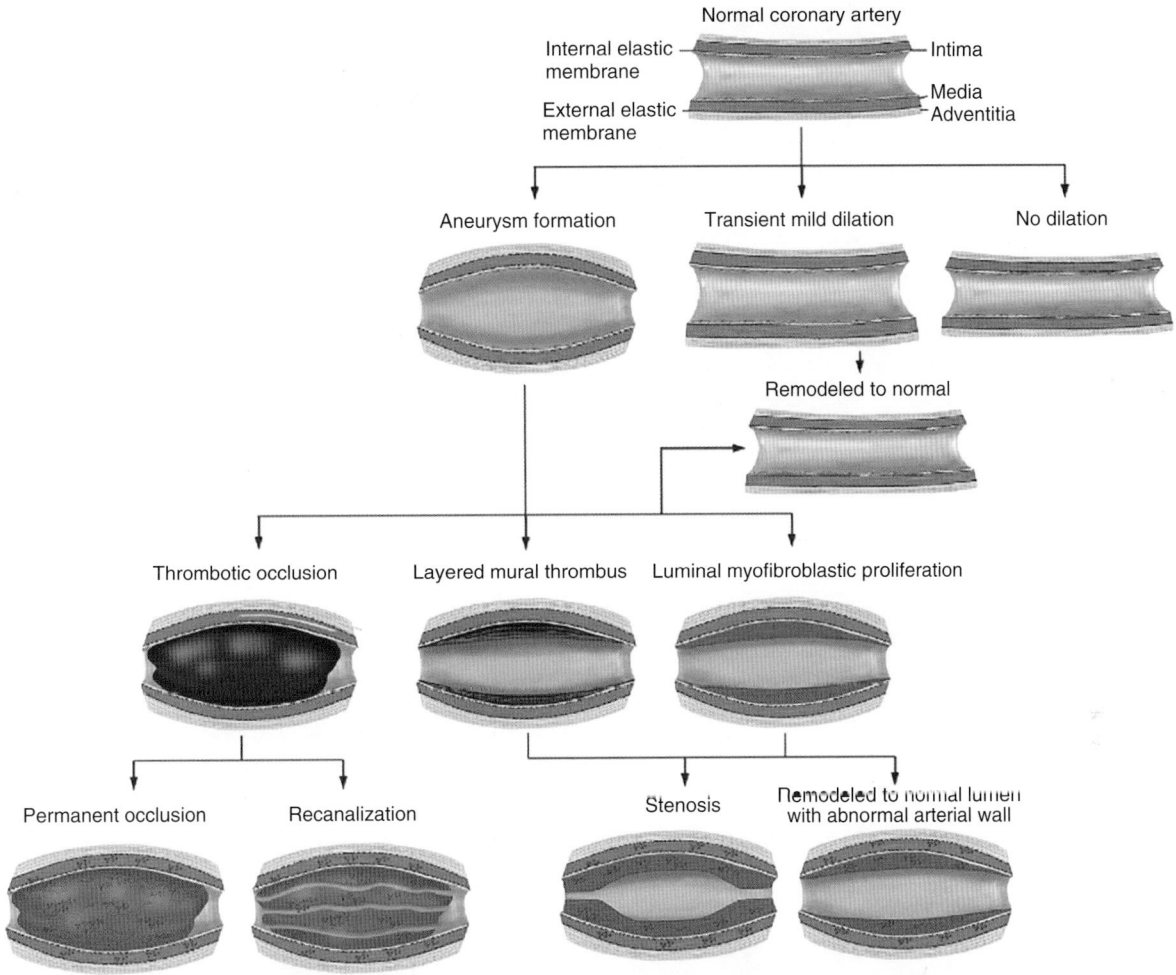

• **Fig. 46.1** Natural history of coronary artery architecture in Kawasaki disease. (Used with permission from J.W. Newburger, H. Kato Kawasaki disease, J.T. Willerson, D.R. Holmes (Eds.), Coronary Artery Disease, Springer-Verlag, London, UK (2015), pp. 581-596. https://link.springer.com/chapter/10.1007/978-1-4471-2828-1_22 (Part of the Cardiovascular Medicine book series (CVM)))

Unfortunately, not all patients with KD present with these criteria. KD should be considered in the differential diagnosis of prolonged unexplained fever. The diagnosis can be supported by clinical laboratory and echocardiographic findings (Fig. 46.3). Infants less than 6 months of age are especially likely to present with incomplete criteria. They are at high risk of delayed diagnosis and coronary artery complications, so a high level of suspicion is needed in infants who may have prolonged fever and irritability as their only manifestation. Children with > 5 days of fever and two or three clinical criteria, or infants with fever for > 7 days without alternative explanation and with evidence of systemic inflammation should have echocardiogram performed. A normal echocardiogram does not rule out KD, as coronary artery dilation or aneurysm is often not detected until after the first week of illness.

Other illnesses that may mimic KD include toxin-mediated disease related to *S. aureus* or streptococcal diseases, enterovirus, adenovirus, measles, parvovirus, Epstein-Barr virus, mycoplasma, rickettsial disease, and the multisystem inflammatory syndrome in children associated with COVID-19 (MIS-C).

These diagnoses should be considered and excluded prior to diagnosis of KD, as the clinical criteria are not specific. Concurrent infection with respiratory viral pathogens does not exclude the diagnosis of KD in children with classic clinical findings. Exudative conjunctivitis, exudative pharyngitis, oral ulcerations, splenomegaly, and vesicobullous or petechial rashes are unusual in KD and should prompt consideration of alternative diagnosis.

Multiple organs and tissues are inflamed during KD and can cause clinical symptoms beyond the diagnostic criteria and coronary complications. Neurologic symptoms include extreme irritability and aseptic meningitis. Gastrointestinal symptoms are common and include abdominal pain, diarrhea, vomiting, and gallbladder hydrops. Urethritis with sterile pyuria is a common genitourinary finding. Arthralgia and arthritis of both small and large joints can be observed in the first 3 weeks of illness.

Cardiovascular manifestations during the acute episode include a hyperdynamic precordium, tachycardia, and a gallop rhythm. Innocent systolic flow murmurs can be accentuated. Rarely, children present with cardiovascular collapse and

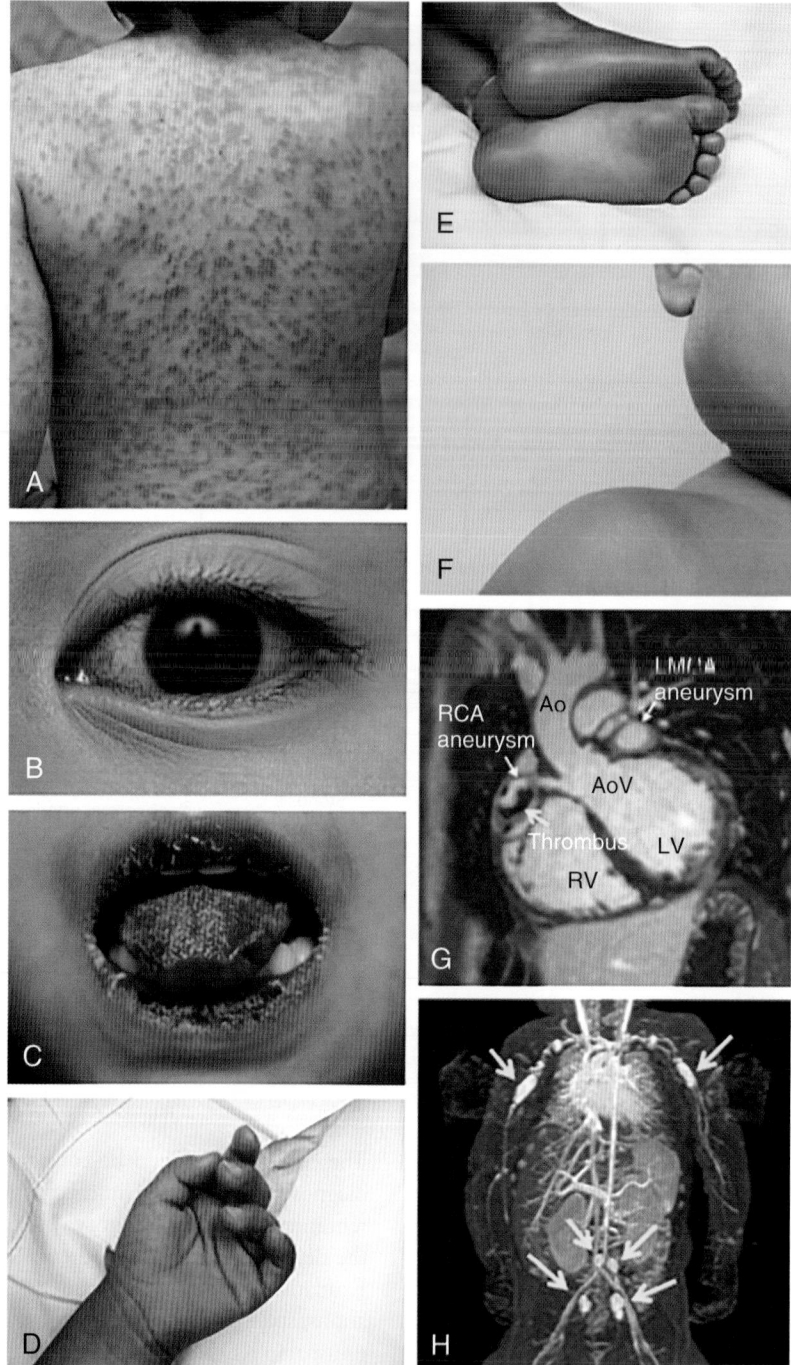

• **Fig. 46.2** **(A)** Rash: maculopapular, diffuse erythroderma, or erythema multiforme-like. **(B)** Conjunctivitis: bulbar conjunctival injection without exudate; bilateral. **(C)** Oral changes: erythema and cracking of lips (cheilitis); strawberry tongue; erythema of oral and pharyngeal mucosa. **(D)** and **(E)** Palmar and plantar erythema: usually accompanied by swelling; resolves with subsequent periungual desquamation in the subacute phase. **(F)** Cervical adenopathy: usually unilateral, node ≥ 1.5 cm in diameter. **(G)** Coronary artery aneurysms: magnetic resonance image of the left ventricular outflow tract showing a giant right coronary artery *(RCA)* aneurysm with non-occlusive thrombus *(yellow arrow)* and a giant left main coronary artery *(LMCA)* aneurysm. **(H)** Peripheral artery aneurysms: magnetic resonance imaging showing aneurysms in the axillary and subclavian arteries and the iliac and femoral arteries *(yellow arrows)*. *Ao*, Aorta; *AoV*, aortic valve; *LV*, left ventricle; *RV*, right ventricle. Patient photographs used with permission from the Kawasaki Disease Foundation, Inc. (Adapted from McCrindle BW, Rowley AH, Newburger JW, et al. Diagnosis, treatment, and long-term management of Kawasaki disease. a scientific statement for health professionals from the American Heart Association. *Circulation.* 2017;135:e927–e999.)

TABLE 46.1   Diagnosis of Classic Kawasaki Disease

Classic KD is diagnosed in the presence of fever for at least 5 days (the day of fever onset is taken to be the first day of fever) together with at least four of the five following principal clinical features. In the presence of four or more principal clinical features, particularly when redness and swelling of the hands and feet are present, the diagnosis of KD can be made with 4 days of fever, although experienced clinicians who have treated many patients with KD may establish the diagnosis with 3 days of fever in rare cases (Fig. 46.2):

1. Erythema and cracking of lips, strawberry tongue, and/or erythema of oral and pharyngeal mucosa

2. Bilateral bulbar conjunctival injection without exudate

3. Rash: maculopapular, diffuse erythroderma, or erythema multiforme-like

4. Erythema and edema of the hands and feet in acute phase and/or periungual desquamation in subacute phase

5. Cervical lymphadenopathy (≥1.5 cm diameter), usually unilateral

A careful history may reveal that one or more principal clinical features were present during the illness but resolved by the time of presentation.

Patients who lack full clinical features of classic KD are often evaluated for incomplete KD (Fig. 46.3). If coronary artery abnormalities are detected, the diagnosis of KD is considered confirmed in most cases.

Laboratory tests typically reveal normal or elevated white blood cell count with neutrophil predominance and elevated acute-phase reactants such as C-reactive protein and erythrocyte sedimentation rate during the acute phase. Low serum sodium and albumin levels, elevated serum liver enzymes, and sterile pyuria can be present. In the second week after fever onset, thrombocytosis is common.

Other clinical findings may include the following:

Cardiovascular

Myocarditis, pericarditis, valvular regurgitation, shock

Coronary artery abnormalities

Aneurysms of medium-sized noncoronary arteries

Peripheral gangrene

Aortic root enlargement

Respiratory

Peribronchial and interstitial infiltrates on chest x-ray

Pulmonary nodules

Musculoskeletal

Arthritis, arthralgia (pleocytosis of synovial fluid)

Gastrointestinal

Diarrhea, vomiting, abdominal pain

Hepatitis, jaundice

Gallbladder hydrops

Pancreatitis

Nervous system

Extreme irritability

Aseptic meningitis (pleocytosis of cerebrospinal fluid)

Facial nerve palsy

Sensorineural hearing loss

Genitourinary

Urethritis/meatitis, hydrocele

Continued

| TABLE 46.1 | Diagnosis of Classic Kawasaki Disease—cont'd |

Desquamating rash in groin

Retropharyngeal phlegmon

Anterior uveitis by slit lamp examination

Erythema and induration at BCG inoculation site

The differential diagnosis includes other infectious and noninfectious conditions, including the following:

Measles

Other viral infections (e.g., adenovirus, enterovirus)

Staphylococcal and streptococcal toxin-mediated diseases (e.g., scarlet fever and toxic shock syndrome)

Drug hypersensitivity reactions, including Stevens-Johnson syndrome

Systemic onset juvenile idiopathic arthritis

With epidemiologic risk factors:

Rocky Mountain spotted fever or other rickettsial infections

Leptospirosis

BCG, Bacillus Calmette-Guérin; *KD,* Kawasaki disease.
Adapted from McCrindle BW, Rowley AH, Newburger JW, et al. Diagnosis, treatment, and long-term management of Kawasaki disease. A scientific statement for health professionals from the American Heart Association. *Circulation.* 2017;135:e927–e999. ©2017 American Heart Association, Inc.

hypotension. The pericardium, myocardium, and endocardium including the valves and coronary arteries all may be inflamed during the acute episode. This can manifest as a pericardial rub with pericardial effusion, valvar dysfunction, and coronary artery aneurysms. KD causes coronary artery aneurysms by 1984 Japanese Ministry of Health criteria in 15% to 25% of patients who are not treated in the acute phase of the disease with high-dose intravenous immunoglobulin (IVIG). Using z-score criteria, the incidence of coronary artery abnormalities during the course of KD is much higher, ~25% in children and ~50% in infants less than age 6 months.[9] Coronary artery enlargement may be observed by echocardiography as early as 1 week from the onset of fever, and may progress further over the next 3–6 weeks.

Laboratory Data

Laboratory values in the acute phase reflect the systemic vasculitis uniformly present early in the disease. Acute-phase reactants, including erythrocyte sedimentation rate and C-reactive protein, are increased markedly. The white blood cell count is elevated with a leftward shift, and a normochromic, normocytic anemia is noted within the first week of illness. Thrombocytosis is usually present by the second week of the disease, often peaking at counts greater than 1,000,000 mm³ in association with hypercoagulability. More rarely, thrombocytopenia can be seen and associated with a more severe clinical course including shock at presentation and coronary artery aneurysms. Hepatocellular inflammation is accompanied by increases in serum transaminases and gamma-glutamyltransferase and mild hyperbilirubinemia. Hypoalbuminemia is also

common. Sterile pyuria and pleocytosis of cerebrospinal fluid or synovial fluid, both with mononuclear cells, are found frequently. Elevated inflammatory markers and three or more abnormal laboratory values can be used to support the diagnosis of incomplete KD.

N-terminal moiety of B-type natriuretic peptide (NT-proBNP) may be elevated in patients with KD, reflective of myocardial involvement; however, cut-point values have not been clearly defined. Biomarkers are an active area of research in the absence of diagnostic test.

Electrocardiography

The electrocardiogram is generally not helpful in KD, but in the acute phase, nonspecific ST-T wave changes are present and the PR interval may be prolonged. These findings are probably related to myocardial inflammation.

Chest Radiography

Chest radiographs are usually unremarkable, but can rarely show pulmonary infiltrates or pulmonary effusions. When chest radiographs show such findings, other potentially explanatory diagnosis should be sought.

Echocardiography

Two-dimensional echocardiography provides excellent visualization of the proximal coronary arteries in young children and is the primary imaging modality. It allows for assessment of coronary artery dimension (Fig. 46.4), ventricular

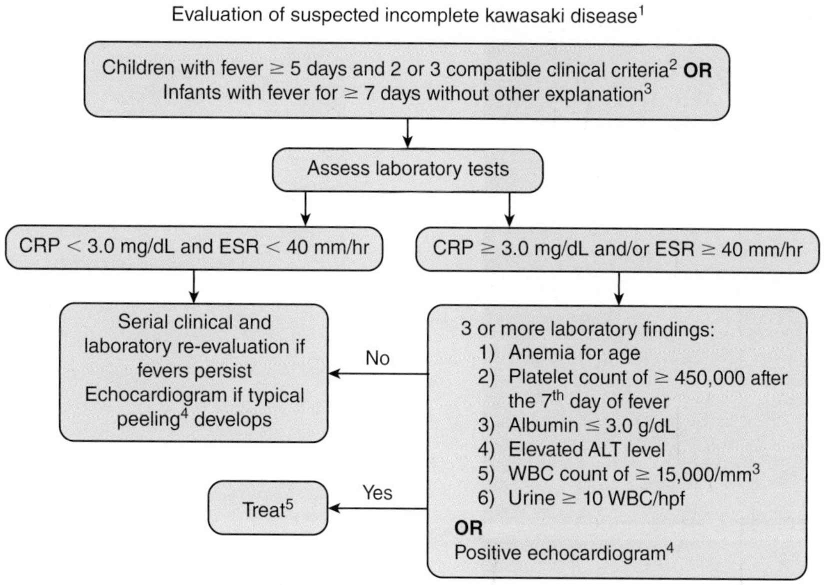

Evaluation of suspected incomplete kawasaki disease[1]

• **Fig. 46.3** Evaluation of suspected incomplete Kawasaki disease. (1) In the absence of a "gold standard" for diagnosis, this algorithm cannot be evidence based but rather represents the informed opinion of the expert committee. Consultation with an expert should be sought any time assistance is needed. (2) Clinical findings of Kawasaki disease are listed in Fig. 46.1. Characteristics suggesting that another diagnosis should be considered include exudative conjunctivitis, exudative pharyngitis, ulcerative intraoral lesions, bulbous or vesicular rash, generalized adenopathy, or splenomegaly. (3) Infants ≤ 6 months of age are most likely to develop prolonged fever without other clinical criteria for Kawasaki disease; these infants are at particularly high risk of developing coronary artery abnormalities. (4) Echocardiography is considered positive for purposes of this algorithm if any of three conditions are met: z-score of left anterior descending coronary artery or right coronary artery ≥ 2.5; coronary artery aneurysm is observed; or three or more features exist, including decreased left ventricular function, mitral regurgitation, pericardial effusion or z-scores in the left anterior descending coronary artery or right coronary artery of 2–2.5. (5) If the echocardiogram is positive, treatment should be given within 10 days of fever onset or after the 10th day of fever in the presence of clinical or laboratory signs, including C-reactive protein *(CRP)* and erythrocyte sedimentation rate *(ESR)* of ongoing inflammation. (6) Typical peeling begins under the nail beds of fingers and toes. *ALT,* Alanine transaminase; *WBC,* white blood cells. (Adapted from McCrindle BW, Rowley AH, Newburger JW, et al. Diagnosis, treatment, and long-term management of Kawasaki disease. a scientific statement for health professionals from the American Heart Association. Reprinted with permission, *Circulation.* 2017;135:e927–e999, ©2017 American Heart Association, Inc.)

systolic function, valvular regurgitation, aortic root dilation, and pericardial effusion. It should be performed as soon as the diagnosis is suspected, but initiation of treatment should not be delayed for the echocardiogram. Sedation may be required in younger children who are uncooperative.

The highest-frequency transducer should be used to visualize all the coronary artery segments. Aneurysms are most often seen in the proximal left anterior descending coronary, proximal right coronary artery, left main coronary artery, left circumflex, and distal right coronary artery. Coronary artery measurements should be made from inner edge to inner edge, and normalized for body surface area as z-scores. Coronary artery dilation is defined as z-score 2 to <2.5, small aneurysm ≥2.5 to <5, medium aneurysm ≥5 to <10, and large or giant aneurysm ≥10 or absolute dimension ≥8mm.[4] Anatomic variations are frequent in the left main coronary artery, where the z-score must be interpreted with caution. The Japanese guidelines are seldom used and define dilation or small aneurysms as a localized dilation of the internal lumen diameter but ≤ 4 mm, or if the child is ≥ 5 years, dilation but with an internal diameter

of a segment measuring 1.5 times that of an adjacent segment. Medium aneurysm is defined as internal diameter > 4 mm but ≤ 8mm or internal diameter 1.5–4 times that adjacent segment. Large or giant aneurysms are defined as internal diameter > 8 mm or > 4 times that of an adjacent segment. The echocardiogram may have limited accuracy for the detection of coronary artery thrombosis, stenosis, or distal coronary aneurysms, which may require computed tomographic angiography, cardiac magnetic resonance imaging, or invasive angiography for assessment.

Echocardiogram/Doppler evaluation should also include assessment of systolic and diastolic ventricular function, regional wall motion, valvular regurgitation (specifically mitral and aortic), aortic root dimension, and pericardial effusion.

Other Imaging Modalities

Historically, selective coronary arteriography has been used for the diagnostic assessment of coronary abnormalities (Fig. 46.5), but given the current technical quality of non-invasive imaging, invasive studies are rarely needed. Advanced coronary imaging,

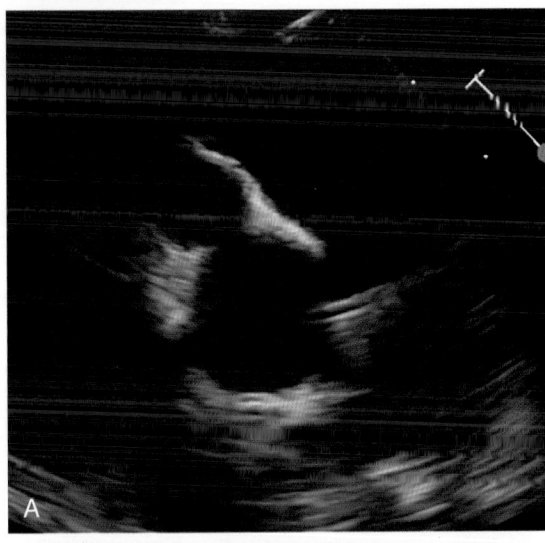

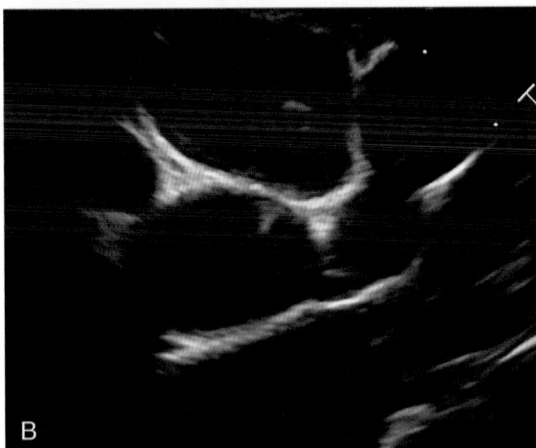

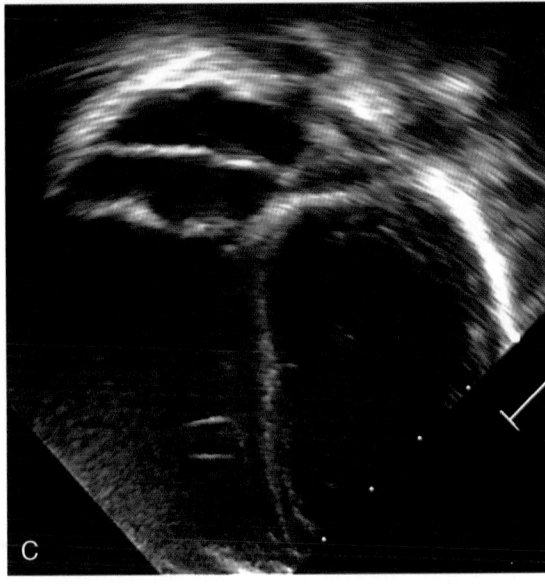

• **Fig. 46.4** Echocardiographic evaluation of coronary arteries. **(A)** Short-axis view demonstrating giant aneurysm of the right coronary artery. **(B)** Short-axis view demonstrating giant aneurysm of the left anterior descending coronary artery. **(C)** Apical view demonstrating aneurysm of the distal right coronary artery. *Circulation.* 2017;135: e927–e999.

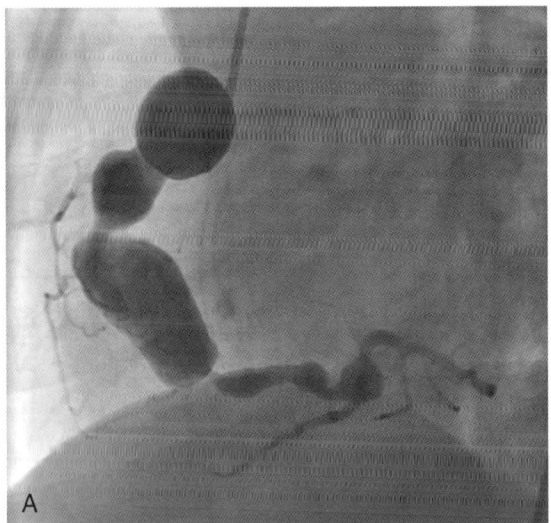

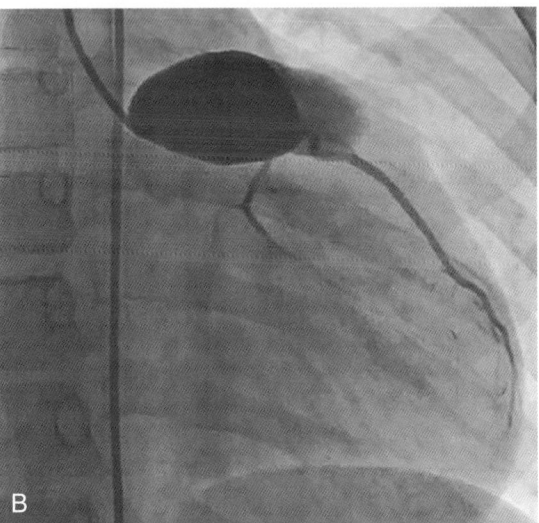

• **Fig. 46.5** Coronary artery angiogram. **(A)** Right coronary artery with multiple giant aneurysms. **(B)** Giant aneurysm of the left coronary artery, with occlusion of the left anterior descending coronary artery. ©2017 American Heart Association, Inc.

either through computed tomographic angiography, cardiac magnetic resonance, or catheterization, is most often reserved for the evaluation of children with large aneurysms. These tests allow for the evaluation of distal coronary arteries, stenosis, thrombosis, and extraparenchymal arteries, particularly the subclavian, axillary, femoral, iliac, renal, and mesenteric arteries, which can also be affected by aneurysms. Cardiac magnetic resonance allows for the evaluation of myocardial scarring and ischemia.

Management

Initial Therapy

Aspirin is a standard therapy for KD, both for its anti-inflammatory and antithrombotic effects. At diagnosis, most clinicians begin moderate-dose (40–60 mg/kg/day, preferred) or high-dose (80–100 mg/kg/day) aspirin divided into four daily doses until defervescence, and then reduce the dose to 3–5 mg/kg/day administered once daily. Low-dose aspirin is usually continued for 6–8 weeks and stopped for patients with normal coronary arteries; it is continued for patients with aneurysms, sometimes in combination with anticoagulants or other antiplatelet agents.

IVIG is beneficial in reducing the frequency of coronary aneurysms and the inflammatory response in the acute phase. Randomized controlled studies and meta-analysis have confirmed the efficacy of high-dose IVIG.[10,11] A single dose of IVIG, 2 g/kg, is administered over 8–12 hours within the first 7–10 days (ideally within 7 days) of onset of fever. It should still be administered after 10 days of fever in patients with persistent fever, ongoing systemic inflammation, and/or coronary artery aneurysms. The mechanism of action of IVIG in KD remains unknown but has generalized anti-inflammatory effects through modulating cytokine levels and production, augmenting T-cell suppressor activity, downregulating antibody synthesis, providing anti-idiotypic antibodies, and inhibiting neutrophil function, with decreasing IL-1ß+ neutrophils. Adverse events may include early reactions that are, in part, related to the rate of infusion, such as spiking fever, shaking chills, and hypotension; anaphylaxis is fortunately very rare. Other common reactions include headache/aseptic meningitis and hemolytic anemia within 5–10 days of infusion in patients with non-type O blood (i.e., type A, B, or AB) due to isoagglutinins. The risk of hemolytic anemia is highest in those who receive greater amounts of IVIG, including more than one dose, and who are highly inflamed.

Primary Adjunctive Therapy

Some patients who are at high risk of coronary artery complications may benefit from primary adjunctive treatment. Risk scores to identify children at high risk of IVIG resistance and coronary complications have been developed.[12,13] While they perform well in Japanese populations, they have limited sensitivity and specificity outside of Japan. A North American risk score identified coronary artery aneurysms at presentation, age < 6 months, Asian race, and C-reactive protein > 13 mg/dL as risk factors for IVIG resistance and coronary artery aneurysms.[14] Other patients at high risk include those who present with shock or macrophage activation syndrome.

Corticosteroids are the most widely used primary adjunctive therapy in patients at high risk of IVIG resistance. Randomized clinical trials in Japan and meta-analysis found that corticosteroids, when used with standard-dose IVIG for initial treatment of KD in high-risk patients, decreased the risk of coronary artery abnormalities and treatment failure. Limitations include the various corticosteroid dosing regimens and the challenge of identifying high-risk patients outside of Japan. One of the most widely used regimens was tested in the Randomized Controlled Trial to Assess Immunoglobulin Plus Steroid Efficacy for Kawasaki Disease (RAISE study), a multicenter, prospective, randomized, open-label, blinded end-points trial to assess the efficacy of IVIG (2 g/kg), aspirin (30 mg/kg/day), and intravenous prednisolone (2 mg/kg/day) for 5 days followed by an oral taper over weeks.[15] In the KAICA trial, primary adjunctive therapy with cyclosporine has also been associated with a lower incidence of coronary artery abnormalities.[16] Both the RAISE and KAICA trials were performed in Japan in children at high risk for aneurysms, heightening power to detect efficacy.

Two primary adjunctive treatment trials using TNF blockers were performed in routine-risk populations in North America. Primary adjunctive therapy with infliximab, compared with conventional therapy, did not show a difference in the rate of treatment failure or coronary artery aneurysms or z-scores at 5 weeks.[17] However, the infliximab group had more rapid improvement of inflammation and fever, as well as a borderline significant effect on the left anterior descending coronary artery z-score at 2 weeks. Primary adjunctive treatment with etanercept showed no effect on treatment resistance overall and no difference between groups in coronary z-scores over time.[18] However, in a subgroup with baseline coronary enlargement, etanercept reduced the progression of coronary dilation.

Intravenous Immunoglobulin Resistance

IVIG resistance is defined as persistent or recrudescent fever at least 36 hours after completion of IVIG infusion, and occurs in 10%–20% of patients.[4] IVIG resistance is a strong risk factor for development of coronary aneurysms, and thus children who fail to respond to initial therapy need additional treatment. There are limited data to guide the choice of therapeutic agents.

Most experts recommend retreatment with IVIG 2 g/kg, based on the dose-response effect of IVIG (class IIa). Other alternatives include corticosteroids or infliximab (class IIb), which have been reported in observational studies to decrease the duration of fever, although have not convincingly demonstrated effects on coronary artery anomalies. The KIDCARE trial was a randomized, 30-site, comparative effectiveness trial of infliximab 10 mg/kg versus a second dose of IVIG for IVIG-resistant KD.[19] Those treated with infliximab had a lower need for additional therapy, less anemia, and shorter hospitalizations, but no difference in coronary artery outcomes. There may be benefits of combining IVIG and corticosteroids. A retrospective study assessed the efficacy of intravenous prednisolone (2 mg/kg tapered over 2 weeks) in addition to IVIG and found lower rates of persistent or recrudescent fever and coronary artery abnormalities.[20] Patients who were retreated with IVIG and corticosteroids had a lower rate of coronary aneurysm 1 month after treatment than those treated with either IVIG or steroids alone (28.7% for patients retreated with IVIG, 30.6% for patients retreated with prednisolone, and 15.9% for those retreated with IVIG and prednisolone).

Cyclosporine, cyclophosphamide, or rarely plasma exchange may be considered in patients refractory to other therapies and with severe coronary artery aneurysms.

Thromboprophylaxis

Coronary artery thrombosis is promoted early in the illness by the presence of active vasculitis with endothelial damage, thrombocytosis, and a hypercoagulable state. Since the peak occurrence for coronary thrombosis is 15 to 45 days from the onset of illness, the current therapeutic recommendation is aspirin 3–5 mg/kg/day for 6–8 weeks. If the echocardiographic findings are normal at that time, aspirin is discontinued; however, in the presence of dilation or aneurysms, aspirin is continued.

For patients with moderate-sized aneurysms, some clinicians consider dual antiplatelet therapy with the addition of clopidogrel, 1 mg/kg/day in a single dose.

Patients with large or giant coronary aneurysms are at particularly high risk for thrombosis from markedly abnormal flow conditions, with low wall sheer stress and stasis, together with activation of platelets, clotting factors, and the endothelium. This can lead to coronary obstruction with subsequent myocardial infarction. Systemic anticoagulation combined with low-dose aspirin is recommended. Warfarin has been most often used, although low-molecular-weight heparin and, more recently, direct oral anticoagulants are alternatives.

Long-term Follow-up

The long-term outcomes are primarily driven by coronary artery anomalies. Surveillance is aimed at identifying changes in coronary artery aneurysms and complications related to thrombosis, stenosis/obstruction, and myocardial ischemia. Both the worst and current coronary artery dimensions are used for management decisions during follow-up (Tables 46.2 and 46.3).

Children without cardiovascular abnormalities during the acute and subacute phases do very well without cardiac

TABLE 46.2	Long-Term Assessment and Counseling Algorithm					
Risk Level	Frequency of Cardiology Assessment*	Assessment for Inducible Myocardial Ischemia†	Type and Frequency of Additional Cardiology Assessment	Cardiovascular Risk Factor Assessment and Management‡	Physical Activity Counseling§	Reproductive Counseling
1: No involvement	May discharge between 4 wk and 12 mo	None	None	Assess at 1 y	Promotion counseling at every visit	Age-appropriate counseling without modification
2: Dilation only	If decreased to normal, discharge between 4 wk to 12 mo; if persistent dilation, reassess every 2–5 y	None	None	Assess at 1 y	Promotion counseling at every visit	Age-appropriate counseling without modification
3.1: Small aneurysm, current or persistent	Assess at 6 mo, then yearly	Assess every 2–3 y	May consider every 3–5 y	Assess at 1 y	Promotion counseling at every visit; restrict contact	Age-appropriate counseling without modification
3.2: Small aneurysm, regressed to normal or dilation only	Assess every 1–3 y (may omit echocardiography)	Assess every 3–5 y	May consider if there is inducible ischemia or ventricular dysfunction	Assess at 1 y, then every 2 y	Promotion counseling at every visit	Age-appropriate counseling without modification
4.1: Medium aneurysm, current or persistent	Assess at 3, 6, and 12 mo, then every 6–12 mo	Assess every 1–3 y	May consider every 2–5 y	Assess at 1 y	Promotion counseling at every visit, restrict contact; self-limit	Precautions for contraception and pregnancy

TABLE 46.2 Long-Term Assessment and Counseling Algorithm—cont'd

Risk Level	Frequency of Cardiology Assessment*	Assessment for Inducible Myocardial Ischemia†	Type and Frequency of Additional Cardiology Assessment	Cardiovascular Risk Factor Assessment and Management‡	Physical Activity Counseling§	Reproductive Counseling
4.2: Medium aneurysm, regressed to small aneurysm	Assess yearly	Assess every 2–3 y	May consider every 3–5 y	Assess yearly	Promotion counseling at every visit; restrict contact; self-limit	Precautions for contraception and pregnancy
4.3: Medium aneurysm, regressed to normal or dilation only	Assess every 1–2 y (may omit echocardiography)	Assess every 2–5 y	May consider if there is inducible ischemia or ventricular dysfunction	Assess every 2 y	Promotion counseling at every visit; restrict contact; self-limit	Precautions for contraception and pregnancy
5.1: Large or giant aneurysm, current or persistent	Assess at 3, 6, 9, and 12 mo, then every 3–6 mo	Assess every 6–12 mo	Baseline within first year, may consider every 1–5 y	Assess every 6–12 mo	Promotion counseling at every visit, restrict contact; self-limit	Precautions for contraception and pregnancy
5.2: Large or giant aneurysms, regressed to medium aneurysm	Assess every 6–12 mo	Assess yearly	May consider every 2–5 y	Assess yearly	Promotion counseling at every visit; restrict contact; self-limit	Precautions for contraception and pregnancy
5.3: Large or giant aneurysm, regressed to small aneurysm	Assess every 6–12 mo	Assess every 1–2 y	May consider every 2–5 y	Assess yearly	Promotion counseling at every visit, restrict contact; self-limit	Precautions for contraception and pregnancy
5.4: Large or giant aneurysm, regressed to normal or dilation only	Assess every 1–2 y (may omit echocardiography)	Assess every 2–5 y	May consider every 2–5 y	Assess every 2 y	Promotion counseling at every visit, restrict contact; self-limit	Precautions for contraception and pregnancy

Yellow indicates a class IIa recommendation (it is reasonable to perform); orange indicates a class IIb recommendation (may be considered).
*To include history and physical examination, echocardiography, and electrocardiography.
†May include stress echocardiography, stress electrocardiography, stress with magnetic resonance perfusion imaging, and stress with nuclear medicine perfusion imaging.
‡General healthy lifestyle counseling should be provided at every visit (may be performed by primary care provider).
§Restrictions for contact apply to patients on anticoagulation or dual antiplatelet therapy; self-limit refers to allowing patients to participate to their reasonable abilities without coercion or pressure to perform or overexert (self, parents, coaches).
Adapted from McCrindle BW, Rowley AH, Newburger JW, et al. Diagnosis, treatment, and long-term management of Kawasaki disease. A scientific statement for health professionals from the American Heart Association. *Circulation.* 2017;135:e927–e999. ©2017 American Heart Association, Inc.

symptoms on long-term follow-up. Patients without coronary involvement can be discharged from cardiology follow-up 4–6 weeks after initial diagnosis.

Most patients with non-giant coronary aneurysms have regression of coronary aneurysms during follow-up (99% for small coronary aneurysms, 92% for moderate aneurysms).[21]

Despite remodeling to a normal internal lumen dimension from myofibroblastic proliferation and/or layering thrombosis, these children do not have normal vascular reactivity and require regular long-term cardiologic follow-up. Most require assessment for myocardial ischemia every 1–5 years, for example by stress testing with myocardial imaging; advanced coronary imaging should be considered in the presence of inducible ischemia or ventricular dysfunction.

Patients with large or giant coronary aneurysm are at the greatest risk of adverse cardiac events during follow-up, including thrombosis and/or stenosis that can lead to

TABLE 46.3	Long-Term Thromboprophylaxis and Medical Therapy Algorithm				
Risk Level	**Low-Dose ASA**	**Anticoagulation (Warfarin or LMWH)**	**Dual Antiplatelet Therapy (ASA + Clopidogrel)**	**Beta-Blocker**	**Statin**
1: No involvement	4–6 wk, then discontinue	Not indicated	Not indicated	Not indicated	Not indicated
2: Dilation only	Indicated until regression to normal	Not indicated	Not indicated	Not indicated	Not indicated
3.1: Small aneurysm, current or persistent	Indicated	Not indicated	Not indicated	Not indicated	May be considered
3.2: Small aneurysm, regressed to normal or dilation only	May be considered	Not indicated	Not indicated	Not indicated	May be considered
4.1: Medium aneurysm, current or persistent	Indicated	Not indicated	May be considered	Not indicated	May be considered
4.2: Medium aneurysm, regressed to small aneurysm	Indicated	Not indicated	May be considered	Not indicated	May be considered
4.3: Medium aneurysm, regressed to normal or dilation only	Reasonably indicated	Not indicated	Not recommended except in the presence of inducible myocardial ischemia	Not indicated	May be considered
5.1: Large and giant aneurysm, current or persistent	Indicated	Reasonably indicated	May be considered in addition to anticoagulation*	May be considered	May be considered
5.2: Large or giant aneurysm, regressed to medium aneurysm	Indicated	Not indicated	Reasonably indicated	May be considered	May be considered
5.3: Large or giant aneurysm, regressed to small aneurysm	Indicated	Not indicated	Not indicated	May be considered	May be considered
5.4: Large or giant aneurysm, regressed to normal or dilation only	Reasonably indicated	Not indicated	Not indicated	Not indicated	May be considered

Green indicates a class I recommendation (should be performed); yellow indicates a class IIa recommendation (it is reasonable to perform); orange indicates a class IIb recommendation (may be considered); and red indicates a class III recommendation (should not be performed).

*May be considered in addition to anticoagulation in the setting of very extensive or distal coronary artery aneurysms, or if history of coronary artery thrombosis.

ASA, Acetylsalicylic acid or aspirin; *LMWH,* low-molecular-weight heparin.

Reprinted with permission from McCrindle BW, Rowley AH, Newburger JW, et al. Diagnosis, treatment, and long-term management of Kawasaki disease. a scientific statement for health professionals from the American Heart Association. *Circulation.* 2017;135:e927–e999. ©2017 American Heart Association, Inc.

coronary occlusion and myocardial infarction. In a large registry of patients with aneurysms, stenosis (>50%) occurred in 20% during follow-up, coronary artery thrombosis in 18%, and major adverse cardiovascular complications in 14%; no patients with non-giant aneurysms had a cardiac event on follow-up.[21] Patients with large or giant aneurysms should generally be followed in cardiology with an echocardiogram every 3 months in the first year, then every 6 months, with yearly assessment for inducible ischemia. This can be performed through stress echocardiogram, stress cardiac magnetic resonance, nuclear medicine myocardial perfusion (Technetium 99m sestamibi [MIBI]) or cardiac positron emission tomography. Exercise stress or

pharmacologic stress can be used in combination with those imaging modalities based on the patient's age and clinical scenario; electrocardiographic testing alone should not be used for assessment of ischemia. Advanced coronary imaging is recommended within the first year for baseline, and then every 1–5 years depending upon current disease severity. In addition to thromboprophylaxis described above, patients with large/giant coronary aneurysms are often treated with beta-blockers, and statins may be considered.[4] Their use is largely extrapolated on the benefits in adults with ischemic heart disease.

Myocardial infarction resulting from complete or near-complete coronary occlusion is an infrequent but important clinical sequela. Infarction tends to occur early in the course with approximately 50% within the first 3 months and 73% in the initial year following onset. A high index of suspicion is needed from parents and caregivers, as many children present without the typical symptoms of angina. Symptoms may include crying, chest pain, shock, abdominal pain, vomiting, dyspnea, and arrhythmia. In the reported series, these symptoms were more common in those > 4 years (83%) than in younger children (17%).

ST-segment elevation myocardial infarction (STEMI) is a medical emergency and prompt restoration of antegrade coronary flow should be attempted. Systemic thrombolysis with anticoagulation or antiplatelet therapy (i.e., abciximab) is often the best option to reduce thrombus burden and allow for rapid recanalization.[22] Some patients may be amenable to percutaneous coronary intervention for recanalization, especially older children in a center with local expertise available. Patients with non-ST-segment elevation myocardial ischemia (non-STEMI) should be treated with systemic anticoagulation and antiplatelet therapy pending advanced coronary imaging to determine the best mean of flow restoration.

Other patients may be asymptomatic or have stable angina and require revascularization. Decisions regarding the need for revascularization are often difficult and based on limited observational data and expert consensus. Data in adults with ischemic heart disease suggest that patients with coronary obstruction and angina can be managed medically without an increased risk of long-term morbidity or myocardial infarction. Patients with symptoms refractory to maximal medical therapy are candidates for revascularization. In addition, patients with stable angina and high-risk coronary artery anatomy may benefit from revascularization, including patients with left main coronary disease, multiple vessel coronary disease with reduction in left ventricular systolic function or diabetes mellitus, or high-risk noninvasive ischemia testing. Asymptomatic patients with ischemia > 10% of myocardial muscle mass may also benefit from revascularization. Fractional flow reserve assessment during an invasive cardiac catheterization may be a useful tool for risk stratification. There are, however, few evidence-based data on indications for coronary intervention in children with KD, and the trade-offs of different management strategies should be discussed among multidisciplinary teams including pediatric and adult cardiologists and cardiac surgeons.

Both coronary artery bypass grafting and percutaneous coronary intervention can be used for revascularization, and the relative risks and benefits of these procedures should be weighed in light of anatomy and technical considerations in individual patients.[23,24] Coronary artery bypass grafting is likely to allow more complete revascularization, and thus should be considered in patients with multivessel coronary involvement, reduced left ventricular systolic function, and/or prior failed percutaneous intervention. Whenever possible, mammary artery grafts should be favored, as they allow growth in children and have a higher rate of patency on

follow-up. Patients with single lesion disease may be candidates for percutaneous revascularization, although the anatomy should be carefully reviewed with an interventional team, including adult cardiologists, to ensure feasibility.

A small proportion of patients with progressive disease despite medical and/or surgical intervention may require cardiac transplantation for severe ventricular dysfunction, i.e., end-stage ischemic cardiomyopathy, and/or ventricular arrhythmias.

References

1. Ae R, Makino N, Kosami K, et al. Epidemiology, treatments, and cardiac complications in patients with Kawasaki disease: the nationwide survey in Japan, 2017-2018. *J Pediatr.* 2020;225: 23-29.
2. Lio K, Matsubara K, Miyakoshi C, et al. Incidence of Kawasaki disease before and during the COVID-19 pandemic: a retrospective cohort study in Japan. *BMJ Paediatr Open.* 2021;5:e001034.
3. Holman RC, Belay ED, Christensen KY, et al. Hospitalizations for Kawasaki syndrome among children in the United States, 1997-2007. *Pediatr Infect Dis J.* 2010;29:483.
4. McCrindle BW, Rowley AH, Newburger JW, et al. Diagnosis, treatment, and long-term management of Kawasaki disease: a scientific statement for health professionals from the American Heart Association. *Circulation.* 2017;135:e927-e999.
5. Zhao QM, Chu C, Wu L, et al. Systemic artery aneurysms and Kawasaki disease. *Pediatrics.* 2019;144:e20192254.
6. Orenstein JM, Shulman ST, Fox LM, et al. Three linked vasculopathic processes characterize Kawasaki disease: a light and transmission electron microscopic study. *PLoS One.* 2012;7: e38998.
7. Gordon JB, Daniels LB, Kahn AM, et al. The spectrum of cardiovascular lesions requiring intervention in adults after Kawasaki disease. *JACC Cardiovasc Interv.* 2016;9:687-696.
8. Dionne A, Ibrahim R, Gebhard C, et al. Coronary wall structure changes in patients with Kawasaki disease: new insights from optical coherence tomography (OCT). *J Am Heart Assoc.* 2015; 4:e001939.
9. Salgado AP, Ashouri N, Berry EK, et al. High risk of coronary artery aneurysms in infants younger than 6 months of age with Kawasaki disease. *J Pediatr.* 2017;185:112-116.
10. Furusho K, Kamiya T, Nakano H, et al. High-dose intravenous gammaglobulin for Kawasaki disease. *Lancet.* 1984;2:1055-1058.
11. Newburger JW, Takahashi M, Burns JC, et al. The treatment of Kawasaki syndrome with intravenous gamma globulin. *N Engl J Med.* 1986;315:341-347.
12. Egami K, Muta H, Ishii M, et al. Prediction of resistance to intravenous immunoglobulin treatment in patients with Kawasaki disease. *J Pediatr.* 2006;149:237-240.
13. Kobayashi T, Inoue Y, Takeuchi K, et al. A prediction of intravenous immunoglobulin unresponsiveness in patients with Kawasaki disease. *Circulation.* 2006;113:2606-2612.
14. Son MBF, Gauvreau K, Kim S, et al. Predicting coronary artery aneurysms in Kawasaki disease at a North American center: an assessment of baseline z scores. *J Am Heart Assoc.* 2017;6:e005378.
15. Kobayashi T, Saji T, Otani T, et al. Efficacy of immunoglobulin plus prednisolone for prevention of coronary artery abnormalities in severe Kawasaki disease (RAISE study): a randomized, open-label, blinded endpoints trial. *Lancet.* 2012;379: 1613-1620.

16. Hamada H, Suzuki H, Onouchi Y, et al. Efficacy of primary treatment with immunoglobulin plus ciclosporin for prevention of coronary artery abnormalities in patients with Kawasaki disease predicted to be at increased risk of non-response to intravenous immunoglobulin (KAICA): a randomised controlled, open-label, blinded-endpoints, phase 3 trial. *Lancet.* 2019;393:1128-1137.

17. Tremoulet AH, Jain S, Jaggi P, et al. Infliximab for intensification of primary therapy for Kawasaki disease: a phase 3 randomised, double-blind, placebo-controlled trial. *Lancet.* 2014;383:1731-1738.

18. Portman MA, Dahdah NS, Slee A, et al. Etanercept with IVIg for acute Kawasaki disease: a randomized controlled trial. *Pediatrics.* 2019;143:e20183675.

19. Burns JC, Roberts SC, Tremoulet AH, et al. Infliximab versus second intravenous immunoglobulin for treatment of resistant Kawasaki disease in the USA (KIDCARE): a randomised, multicenter comparative effectiveness trial. *Lancet Child Adolesc Health.* 2021;5:852-861.

20. Kobayashi T, Kobayashi T, Morikawa A, et al. Efficacy of intravenous immunoglobulin combined with prednisolone following resistance to initial intravenous immunoglobulin treatment of acute Kawasaki disease. *J Pediatr.* 2013;163:521-526.

21. McCrindle BW, Manlhiot C, Newburger JW, et al. Medium-term complications associated with coronary artery aneurysms after Kawasaki disease: a study from the International Kawasaki Disease Registry. *J Am Heart Assoc.* 2020;9:e016440.

22. Burns JC, El-Said H, Tremoulet AH, et al. Management of myocardial infarction in children with giant coronary artery aneurysms after Kawasaki disease. *J Pediatr.* 2020;221:230-234.

23. Tsuda E, Kitamura S, Cooperative study group of Japan. National survey of coronary artery bypass grafting for coronary stenosis caused by Kawasaki disease in Japan. *Circulation.* 2004;110:1161-1166.

24. Akagi T, Ogawa S, Ino T, et al. Catheter interventional treatment in Kawasaki disease a report from the Japanese Pediatric Interventional Cardiology Investigation group. *J Pediatr.* 2000;137:181-186.

47

Lyme disease, COVID-19, and Myocarditis

AUDREY DIONNE AND CATHERINE ALLAN

KEY LEARNING POINTS

- Lyme disease is a tick-borne illness that can include cardiac involvement with atrioventricular block and/or myopericarditis in the early disseminated phase of the disease.
- Pediatric patients with COVID-19 infection are at risk of multisystem inflammatory syndrome in children, which is characterized by fever, elevated inflammatory markers, and multisystem organ involvement. Cardiac complications are common and include ventricular dysfunction,

coronary artery aneurysm, arrhythmias, and pericardial effusion.
- Myocarditis is an inflammatory disease of the myocardium that can cause subclinical disease or manifest as cardiogenic shock, malignant arrhythmias, and sudden cardiac death. Infectious etiologies are most common in children. Outcomes span from complete recovery to cardiomyopathy, heart transplant, and death.

Lyme Disease

Lyme disease is a tick-borne illness caused by species in the spirochete family *Borreliaceae*. Lyme disease has a broad range of manifestations, including Lyme carditis in a minority of children. The most common cardiac manifestation is atrioventricular (AV) block, which is usually self-limited, although it may require temporary pacing.

Epidemiology

Lyme disease is the most common tick-borne infection in the United States with > 250,000 confirmed cases from 2010 to 2019. It is usually found in forested regions, with most cases from the Northeast.

Lyme carditis occurs in approximately 1% of adults with Lyme disease based on surveillance data in the United States from 2008 to 2018. Earlier studies reported higher rates (4–10%), although that may be related to improved recognition and treatment of early Lyme disease in recent years. Boys are affected more frequently with a 3:1 male predominance. No studies have evaluated the risk of carditis in children versus adults. Carditis can be prevented with antibiotic therapy, highlighting the importance of early recognition and treatment.

Pathophysiology

In North America, *Borrelia burgdorferi* is the motile, spiral spirochete primarily responsible for Lyme disease; *Borrelia afzelii* and *Borrelia garinii* are predominant in Europe and Asia. *Borrelia* species cause infection by migrating through tissues, disseminating in the blood, adhering to host cells, and evading immune clearance.

Clinical Manifestations

The clinical manifestations of Lyme disease depend on the stage of illness. Early localized disease is characterized by a single erythema migrans lesion appearing at the site of the tick bite, usually within 7 to 14 days after the bite (Fig. 47.1).[1] Erythema migrans is the only manifestation that permits clinical diagnosis without laboratory confirmation. Serologic testing is not sufficiently sensitive early in the disease.

Early disseminated disease occurs weeks to several months after the tick bite if not recognized and treated. Clinical manifestations include multiple erythema migrans, cranial nerve palsy, meningitis, and carditis. Systemic signs and symptoms, including fever, fatigue, headache, and arthralgia are also common.

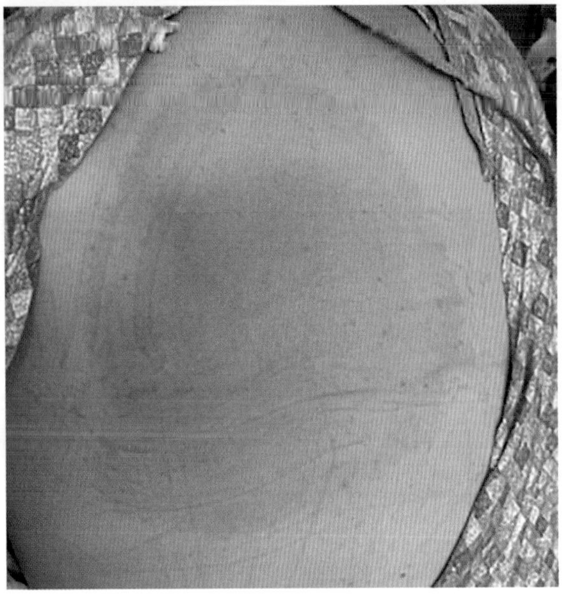

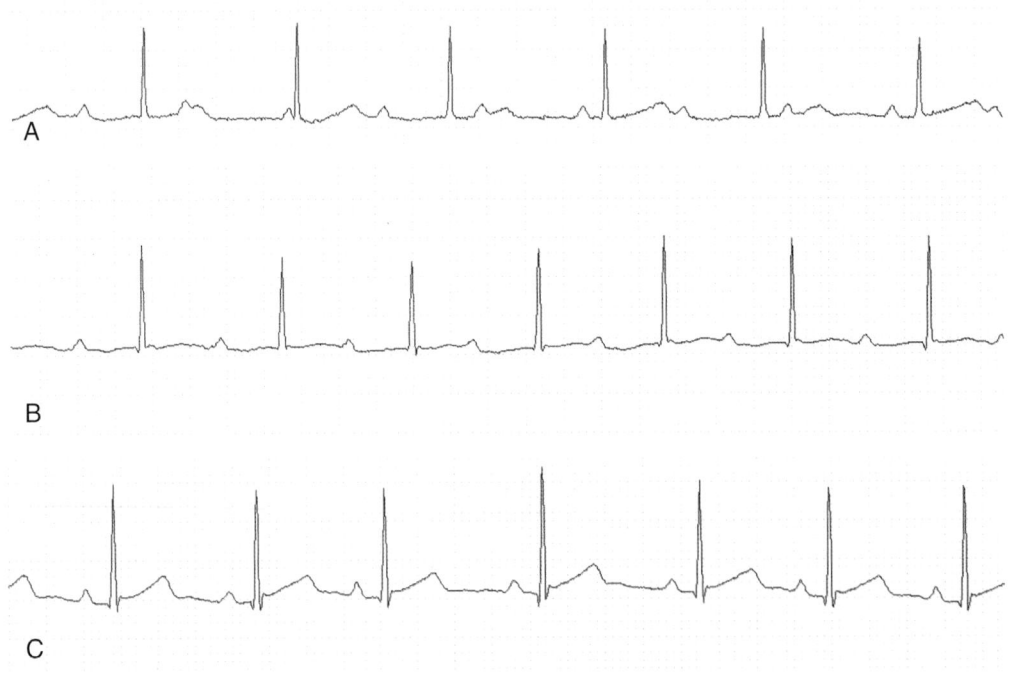

• **Fig. 47.1** Erythema migrans lesion in a patient with Lyme carditis and atrioventricular block.

Late Lyme disease occurs weeks to months after initial infection, and most often presents with arthritis.

Lyme Carditis

Cardiac disease can be isolated or occur with other features of early Lyme disease. In a small series, erythema migrans was found in 75% of patients with carditis, joint involvement in 65%, and meningoencephalitis in 35%.[2] Patients with cardiac involvement may be asymptomatic or complain of lightheadedness, syncope, shortness of breath, palpitations, or chest pain.

AV block is the most common manifestation of Lyme carditis, occurring in 77–87% of patients with carditis (Fig. 47.2).[3] Conduction abnormalities can progress and fluctuate rapidly from first-degree AV block to complete AV block. Patients with a PR interval greater than 300 ms are at the highest risk of progression.[2] Approximately half of patients with carditis develop complete AV block, most of whom are symptomatic. The conduction delay typically occurs in the AV node, above the bundle of His. Abnormalities can occur throughout the His-Purkinje system, however, and manifest as sinoatrial node dysfunction, interatrial block, fascicular block, and bundle branch block.

Myopericarditis has also been described in Lyme disease although it is often mild and self-limited. Most frequently this is observed as nonspecific ST- and T-wave changes on electrocardiogram (ECG). Small pericardial effusions can also be seen. Rarely, patients may have more severe myocardial inflammation leading to systolic ventricular dysfunction and sudden death. In a case series of 33 patients with Lyme carditis, 4 patients had associated ventricular dysfunction, 3 of whom required mechanical ventilation, inotropic support, and temporary pacing.[4]

• **Fig. 47.2** Sequential electrocardiograms from a patient with resolving Lyme carditis showing **(A)** complete atrioventricular block with narrow junctional escape; **(B)** marked first-degree atrioventricular block with PR interval 342 ms; and **(C)** normal atrioventricular conduction and PR interval.

Diagnostic Testing

Serology

The diagnosis of Lyme disease can be made with an enzyme-linked immunosorbent assay (ELISA) and confirmed with Western blot analysis. When performed for early disseminated disease 1–2 months after the initial infection, most patients have positive serologic responses. Thus, if negative, alternative diagnoses should be strongly considered. Seropositivity, including IgM, can persist for years after Lyme infection and should be interpreted in the clinical context.

Electrocardiogram

ECG should be considered in all patients with evidence of Lyme disease as up to half of the patients with carditis may be asymptomatic. First-degree AV block is most common, and higher-grade AV block is frequent. Other findings consistent with carditis include ST- and T-wave changes, ventricular enlargement, QTc prolongation, and arrhythmias.

Echocardiogram

Echocardiogram to evaluate ventricular size and function, valvar function, and pericardial effusion should be considered in selected patients with Lyme disease and cardiac symptoms or concerns for carditis.

Management

The goal of therapy for Lyme disease is to decrease the duration of symptoms and the risk of acute and long-term complications. Acute complications, including third-degree AV block, may be life-threatening if not treated.

Selected asymptomatic patients with PR interval < 300 ms may be treated as outpatients with doxycycline, amoxicillin, or cefuroxime for 14–21 days. However, given the risk of progression of disease after presentation, patients with cardiac symptoms, PR interval > 300 ms, and/or second- or third-degree AV block or other arrhythmias, should be hospitalized for monitoring and treatment.[5]

Patients should be monitored on cardiac telemetry, usually for an additional 24–48 hours after PR interval is < 300 ms. Intravenous ceftriaxone (50–75 mg/kg or 2 g daily in adults) is the first-line therapy for inpatient treatment; alternatives include cefotaxime and penicillin G. Patients should be treated with intravenous antibiotics until resolution of high-grade AV block and PR interval < 300 ms, after which they can be transitioned to oral antibiotics to complete a 14- to 21-day course. However, these recommendations are based on small case series, and no trials have compared different antibiotic regimens or the superiority of intravenous over oral antibiotics.

Pacing via a temporary transvenous pacing lead should be considered for patients with evidence of high-grade AV block with or without cardiac symptoms. Pacing is typically needed only transiently, with improvement in high-grade AV block usually seen within 1 week and resolution of conduction abnormalities in 3–42 days.

Coronavirus Disease 2019

In late 2019, the novel coronavirus, severe acute respiratory syndrome coronavirus 2 (SARS-CoV-2), rapidly spread resulting in a global pandemic. The illness it causes, coronavirus disease 2019 (COVID-19), ranges from asymptomatic to life-threatening, with children overall more likely to have asymptomatic or milder disease than adults. However, a small percentage of children with symptomatic COVID-19 manifest clinically significant cardiovascular involvement.

Epidemiology

In the first 2 years of the pandemic, more than 13 million cases of COVID-19 occurred in children < 18 years, accounting for 19% of the cumulative total of COVID-19 cases. The number of reported cases is likely an underestimate given the number of asymptomatic or non-reported cases from home testing. Approximately 75% of children and adolescents tested in schools were seropositive for SARS-CoV-2, higher than seroprevalence in adults which is 33% to 64%.

Underrepresented racial and ethnic groups appear to be disproportionately affected by SARS-CoV-2 infection and its morbidities. Hospitalization rates have been 2.2–2.5 times greater among non-Hispanic American Indian/Alaska Native children, non-Hispanic Black children, and Hispanic/Latino children compared with non-Hispanic White children (158.5–179.2 vs. 72 per 100,000 population).

Clinical Manifestations

To date, data from large electronic medical records in the United States demonstrate that of children with SARS-CoV-2 infection, approximately two-thirds are asymptomatic, approximately one-third have mild COVID-19 related symptoms, 5% have moderate symptoms (e.g., pneumonia, gastroenteritis, dehydration), and 2% have severe disease requiring intensive care unit (ICU) admission.

Frequently reported symptoms include fever, cough, shortness of breath, myalgia, rhinorrhea, sore throat, headache, nausea/vomiting, abdominal pain, diarrhea, and loss of smell or taste. Children with underlying medical conditions are at greater risk for severe disease. The most frequent underlying medical conditions in children admitted to the ICU with COVID-19 include chronic pulmonary disease, obesity, neurologic and developmental conditions, and cardiovascular conditions. The median duration of illness is 6 days (interquartile range, 3–11 days), although clinical deterioration can occur suddenly during the course and prompt urgent re-evaluation.

Cardiovascular involvement was documented in 12% of patients with acute severe COVID-19, including ventricular dysfunction (12%), pericardial effusion (5%), coronary artery aneurysm (1%), and arrhythmias (1%).[6]

Multisystem Inflammatory Syndrome in Children

Multisystem inflammatory syndrome in children (MIS-C) is a rare but serious complication of SARS-CoV-2 infection. It is characterized by fever, elevated inflammatory markers, multisystem organ involvement, and evidence of recent SARS-CoV-2 infection (Table 47.1).

Epidemiology

MIS-C occurs 2–5 weeks following COVID-19 infection. It is relatively rare with incidence of approximately 3 per 10,000 individuals aged < 21 years with COVID-19, although this is probably an overestimate given that many children are likely to be either asymptomatic or not tested for SARS-CoV-2 infection. Black and Hispanic children have been disproportionately affected by MIS-C. The incidence of MIS-C may continue to evolve as more of the population is vaccinated against COVID-19 and/or has been previously exposed to the virus.

Clinical Manifestations

MIS-C has been reported in children of all ages (although rarely in adults), with a median age of 8–11 years. Signs and symptoms include fever (100%), gastrointestinal (abdominal pain, vomiting, diarrhea; 60–100%), mucocutaneous (rash, conjunctivitis, red or swollen lips, strawberry tongue; 30–81%), cardiorespiratory (40–65%), and/or neurologic (headache, lethargy, confusion; 29–58%).[7] Dermatologic or mucocutaneous symptoms are most common in children aged 0–5 years, while cardiac and neurologic involvement are seen more often in older children and teenagers.

Clinical signs of shock are frequent and found in 32–76% of patients, often a combination of both vasodilatory and cardiogenic. Cardiac involvement is reported in 40–80% of patients. Respiratory symptoms are less frequent than in acute COVID-19 and may be secondary (e.g., cardiogenic pulmonary edema). Acute respiratory failure requiring non-invasive or invasive ventilation is found in 28–52% of patients. Mucocutaneous symptoms are frequent; 22–64% of patients with MIS-C meet complete criteria for Kawasaki disease. Although the features of the two diseases overlap, they are distinct conditions. Patients with Kawasaki disease are typically younger, whereas patients with MIS-C have more intense inflammation, are more likely to have gastrointestinal and neurologic symptoms, and more likely to present with myocardial dysfunction and shock. Other frequently observed organ dysfunction includes acute kidney injury (typically mild; 8–52%), hepatitis or hepatomegaly (5–21%), and encephalopathy, seizures, coma, or meningoencephalitis (6–7%).

Patients with MIS-C can be critically ill and may require ICU admission (80%), inotropic support (50%), and mechanical ventilation (20%). Despite the initial severity of illness, most patients recover, with hospital discharge after a median of 7 days.[7]

Cardiovascular Involvement

Cardiovascular injury in children with COVID-19 is incompletely understood but likely involves multiple mechanisms. It is hypothesized that COVID-19 has direct cardiomyocyte toxicity leading to microvascular dysfunction, dysregulated inflammation, and coagulopathy. MIS-C can affect the myocardium, coronary arteries, and conduction system, and can manifest as ventricular dysfunction, pericardial effusion, coronary artery dilation, aneurysms, and arrhythmias (Fig. 47.3).

Ventricular dysfunction was found in 38% of patients in a large registry and noted to be severe (ejection fraction < 30%) in 5% of patients.[7] Diastolic dysfunction was also noted in most patients with MIS-C and was worse in those with elevated troponin level and/or brain natriuretic peptide (BNP).[8] Reassuringly, almost all patients had recovery of ventricular function at a median of 4 days.

Coronary aneurysms have been reported in 0%–25% of patients with MIS-C. It remains under debate whether these represent true aneurysms with destruction of the arterial wall versus extreme vasodilation from cytokine storm. In the "Overcoming COVID-19" cohort, patients with coronary

TABLE 47.1	Case Definition for Multisystem Inflammatory Syndrome in Children From the Center for Disease Control and Prevention

Individual aged < 21 years

Fever ≥ 38.0°C for ≥ 24 hours or report of subjective fever lasting ≥ 24 hours

Laboratory evidence of inflammation including, but not limited to, one or more of the following: an elevated C-reactive protein, erythrocyte sedimentation rate, fibrinogen, procalcitonin, D-dimer, ferritin, lactic acid dehydrogenase, or interleukin 6, elevated neutrophils, reduced lymphocytes, and low albumin

Evidence of clinically severe illness requiring hospitalization

Multisystem (≥2) organ involvement (cardiac, renal, respiratory, hematologic, gastrointestinal, dermatologic, and/or neurological)

No alternative plausible diagnosis

Positive for current or recent SARS-CoV-2 infection by reverse transcription-polymerase chain reaction, serology, or antigen test; or exposure to a suspected or confirmed COVID-19 case within the 4 weeks prior to the onset of symptoms

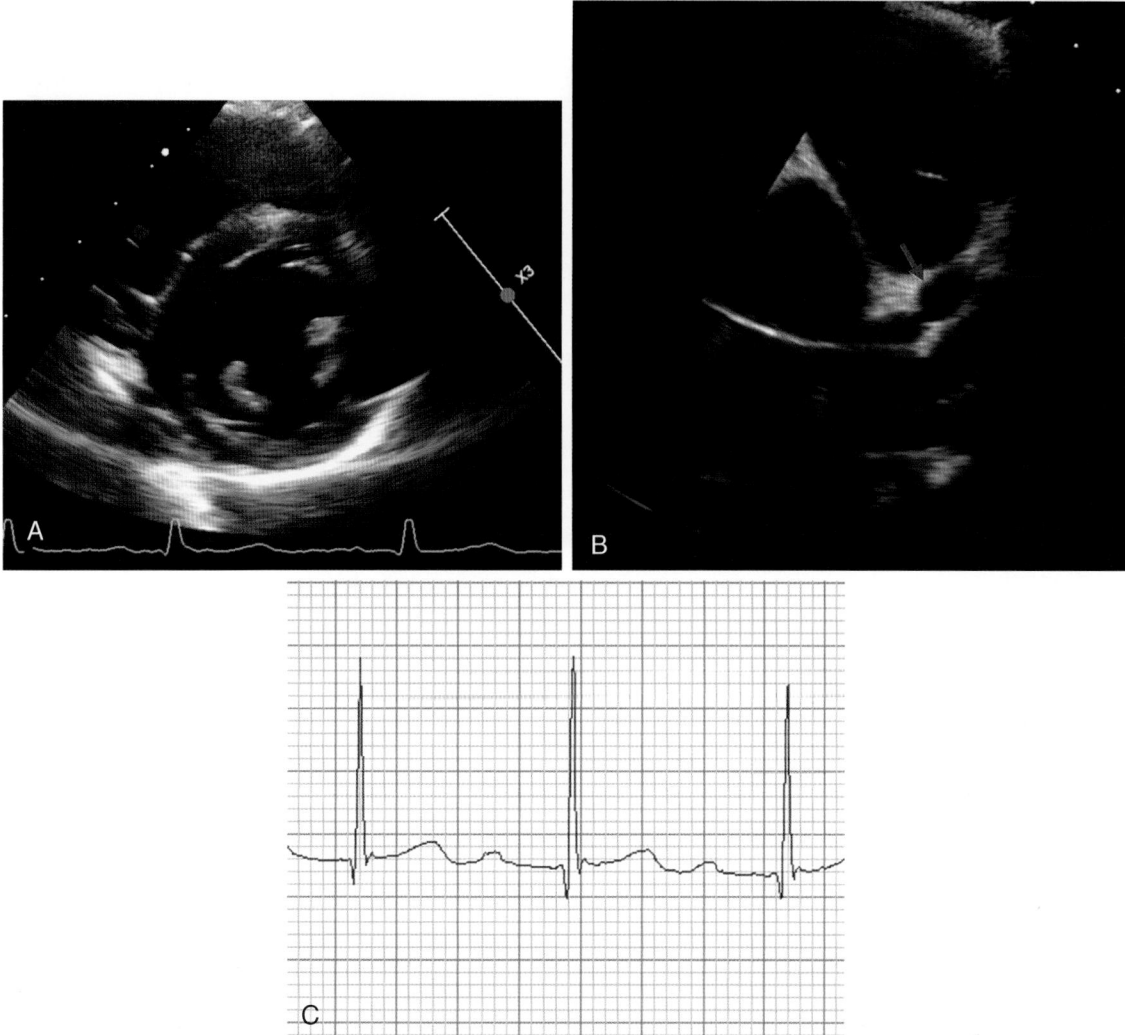

• **Fig. 47.3** Cardiac complications in multisystem inflammatory syndrome in children (MIS-C) include **(A)** ventricular dysfunction, **(B)** coronary artery aneurysm, and **(C)** atrioventricular block and arrhythmias.

aneurysms were mild in 93% (z-score < 5) and moderate in 7% (z-score between 5 and 10). Giant aneurysms have been reported in small case series. Follow-up of a small number of patients showed resolution of coronary artery aneurysm (z-score < 2.5) by 30 days in 79% of patients and by 90 days in all patients.[6]

In a small series of patient who underwent cardiac magnetic resonance imaging (MRI) within 30 days of diagnosis of MIS-C, half had myocardial edema and one patient had late gadolinium enhancement. Ejection fraction and strain values on MRI did not correlate with persistent myocardial edema, scarring, age or timing of presentation.[9] The long-term changes on cardiac MRI after MIS-C remain unknown.

ECG changes are found in approximately two-thirds of patients, most frequently prolongation of PR, QRS, and QTc intervals.[10] ECG changes may manifest midway through hospitalization, highlighting the need for ongoing monitoring. PR prolongation was the most frequently encountered conduction delay in approximately 20%–30% of patients, with persistent first-degree AV block in 12% of patients at hospital discharge. Higher-grade AV block has

been described in patients with more severe illness course including shock and ventricular dysfunction; it is typically preceded by first-degree AV block.[11] Monitoring on telemetry is recommended for these patients due to the risk of progression. Higher-grade AV block was typically transient, lasting 1–6 days. No patients required medications or pacing for AV block.

Tachyarrhythmias, most common in older and sicker patients, were found in approximately 1.7% of patients with MIS-C, and included atrial (44%), junctional (14%), and ventricular arrhythmias (60%). Furthermore, 60% of arrhythmias required intervention including antiarrhythmic medication, cardioversion, cardiopulmonary resuscitation, and/or extracorporeal membrane oxygenation (ECMO).

Diagnostic Testing

Laboratory Testing

Laboratory testing includes inflammatory markers (C-reactive protein, erythrocyte sedimentation rate, D-dimer, fibrinogen, ferritin, procalcitonin, albumin); cardiac markers (BNP, troponin); and indicators of other organ involvement (liver enzymes, renal function). Lymphocytopenia, neutrophilia, mild anemia, and thrombocytopenia are frequent findings on complete blood count.

Testing should also include polymerase chain reaction (PCR) and serology for SARS-CoV-2. Most patients have positive serologies with negative PCR; however, 30–35% are positive on both tests. Clinical history and exposure to COVID-19 remain important, as some patients may have negative serologies, and incidental positive serologies unrelated to current presentation may occur.

Additional infectious testing for viral and bacterial pathogens may be considered based on clinical presentation.

Chest Radiograph

Chest radiographs are normal in many patients though some may reveal pleural effusion(s), ground-glass opacities, patchy consolidation, and/or atelectasis.

Electrocardiogram

ECG should focus on evaluation of intervals (PR, QRS, QT, QTc), atrial or ventricular hypertrophy, repolarization abnormalities, and arrhythmias. Screening ECG should be performed every 48 hours given the risk of arrhythmias and AV block, which may not be present at the time of hospital admission.

Echocardiogram

Echocardiogram, performed at the time of diagnosis and prior to hospital discharge, should focus on evaluation of systolic and diastolic ventricular function, valvar function, coronary artery dimensions, and presence of pericardial effusion. Patients with significant dysfunction or coronary aneurysm may need more frequent evaluations.

Cardiac Magnetic Resonance Imaging

Cardiac MRI should focus on assessment of ventricular systolic function, myocardial edema (T2-weighted imaging), hyperemia and capillary leakage (myocardial early gadolinium enhancement), necrosis and fibrosis (late gadolinium enhancement), coronary artery dimensions, and presence of pericardial effusion. Cardiac MRI can be considered acutely in hemodynamically stable patients with ventricular dysfunction and arrhythmia, or during follow-up prior to return to sports.

Management

Treatment of MIS-C evolved rapidly through the course of the COVID-19 pandemic and has included the use of intravenous immunoglobulin (IVIG), glucocorticoids, and biologic agents such as interleukin 1 receptor antagonist (i.e., anakinra), tumor necrosis factor inhibitors (i.e., infliximab), and anti-interleukin 6 therapies (i.e., tocilizumab). Glucocorticoids were introduced due to the appreciation of the highly inflammatory nature of MIS-C and decreased concerns regarding potentiation of viral replication.

Evidence regarding efficacy of IVIG and glucocorticoids has been conflicting. The "French COVID-19 Paediatric Inflammation Consortium," a retrospective study utilizing a propensity score analysis comparing IVIG to IVIG and corticosteroids, showed a lower risk of persistent or recrudescent fever as well as decreased need for second-line therapy, hemodynamic support, left ventricular dysfunction, and ICU length of stay with IVIG and corticosteroids.[12] The "Overcoming COVID-19" network similarly showed improved short-term cardiovascular outcomes (improved left ventricular ejection fraction and lower vasopressor requirement measured at $\geq$ 2 days) for patients treated with IVIG plus corticosteroids compared with those treated with IVIG alone.[13] In contrast, there were no significant differences in composite outcome of inotropic support, mechanical ventilation, or death in the International BATS cohort across treatment groups (IVIG, IVIG with glucocorticoids, or glucocorticoids alone).[14] Potential reasons for discrepant findings include differences in cohort definitions (CDC versus WHO) and in markedly higher illness severity in the "Overcoming COVID-19" cohort.

Based on current evidence, recommendations from the American College of Rheumatology include a stepwise progression of immunomodulatory therapies with high-dose IVIG in all patients and adjunctive steroids in patients with shock, organ-threatening disease, or non-responders. Anakinra is suggested for patients refractory to IVIG and steroids.

Anticoagulation therapy is another important component of treatment given the high risk of thrombotic events in patients with COVID-19. Pediatric data demonstrate thrombotic events in 6.5% of patients with MIS-C versus 2.1% in acute COVID-19. Risk factors for thrombosis included age > 12 years, cancer, and presence of a central venous catheter. Expert consensus guidelines recommend the use of low-dose aspirin in all patients with suspected or confirmed MIS-C. For patients with giant coronary artery aneurysm, moderate to severe ventricular dysfunction, arrhythmias, documented thrombosis, or significantly elevated D-dimer, therapeutic anticoagulation, most often with low-molecular-weight heparin or apixaban, is added to aspirin.

Follow-Up

Glucocorticoids are typically weaned over 2–4 weeks. Complete blood count and inflammatory markers are routinely performed every 3–5 days during the wean to ensure ongoing normalization of inflammation.

ECG and echocardiogram should be considered at 7–10 days and 4–6 weeks following discharge. Holter monitor may be appropriate during outpatient follow-up for patients with history of arrhythmia during acute hospitalization.

The majority of patients have improvement and normalization in cardiac testing prior to hospital discharge or during early follow-up. Some patients with significant cardiac involvement may require more frequent monitoring.

Due to the high rate of myocardial involvement in MIS-C, either clinical or subclinical, all patients should be restricted from vigorous physical activity for a minimum of 2 weeks. Patients with evidence of cardiac involvement should be restricted for 3–6 months. Exercise stress test and/or cardiac MRI should be considered prior to return to sports.

Although data to date suggest rapid recovery after hospital discharge, the long-term sequelae of MIS-C remain unknown. At this time, we see patients 1 year after diagnosis and discharge them for follow-up if all testing is normal.

Myocarditis

Myocarditis is an inflammatory disease of the myocardium with multiple causes including infectious agents, toxins, hypersensitivity reactions, and systemic disorders. Presentation can vary widely, from subclinical disease to cardiogenic shock, arrhythmias, and sudden cardiac death.

Epidemiology

Myocarditis is considered to be rare, with an estimated annual incidence of 1 to 2 per 100,000 children. This is likely an underestimate, however, due to the presence of subclinical disease, non-specific symptoms, and diagnostic challenges. The incidence is as high as 10–20% in autopsy series of infants and children who experienced sudden death.

Pathophysiology

The causes of myocarditis are summarized in Table 47.2. Management and prognosis vary widely depending on specific etiology; the following sections refer to viral or idiopathic myocarditis unless otherwise noted.

A variety of infectious agents have been associated with myocarditis, most often viruses.[15] Parvovirus B19 and human herpesvirus are most frequently identified from PCR analysis of myocardial tissue and are now more common than adenovirus and enterovirus. More recently, SARS-CoV-2 infection has been associated with myocarditis, especially in children who develop MIS-C following COVID-19 infection. Rare infectious causes of myocarditis include bacteria, fungi, protozoa, and helminths.

Myocarditis can be a complication of autoimmune disease such as systemic lupus erythematosus, granulomatosis with polyangiitis, giant cell arteritis, and Takayasu arteritis. Myocarditis, pericarditis, or both can be found in up to 10% of children with systemic lupus erythematosus and may be a presenting symptom. Giant cell myocarditis, though rare in pediatrics, is a severe type of autoimmune myocarditis associated with systemic disorder in 20% of cases.

Hypersensitivity myocarditis, characterized by eosinophilic infiltrate on biopsy, is most commonly associated with medication, but can also occur with toxins, infections, and malignancies. It often presents with acute rash, fever, and peripheral eosinophilia.

TABLE 47.2	Causes of Myocarditis

Viral: adenovirus, arbovirus, coxsackie A and B virus, cytomegalovirus, dengue, echovirus, hepatitis B and C, herpesvirus (cytomegalovirus, human herpesvirus 6, Epstein-Barr virus), HIV, influenza A and B, mumps, parvovirus, poliovirus, rabies, rubella, rubeola, varicella, variola, yellow fever, chikungunya, respiratory syncytial, coronavirus

Bacterial: actinomycosis, bartonella, brucellosis, *Burkholderia pseudomallei*, chlamydia, cholera, clostridial, diphtheria (*Corynebacterium diphtheria*), gonococcus, haemophilus, legionella, meningococcal, mycoplasma, nocardia, pneumococcus, psittacosis, salmonella, staphylococcus, streptococcus, tetanus, tuberculosis, tularemia (*Francisella tularensis*)

Spirochetal: Lyme disease, syphilis, leptospirosis, relapsing fever, *Borrelia recurrentis*

Mycotic: actinomyces, aspergillosis, blastomycosis, candidiasis, coccidioidomycosis, cryptococcosis, histoplasmosis, mucormycosis, nocardia, sporotrichosis

Rickettsial: *Coxiella burnetii*, *Rickettsia prowazekii*, *Rickettsia rickettsii* (Rocky Mountain spotted fever), typhus

Protozoal: amebiasis, balantidiasis, leishmaniasis, malaria, toxoplasmosis, *Trypanosoma cruzi* (Chagas disease), *Trypanosoma brucei*

Helminthic: ascariasis, echinococcosis, filariasis, paragonimiasis, schistosomiasis, strongyloidiasis, trichinosis

Cardiotoxins: alcohol, anthracyclines, arsenic, carbon monoxide, catecholamines, cocaine, cyclophosphamide, heavy metals (copper, lead, iron), radiation

Hypersensitivity reactions: aminophylline, antibiotics (beta-lactams, tetracyclines, fluoroquinolones, vancomycin, macrolids, isoniazid, sulfonamides), central nervous system agents (benzodiazepines, carbamazepine, clozapine, methyldopa, phenytoin, tricyclic antidepressant), colchicine, diuretics (thiazide, loop), dobutamine, insect bites (bee, wasp, spider, scorpion), lidocaine, lithium, phenylbutazone, snake bites, tetanus toxoid, vaccinations (e.g., vaccinia, coronavirus mRNA vaccines)

Systemic disorders: celiac disease, collagen-vascular diseases, granulomatosis with polyangiitis, hypereosinophilia, inflammatory bowel disease (Crohn's disease, ulcerative colitis), Kawasaki disease, sarcoidosis, thyrotoxicosis

Clinical Manifestations

The clinical presentation of myocarditis is highly variable and often non-specific; it requires a high index of suspicion for diagnosis.

Frequent symptoms at presentation include fatigue (25–70%), shortness of breath (35–69%), fever (31–58%), nausea/vomiting and abdominal pain (28–48%), rhinorrhea (38–44%), chest pain (24–42%), cough (17–44%), palpitations (16%), and diarrhea (8%).[16] Symptoms at presentation usually reflect a viral prodrome, observed in two-thirds of patients, manifestations of congestive heart failure, and/or arrhythmias. As these symptoms may be nonspecific and found in many common pediatric diseases, incorrect initial diagnosis is common. Rarely, patients may present with sudden cardiac death.

Physical examination can reveal evidence of low cardiac output and shock due to ventricular dysfunction; these include hypotension, poor pulses and perfusion, hepatomegaly, and altered mental status. A gallop may be heard in this setting. If present, murmurs may reflect flow or functional AV valve insufficiency. In the setting of a pericardial effusion, a friction rub or distant heart sounds may be appreciated. Tachycardia is frequent and non-specific but should raise suspicion when out of proportion to the degree of fever. Respiratory findings, including tachypnea, retractions, and rales are frequent, and can be related to associated respiratory viral illness or pulmonary edema.

Diagnostic Testing

Laboratory Testing

Cardiac biomarkers, including troponin and creatinine kinase, reflect myocardial injury and are elevated in most patients with myocarditis. Both lack sensitivity and specificity, however, and should be interpreted within the context of the overall clinical presentation. Troponin levels can help distinguish chronic dilated cardiomyopathy from myocarditis, although there is overlap between both groups and no diagnostic cut-off level has been established. Troponin levels have not correlated with ventricular dysfunction or arrhythmias. They are associated with worse outcomes, however, specifically the need for ECMO and mortality.

BNP and N-terminal pro-BNP (NT-proBNP), though not specific for myocarditis, are often elevated in affected patients and can help distinguish between respiratory and cardiac cause for symptoms; levels have been associated with cardiac dysfunction, need for cardiopulmonary resuscitation, and need for mechanical circulatory support (MCS).

Other laboratory findings include elevation of non-specific inflammatory markers such as C-reactive protein, erythrocyte sedimentation rate, and white blood cell count. Blood gases, lactate level, and markers of renal and hepatic function may be useful to assess for evidence of inadequate systemic perfusion and end-organ dysfunction and/or direct viral injury.

Chest Radiograph

Findings on chest radiograph can include cardiomegaly, pulmonary vascular congestion, and/or pleural effusion in approximately half of patients. It is not uncommon for chest radiographs to appear remarkably normal on initial presentation in patients with acute fulminant disease.

Electrocardiogram

ECG changes are frequent and include sinus tachycardia, non-specific ST-segment changes, T-wave inversion, ST-segment elevation and low-voltage QRS complexes. ST-segment changes can be diffuse, or in a defined coronary distribution with pattern of infarction or injury. Pericarditis may manifest with diffuse ST-segment elevation and PR depression. AV block and tachyarrhythmias (e.g., atrial tachycardia, ventricular tachycardia) are seen in up to 44% of children with myocarditis and are associated with worse outcomes, including need for MCS, transplant, or death.[17]

Echocardiogram

Echocardiographic findings may include decreased ventricular systolic function with or without regional wall motion abnormalities, left ventricular enlargement, thickened myocardium due to myocardial edema, pericardial effusion, intracardiac thrombus, and functional valvar regurgitation.

Cardiac Magnetic Resonance

Cardiac MRI can demonstrate myocardial inflammation and necrosis; it is increasingly used for diagnosis of myocarditis. Cardiac MRI is a noninvasive test; however, it requires sedation and intubation in infants and young children which adds significant risk in sick patients with minimal hemodynamic reserve.

The Lake Louise criteria are a consensus definition for diagnosis of myocarditis in adults based on MRI findings (Table 47.3). Diagnosis is made if two of three criteria are fulfilled, including: (1) increased T2 signal intensity consistent with edema; (2) increased early myocardial contrast enhancement relative to skeletal muscle consistent with hyperemia in gadolinium-enhanced T1-weighted images; and (3) presence of late gadolinium enhancement in T1-weighted images consistent with necrosis or scar (Fig. 47.4). Pediatric experience is limited to small series.[18]

Endomyocardial Biopsy

Direct tissue examination remains the goal standard for diagnosis of myocarditis. The Dallas criteria established light microscopy standard histopathologic criteria.[19] Active myocarditis is defined as an inflammatory infiltrate of the myocardium with myocyte necrosis not typical of the ischemic damage associated with coronary heart disease. Infiltrates are usually mononuclear but may be neutrophilic or eosinophilic. Borderline myocarditis is diagnosed in the presence of lymphocytic infiltration without myocyte destruction.

TABLE 47.3	Lake Louise Criteria for Myocarditis	
Original Lake Louise criteria Any 2 out of 3 main criteria		Updated Lake Louise criteria 2 out of 2 main criteria
Main Criteria		**Main Criteria**

T2W imaging
    Regional high T2 SI
    or
    Global T2 SI ratio ≥ 2.0 in T2W MRI images
		T2-based imaging
		    Regional high T2 SI
		    or
		    Global T2 SI ratio ≥ 2.0 in T2W MRI images
		    or
		    Regional or global increase of myocardial T2 relaxation time

Early gadolinium enhancement
    SI ratio myocardium/skeletal muscle (EGE ratio) of ≥ 4.0
        in EGE images
		T1-based imaging
		    Regional or global increase of native myocardial T1 relax-
		        ation time or ECV
		    or
		    Areas with high SI in a non-ischemic distribution pattern in
		        LGE images

Late gadolinium enhancement (LGE)
    Areas with high SI in a non-ischemic distribution pattern
        in LGE images		

Supportive Criteria		*Supportive Criteria*
Pericardial effusion in cine MRI images		Pericardial effusion in cine MRI images
Systolic LV wall motion abnormality in cine MRI images		High signal intensity of the pericardium in LGE images, T1-mapping or T2-mapping
		Systolic LV wall motion abnormality in cine MRI images

EGE, Early gadolinium enhancement; *ECV,* extracellular volume; *LV,* left ventricle; *MRI,* magnetic resonance imaging; *SI,* signal intensity; *T2W,* T2-weighted.

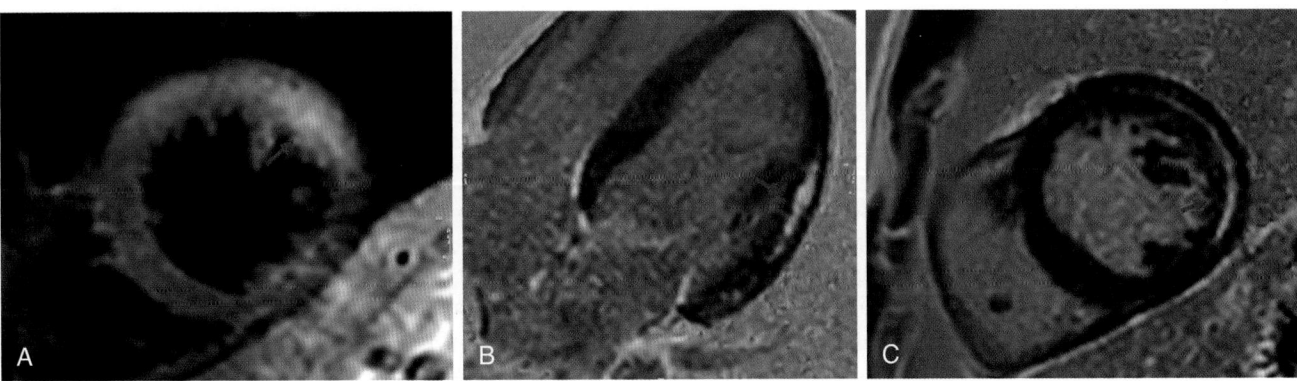

• **Fig. 47.4** Cardiac magnetic resonance imaging in a patient with acute myocarditis. **(A)** Short-axis view at the mid-ventricular level showing increased signal in the lateral wall of the left ventricle on T2-weighted imaging consistent with myocardial edema. **(B)** Four-chamber view showing mid-wall late gadolinium enhancement of the lateral wall of the left ventricle, consistent with myocardial injury. **(C)** Short-axis view at the mid-ventricular level showing mid-wall late gadolinium enhancement of the lateral wall of the left ventricle.

The sensitivity of endomyocardial biopsy is limited by the focal and transient nature of the inflammatory process, with diagnosis by biopsy in fewer than 20–50% of children with suspected disease. Additional testing with immunohistochemistry and viral genome analysis has increased the diagnostic yield of endomyocardial biopsy to 63% of patients. Endomyocardial biopsy is used selectively given the high risk of adverse events and often reserved for patients who require catheterization for another reason. Reported rates of complications are 1–16% but can be as high as 30–40% in infants.[20] The most frequent complication is perforation of the right ventricle, more likely in patients requiring inotropic support, or fewer than 10 kg. Other complications include arrhythmias, pneumothorax, and flail tricuspid leaflet.

Management

Management of myocarditis during the acute phase includes hemodynamic support, treatment of arrhythmias, and immunomodulatory therapy.

All patients should be carefully monitored, including cardiorespiratory monitoring and continuous rhythm monitoring, as clinical status may quickly deteriorate. The sickest patients may require management in ICUs, and/or transfer to a center that provides MCS and transplantation. Early triage is imperative as overall prognosis is very good with timely support of the circulation including, in some cases, ECMO or ventricular assist device (VAD).

Patients with depressed ventricular function may require pharmacologic management of heart failure, which can include diuretics, afterload reducing agents, inotropic support, mechanical ventilation, and/or MCS. Vasoactive agents are used to manage low cardiac output, hypotension, and cardiogenic shock. Positive pressure ventilation can improve cardiac function by reducing left ventricular afterload. Sedation and intubation may have additional benefits to reduce metabolic demand, although induction of anesthesia carries significant risk of hemodynamic deterioration and cardiac arrest in this population. Children with cardiogenic shock refractory to these interventions are likely to require MCS. In a multicenter registry, ECMO or VAD was required in 23% of children. In patients with MCS, survival to hospital discharge was 60%, with 3–16% requiring MCS as a bridge to transplantation.[21] An oral heart failure regimen can be used once the patient is beyond the acute stage of illness.

Arrhythmias occur in approximately half of patients with acute myocarditis, and most often include complete heart block and ventricular arrhythmia.[17] Their presence is associated with an eight-fold increase in risk for MCS, heart transplantation, or death. An individualized approach is required due to the multiple different arrhythmias and mechanisms that can be seen. Prompt treatment is required due to the potential hemodynamic impact, although caution is also needed due to the side effects of antiarrhythmic treatment (e.g., cardiac depressant, vasodilatory, pro-arrhythmic). Patients with complete heart block may require temporary pacing although this rhythm is often a harbinger of cardiovascular collapse refractory to pacing strategies. The clinician's focus should remain on supporting and protecting end-organ function during the fulminant course of the disease; MCS should be considered early in any patient demonstrating a malignant arrhythmia.

Immunomodulatory Treatment

Immunomodulatory treatment is often used for the treatment of acute myocarditis even though there is limited data regarding efficacy in pediatrics. In multicenter observational studies, IVIG was used in 70% of patients and glucocorticoids in 20% to 30%.

IVIG has anti-inflammatory, antiviral, and immunomodulatory effects. Despite limited data on efficacy, IVIG is generally recommended due to the considerable risk of death and morbidity with myocarditis and the therapy's limited side-effect profile. Observational studies suggest improved survival in patients treated with IVIG, although this was no longer significant after adjusting for confounders.[22,23] Limitations to studies include small sample sizes, diagnosis ascertainment, and limited clinical information from large registries. A pediatric randomized controlled trial did not show statistical difference in transplant-free survival but demonstrated higher left ventricular ejection fraction in patients treated with IVIG.

An infusion of 2 g/kg IVIG is recommended, with dose divided over 2 days if there is concern about the volume load in patients with significant dysfunction.

The data on glucocorticoids are also limited in pediatrics, and their use is generally reserved for patients with associated systemic autoimmune or inflammatory conditions or those who are refractory to IVIG. Large studies and meta-analysis have not demonstrated survival benefits with the use of steroids for patients with viral or idiopathic myocarditis, though some data suggest that patients treated with steroids may have greater improvement in left ventricular ejection fraction.[24] Although rare in children, giant cell myocarditis, sarcoidosis, and eosinophilic myocarditis are known to respond to corticosteroids. Treatment for myocarditis associated with a systemic autoimmune condition should target the underlying disease in collaboration with rheumatology.

Antiviral medications have not been rigorously tested for the treatment of myocarditis. Given their known beneficial effects in noncardiac infections, however, it is reasonable to consider for treatment when an active viral infection is found.

Prognosis

The course of myocarditis is highly variable; outcomes range from complete recovery, to progression to chronic dilated cardiomyopathy, to death or transplantation. While complete recovery of ventricular function is seen in approximately half of patients at 3-year, and 70% at 6-year follow-up, the process is gradual, with most still showing ventricular dysfunction at hospital discharge.[25] Approximately 27–40% of patients progress to dilated cardiomyopathy. Transplantation is reported in approximately 5–20% of patients and death in 6–7% over 3-year follow-up. Factors associated with increased risk of death include fulminant presentation, severely depressed left ventricular systolic function, need for MCS, need for inotropes, tachyarrhythmias, and peak BNP level $> 10,000$ pg/mL. Mortality is most common during the acute illness, with late deaths occasionally seen due to persistent ventricular dysfunction, refractory heart failure, or complications of heart transplantation. MCS may be required as a bridge to transplantation.

Follow-Up

Regular follow-up with ECG and echocardiography is recommended for patients after acute myocarditis and tailored based on the degree of ventricular dysfunction at the time of discharge. Controversies exist around the duration of heart failure medication and need for repeat endomyocardial biopsy and/or cardiac MRI.

Guidelines recommend exercise and activity restriction for a minimum of 3–6 months in children with myocarditis. This is based on the association of myocarditis with cardiac sudden death, especially with exercise. The risk of sudden death may not correlate with the severity of myocardial inflammation and ventricular function; however, patients should be restricted from exercise until normalization of laboratory and imaging data. Testing with 24-hour Holter monitor and exercise stress test should be considered prior to return to sport.

References

1. Steere AC. Lyme disease. *N Engl J Med*. 1989;321:586.
2. Steere AC, Batsford WP, Weinberg M, et al. Lyme carditis: cardiac abnormalities of Lyme disease. *Ann Intern Med*. 1980;93:8-16.
3. McAlister HF, Klementowicz PT, Andrews C, et al. Lyme carditis: an important cause of reversible heart block. *Ann Intern Med*. 1989;110:339-345.
4. Costello JM, Alexander ME, Greco KM, et al. Lyme carditis in children: presentation, predictive factors, and clinical course. *Pediatrics*. 2009;123:e835-e841.
5. Lantos PM, Rumbaugh J, Bockenstedt LK, et al. Clinical practice guidelines by the Infectious Diseases Society of America, American Academy of Neurology, and American College of Rheumatology: 2020 guidelines for the prevention, diagnosis and treatment of Lyme disease. *Clin Infect Dis*. 2021;96:262-273.
6. Feldstein LR, Tenforde MW, Friedman KG, et al. Characteristics and outcomes of US children and adolescents with multisystem inflammatory syndrome in children (MIS-C) compared with severe acute COVID-19. *JAMA*. 2021;325:1074-1087.
7. Feldstein LR, Rose EB, Horwitz SM, et al. Multisystem inflammatory syndrome in US children and adolescents. *N Engl J Med*. 2020;383:334-346.
8. Matsubara D, Kauffman HL, Wang Y, et al. Echocardiographic findings in pediatric multisystem inflammatory syndrome associated with COVID-19 in the United States. *J Am Coll Cardiol*. 2020;76:1947-1961.
9. Theocharis P, Wong J, Pushparajah K, et al. Multimodality cardiac evaluation in children and young adults with multisystem inflammation associated with COVID-19. *Eur Heart J Cardiovasc Imaging*. 2021;22:896-903.
10. Regan W, O'Byrne L, Stewart K, et al. Electrocardiographic changes in children with multisystem inflammation associated with COVID-19: associated with coronavirus disease 2019. *J Pediatr*. 2021;234:27-32.e2.
11. Dionne A, Mah DY, Son MBF, et al. Atrioventricular block in children with multisystem inflammatory syndrome. *Pediatrics*. 2020;146:e2020009704.
12. Ouldali N, Toubiana J, Antona D, et al. Association of intravenous immunoglobulins plus methylprednisolone vs immunoglobulins alone with course of fever in multisystem inflammatory syndrome in children. *JAMA*. 2021;325:855-864.
13. Son MBF, Murray N, Friedman K, et al. Multisystem inflammatory syndrome in children – initial therapy and outcomes. *N Engl J Med*. 2021;385:23-34.
14. McArdle AJ, Vito O, Patel H, et al. Treatment of multisystem inflammatory syndrome in children. *N Engl J Med*. 2021;385:11-22.
15. Mahrholdt H, Wagner A, Deluigi CC, et al. Presentation, patterns of myocardial damage and clinical course of viral myocarditis. *Circulation*. 2006;114:1581-1590.
16. Law YM, Lal AK, Chen S, et al. Diagnosis and management of myocarditis in children. *Circulation*. 2021;144:e123-e135.
17. Miyake CY, Teele SA, Chen L, et al. In-hospital arrhythmia development and outcomes in pediatric patients with acute myocarditis. *Am J Cardiol*. 2014;113:535-540.
18. Banka P, Robinson JD, Uppu SC, et al. Cardiovascular magnetic resonance techniques and findings in children with myocarditis: a multicenter retrospective study. *J Cardiovasc Magn Reson*. 2015;17:96.
19. Aretz HT, Billingham ME, Edwards WD, et al. Myocarditis: a histopathologic definition and classification. *Am J Cardiovasc Pathol*. 1987;1:3-14.
20. Brighenti M, Donti A, Giulia Gagliardi M, et al. Endomyocardial biopsy safety and clinical yield in pediatric myocarditis: an Italian perspective. *Catheter Cardiovasc Interv*. 2016;87:762-767.
21. Rajagopal SK, Almond CS, Laussen PC, et al. Extracorporeal membrane oxygenation for the support of infants, children and young adults with acute myocarditis: a review of the extracorporeal life support organization registry. *Crit Care Med*. 2010;38:382.
22. Yen CY, Hung MC, Wong YC, et al. Role of intravenous immunoglobulin therapy in the survival rate of pediatric patients with acute myocarditis: a systematic review and meta-analysis. *Sci Rep*. 2019;9:10459.
23. Robinson J, Hartling L, Vandermeer B, et al. Intravenous immunoglobulin for presumed viral myocarditis in children and adults. *Cochrane Database Syst Rev*. 2020;8:CD004370.
24. Chen HS, Wang W, Wu SN, Lio JP. Corticosteroids for viral myocarditis. *Cochrane Database Syst Rev*. 2013;2013:CD004471.
25. Gagliardi MG, Bevilacqua M, Bassano C, et al. Long term follow-up of children with myocarditis treated by immunosuppression and of children with dilated cardiomyopathy. *Heart*. 2004;90:1167-1171.

48

Cardiomyopathies

JESSICA C. GARBERN AND DANIEL QUIAT

KEY LEARNING POINTS

- Dilated cardiomyopathy (DCM), the most common form of pediatric cardiomyopathy, has a wide range of primary and secondary causes but is most often idiopathic.
- Left ventricular non-compaction (LVNC) can be associated with normal cardiac structure and function or other cardiomyopathy phenotypes, and clinical outcomes mirror those of the associated cardiomyopathy.
- Hypertrophic cardiomyopathy (HCM) is a diagnosis of exclusion which benefits from care at specialized centers

- to provide up-to-date evidence on genetic and clinical risks and engage in shared decision-making on management options.
- Restrictive cardiomyopathy (RCM) is a rare diagnosis with poor prognosis that benefits from early consideration of heart transplantation.
- Genetic counseling is increasingly important in diagnosis and management of pediatric cardiomyopathies as molecularly targeted and gene-specific therapies become available.

Introduction

Cardiomyopathies are diseases of the heart muscle that are diverse in etiology. Pediatric cardiomyopathies have an incidence of 1.1–1.5 per 100,000 per year.[1] Cardiomyopathies can be genetic or caused by exposure to toxins or infectious agents, ischemia, or conduction abnormalities. Dilated and hypertrophic cardiomyopathies (DCM and HCM, respectively) are the most common forms of cardiomyopathy, and our understanding of the genetic heterogeneity leading to these disorders continues to evolve. Left ventricular non-compaction (LVNC) and restrictive cardiomyopathies (RCM) are less common but can have overlapping phenotypes with dilated or hypertrophic forms. In this chapter, we review key features, diagnostic considerations, and management approaches for DCM, HCM, LVNC, and RCM in the pediatric population.

Dilated Cardiomyopathy

Definition and Epidemiology

DCM is characterized by dilation and impaired systolic function of the left ventricle (LV) or both ventricles, typically in the absence of ischemia, abnormal loading conditions, or physiologic insult (e.g., sepsis).[2] Diagnostic criteria

include reduced measures of ventricular function combined with increased ventricular volumes normalized for age and body surface area (left ventricular end-diastolic diameter [LVEDD] and left ventricular end-systolic diameter [LVESD] z-scores > 2) on cardiac imaging.[2] It is the most common form of cardiomyopathy in children, accounting for at least 50% of cases, and has a population incidence of 0.58 per 100,000 children.[3] DCM has numerous etiologies, clinical manifestations, and outcomes that vary depending on the underlying cause and patient specific factors. DCM can be classified as primary or secondary, depending on if the underlying mechanism is intrinsic to the cardiomyocyte or in response to an external insult.[2] Primary DCM includes genetic etiologies such as sarcomeric gene mutations, mitochondrial diseases, neuromuscular disorders, and other genetic mechanisms (Table 48.1). Secondary DCM encompasses inflammatory, infectious, endocrine, toxic, metabolic, nutritional, hemodynamic (structural heart disease), arrhythmic, and ischemic causes.[2] In some cases, such as DCM in the presence of structural heart disease, it can be difficult to discern if the DCM phenotype is caused by a primary myocardial defect or coexistent hemodynamic factors. Approximately one-third of pediatric DCM cases have an identifiable etiology, with neuromuscular disease and myocarditis being the most common causes, and the remaining two-thirds of cases categorized as idiopathic.[4]

TABLE 48.1	Classification of Pediatric Dilated Cardiomyopathy Etiologies[2]	
Classification	**Subtype**	**Examples/Comments**
Primary DCM	Genetic	Sarcomeric, mitochondrial, neuromuscular, laminopathies
	Familial	Genotype positive or genotype negative with suggestive family history
	Idiopathic	A diagnosis of exclusion
Secondary DCM	Inflammatory	Viral myocarditis or other infectious myocarditis, autoimmune disease, hypersensitivity reactions
	Toxin-mediated	Anthracycline drugs, iron, lead, cobalt, arsenic, radiation
	Metabolic disorders	Endocrinopathies: thyroid disease, catecholamine-producing neoplasm, diabetes
		Fatty acid oxidation disorders: carnitine deficiency, malonyl coenzyme decarboxylase deficiency
		Glycogen storage disorders: type II (Pompe disease), type IV (Andersen disease)
		Lysosomal storage disorders: Gaucher disease, mucopolysaccharidoses, sphingolipidoses
	Nutritional disorders	Thiamine deficiency, selenium deficiency, protein malnutrition (Kwashiorkor)
	Ischemic injury	Coronary anomalies (ALCAPA), coronary injury, myocardial infarction
	Structural heart disease	Valvular disease
	Heart rhythm disorders	Tachycardias (SVT, PJRT), pacing-induced cardiomyopathy
	Pulmonary disease	Pulmonary hypertension leading to RV dilation and dysfunction

ALCAPA, Anomalous left coronary from the pulmonary artery; *DCM*, dilated cardiomyopathy; *PJRT*, permanent junctional reciprocating tachycardia; *RV*, right ventricle; *SVT*, supraventricular tachycardia.

Adapted from Lipshultz SE, Law YM, Asante-Korang A, et al. Cardiomyopathy in children: classification and diagnosis: a scientific statement from the American Heart Association. *Circulation.* 2019;140:e9–e68. ©2019 American Heart Association, Inc.

Genetics and Pathophysiology

The genetic basis of isolated DCM has considerable overlap with other forms of cardiomyopathy.[5] Nineteen genes (*ACTC1, ACTN2, BAG3, DES, DSP, JPH2, FLNC, LMNA, MYH7, NEXN, PLN, RBM20, SCN5A, TNNC1, TNNI3, TNNT2, TPM1, TTN, VCL*) demonstrate high-level evidence as causing isolated DCM[5] but are associated with a minority of cases. Many of these genes encode proteins that are integral to cardiomyocyte contractility and cytoskeletal integrity, with the largest fraction of genes contributing to formation of the sarcomere (*ACTC1, ACTN2, FLNC, MYH7, TNNC1, TNNI3, TNNT2, TPM1, TTN*). Pathogenic variants in DCM genes are most frequently autosomal dominant.[5] Variants may be transmitted from affected or unaffected parents or arise *de novo* (not inherited from either parent), especially in younger patients. Certain DCM genotypes are associated with a distinct age of disease onset. For example, truncating variants in *TTN* are responsible for 10%–20% of adult-onset DCM but are infrequently identified in infants and young children.[6] Mutations in *MYH7* are the predominant genetic cause of isolated DCM in infancy but also present in older children and adults.[6] Most genetic forms of DCM have indistinguishable cardiac

phenotypes of LV dysfunction and dilation, but several genes are associated with a higher burden of arrhythmia and conduction system disease (*LMNA, SCN5A, DES, FLNC*).[2] A rare recessive form of cardiomyopathy due to biallelic mutations in *ALPK3* can present with severe DCM in infancy and progress to HCM. Several important genetic forms of DCM are X-linked (*DMD, TAZ, EMD, LAMP2*)[2] and are discussed in detail in the section on dystrophinopathies. Genetic testing by targeted cardiomyopathy gene panels identifies a likely pathogenic or pathogenic variant in approximately 30% of idiopathic primary DCM cases; broader genetic testing with whole exome sequencing or whole genome sequencing is currently of limited additional diagnostic yield.[7]

The variety of causes that can eventuate in DCM suggests that the disorder is the final common pathway for intrinsic and extrinsic insults to cardiomyocyte function. One potential pathologic mechanism shared by many causes of DCM is reduced cardiomyocyte contractility. Many DCM mutations either directly disrupt sarcomere function or affect coordinated transmission of force across the cardiac mass by disrupting the cytoskeleton.[5] Secondary causes of DCM reduce contractility by causing cardiomyocyte injury or death. In response to decreased contractility, the myocardium undergoes pathological remodeling marked by cardiomyocyte hypertrophy, myocyte apoptosis and loss, and varying degrees of fibrosis. This results in a ventricle with eccentric hypertrophy, poor contractility, increased volume load, and increased myocardial oxygen demand.

Clinical Presentation

Patients with DCM may remain well compensated and asymptomatic for a period of time. Patients who present with symptomatic DCM most often exhibit similar age-related signs of decompensated heart failure regardless of the underlying cause of the ventricular dysfunction. The clinical presentation of decompensated heart failure in various age groups is discussed in detail in Chapter 53. Extracardiac symptoms may provide important diagnostic information, with myocarditis, neuromuscular disorders, mitochondrial/metabolic disorders, and secondary causes of DCM having a range of presenting symptoms related to the underlying cause.

Diagnostic Evaluation

Physical Exam

Physical findings depend on the severity of clinical compromise. Patients with mild ventricular dysfunction can present with reduced exercise capacity but no abnormal physical findings. Congestive heart failure (CHF) is nearly always accompanied by tachypnea and tachycardia. Intercostal retractions are a common finding in infants and young children, but in contrast to adults, pulmonary auscultation rarely reveals rales, even when frank pulmonary edema is present on chest radiograph. The cardiac impulse is often displaced laterally and is diffuse. Gallop rhythm with a third heart sound is common, as is a murmur of mitral regurgitation. Peripheral pulses are often weak and can be difficult to palpate, reflecting a narrow pulse pressure and hypotension. Neck vein distention and peripheral edema are almost never detected in infants but become more common with age. Cool extremities and poor capillary refill may be seen, particularly in infants. Peripheral cyanosis is noted only in the presence of severe compromise. Hepatomegaly is a seminal finding and can be massive in infants, changing rapidly in response to therapy. Careful observation for extracardiac findings, such as hypotonia and developmental delays, may provide important clues to neuromuscular or metabolic etiologies of DCM.

Radiographic Findings

Cardiomegaly on chest radiograph may be the only finding in asymptomatic LV dysfunction, but the sensitivity and specificity of this finding is quite poor in children. Cardiomegaly, pulmonary venous congestion, pulmonary edema, atelectasis, and pleural effusions are key radiographic findings, depending on severity.

Electrocardiography

The electrocardiogram (ECG) shows sinus tachycardia in most patients. Non-specific ST-T wave changes and left ventricular hypertrophy (LVH) are noted in about half of patients, with atrial and right ventricular hypertrophy in 25%. Nearly 50% of patients have arrhythmias detectable by Holter monitoring at the time of presentation, including atrial fibrillation and flutter, ventricular ectopic beats, and non-sustained ventricular tachycardia (NSVT). DCM must be differentiated from tachycardia-induced cardiomyopathy, a process that can have a similar presentation but frequently resolves with arrhythmia control.

Echocardiography

The diagnostic findings on echocardiogram are a dilated LV with diminished systolic performance (Fig. 48.1). Dysfunction is global although moderate regional variation in wall motion is usually present. Quantitative assessment of systolic and diastolic functional parameters and ventricular morphology is diagnostically and prognostically useful. Pericardial effusions are frequent. Intracardiac thrombi have been reported in as many as 23% of children, although rarely in infants. Color flow and spectral Doppler are useful for assessment of mitral regurgitation and diastolic function. The echocardiogram is equally critical for excluding valvar and structural cardiac disease. The diagnosis of anomalous origin of the left coronary artery from the pulmonary artery (ALCAPA) should be excluded by imaging and color flow doppler.

Cardiac Magnetic Resonance Imaging

Cardiac magnetic resonance imaging (MRI) provides an accurate method of measuring left and right ventricular volumes, masses, and ejection fractions, especially in patients with poor echocardiographic windows. The spatial distribution and extent of cardiac fibrosis can be assessed by late gadolinium enhancement (LGE) and can be helpful in differentiating DCM from ischemic heart disease (see Chapter 10). Cardiac MRI is also useful in evaluating for myocarditis. The primary limitations relate to exclusion of patients with pacemakers, the safety of which is not established, and the need for anesthesia in young children.

Cardiac Catheterization

Cardiac catheterization is performed primarily for endomyocardial biopsy (EMB) when the detection of known causes of DCM will inform management and prognosis. This includes histologic or molecular (polymerase chain reaction) evidence of myocarditis and other infiltrative disorders, such as histiocytoid cardiomyopathy of infancy, which although rare, can only be diagnosed by histology. Identification of myocarditis on EMB can be associated with a more favorable prognosis, including the potential for complete recovery. Occasionally the possibility of a coronary anomaly remains in doubt, in which case coronary angiography. is necessary. Assessment of hemodynamics is rarely useful for patient management but has important prognostic implications; it is needed to assess candidacy for transplantation, particularly measurements of pulmonary artery pressure and pulmonary vascular resistance (PVR).

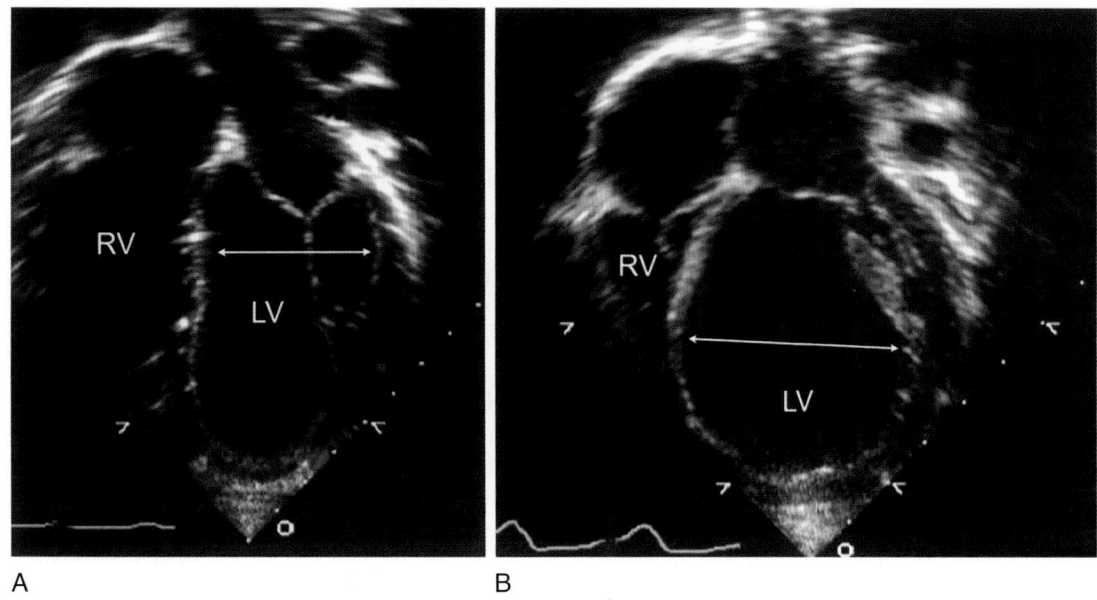

• **Fig. 48.1** Comparison of ventricular configuration in the normal left ventricle (*LV*) **(A)** and dilated cardiomyopathy **(B)** in apical, transverse echocardiographic imaging. In the normal heart, the size of the right ventricle (*RV*) is similar to that of the LV, and the transverse width of the LV *(arrow)* is about two-thirds the long-axis dimension. In patients with dilated cardiomyopathy, the LV dilates more than the RV, and the ventricle is more spherical with a transverse dimension *(arrow)* that is nearly as great as the long-axis dimension.

Familial Screening and Genetic Testing

As most inherited forms of DCM are autosomal dominant, first-degree relatives of an individual with primary DCM should undergo clinical evaluation with a screening echocardiogram. A thorough, three-generation family history should also be obtained. Genetic testing is recommended as part of the routine evaluation of DCM probands (first person to seek medical attention for the condition),[8] and should be performed following appropriate genetic counseling and in consultation with providers trained in interpretation of genetic testing results. Variants classified as pathogenic or likely pathogenic can be used for cascade screening of at-risk family members without a DCM phenotype, and inform the need for additional follow-up. Genetic and clinical screening is also important in many X-linked forms of DCM, such as Duchenne muscular dystrophy (DMD), where genotype-positive carriers are at increased risk for abnormal cardiac function.[9] Finally, patients of child-bearing age with a suspected genetic DCM should be counseled about recurrence risk.

Management

Medications

Medical management of DCM is primarily focused on heart failure–directed therapy, discussed in detail in Chapter 53. Disease-specific therapeutic considerations for DMD are discussed below.

Implantable Cardioverter-Defibrillator Placement

DCM has a lower overall rate of sudden cardiac death (SCD) than other forms of pediatric cardiomyopathy.[10]

Younger age at diagnosis, increased LV dilation, and LV posterior wall thinning have been associated with SCD risk in DCM.[10] In addition, certain genetic causes of DCM (*LMNA*, *FLNC*) are associated with higher arrhythmic burden and risk of SCD,[1] and there can be considerable phenotypic overlap between DCM and arrhythmogenic cardiomyopathies (see Chapter 20). Patients who experience a cardiac arrest or high-grade arrhythmia are candidates for placement of a secondary prevention implantable cardioverter-defibrillator (ICD), and those with high-risk features may warrant consideration of a primary prevention ICD.

Outcomes

The natural history of DCM is quite variable, depending on the etiology and severity of cardiac compromise. Arrhythmias, CHF, and death can be seen during any stage of the disease. The clinical course can be a rapid and unremitting progression to cardiogenic shock and death, transient dysfunction with full recovery and few or no symptoms, or any course in between these extremes. Regardless of the initial presentation, patients with persistent dysfunction remain at risk for progressively impaired cardiac function, CHF, and death. Reported 5-year transplant-free survival rates in children with DCM range from 50% to 75%,[1,2] with clinical outcomes varying widely by etiology. Many patients with DCM due to myocarditis demonstrate improvement and even complete recovery of cardiac function (see Chapter 47 on myocarditis). Children with idiopathic DCM, CHF symptoms at presentation, and worse measures of LV function have worse transplant-free survival.

Specific Subtypes of DCM

Dystrophinopathies

The identification of mutations in the dystrophin gene (*DMD*) as the molecular basis for DMD was the initial stage in the recognition of a wide clinical spectrum of disease associated with dystrophin gene mutations. The term "dystrophinopathy" describes disorders unified by a defect in the dystrophin gene that range from classic DMD to asymptomatic mild elevation of serum creatine kinase. The disorders include Duchenne and Becker muscular dystrophy, congenital muscular dystrophy, various forms of limb-girdle muscular dystrophy, X-linked DCM, and carriers of the Duchenne and Becker muscular dystrophy–associated mutations. The dystrophinopathies are one of the several forms of cardiomyopathy that manifest X-linked recessive inheritance, including Barth syndrome secondary to defects in *TAZ* gene, X-linked variants of Emery-Dreifuss muscular dystrophy (*EMD* and *FHL1* genes), Danon disease (*LAMP2* gene), and McLeod syndrome (*XK* gene). Dystrophin is localized to the intracellular plasma membrane of striated muscle cells and functions to maintain the integrity of membrane-associated glycoprotein complexes and the sarcolemma. In the absence of dystrophin, there is increased susceptibility of the sarcolemma to mechanical injury during the application of contractile force. Dystrophin is absent in nearly all patients with the Duchenne phenotype but in Becker dystrophy there can be either reduced quantities of a normal protein or normal quantities of a structurally abnormal protein. The severity of the phenotype is directly related to the quantity of functional dystrophin that is expressed. In addition to skeletal muscle, dystrophin is present in neurons, smooth muscle, and cardiac muscle; the dystrophinopathies may have clinical findings due to the dystrophin deficiency in these other tissues, such as cognitive deficits and cardiomyopathy in DMD. Despite this, involvement in the various tissues is non-uniform, such as the case of X-linked DCM that is associated with severe myocardial dysfunction but normal skeletal muscle strength.

Duchenne Muscular Dystrophy

With an incidence of about 30 per 100,000 live births, the Duchenne form of muscular dystrophy is the most common and most severe type of childhood progressive muscular dystrophy. The mode of inheritance is X-linked recessive, with approximately two-thirds of mothers of affected boys being carriers and the remaining one-third of mutations arising *de novo*. Although serum levels of creatine kinase and other sarcoplasmic enzymes are elevated from birth, the first clinical manifestation is weakness that becomes apparent when the child begins to walk, or between 2 and 6 years of age at the latest. Weakness progresses to an inability to walk by the end of the first decade, with the development of contractures and severe kyphoscoliosis in the later stages.

Invariably there is an associated cardiomyopathy, although this is usually masked by the consequences of the skeletal myopathy. Patients may sustain mild to moderate left ventricular dysfunction for a long period of time, but with the onset of moderate to severe dysfunction, the rate of myocardial deterioration escalates, progressing rapidly to CHF and death. Death is predominantly related to respiratory insufficiency, CHF, or sudden death. The life expectancy of patients with DMD has increased with improvements in medical care, and patients born after 1990 frequently survive into adulthood with a median life expectancy of 28 years.[11]

Electrocardiographic findings in a patient with DMD are characterized by tall, narrow R waves in the anterior precordial leads and deep, narrow Q waves in the lateral leads. Because these electrocardiographic findings resemble the changes associated with posterior and lateral infarction, selective scarring in the posterobasal myocardium has been suggested as the basis for the Q waves and right axis shift. Abnormalities of rhythm and conduction are also common. Persistent or labile sinus tachycardia is present from early in the disease. Tachycardia can progress with age, in contrast to the normal age-related fall in heart rate. The elevated heart rate does not appear to be closely related to the coexistence of systolic dysfunction, and is seen both in subjects with abnormal and those with preserved ventricular performance. Atrial flutter is commonly encountered in the preterminal stages of DMD. Ventricular arrhythmias with a risk of sudden death are seen more commonly in patients with severe cardiomyopathy. Routine surveillance for arrhythmia in patients in the late stage of disease is recommended.[9]

Most studies of ventricular function have noted abnormal systolic function with progressive abnormalities over time. Abnormal systolic function is rarely present before age 10 years, but increases in prevalence thereafter and is virtually universal after age 18 years. Skeletal and cardiac involvement in DMD can progress at different rates, thus cardiac function should be independently assessed by functional imaging (echocardiography or cardiac MRI). At least 25% of subjects cannot be adequately evaluated by ultrasound once the non-ambulatory phase of the disease is reached, and cardiac MRI is particularly useful in providing detailed information about ventricular size and function in the older patients.

To date, therapy for the cardiomyopathy associated with DMD has been largely non-specific. Early treatment with angiotensin-converting enzyme inhibitors (ACEi) has been demonstrated to delay the onset and progression of left ventricular systolic dysfunction, and guidelines recommend initiation of ACEi or angiotensin receptor blockers (ARB) therapy prior to 10 years of age.[9] Similarly, the mineralocorticoid receptor antagonist, eplerenone, has been shown to attenuate decline in ventricular function in prospective studies.[9] Systemic corticosteroids are often used as a disease-modifying therapy and may also improve cardiac outcomes. The development of specific therapeutics for DMD is an active area of research. Newer oligonucleotide therapeutics target the underlying genetic mechanisms of DMD by increasing dystrophin gene expression, either by inducing exon skipping (eteplirsen) or preventing usage of a premature stop codon (ataluren). They have been demonstrated to increase dystrophin expression in a dose-dependent manner but have limited efficacy data. Additional efforts in gene therapy using viral vectors to deliver a gene copy of a smaller dystrophin ortholog, termed microdystrophin, and genome editing using CRISPR/Cas9 to promote exon skipping, are active areas of research.

Becker Muscular Dystrophy

Dystrophin mutations in Becker muscular dystrophy result in production of a semi-functional dystrophin molecule, and result in a clinical course with later onset and slower progression than in DMD. Cardiac involvement can be detected during adolescence and eventually affects nearly all patients. Female carriers also have a high incidence of cardiac involvement, although usually less severe.[9] There is a striking absence of correlation between the degree of skeletal muscle weakness and the severity of the cardiomyopathy. Systolic dysfunction similar in magnitude to that seen in DMD can be identified in children with Becker muscular dystrophy prior to the onset of significant skeletal muscle impairment. In teenagers, the clinical picture may be dominated by a severe, symptomatic cardiomyopathy. Evaluation and management are similar to that for DMD.

Doxorubicin Cardiomyopathy

The anthracycline drug doxorubicin (Adriamycin) is a key antineoplastic drug in treatment of many pediatric cancers. In tandem with significant improvements in long-term outcomes, doxorubicin-associated cardiomyopathy has emerged as an important clinical problem for childhood cancer survivors. The pathogenesis of doxorubicin cardiotoxicity is thought to involve the generation of reactive oxygen species, either via direct iron-dependent hydroxyl free radical formation by doxorubicin and/or as a secondary consequence of DNA damage induced by doxorubicin's primary mechanism of action, inhibition of type II topoisomerase. The cardioselectivity of these actions may reflect an enhanced susceptibility of the heart to oxidant stress due to a high rate of oxidative metabolism. The clinical toxicity of the anthracyclines can be divided into acute, early, and late presentations. Clinically, the most significant problems relate to a late, dose-related cardiomyopathy. Acute toxicity can manifest as arrhythmias, transient left ventricular dysfunction, and pericarditis/myocarditis syndrome, but often improves with cessation of therapy. Early (within 1 year of treatment) and late toxicity can manifest as both systolic and diastolic ventricular dysfunction and the development of heart failure. The incidence of clinical CHF is related to cumulative dose in a non-linear fashion, and adult survivors of childhood cancer have a five-fold higher relative risk of CHF if treated with > 250 mg/m^2 cumulative dose of anthracyclines.[12] Numerous clinical studies have identified risk factors that place patients at increased risk for the adverse cardiac effects of doxorubicin. Patients younger than 4 years of age are at increased risk and females are at higher risk on a dose-matched basis; however, the factor found consistently to bear the strongest relationship to the incidence of cardiotoxicity is the total cumulative dose.[2] The relationship between total cumulative dose of doxorubicin and symptomatic cardiotoxicity is non-linear with an inflection point somewhere between 400 and 600 mg/m^2. Historically, recognition of the dose-related nature of early-onset CHF resulted in modification of chemotherapeutic protocols to a nearly universal limitation of cumulative dose of less than 450 mg/m^2. This successfully reduced cardiac complications to 1% or less. Dexrazoxane, an iron-chelating agent that prevents accumulation of oxygen free radicals, has been used to protect against cardiotoxic effects of anthracyclines. Dexrazoxane has been shown to reduce biomarkers of cardiac injury in children and to be particularly beneficial in patients with malignancies that require treatment with high-dose anthracyclines.[2] Given the lifelong risk of cardiac sequelae, children and adults treated with anthracycline chemotherapeutics warrant regular follow-up, including routine functional cardiac assessment by echocardiography or cardiac MRI.[2]

Iron-Overload Cardiomyopathy

Myocardial injury due to excess iron deposition is associated with hereditary hemochromatosis and also as a consequence of chronic transfusion therapy in a number of disorders including thalassemia, sickle cell anemia, aplastic anemia, myelodysplastic syndromes, and chronic renal failure.[2] During childhood, iron overload is seen primarily in conjunction with transfusion therapy. Although children who receive adequate transfusion therapy grow and develop normally with substantially improved survival, outcomes are ultimately limited by the toxicity of the resultant cumulative iron overload. Lifelong transfusion therapy, extravascular hemolysis, and increased intestinal absorption of iron result in systemic iron accumulation with secondary multiorgan injury. Symptomatic involvement is rare in childhood, but myocardial dysfunction limits survival with death from CHF in the latter half of the second decade if iron accumulation is not treated.[2] MRI is used routinely for monitoring of cardiac iron accumulation. The relaxation parameter T2* is inversely related to cardiac iron deposition and is predictive of risk for developing heart failure.[2,13] Numerous studies have noted reversal of cardiac dysfunction and improvement in event-free cardiac survival in patients treated with chelation therapy, and clinical management of iron overload is focused on prophylactic and therapeutic iron chelation.

Left Ventricular Non-compaction Cardiomyopathy

LVNC, also referred to as left ventricular hypertrabeculation, is marked by the presence of prominent ventricular trabeculations with deep intertrabecular recesses, most often located in the left ventricular apex[2] (Fig. 48.2). It is thought to result from failure of the proliferating trabecular myocardium of the embryonic heart to undergo compaction and form the compact myocardial layer.[1] LVNC can be an isolated finding in asymptomatic individuals with normal ventricular size and systolic function, concomitant with other cardiomyopathy phenotypes (DCM, HCM, RCM),[2] or associated with congenital heart disease, especially Ebstein anomaly of the tricuspid valve. LVNC is frequently seen in large studies of adults by cardiac MRI, especially in those who participate in vigorous exercise, suggesting that a degree of hypertrabeculation is non-pathological.[14] Specific diagnostic criteria related to the number of trabeculae, the relative thickness of the compact and non-compact layers of the myocardium, and flow within intertrabecular recesses on color Doppler have been developed to identify pathological LVNC. LVNC cardiomyopathy is the third most common form of cardiomyopathy in the pediatric population,[3] with the LVNC/DCM phenotype being most common. Clinical findings, management, and outcomes of LVNC typically mirror the predominant cardiomyopathy phenotype.[2] Ventricular systolic dysfunction and arrhythmia with or without co-occurring ventricular dysfunction are associated with increased mortality in LVNC.[1] Although patients with LVNC and normal ventricular function may be at risk for development of systolic or diastolic dysfunction, currently it is not known how frequently or how rapidly this transition takes place.

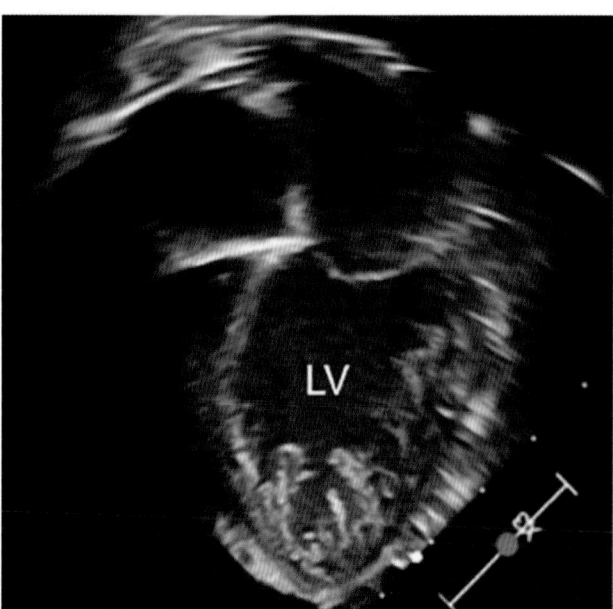

• **Fig. 48.2** Apical transverse end-diastolic echocardiographic image in a patient with left ventricular non-compaction and dilated cardiomyopathy. The smooth surface of the LV interventricular septum contrasts with the finger-like projections of myocardium from the apical and lateral free wall into the LV cavity. *LV,* Left ventricle.

Hypertrophic Cardiomyopathy

Definition and Epidemiology

HCM is a diagnosis of exclusion, with the presence of LVH without another identifiable physiologic, metabolic, or genetic cause. In children, HCM is defined as having a maximum end-diastolic LV wall thickness with a z-score ≥ 2.5 standard deviations above the mean (adjusted to body surface area) in any location of the LV wall without an identifiable secondary cause of LVH.[15] In adults, the maximum end-diastolic LV wall thickness threshold for HCM is ≥ 15 mm.[15] In individuals with a family history of HCM or with a known gene mutation, an LV wall thickness z-score ≥ 2 in children or 13–14 mm in adults may be considered diagnostic.[15]

The prevalence of HCM is ~1:200 to 1:500, although the number of individuals diagnosed with HCM is much lower, as many individuals are asymptomatic.[16] The genetic causes of HCM are currently known in approximately 60% of patients.[7] Age of presentation can range from infancy to late adulthood.[17]

For clarity, the term HCM is used to describe isolated LVH arising from a primary cardiac mechanism and will exclude systemic disorders that can lead to LVH. Syndromes and metabolic disorders with multisystem involvement and associated LVH can mimic HCM ("HCM phenocopies") but should not be referred to as HCM per current nomenclature given their different prognoses and management.[15]

Genetics and Pathophysiology

HCM is a genetically heterogeneous disease with a common clinical phenotype. HCM is most commonly caused by a mutation in a gene encoding a sarcomeric protein. Eight genes associated with sarcomere formation are considered definitively causative of HCM (*MYBPC3, MYH7, TNNT2, TNNI3, TPM1, ACTC1, MYL3,* and *MYL2*).[18] Mutations in non-sarcomere genes can also cause HCM, such as in genes encoding proteins associated with mechanosensory signaling (e.g., *CSRP3*) or excitation-contraction coupling (e.g., *JPH2*).[7] Pathogenic mutations for HCM are usually inherited in an autosomal dominant pattern, with *de novo* mutations common.

While genetic causes of HCM are diverse, there is a common pathogenesis of the clinical phenotype in most cases. Most genetic defects lead to a missense mutation in a sarcomere protein, leading to abnormal function of sarcomeres.[18] Abnormal sarcomere function leads to activation of stress-response pathways within cardiomyocytes which promote cardiomyocyte hypertrophy and myocyte disarray.[19] These stress pathways also likely contribute to myocardial inflammation and increased interstitial fibrosis in HCM.[19]

Septal hypertrophy leads to anterior displacement of the mitral valve and dynamic left ventricular outflow tract obstruction (LVOTO), present at rest in approximately one-third of patients.[19] HCM hearts have reduced coronary flow reserve due to coronary artery narrowing (from smooth muscle cell hyperplasia), myocardial bridging (congenital variant where muscle bands overlay epicardial coronary arteries causing systolic compression of a coronary artery), and/or decreased coronary perfusion from elevated diastolic pressures, leading to myocardial ischemia.[15] Apical myocardial ischemia can result in the formation of LV aneurysms, which increase the risk of ventricular arrhythmias and systolic dysfunction.[15] Interstitial fibrosis leads to diastolic dysfunction and subsequent left atrial enlargement, which itself is a risk factor for atrial fibrillation.[19] Ventricular arrhythmias are seen in 20%–30% of patients and are a risk factor for SCD.[19]

Phenotype variability can be seen within families with the same primary genetic cause of HCM, with individuals presenting at different ages and/or with varying degrees of severity. This variability in penetrance is thought to be due to environmental factors and/or genetic modifiers that are not causative of HCM but can influence the phenotype of HCM in an individual.[19]

Clinical Presentation

Many patients with isolated HCM are asymptomatic at diagnosis and are identified during screening due to a known family history, during evaluation of a new murmur, or during workup for an abnormal ECG.

Presenting symptoms can include dyspnea on exertion, fatigue, chest pain, syncope/presyncope, palpitations, or SCD. Chest pain is often angina-like and exercise-induced, but it can also be atypical, occurring at rest. Palpitations and syncope are more common in adults; syncope is less common in children with HCM but is associated with an increased risk of SCD when observed. Patients with advanced disease can progress to a DCM phenotype with CHF symptoms such as orthopnea and edema, although this usually does not occur until adulthood.

While signs and symptoms of CHF can occur with infantile HCM (i.e., respiratory distress and failure to thrive), infants with these symptoms more likely have a metabolic or syndromic cause for their LVH (e.g., Noonan syndrome). It is particularly important to rule out syndromic and metabolic causes of LVH in this age group as the prognosis and management can be quite different depending on the underlying etiology of LVH (see Differential Diagnosis below).

Diagnostic Evaluation

Initial evaluation involves a history and physical exam, ECG, and an echocardiogram. After echocardiographic diagnosis of HCM (and exclusion of other causes of LVH), additional testing such as an exercise test, stress echocardiography, Holter monitor, and cardiac MRI (as age-appropriate) is typically performed to assess risk of SCD and guide management.

Physical Exam

Physical exam findings in HCM (in the absence of CHF) relate to dynamic LVOTO and are absent in patients without obstruction. Individuals with early or mild forms of HCM may have a completely normal physical exam. Many patients without a known family history present first with a new murmur, while patients with advanced disease may present with signs and symptoms of CHF.

Infants with HCM can present with tachypnea, increased work of breathing, and/or hepatomegaly. They can be underweight due to poor feeding and growth. On cardiac exam, they often have a hyperdynamic precordium with a systolic ejection murmur from LVOTO.

Older children, adolescents, and adults with LVOTO may also have a hyperdynamic precordium, with apical and parasternal cardiac impulses that are augmented and sometimes displaced laterally. The point of maximum impulse may be bifid (due to a forceful atrial contraction) or trifid ("triple ripple" due to forceful atrial contraction plus a double systolic impulse in patients with dynamic LVOTO).[15] A double pulsation of the carotid pulse ("pulsus bisferiens") can also be encountered. Parasternal and carotid systolic thrills are frequent in patients with LVOTO.

On auscultation, an S4 gallop can be heard as a consequence of the non-compliant LV.[15] The characteristic murmur of HCM is a harsh, crescendo-decrescendo systolic ejection murmur, typically heard best along the left sternal border, audible when there is LVOTO (defined as a peak LVOT gradient of $\geq$ 30 mm Hg).[15] Because LVOTO is dynamic, many individuals have lower resting gradients, and provocation maneuvers may be needed to elicit a murmur in these patients; these include actions that increase contractility (e.g., exercise), decrease preload (e.g., standing, Valsalva maneuver), or decrease afterload (e.g., amyl nitrate inhalation).[15] In contrast, maneuvers that increase preload (e.g., squatting or passive leg raise, which both increase preload by increasing venous return to the heart) or increase afterload (e.g., hand grip) will decrease LVOTO with HCM and therefore the murmur will soften.[15] A systolic, rumbling murmur due to mitral regurgitation can sometimes be heard, but this can be difficult to separate from the outflow murmur as it is typically lower in intensity.

Electrocardiography

A 12-lead ECG should be performed routinely as it can detect evidence of LVH as well as arrhythmias. Up to 25% of patients with HCM have normal ECG findings.[15] The most common abnormalities seen on a 12-lead ECG are LVH, ST-segment and T wave abnormalities, and abnormal Q waves. The presence of pre-excitation may indicate an HCM phenocopy, such as a PRKAG2 cardiomyopathy or Danon disease which can cause LVH and Wolff-Parkinson-White syndrome.[15]

Echocardiography

The transthoracic echocardiogram (TTE) is the primary tool used to diagnose and monitor HCM (Fig. 48.3) as it permits non-invasive assessment of wall thickness, chamber dimensions, systolic and diastolic function, LVOTO, presence of an LV apical aneurysm, and valvar insufficiency (especially of the mitral valve). A TTE should be performed at least once a year in children and adolescents. In asymptomatic adults, a TTE can be performed every 1–2 years or longer if clinically stable.

Echocardiographic parameters that should be evaluated include LV morphology, LV diastolic wall thickness, LV ejection fraction, peak instantaneous LV outflow tract gradient, LV diastolic function, mitral valve morphology (and whether systolic anterior motion of the mitral valve is present), degree of mitral regurgitation, and left atrial size. Transesophageal echocardiogram is not used during routine evaluation but can be used to guide interventions such as alcohol septal ablation or surgical myectomy, or if improved imaging of the mitral valve is required.[15]

Ambulatory ECG Monitoring

Ambulatory ECG monitoring with a 24- or 48-hour Holter monitor should be performed every 1–2 years to evaluate for baseline arrhythmias.[15] The presence of NSVT increases the risk of SCD, particularly in individuals < 35 years of age and/or in individuals with higher rates or longer duration of NSVT.[15] Monitors capable of longer observation periods (e.g., patch monitors or implantable monitors) may be more sensitive in detecting episodic NSVT and may be useful in individuals who report intermittent palpitations.[15] Atrial fibrillation is uncommon in children but can be seen in up to 50% of adult patients with HCM.[15]

Exercise Stress Testing

Exercise testing is typically performed every 2–3 years to assess functional capacity in conjunction with a stress echocardiogram; either treadmill or bicycle ergometry can be used.[15] Children younger than 7–8 years of age are not often able to cooperate with this test to obtain meaningful results, thus this would be reserved for older children, adolescents, and adults. An abnormal blood pressure response to exercise (considered to be the absence of an increase in systolic blood pressure [SBP] by ≥ 20 mm Hg during exercise compared with baseline or a decrease in SBP by > 20 mm Hg from peak SBP during exercise) is associated with increased risk of SCD in individuals ≤ 40 years old.[15] High-grade arrhythmias may also be elicited in some patients, with a negative prognostic implication.

Stress Echocardiography

Stress echocardiograms in conjunction with exercise stress testing in older children, adolescents, and adults may be considered every 2–3 years or sooner if symptoms arise.[15] Because LVOTO is dynamic, many patients with obstructive lesions may be missed on a resting echocardiogram. Symptoms generally occur when the LVOT gradient is > 50 mm Hg. Provocative maneuvers such as performing a Valsalva or changing from a squatting to standing position can reveal LVOTO.

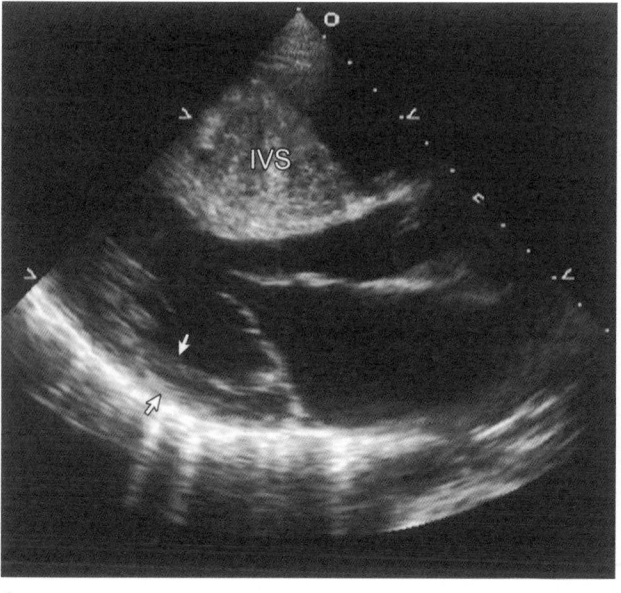
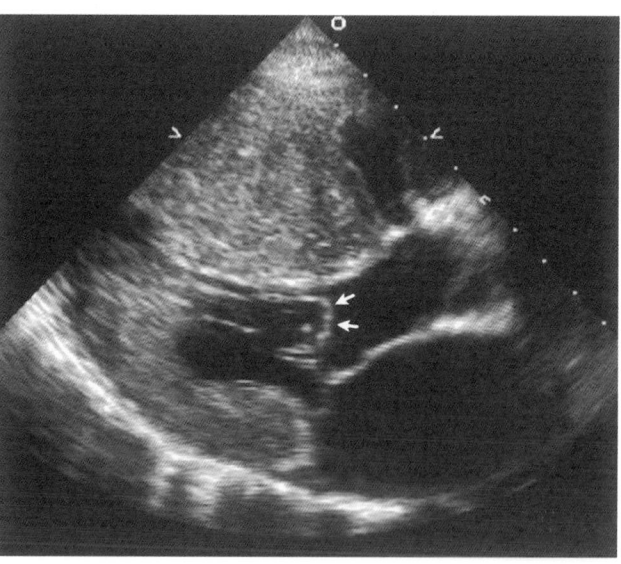

A   B

• **Fig. 48.3** Parasternal long-axis image of a patient with familial sarcomeric hypertrophic cardiomyopathy. **(A)** The marked increase in IVS thickness compared with posterior wall thickness *(arrows)* is seen on this late diastolic frame, and the mitral valve leaflets are in a neutral, nearly closed position. **(B)** Dynamic left ventricular outflow obstruction is illustrated. During ejection, the anterior mitral leaflet moves into apposition with the IVS and buckles anteriorly *(arrows)*, nearly obliterating the left ventricular outflow tract. *IVS,* Interventricular septum.

Cardiac Magnetic Resonance Imaging

Cardiac MRI is a useful tool to measure myocardial mass, wall thickness, regional hypertrophy, differences in regional systolic function, presence of apical aneurysms, and fibrosis. It can be particularly helpful in patients with limited echocardiographic windows and to evaluate for evidence of myocardial fibrosis in regions with LGE. The percentage of the LV mass occupied by fibrosis is a prognostic factor for SCD, and this value is included in some algorithms to guide decision-making on placement of an ICD ($\geq$ 15% LGE increases SCD risk by two-fold).[15] Current guidelines recommend a cardiac MRI at initial diagnosis followed by serial MRI approximately every 3–5 years, depending on individual circumstances.[15] In asymptomatic children, cardiac MRI is often deferred until adolescence due to adequate echocardiographic windows, difficulties in performing an unsedated MRI, and concerns for gadolinium deposition in the brain with unclear long-term consequences.

Cardiac Computed Tomography

Cardiac computed tomography (CT) is not typically performed during routine diagnosis or evaluation of HCM. However, as with CMR, it can provide high spatial resolution of regional hypertrophy and can be helpful in patients with limited echocardiographic windows in whom MRI is contraindicated.[15]

Cardiac Catheterization

Invasive hemodynamic assessment with or without angiography via cardiac catheterization is not performed routinely during evaluation of HCM but may be considered in select cases. Patients with symptoms out of proportion to LVOT gradients on non-invasive imaging or with concomitant valvar aortic stenosis may benefit from invasive hemodynamic assessment to quantify LVOTO, cardiac output, and filling pressures.[15] Coronary angiography is recommended in patients prior to undergoing alcohol septal ablation or in patients at risk for atherosclerotic disease prior to undergoing surgical myectomy.[15]

Genetic Testing

Genetic testing can guide diagnosis and management of HCM. A comprehensive family history (spanning three or more generations) should be obtained at diagnosis. Pre-test counseling should discuss risks and benefits of performing genetic testing, and post-test counseling should review the results and implications to engage in a shared decision-making process.[15] When performed, genetic testing of a proband should include a panel of genes known to be strongly associated with HCM. Some panels may also include genes that cause HCM phenocopies such as glycogen storage diseases or RASopathies but have different management from isolated HCM.[15]

Genetic testing reveals a pathogenic or likely pathogenic mutation in ~60% of probands with HCM.[15] In this case, first-degree relatives may be offered cascade testing, where relatives are tested only for the disease-causing variant found in the affected family member.[15] Such testing may reveal additional at-risk genotype-positive, phenotype-negative individuals who require lifelong surveillance.[15] Genotype-negative family members can be discharged from repeated surveillance for HCM.[15] Genetic results can also be used in prenatal counseling to discuss disease transmission risk and to help families understand reproductive options including pre-implantation screening.[15]

If a cardiomyopathy panel in a proband does not reveal a pathogenic/likely pathogenic mutation, further genetic testing is not recommended, as there is currently low diagnostic yield with exome sequencing or whole genome sequencing.[15] If a variant of unknown significance (VUS) is identified, this is not considered clinically actionable, but clinical judgment is used to determine whether additional family members should be tested for the same variant.[15] VUS classifications can change and new genes may be identified; thus, evaluation with a provider experienced in cardiovascular genetics should be performed every few years to discuss if further genetic testing is warranted or if interpretation of prior results has changed.[15]

Family Screening

All first-degree relatives of individuals with HCM should be screened with an ECG and echocardiogram. If no genetic testing is performed or if genetic results are inconclusive, all first-degree relatives of the proband should have an ECG and echocardiogram performed every 1–2 years in children and adolescents, and every 3–5 years in adults.[15]

Preclinical HCM (Genotype-Positive, Phenotype-Negative)

Genotype-positive, phenotype-negative individuals with preclinical HCM should have a periodic evaluation with an ECG and echocardiogram to assess for phenotype conversion (~ every year during the peri-adolescent period), as HCM can present through mid-to-late adulthood.[15] Because the risk of SCD is low in genotype-positive, phenotype-negative individuals, these individuals are not restricted from competitive athletics.[15]

Management

In patients with asymptomatic, non-obstructive HCM, medications are not typically used as current pharmacologic therapies address symptoms but not the underlying cause of HCM. It should also be emphasized that patients with HCM are preload-dependent and thus should ensure adequate hydration and avoid vasodilators and high-dose diuretics.

Medications

In patients with symptoms due to LVOTO (e.g., chest pain, exercise intolerance), beta-blockers are considered first-line therapy.[15] Calcium channel blockers (e.g., diltiazem, verapamil) can also provide symptomatic benefit in patients with obstructive HCM; adverse effects from vasodilation may limit their use but can be helpful in patients who do not tolerate beta-blockers.[15] Disopyramide may be considered but should be used in combination with an atrioventricular (AV) nodal blocking agent (e.g., beta blocker, calcium channel blocker) to avoid the potential for rapid conduction through the AV node during atrial arrhythmias.[15]

Beta-blockers or calcium channel blockers may also be helpful for patients with non-obstructive HCM with symptoms of dyspnea or chest pain attributed to diastolic dysfunction, myocardial ischemia, or heart failure.[15] Heart failure from systolic dysfunction can be seen in advanced disease (uncommon in children) and should be managed per current guidelines for heart failure with reduced ejection fraction.[13] Conservative use of diuretics may be appropriate to treat volume overload, if present.[15]

Septal Ablation or Surgical Myectomy

Septal ablation or surgical myectomy can be performed at experienced centers in patients with symptoms not relieved by medical therapy, but while they may improve symptoms, it is unclear if these maneuvers change the risk of SCD.[15] Septal ablation by transcatheter septal infusion of alcohol reduces septal thickness and relieves LVOTO, which may result in symptom improvement. Adverse effects can include transient or permanent heart block, distal infarction, or ventricular arrhythmias.[17] Surgical myectomy may be considered in patients with debilitating symptoms not relieved by maximum medical therapy; however, gradient alone should not determine surgical referral. Myectomy is considered effective at relieving LVOTO and may reverse left atrial remodeling with low perioperative morbidity and mortality.[17] This may be performed in conjunction with mitral valve repair or remodeling to facilitate relief of LVOTO.[17]

Arrhythmias

Individuals with a history of ventricular tachycardia (VT) are considered at higher risk of SCD and should be considered candidates for ICD placement (see below). Beta-blockers are first-line therapy for children and adults with HCM and VT.[13] If beta-blockers are ineffective at suppressing VT, antiarrhythmics such as amiodarone or dofetilide can be considered.[15] Catheter ablation or sympathetic denervation can be considered in children with poorly controlled VT.[15] Heart transplantation may be considered for intractable VT.[15] Atrial fibrillation does not occur often in children with HCM but is common in adults. Therapy for atrial fibrillation involves anticoagulation therapy, symptom control with medications to control rate and/or rhythm, and consideration of catheter or surgical ablation.[15]

Risk Stratification of SCD and Considerations for ICD Placement

SCD is the most devastating outcome from HCM although the incidence is relatively low; heart failure and atrial fibrillation are more common complications of HCM across all ages.[17] The risk for SCD in HCM across all ages is ~0.9% per year, which has decreased in the past two decades to 0.5% per year with appropriate use of ICDs in individual considered at high risk for SCD.[17] Children have a higher risk for SCD than adults, possibly reflecting more severe disease presenting at younger ages, with current estimates of SCD incidence during childhood between 0.8% and 2% per year.[20]

Predictive risk calculators are available to assess the relative risk of SCD in adult patients and similar calculators are being developed for the pediatric population.[15] Although there is a higher risk of SCD in the pediatric population, ICDs also have a higher risk of complications in children (e.g., inappropriate discharge, lead fracture, need for battery replacement), thus individualized discussions detailing the risks and benefits are essential. Current guidelines recommend ICD placement in individuals with a personal history of aborted SCD, ventricular fibrillation, or sustained VT. ICD placement is also reasonable in patients with other risk factors considered high risk for SCD (Table 48.2).[15]

TABLE 48.2	Recommendations for Implantable Cardioverter-Defibrillator Placement in Hypertrophic Cardiomyopathy[15]			
ICD Recommended	**ICD Reasonable**	**ICD Considered**	**ICD not Recommended**
• Personal history of prior aborted SCD, VF, or sustained VT	At least one of the following: • Family history of SCD • Massive LVH (≥30 mm)* • Unexplained syncope • Apical aneurysm • LV ejection fraction ≤ 50% For children: • History of NSVT**	• Extensive LGE on cardiac MRI For adults: • Personal history of NSVT (higher risk with history of longer or faster runs of NSVT)	• No high-risk factors for SCD present (i.e., no risk factors listed under ICD recommended, ICD reasonable or ICD considered columns)

*In children, massive LVH can be considered when absolute end-diastolic LV wall thickness ≥ 30 mm or z-score ≥ 20 with no other risk factors or z-score ≥ 10 with other risk factors present.

**Non-sustained VT defined as ≥ 3 consecutive ventricular beats at rate ≥ 120 bpm and lasting ≤30 seconds.

HCM, Hypertrophic cardiomyopathy; *ICD,* implantable cardioverter-defibrillator; *LGE,* late gadolinium enhancement; *LV,* left ventricular; *LVH,* left ventricular hypertrophy; *MRI,* magnetic resonance imaging; *NSVT,* non-sustained VT; *SCD,* sudden cardiac death; *VF,* ventricular fibrillation; *VT,* ventricular tachycardia.

Lifestyle Considerations

Recreational exercise of mild-to-moderate intensity is encouraged in patients with HCM to maintain overall cardiovascular health.[15] Adequate hydration should be maintained, particularly in those with LVOTO. Children with HCM may be permitted to participate in the physical education curriculum at school but should not be graded on performance.[15]

The risk of SCD with competitive sports participation is unclear. For athletes, participation in competitive sports requires a comprehensive evaluation and shared discussion of potential risks and benefits. Competition in low-intensity sports is generally considered reasonable.[15] Individualized discussion with an experienced provider is important when considering participation in competitive athletics of moderate-to-high intensity due to the potential increased risk of SCD.[15] Placement of a primary prevention ICD in athletes who do not otherwise meet criteria for ICD placement solely to permit sports participation is not recommended.[15]

Differential Diagnosis

The differential diagnosis for an individual with a new diagnosis of LVH includes physiologic causes (e.g., athlete's heart, hypertension), and a number of syndromes (such as RASopathies) and metabolic disorders (such as Fabry disease or Danon disease) with known genetic causes.

Athlete's Heart

Athletes who engage in high-intensity exercise, particularly endurance athletes, can develop physiologic concentric LVH known as "athlete's heart" that can be challenging to distinguish from mild cases of isolated, genetically caused HCM. There are some features that can help distinguish athlete's heart from HCM; this is important in understanding an individual's risk for SCD and determining subsequent management (Table 48.3).[21]

A minority of athletes can have LV wall thicknesses in the "gray zone," in between the upper limits of normal and the lower limit considered for a diagnosis of HCM, which is a challenging clinical conundrum.[21] Detraining is one approach that can be used to distinguish between athlete's heart and HCM, where individuals in the "gray zone" are asked to refrain from exercise for 2–3 months to see if there is regression of LVH. Athletes with concomitant HCM would have sustained LVH, while physiologic LVH regression can be detected by ~6 weeks of exercise abstinence.[21] Understandably, this period of detraining can be challenging to fully implement in elite athletes and is generally reserved for those truly in the "gray zone" for which other diagnostic methods are inconclusive.

Inherited Syndromes with Associated LVH

There are numerous syndromic conditions associated with LVH. RASopathies (including Noonan, Costello, and cardiofaciocutaneous syndromes) can lead to biventricular hypertrophy and CHF during infancy.[22] Mutations in the phospholamban (*PLN*) gene can cause LVH or other primary cardiac disease such as arrhythmogenic right ventricular cardiomyopathy or DCM.[18] Alpha-actinin-2 (*ACTN2*) mutations are also associated with LVH and other cardiac phenotypes including LVNC or arrhythmias.[18] Timothy syndrome, caused by a mutation in CACNA1c, is associated with biventricular hypertrophy that can present in infancy, long QT syndrome, SCD, autism, and syndactyly; however, certain CACNA1c mutations (Arg518Cys and Arg518His) cause only cardiac defects.[18] Mutations in desmin (*DES*), four and a half LIM domain protein 1 (*FHL1*) (causing Emery-Dreifuss muscular dystrophy), or filamin C (*FLNC*) lead to skeletal myopathies but can be associated with LVH that precedes skeletal muscle weakness in some individuals.[18]

Inherited Metabolic Disorders with Associated LVH

Inherited metabolic disorders, including glycogen storage disorders (e.g., Pompe disease, Forbes disease, PRKAG2

TABLE 48.3 Parameters That Can Help Distinguish Athlete's Heart From Hypertrophic Cardiomyopathy[21]

Parameter	Athlete's Heart	HCM
LV wall thickness	Adults: Women: ≤10–11 mm Men: ≤12–14 mm Children: z-score < 2	Adults: >15 mm Children: z-score > 2.5
LVH pattern	Concentric	Asymmetric
LV mass:volume ratio	Normal	Elevated
Diastolic function	Normal	Impaired
LGE on cardiac MRI	None	Present
Detraining	Regression of LVH	Sustained LVH

HCM, hypertrophic cardiomyopathy; *LGE*, late gadolinium enhancement; *LV*, left ventricular; *LVH*, left ventricular hypertrophy; *MRI*, magnetic resonance imaging.

cardiomyopathy, Danon disease), lysosomal storage disorders (e.g., Anderson-Fabry disease), and mitochondrial diseases (e.g., Friedreich's ataxia), are considered HCM phenocopies due to LVH mimicking isolated HCM.[23] Appropriate genetic diagnosis is essential to provide therapies, such as enzyme replacement, targeted at the underlying disease mechanism.

Diseases caused by a mutation in the mitochondrial genome are maternally inherited and can affect multiple systems, in particular, skeletal muscle, the heart, and the central nervous system.[23] Mild, non-obstructive, concentric LVH is seen in ~25% of patients.[23]

Other Causes of LVH

Physiologic and non-inherited causes of LVH should also be considered in the differential diagnosis of HCM. In addition to athlete's heart, other physiologic causes of LVH include hypertension and valvular heart disease. Concentric LVH is often seen in individuals with chronic renal failure due to a combination of pressure and volume overload. A number of metabolic derangements are associated with LVH, including hyperthyroidism, hypoglycemia, and catecholamine-secreting tumors. Infants born to a diabetic mother can also have LVH that resolves over the first few months of life.

Prognosis and Outcomes

Many individuals with HCM are asymptomatic and have a normal life expectancy.[15] Individuals with two or more pathogenic mutations in sarcomeric genes tend to present earlier and have higher risk for adverse outcomes.[7] We do not yet have the ability to predict an individual's risk for adverse events based solely on the specific gene mutation.[15] Approximately 30%–40% of individuals with HCM will experience an adverse outcome with one or more of a sudden death event, symptoms limiting activity (due to LVOTO or CHF from systolic or diastolic dysfunction), or atrial fibrillation.[15] With current management guidelines, the mortality rate of HCM is less than 1% per year, due in large part to appropriate referral for ICD placement in individuals at increased risk for SCD.

Future Directions

Emerging therapies aim to target the underlying molecular mechanisms leading to the clinical phenotype of HCM. Mavacamten is a small molecule inhibitor of cardiac myosin that has been shown to reduce LVOTO and improve echocardiographic parameters of diastolic function in the EXPLORER-HCM clinical trial.[24] Gene therapies that either overexpress normal protein, suppress abnormal protein production, or perform gene editing may correct the clinical phenotype of HCM.[24] Further testing is necessary to ensure safety and efficacy before these approaches can be considered for clinical use.

Restrictive Cardiomyopathy

Definition and Epidemiology

RCM is a rare form of cardiomyopathy accounting for ≤ 5% of pediatric cardiomyopathy diagnoses.[23] It is characterized primarily by severe diastolic dysfunction with elevated end-diastolic ventricular filling pressures and atrial enlargement; one or both ventricles can be affected. Systolic function is usually normal but can be mildly reduced. Approximately one-third of patients with RCM also have some degree of LVH, leading to a mixed RCM/HCM phenotype.[1]

Genetics and Pathophysiology

RCM can be caused by a primary cardiac gene defect or secondarily by infiltrative diseases. Familial RCM (seen in ~25%–30% of cases) can be inherited in an autosomal dominant, autosomal recessive, X-linked, or mitochondrial pattern.[1] Sarcomere or other muscle-specific genes associated with RCM include *DES, MYBPC3, MYH7, MYL3, TNNI3, TNNT2,* and *TPM1*.[25] Infiltrative and inflammatory diseases that can cause RCM include scleroderma, amyloidosis, sarcoidosis, and hemochromatosis, but these are rare causes of RCM in children.[1] A history of radiation can also increase the risk of RCM.[25] Atrial enlargement increases the risk of arrhythmias, thrombosis, and stroke.[1]

Clinical Presentation

Patients with RCM often present with signs and symptoms of heart failure or arrhythmic events. Symptoms can include dyspnea, exercise intolerance, edema, syncope, or SCD.[1] Symptoms can be progressive over a period of months to years, and age at diagnosis can range from infancy to adulthood.[1]

Diagnostic Evaluation

Physical Exam

Physical exam findings are consistent with those seen in decompensated heart failure including a gallop rhythm on cardiac auscultation, jugular venous distension, hepatomegaly, peripheral edema, and ascites.[25] A loud pulmonic valve closure (P2) can be auscultated in the presence of pulmonary hypertension.[25]

Diagnostic Testing

A 12-lead ECG can show left and/or right atrial enlargement, ST-T wave abnormalities and ST-segment depression, conduction abnormalities, or ventricular hypertrophy.[25] Ambulatory ECG monitoring can be helpful in identifying underlying arrhythmias, seen in ~15% of children with RCM.[25] Chest radiography may demonstrate cardiomegaly with atrial enlargement and pulmonary venous congestion.[25]

Echocardiography usually reveals marked dilation of one or both atria and parameters consistent with impaired diastolic function (Fig. 48.4).[25] Systolic function is often

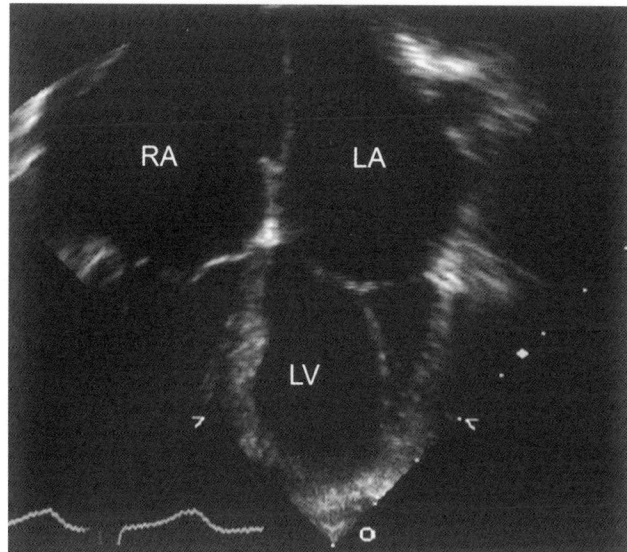

• **Fig. 48.4** Apical transverse end-diastolic echocardiographic image in a patient with restrictive cardiomyopathy. The left atrium *(LA)* and right atrium *(RA)* are markedly dilated and often exceed the size of the left ventricle *(LV)*.

normal but can be mildly depressed in those with more advanced disease.[25] There may be mild LVH but many have a normal LV wall thickness.[25] Cardiac MRI is not always performed but can be helpful to distinguish between constrictive pericarditis (rare in children) and infiltrative forms of RCM.[1]

Cardiac catheterization should be performed at diagnosis to measure left and right ventricular filling pressures, evaluate for pulmonary hypertension, and quantify PVR to determine candidacy for possible orthotopic heart transplantation; individuals with a high PVR may not be transplant candidates.[25] EMB is usually non-diagnostic but may be performed if imaging or genetic testing do not reveal an underlying disease mechanism.

Management

Medical therapies are currently inadequate to effectively treat RCM. Individuals with pulmonary or systemic venous congestion may benefit from low-dose diuretic use, but patients with RCM are preload-dependent, thus excessive diuresis should be avoided.[1] Anticoagulation should be used to reduce the risk of thromboembolic events.[1] Antiarrhythmic medications or ICD placement may be considered for patients with recurrent arrhythmic events, but it is not clear that these treatments affect outcomes.[1] Because there is a limited ability to augment stroke volume, patients may not tolerate ACEi or beta-blockers; inpatient observation should be considered when initiating treatment.[25]

Due to lack of adequate medical therapies, heart transplantation is currently considered definitive therapy for RCM. Survival times after cardiac transplantation exceed survival times for the natural history of RCM from diagnosis. Early consideration for heart transplantation is usually recommended, prior to development of irreversible pulmonary vascular disease.[25] Some groups may recommend listing patients for transplant at the time of RCM diagnosis, even in asymptomatic patients, given the poor prognosis for untreated RCM and long waitlist times.[25]

Prognosis and Outcomes

Prognosis is poor for patients with RCM, with a 5-year survival rate of 68% from the time of diagnosis in children.[1] Cause of death is most commonly due to CHF but SCD is not uncommon.[25] Transplant-free survival is 22% at 5 years in children with isolated RCM; those with a mixed RCM/HCM phenotype have better outcomes with a transplant-free survival rate of 68% at 5 years.[1] Post-transplant survival is 77% at 5 years in children, which is similar to survival rates for those who receive a heart transplantation for other indications.[1]

Future Directions

Improved risk assessment models to understand who would benefit from early transplantation are needed to optimize timing prior to development of fixed PVR. Personalized medicine approaches that target molecular mechanisms leading to disease and gene therapies that can correct underlying defects may be possible in the future.

References

1. Lee TM, Hsu DT, Kantor P, et al. Pediatric cardiomyopathies. *Circ Res*. 2017;121:855-873.
2. Lipshultz SE, Law YM, Asante-Korang A, et al. Cardiomyopathy in children: classification and diagnosis: a scientific statement from the American Heart Association. *Circulation*. 2019;140:e9-e68.
3. Lipshultz SE, Sleeper LA, Towbin JA, et al. The incidence of pediatric cardiomyopathy in two regions of the United States. *N Engl J Med*. 2003;348:1647-1655.
4. Towbin JA, Lowe AM, Colan SD, et al. Incidence, causes, and outcomes of dilated cardiomyopathy in children. *JAMA*. 2006;296:1867-1876.
5. Jordan E, Peterson L, Ai T, et al. Evidence-based assessment of genes in dilated cardiomyopathy. *Circulation*. 2021;144:7-19.
6. Pugh TJ, Kelly MA, Gowrisankar S, et al. The landscape of genetic variation in dilated cardiomyopathy as surveyed by clinical DNA sequencing. *Genet Med*. 2014;16:601-608.
7. Ware SM, Wilkinson JD, Tariq M, et al. Genetic causes of cardiomyopathy in children: first results from the pediatric cardiomyopathy genes study. *J Am Heart Assoc*. 2021;10:e017731.
8. Hershberger RE, Givertz MM, Ho CY, et al. Genetic evaluation of cardiomyopathy: a clinical practice resource of the American College of Medical Genetics and Genomics (ACMG). *Genet Med*. 2018;20:899-909.
9. Birnkrant DJ, Bushby K, Bann CM, et al. Diagnosis and management of Duchenne muscular dystrophy, part 2: respiratory, cardiac, bone health, and orthopaedic management. *Lancet Neurol*. 2018;17:347-361.

10. Pahl E, Sleeper LA, Canter CE, et al. Incidence of and risk factors for sudden cardiac death in children with dilated cardiomyopathy: a report from the Pediatric Cardiomyopathy Registry. *J Am Coll Cardiol.* 2012;39:607-615.

11. Broomfield J, Hill M, Guglieri M, et al. Life expectancy in Duchenne muscular dystrophy: reproduced individual patient data meta-analysis. *Neurology.* 2021;97:e2304-e2314.

12. Mulrooney DA, Yeazel MW, Kawashima T, et al. Cardiac outcomes in a cohort of adult survivors of childhood and adolescent cancer: retrospective analysis of the Childhood Cancer Survivor Study cohort. *BMJ.* 2009;339:b4606.

13. Pennell DJ, Udelson JE, Arai AE, et al. Cardiovascular function and treatment in beta-thalassemia major: a consensus statement from the American Heart Association. *Circulation.* 2013;128:281-308.

14. Ross SB, Jones K, Blanch B, et al. A systematic review and meta-analysis of the prevalence of left ventricular non-compaction in adults. *Eur Heart J.* 2020;41:1428-1436.

15. Ommen SR, Mital S, Burke MA, et al. 2020 AHA/acc guideline for the diagnosis and treatment of patients with hypertrophic cardiomyopathy: a report of the American College of Cardiology/American Heart Association Joint Committee on Clinical Practice Guidelines. *J Am Coll Cardiol.* 2020;76:e159-e240.

16. Maron BJ, Desai MY, Nishimura RA, et al. Diagnosis and evaluation of hypertrophic cardiomyopathy: JACC state-of-the-art review. *J Am Coll Cardiol.* 2022;79:372-389.

17. Maron BJ, Desai MY, Nishimura RA, et al. Management of hypertrophic cardiomyopathy: JACC state-of-the-art review. *J Am Coll Cardiol.* 2022;79:390-414.

18. Ingles J, Goldstein J, Thomson C, et al. Evaluating the clinical validity of hypertrophic cardiomyopathy genes. *Circ Genom Precis Med.* 2019;12:e002460.

19. Marian AJ, Braunwald E. Hypertrophic cardiomyopathy: genetics, pathogenesis, clinical manifestations, diagnosis, and therapy. *Circ Res.* 2017;121:749-770.

20. Norrish G, Kaski JP. The risk of sudden death in children with hypertrophic cardiomyopathy. *Heart Fail Clin.* 2022;18:9-18.

21. Brosnan MJ, Rakhit D. Differentiating athlete's heart from cardiomyopathies: the left side. *Heart Lung Circ.* 2018;27:1052-1062.

22. Monda E, Rubino M, Lioncino M, et al. Hypertrophic cardiomyopathy in children: pathophysiology, diagnosis, and treatment of non-sarcomeric causes. *Front Pediatr.* 2021;9:632293.

23. Sankaranarayanan R, Flemming EJ, Garratt CJ. Mimics of hypertrophic cardiomyopathy: diagnostic clues to aid early identification of phenocopies. *Arrhythm Electrophysiol Rev.* 2013;2:36-40.

24. Helms AS, Thompson AD, Day SM. Translation of new and emerging therapies for genetic cardiomyopathies. *JACC Basic Transl Sci.* 2022;7:70-83.

25. Denfield SW, Webber SA. Restrictive cardiomyopathy in childhood. *Heart Fail Clin.* 2010;6:445-452, viii.

49
Pericardial Disease

DAVID KANE AND ROGER E. BREITBART

KEY LEARNING POINTS

- Idiopathic acute pericarditis (presumed to have a viral etiology) is the most common form of pericardial disease.
- More than 15% of patients with acute idiopathic pericarditis will have recurrent symptoms sometime after the initial episode. Recurrence is more common among those treated with steroids.
- Pericardial effusion can result in tamponade. Physical exam and echocardiography are used to determine when

an effusion has become significant enough to warrant drainage.
- Constrictive pericarditis is rare in young patients, but must be distinguished from restrictive cardiomyopathy.
- In the rare patient with partial congenital defects in the pericardium, the heart can herniate through the defect resulting in epicardial coronary compression.

Introduction

Pericardial diseases involve the pericardial membranes and fluid space surrounding the heart. They include congenital abnormalities, primary inflammatory and infectious processes, secondary reactive processes, and chronic conditions. The pericardium is an avascular sac comprising inner visceral and outer parietal layers. The visceral layer serves as the epicardium and reflects on itself at the level of the great vessels to form an outer serosal layer that adheres to the fibrosa, creating the parietal pericardium. In adults, this potential space typically contains 15–50 mL of serous fluid. The role of the pericardium is to fix the heart in position and to provide lubrication for beating motion.[1] This chapter presents an overview of pericardial conditions pertinent to pediatric practice but it is, of necessity, not exhaustive.

Pericarditis

Inflammation of the pericardium is the most common form of pericardial disease and is described as acute, recurrent, or chronic when lasting greater than 3 months.[2] Inflammatory infiltration of the pericardial membranes is further characterized as with (effusive) or without (noneffusive) excess pericardial fluid.[1] Acute pericarditis is most often idiopathic but thought to be triggered by preceding viral infection. Other etiologies are numerous, outlined in Table 49.1. Pericardial inflammation may be an isolated condition or part of a systemic disease process such as autoimmune disorders and metabolic conditions. Malignancy and complications

from its treatment such as chemotherapy and radiation can also result in acute pericarditis.

Acute pericarditis typically presents with a combination of chest pain, pericardial friction rub, electrocardiogram (ECG) changes, and pericardial effusion.[2,3] Chest pain in pericarditis is often characterized as sharp and acute in onset, worse in the supine position. Leaning forward in an upright seated position may bring pain relief. Fever is common in viral and bacterial pericarditis. Patients with bacterial pericarditis are often ill appearing and may present with shock and a septic circulation. A pericardial friction rub may be noted on physical examination due to the two inflamed layers of the pericardium creating the characteristic sound on auscultation.[2]

In the setting of pericardial inflammation, the ECG often goes through a sequence of changes beginning with PR segment deflection and diffuse ST segment elevation, followed by T-wave flattening, inversion, and eventual normalization over the ensuing weeks (Fig. 49.1). Electrical alternans is an ECG finding where the QRS complex amplitude or axis alternates, presumed to be due to the heart "swinging" in the pericardial space.[2] Chest radiography may be normal, but an enlarged cardiac silhouette, pleural effusions, or pulmonary vascular congestion can be seen. Laboratory testing demonstrates elevated inflammatory markers in 80% of cases, while troponin values are elevated in upwards of 30% of cases, representing myopericarditis.[3,4] Echocardiography is essential in the diagnostic evaluation of acute pericarditis, to determine whether there is a pericardial effusion (Fig. 49.2), and whether there are

TABLE 49.1	Etiologies of Pediatric Acute Pericarditis and Pericardial Effusion

Idiopathic (Probably Viral)

Infection
Bacterial
  Neisseria meningitidis
  Hemophilus influenza
  Staphylococcus aureus
  Mycobacterium tuberculosis
  Borrelia burgdorferi
  Other bacteria, including obligate intracellular species
Viral
  Coxsackie virus
  Cytomegalovirus
  Human immunodeficiency virus
  Other viruses
Fungal
  Candida
  Other
Parasitic
  Toxoplasma gondii
  Other
Connective Tissue Disease and Vasculitis
Systemic lupus erythematosus
Rheumatoid arthritis
Rheumatic fever
Inflammatory bowel disease
Kawasaki disease
Other vasculitides and connective tissue syndromes
Other Etiologies
Postpericardiotomy syndrome
Renal failure, including uremia and chronic dialysis
Malignancy, especially leukemia and lymphoma
Graft-versus-host disease
Pneumonia
Myxedema
Drug, especially mesalamine
Trauma, including hemopericardium
Extravasation from indwelling central venous catheters,
  especially in low-birth-weight neonates
Other

Adapted from Spodick DH. The Pericardium: A Comprehensive Textbook. New York: Marcel Dekker, 1997.[18]

echocardiographic findings consistent with tamponade. Approximately 60% of patients with acute pericarditis will have a pericardial effusion.[2,3] Additional diagnostic imaging is often unnecessary. Cardiac magnetic resonance (CMR) is at times used when concerns for myocardial involvement exist. Late gadolinium enhancement (LGE) can provide accurate assessment of pericardial inflammation with high sensitivity. Patients with higher levels of pericardial LGE may have increased risk of complications and reduced clinical remission rates.[3]

When acute pericarditis is part of a systemic disease process, treatment is focused on the causal disease such as malignancy or renal failure. However, treatment for postviral or idiopathic acute pericarditis begins with nonsteroidal anti-inflammatory drugs (NSAIDs). Although NSAIDs have not been studied as monotherapy in a randomized controlled trial, they are recommended based on clinical experience.

Ibuprofen, indomethacin, and ketorolac have been widely used. The duration of NSAID therapy is not well outlined, but is typically based on the resolution of signs (effusion) and symptoms, as well as of laboratory evidence of inflammation.[3-5] Colchicine is an anti-inflammatory medication commonly used for acute pericarditis. A 3-month course of colchicine in adults reduced symptom persistence, recurrence, and hospitalization rates compared with patients receiving NSAIDs alone in acute pericarditis.[6-8] The use of colchicine can be limited due to gastrointestinal side effects reported in 5–8% of patients. Anti-inflammatory therapies are often tapered, monitoring symptoms, inflammatory markers, and effusions by echocardiography to help guide the dosing reductions.[3,9] Corticosteroids for acute pericarditis have been shown to increase the risk of recurrence and are therefore often avoided as first-line therapy.[7,10] However, corticosteroids are very effective in treating patients who have failed initial treatment with NSAIDs and colchicine. In these patients with standard treatment failure, immunomodulators are often used to limit steroid use.[9]

Recurrent Pericarditis

It has been reported that 15–50% of patients with acute pericarditis experience recurrence after resolution of their original symptoms, thought related to incomplete treatment of the initial episode.[4,11,12] Risk factors for recurrence include history of treatment with corticosteroids, prior recurrence, and female sex. Also, patients who had a nonidiopathic or nonviral cause for acute pericarditis (bacterial, malignancy) are at higher risk for recurrence.[9,13] The signs and symptoms of recurrent pericarditis are often similar to those at the initial presentation.[7,12,14]

Treatment of recurrent pericarditis should include colchicine and may require initiation or re-initiation of corticosteroids, often extremely effective in controlling these flares of inflammation.[7] Steroids should be tapered slowly with close monitoring of inflammatory markers. Other immunomodulatory agents have been studied in this population. IL-1 blockade (anakinra) is effective at treating recurrent pericarditis and reducing corticosteroid treatment.[3,15] Azathioprine, methotrexate, and mycophenolate mofetil have also shown efficacy in these patients.[3,9]

Post-Pericardiotomy Syndrome

Pericarditis may develop following cardiac surgery (post-pericardiotomy syndrome), myocardial infarction (Dressler syndrome), and chest trauma. Post-pericardiotomy syndrome is thought to result from an immune-mediated process that is initiated by pericardial or pleural injury and bleeding following cardiac surgery. The majority of patients present in the first month following surgery. The clinical features are similar to acute pericarditis.[16] Patients with trisomy 21 and those who underwent heart transplant, systemic to pulmonary shunt, or atrial septal defect closure were noted to have increased risk for post-pericardiotomy

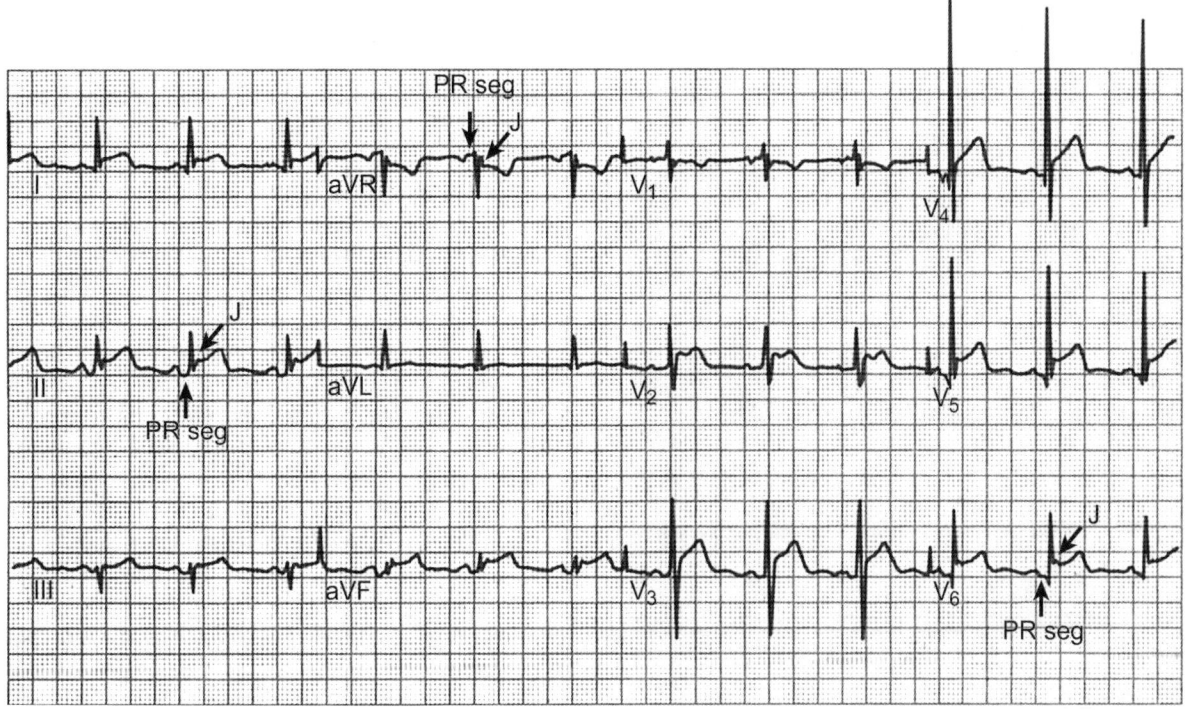

• **Fig. 49.1** Electrocardiogram showing changes pathognomonic of acute pericarditis, including widespread J-point and ST-segment elevation and deflection of the PR segments in the direction opposite that of the P wave, generally PR depression with upright P waves. (Adapted from Spodick DH. Pericardial Diseases. In: Braunwald E, Zipes DP, Libby P, eds. *Heart Disease*, 6th ed, ch 50. Philadelphia, W.B. Saunders, 2001: 1823, with permission.)

syndrome.[17] The diagnosis is made in patients who have had cardiac injury or intervention and develop fever without an alternative cause, chest pain, a friction rub, a pericardial or pleural effusion, and elevated systemic inflammatory markers. Treatment is analogous to acute pericarditis as NSAIDs and colchicine are recommended, while corticosteroids are at times used for NSAID treatment failure.[2] The COPPS trial demonstrated a reduction in the incidence of post-pericardiotomy syndrome in adults who received colchicine prophylaxis following surgery.[12] However, colchicine prophylaxis has not been widely adopted for children as the incidence of post-pericardiotomy is relatively low, treatment quite effective, and colchicine-associated gastrointestinal side effects not infrequent.

Noninflammatory Pericardial Effusions

In addition to the exudate in effusive pericarditis, blood, chyle, and transudative serous fluid can accumulate in the pericardial space. Hemopericardium can develop from aortic dissection/rupture, penetrating chest trauma, or cardiac perforation during a procedure. Rarely, chylous fluid from lymphatic obstruction or thoracic duct injury can result in a pericardial effusion. Disorders that cause right atrial hypertension can impair myocardial venous drainage in the coronary sinus and Thebesian veins, altering hydrostatic pressure, and leading to transudative fluid accumulation in the pericardial space. Examples include hydrops fetalis,

pulmonary artery hypertension, and congestive heart failure. A rare complication from a central venous catheter is migration or malposition into the pericardial space, where medication, colloid, or non-colloidal fluids can be inadvertently delivered resulting in an effusion.

Tamponade

Cardiac tamponade is a potentially life-threatening complication of pericardial effusion. Rapid accumulation of fluid is more likely to result in tamponade physiology. The physical exam features of tamponade include tachycardia, pulsus paradoxus, and the features of Beck's triad—hypotension, jugular venous distention, and muffled heart sounds with auscultation. Pulsus paradoxus is defined by a decrease in systolic blood pressure of at least 10 mm Hg with inspiration during manual blood pressure auscultation. Decreased systemic output with inspiration can be seen on arterial blood pressure monitoring and at times on pulse oximetry plethysmography waveforms (Fig. 49.3). Ultimately, in tamponade physiology, the increased intrapericardial pressure impairs chamber compliance resulting in exaggerated ventricular interdependence. As inspiration increases venous return on the right side, it results in reduced diastolic filling on the left side compromising systemic cardiac output (see Fig. 49.4 for further description).[1–5]

Signs and symptoms of incipient tamponade include dyspnea, tachypnea, tachycardia, poor perfusion, and concern

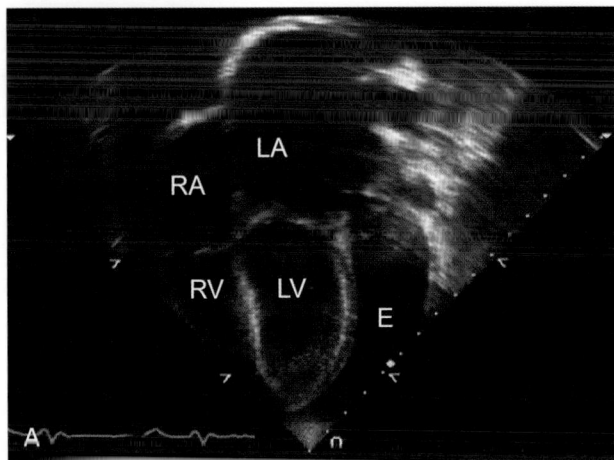

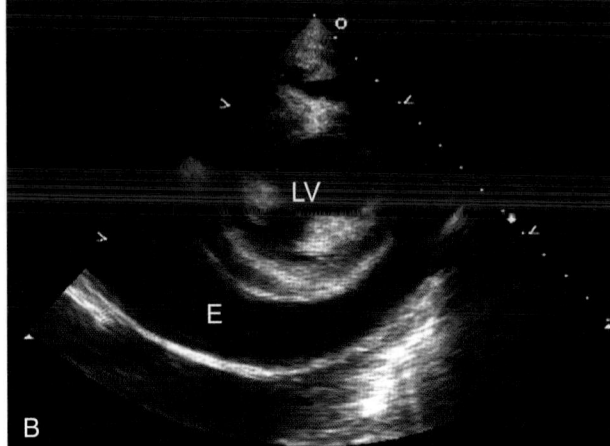

• **Fig. 49.2** Echocardiogram of a patient with a large, circumferential pericardial effusion (E). **(A)** Apical four-chamber view including the right atrium (RA), left atrium (LA), right ventricle (RV), and left ventricle (LV). **(B)** Parasternal short-axis view. (Adapted from Breitbart RE. Chapter 27: Pericardial Diseases. In: Keanne JF, Lock JE, Fyler DC, eds. *Nadas' Pediatric Cardiology*, 2nd edn. Elsevier; 2006. pp. 459–466.)

for shock. Although cardiac tamponade is a clinical diagnosis, exaggerated respirophasic variation of atrioventricular valve inflow or semilunar valve outflow are echocardiographic findings suggestive of tamponade physiology. Right atrial or right ventricular collapse can also be seen, the result of elevated intrapericardial pressure.

Cardiac tamponade is life-threatening and should be treated emergently. Medical management is of limited benefit, but intravascular volume expansion may help cardiac filling and output transiently while preparing for pericardial drainage. Definitive treatment is accomplished by percutaneous pericardiocentesis, or in some cases open surgical drainage. The standard approach to percutaneous drainage is from a subxiphoid approach, but the pericardial space can be entered from a non-subxiphoid approach where the fluid collection is maximal. Ultrasound and fluoroscopy are used to help guide percutaneous needle aspiration, and often a guidewire is used to allow for placement of a pericardial drain. Pericardiocentesis is typically performed to alleviate cardiac tamponade, but it can be done for diagnostic evaluation when there is clinical concern for tuberculous, bacterial, or neoplastic pericarditis.[9] Pericardial fluid is generally sent for routine chemistry and cell count as well as culture, Gram stain, and pathologic evaluation to help determine etiology.

For patients with recurrent pericardial effusions, a pericardial "window" can be created thoracoscopically to allow fluid to drain from the pericardial space to the chest. This approach does not treat the underlying etiology of an effusion, but attempts to reduce the risk of cardiac tamponade.

Constrictive Pericardial Disease

Chronic inflammation or scarring of the pericardium can lead to constrictive pericarditis, as the pericardium loses its elasticity and the two layers fuse together. Diastolic compliance of the ventricles is impaired resulting in elevated filling pressures that can produce signs of both left and right heart failure. However, the clinical presentation of right atrial hypertension is more common. Constrictive pericarditis is a rare disease entity in pediatrics, but can be a complication of recurrent pericarditis, infection (especially tuberculous pericarditis), prior radiation therapy, malignancy, and post cardiac surgery.[19,20]

The diagnosis of constrictive pericarditis is often based on physical exam features of right heart failure in a patient with prior pericardial disease. Symptoms include fatigue, anorexia, exercise intolerance, and dyspnea, while the physical exam may demonstrate jugular venous distention and

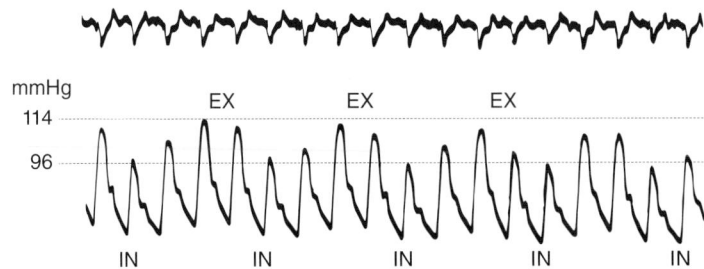

• **Fig. 49.3** Brachial artery pressure tracing demonstrating pulsus paradoxus, with the corresponding electrocardiogram above. The systolic pressures at end inspiration (IN), 96 mm Hg, and peak expiration (EX), 114 mm Hg, differ by 18 mm Hg, which is the magnitude of the pulsus. (Adapted from Spodick DH. The Pericardium: A Comprehensive Textbook. New York: Marcel Dekker, 1997, with permission.)[18]

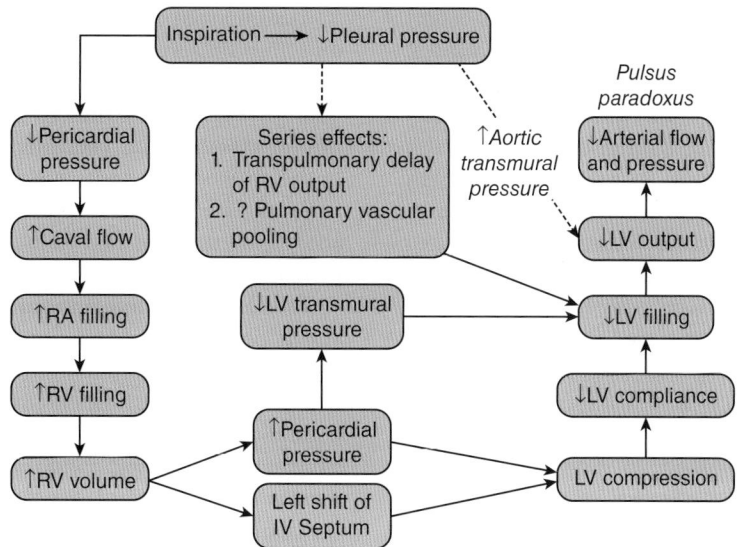

• **Fig. 49.4** Physiology of pulsus paradoxus. Responses to inspiratory reduction of pleural pressure combine to produce the inspiratory fall in left ventricular *(LV)* output and arterial systolic pressure. *RV,* Right ventricular. (Adapted from Spodick DH. The Pericardium: A Comprehensive Textbook. New York: Marcel Dekker, 1997, with permission.)[18]

hepatomegaly. In approximately half of patients with constrictive pericarditis, a pericardial "knock" has been reported on auscultation.[3]

Echocardiographic features of diastolic dysfunction contribute to the diagnosis of constrictive pericarditis. These include abnormal mitral valve inflow velocities (E/A > 1 and deceleration < 150 ms). Interventricular dependence can result in a diastolic septal bounce and respirophasic septal shift. Respiratory variation in mitral inflow is prominent in constrictive disease as the velocities increase during expiration. The most specific echocardiographic sign is expiratory hepatic vein diastolic flow reversal.[3,21,22]

CMR and computed tomography (CT) may assist in the diagnosis of constrictive pericarditis. Accurate determinations of diffuse or localized pericardial thickening can be made by CMR, while cardiac CT detects small amounts of pericardial calcification (Fig. 49.5). Additional imaging findings of inferior vena cava, right atrial, and hepatic vein dilation are also noted with abnormal diastolic filling conditions.[20-22]

When a diagnosis of constrictive pericarditis remains unclear following non-invasive imaging, cardiac catheterization is often performed to evaluate hemodynamics. Features of constriction include elevation of diastolic filling pressures in the left and right ventricles with equalization (<5 mm Hg difference), prominent rapid diastolic filling in

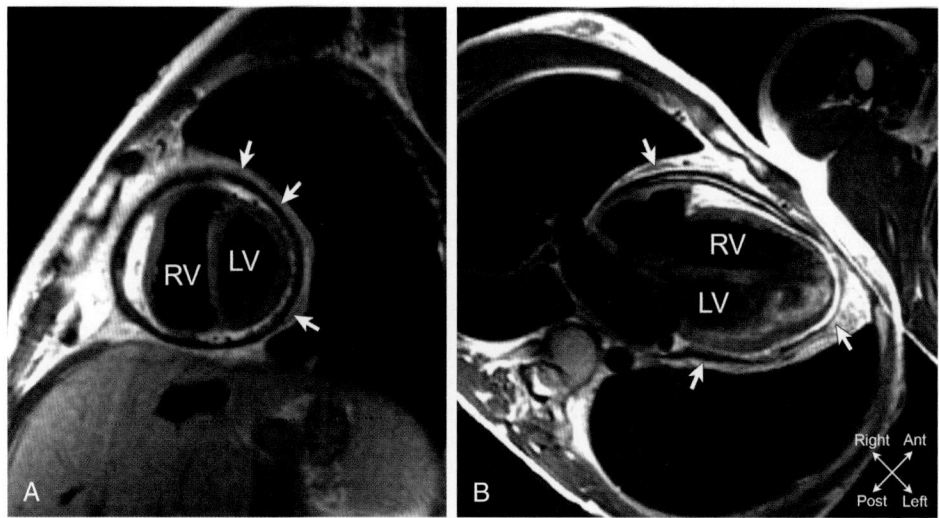

• **Fig. 49.5** Magnetic resonance images of a patient with a constrictive pericardium *(arrows)* encasing the right *(RV)* and left *(LV)* ventricles. **(A)** Parasagittal cut. **(B)** Axial cut. (Adapted from Breitbart RE. Chapter 27: Pericardial Diseases. In: Keanne JF, Lock JE, Fyler DC, eds. *Nadas' Pediatric Cardiology*, 2nd edn. Elsevier; 2006: pp. 459–466.)

both ventricles with characteristic pressure tracing commonly referred to as the square root sign, reduced cardiac output, and an exaggerated decrease in systolic blood pressure during inspiration as shown in Fig. 49.6.[5,20] Constrictive pericardial disease can be challenging to distinguish from restrictive cardiomyopathy as they both result in right and left heart non-compliance. However, in constrictive disease respirophasic alterations in cardiac output exist due to the enhanced ventricular interactions from an encased pericardium as seen in Fig. 49.6. The diastolic filling changes that occur during the respiratory cycle affect cardiac output in constrictive disease but not in restrictive disease.[20]

Treatment of constrictive pericarditis is generally based on symptom severity. Initial medical management focuses on treating any residual inflammation that may be present while attempting to carefully diurese and reduce diastolic filling pressures. Heart rate control with beta-blockers can be helpful in some patients with tachycardia. However, patients with New York Heart Association (NYHA) class III or IV symptoms that do not respond to medical therapy may benefit from surgical pericardiectomy. This surgery is associated with a significant mortality risk (6%–12%) and at times the efficacy is limited, which is why it is often considered as a last alternative.[2,20]

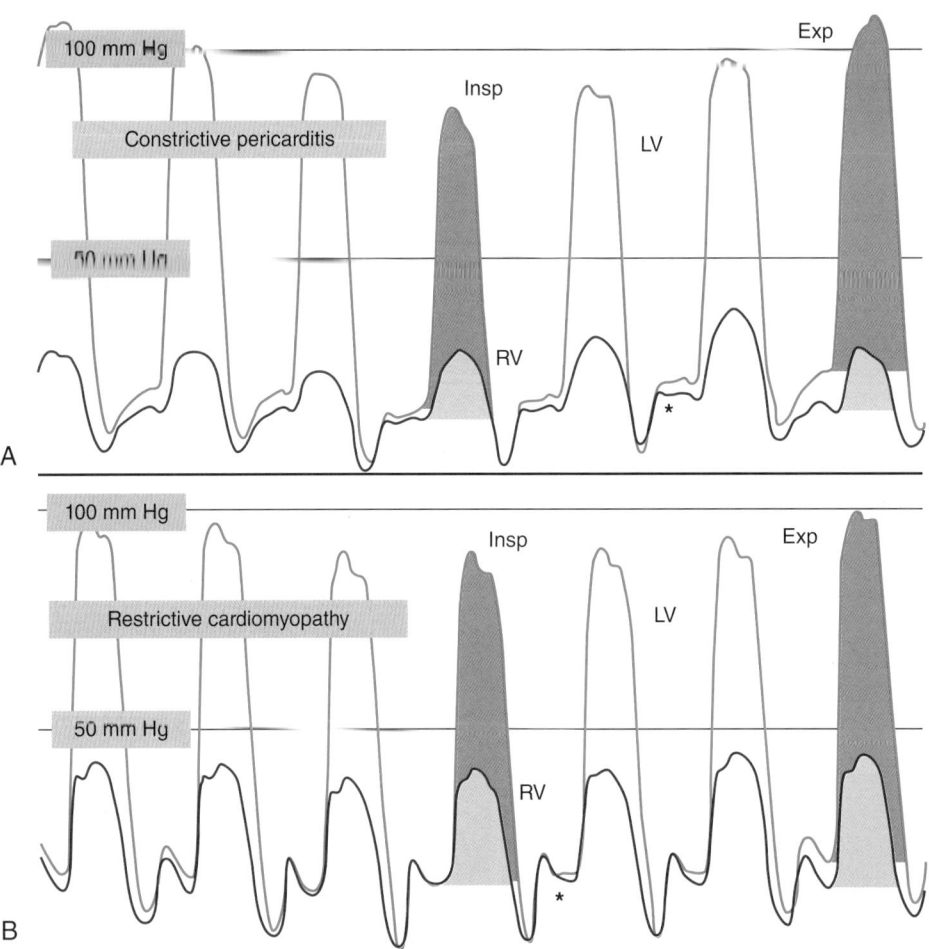

(**Top**) Left ventricular (LV) (**blue**) and right ventricular (RV) (**red**) hemodynamic pressure tracings in constrictive pericarditis. End-diastolic filling pressures are elevated and a "square root" sign is present on both pressure tracings (*). Enhanced ventricular interdependence is present, demonstrated by visualization of the systolic area index; RV (**gray**) and LV (**dark gray**) areas under the curve are shown for both inspiration (Insp) and expiration (Exp). During inspiration, there is an increase in the area of the RV pressure curve and decrease in the area of the LV pressure curve. (**Bottom**) LV and RV pressure tracings in restrictive cardiomyopathy. Although end-diastolic filling pressures are elevated and a square root sign (*) is present, there is no evidence of enhanced ventricular interdependence, with parallel changes in LV and RV pressure curve areas.

• **Fig. 49.6** Intracardiac pressure recordings in patients with constrictive pericarditis (**A**) and restrictive cardiomyopathy (**B**). Left ventricular *(LV) (blue)* and simultaneous right ventricular *(RV) (red)* pressure tracings, demonstrating the "square root" sign *(*)* with dip and rapid rise in early diastole. The darkly shaded regions represent the LV systolic area under the curve *(AUC)*, while the lightly shaded regions represent the RV systolic AUC. In constrictive pericarditis, the enhanced interventricular dependence is demonstrated as the LV AUC increases while RV AUC is simultaneously reduced during expiration. In contrast, the RV and LV AUC in restrictive cardiomyopathy increase proportionally during expiration. (Used with permission from: Geske JB, Anavekar NS, Nishimura RA, et al. Differentiation of constriction and restriction. *J Am Coll Cardiol.* 2016;68:2329–2347.)

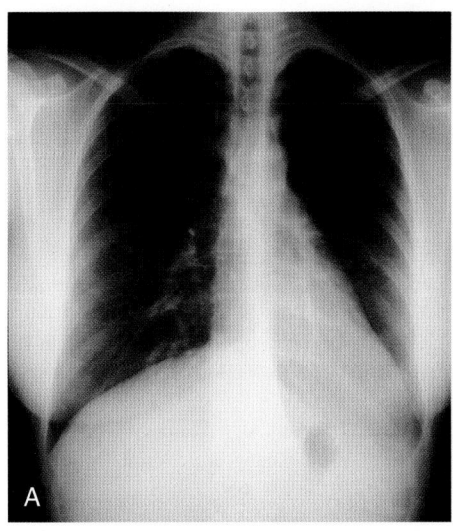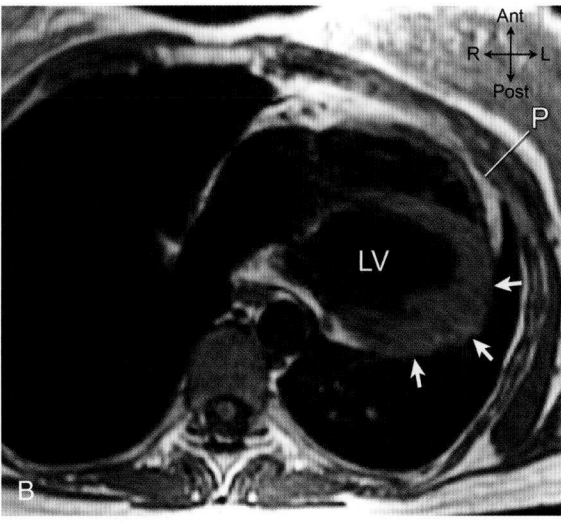

• **Fig. 49.7** Images of a patient with congenital absence of the left pericardium. **(A)** Chest radiograph showing leftward displacement of the cardiac apex. **(B)** Magnetic resonance image showing that the pericardium *(P)* is absent posterolaterally *(arrows)* around the left ventricle *(LV)* in an axial cut. (Adapted from Breitbart RE. Chapter 27: Pericardial Diseases. In: Keanne JF, Lock JE, Fyler DC, eds. *Nadas' Pediatric Cardiology*, 2nd edn. Elsevier; 2006: pp. 459–466.)

Congenital Partial or Complete Absence of the Pericardium

Congenital absence of the pericardium is rare with reported incidence of 0.004% and is described as complete or partial.[3] During fetal development, a disturbance of pleuropericardial membrane fusion can result in this congenital defect.[23] The majority of cases (70%) comprise absence of the left sided pericardium, while absence of the right (17%) and bilateral defects (9–13%) are much less common. Defects have been associated with other congenital heart lesions such as atrial septal defects and tetralogy of Fallot.[21,23] Patients are often asymptomatic, making the diagnosis one that is often made incidentally. However, in patients with partial defects, the heart can herniate through the defect resulting in epicardial coronary compression. The diagnosis should be considered when there is leftward cardiac malposition on chest radiograph (so-called "Snoopy" sign), and on echocardiography when the apical imaging windows are much more leftward and posterior than usual. CMR and CT are the best imaging modalities to make this diagnosis (Fig. 49.7). Partial defects are often repaired in symptomatic patients either with patch closure of the pericardium or, instead, total pericardiectomy, while complete defects tend to remain asymptomatic.[23] Trauma including acute deceleration in a motor vehicle accident can rupture the pericardium and produce features similar to congenital absence.[24]

Pericardial Cysts and Masses

Pericardial cysts are rare mediastinal masses with a reported incidence of 1 in 100,000.[2,21] Cysts differ from pericardial diverticula in that they do not communicate with the pericardial space. They are often isolated and detected incidentally on chest radiograph. In addition to echocardiography, cross-sectional imaging is performed to delineate the anatomic relationships and differentiate pericardial from bronchogenic, thymic, and enteric cysts. Pericardial cysts can cause mass effects on mediastinal structures. If treatment is deemed necessary, it is often with percutaneous aspiration or surgical resection.[2]

Primary pericardial tumors including mesotheliomas, sarcomas, lipomas, hemangioma, and teratomas are rare. Metastatic tumors to the pericardium are more common in adults, but remain rare in pediatrics. Thoracic malignancies can locally invade the pericardium and are often imaged with cardiac CT or CMR as opposed to echocardiography.[21]

References

1. Breitbart RB. Pericardial diseases. In: Keane JF, Lock JE, Fyler DC, eds. *Nadas' Pediatric Cardiology*. 2nd ed. Philadelphia: Saunders Elsevier; 2006:459-466.
2. Adler Y, Charron P, Imazio M, et al. 2015 ESC Guidelines for the diagnosis and management of pericardial diseases. *Eur Heart J.* 2015;36:2921-2964.
3. Chiabrando JG, Bonaventura A, Vecchie A, et al. Management of acute and recurrent pericarditis. *J Am Coll Cardiol.* 2020;75:76-92.
4. Imazio M, Brucato A, Barbieri A, et al. Good prognosis for pericarditis with and without myocardial involvement. *Circulation.* 2013;128:42-49.
5. Imazio M, Gaita F, LeWinter M. Evaluation and treatment of pericarditis. *JAMA.* 2015;314:1498-1506.
6. Imazio M, Adler Y. Treatment with aspirin, NSAID, corticosteroids, and colchicine in acute and recurrent pericarditis. *Heart Fail Rev.* 2013;18:355-360.

7. Imazio M, Bobbio M, Cecchi E, et al. Colchicine in addition to conventional therapy for acute pericarditis: results of the COlchicine for acute PEricarditis (COPE) trial. *Circulation.* 2005;112:2012-2016.

8. Imazio M, Brucato A, Cemin R, et al. A randomized trial of colchicine for acute pericarditis. *N Engl J Med.* 2013;369:1522-1528.

9. Imazio M, Spodick DH, Brucato A, Trinchero R, Adler Y. Controversial issues in the management of pericardial diseases. *Circulation.* 2010;121:916-928.

10. Lotrionte M, Biondi-Zoccai G, Imazio M, et al. International collaborative systematic review of controlled clinical trials on pharmacologic treatments for acute pericarditis and its recurrences. *Am Heart J.* 2010;160:662-670.

11. Imazio M, Brucato A, Pluymaekers N, et al. Recurrent pericarditis in children and adolescents: a multicentre cohort study. *J Cardiovasc Med.* 2016;17:702-712.

12. Imazio M, Trinchero R, Brucato A, et al. Colchicine for the prevention of the post-pericardiotomy syndrome (COPPS): a multicentre, randomized, double-blind, placebo controlled trial. *Eur Heart J.* 2010;31:2749-2754.

13. Imazio M, Brucato A, Cemin R, et al. Colchicine for recurrent pericarditis (CORP): a randomized trial. *Ann Intern Med.* 2011; 155:409-414.

14. Imazio M, Belli R, Brucato A, et al. Efficacy and safety of colchicine for treatment of multiple recurrences of pericarditis (CORP-2): a multicenter, double-blind, placebo controlled randomized trial. *Lancet.* 2014;383:2232-2237.

15. Brucato A, Imazio M, Gatorno M, et al. Effect of anakinra on recurrent pericarditis among patients with colchicine resistance and corticosteroid dependence. *JAMA.* 2016;316:1906-1912.

16. Imazio M, Brucato A, Rovere ME, et al. Contemporary features, risk factors, and prognosis of the post-pericardiotomy syndrome. *Am J M Cardiol.* 2011;108:1183-1187.

17. Elias MD, Glatz AC, Cohen MS, et al. Prevalence and risk factors for pericardial effusions requiring readmission after pediatric cardiac surgery. *Pediatr Cardiol.* 2017;38:484-494.

18. Spodick DH. *The Pericardium: A Comprehensive Textbook.* New York: Marcel Dekker, Inc.; 1997.

19. Imazio M, Brucato A, Maestroni S, et al. Risk of constrictive pericarditis after acute pericarditis. *Circulation.* 2011;124: 1270-1275.

20. Geske JB, Anavekar NS, Nishimura RA, Oh JK, Gersh BJ. Differentiation of constriction and restriction. *J Am Coll Cardiol.* 2016;68:2329-2347.

21. Yared K, Baggish AL, Picard MH, Hoffmann U, Hung J. Multimodality imaging of pericardial diseases. *JACC Cardiovasc Imaging.* 2010;3:650-659.

22. Klein AL, Abbara S, Agler DA, et al. American Society of Echocardiography clinical recommendations for multimodality cardiovascular imaging of patients with pericardial disease: endorsed by the Society for Cardiovascular Magnetic Resonance and Society of Cardiovascular Computed Tomography. *J Am Soc Echocardiogr.* 2013;26:965.e15 1012.e15.

23. Iglesias PC, Pascual FA, de la Torre LA, et al. Pericardial agenesis. *Ann Pediatr Cardiol.* 2021;14:119-121.

24. Hetherman D, Malka K, Schanzer A, Wallace EC, Kane D, Breitbart R. Endovascular repair of traumatic aortic pseudoaneurysm and delayed presentation of pericardial rupture with cardiac herniation in pediatric trauma. *Clin Surg.* 2017;2:1673.

50

Infective Endocarditis

SHARON E. O'BRIEN AND SUSAN F. SALEEB

KEY LEARNING POINTS

- Endocarditis in pediatric patients is predominantly related to congenital heart disease or indwelling catheters/devices and carries high morbidity and mortality; familiarity with signs and symptoms allows prompt recognition and management.
- The accurate diagnosis and treatment of endocarditis are heavily dependent on blood/tissue culture results; obtaining sufficient blood cultures prior to initiation of antibiotic therapy in appropriate cases is key.
- Endocarditis can lead to serious life-threatening complications that may require surgical intervention to increase chances of survival.

- In 2007, the American Heart Association updated guidelines on the use of antibiotics for the prevention of infective endocarditis, resulting in the cessation of antibiotic prophylaxis for the majority or patients and procedures. Only those patients and procedures with highest risk for poor outcomes from endocarditis are recommended to receive prophylaxis.
- Attention to good oral hygiene with regular brushing, flossing, and dental visits is thought to be the most impactful measure for preventing endocarditis.

Introduction

Infective endocarditis (IE), although uncommon in pediatrics, carries a high morbidity and mortality and therefore is imperative to diagnose and treat promptly. All providers should have a familiarization with this disease process, since the earliest signs and symptoms may be presented to the primary care provider, neonatologist, or cardiologist. The condition involves infection of the endocardium, the valves of the heart, and/or prosthetic cardiac material/devices, with most patients having an identifiable risk factor such as structural heart disease or indwelling catheters or devices. Although commonly referred to as bacterial endocarditis, fungi can also infect the endocardial surface, is increasing in incidence, and has a poor prognosis. At times, no identifiable organism will be identified, a condition referred to as culture-negative endocarditis.

With medical advancements over the past half-century including the use of prosthetic material and indwelling lines, survival of patients with congenital heart disease (CHD) has increased, and with it the overall incidence of IE. Changes in patient characteristics, causative organisms, medical therapies, and prophylaxis recommendations have also occurred. Given the complexity of the disease process, a multi-specialty approach including cardiology, infectious disease,

cardiothoracic surgery, radiology, and interventionalists is often warranted. Recognition and management of complications of IE are crucial to optimal patient outcomes. Despite advancements in treatment, mortality for this condition remains at 5–10%.[1]

Epidemiology

IE occurs less frequently in children than in adults with an incidence of 0.05–0.12 cases per 1000 pediatric admissions as estimated by one multicenter US study conducted between 2003 and 2010.[1,2] With the decreased incidence of rheumatic fever in developed countries, cardiac malformation is now the major risk factor for IE in children > 2 years old with an incidence of 6.1 first-cases/1000 children with CHD from birth to 18 years.[3] Since the 1980s, some studies have indicated an increase in overall frequency of endocarditis in children, with a shift toward those with previous cardiac surgery. This trend mirrors increased rates of hospitalized newborns with indwelling catheters and increased survival of children with repaired CHD.[4]

Certain cardiac lesions present the highest risk of IE including cyanotic lesions, endocardial cushion defects, and left-sided lesions. One study highlights increased risk of IE

615

within the first 6 months of surgery (during endothelialization), or a need for surgery at age < 3 years, suggesting more complex CHD. There does not appear to be a difference in incidence between boys and girls in the pediatric population.[3] There are increasing numbers of patients without CHD who are developing IE representing approximately 8–10% of cases. Those are often in association with indwelling venous catheters, involve the mitral or aortic valve, and are due to *Staphylococcus aureus* (*S. aureus*) bacteremia. In contrast to adults, intravenous (IV) drug use and degenerative heart disease are not frequent predisposing factors of IE in the pediatric population.[1]

The vast majority of organisms causing IE are gram-positive cocci that include staphylococci, viridans group streptococci (VGS), β-hemolytic streptococci, and enterococci. Many recent studies have shown that *S. aureus* has now replaced VGS as the most common organism causing IE and is definitely the most common organism in acute endocarditis. According to one pediatric study, *S. aureus* was the most prevalent cause of IE (57%), followed by VGS (20%) and coagulase-negative staphylococci (14%). Together, these organisms accounted for > 90% of IE.[4] *Staphylococcus aureus* appears to be the most common organism in those patients without underlying heart disease or those with prosthetic valves, whereas VGS is the most common organism in patients with underlying heart conditions.[5] Fungal IE has a prevalence of 1–10% and is increasing in incidence.[6] The rising rate of fungal IE may be related to increasing use of intracardiac devices and central venous catheters, the latter particularly in hospitalized infants. Fungal IE carries a particularly high mortality rate of ~50%.[7]

Pathophysiology

The development of IE is the result of complex interactions between damaged endothelium, blood-borne pathogens, fibrin, and platelets. The initial step is disruption of the endothelial surface by a turbulent jet of blood flow, abrasion from an indwelling catheter or device, or surgical intervention. In general, cardiac defects that include prosthetic material and high-velocity flow jets are at the highest risk of developing IE. Patients with palliative shunts and conduits have been found to be the largest group at risk.[8] Normal endothelium is not prone to pathogen adhesion. Since damaged endothelium activates thrombogenesis, fibrin and platelets are deposited at this site and form a nonbacterial thrombotic endocarditis (NBTE).

Transient bacteremia or fungemia leads to colonization of the NBTE. Transient bacteremia is frequent following manipulation of the teeth and periodontal tissue, as well as during routine daily activities such as chewing, flossing, or brushing of teeth.[9] These everyday activities can present frequent, low-grade bacteremia and likely account for the majority of bacterial seeding leading to IE.[10] Following colonization of NBTE, commonly known as a vegetation, there is subsequent deposition of fibrin and platelets, which

further protects the pathogen from phagocytosis and other host defenses. Vegetations when large enough can become unstable and embolize involving other organs, including the brain, lungs, spleen, and kidneys.

Gram-positive cocci, which are the most common pathogens of both native and prosthetic valve infections, express multiple adhesins which are critical virulence factors allowing for initiation and propagation of IE. Adhesins can act in numerous ways, sometimes promoting direct pathogen adhesion to host cell structures or by forming a biofilm.[1] Biofilms are particularly important in prosthetic valve endocarditis and present a complex environment for pathogens to attach and thrive on device surfaces. Host immune cells and antimicrobial agents have difficulty penetrating this biofilm leading to reduced effectiveness in killing off bacteria and subsequently an increased risk of infection relapse. These adhesins are not only important to the initial adherence of the bacteria but may also play a role in enhancing invasion into the host cell. This is an important area of research as new tools for prevention and treatment of IE are developed.

It is important to recognize that the mouth is an important source of bacteremia and emphasis on good oral hygiene is critical to the prevention of IE. In 2007, the American Heart Association (AHA) revised its guidelines on the use of antibiotic prophylaxis against IE. Those recommendations included the cessation of antibiotic prophylaxis prior to dental procedures for most patients with the exception of those with underlying heart conditions thought to be at the highest risk of IE and adverse outcomes.[9] The teeth and oral mucosa are home to numerous bacteria, which differ depending on the age of the child. A healthy child's mouth contains viridans group streptococcus, *Neisseria*, *Staphylococcus*, and *Haemophilus* species. In the absence of good oral hygiene, pathogenic bacteria build, leading to gingival inflammation and increased risk of bacterial invasion. In the healthy oral cavity, the gingival crevicular mucosa provides a barrier against development of bacterial seeding of the bloodstream. The gingiva is the likely source of all transient bacteremia from the oral cavity whether through gingival manipulation in the dental office or through normal daily activities such as chewing, brushing, and flossing.

Diagnosis

The clinical presentation of IE in children will vary based on several factors, including age, the presence or absence of CHD, prior surgical or catheter-based interventions, prosthetic material used, location of infection, particular organism involved, and the sequelae of IE. The most common IE presentation is subacute, in which children can manifest an indolent course with protracted fever, malaise, myalgia, arthralgia, weight loss, rigors, and diaphoresis. Less commonly, acute IE can present with spiking fever, respiratory distress, and circulatory instability, often necessitating urgent intervention. The most concerning organisms associated with acute IE are *S. aureus* and *Streptococcus pneumoniae*, both with the potential for rapid tissue destruction.[1]

Physical exam findings will vary based on the hemodynamic effect of the infection. New or exacerbated valve regurgitation can present with a murmur and may spur development of congestive heart failure. Prosthetic valve infection notoriously presents with rapid-onset valve obstruction and resultant ventricular dysfunction; valve regurgitation is also common. Progressive cyanosis may ensue from infection of systemic-to-pulmonary shunt. Systemic and/or pulmonary emboli can occur based on location of the infection and underlying circulation, including right-to-left shunting associated with cyanotic lesions. Children with neurologic emboli can present with headache, seizure, and altered mental status. Mycotic aneurysms, although rare, can be catastrophic. Systemic emboli to abdominal organs may present with ischemic enterocolitis, splenic infarct, or renal insufficiency. Respiratory symptoms may signal septic pulmonary embolization. Some immune-mediated findings in IE, including Janeway lesions, Roth spots, and Osler nodes are less common in infants and children than in adults.[1]

As noted, rates of IE in neonates is rising, particularly in premature infants requiring indwelling catheters.[1] Neonates may present with a sepsis-like picture, sometimes without fever, complicating the diagnosis. Congestive heart failure and low cardiac output may ensue, with extracardiac manifestations related to septic emboli being common, presenting as pneumonia, meningitis, or osteomyelitis. *S. aureus* bacteremia is most commonly associated with indwelling catheters and can cause rapid destruction of heart valves and abscess formation. Fungal endocarditis, particularly *Candida* species, can present similarly, particularly in neonates. Fewer than one-third of neonatal IE cases occur in those with CHD. Mortality rates from IE are formidable, particularly fungal infection, necessitating a high index of suspicion for

IE in sick, hospitalized neonates to allow for earliest possible treatment.[1]

Organism identification through blood cultures is paramount to accurate diagnosis and management. Serial, large-volume cultures (1–3 mL for infants and young children, 5–7 mL for older children) are obtained over days, ideally from different puncture sites. As bacteria are shed continuously in IE, cultures can be drawn irrespective of fever cycle. Fastidious and slow-growing organisms require prolonged culture duration. Fungal cultures should be sent in high-risk cases including neonates with indwelling catheters, immunocompromised, and those with prolonged hospitalization.

For stable patients, multiple cultures are obtained prior to the initiation of antibiotics, whereas rapid, broad-spectrum antibiotic administration is necessary in those presenting with fulminant disease, concurrent with blood culture acquisition. Markers of inflammation, including erythrocyte sedimentation rate and C-reactive protein, are frequently elevated. Procalcitonin levels can become quite elevated in IE, a marker of bacterial infection. Anemia may result from hemolysis or secondary to chronic disease. Electrocardiographic changes may include ectopy or development of heart block, the latter of which can signify abscess formation, a serious and sometimes life-threatening complication.[1]

The modified Duke criteria are used to determine probability of IE based on presenting findings, cultures, and imaging (Table 50.1)[10-12] The modified Duke criteria have been demonstrated to be sensitive for the diagnosis of IE in children and adolescents, though some limitations exist. As CHD is a risk factor for IE, CHD itself is incorporated into the minor criteria as a "predisposing cardiac condition." This increases the likelihood of a CHD patient with fever and suggestive echocardiographic changes being diagnosed with IE, even in the absence of positive blood cultures, the mainstay of IE diagnosis.[10,13,14] Similarly, increased use of

TABLE 50.1 Definition and Criteria for Infective Endocarditis (IE) Diagnosis Based on Modified Duke Criteria

Definition of endocarditis	Definite	**Pathologic criteria:** • Microorganisms demonstrated by culture or histologic examination of a vegetation, a vegetation that has embolized, or an intracardiac abscess specimen; OR • Pathologic lesions; vegetation or intracardiac abscess confirmed by histologic examination showing active endocarditis **Clinical criteria:** • 2 major criteria, OR • 1 major criterion and 3 minor criteria, OR • 5 minor criteria
	Possible	• 1 major criterion and 1 minor criterion, OR • 3 minor criteria
	Rejected	• Firm alternate diagnosis explaining evidence of infective endocarditis; OR • Resolution of infective endocarditis syndrome with antibiotic therapy for < 4 days; OR • No pathologic evidence of infective endocarditis at surgery or autopsy, with antibiotic therapy for ≤ 4 days; OR • Does not meet criteria for possible infective endocarditis, as above

Continued

TABLE 50.1 Definition and Criteria for Infective Endocarditis (IE) Diagnosis Based on Modified Duke Criteria—cont'd

Criteria	Major criteria	• Blood culture positive for IE

• Blood culture positive for IE
  • Typical microorganisms consistent with IE from 2 separate blood cultures:
    • Viridans streptococci, *Streptococcus bovis*, HACEK* group, *Staphylococcus aureus*; OR
    • Community-acquired enterococci, in the absence of a primary focus
  OR
  • Microorganisms consistent with IE from persistently positive blood cultures, defined as follows:
    • At least 2 positive cultures of blood samples drawn > 12 hours apart; OR
    • All of 3 or a majority of ≥ 4 separate cultures of blood (with first and last sample drawn at least 1 hour apart)
  OR
  • Single positive blood culture for *Coxiella burnetii* or antiphase I IgG antibody titer > 1:800

• Evidence of endocardial involvement

• Echocardiogram positive for IE (TEE recommended in patients with prosthetic valves, rated at least "possible IE" by clinical criteria, or complicated IE [paravalvular abscess]; TTE as first test in other patients), defined as follows:
  • Oscillating intracardiac mass on valve or supporting structures, in the path of regurgitant jets, or on implanted material in the absence of an alternative anatomic explanation; OR
  • Abscess; OR
  • New partial dehiscence of prosthetic valve; OR

• New valvular regurgitation (worsening or changing of pre-existing murmur not sufficient)

Minor criteria

• Predisposition, predisposing heart condition or injection drug use

• Fever, temperature > 38°C

• Vascular phenomena, major arterial emboli, septic pulmonary infarcts, mycotic aneurysm, intracranial hemorrhage, conjunctival hemorrhages, and Janeway's lesions

• Immunologic phenomena: glomerulonephritis, Osler nodes, Roth spots, and rheumatoid factor

• Microbiological evidence:
  • Positive blood culture but does not meet a major criterion as noted above, OR
  • Serological evidence of active infection with organism consistent with IE

• Echocardiographic minor criteria eliminated

*HACEK group includes: *Haemophilus* species, *Aggregatibacter actinomycetemcomitans*, *Cardiobacterium hominis*, *Eikenella corrodens*, and *Kingella kingae*.
TEE, Transesophageal echocardiography; *TTE*, transthoracic echocardiogram.
Modified from Li JS, Sexton DJ, Mick N, et al. Proposed modifications to the Duke criteria for the diagnosis of infective endocarditis. *Clin Infect Dis*. 2000;30:633–638.

indwelling catheters and associated *S. aureus* bacteremia, a major criteria, can overestimate IE rates, particularly when positive cultures persist while the catheter remains *in situ*.[15] On the contrary, considering children present less frequently with immunologic findings associated with IE, minor criteria may not be met with the same frequency as in adults.

Echocardiography is first-line imaging in suspected IE, both for vegetation identification as well as for assessment and monitoring of associated hemodynamic complications. Improved acoustic windows in children may allow for IE diagnosis by transthoracic echocardiogram (TTE; Fig. 50.1), though TTE is often insufficient in the assessment of prosthetic valve IE. In a series of pediatric-sized patients (<60 kg) with definite IE by modified Duke criteria, TTE was 97% sensitive in detecting endocarditis compared with 70% in larger patients; 62% had CHD, 41% had previous cardiac surgery, and no patients had prosthetic valves.[16]

The modified Duke criteria recommends transesophageal echocardiography (TEE) in all patients with prosthetic valves. TEE has higher spatial resolution, allowing for superior assessment for prosthetic valve vegetation, perivalvular leakage or dehiscence, and abscess formation.[17] Anterior structures, such as reconstructed right ventricular outflow tracts, remain a challenge for TEE visualization. Intracardiac echocardiogram (ICE) is emerging as a novel tool in the diagnosis of IE. Early reports of ICE in adults demonstrate enhanced visualization of implanted electronic devices as well as prosthetic valves (Fig. 50.2) when other echocardiographic modalities are nondiagnostic. ICE has been used anecdotally in adolescents.[1]

If clinical suspicion remains for IE despite echocardiography being negative, additional imaging should be pursued. Cardiac computed tomography (CT) and CT angiography (CTA) can be used adjunctively in the assessment of

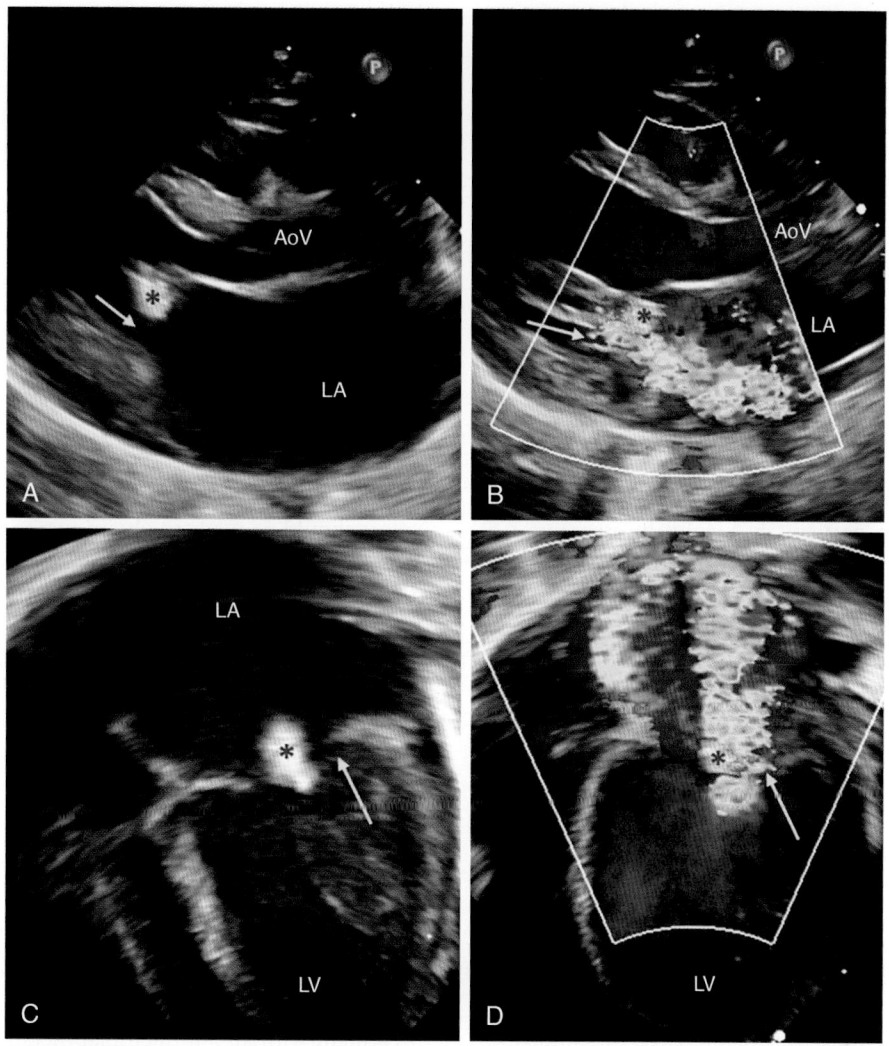

• **Fig. 50.1** Parasternal long-axis (A, B) and apical (C, D) transthoracic echocardiogram views demonstrate a vegetation (*) on the anterior leaflet of the mitral valve in a newborn with *Staphylococcus aureus* bacteremia. A perforation is shown in the leaflet (*yellow arrow,* A and C) through which can be seen severe mitral regurgitation (*yellow arrow,* B and D). *AoV,* Aortic valve; *LA,* left atrium; *LV,* left ventricle;

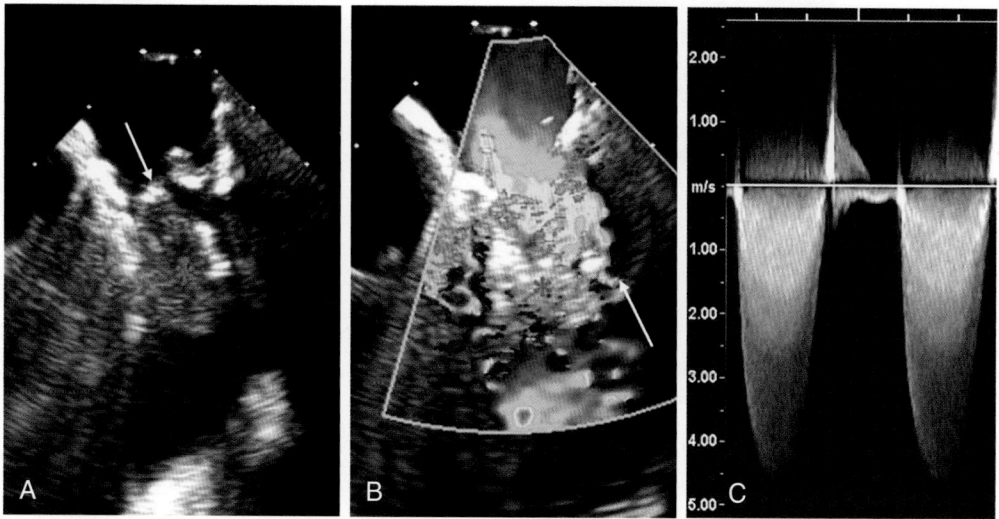

• **Fig. 50.2** Intracardiac echocardiogram (ICE) in a patient with right ventricle to pulmonary artery (RV-PA) conduit and subsequent transcatheter pulmonary valve replacement. ICE demonstrates (A, B) a large vegetation (*) attached to the prosthetic valve leaflet (*arrow,* A) and filling the RV-PA conduit. With color flow Doppler (B), the vegetation is seen to cause obstruction (*arrow,* B) with a resultant outflow gradient of > 80 mm Hg (C).

IE, particularly involving prosthetic material. CT offers improved visualization of the extent of infection, including abscess or fistula formation, valve dehiscence, or pseudoaneurysm development. Similarly, CT can assess for embolic phenomena in the lungs or systemic circulation, all factors that may indicate the need for surgical intervention. When surgery is indicated in the management of IE, CTA can allow for noninvasive coronary artery imaging for procedural planning. Exposure to ionizing radiation, particularly for young children, needs to be considered when choosing CT.[17]

Functional imaging can be performed using F-fluorodeoxyglucose positron emission tomography/computed tomography (FDG-PET/CT), which targets inflammatory cells (macrophages, neutrophils, and lymphocytes) as they congregate at the site of infection or inflammation. FDG-PET/CT has proven particularly helpful in assessment of cardiac device infection, including prosthetic valves, implanted electronic devices (Fig. 50.3), and left ventricular assist devices. Whole-body scans can detect embolic phenomena that may not otherwise be recognized and would affect management.[17] In adults, FDG-PET/CT increased diagnostic sensitivity of prosthetic valve endocarditis from 52–70% to 91–97% without compromising specificity, when used as an additional major criterion to the modified Duke Criteria.[18,19] FDG-PET/CT is not recommended within 3 months of cardiac surgical implantation given potential of false-positive results related to inflammatory changes.

Treatment

Principles of antimicrobial treatment of IE are similar in children and adults. Determination of antibiotic choice, dose, and duration is dependent on a number of factors including organism involved, previous antibiotic treatment, site of infection, native versus prosthetic material, recent invasive procedures, acute versus subacute infection, and high-risk populations. Recommendations regarding treatment can change frequently; therefore, a multidisciplinary approach with input from cardiology, infectious diseases, laboratory medicine, and pharmacy should be sought. For patients with negative blood cultures and who are not severely ill, it is reasonable to withhold antibiotics for 48 hours while additional blood cultures are obtained. Similarly, it may be reasonable to stop antibiotics that were started fewer than 4 days earlier to obtain the appropriate blood cultures.

In some cases, antibiotic therapy is warranted prior to having blood culture results. This is most common in those patients with high-risk of endocarditis or presenting with signs/symptoms of acute endocarditis. In these cases, every effort should be made to obtain two to three blood cultures prior to initiation of antibiotics. When initial empirical therapy is warranted and a native valve or "late" prosthetic valve (>1 year after surgery) is involved, a combination of ampicillin/sulbactam and an aminoglycoside is usually recommended, with or without vancomycin. Rifampin should be added in cases of prosthetic valve involvement. For empirical treatment of nosocomial IE associated with a vascular catheter or "early" (<1 year after surgery) prosthetic valve, vancomycin plus gentamicin plus cefepime or ceftazidime should be used. Again, rifampin should be added if a prosthetic valve is present.[1,20] Once the infecting organism is identified, antibiotic therapy can be tailored appropriately.

Culture-negative endocarditis can occur in pediatrics, but is rare, representing ~5% of IE cases in the United States. The most common causes of culture-negative IE are prior treatment with an antimicrobial therapy and infection with organisms that are difficult to culture, including fastidious or HACEK organisms (*Haemophilus* species, *Aggregatibacter*

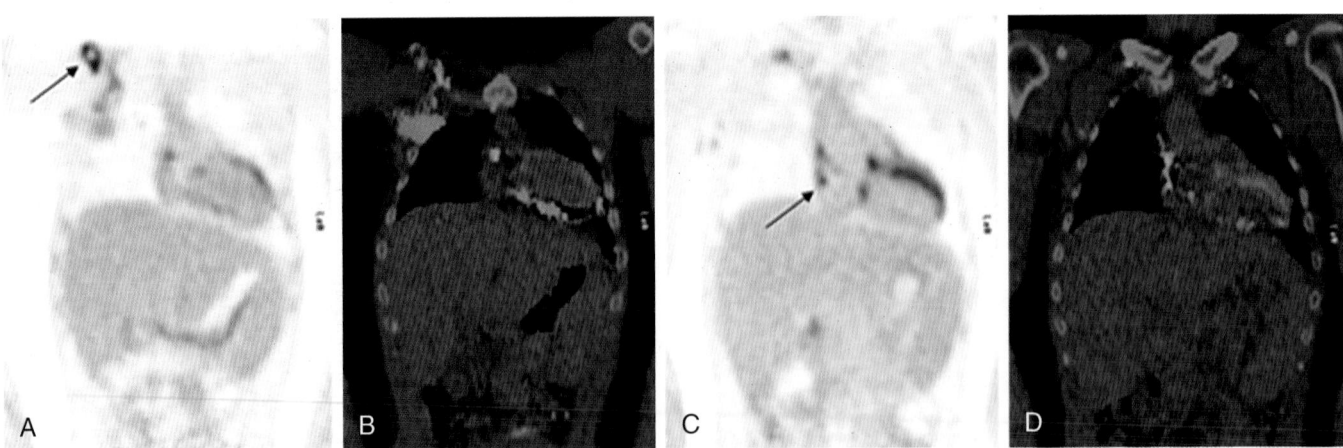

• **Fig. 50.3** Coronal[18] F-FDG PET (A, C) and fused[18] F-FDG PET/CT (B, D) images show circumferential increased FDG uptake around a subcutaneous abscess in the right upper chest (*arrow*, A) at the site of dual chamber transvenous pacemaker insertion in the right subclavian vein (B). Abnormal uptake is also seen associated with the atrial and ventricular pacemaker leads (*arrow*, C), concerning for extension of infection along the implanted pacemaker leads. Abnormal uptake was also seen around the pacemaker device (not shown) and the constellation of findings resulted in removal of the pacemaker device and leads with prolonged antibiotic therapy for polymicrobial infection.

actinomycetemcomitans, *Cardiobacterium hominis*, *Eikenella corrodens*, and *Kingella kingae*). Fungal infections can be difficult to diagnose given lower sensitivity of blood cultures for yeast. Making laboratory staff aware when fastidious or unusual organisms are suspected can improve chances of identification; separate cultures with specialized media may be appropriate in certain clinical situations.[1]

The general approach to IV antimicrobial treatment is described below.[1,21] Recommendations regarding treatment can change frequently. Collaboration between cardiology, infectious disease specialists, and pharmacy is recommended in determining appropriate antimicrobial therapy.

Native Valve Endocarditis

- Viridans group streptococcus/streptococcus gallolyticus
  - Penicillin (PCN) susceptible (MIC < 0.1 mcg/mL): PCN G, or ampicillin or ceftriaxone for 4 weeks. Adult patients can be treated with a 2-week course of PCN G or ceftriaxone PLUS gentamicin.
  - PCN relatively resistant (MIC > 0.1 to < 0.5 mcg/mL): PCN G, or ampicillin or ceftriaxone for 4 weeks PLUS gentamicin for the first 2 weeks of treatment
  - β-lactam-intolerant patients:
    - PCN susceptible: vancomycin (only in patients allergic to PCN and cephalosporins, adjust dose to trough level) for 4 weeks
    - PCN relatively resistant: vancomycin PLUS gentamicin for 4 weeks
- Enterococci: PCN and gentamicin susceptible
  - No contraindication to aminoglycoside
    - PCN G or ampicillin PLUS gentamicin for 4–6 weeks
  - Contraindication to aminoglycoside
    - Ceftriaxone PLUS ampicillin for 6 weeks if aminoglycoside cannot be used due to renal impairment, cranial nerve VIII dysfunction, or inability to obtain serum concentrations AND if the organism is not *Enterococcus faecium*
- Staphylococcus (*S. aureus* or coagulase-negative staphylococcus)
  - Methicillin sensitive
    - Nafcillin or oxacillin or cefazolin for 4–6 weeks
  - Methicillin resistant
    - Vancomycin for 6 weeks
- HACEK
  - Monotherapy
    - Ceftriaxone or cefotaxime for 4 weeks
  - Combination therapy
    - Ampicillin/sulbactam PLUS gentamicin for 4 weeks
- Fungal: medical therapy alone is generally unsuccessful outside of the neonatal age group
  - Amphotericin B with or without flucytosine
  - Fluconazole for long-term suppressive therapy may be needed
- Culture negative: infectious disease specialist should be consulted

- Ampicillin/sulbactam PLUS gentamicin for 4–6 weeks
- Vancomycin (for those unable to tolerate PCN) PLUS gentamicin PLUS ciprofloxacin for 4–6 weeks

Prosthetic Valve Endocarditis

- Viridans group streptococcus/*Streptococcus gallolyticus*
  - PCN susceptible:
    - PCN G, ampicillin or ceftriaxone for 6 weeks PLUS gentamicin for the first 2 weeks of therapy
  - PCN relatively resistant:
    - PCN G or ampicillin or ceftriaxone PLUS gentamicin for 6 weeks
  - β-lactam-intolerant patients
    - Vancomycin for 6 weeks PLUS gentamicin for first 2 weeks
- Enterococci: PCN and gentamicin susceptible
  - No contraindication to aminoglycoside
    - PCN G or ampicillin PLUS gentamicin for 4–6 weeks
  - Contraindication to aminoglycoside
    - Ceftriaxone PLUS ampicillin for 6 weeks if aminoglycoside cannot be used due to renal impairment, cranial nerve VIII dysfunction, or inability to obtain serum concentrations AND if the organism is not *Enterococcus faecium*
- *Staphylococcus*
  - Methicillin sensitive
    - Nafcillin or oxacillin or cefazolin for ≥ 6 weeks PLUS rifampin ≥ 6 weeks PLUS gentamicin for the first 2 weeks
  - Methicillin resistant
    - Vancomycin for ≥ 6 weeks PLUS rifampin ≥ 6 weeks PLUS gentamicin for the first 2 weeks
- HACEK
  - Monotherapy
    - Ceftriaxone (preferred) or cefotaxime (or other third- or fourth-generation cephalosporin) for 6 weeks
  - Combination therapy
    - Ampicillin/sulbactam (if susceptible) PLUS gentamicin for 6 weeks
- Fungal: medical therapy alone is generally unsuccessful outside of the neonatal age group
  - Amphotericin B with or without flucytosine
  - Fluconazole for long-term suppressive therapy may be needed
- Culture negative: infectious disease specialist should be consulted
  - Early (≤1 year since placement)
    - Vancomycin (for 6 weeks) PLUS gentamicin (for first 2 weeks) PLUS cefepime (for 6 weeks) PLUS rifampin (for 6 weeks)
  - Late (>1 year since placement)
    - Ampicillin/sulbactam PLUS gentamicin for 6 weeks or
    - Vancomycin (for those unable to tolerate PCN) PLUS gentamicin PLUS ciprofloxacin for 6 weeks

Bacteremia generally resolves within days of initiation of antibiotic therapy, although *S. aureus* bacteremia may persist longer than streptococcal bacteremia. *S. aureus* bacteremia associated with central venous catheters may not resolve until the central catheter is removed. Prolonged therapy with bactericidal, rather than bacteriostatic, antibiotic drugs for 4–6 and sometimes 8 weeks are generally recommended given that high concentrations of bacteria can exist in a protected sheath of fibrin and platelets. In these instances, there is decreased bacterial cell metabolism and cell division, which makes β-lactams and other antibiotics that act on the cell wall less effective. Home IV therapies are reasonable in a select group of patients.

Complications and Surgical Consideration

Infectious endocarditis can lead to life-threatening complications including congestive heart failure, progressive valvular dysfunction, periannular extension of infection, myocardial dysfunction, obstruction of shunts or conduits, prosthetic valve dysfunction, sinus of Valsalva rupture, pericardial effusion, and septic emboli. These may require early surgical intervention to increase likelihood of survival and preserve ventricular function. In general, the degree of illness should not be a limitation to surgery, since deferring surgery may have a devastating outcome. According to the 2015 update on infective endocarditis in childhood, the most common clinical factors constituting high risk for complications of IE include: 1) cyanotic congenital heart defects 2) history of a prosthetic cardiac valve 3) presence of systemic-to-pulmonary artery shunts 4) IE involving left-sided structures 5) previous history of IE 6) IE involving s. aureus or fungal infection 7) symptoms persisting for longer than 3 months 8) inadequate response to antimicrobial treatment. Imaging findings that suggest the need for surgical intervention would include persistent vegetation after embolization, large vegetations, particularly if mobile and/or > 10 mm, increasing vegetation size despite adequate therapy, valvular dysfunction with signs of ventricular failure, heart failure unresponsive to medical therapy, valve perforation, rupture or dehiscence, and development of new heart block suggesting perivalvular extension. Other important factors leading to consideration of surgical management include persistent bacteremia despite appropriate medical therapy, infected prosthetic material, mycotic aneurysms, and ventricular septal aneurysms.

Congestive heart failure, one of the more common complications of IE, can result from worsening valve regurgitation and be associated with ventricular dysfunction, which is a poor prognostic factor. Surgical intervention in patients with moderate to severe heart failure improves likelihood of survival and preserves cardiac function.[1] Prosthetic valves, shunts, or conduits are a risk for obstruction, dehiscence, periannular extension, and emboli. Frequently the infection cannot be eradicated without surgical intervention, particularly when fungal endocarditis exists.

Periannular extensions of infection can cause or worsen congestive heart failure and is of greatest risk with IE of the aortic valve. Periannular infections can lead to fistulous tracts between cardiac chambers, vessels, or into the pericardium. These infections do not respond well to medical management alone and frequently require surgical intervention to eradicate.

Embolization of septic vegetations is one of the most important extracardiac complications of IE. Larger vegetations (>10 mm), particularly when mobile, are more likely to embolize than smaller vegetations, left-sided vegetations more than right-sided, and vegetations involving the anterior leaflet of the mitral valve are more likely to embolize than vegetations of the aortic valve. In general, there is a higher risk of embolization early in the disease or with rapid growth of the vegetation. Staphylococci, fungi, and pneumococci carry a high risk of embolization. Infarcts and/or abscesses of target organs can develop and the cerebral, pulmonary, coronary, splenic, renal, or peripheral arteries can all be affected by embolization. Mycotic aneurysms can develop in systemic, pulmonary, or cerebral arteries, which are particularly concerning, and surgical intervention may be required to avoid rupture. Other complications of IE include glomerulonephritis (as a result of immune complex deposition), rhythm abnormalities, and pericardial effusion.

Prevention

Beginning in 1955, antibiotic prophylaxis prior to invasive procedures was recommended as a means of preventing IE. However, these recommendations were generally the result of expert opinion and a conservative approach to prevent life-threatening infections. The quality of evidence was limited, since they were based on predominantly case-controlled studies, not grounded on well-designed randomized clinical trials. The rationale was challenged by the fact that only 20% of cases were actually related to a preceding invasive procedure eligible for prophylaxis and only 50% of cases were in patients with CHD which would have warranted prophylaxis.[1] One 2017 Taiwanese study demonstrated that dental procedures did not increase risk of IE (in comparison with atrial septal defects, a known low-risk group for IE) irrespective of antibiotic usage.[22]

IE is much more likely to result from transient bacteremia related to daily activities such as chewing, brushing, and flossing. Prophylaxis was thus viewed as perhaps being able to prevent a very small number of cases at potentially high cost. Adverse reactions to antibiotic prophylaxis were recognized including anaphylaxis in 15–25/1 million patients who received prophylaxis. No known history of allergy to PCN was present in 64%.[9]

There was also increasing concern about the risk of dispensing so many doses of antibiotics, which could contribute to the development of antibiotic resistance a high cost for small benefit. Emphasis on good oral hygiene was recognized as potentially being more impactful in the prevention of IE than antibiotic prophylaxis. Subsequent topic reviews by professional societies, including the AHA, resulted in the revision of guidelines, including the cessation of antibiotic prophylaxis for the majority of patients and procedures.

In 2007, the AHA updated guidelines on the use of antibiotics for the prevention of IE.[9] These recommendations decreased significantly the number of underlying conditions considered appropriate for antibiotic prophylaxis to just four categories thought to present the highest risk (Table 50.2).

The list of procedures appropriate for prophylaxis was also revised, resulting in the removal of genitourinary (GU) and gastrointestinal (GI) procedures (Table 50.3). Enterococci are part of the normal flora of the GI tract and are the only organism from the GI tract likely to cause IE. There are no published data that show a conclusive link between GI/GU procedures and IE. Additionally, there are no studies to demonstrate that antibiotic prophylaxis prevents IE associated with GI/GU procedures. For patients with conditions in Table 50.2 who have

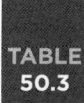

TABLE 50.3 Procedures for Which Endocarditis Prophylaxis Is Reasonable for Patients With Underlying Cardiac Conditions Associated With the Highest Risk of Adverse Outcomes From Infective Endocarditis as Noted in Table 50.2[9]

- Dental procedures which involve manipulation of gingival tissues or periapical region of teeth or perforation of oral mucosa

- Respiratory tract procedures that involve incision or biopsy of the respiratory mucosa including tonsillectomy and adenoidectomy

- Procedures on infected skin, skin structures, or musculoskeletal tissue

TABLE 50.2 Conditions in Which Endocarditis Prophylaxis Is Recommended

- Prosthetic cardiac valve/prosthetic material used for cardiac valve repair

- Previous infective endocarditis (IE)

- Congenital heart disease (CHD):
  - Unrepaired cyanotic CHD, including palliative shunts and conduits
  - Completely repaired CHD with prosthetic material or device (whether by surgery or catheterization) during the first 6 months after the procedure (to allow for endothelialization)
  - Repaired CHD with residual defects at the site or adjacent to the site of prosthetic patch or prosthetic device (because of inhibited endothelialization)

- Cardiac transplantation recipients who develop cardiac valvulopathy

GI/GU infections or who receive antibiotics to prevent wound infections or sepsis from a GI/GU procedure, it may be reasonable to include an agent against enterococcus in the regimen. The antibiotic regimen currently recommended prior to dental and respiratory procedures for prevention of IE is outlined in Table 50.4. Recommendations may change over time, and confirming most up-to-date guidance is advised.

For procedures involving infected skin, skin structures, or musculoskeletal tissue, treatment regimen should include an agent against staphylococci and β-hemolytic streptococcus such as an antistaphylococcal PCN or cephalosporin. For patients who cannot tolerate β-lactam or who have a methicillin-resistant staphylococcus, vancomycin may be used. Of note, as of 2021, clindamycin is no longer recommended for antibiotic prophylaxis for dental procedures.[9] Patients receiving chronic antibiotics should receive an antibiotic from a different class for prophylaxis. Although tattooing and piercings are not procedures for which prophylaxis

TABLE 50.4 Antibiotic Regimen for Dental or Respiratory Procedures for Prevention of Infective Endocarditis[23]

Situation	Antibiotic	Children	Adults
Oral	Amoxicillin	50 mg/kg, max dose 2 g	2 g
Unable to take oral medication	Ampicillin OR Cefazolin or ceftriaxone	50 mg/kg IM or IV, max 2 g 50 mg/kg IM or IV, max 1 g	2 g 1 g
Allergic to penicillin or ampicillin	Cephalexin*,# OR Azithromycin OR Clarithromycin OR Doxycycline	50 mg/kg, max 2 g 15 mg/kg, max 500 mg 15 mg/kg, max 500 mg 2.2 mg/kg, max 100 mg	2 g 500 mg 100 mg
Unable to take oral medication and allergic to penicillin or ampicillin	Cefazolin or ceftriaxone	50 mg/kg IM or IV	1 g

*Cephalosporins should not be used in patients with history of anaphylaxis, angioedema, or urticaria with penicillin or ampicillin.
#Or other first- or second-generation cephalosporin in equivalent pediatric or adult dosage.

is recommended, they are generally discouraged in patients with conditions in Table 50.2 due to the risk of developing skin infections, possible bacteremia and seeding of the heart.

Based on a 2021 AHA Scientific Statement, there appears to be good general awareness of the 2007 guidelines, but there is variable adherence to the recommendations.[23] According to one large study, the new recommendations resulted in a decrease in prophylaxis prescribing overall by ~20% in high-risk individuals, 64% in moderate-risk, and 52% in low-risk individuals.[24]

Since the 2007 revision of the guidelines, there have been a number of observational, population-, or health system-based studies to assess the impact of the new recommendations. Some studies have suggested a trend toward an increase in the overall incidence of IE, while others have implied no change in pediatric IE admissions.[2] In a review assessing the impact of prophylaxis before dental procedures following the new 2007 guidelines, there is no convincing evidence of an increase in cases of viridans group streptococcus IE in any risk group.[23]

It is interesting to note that in 2008, the United Kingdom's National Institute for Health and Clinical Excellence (NICE) recommended the cessation of antibiotic prophylaxis for dental procedures in all people at risk for IE. A 2018 analysis of the impact of that decision revealed a 79% decrease in prescriptions with a statistically significant increase in the number of IE cases in both moderate- and high-risk cases beginning in March 2008.[24,25]

A prospective, double-blind, placebo-controlled, randomized study would be required to accurately assess the efficacy of antibiotic prophylaxis in preventing IE in various patient populations in various clinical situations. As we continue to promote recommendations with imperfect data, shared decision-making between patient and care provider is important. Continued focus on good oral care is vital to cardiac health, and discussion of daily brushing and flossing regimen, regular dental exams, and current recommendations for IE prophylaxis need to be a part of each provider visit.

References

1. Bayer AS, Bolger AF, Taubert KA, Wilson W, Steckelberg J, Karchmer AW, Levison M, Chambers HF, Dajani AS, Gewitz MH, Newburger JW, Gerber MA, Shulman ST, Pallasch TJ, Gage TW, Ferrieri P. Diagnosis and management of infective endocarditis and its complications. *Circulation.* 1998;98:2936-2948.
2. Pasquali SK, He X, Mohamad Z, et al. Trends in endocarditis hospitalizations at US children's hospitals: impact of the 2007 American Heart Association Antibiotic Prophylaxis Guidelines. *Am Heart J.* 2012;163:894-899.
3. Rushani D, Kaufman JS, Ionescu-Ittu R, et al. Infective endocarditis in children with congenital heart disease: cumulative incidence and predictors. *Circulation.* 2013;128:1412-1419.
4. Day MD, Gauvreau K, Shulman S, et al. Characteristics of children hospitalized with infective endocarditis [published correction appears in *Circulation.* 2010 Nov 23;122(21):e560]. *Circulation.* 2009;119:865-870.
5. Gupta S, Sakhuja A, McGrath E, et al. Trends, microbiology, and outcomes of infective endocarditis in children during 2000-2010 in the United States. *Congenit Heart Dis.* 2017;12:196-201.
6. Giamarellou H. Nosocomial cardiac infections. *J Hosp Infect* 2002;50:91-105.
7. Pappas PG, Kauffman CA, Andes D, et al. Clinical practice guidelines for the management of candidiasis: 2009 update by the Infectious Diseases Society of America. *Clin Infect Dis.* 2009;48:503-535.
8. Saiman L, Prince A, Gersony WM. Pediatric infective endocarditis in the modern era. *J Pediatr.* 1993;122:847-853.
9. Wilson W, Taubert KA, Gewitz M, et al. Prevention of infective endocarditis: guidelines from the American Heart Association: a guideline from the American Heart Association Rheumatic Fever, Endocarditis, and Kawasaki Disease Committee, Council on Cardiovascular Disease in the Young, and the Council on Clinical Cardiology, Council on Cardiovascular Surgery and Anesthesia, and the Quality of Care and Outcomes Research Interdisciplinary Working Group [published correction appears in *Circulation.* 2007 Oct 9;116(15):e376-7]. *Circulation.* 2007;116:1736-1754. doi:10.1161/CIRCULATIONAHA.106.183095.
10. Tissières P, Gervaix A, Beghetti M, et al. Value and limitations of the von Reyn, Duke, and modified Duke criteria for the diagnosis of infective endocarditis in children. *Pediatrics.* 2003;112:e467
11. Durack DT. Proposed modifications to the Duke criteria for the diagnosis of infective endocarditis. *Clin Infect Dis.* 1994; 30:200-209.
12. Li JS, Sexton DJ, Mick N, et al. Proposed modifications to the Duke criteria for the diagnosis of infective endocarditis. *Clin Infect Dis.* 2000;30:633-638.
13. Snygg-Martin U, Giang KW, Dellborg M, et al. Cumulative Incidence of infective endocarditis in patients with congenital heart disease: a nationwide, case-control study over nine decades. *Clin Infect Dis.* 2021;73:1469-1475.
14. Coward K, Tucker N, Darville T. Infective endocarditis in Arkansan children from 1990 through 2002. *Pediatr Infect Dis J.* 2003;22:1048-1052.
15. Bendig EA, Singh J, Butler TJ, et al. The impact of the central venous catheter on the diagnosis of infectious endocarditis using Duke criteria in children with Staphylococcus aureus bacteremia. *Pediatr Infect Dis J.* 2008;27:636-639.
16. Penk JS, Webb CL, Shulman ST, et al. Echocardiography in pediatric infective endocarditis. *Pediatr Infect Dis J.* 2011;30: 1109-1111.
17. Dilsizian V, Budde RPJ, Chen W, et al. Best practices for imaging cardiac device-related infections and endocarditis: A JACC: Cardiovascular Imaging Expert Panel Statement. *JACC Cardiovasc Imaging.* 2022;15:891-911.
18. Pizzi MN, Roque A, Fernández-Hidalgo N, et al. Improving the diagnosis of infective endocarditis in prosthetic valves and intracardiac devices with 18F-fluordeoxyglucose positron emission tomography/computed tomography angiography: initial results at an infective endocarditis referral center. *Circulation.* 2015; 132:1113-1126.
19. Saby L, Laas O, Habib G, et al. Positron emission tomography/computed tomography for diagnosis of prosthetic valve endocarditis: increased valvular 18F-fluorodeoxyglucose uptake as a novel major criterion. *J Am Coll Cardiol.* 2013;61:2374-2382.
20. Calza L, Manfredi R, Chiodo F. Antibiotic therapy for infective endocarditis in childhood. *J Pediatr Pharmacol Ther.* 2006;11: 64-91.

21. O'Brien SE. *"Infective Endocarditis in Children."* UpToDate; 2019. Available at: www.uptodate.com.

22. Sun LC, Lai CC, Wang CY, et al. Risk factors for infective endocarditis in children with congenital heart diseases: a nationwide population-based case control study. *Int J Cardiol.* 2017;248: 126-130.

23. Wilson WR, Gewitz M, Lockhart PB, et al. Prevention of viridans group streptococcal infective endocarditis: a scientific statement from the American Heart Association [published correction appears in *Circulation.* 2021 Aug 31;144(9):e192] [published correction appears in *Circulation.* 2022 Apr 26;145(17):e868]. *Circulation.* 2021;143:e963-e978.

24. Thornhill MH, Gibson TB, Cutler E, et al. Antibiotic prophylaxis and incidence of endocarditis before and after the 2007 AHA recommendations. *J Am Coll Cardiol.* 2018;72:2443-2454.

25. Thornhill MH, Dayer MJ, Forde JM, et al. Impact of the NICE guideline recommending cessation of antibiotic prophylaxis for prevention of infective endocarditis: before and after study. *BMJ.* 2011;342:d2392.

51

Cardiac Masses

REBECCA S. BEROUKHIM, TAL GEVA, EDWARD P. WALSH, AND MEENA NATHAN

KEY LEARNING POINTS

- Cardiac masses encompass a wide range of histologic subtypes and clinical behaviors.
- Evaluation and management of cardiac masses will vary based on presentation and histology.
- Cardiac magnetic resonance imaging is particularly useful in the evaluation of cardiac masses because of its ability to identify tissue characteristics.

- A high percentage of children with cardiac masses have an associated genetic abnormality. Genetic testing can be helpful for diagnosis, prognosis, and counseling.
- Mobile cardiac masses involving the left heart structures are at high risk for embolization, and strong consideration should be given to surgical resection.

Introduction

Cardiac masses are abnormal growths of normal or abnormal tissue found within the heart or pericardium, and can be categorized as either tumors or non-neoplastic masses. Cardiac tumors (benign and malignant) are caused by an abnormal neoplastic proliferation of tissue, and may arise from a variety of cellular precursors. The most common cardiac tumors in children include rhabdomyoma (muscle), fibroma (fibrous tissue), hemangioma (vascular), lipoma (fat), paraganglioma (neuroendocrine), and teratoma (ectopic, of germ cell lineage). While most cardiac tumors in children are benign, primary and secondary malignant cardiac tumors can occur. Non-neoplastic cardiac masses are exceedingly rare; e.g., pericardial cysts, inflammatory masses, and vascular malformations arising from malformed tissues composed of venous, arterial, or lymphatic tissues. Because of the wide range in cellular origin and location, each mass carries a unique phenotype. Accordingly, clinical presentations, prognoses, and treatment strategies vary among patients.

Incidence

Cardiac tumors in children are rare, with an incidence of up to 0.08% in autopsy studies.[1] The advent of echocardiography has significantly improved detection rate, with a reported incidence of 0.32% of first-time echocardiograms.[1] Of these, over 50% are diagnosed in the first year of life.

The relative frequencies of primary cardiac masses among patients from the New England area treated at Boston Children's Hospital from 1990 to 2020 are outlined in Table 51.1. Rhabdomyoma is the most common cardiac tumor diagnosed during fetal life and childhood, accounting for 60% of all cardiac tumors in children. With a birth incidence of tuberous sclerosis of 1 in 6000–10,000, and an 80% prevalence of rhabdomyomas among infants with tuberous sclerosis, the estimated incidence of rhabdomyoma is approximately 1 in 8000–13,000 newborns. Fibromas are the second most common tumor, accounting for 9% of cardiac tumors in children. Cardiac myxoma is the third most common tumor in children, and the most common primary cardiac tumor in adults with a slight female predominance.

Primary tumors of the heart are usually benign, with a low incidence of primary cardiac malignant tumors. However, ~1.6% of malignant solid tumors in children have cardiac involvement from either distant metastasis, direct extension of the tumor into the heart, with a smaller proportion of primary cardiac tumors.[2] Non-malignant cardiac tumors may cause obstruction to blood flow, valve dysfunction, ventricular dysfunction, arrhythmias, and embolic complications. Arrhythmias are commonly associated with fibromas and rhabdomyomas. In a review of 173 patients with various cardiac tumors, 64% of fibromas and 24% of rhabdomyomas had clinically significant arrhythmias at some point (Table 51.2).[3]

TABLE 51.1 Frequencies of Cardiac Tumors and Masses for Patients From the New England Region Treated at Boston Children's Hospital From 1990 to 2020

Mass Type	N (%)
Total	191
Rhabdomyoma	115 (60%)
Fibroma	18 (9%)
Myxoma	13 (7%)
Malignant	8 (4%)
Pericardial cyst	7 (4%)
Hemangioma	6 (3%)
Inflammatory myofibroblastic tumor or inflammatory pseudotumor	3 (2%)
Lipoma	2 (1%)
Teratoma	2 (1%)
Blood cyst	2 (1%)
Myofibroma	1 (<1%)
Lymphatic malformation	1 (<1%)
Neurofibroma	1 (<1%)
Papillary fibroelastoma	1 (<1%)
Paraganglioma	1 (<1%)
Endodermal sinus tumor	1 (<1%)
Unknown tissue diagnosis	9 (5%)

Diagnosis and Management of Cardiac Masses in Children:

Cardiac mass characteristics and clinical manifestations are described below. Identification, characterization, and management of a new cardiac mass on echocardiography may be daunting, because of the wide range of not only clinical presentation but also pathology. Fig. 51.1 provides a decision tree based on the acuity of clinical presentation and course, and outlines the potential for life-threatening sequelae such as embolization, malignant arrhythmias, or malignant transformation or spread.[4]

Subtypes of Cardiac Masses

Rhabdomyoma

Cardiac rhabdomyoma is a hamartoma of striated cardiac muscle. Gross pathology reveals a circumscribed but non-encapsulated mass that is millimeters to centimeters in size.[5] Multiple rhabdomyomas, often involving different cardiac chambers, are common. The tumors typically originate from the right or left ventricular myocardium, with intracavitary protrusions that can result in inflow or outflow tract obstruction. The cells contain glycogen, and strands of cytoplasm extend to the periphery of the cell, giving the appearance of a "spider cell." Rhabdomyomas are associated with the tuberous sclerosis complex in a majority of newly diagnosed cases, including nearly all patients with multiple tumors, and some patients with solitary ventricular tumors. The tuberous sclerosis complex is a dominantly inherited

TABLE 51.2 Arrhythmias by Tumor Type in a Review of 173 Cardiac Tumors at Boston Children's Hospital

	All Tumors	Rhabdomyoma	Fibroma	Myxoma	Vascular	Teratoma	Lipoma	Other
Patients, n	173	106	25	14	6	4	3	15
Clinically significant arrhythmia	42 (24%)	17 (16%)	16 (64%)	1 (7%)	1 (17%)	0	0	7 (47%)
Cardiac arrest/VF	4 (2%)	–	2 (10%)	–	1 (17%)	–	–	1 (6%)
VT	27 (16%)	6 (6%)	16 (64%)	1 (7%)	–	–	–	4 (27%)
WPW/sustained SVT	2 (1%)	2 (2%)	–	–	–	–	–	–
WPW/ no SVT	9 (5%)	8 (8%)	–	–	–	–	–	1 (7%)
Non-WPW sustained SVT	9 (5%)	5 (5%)	–	–	–	–	–	5 (33%)
Low-grade arrhythmia	15 (9%)	13 (12%)	1 (4%)	1 (7%)	–	–	–	–
Any arrhythmia (low-grade + clinically significant)	57 (33%)	57 (33%)	17 (68%)	2 (14%)	1 (17%)	0	0	7 (47%)

SVT, Supraventricular tachycardia; *VF,* ventricular fibrillation; *VT,* ventricular tachycardia; *WPW,* Wolff-Parkinson-White.
With permission from Miyake CY, Del Nido PJ, Alexander ME, et al. Cardiac tumors and associated arrhythmias in pediatric patients, with observations on surgical therapy for ventricular tachycardia. *J Am Coll Cardiol.* 2011;58:1903–1909.

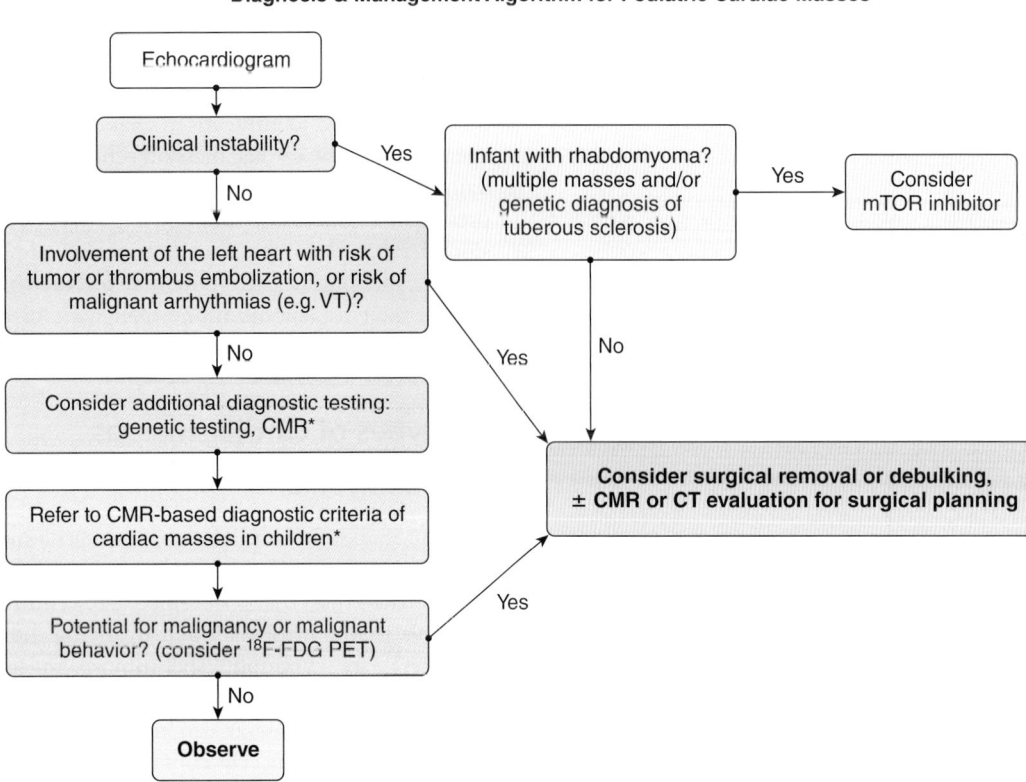

Diagnosis & Management Algorithm for Pediatric Cardiac Masses

• **Fig. 51.1** Suggested diagnosis and management algorithm for pediatric cardiac masses. *18F-FDG,* 18F-fluorodeoxyglucose; *CMR,* cardiovascular magnetic resonance; *mTOR,* mammalian target of rapamycin; *PET,* positron emission tomography; *VT,* ventricular tachycardia. (Borrowed with permission from Beroukhim RS, Ghelani S, Ashwath R, et al. Accuracy of cardiac magnetic resonance imaging in diagnosing pediatric cardiac masses: A multicenter study. *JACC Cardiovasc Imaging.* 2021.)

disorder affecting multiple organ systems, including the brain, skin, kidneys, heart, and other organs, and patients can have variable associated neurologic abnormalities including seizures and developmental delay. About two-thirds of newborns with a diagnosis of tuberous sclerosis have cardiac rhabdomyomas.[6]

Rhabdomyomas commonly present during fetal life or early childhood. Fetal presentation is usually either as a single or as multiple cardiac masses detected on prenatal ultrasound, with or without fetal arrhythmia. The size and number of tumors are variable, ranging from small solitary tumors that grow proportionally with fetal size until the third trimester, to multiple atrial and ventricular tumors that, in some cases, can cause hemodynamic compromise and fetal demise. Development of fetal hydrops and death may be related to obstruction of ventricular inflow/outflow, arrhythmias, extrinsic compression of coronary arteries, and loss of functional myocardium. A diagnosis of tuberous sclerosis can be inferred prenatally when cerebral masses are identified in fetal brain ultrasound or MRI in a fetus with cardiac tumors, adding more certainty to the diagnosis of cardiac rhabdomyoma.[7] Postnatally, rhabdomyomas are commonly asymptomatic without physiologic sequelae; however they may be associated with hemodynamic disturbances such as inflow/outflow obstruction or arrhythmias.

In a study by Miyake et al,[3] 16% of patients with rhabdomyomas had clinically significant arrhythmias, involving predominantly supraventricular mechanisms (Table 51.2). Arrhythmias are most common during infancy or early childhood, and often resolve as the tumor regresses.

Imaging

When multiple tumors are identified by echocardiogram, or the patient has a confirmed diagnosis of tuberous sclerosis, a diagnosis of rhabdomyoma can be made by echocardiography alone. The finding of multiple echobright intramyocardial masses is typical (Fig. 51.2). Tumors can protrude into the cardiac chambers (usually the ventricles) causing inflow or outflow obstruction. In the setting of a solitary tumor, cardiovascular magnetic resonance imaging (CMR) can differentiate rhabdomyoma from other common tumors of childhood, including fibroma and hemangioma.[4]

Management

Rhabdomyomas will naturally regress over time, so patients should be managed expectantly in the absence of severe cardiac symptoms, such as heart failure or arrhythmias.[8] Given the strong association with tuberous sclerosis, comprehensive genetics evaluation should be considered in any patient diagnosed with rhabdomyoma. In patients with

Rhabdomyomas **Fibroma**

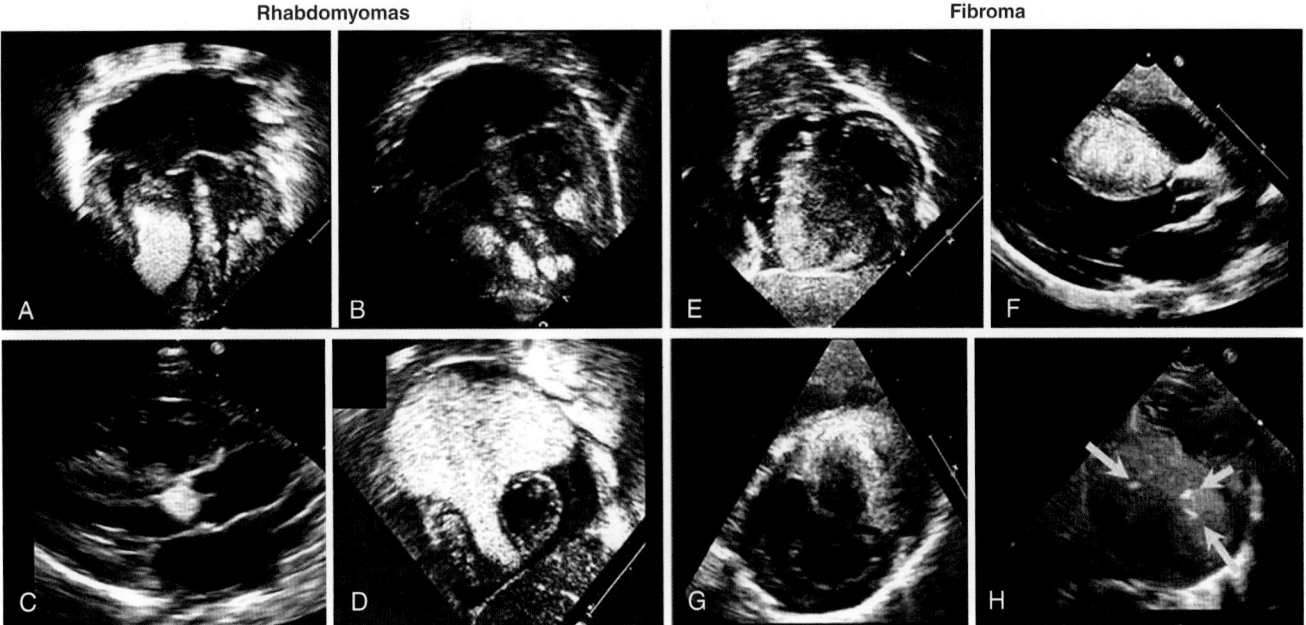

• **Fig. 51.2** Echocardiogram appearance of rhabdomyomas (**A–D**) and fibroma (**E–H**). Rhabdomyomas are typically homogenous and echo-bright, arise from the myocardium, and protrude into the cavity or over the epicardial surface of the heart. Fibromas are intramyocardial (best seen in **F**), and may have calcifications (*blue arrows*, **H**).

severe inflow or outflow tract obstruction, resection has historically proven effective in reducing the degree of obstruction. However, based on multiple case reports demonstrating rapid reduction in size and hemodynamic burden of rhabdomyomas, oral mammalian target of rapamycin (mTOR) inhibitors (e.g., sirolimus and everolimus) are becoming first-line therapy. To better define clinical efficacy, the ORACLE trial is a randomized multicenter clinical trial assessing the efficacy of everolimus as a therapy for symptomatic cardiac rhabdomyoma.[9] Case reports note minimal side effects of these medications, and although tumor rebound has been reported after cessation of therapy, most patients remained hemodynamically stable.[10] Transplacental sirolimus therapy has also shown promise in treating fetal rhabdomyomas complicated by supraventricular tachycardia and hydrops.[11] The mTOR inhibitors have also been used successfully to treat rhabdomyoma-associated arrhythmias in neonates and children.[12] Given that arrhythmias associated with rhabdomyomas tend to resolve with tumor regression, it is reasonable to attempt medical management with antiarrhythmic drugs and mTOR inhibitor therapy before more invasive therapies such as catheter ablation or tumor resection are initiated.[9]

Fibroma

Fibroma is a benign tumor of fibroblasts, composed of hyalinized collagen and elastic tissue.[5] In infants and children, the tumors are fibroblast-rich with paucity of mitotic activity and have small areas of entrapped myocardium; however in adults, the tumors are mostly acellular and composed primarily of collagen. Microscopic areas of calcification,

and regions of necrosis have also been observed. Gross pathology reveals a well-circumscribed, non-encapsulated, solitary tan-colored mass that can exceed 10 cm in size. On cut section, there is a classic "whorled" pattern.

Clinical Manifestations

While fibromas are more common in the prenatal and pediatric population, they can span the age spectrum from fetus to adulthood. Postnatally, symptoms include atrial and ventricular arrhythmias, heart failure due to ventricular dysfunction, mitral regurgitation, or inflow/outflow obstruction, compression of pulmonary veins, airways and lung tissue, and sudden death. About a third of fibromas are found incidentally in asymptomatic patients. Fibromas can be associated with Gorlin syndrome, a disorder caused by an autosomal dominant mutation in PTCH1, a tumor suppressor gene which has been mapped to chromosome band 9q22.3.[13]

Ventricular arrhythmias are frequently seen in patients with fibromas, and often the presenting clinical manifestation. In a study by Miyake et al.,[3] ventricular tachycardia (VT) and/or cardiac arrest were documented in more than half of the patients with ventricular fibroma (Table 51.2). The mechanism of arrhythmia and sudden cardiac death is thought to be related to areas of entrapped interdigitating myocardium within the tumor that slow conduction thus enabling re-entrant tachycardia, not dissimilar to the mechanism of ventricular arrhythmia related to fibrous scar following myocardial infarction.[14] Ventricular fibroma has a characteristic appearance on ECG: inverted T wave in leads I, aVL, and in the left precordial leads (V1 through V6) (Fig. 51.3).

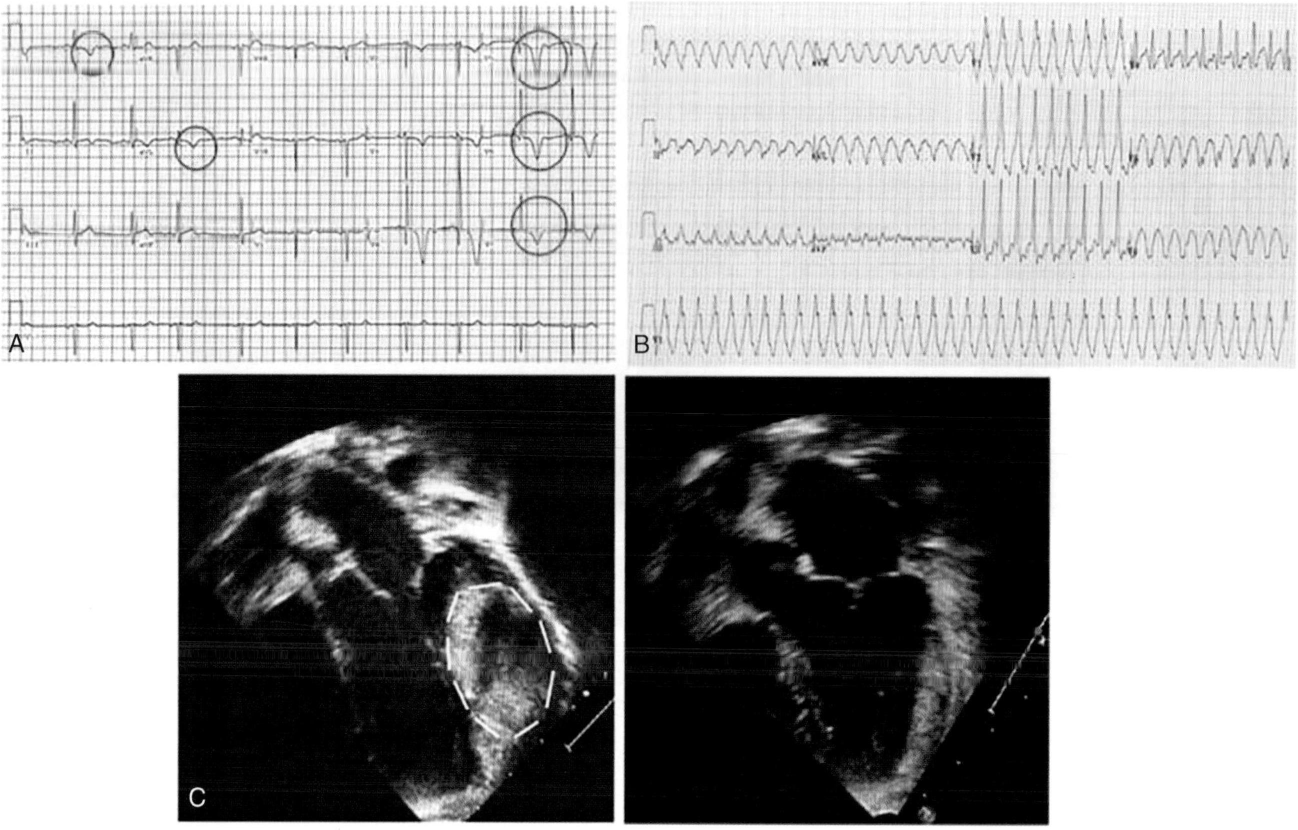

• **Fig. 51.3** Patient with a left ventricular fibroma. Common electrocardiographic changes in this patient and a majority of patients demonstrating T-wave inversions in the left lateral leads **(A)**, electrocardiogram of this patient in ventricular tachycardia **(B)**, and preoperative and postoperative echocardiographic images of the same patient after resection of a large left lateral ventricular fibroma **(C)**. (With permission from Miyake CY, Del Nido PJ, Alexander ME, et al. Cardiac tumors and associated arrhythmias in pediatric patients, with observations on surgical therapy for ventricular tachycardia. *J Am Coll Cardiol*. 2011;58:1903–1909.)

Fibromas may increase in size during late gestation, reaching maximal size around birth and early infancy, and generally do not shrink during childhood. In most cases tumor size remains unchanged; however, as the patient grows the tumor appears smaller relative to body size. Ventricular arrhythmias may persist, though may become clinically less significant with increasing age.[3]

Imaging

By chest radiography, fibromas may be evident as an abnormal ventricular contour with or without areas of punctate calcifications. By echocardiography, fibromas are large, intramyocardial, echobright masses with a hypoechoic core, commonly involving the wall of the left ventricle or interventricular septum. However, fibromas may involve all cardiac chambers. They differ from rhabdomyomas in that they do not protrude into the cavity of the heart but instead protrude onto the epicardial surface of the heart (Fig. 51.2). Fibromas may be massive in size, and major coronary artery branches sometimes course over the epicardial surface, sometime penetrating the tumor mass (Figs. 51.4 and 51.5). They have a homogenous appearance and may cause substantial hemodynamic compromise, including ventricular dysfunction, inflow or outflow obstruction, or valve dysfunction, usually mitral regurgitation. By CMR, fibroma is a large intramyocardial tumor in the ventricular septum or free wall with a well-defined border and a characteristic late gadolinium enhancement pattern.[4] Because of the high diagnostic accuracy by CMR, biopsy is usually not indicated.[4] CMR images are particularly useful in creation of 3D models for surgical planning, as they provide a spatial map of not only the tumor location but also details of surrounding cardiac structures and coronary arteries and their relationship to the tumor.

Management

Because fibroma is a benign tumor, the approach to management is based on clinical features. Thus, management is directed at treatment of symptoms, arrhythmias, and local complications associated with the tumor. Patients who present with clinically significant arrhythmias or hemodynamic instability initially require appropriate medical management. Heart transplantation has been performed in patients with massive tumors in whom surgery was not considered feasible; however, extensive surgical debulking or complete/near-complete tumor resection is the treatment of choice in the majority of cases where surgery is indicated. Postoperatively, most arrhythmias resolve.[3] In our earlier experience, where indication for surgical treatment was VT, 13 patients

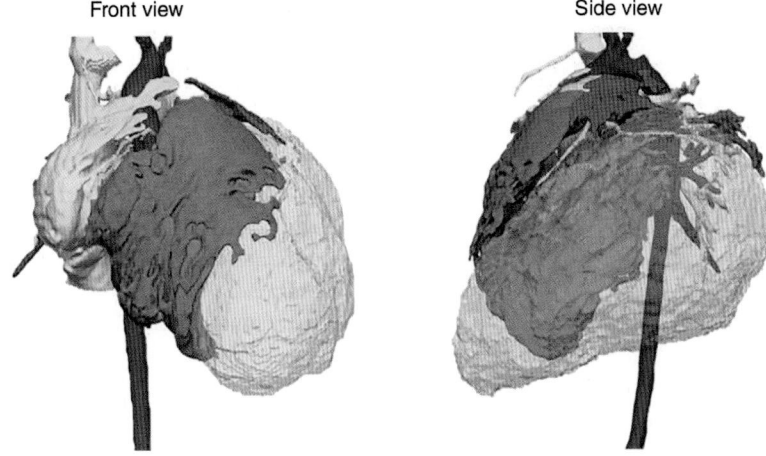

Front view

Side view

• **Fig. 51.4** A 3D model of a massive left ventricular fibroma *(gray color)*. The tumor is compressing the left ventricle *(dark orange)*. Coronary arteries are seen coursing over the tumor *(bright green)* and through the center of the tumor *(light blue)*.

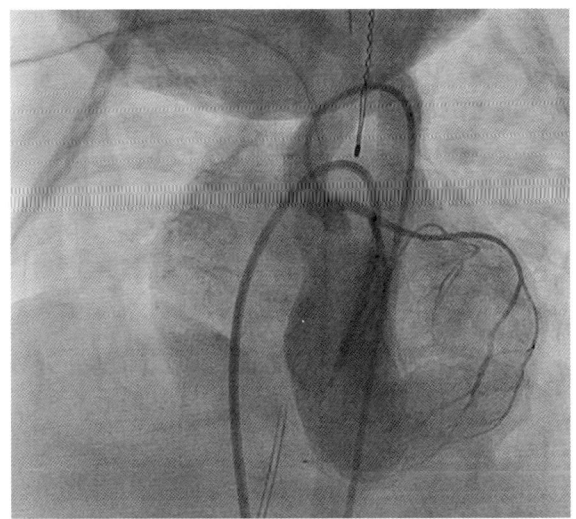

• **Fig. 51.5** Simultaneous ventricular and coronary artery angiography in a child with a left ventricular fibroma illustrates major coronary artery branches coursing over the epicardial surface of the tumor.

underwent resection, leaving behind portions of tumor if important coronary arterial branches were involved. There were no postoperative deaths, and VT was eliminated in all cases.[3] However, our recent experience with 46 patients (El Assaad et al.[15]) identified recurrence of clinical VT in two patients, and a positive postoperative ventricular stimulation study in another. Two of these cases were treated with implantable cardioverter defibrillator, although neither has required an appropriate shock at the time of data collection in 2022. The third case is being treated medically. In light of this, we have modified our practice to include rigorous preoperative and postoperative electrophysiologic assessment, with additional mapping in the operating room in selected cases. Following surgery, regional wall motion abnormalities at the site of resection, increased LV volume, and reduced LV systolic function may persist.[16] Because of the association with Gorlin syndrome and heritable,

autosomal dominant PTCH1 gene mutations, we recommend genetic evaluation in any child or adult diagnosed with fibroma.

Myxoma

Cardiac myxoma is a neoplasm of multipotent mesenchymal cells of endocardial origin, consisting of myxoma cells, described as stellate to plump, cytologically bland mesenchymal cells, set in a myxoid stroma.[17] The gross appearance is variable. Macroscopically, they are white, gray-white, yellowish, or brownish and measure 1–15 cm in dimension. They are usually gelatinous, but may also have regions with hard consistency. The surface may be lobular, smooth, or villous and frondlike. The tumor, while usually pedunculated with a short stalk, may also be sessile.[17] About 75% arise from the left atrium; the remainder arise from the right atrium, right or left ventricles, or from multiple chambers.[18] Approximately 80% of left atrial myxomas arise directly from the fossa ovalis.[17] Focal areas of hemorrhage, calcification, fibrosis, and necrosis have been reported.[17] On gross inspection, myxomas may be covered by thrombus.[18] In a series of 112 myxomas, 64% were deemed histologically "active," i.e., with a dense myxoma cell population, compared with 36% that were "inactive," or with sparse cell concentration and calcification or ossification. In that cohort, all recurrences (5%) occurred in tumors that were "active" with poorly differentiated cells.[17] While cardiac myxomas are considered histologically benign, they can recur locally after resection, or embolize throughout the arterial tree, particularly in the cerebral circulation, manifesting as aneurysms or local areas of obstructing tumor mass in embolized territory, resulting in life-threatening adverse events such as stroke or sudden death.[17]

Clinical Manifestations

It is important to note that there are no pathognomonic signs in the clinical presentation of cardiac myxomas, and that symptoms depend on location, size, and mobility of the tumors.[18] Approximately 10% of cases are asymptomatic, with variable modes of presentation in the remainder. The following triad of symptoms has been described in some patients with cardiac myxoma: (1) symptoms secondary to valvular obstruction; (2) systemic emboli, commonly involving arteries of the central nervous system, but also in other systemic arteries such as the aortic bifurcation, retinal arteries, and coronary arteries; and (3) nonspecific constitutional signs and symptoms, including myalgia, muscle weakness, arthralgia, fever, weight loss, anemia, and elevated sedimentation rate. The constitutional symptoms are thought to be related to an immunologic response to the tumor. Smooth surfaced myxomas are more likely to present with constitutional symptoms, whereas friable, irregular, or villous tumors tend to embolize.[18] There is no clear association between the size of the tumor and clinical symptoms.

About 10% of patients with cardiac myxoma have the Carney complex, which is a neuroendocrine-cardiac syndrome characterized by (1) familial recurrent myxoma; (2) pigmented skin lesions, schwannomas, and multiple recurrent mucocutaneous myxomas; and (3) various endocrine overactivity and neoplasms.[19] About 67% of patients with Carney complex have cardiac myxomas.[19] Mutations in the gene encoding PRKAR1, a tumor suppressor gene, are often present in patients with Carney complex.[19]

About two-third of the patients with cardiac myxoma have abnormal findings on electrocardiogram: left atrial enlargement being the commonest, followed by ST-segment abnormalities, ventricular hypertrophy, micro-voltage, and extrasystoles.[17]

Imaging

Chest radiograph findings vary depending on the size and location of the tumor, and may include left atrial enlargement, intracardiac calcifications, pulmonary vascular congestion, enlarged pulmonary artery, cardiomegaly, and pleural effusion.

Echocardiography is the screening modality of choice for identifying a myxoma. The classic appearance is that of a pedunculated left atrial mass that moves in and out of the mitral valve orifice during the cardiac cycle (Fig. 51.6). Cardiac myxoma has a variable appearance on CMR imaging depending on the fraction of vascularity, myxomatous elements, chronic hemorrhage, fibrosis, and cystic changes. The two independent predictors of myxoma by CMR in the pediatric population includes (1) endocardial location and (2) high signal intensity on cine SSFP.[4]

Management

Given the high risks of embolization and sudden death, prompt surgical excision is indicated.[17,18] Tumor resection is generally straightforward, particularly if mass is pedunculated, and carries low risk for operative mortality.[17,18] Full-thickness excision of the tumor base is recommended to avoid local recurrence, reported in ~5% of cases.[17,18] Valvuloplasty or valve replacement may be indicated if a valve has sustained significant damage from the tumor.[18]

Hemangioma and Other Vascular Anomalies

Cardiac hemangioma is the most common type of vascular anomaly of the heart. Vascular anomalies of the heart can

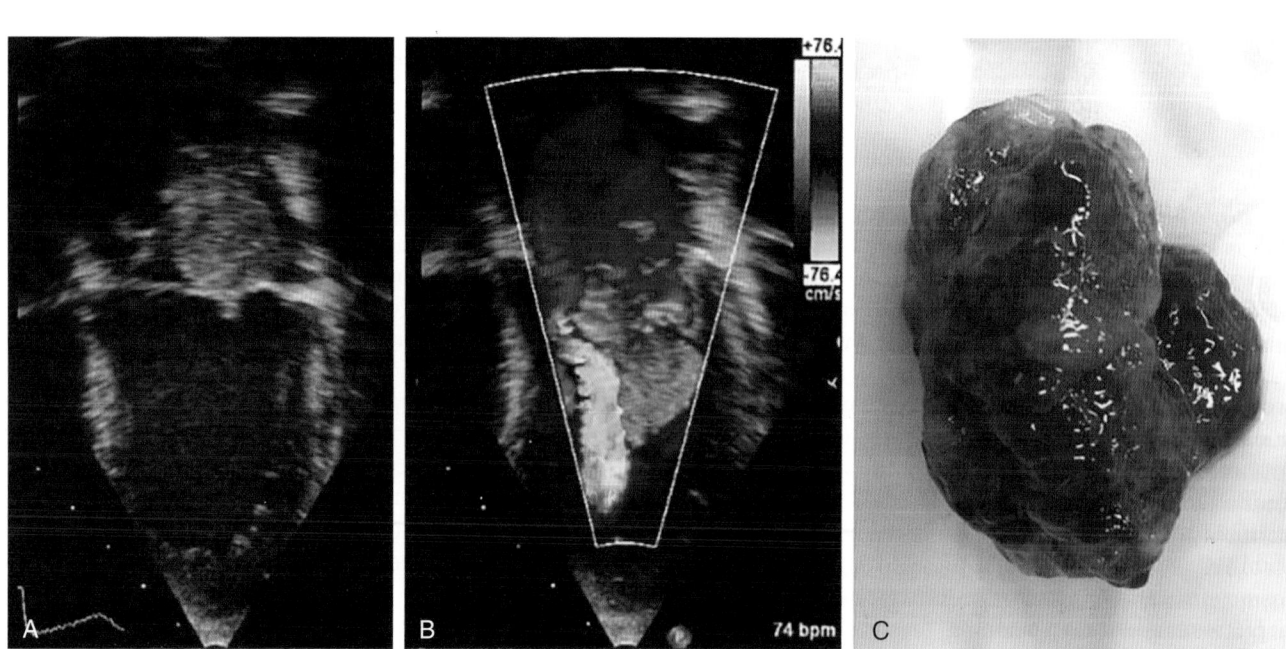

• **Fig. 51.6** Atrial myxoma. By echocardiography, the mass flops between the left atrium and ventricle throughout the cardiac cycle, obstructing mitral valve inflow **(A, B)**. Myxomas have a variable appearance on gross pathology. This tumor has a lobular, smooth surface with a gelatinous appearance and regions of hemorrhage **(C)**.

be divided into two major categories: vascular tumors (including hemangioma) and vascular malformations. Because of historical variations in nomenclature, the International Society for the Study of Vascular Anomalies (ISSVA) was developed in 1996; despite this, misclassification of vascular anomalies is common. The ISSVA can be referenced online for the most up-to-date classification system available (www.issva.org).

Cardiac hemangiomas (congenital, infantile, and intramuscular) involve proliferation of endothelial cells of blood vessels, and are histologically similar to hemangiomas in other regions of the body. As different subtypes of cardiac hemangioma are difficult to distinguish in the absence of histologic data, and because of challenges with misclassifications, the natural history of the subtypes of cardiac hemangioma have not been well delineated. In general, they may involve the endocardium, myocardium, or epicardium, and can develop in any location within the heart.[20] On gross pathology, they appear red and hemorrhagic.

Clinical Presentation

Cardiac hemangiomas can present at any age, but are more commonly found prenatally, in infants, and in children.[4] Clinical presentations vary according to patient age and anatomic location. Prenatally, they present as a cardiac mass during routine obstetric ultrasound examination. Neonatal hemangiomas commonly cause pericardial effusion and tamponade, but patients may also present with arrhythmias, syncope, congestive heart failure, and sudden death.[20] Older children and adults are asymptomatic and diagnosis is often incidental.[20]

Imaging

Hemangiomas diagnosed in the neonatal period commonly arise from the right atrium, but more likely involve other cardiac chambers beyond the neonatal period.[4] Echocardiography is useful in documenting the presence and location of the tumor, and occasionally demonstrates vascular channels within the tumor. However, CMR imaging is diagnostically more useful in distinguishing vascular from nonvascular tumors because of the characteristic avid perfusion on first-pass perfusion imaging in vascular tumors. However, current CMR techniques do not allow reliable distinction among benign vascular tumors, malignant vascular tumors, vascular malformations, and other tumors with rich vascular supply.[4]

Management

Natural history of cardiac hemangiomas is unpredictable given that non-invasive imaging cannot reliably identify which tumors have malignant characteristics. Therefore, surgical resection is recommended and usually has favorable outcomes. As incomplete resection may lead to local recurrence, when technically feasible, the tumors should be completely resected to minimize this risk of recurrence.

Lymphatic Malformation

Classification

Lymphatic malformations are vascular anomalies involving the lymphatic system. As with other vascular anomalies, the nomenclature of lymphatic malformations has varied in the literature, such that many have been misclassified as tumors ("lymphangioma"). Although many of these malformations are not strictly defined as tumors (e.g., no neoplastic process), there are rare malignant tumors of lymphatic origin (e.g., lymphangiomyomatosis and kaposiform lymphangiomatosis). Gross pathology reveals a soft, spongy or firm mass.[21] The mass typically has multiloculated cystic cavities containing lymphatic fluid, divided by septa of variable thickness, and importantly, does not communicate with the normal lymphatic system. Lymphatic malformations in an intrapericardial location may ooze lymph into the pericardial space, resulting in chylous pericardial effusion.[21] By histology, lymphatic malformations have characteristic flat endothelial cells, disorganized smooth muscle cells, lymphoid aggregates, and typically stain positive on D2-40 or LYVE-1 stains.

Clinical Presentation

Cardiac lymphatic malformations vary in their presentation depending on the size of the mass and location. They may present as an incidental finding on chest radiography or may cause congestive heart failure, respiratory distress, syncope, embolic complications, arrhythmias, palpitations, or, more commonly, cardiac tamponade from mass effect or pericardial effusion.[21]

Imaging

Noninvasive imaging—echocardiography, CT, and CMR—demonstrates a multilocular cystic mass in either a pericardial or intracardiac location, and may encase a coronary artery. The mass typically causes compression of adjacent cardiac structures and may be associated with pericardial effusion with or without tamponade. Lymphatic malformations are usually avascular with typical characteristics on CMR and CT imaging.

Management

Treatment of cardiac lymphatic malformations depends on the location of the mass, the degree of involvement with adjacent cardiac structures, and the clinical presentation. In patients with cardiac tamponade, immediate relief of the chylous pericardial effusion is recommended and can establish the diagnosis. A cautious management approach, including involvement of a team specialized in vascular malformations, is advised. In asymptomatic patients without evidence of associated hemodynamic abnormalities, close observation may be considered, particularly for patients with coronary artery involvement. Malformations that are incompletely resected are at risk for persistent chylous drainage, resulting in prolonged pericardial or pleural effusions, and recurrence; thus complete resection is advised if feasible.

Intrapericardial Teratoma

Classification

Intrapericardial teratomas belong to the family of germ cell tumors, comprising benign or malignant tumors derived from primordial germ cells.[5] The gross appearance is an encapsulated, lobulated, cystic mass with fluid-filled cavities of various sizes intermingled with solid areas. Components from all three germ cell layers (endoderm, mesoderm, and ectoderm) coexist and often include neuroglia, cartilage, bone, smooth muscle, skeletal muscle, liver, intestine, pancreas, and glandular tissue. A small percentage may be classified as malignant based on histologic characteristics and mitotic activity.

Clinical Presentation

Prior to the era of fetal echocardiography, patients presented in the newborn period with clinical symptoms of respiratory distress, cyanosis, and congestive heart failure related to pericardial effusion and/or cardiac compression from the tumor. Numerous fetal cases have been described with a mean age at diagnosis of 28 weeks' gestation.[22] The tumors are commonly missed at second trimester ultrasound examinations, and grow rapidly between 20 and 40 weeks gestation when cellular differentiation occurs. By the third trimester, almost 50% of fetuses develop pericardial effusion, hydrops, or tamponade.[22] Intrapericardial teratomas may occasionally be identified in asymptomatic older children and adults.

Imaging

Intrapericardial teratoma typically comprises a large mass, usually located adjacent to the right atrium with cystic components.[4] There is classically a fibrous attachment to the aorta, containing the blood supply to the tumor. Rarely, the tumor attaches to the pulmonary trunk or presents as an intracardiac mass.[5] As with other tumors, the clinical signs relate to the size and location of the tumor. Often, tumors cause extrinsic compression of the right atrium and/or superior vena cava, with associated low cardiac output, pericardial effusion, and fetal hydrops.

Management

For prenatally diagnosed intrapericardial teratomas, management depends on the presence or absence of hydrops. In the fetus with hydrops, pericardiocentesis is recommended to reduce the risk of *in utero* fetal demise and allow for lung development. If hydrops is absent, the pregnancy can be carried to term, with prompt early postnatal resection. Postnatal resection within the first few days of life is recommended as unresected teratomas can grow rapidly in size. Resection, in addition to addressing cardiorespiratory symptoms, can prevent malignant transformation.[6] Most surgeries can be performed without the use of cardiopulmonary bypass, unless the tumor involves the aorta or an adjacent cardiac structure. In a review of prenatally diagnosed intrapericardial teratoma, the overall hospital mortality,

including fetal demise, was 16/38 or 42% (13 deaths, 1 death after fetal surgery, 1 tumor recurrence causing death, and 1 termination of pregnancy).[22] Fetal hydrops was associated with a higher rate of mortality; pericardiocentesis was associated with a lower rate of mortality (0/15 non-survivors had pericardiocentesis compared with 10/22 survivors).[22]

Papillary Fibroelastoma

Classification

Papillary fibroelastoma is a primary valvular tumor, originating from cardiac valvular endocardium. The tumor contains collagen, elastic fibers, and smooth muscle. They measure from millimeters to centimeters in dimension, and can arise from either the atrioventricular valves or semilunar valves.[23] On the mitral and tricuspid valves, the tumors usually occur on the atrial aspect of the valve, whereas they may occur with equal frequency on either the ventricular or arterial side of the semilunar valves.[23] The tumors may also have attachments to the chordae tendineae, papillary muscles, or ventricular endocardial surface. The gross appearance is that of filiform threads attached to the endocardium, either sessile or connected by a short pedicle. When suspended in water, they may have the appearance of a sea anemone.[23] On histology, the strands have a central core of collagen that is continuous with the valve leaflet. The core is surrounded by a myxomatous matrix, with an outer layer of elastin.[23] It has been suggested that this lesion is a hamartoma of subvalvar apparatus (as its histology is similar to that of normal chordae tendineae) versus a proliferative response to mechanical injury.[23]

Clinical Presentation

Given its rare occurrence in children, the clinical presentation of papillary fibroelastoma is limited to case reports. It can present either as an incidental finding in an asymptomatic patient, or present with right heart obstruction, myocardial infarction, cardiac failure, or embolic events (including stroke and neurologic symptoms associated with tumor embolization).

Imaging

Echocardiography may show one or more round, homogenous, echogenic masses attached to a valve. The appearance has also been described as multiple masses attached to thin stalks, similar to a string of beads. On CMR, characteristic findings include a pedunculated, mobile, endocardial or valvular mass.[4]

Management

Given the high risk of embolization, surgical excision of papillary fibroelastoma is indicated. In some cases, excision may have to be limited to surgical debulking to avoid injury to valve leaflets and resulting valvar incompetence. In cases with significant valve destruction, valve replacement maybe required.

Inflammatory Myofibroblastic Tumor

Classification

Inflammatory myofibroblastic tumor (IMT) is a rare tumor found in nearly all sites of the body. Although IMT is a distinct entity based on anaplastic lymphoma kinase (ALK) expression, it has previously been called inflammatory pseudotumor, plasma cell granuloma, and pseudosarcomatous fibromyxoid tumor.[4] The pathogenesis may be related to an exaggerated immunologic response to prior injury, inflammation, or infection. It is considered a benign tumor/low-grade neoplasm.[24] Macroscopically, the tumor may be firm, fleshy, or gelatinous, with a white or tan cut surface, and may comprise either a single dominant polyp or appear multilobulated to filiform. Histologic appearance is similar to a chronic inflammatory infiltrate and may include areas of calcification, hemorrhage, and necrosis. In some cases, IMT may evolve into a higher-grade malignant lesion with nuclear atypia, mitosis, and/or necrosis.[24] Although IMT arises primarily from the endocardial surface of the cardiac chambers or valves, it is histologically distinct from myxoma and papillary fibroelastoma.

Clinical Presentation

The clinical presentation varies according to tumor location and immunologic profile. Patients may present with systemic inflammatory symptoms including fever, weight loss, anemia, thrombocytopenia, hypergammaglobulinemia, and elevated inflammatory markers. Shortness of breath, pulmonary embolism, recurrent neurologic symptoms due to systemic embolism, heart murmur, syncope, chest pain, and sudden death have also been reported.

Incidence

Cardiac IMT is extremely rare, and most of the cardiac IMT cases described in the literature involve children or young adults.

Imaging

The imaging features of IMT are variable and non-specific, possibly because of the wide range in size, location, gross appearance, and histologic makeup. However, IMTs are likely to demonstrate metabolic activity on ^{18}F-FDG PET imaging.[4]

Management

Complete surgical resection of cardiac IMT is advised for reasons that include a strong association with systemic inflammatory symptoms and risk of sudden cardiac death, as well as the risk of local recurrence and malignant transformation. In some cases, surgical resection has been curative.[25] In situations with extensive tumor involvement or recurrence, cardiac transplantation may be recommended.

Malignant Cardiac Tumors

Classification

Primary and secondary cardiac malignancies are exceptionally rare in the pediatric population, and are typically associated with poor prognosis. In a series of 3641 children with solid malignancies, Chan et al.[2] reported 59 patients (1.6%) with cardiac involvement. Of those, 45 had distant metastasis to the heart and 14 had direct extension or primary location of the tumor in cardiac chambers and/or great veins.[2] In children, sarcomas are the most common type of primary malignant cardiac tumor. The frequencies of malignant cardiac tumors and mode of entry to the heart in children from the New England area treated at Boston Children's Hospital from 1990 to 2020 include the following: hepatocellular carcinoma ($N = 2$; intravascular extension), unspecified sarcoma ($N = 2$, direct invasion), leukemia, Ewing sarcoma, rhabdomyosarcoma, and osteosarcoma ($N = 1$ each; metastasis).

Clinical Presentation

The clinical presentation of a malignant cardiac tumor relates to tumor size and location. Symptoms are generally nonspecific and vary from a heart murmur in an asymptomatic child to fevers, lethargy, lightheadedness, dyspnea, heart failure, arrhythmia, stroke, and sudden death. Because most malignant cardiac tumors in children have metastasized from another location, patients will often have a prior history of malignancy. Malignant tumors have a lower rate of survival than histologically benign tumors and masses (Fig. 51.7).[4]

Imaging

Imaging characteristics of malignancy include: (1) history of extracardiac malignancy; and (2) infiltrative appearance, defined as (a) crossing an annular or tissue plane within the heart; (b) involving both cardiac and extracardiac structures; or (c) appearance of linear growth through a large vessel such as the superior or inferior vena cava. By CMR, malignant tumors are often hyperintense on T2-weighted imaging.[26]

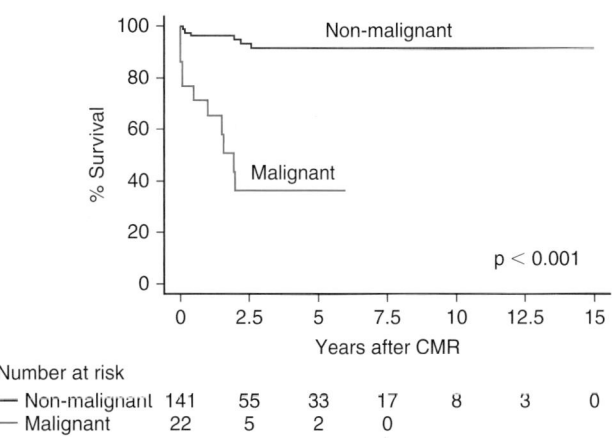

• **Fig. 51.7** Kaplan-Meier estimates of survival following CMR examination for malignant and non-malignant tumors. Lower survival was found for patients with malignant tumors ($P < .001$). *CMR,* Cardiac magnetic resonance. (Borrowed with permission from Beroukhim RS, Ghelani S, Ashwath R, et al. Accuracy of cardiac magnetic resonance imaging in diagnosing pediatric cardiac masses: a multicenter study. *JACC: Cardiovasc Imaging.* 2021.)

Management

Treatment of cardiac malignant tumors is dictated by the nature of the primary tumor. In general, most malignant cardiac tumors are fairly aggressive with a poor prognosis, and treatment is palliative in nature. In some cases, surgical resection with chemotherapy or heart transplantation is offered. For patients with symptomatic pericardial effusion associated with a malignant cardiac tumor, pericardiocentesis or pericardial window can be a temporizing palliative measure.

References

1. Isaacs Jr H. Fetal and neonatal cardiac tumors. *Pediatr Cardiol.* 2004;25:252-273.
2. Chan HS, Sonley MJ, Moes CA, et al. Primary and secondary tumors of childhood involving the heart, pericardium, and great vessels: a report of 75 cases and review of the literature. *Cancer.* 1985;56:825-836.
3. Miyake CY, Del Nido PJ, Alexander ME, et al. Cardiac tumors and associated arrhythmias in pediatric patients, with observations on surgical therapy for ventricular tachycardia. *J Am Coll Cardiol.* 2011;58:1903-1909.
4. Beroukhim RS, Ghelani S, Ashwath R, et al. Accuracy of cardiac magnetic resonance imaging diagnosis of pediatric cardiac masses: a multicenter study. *JACC Cardiovasc Imaging.* 2022;15:1391-1405.
5. Becker AE. Primary heart tumors in the pediatric age group: a review of salient pathologic features relevant for clinicians. *Pediatr Cardiol.* 2000;21:317-323.
6. Roach ES, Sparagana SP. Diagnosis of tuberous sclerosis complex. *J Child Neurol.* 2004;19:643-649.
7. Fesslova V, Villa L, Rizzuti T, et al. Natural history and long-term outcome of cardiac rhabdomyomas detected prenatally. *Prenat Diagn.* 2004;24:241-248.
8. Dereddy NR, Sett SS, Krishnan U. Resection of ventricular rhabdomyomas in infants presenting with cardiac failure. *Cardiol Young.* 2008;18:635-637.
9. Stelmaszewski EV, Parente DB, Farina A, et al. Everolimus for cardiac rhabdomyomas in children with tuberous sclerosis. The ORACLE study protocol (everOlimus for caRdiac rhAbdomyomas in tuberous sCLErosis): a randomised, multicentre, placebo-controlled, double-blind phase II trial. *Cardiol Young.* 2020;30:337-345.
10. Wagner R, Riede FT, Seki H, et al. Oral everolimus for treatment of a giant left ventricular rhabdomyoma in a neonate: rapid tumor regression documented by real time 3D echocardiography. *Echocardiography.* 2015;32:1876-1879.
11. Barnes BT, Procaccini D, Crino J, et al. Maternal sirolimus therapy for fetal cardiac rhabdomyomas. *N Engl J Med.* 2018;378:1844-1845.
12. Ninic S, Kalaba M, Jovicic B, et al. Successful use of sirolimus for refractory atrial ectopic tachycardia in a child with cardiac rhabdomyoma. *Ann Noninvasive Electrocardiol.* 2017;22:e12435.
13. Gorlin RJ. Nevoid basal cell carcinoma (Gorlin) syndrome. *Genet Med.* 2004;6:530-539.
14. Carreon CK, Sanders SP, Perez-Atayde AR, et al. Interdigitating myocardial tongues in pediatric cardiac fibromas: plausible substrate for ventricular tachycardia and cardiac arrest. *JACC Clin Electrophysiol.* 2019;5:563-575.
15. El Assaad I, Jurow K, Dasgupta S, et al. Ventricular arrhythmias after fibroma resection: Are patients still at risk? *Heart Rhythm.* 2023;20(2):243–249.
16. Beroukhim RS, Geva T, Del Nido P, et al. Risk factors for left ventricular dysfunction following surgical management of cardiac fibroma. *Circ Cardiovasc Imaging.* 2021;14:e011748.
17. Pinede L, Duhaut P, Loire R. Clinical presentation of left atrial cardiac myxoma: a series of 112 consecutive cases. *Medicine (Baltimore).* 2001;80:159-172.
18. Markel ML, Waller BF, Armstrong WF. Cardiac myxoma: a review. *Medicine (Baltimore).* 1987;66:114-125.
19. Shetty Roy AN, Radin M, Sarabi D, Shaoulian E. Familial recurrent atrial myxoma: Carney's complex. *Clin Cardiol.* 2011;34:83-86.
20. Kojima S, Sumiyoshi M, Suwa S, et al. Cardiac hemangioma: a report of two cases and review of the literature. *Heart Vessels.* 2003;18:153-156.
21. Zakaria RH, Barsoum NR, El-Basmy AA, et al. Imaging of pericardial lymphangioma. *Ann Pediatr Cardiol.* 2011;4:65-67.
22. MacKenzie S, Loken S, Kalia N, et al. Intrapericardial teratoma in the perinatal period. Case report and review of the literature. *J Pediatr Surg.* 2005;40:e13-e18.
23. Fletcher CDM. *Diagnostic Histopathology of Tumors.* Edinburgh, New York: Churchill Livingstone; 1995.
24. Burke A, Li L, Kling E, et al. Cardiac inflammatory myofibroblastic tumor: a "benign" neoplasm that may result in syncope, myocardial infarction, and sudden death. *Am J Surg Pathol.* 2007;31:1115-1122.
25. Bao M, Zheng C, Zhang H, et al. Inflammatory myofibroblastic tumor of the left atrium in infant. *Int J Cardiol.* 2016;222:965-967.
26. Beroukhim RS, Prakash A, Valsangiacomo Buechel ER, et al. Characterization of cardiac tumors in children by cardiovascular magnetic resonance imaging a multicenter experience. *J Am Coll Cardiol.* 2011;58:1044-1054.

Special Problems/ Diagnosis and Therapy

52

Evaluating Murmurs, Chest Pain, and Syncope

SHANNON LYON, MARK E. ALEXANDER, AND SARAH D. DE FERRANTI

KEY LEARNING POINTS

- Murmurs are common, present in at least half of all children at some point during childhood, and innocent murmurs are often transient.
- Innocent murmurs are typically short, < 3/6 intensity, well localized, often along the left sternal border, and are not accompanied by thrills, cyanosis, or other cardiac symptoms.
- Chest pain in children is largely noncardiac in origin; common etiologies may include musculoskeletal pain, gastroesophageal reflux, or pulmonary processes such as asthma.

- Identifying red flags for cardiac chest pain, such as exercise-induced pain or underlying congenital heart disease, is important in initial assessment.
- Syncope is another common reason for referral to the cardiology clinic; prodromal symptoms such as dizziness, vision change, and nausea are common in vasovagal syncope.
- Syncope during peak exertion, in response to auditory or emotional triggers, or without prodromal symptoms is worrisome for cardiac pathology.

A mainstay of the practice of pediatric cardiology is the evaluation of murmurs, chest pain, and syncope, which, combined with palpitations, makes up the "bread and butter" of ambulatory pediatric cardiology evaluations. Differentiation of the few patients with underlying pathology from the many with benign conditions, or no disease whatsoever, is the focus of this chapter. The incidence of newly recognized and newly acquired heart disease has a marked increase in neonates and infants. The sharp decline in new diagnoses after infancy results in practice patterns that permit more focused use of echocardiography and more advanced cardiac diagnostic testing in the older child.

Murmurs

The differentiation of innocent from pathologic murmurs is a leading cause for referral to a pediatric cardiologist. Innocent heart murmurs occur in the absence of cardiac pathology and are noted in about half of all children.[1] This contrasts to the low incidence of congenital heart disease, which is found in 12.3 per 1000 births in high-income North America.[2] Murmurs generally can be evaluated using history and skilled physical examination including auscultation and electrocardiography.

Prevalence of Murmurs

The reported prevalence of murmurs in the neonatal period varies from 0.6% to 8.6%,[3] though the prevalence can be higher depending on the timing of the exam and level of training of the examiner. In a study of otherwise healthy children from birth through 14 years of age, a benign systolic murmur was heard in about half.[1] Even in reviews of patients seen in pediatric cardiology referral centers, most children newly referred for an evaluation of a murmur have no significant heart disease.[4] At Boston Children's Hospital, the evaluation of murmurs accounts for 7.7% of all outpatient clinic visits; between the years 2021 and 2022, this equated to 2310 of 30,084 patients seen in the outpatient clinic.

Clinical Manifestations

General Characteristics of Innocent Murmurs

Innocent murmurs occur in systole, with the exception of the venous hum, which is continuous. Whereas pathologic murmurs may be of any length, innocent murmurs are usually brief, peaking in the first half of systole and are typically less than a grade 3/6 in intensity. The murmur's intensity often changes with position and, occasionally, from examination to examination. The quality of the innocent murmur is often vibratory and musical, or sometimes blowing, in contrast to the harsh quality of many pathologic murmurs. Innocent murmurs are often well localized, usually along the left sternal border. With the exception of venous hums, there are no innocent thrills. Cyanosis should never accompany an innocent murmur. The most common innocent heart murmurs are described below.

Still's Murmur

The Still's murmur is most commonly heard in patients between the ages of 2 and 7 years.[5] Characteristically, it is a grade 1–2/6, vibratory, buzzing, or twanging systolic ejection murmur. It is usually maximal between the third intercostal space, left lower sternal border, and apex; is louder in the supine position than in the seated position; and is characteristically louder with exercise, excitement, or fever. It usually resolves in adolescence. The association of Still's murmur with false chordae tendineae in the left ventricle is debated, with some authors finding a strong relationship and others finding a high prevalence of both Still's murmurs and false tendons in healthy hearts but no association. Individuals with Still's murmurs have been reported to have a significantly smaller mean ascending aortic diameter relative to body surface area, with higher average peak velocities in the ascending and descending aorta than are found in children and young adults without murmurs. These observations suggest that the origin of Still's murmur may be related to a small aortic root and ascending aortic diameter with concomitant high-velocity flow across the left ventricular outflow tract and ascending aorta.[4]

Innocent Pulmonary Flow Murmur

The pulmonary flow murmur may be heard in children of any age and frequently occurs in children with asthenic builds who have narrow anteroposterior diameters. The murmur is identical in quality to the murmur of an atrial septal defect due to increased flow through the normal pulmonic valve but associated with a normal second sound. It is a grade 1–2/6, blowing, rather high-pitched murmur that peaks in the first half of systole and is maximal in intensity in the second left intercostal space, without wide transmission. Like the Still's murmur, it is louder when the patient is in the supine position and is accentuated by exercise, fever, or excitement.[5]

Physiologic Pulmonary Artery Branch Stenosis of the Newborn

Physiologic pulmonary artery branch stenosis or peripheral pulmonary artery stenosis is heard in the newborn period as a low-frequency systolic ejection murmur maximal in the lateral chest, axillae, and occasionally the back, but is heard less well over the precordium itself. This murmur generally wanes by age 6 months and is believed to be caused by turbulence from the relative discordance in size between the larger main pulmonary artery and smaller branch pulmonary arteries.[6] If this murmur persists past 6 months of age, underlying pulmonary artery pathology as well as lesions, such as atrial septal defects, which increase flow through the pulmonary arteries should be investigated.

Cervical Venous Hum

The cervical venous hum is a continuous, low-frequency murmur with diastolic accentuation that is heard most frequently in children aged between 3 and 6 years, though it can be heard in older children as well.[5] It is located in the low anterior part of the neck, more often on the right than the left. The murmur is loudest with the patient in the sitting position and disappears or diminishes in the supine position. Usually the venous hum is accentuated by turning the patient's head away from the side of the murmur and elevating the chin. The murmur may be obliterated by pressing lightly over the jugular vein with the stethoscope or a finger.[5] The mechanism of the venous hum has not been definitively delineated, although it has been postulated to be secondary to turbulence of venous flow in the jugular veins.

Supraclavicular Arterial Bruit

The supraclavicular arterial bruit is a crescendo–decrescendo systolic murmur heard best just above the clavicles, usually on the right side more than on the left. It radiates better to the neck than below the clavicles and, very occasionally, can generate a faint carotid thrill. The bruit may be accentuated by exercise but is not affected by posture and respiration. It can be distinguished from the murmur of aortic stenosis by the disappearance of the supraclavicular murmur with the maneuver of hyperextension of the shoulders or compression of the subclavian artery against the first rib. Supraclavicular systolic murmurs have been postulated to arise from the major brachiocephalic arteries near their aortic origins at the site of caliber change of these vessels.

Distinguishing Innocent From Pathologic Murmurs

A comprehensive approach, taking into account the family history, patient history including signs and symptoms, physical exam, and vital signs, is needed to distinguish innocent from pathologic murmurs. Certain features increase the likelihood of a murmur being pathologic, including a first-degree relative with congenital heart disease, an abnormal fetal echocardiogram, an underlying genetic disorder associated with congenital heart disease, patient age less than 1 year, or symptoms such as cyanosis, respiratory distress, feeding difficulties, diaphoresis, syncope, or exertional chest pain. Murmurs with certain characteristics, such as being ≥ grade 3 in intensity, increased intensity in the upright position, holosystolic, maximum intensity at the left upper sternal border, harsh or blowing quality, or a diastolic murmur, may be more likely to be pathologic.[4] Similarly, the presence of an abnormal S2, a click, thrill, or S3 or S4 gallop rhythm is more likely to be pathologic. Other physical exam findings such as diminished femoral pulses, bounding pulses, hepatomegaly, or abnormal vital signs such as tachycardia or ≥ 10 point blood pressure gradient between upper and lower extremities can increase the suspicion of congenital heart disease.

Diagnostic Testing

Diagnostic testing should be tailored to the clinical situation. Most children older than 1 year of age can be evaluated with history, physical examination, and an electrocardiogram (ECG) alone. In patients newly diagnosed with a heart murmur, it may be more cost-effective for pediatricians to refer patients to pediatric cardiologists for clinical evaluation than to order two-dimensional echocardiograms prior to referral.[7] Heart disease is seldom diagnosed when a pediatric cardiologist orders an echocardiogram if patients are older than age 6 weeks with innocent-sounding murmurs and have no worrisome signs or symptoms. Conversely, the threshold for performing a two-dimensional echocardiogram should be low when structural heart disease is suspected by a pediatric cardiologist because of young age or worrisome history, signs, symptoms, or abnormalities on electrocardiography or chest radiography. This aligns with general guidelines for appropriate use criteria for echocardiograms.[8]

Management

For children in whom the diagnosis of innocent murmur is made clinically, the authors do not recommend reevaluation unless some uncertainty exists (e.g., because of suboptimal patient cooperation or a possible abnormality on a diagnostic test). It is of utmost importance to reassure the family of a child with an innocent murmur. The label of heart disease may have adverse emotional effects on the child and the family. Even temporary mislabeling may increase the morbidity from cardiac non-disease. If underlying cardiac pathology is detected, management is tailored to the specific diagnosis.

Prognosis

A study assessing the 20-year follow-up of patients diagnosed with an innocent murmur during childhood revealed that only 4/96 patients had heart disease in adulthood, and even in those rare patients the pathology was not definitely related to the murmur heard during childhood.[9] Children diagnosed with an innocent murmur of childhood are expected to have a normal life expectancy with no complications related to the murmur.

Chest Pain

After murmurs, chest pain in children and adolescents is the most frequent symptom leading to referral to a pediatric cardiologist. At Boston Children's Hospital, 1597 of 30,084 clinic visits between 2021 and 2022 were for the evaluation of chest pain, accounting for 5.3% of outpatient clinic visits. Cardiac origins of chest pain in children are infrequent;

however, accurate assessment of the clinical presentation is essential so that pathology is not overlooked (Table 52.1). By the time a patient reaches the cardiologist, the anxiety level of the family is high, reinforced by knowledge that cardiac causes of chest pain in older individuals can be life-threatening. Therefore, appropriate care for this group of patients must address not only the etiology but also provide reassurance about the nature of what is often a self-limited condition.

Epidemiology

Depending on the point of entry to the medical system, the prevalence of chest pain varies in children, but is a common presenting complaint in this age group. Cardiac etiology of chest pain in patients referred to Boston Children's Hospital cardiology clinic was found in only 41 patients over a 10-year follow-up period.[10] Further, a review of patients discharged from this cardiology clinic with the diagnosis of benign chest pain found that there were no deaths due to cardiac etiology within a median follow-up period of 4.4 years.[11]

Etiology

Noncardiac Causes of Chest Pain

Musculoskeletal

Pain attributable to the chest wall is the most common explanation in the pediatric age range, seen in as many as a third of patients, and may involve connective, bony, or muscular tissue. The underlying cause can be traumatic or atraumatic. Costochondritis related to inflammation at the costochondral junction is a common explanation for chest pain, particularly in adolescents, and can be traced to traumatic strain in athletes or lifting of relatively heavy objects.[12] Precordial catch syndrome is generally sharp pain of short duration and unclear etiology isolated to the left lower sternal border or apex that is sometimes exercise induced and may recur. Some patients are able to relieve the pain with deep inspiration. Slipping rib syndrome is pain caused by trauma or tension on the fibrous connections to the 8th, 9th, or 10th ribs. These ribs are not attached to the sternum but to each other, and with unrestrained motion of a rib, pain is produced by irritation of the intercostal nerves. The pain can be sharp or dull and is sometimes reproducible. The sternum itself can be the source of chest pain with an uncommon condition known as hypersensitive xiphoid that improves spontaneously. Pectus deformities of the chest wall can be associated with occasional pain that may be accentuated by exercise. Traumatic chest pain is very common in adolescents related to muscular strain or tears, rib fractures, or spasm. Such pain is almost always self-limited.

Pulmonary

Underlying pulmonary pathology leads to chest pain in a variety of settings. Chest pain is a frequent presenting symptom after a pulmonary embolus. The pain may be pleuritic, but this is not always the case. Associated signs

TABLE 52.1 Cardiac and Non-Cardiac Etiologies, Clinical Clues, and Exam Findings

Etiology	Clinical History	Exam Findings	Initial Testing
Cardiac			
Myocardial			
Hypertrophic cardiomyopathy	• Chest pain with exertion • Syncope • Positive family history	• Systolic murmur (LVOT obstruction and mitral regurgitation)	• ECG with LVH, ST-segment or T-wave abnormalities • Echo with septal hypertrophy
Dilated cardiomyopathy	• Decreased exercise tolerance • Syncope • Positive family history	• Gallop rhythm	• ECG with increased left ventricular forces, T-wave abnormalities • Echo with left ventricular dilation +/− diminished function
Myocarditis	• Fever • Acute onset of symptoms • +/− heart failure symptoms	• Tachycardia • Tachypnea • +/− arrhythmia • Shock, if severe	• Diffuse ST-segment changes • T-wave abnormalities • Elevated troponin
Valvular			
Severe aortic valve stenosis or subvalvar left ventricular outflow obstruction	• Chest pain with exertion • Syncope	• Systolic ejection murmur	• LVH or left ventricular strain
Coronary			
Coronary ischemia	• Anginal chest pain • Chest pain with exertion Predisposing conditions: • Surgical manipulation of coronary arteries • Heart transplant • Kawasaki disease • William's syndrome • Homozygous familial hypercholesterolemia • Cocaine use • Significant chest wall trauma	• Tachycardia • Tachypnea	ECG findings: • ST depressions/elevations • T-wave changes • Q waves Labs: • Elevated troponin
Pericardial			
Pericarditis	• Sharp pleuritic chest pain improved by leaning forward	• Tachycardia • Pericardial friction rub	• Diffuse ST-segment elevations • PR depression
Aortic			
Aortic Dissection	• Sudden severe chest pain +/− radiation to the back	• Tachycardia • Tachypnea	• ST-segment elevation or depression • T-wave abnormalities • Q waves
Musculoskeletal			
Costochondritis	• Chest pain at rest or both at rest and with activity • Intermittent or persistent pain for days to weeks	• Chest pain may be reproducible on exam	Normal ECG
Precordial catch	• Sharp pain at rest • Resolves within seconds to minutes • May be associated with inspiration	Normal exam	Normal ECG

TABLE 52.1	Cardiac and Non-Cardiac Etiologies, Clinical Clues, and Exam Findings—cont'd		
Etiology	**Clinical History**	**Exam Findings**	**Initial Testing**
Pulmonary			
Pulmonary embolus	• +/– pleuritic chest pain • Dyspnea • Cough • +/– hemoptysis • Syncope • Predisposing factors (extreme inactivity, broken bone, clotting propensity, OCPs, COVID-19, etc.) • Prosthetic pulmonary/tricuspid valves	• Tachycardia • +/– loud S2	ECG: • Right ventricular hypertrophy or strain • Computed tomography pulmonary angiogram protocol • D-dimer
Reactive airway disease	• History of allergies or asthma • Chest pain or tightness at rest or with activity • Improves with bronchodilator	• Normal exam or • Wheezing, tachypnea, tachycardia	Normal ECG
Pneumonia	• Fever • Dyspnea • Cough	• Tachypnea • Febrile • Diminished breath sounds or crackles	Normal ECG
Pneumothorax	• Acute dyspnea and chest pain • History of Marfan syndrome, Ehlers-Danlos syndrome, or alpha-1 antitrypsin deficiency	• Normal or decreased breath sounds	• Normal ECG • Normal troponin and D-dimer • CXR
Gastrointestinal			
Gastroesophageal reflux	• Burning pain in retrosternal region • Temporally associated with meals • Regurgitation of gastric content into mouth	• Normal exam	Normal ECG
Peptic ulcer disease	• Upper abdominal pain • Occurs several hours after a meal	• Normal exam	Normal ECG

CXR, Chest x-ray; *ECG,* electrocardiogram; *LVH,* left ventricular hypertrophy; *LVOT,* left ventricular outflow tract; *OCPs,* oral contraceptive pills.
Adapted from Friedman KG, Alexander ME. Chest pain and syncope in children: A practical approach to the diagnosis of cardiac disease. *J Pediatr.* 2013;163:896.

and symptoms may include dyspnea, cough, hemoptysis, and tachycardia. If the pulmonary embolus is large, a patient may present with shock or syncope. Although uncommon, a family history of hypercoagulability may provide insight into the diagnosis. Reactive airway disease causes pain related to strain from persistent cough, dyspnea, or pneumothorax. In particular, exercise-induced bronchospasm is present in many children and adolescents, limiting their ability to participate in sports. Pretreatment with bronchodilator therapy may avert recurrent episodes. Pneumonia is associated with chest pain in many patients in the setting of acute febrile illness. Pleural disease is associated with chest pain that may be acute in onset, accentuated by inspiration and prolonged in duration. Pleural effusion is most frequently of infectious origin but can also be produced by systemic inflammatory

conditions or malignancy. Pleural irritation can also result from pneumothorax producing inspiratory pain; however, the pain can also be referred to the shoulder from diaphragmatic irritation. Pneumothorax can present spontaneously in Marfan syndrome and cystic fibrosis, or it may follow trauma.

Acute Chest Syndrome
Sickle cell disease is associated with acute chest syndrome, an important cause of death in this group of patients and frequently responsible for hospital admissions. It is defined as a new pulmonary infiltrate in addition to a fever, chest pain, tachypnea, wheezing, or cough. The etiology of the pain remains unclear, with episodes attributed to fat embolism, infection, or bony infarction.

Gastrointestinal

Chest pain may derive from a number of common gastrointestinal conditions. Gastroesophageal reflux with esophagitis produces a burning sensation in the retrosternal area, sometimes exacerbated by supine positioning. Signs of reflux in infants include arching of the back with feeding, spitting or recurrent vomiting, and respiratory changes related to aspiration, including wheezing and rhonchi. Peptic ulcer disease most frequently associated with *Helicobacter pylori* infection can be an important source of pain localized to the epigastric region or lower chest. Spasm of the esophagus can produce marked chest pain. When a possible gastrointestinal source of pain is suspected, evaluation of both motility and tissue involvement is warranted using manometry and endoscopy with biopsy.

Breast

Breast-related etiology of chest pain is a rare but potential source of pain in children. Infections, pubertal or menstrual change, and pregnancy in females may lead to breast discomfort. Gynecomastia in males may also lead to discomfort.

Psychogenic

Among pediatric patients presenting to a cardiology clinic with chest pain, a substantial number have symptoms that are psychogenic in origin. The history can pinpoint a preceding event that can act as a trigger for the pain, including death of a friend or family member, divorce or separation, illness or trauma in a family member, or depression. Chest pain can present as a symptom in hyperventilation syndrome. Despite the inclination to ascribe the complaint to a nonorganic cause, the provider must consider the social setting. Family members are generally very anxious about the possibility of underlying organ pathology and may not be ready to accept an alternate explanation. Often, reassurance about the anticipated benign outcome is helpful. Adolescents with chest pain frequently believe they have heart disease and tend to change their lifestyle as a result. In some cases, it may be necessary to obtain some non-invasive testing to provide support for the absence of underlying disease. Several encounters may allow the development of trust and rapport so that the family is more amenable to a diagnosis of psychogenic origin and likely to seek further counseling if necessary.

Cardiac Causes of Chest Pain

Myocardial

Cardiomyopathy, either hypertrophic or dilated, is associated with chest pain. The pain is the result of imbalance between myocardial demand and cardiac output. In the former case, marked increase in myocardial oxygen demand exceeds coronary flow during exercise, resulting in angina. Mid-cavitary obstruction exacerbates the imbalance, leading to increased myocardial work and myocardial oxygen consumption. Coronary artery compression produced by myocardial bridging may cause myocardial ischemia and

angina in patients with hypertrophic cardiomyopathy.[13] In dilated cardiomyopathy, the muscle mass is decreased, but the capacity of the heart to deliver adequate coronary blood flow is impaired by diminished stroke volume. Acute myocarditis generally of viral origin may present with chest pain, usually the result of concomitant pericarditis.

Valvular

Severe aortic valve or subaortic obstruction produces chest pain due to limitation of cardiac output during exercise in the setting of left ventricular hypertrophy. The supply–demand mismatch is similar to that of hypertrophic cardiomyopathy. Mitral regurgitation can be the source of chest pain when severe, related to volume overload of the left ventricle producing increased myocardial work with limited output due to the large regurgitant fraction of blood. Although more likely to occur as a chronic condition, the onset of mitral regurgitation can be acute after ruptured chordae tendineae in individuals with mitral valve prolapse or connective tissue disease. Less acute and poorly understood is the pain that has been associated in a small percentage of patients with mitral valve prolapse, which may in fact be unrelated to this condition.

Pericardial

Acute inflammation of the pericardium, or pericarditis, is frequently accompanied by chest pain thought to result from opposition of the inflamed parietal and visceral pericardial surfaces. The underlying cause can be viral, bacterial, autoimmune, or related to operative procedures in which the pericardium is entered. In the presence of effusion, the pericardial surfaces are separated so that the pain is diminished or absent.

Coronary

Kawasaki disease results in coronary aneurysms in 25% of those not treated early in the course with intravenous γ-globulin and in 4% of those receiving treatment before 10 days from the onset of fever. Giant aneurysm (> 8 mm in absolute diameter or z-score ≥ 10) formation puts patients at risk for late progressive stenosis at the distal or proximal end of the aneurysm. Exercise produces chest pain in those with critical narrowing.[14] Uncommonly, coronary artery abnormalities of congenital origin produce chest pain during exercise, which is thought to be related to compression of an artery between the aortic and pulmonic roots or insufficient coronary flow through an acutely angled takeoff or slit-like origin of the artery or spasm of the artery.[15] Rarely, the left coronary artery may arise from the pulmonary artery, a condition that presents in infancy with heart failure after left ventricular infarction, but it can remain silent until later in childhood when symptoms of pain with exercise may prevail.

Aortic

Aortic dissection is characterized by a sharp, severe, tearing pain that may be localized to the chest or back. Certain conditions including Marfan syndrome, Turner syndrome, type IV Ehlers-Danlos syndrome, and familial aortopathies carry an increased risk of aortic dissection. Sinus of Valsalva aneurysms are rare and typically due to a congenital weakness in the junction between the aortic media and annulus fibrosis. They can rupture unexpectedly into the right atrium or ventricle and present with chest pain or arrhythmias and sudden death.

Rhythm Abnormalities

Children with supraventricular tachycardia may complain of chest pain during acute events. The pain may be the result of coronary ischemia related to diminished ventricular diastolic filling and low cardiac output. More commonly, younger children may describe the discomfort of the palpitations as pain. Ventricular tachycardia producing chest pain is rare, and is most commonly seen in patients who have undergone repair or palliation of congenital lesions, as well as individuals with cardiomyopathy, long QTc syndrome, or severe electrolyte disturbances.

Clinical Evaluation

History

More than any other component of the clinical assessment of chest pain, the history is most critical because careful exploration of the present illness can often identify the cause of chest pain. A primary goal in obtaining this history is ruling out life-threatening etiologies of chest pain. If possible, the history should be obtained from the patient rather than the parents, who may be prone to overlay related to their personal experiences or anxiety. The patient should establish total duration of the symptom from the first episode. In many circumstances, chest pain is present for many months if not years before parents seek input, supporting a noncardiac cause. The manner of onset, whether acute or chronic, gradual or sudden, may suggest an etiology, with cardiac causes more acute in nature. Precipitating and predisposing factors provide insight, such as pain occurring with physical exertion (cardiac or musculoskeletal), injury or strain (musculoskeletal), response to rest or analgesics (musculoskeletal), emotional circumstances related to family disruption, school difficulties, illness of a friend or relative, or depression (psychogenic). Association with fever, chills, or rigors may indicate infectious etiology, which may originate from the pulmonary (pneumonia, bronchitis, etc.), cardiac (endocarditis—though chest pain is not the salient feature, pericarditis, myocarditis), or gastrointestinal system. The characteristics of the symptom should be detailed with a subjective description of the pain (i.e., squeezing, sharp, dull, aching, cramping), and the patient should locate the pain by pointing directly to the site of greatest intensity and then areas of possible radiation.

Anginal chest pain is generally substernal, crushing, and may radiate to the left arm or jaw. There may be associated nausea, diaphoresis, or dyspnea. Severe crushing pain radiating to the back is experienced with aortic dissection. Subcostal pain is generally chest wall related. The intensity

of the pain should be estimated using a scale of 1 to 10, with the lower and upper ranges defined for reference. The temporal nature of the episode should be identified as continuous, constant, intermittent, or recurrent. Aggravating and relieving factors may provide insight about the nature of the cause with respect to exertion, position, meals, or breathing. The course of the symptoms since initial presentation may indicate that the process is improving or progressing. It is often helpful to ask patients if they are worried about the pain, and if so, why—a line of questioning that can help to disclose emotional factors influencing the symptoms. Associated symptoms may be helpful clues, including palpitations, dizziness, syncope, metallic taste, nausea, vomiting, fatigue, fever, cough, coryza, shortness of breath, and orthopnea or dyspnea on exertion. The family history can identify other individuals with possible connective tissue disease or congenital heart disease.

Physical Examination

The appearance of the patient may suggest a connective tissue disorder in a tall individual with dolichocephaly and pectus excavatum or carinatum. The costochondral junctions and sternum should be palpated to elicit tenderness in all patients. Auscultation may identify wheezing associated with reactive airway disease or rales found with pneumonia or congestive failure. The cardiac assessment may suggest underlying heart disease by its hyperdynamic quality and displacement of the point of maximal intensity in patients with volume-overloaded lesions. A palpable thrill along the left sternal border, at the base bilaterally, and the suprasternal notch supports left ventricular outflow tract obstruction. An apical or parasternal heave is associated with left or right ventricular hypertrophy, respectively. On auscultation, underlying cardiac disease may be heralded by the presence of a loud S_2 associated with pulmonary hypertension, whereas muffled heart sounds are found in moderate to large pericardial effusions. Systolic clicks are noted with bicuspid aortic valves or mitral valve prolapse. The harsh systolic ejection murmur of valvar or subvalvar aortic stenosis is heard along the left sternal border with radiation to the base and neck. Mitral regurgitation is heard at the apex with radiation to the left axilla, although murmurs associated with posterior mitral leaflet abnormalities may be heard at the left mid to upper sternal border, related to a more anteriorly and superiorly directed regurgitant jet. Aortic regurgitation of at least mild to moderate degree produces a regurgitant murmur radiating from the right base, down the left lower sternal border toward the apex. S_3 gallops are heard in the presence of at least moderate mitral regurgitation or dilated cardiomyopathy, whereas S_4 gallops, although far less common, are noted in hypertrophic cardiomyopathy or severe aortic stenosis. A friction rub is often present with acute pericarditis.

Electrocardiogram

The ECG is of occasional benefit in the assessment of the patient with chest pain. A short PR interval and delta wave on ECG identifies the presence of an accessory bypass tract that can support supraventricular tachycardia in the patient who complains of chest pain with fast heart rate. Left ventricular hypertrophy is sometimes seen in patients with hypertrophic cardiomyopathy, moderate to severe aortic valve stenosis, subaortic stenosis, or aortic regurgitation and dilated cardiomyopathy. Long QTc interval may suggest the possibility of ventricular tachyarrhythmia. An infarct pattern can be present in anomalous left coronary artery from the pulmonary artery or rarely in Kawasaki disease. In pericarditis, PR depression and diffuse T-wave abnormalities are common.

Chest X-Ray

As with the ECG, chest x-rays are helpful in a limited number of those presenting with chest pain and therefore can be used selectively. In the patient with myocarditis, pericarditis, dilated cardiomyopathy, or aortic regurgitation of at least moderate degree, the x-ray may show cardiac chamber enlargement. A dilated ascending aorta can be present in those with Marfan syndrome. Reactive airway disease produces air trapping with hyperexpansion of the lung fields and flattened diaphragms. Pleural effusions or infiltrates are noted in infectious processes, and peripheral lung field abnormalities may be suggestive of pulmonary embolus. Spontaneous pneumothorax producing chest pain is readily recognized by radiograph.

Echocardiography

The echocardiogram is a useful modality if applied prudently in the assessment of the patient with chest pain; fortunately most patients do not have underlying heart disease. Echo can make the diagnosis of hypertrophic cardiomyopathy with or without left ventricular outflow tract obstruction. The left ventricular function is reduced in dilated cardiomyopathy and with myocarditis with reduced ventricular function. Pericardial fluid is easily identified, and in the setting of large effusions, tamponade physiology is marked by atrial wall collapse and variability of the Doppler flow velocity across the mitral valve or in the descending thoracic aorta. In Marfan syndrome, the aortic dimensions can be markedly increased; associated findings include mitral valve prolapse with or without mitral regurgitation and aortic regurgitation related to a dilated aortic root. Coronary artery dilation or aneurysm formation is virtually pathognomonic for Kawasaki disease in a patient with a history of a prolonged febrile illness. Patients with giant aneurysms are at particular risk for stenotic lesions at late follow-up. Although echo identification of these stenoses is difficult, chest pain in the presence of giant aneurysms should prompt further workup for coronary ischemia. The course and distribution of rare congenital coronary abnormalities predisposing to exertional chest pain can be visualized by echo, including single right or left coronary arteries.

Exercise Testing

In most patients with chest pain, exercise testing is not necessary. In some cases, rhythm abnormalities such as supraventricular tachycardia are unmasked during exercise testing. Ventricular arrhythmias can either suppress with exercise (generally thought to have benign implications) or degenerate during testing, potentially correlating with the patient's symptoms. When ischemia is suggested by history, treadmill exercise testing combined with stress echo can be useful, particularly in specific populations such as those with surgically reimplanted coronary arteries, coronary anomalies secondary to Kawasaki disease, and post-transplant vasculopathy.[16] In some cases, although the clinician is convinced that chest pain is unrelated to underlying heart disease or exercise-induced bronchospasm, exercise testing may be helpful to reassure an anxious family about the benign nature of the pain.

Syncope

Definition

Syncope is the transient and abrupt loss of consciousness resulting from a decrease in cerebral blood flow, resulting in a collapse with prompt and spontaneous recovery. Presyncope is characterized by symptoms including dizziness and visual changes that suggest an impending faint but that do not progress sufficiently to result in collapse. Although the etiology of syncope in children is usually benign and related to vasomotor instability, it is critical to differentiate benign syncope from life-threatening etiologies, which may be cardiac in origin.

Incidence

Syncope is common, with 30–50% of the population experiencing at least one syncopal event during childhood and adolescence.[17] Between the years 2021–2022, 1114 of 30,084 patients were evaluated in Boston Children's Hospital outpatient cardiology clinic for syncope, accounting for 3.7% of outpatient visits. Adolescent females are more often affected than adolescent boys.[17] Breath-holding spells are seen in up to 5% of toddlers, with boys and girls being equally affected.[18] The incidence of syncope in adulthood remains stable around 3–6 per 1000 person years with a distinct rise to 11 per 1000 person years at the age of 70 years.[19]

This high incidence of syncope contrasts with the exceptionally low incidence of cardiac-mediated syncope. In 480 patients referred to a pediatric cardiology practice for syncope, 22 (5%) had cardiac syncope. Of those, 21 were identified either by the historical linkage to exercise (10 of 153, 6%), abnormal ECG,[20] a concerning family history of arrhythmia, or abnormal physical examination.

Etiologies

Cardiac Syncope

Cardiac syncope occurs secondary to combinations of obstruction to left ventricular filling, obstruction to left ventricular outflow, or ineffective left ventricular contraction

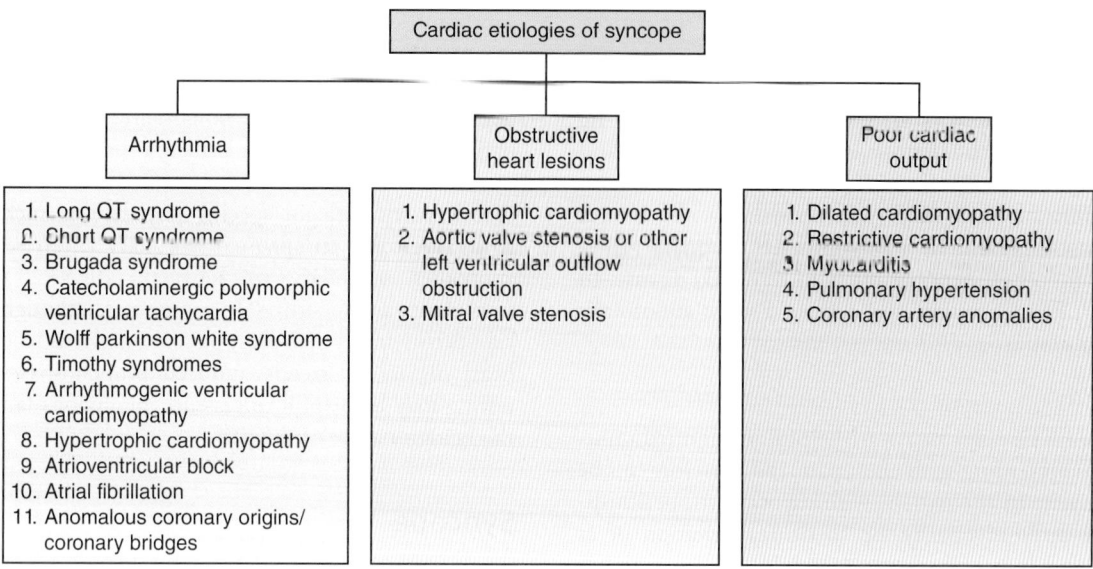

• **Fig. 52.1** Cardiac etiologies of syncope.

(Fig. 52.1). Details regarding these conditions will be discussed elsewhere in this text, but it is critical to recognize features of cardiac syncope to ensure thorough evaluation. Many (probably most) of the cases of cardiac syncope in childhood occur in people with previously diagnosed cardiac disease. History, abnormal ECG, or abnormal echocardiogram quickly clarifies the classification in most cases.

Clinical Features

Characteristics associated more commonly with cardiac syncope include syncope during exertion, a brief prodrome or lack of prodromal symptoms, injury, incontinence, syncope in the supine position, an abnormal cardiac exam, family history of inherited arrhythmias or sudden death, and presence of congenital heart disease.[17] Palpitations are sometimes noted but are not diagnostic in any clear fashion. While these features increase suspicion for cardiac syncope, none are diagnostic. When there is significant residual of confusion, disorientation, or need for CPR, the event is best classified as aborted sudden cardiac death. For transient events, recovery is similarly rapid. Indeed, the responses to arrhythmias and other transient impairments in cardiac output are in part determined by the effectiveness of baroreflex controls. Hence, the most critical distinction is whether there is historical or exam evidence of heart disease.

Autonomic Syncope

Autonomic syncope goes by many names, some of them emphasizing the dominant line of disordered cardiac and vascular regulation that results in symptoms. These include vasovagal syncope, cardio-inhibitory syncope, pallid breath-holding spells (or reflex anoxic seizures), vasodepressor syncope, postural orthostatic tachycardia syndrome (POTS), and many others. Although there are clear distinctions between both the clinical manifestations and the patients who demonstrate each subtype of physiology, we prefer the

summary terminology of neurally mediated or neurocardiogenic syncope, which emphasizes the interrelationships between each kind of syncope.

Vasovagal Syncope

Vasovagal syncope, the most common cause of syncope,[17] is caused by exaggerated physiologic responses to maintain adequate blood pressure. A complex series of hemodynamic changes occur leading up to the syncopal event. The initial change from the supine or seated to standing position results in 500–1000 mL of blood pooling to the lower half of the body. As this occurs, cardiac output decreases, as the heart rate has not yet compensated for this change in stroke volume. In children, though, there is a marked increase in heart rate during these initial hemodynamic changes. As a compensatory measure, the diastolic blood pressure rises due to baroreflex-mediated vasoconstriction of the peripheral vessels, which allows more blood to be directed back to the heart. After these changes, there is a fall in the systolic blood pressure and cardiac output. An increase in systemic vascular resistance is mediated by continued baroreflex-mediated vasoconstriction of peripheral arterioles. Next, there is a fall in cerebral blood flow velocity. Prior to the syncopal event, the systolic blood pressure falls further, accompanied by a decrease in heart rate and blood pressure variability. Autonomic activation and cerebral hypoperfusion lead to symptoms such as flushing, nausea, and vision change. When the systolic blood pressure falls sufficiently, a syncopal event occurs. The blood pressure recovers and heart rate normalizes in a matter of seconds as more blood flows into the central venous system and right heart, leading to recovery from the event.[21]

Clinical Features

Typical prodromal symptoms associated with vasovagal syncope include visual field changes, dizziness or lightheadedness, nausea, headache, diaphoresis or feeling hot or clammy, and palpitations. The syncopal event is short in duration, lasting less than 1–2 minutes. After the event, the individual may continue to feel somewhat dizzy, remain pale for minutes and is typically exhausted, often is diaphoretic and clammy, sometimes with a headache. Symptoms usually occur with position change to the standing position or when standing for a prolonged period, particularly in a hot environment. Individuals may experience vasovagal syncope after exercise, but any syncopal event which occurs during maximal exertion deserves complete evaluation for cardiac etiology. Vasovagal syncope can also occur in relation to a trigger such as pain, emotional stress, or the sight of blood. For single episodes, the only important reason for referral is parental or patient anxiety.

Postural Orthostatic Tachycardia Syndrome

POTS is defined as symptoms of orthostatic intolerance associated with an increase in heart rate of $\geq$ 40 bpm occurring within the first 10 minutes of standing or head-up tilt without associated hypotension. The orthostatic intolerance may or may not culminate in a syncopal event. The criteria to consider this diagnosis is more stringent in adolescents than the adult criteria of orthostatic pulse change of $\geq$ 30 bpm[22] and requires careful evaluation for alternative disease, including eating disorders. Among typical low-severity syncope, orthostatic heart rate increases of up to 35 bpm are common during a rapid 3-minute office screen for orthostasis. Orthostatic hypotension, in contrast, is quite rare.

Clinical Features
While syncopal events are rare in these patients, individuals may have recurrent presyncopal symptoms that may manifest as palpitations or exercise intolerance. These may include vision change, nausea, lightheadedness, and palpitations when assuming the upright position or when standing for prolonged periods of time. Like other syncope patients, there is an adolescent female dominance. Common conditions or symptoms that may occur concurrently include anxiety, especially a hyperawareness of somatic sensations, cognitive dysfunction, gastrointestinal disturbances, sleep disturbances, and headache. Recognition can guide subsequent diagnostic and therapy choices.

Exercise-Induced or Exercise-Associated Syncope

The rare deaths that have been reported in adolescents with syncope invariably highlight that syncope with exercise is a worrisome finding. Hypertrophic, dilated, and electrical myopathies all can present with exercise-associated syncope with no prior symptoms. All patients with syncope associated with exercise deserve prompt cardiac referral and additional testing with at least an echocardiogram if no diagnosis is apparent on initial evaluation.

Exercise also represents an almost optimal trigger for neurally mediated syncope. Particularly with highly dynamic sports like distance running, the cardiovascular response to

exercise is to vasodilate, increase sympathetic output, and shift blood flow to the legs. During running, the skeletal muscle pump action of the leg muscles enhances venous return, facilitating increased cardiac output. Immediately after exertion, that pump function is decreased or absent and can permit the same reflex responses seen in any other example of venous pooling. When an initial evaluation does not identify clear heart disease, most cases of exercise-induced syncope can eventually be demonstrated to be some form of neurally mediated syncope.[23]

Breath-Holding Spells

These events typically occur in toddlers and are relatively common, affecting 0.1–4.6% of healthy children.[18] These are benign, though often frightening, events, and while the mechanism of syncope as a result of breath-holding is not clearly defined, it may be similar to neurally mediated syncope which occurs in adolescents and adults. A combination of diminished venous return and an enhanced adrenergic state (a prolonged cry in combination with anger/irritability) mimics conditions that elicit syncope in adults (tilt table test with administration of isoproterenol). Overstimulation of parasympathetic activity is a key driver, and studies have shown a hypersensitive cardio-inhibitory response to ocular compression in children who have had breath-holding spells.[18]

Clinical Features
This is a generally stereotypical syndrome of paroxysmal collapse in toddlers. In the typical spell, a trivial physical or emotional trauma triggers an aborted cry, opisthotonic stiffening, and pallor that resolves over 10–60 seconds, usually followed by several minutes of sleepiness. The syncopal event may occur up to 30 seconds after the minor triggering event and is due to sinus bradycardia. Rarely, such spells trigger true seizures. They contrast and overlap with classic breath-holding spells, with ongoing crying with cyanosis, breath-holding, and then symptoms. Onset is typically between age 6 months and 18 months, with termination in more than 65% of cases by age 5 years and in the vast majority by age 8 years.[18]

Diagnostic Evaluation

Similar to the experience in evaluating heart murmurs in the minimally symptomatic child, the diagnosis of autonomic syncope can be confidently made in most children with a detailed history, physical examination, and ECG.

The history is the critical test and focuses on triggers, presyncopal symptoms that can serve as both clues to the physiology and a proxy for therapy efforts, and some assessment of the severity of symptoms. A 10-point visual analogue scale (0, no symptoms, 10 constant dizziness and recurrent syncope) allows rapid self-assessment and a quick way to track symptoms over time. Family history focuses on a history of sudden unexpected death before age 40, congenital deafness, or cardiomyopathy, all of which are worrisome, and the common history of recurrent adolescent or toddler syncope that was outgrown.

Physical examination can be focused but should be designed to offer several opportunities for identifying anatomic and physiologic abnormalities. While there is no consensus that all patients with syncope require formal orthostatic vital signs, auscultation with isometrics and while the patient is both supine and after standing permits examining for orthostatic pulse and for transient murmurs from dynamic subaortic stenosis and mitral valve prolapse. A brief neurologic examination and examination for joint hypermobility (such as a Beighton score) can identify contributing physiology. Focused history and examination should explore signs and symptoms of systemic disease, connective tissue disorders like Marfan syndrome, and underlying eating disorders.

Regarding breath-holding spells in toddlers, when isolated and typical, management is typically driven by the primary care physician with little formal investigation. When recurrent, evaluation for anemia, arrhythmia, and epilepsy is appropriate. Recurrent pallid breath holding spells (also called reflex anoxic seizures or "white syncope") may motivate extended rhythm monitoring. Although the level of bradycardia can be quite impressive, most toddlers have infrequent episodes that resolve without specific therapy.

Electrocardiography

The ECG is examined for left ventricular hypertrophy, Wolff-Parkinson-White syndrome, atrioventricular and interventricular conduction defects, and a prolonged QT interval. The ECG is an imperfect screen for hypertrophic cardiomyopathy and has no value in screening for most coronary anomalies that present after the first year of life. It is not surprising to see somewhat prominent respiratory sinus arrhythmia. For patients with combinations of borderline ECGs or worrisome family histories, ECGs on siblings and parents are useful tools. Ambulatory ECG monitoring, including 24-hour Holter monitors, portable event monitoring, and, rarely, implantable loop recorders, can each be useful in correlating clinical symptoms with arrhythmias, although, like echocardiograms, the primary yield is demonstrating the absence of serious disease. The ECG immediately following a faint is more likely to have mildly increased QTc.[24]

Echocardiography

Routine echo screening for syncope referred to pediatric cardiology has a low yield, with incidental findings noted in 11%, determined to be unrelated to the syncopal event.[25] Even with relatively precise indications, cardiologists will obtain echocardiograms in 20% or more of patients with benign-appearing syncope so that the burden of incidental findings has the potential to be substantial. A careful echocardiographic examination, including examination of the coronary origins,[26] is indicated when the history, physical, ECG, or family history is suggestive of cardiac disease or

cardiac syncope, or when the frequency of the episodes is becoming worrisome.

Cardiac Computed Tomography and Cardiac Magnetic Resonance Imaging

Cardiac magnetic resonance imaging (CMRI) or cardiac computed tomography (CT) can be useful in the rare events that cardiac syncope is suspected and anatomy is not fully delineated by echocardiography. Specifically, in cases concerning for anomalous origin of a coronary artery (syncopal or presyncopal events during exertion with lack of prodromal symptoms), a cardiac CT can identify coronary artery origins and assess for areas of narrowing or compression. For patients in whom hypertrophic cardiomyopathy is suspected and echocardiography is inconclusive, CMRI can help clarify the diagnosis. CMRI also plays a role in the diagnosis of arrhythmogenic cardiomyopathy, which may present with cardiac syncope and is discussed in detail elsewhere in this text.

Cardiac Catheterization

For patients with structurally and functionally normal hearts by echocardiogram, nondiagnostic or normal ECGs, and unrevealing ambulatory monitoring, there is little to no yield in cardiac catheterization, even if it includes programmed electrical stimulation. Most pediatric echocardiography laboratories can adequately image the coronaries to exclude anomalous coronaries. Other diagnoses are effectively excluded by echocardiogram or may require drug challenges.

For patients with congenital heart disease, particularly those with combinations of syncope, palpitations, nonsustained ventricular tachycardia, or other arrhythmias, cardiac catheterization, including programmed atrial and ventricular stimulation and appropriate hemodynamic evaluation, may be indicated. The role of catheterization in evaluating arrhythmia risk in patients with cardiomyopathy remains poorly defined.

Other Studies

Head-up tilt testing is an effective way to recreate neurally mediated syncope and can be effectively performed in adolescents. Unfortunately, these same maneuvers can induce syncope in completely asymptomatic adolescent volunteers,[27] of whom up to 40% will have presyncopal symptoms with a 70-degree tilt.

Because of the high incidence of false-positive results, head-up tilt testing cannot be viewed as a diagnostic test. Rather, it should be used as confirmatory test or a physiologic probe. At Boston Children's Hospital and many other larger pediatric centers, use of head-up tilt testing has declined, so the test has evolved as an infrequently used tool for exploring challenging and recurrent symptoms.

Treadmill exercise testing has a poorly defined role in evaluating patients with syncope. It has advantages of being relatively nonthreatening, easy to obtain, and a reasonable screen for a number of occult arrhythmias. In some series, as many as 15% to 20% of syncope patients recreated their symptoms during or immediately after exercise. At Boston Children's Hospital, exercise testing is obtained more frequently than head-up tilt testing in patients with problematic syncope, although it is still performed in less than 5% of patients with syncope.

Management

For cardiac syncope, therapy is directed at the underlying disorder. For autonomic syncope, the episodic, self-resolving nature of the disorder contributes to inadequate double-blind, placebo-controlled data regarding therapeutic choices in adults and even fewer data in children. Therapy recommendations are based on limited series, more limited trials, and rational planning based on the clinical physiology.

Nonpharmacologic, Non-Device Therapy

The episodic nature of syncope, its benign natural history, and the lack of perfect drug therapy lead to an initial non-pharmacologic approach. Education regarding the nature of syncopal events and ways to either prevent or abort spells represents the cornerstone of therapy. Most patients will have significant relief with a combination of aggressive hydration, including increased fluid, decreased caffeine, and increased sodium intake, and antigravity maneuvers, including isometric leg or arm contractions, staged shifts from supine to upright, squatting or lying down with onset of presyncopal symptoms, and use of compression stockings. Upright, weight-bearing aerobic exercise may also be beneficial.

For many cases of situational syncope, behavioral therapy is critical. When patients will not accept a purely behavioral approach, many accept a combined approach of modest medical therapy along with a cognitive-behavioral approach through psychiatry.

Pharmacologic Therapy

Pharmacologic management focuses on volume enhancement, limiting excessive catecholamine drive, blood pressure augmentation, and rarely anticholinergic therapy. In refractory cases, the effects of these agents appear at least additive, and many have been used in combination. When drug therapy is needed, therapy is typically continued for about 1 year, followed by trials of decreasing therapy.

Fludrocortisone is typically a first-line agent, though its effectiveness in pediatric patients is unclear. An essentially pure mineralocorticoid, fludrocortisone appears to work by increasing blood volume by enhancing sodium renal reabsorption. Advantages include rare side effects, once-daily dosing, and low cost. Disadvantages include slow onset of action and, particularly with higher doses, the potential for chronic hypokalemia or chronic hypertension, although the incidence of those side effects is low. Low doses, by themselves, are ineffective for severe postural tachycardia symptoms. There is only one small pediatric randomized control trial, which demonstrated that children with recurrent syncope had more improvement on placebo than fludrocortisone and salt.

Though the use of beta-blockers is relatively common in the management of pediatric syncope, evidence is lacking to prove their benefit.[28] The use of beta-blockers for syncope aims at decreasing excessive catecholamine stimulation and hence blunting catecholamine-mediated vasodilation and, potentially, cardiac sensory triggers associated with a hyperdynamic, underfilled left ventricle.

Midodrine hydrochloride is a unique prodrug that is metabolized into a peripherally active direct α_1 agonist. Small randomized control trials demonstrate a benefit in symptom reduction in those with vasovagal syncope.[29] Side effects are related to its direct drug effects and include piloerection, scalp itching, and, rarely, urinary symptoms. Advantages of midodrine include its direct and rapid action, allowing titration when required, and the very narrow therapeutic effect. Disadvantages include a short duration of action (3–5 hours) and high cost, limiting its use to highly symptomatic and highly motivated patients.

Ivabradine is a newer agent that may improve symptoms related to POTS. This medication acts on the I_f or "funny" current highly expressed within the sinoatrial node to slow the heart rate. A randomized, double-blinded placebo control trial of 22 patients demonstrated that ivabradine lowers heart rate and improves quality of life in patients with hyperadrenergic POTS.[30]

For highly refractory syncope with documented, clinical pauses, both ventricular and dual-chamber pacing have been effective at decreasing, but not eliminating, symptoms. The published pediatric experience is very limited, and at Boston Children's Hospital, this was the indication for pacing in approximately 2% of pacemakers, meaning one has been placed for this indication every 1–3 years.

Prognosis

Autonomic syncope is not associated with increased risk for mortality. Toddlers with breath-holding spells are more likely to have autonomic syncope than adolescents, but symptoms resolve in most by age 4 years. Most adolescents, even those most disabled, appear to outgrow their episodes over several years. For teens, improvement may result from effective use of behavioral and physical approaches to their symptoms.

References

1. Epstein N. The heart in normal infants and children; incidence of precordial systolic murmurs and fluoroscopic and electrocardiographic studies. *J Pediatr.* 1948;32:39-45.
2. Tsao CW, Aday AW, Almarzooq ZI, et al. Heart disease and stroke statistics—2022 update: a report from the American Heart Association. *Circulation.* 2022;145:e153-e639.
3. Yoon SA, Hong WH, Cho HJ. Congenital heart disease diagnosed with echocardiogram in newborns with asymptomatic cardiac murmurs: a systematic review. *BMC Pediatr.* 2020;20:322.

4. McCrindle BW, Shaffer KM, Kan JS, et al. Cardinal clinical signs in the differentiation of heart murmurs in children. *Arch Pediatr Adolesc Med*. 1996;150:169-174.

5. Fogel DH. The innocent systolic murmur in children: a clinical study of its incidence and characteristics. *Am Heart J*. 1960;59:844-855.

6. Danilowicz DA, Rudolph AM, Hoffman JI, et al. Physiologic pressure differences between main and branch pulmonary arteries in infants. *Circulation*. 1972;45:410-419.

7. Danford DA, Nasir A, Gumbiner C. Cost assessment of the evaluation of heart murmurs in children. *Pediatrics*. 1993;91:365-368.

8. American College of Cardiology Foundation Appropriate Use Criteria Task Force, American Society of Echocardiography, American Heart Association, et al. ACCF/ASE/AHA/ASNC/HFSA/HRS/SCAI/SCCM/SCCT/SCMR 2011 appropriate use criteria for echocardiography: a report of the American College of Cardiology Foundation Appropriate Use Criteria Task Force, American Society of Echocardiography, American Heart Association, American Society of Nuclear Cardiology, Heart Failure Society of America, Heart Rhythm Society, Society for Cardiovascular Angiography and Interventions, Society of Critical Care Medicine, Society of Cardiovascular Computed Tomography, Society for Cardiovascular Magnetic Resonance American College of Chest Physicians. *J Am Soc Echocardiogr*. 2011;24:229-267.

9. Marienfeld CJ, Telles N, Silvera J, et al. A 20-year follow-up study of "innocent" murmurs. *Pediatrics*. 1962;30:42-48.

10. Kane DA, Fulton DR, Saleeb S, et al. Needles in hay: chest pain as the presenting symptom in children with serious underlying cardiac pathology. *Congenit Heart Dis*. 2010;5:366-373.

11. Saleeb SF, Li WY, Warren SZ, et al. Effectiveness of screening for life-threatening chest pain in children. *Pediatrics*. 2011;128:e1062-e1068.

12. Brown RT. Costochondritis in adolescents. *J Adolesc Health Care*. 1981;1:198-201.

13. Yetman AT, McCrindle BW, MacDonald C, et al. Myocardial bridging in children with hypertrophic cardiomyopathy: a risk factor for sudden death. *N Engl J Med*. 1998;339:1201-1209.

14. McCrindle BW, Rowley AH, Newburger JW, et al. Diagnosis, treatment, and long-term management of Kawasaki disease: a scientific statement for health professionals from the American Heart Association. *Circulation*. 2017;135:e927-e999.

15. Basso C, Maron BJ, Corrado D, et al. Clinical profile of congenital coronary artery anomalies with origin from the wrong aortic sinus leading to sudden death in young competitive athletes. *J Am Coll Cardiol*. 2000;35:1493-1501.

16. Ermis P. Stress echocardiography: an overview for use in pediatric and congenital cardiology. *Congenit Heart Dis*. 2017;12:624-626.

17. Writing Committee M, Shen WK, Sheldon RS, et al. 2017 ACC/AHA/HRS guideline for the evaluation and management of patients with syncope: a report of the American College of Cardiology/American Heart Association Task Force on Clinical Practice Guidelines and the Heart Rhythm Society. *Heart Rhythm*. 2017;14:e155-e217.

18. Leung AKC, Leung AAM, Wong AHC, Hon KL. Breath-holding spells in pediatrics: a narrative review of the current evidence. *Curr Pediatr Rev*. 2019;15:22-29.

19. Soteriades ES, Evans JC, Larson MG, et al. Incidence and prognosis of syncope. *N Engl J Med*. 2002;347:878-885.

20. Ritter S, Tani LY, Etheridge SP, et al. What is the yield of screening echocardiography in pediatric syncope? *Pediatrics*. 2000;105:E58.

21. Jardine DL, Wieling W, Brignole M, et al. The pathophysiology of the vasovagal response. *Heart Rhythm*. 2018;15:921-929.

22. Freeman R, Wieling W, Axelrod FB, et al. Consensus statement on the definition of orthostatic hypotension, neurally mediated syncope and the postural tachycardia syndrome. *Clin Auton Res*. 2011;21:69-72.

23. Sakaguchi S, Shultz JJ, Remole SC, et al. Syncope associated with exercise, a manifestation of neurally mediated syncope. *Am J Cardiol*. 1995;75:476-481.

24. Van Dorn CS, Johnson JN, Taggart NW, et al. QTc values among children and adolescents presenting to the emergency department. *Pediatrics*. 2011;128:e1395-e1401.

25. Paris Y, Toro-Salazar OH, Gauthier NS, et al. Regional implementation of a pediatric cardiology syncope algorithm using standardized clinical assessment and management plans (SCAMPS) methodology. *J Am Heart Assoc*. 2016;5:e002931.

26. Stefanelli CB, Stevenson JG, Jones TK, et al. A case for routine screening of coronary artery origins during echocardiography: fortuitous discovery of a life-threatening coronary anomaly. *J Am Soc Echocardiogr*. 1999;12:769-772.

27. Lewis DA, Zlotocha J, Henke L, et al. Specificity of head-up tilt testing in adolescents: effect of various degrees of tilt challenge in normal control subjects. *J Am Coll Cardiol*. 1997;30:1057-1060.

28. 2018 ESC Guidelines for the diagnosis and management of syncope. *Rev Esp Cardiol (Engl Ed)*. 2018;71:837.

29. Sheldon R, Faris P, Tang A, et al. Midodrine for the prevention of vasovagal syncope: a randomized clinical trial. *Ann Intern Med*. 2021;174:1349-1356.

30. Taub PR, Zadourian A, Lo HC, et al. Randomized trial of ivabradine in patients with hyperadrenergic postural orthostatic tachycardia syndrome. *J Am Coll Cardiol*. 2021;77:861-871.

53

Congestive Heart Failure

PAUL ESTESO AND TAJINDER SINGH

KEY LEARNING POINTS

- Heart failure is a clinical syndrome characterized by vascular congestion with elevated filling pressures and compromised perfusion. Management is characterized by well-defined phases:
- On presentation, most patients are acutely decompensated and require stabilization to normalize physiology. This may include use of oral and intravenous medications, respiratory support, sedation, and additional therapies.
- Once stabilized, patients should be transitioned, when possible, to medications demonstrated to improve heart function, decrease heart failure mortality, and encourage

reverse remodeling. Examples include angiotensin-converting enzyme inhibitors, mineralocorticoid receptor antagonists, and beta-blockers. These should be uptitrated to goal therapeutic doses and supplemented with medications intended to improve symptoms (e.g., diuretics) while monitoring volume status and perfusion.
- Over the long term, patients need ongoing monitoring and weight-based titration of medications. When heart failure is refractory to medical management, patients may require additional advanced therapies such as mechanical circulatory support and heart transplantation.

Definition

Heart failure (HF) is a clinical syndrome resulting from the heart's inability to provide for the body's hemodynamic and metabolic demands while maintaining normal filling pressures. It is usually associated with structural and/or functional cardiac abnormalities and is characterized acutely by low cardiac output and/or congestion, and chronically by growth failure.[1]

Epidemiology

The reported incidence of pediatric HF ranges from 0.87 to 7.4 cases per 100,000 children per year.[2] The incidence varies by factors such as age, country, and socioeconomic status, among others. For example, rheumatic heart disease and unrepaired congenital heart disease (CHD) are common causes of HF in developing countries, whereas cardiomyopathies and repaired CHD are more common in developed countries. In the United States, the rate of hospitalization for HF has doubled between 2004 and 2018, with 94% of hospitalized patients having CHD.[3]

Etiology

HF may ensue when normal hemodynamic demands are imposed on abnormal myocardium (e.g., cardiomyopathy),

when volume or pressure overload are imposed on normal myocardium (e.g., left-to-right shunts or obstructive lesions), or when a combination of the two occurs. The distinction as to the absence or presence of systemic ventricular dysfunction and consideration of the etiology (Tables 53.1 and 53.2) are fundamental to the management of HF in children. For most forms of unrepaired CHD, repair of the underlying anatomic abnormality ameliorates the HF syndrome. Children with HF due to systemic ventricular dysfunction, such as those with cardiomyopathy, or those with repaired CHD in the absence of residual lesions, need medical HF therapy to optimize symptoms and ventricular function.

Structural Heart Disease with Normal Ventricular Function

Two hemodynamic abnormalities, volume overload and pressure overload, prevalent in children with CHD may lead to HF. Volume overload is usually due to left-to-right shunt lesions (e.g., large ventricular septal defect) or valvar regurgitation. Children with volume overload may present with clinical HF despite normal ventricular function. Pressure overload arises from outflow obstruction, and when severe, can lead to inadequate cardiac output. Depending on the severity and chronicity, outflow obstruction can be

TABLE 53.1	Causes of Heart Failure in Infants and Children with Preserved Ventricular Function

Volume Overload

Left-to-Right Shunting

Septal defect (VSD, CAVC, rarely ASD)

Patent ductus arteriosus

Totally anomalous pulmonary venous return

Aortopulmonary window

Single ventricle (especially with excessive pulmonary blood flow)

Valvular insufficiency

Non-Cardiac Causes

Arteriovenous malformation

Fluid overload

Anemia

Twin-twin transfusion

Pressure Overload

Left-Sided

Aortic stenosis

Aortic coarctation

Systemic hypertension

Right-Sided

Pulmonary valve stenosis

Pulmonary vein stenosis

Pulmonary hypertension

Mitral stenosis

ASD, Atrial septal defect; *CAVC,* complete atrioventricular canal defect; *VSD,* ventricular septal defect.

TABLE 53.2	Causes of Heart Failure in Infants and Children with Ventricular Dysfunction

Structurally Normal Heart

Cardiomyopathy

Myocarditis

Myocardial Infarction/Ischemia

Anomalous left coronary artery arising off the pulmonary artery (ALCAPA)

Kawasaki disease with coronary artery aneurysm

Coronary vasculitis

Premature atherosclerotic coronary artery disease (genetic dyslipidemia)

Arrhythmogenic

Complete heart block

Supraventricular tachycardia

Ventricular tachycardia

Ventricular pacing induced dysfunction

Non-Cardiac Causes

Sepsis

Renal failure

Respiratory disorders

HIV infection

Systemic Lupus Erythematosus

Iron overload

Drug/toxin exposure (e.g., anthracyclines)

Metabolic disease and endocrinopathies (may present with preserved ventricular function)

Congenital Heart Disease (CHD)

Complex CHD with concurrent ventricular dysfunction

Surgically corrected CHD with late ventricular dysfunction ("burnt-out" CHD)

asymptomatic, when mild and chronic, or lead to decompensated HF or cardiovascular collapse, when acute and severe (such as occurs with a saddle pulmonary embolus). The presence of significant outflow obstruction is of critical importance in the neonatal period as the ductus arteriosus closes and unmasks significant obstructive lesions such as aortic or pulmonary stenosis, or coarctation of the aorta. Systemic and pulmonary hypertension may also lead to chronic ventricular pressure overload. When obstruction to venous pathways is present, congestion and elevated filling pressures predominate.

Structurally Normal Heart with Ventricular Dysfunction

Cardiomyopathy is the most common cause of HF among children with a structurally normal heart with an incidence of approximately 1 case per 100,000 children per year.[4]

Dilated cardiomyopathy (DCM) accounts for just over 50% of cases, hypertrophic cardiomyopathy (HCM) accounts for most remaining cases, with a small proportion of patients having either restrictive cardiomyopathy (RCM) or arrhythmogenic cardiomyopathy (ACM).[5] Left ventricular (LV) systolic dysfunction (impaired ejection) is the predominant physiologic derangement in children with DCM, although it is often associated with secondarily elevated filling pressures. Children with HCM usually have preserved systolic function except those presenting in infancy, who often have systolic dysfunction. Children with RCM usually present with diastolic HF due to impaired ventricular filling with elevated filling pressures but normal systolic function. The presence of dysfunction in patients with ACM is variable.

Myocarditis, cardiotoxic medications, myocardial ischemia, and arrhythmias can cause HF in children. Myocarditis has an annual incidence of 1–2 cases per 100,000 children and usually presents with LV systolic dysfunction.[6] Viral infections are the most common causes of myocarditis. In children with newly diagnosed ventricular dysfunction with a structurally normal heart, consideration of myocarditis is of importance given relatively better long-term outcomes compared to children with cardiomyopathy.[7] Anthracyclines, used to treat children with cancer, are an important cause of ventricular dysfunction and HF in developed countries. Their effects can be acute or chronic and delayed, especially in those who have undergone chest radiation.[8] Myocardial ischemia is an uncommon cause of ventricular dysfunction and HF in children. Anomalous origin of the left coronary artery from pulmonary artery is an important diagnosis to be considered in infants with HF; it is amenable to surgical correction with excellent long-term prognosis. Children with Kawasaki disease and coronary aneurysms are at a particularly high risk of coronary thrombus and require management and surveillance to manage ischemic risk. Arrhythmias, such as complete heart block, or atrial and ventricular tachyarrhythmias, can lead to ventricular dysfunction and HF. Successful management of the arrhythmia typically leads to recovery of ventricular function, though some require medical therapy for HF in the short term.

Ventricular dysfunction and HF may occur in association with systemic diseases. Examples include HIV infection, acute rheumatic fever (usually with valvar dysfunction), sepsis (septic shock), renal disease (severe renal hypertension or chronic kidney disease), and inflammatory conditions (systemic lupus erythematosus). Metabolic disorders associated with inborn errors of metabolism and mitochondrial function, or myocardial iron deposition, as seen in hemochromatosis or thalassemia, may also cause ventricular dysfunction. Right ventricular failure due to pulmonary hypertension may be seen as a consequence of primary pulmonary conditions, as well as in systemic diseases.

Congenital Heart Disease with Ventricular Dysfunction

Ventricular dysfunction in children with CHD may be due to the hemodynamic consequence of the unrepaired defect, residual lesions in patients who have undergone repair, long-term effects of the CHD such as arrhythmias, history of ventriculotomy, or the result of surgical complication. A small proportion of patients with CHD may also have abnormal myocardium. Notably, an analysis of the single-ventricle reconstruction randomized controlled trial (RCT) at 6 years revealed that 14.3% of patients surviving to hospital discharge without heart transplantation after a Norwood operation develop severe HF, with half of those dying by 6 years of age.[9] As surgical and postoperative critical care techniques evolve, patients with increasingly

complex CHD are surviving longer, and the proportion of HF patients with CHD continues to increase.

Pathophysiology

Under normal conditions, a fall in blood pressure is detected by the central arterial baroreceptors and leads to activation of the sympathetic nervous system (SNS). This results in tachycardia, stimulation of myocardial contractility, and regional vasoconstriction. Furthermore, any decrease in renal perfusion leads to stimulation of the juxta-glomerular apparatus with activation of the renin-angiotensin-aldosterone system (RAAS), resulting in systemic vasoconstriction as well as sodium and fluid retention. The rise in vascular tone and volume improves cardiac filling and restores cardiac output through utilization of preload reserve. These finely tuned physiologic mechanisms maintain pressure, flow, and vascular volume within narrow limits.

In HF, there is diminished cardiac capacity and preload reserve recruitment is unable to restore cardiac output to normal without a significant rise in filling pressures. Thus, the symptoms of HF, due to fluid overload and low cardiac output, ensue. The SNS and RAAS are critical to maintaining adequate cardiac output, but sustained activation of these systems is maladaptive and worsens the circulatory disorder. Chronic activation of the RAAS leads to myocyte fibrosis, apoptosis, and pathologic remodeling. Chronic activation of the SNS leads to reduction in norepinephrine stores and in β-adrenergic receptor density, impairing inotropic reserve. Chronically elevated filling pressure also stimulates ventricular remodeling (dilation and dysfunction) by increasing diastolic capacitance at the expense of elevated systolic wall stress and myocardial oxygen consumption.[10]

Categorization

Understanding of the longitudinal trajectory and associated management of patients with HF is aided using stage and severity criteria. The stages of pediatric HF proceed from patients at risk for HF (stage A), to those with pre-HF, defined as structural or functional abnormalities with no current or previous HF symptoms (stage B), to those with current or previous medication responsive HF (stage C), and finally to medication refractory or end-stage HF (stage D) (Fig. 53.1).[11]

The symptomatic stages of HF are further subdivided for those over 6 years of age by New York Heart Association, and, for young children, by the Ross functional classifications (Table 53.3). Class I patients are asymptomatic, while increasing functional class refers to patient who become symptomatic with decreasing demand. Class IV patients are symptomatic at rest.

Presentation

The presenting signs and symptoms of HF are due to low cardiac output and vascular congestion from elevated left

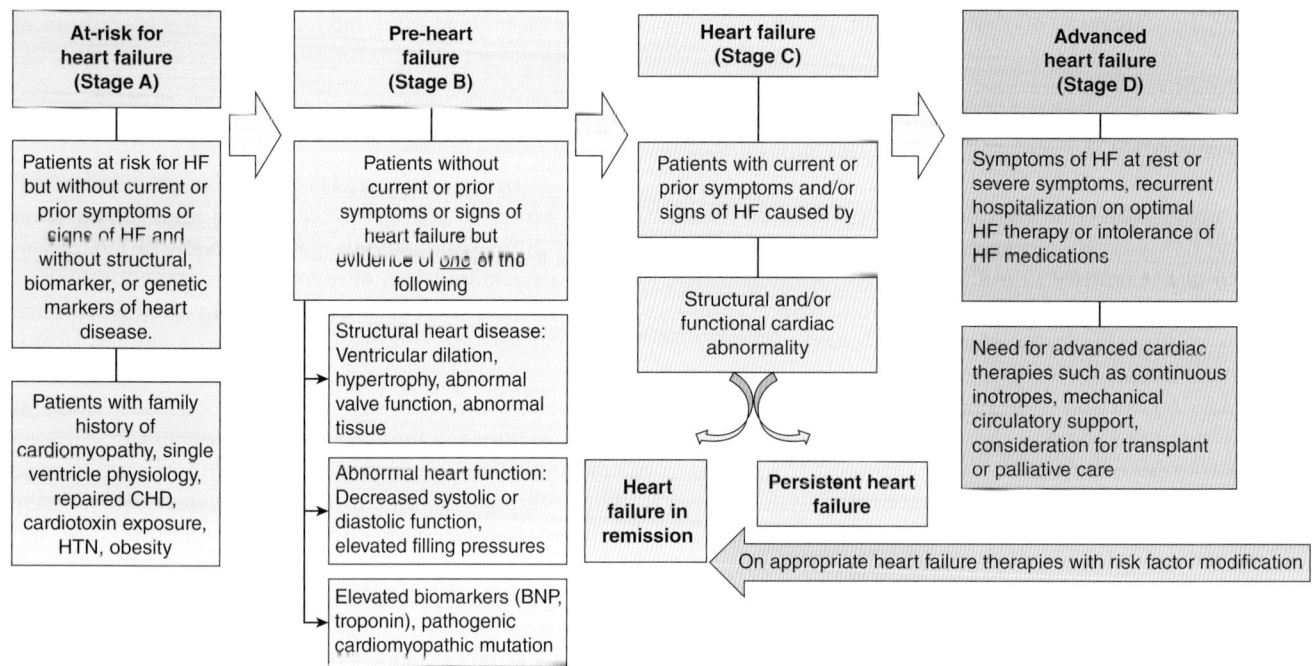

• **Fig. 53.1** Stages of pediatric heart failure. *BNP,* Brain natriuretic peptide; *CHD,* congenital heart disease; *HF,* heart failure; *HTN,* hypertension. (Adapted from Bozkurt B, Coats A, Tsutsui H, et al. Universal definition and classification of heart failure. *J Card Fail.* 2021;27:387–413.)

TABLE 53.3 Functional Classification of Pediatric and Adult Heart Failure

	New York Heart Association	Ross
Class I	No limitations of physical activity	No limitations or symptoms
Class II	Fatigue, palpitations, dyspnea, or angina during moderate exercise	Infants: Mild tachypnea or diaphoresis with feeding Older children: Mild to moderate dyspnea on exertion
Class III	Symptoms with minimal exertion that interfere with normal daily activity	Infants: Growth failure and marked tachypnea on exertion Older children: Marked dyspnea on exertion
Class IV	Symptoms at rest that worsen with exertion	Symptoms at rest such as tachypnea, retractions, grunting, or diaphoresis

Adapted from Kirk R, Dipchand AI, Rosenthal DN, et al. The International Society for Heart and Lung Transplantation Guidelines for the management of pediatric heart failure: Executive summary. [Corrected]. *J Heart Lung Transplant.* 2014;33:888–909.

atrial and/or right atrial pressures. Tachycardia is a reflexive response to diminished stroke volume in an attempt to maintain cardiac output. Presentation is often age specific. In infants, respiratory and feeding difficulties are most salient; they include prolonged feeding times, sweating, increased work of breathing, and emesis secondary to intestinal congestion and decreased perfusion. Failure to thrive is a marker of chronic HF. On examination, tachycardia and tachypnea are common findings. With severe HF, nasal flaring, intercostal retractions, and grunting may be seen. Occasionally, chest auscultation reveals wheezing, however, rales are rare. Edema is often not apparent, with the exception of hepatomegaly. Cool extremities, slow capillary refill, weak pulses, low arterial blood pressure, and narrow pulse pressures are signs of low cardiac output and may signal potential cardiovascular collapse.

Presentation in the older child more closely resembles that of adults. Exertional dyspnea is common and correlates with the degree of HF. Fatigue may lead these children to gravitate towards sedentary activities. On physical examination, children with mild HF may not be in any distress, whereas those with severe HF may be dyspneic at rest. Children in chronic failure may appear malnourished, while those with advanced HF are usually tachycardic and tachypneic. Cool extremities, pallor, poor capillary refill, and hypotension suggest low cardiac output. Hepatomegaly and peripheral edema, especially around the eyelids, may be present due to elevated right atrial pressure. Some patients have ascites, pericardial, and pleural effusions. A gallop rhythm may be present. Pulsus alternans, when present, suggests severe LV systolic dysfunction and is characterized by alternating strong and weak (or absent) pulse volume.

Evaluation

A complete diagnosis of HF requires a combination of clinical, imaging, and laboratory assessment. Clinical diagnosis should lead to laboratory evaluation of end-organ perfusion (renal function, hepatic function, troponin), brain natriuretic peptide (BNP) (elevated in HF), anemia, and iron deficiency (a common finding in HF). A detailed family history and genetic testing are important in evaluating children with suspected cardiomyopathy and systemic disorders. Evaluation of metabolic and thyroid function should be included in the screening of these patients.

Echocardiographic evaluation is necessary to evaluate for the presence or absence of CHD, ventricular, and valve function. Evaluation of possible exacerbating factors and underlying etiologies should be pursued. Chest radiography is useful for assessing heart size, pulmonary congestion, and pulmonary processes such as pneumonia or effusions. Electrocardiogram (ECG) is useful to assess rhythm (e.g., sinus tachycardia, tachyarrhythmia, or heart block) and presence/absence of ischemia, chamber enlargement, and ventricular hypertrophy. In patients with acute decompensated HF and severe cardiorespiratory compromise, prompt treatment to restore a stable circulation should be prioritized. Given the possibility of ductal-dependent lesions, neonates presenting with unexplained shock should be started on prostaglandin infusion to reestablish patency of the ductus arteriosus.

Additional Evaluation

Continuous heart rate monitoring (inpatient telemetry or ambulatory ECG monitoring) helps in evaluating the presence and prevalence of arrhythmia. Additional tests that may be useful in selected patients include cardiac catheterization, magnetic resonance imaging (MRI), and exercise testing. Cardiac catheterization allows measurement of cardiac output and filling pressures, assessment of pulmonary hypertension, pulmonary vascular resistance (PVR), and vasoreactivity which may be used to guide therapy, and determination of candidacy for ventricular assist device (VAD) and heart transplantation if indicated. In the evaluation of clinical myocarditis, it provides the opportunity for an endomyocardial biopsy. Coronary angiography is of critical importance in evaluating coronary anomalies. Furthermore, catheterization-based interventions (e.g., coiling of collateral vessels, relief of vascular or valvar stenoses) may have therapeutic roles in some patients with HF. Cardiac MRI may be useful in the assessment of anatomy, ventricular function, myocarditis, quantification of fibrosis, and presence of iron overload. Exercise testing may be helpful in determining functional capacity and risk of exercise-induced arrhythmia or ischemia.

Daily Assessment

Clinical evaluation of patients with HF should focus on assessment of perfusion (cardiac output) and fluid overload (Fig. 53.2).[12] In hospitalized patients, this includes daily measurement of 24-hour fluid intake, urine output, and morning post-void weight. Changes in signs, symptoms, and monitored data are helpful in placing patients on the congestion (wet or dry), and perfusion (cold or warm) scales, which may then be used to modify medical therapy. In outpatients, daily morning post-void weight may be useful for guiding adjustments in diuretic therapy.

Management

The focus of this section is management of HF patients with systemic ventricular dysfunction. The goals of therapy are to improve patient symptoms, promote ventricular reverse remodeling (reduce ventricular dilation and improve function), and to improve survival. Prompt identification of precipitating factors and anatomic lesions, if present, is important since intervention may be warranted. There are similarities in pediatric patients with regards to hemodynamics (elevated filling pressures, low cardiac output), pathophysiology (activation of SNS and RAAS), and phenotype (ventricular dilation, systolic dysfunction) to adults with HF. Furthermore, due to the low prevalence in children, the pharmacologic treatment of pediatric HF is extrapolated from large, RCTs in adults.

Management of adults with HF is often referred to as guideline-directed medical therapy (GDMT) and is based on a guideline document published by the American Heart Association and the American College of Cardiology.[13] GDMT emphasizes medical therapy demonstrated to improve survival as shown in large RCTs (Fig. 53.3).[14] The recommendations correspond to patients at different HF stages: no therapy in stage A, afterload reduction in stage B,

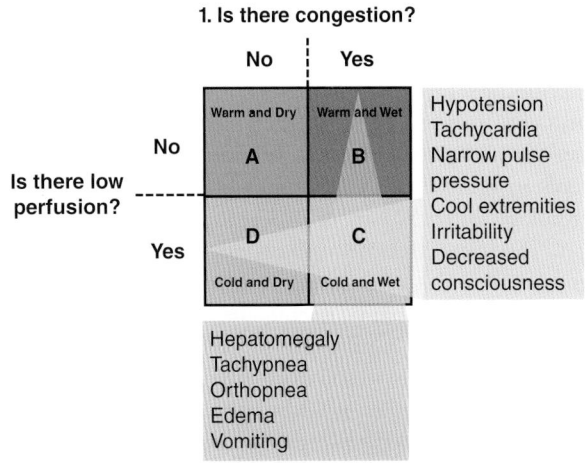

• **Fig. 53.2** Bedside assessment of pediatric heart failure. (Adapted from Kantor PF, Lougheed J, Dancea A, et al. Presentation, diagnosis, and medical management of heart failure in children: Canadian Cardiovascular Society Guidelines. *Can J Cardiol.* 2013;29:1535–1552.)

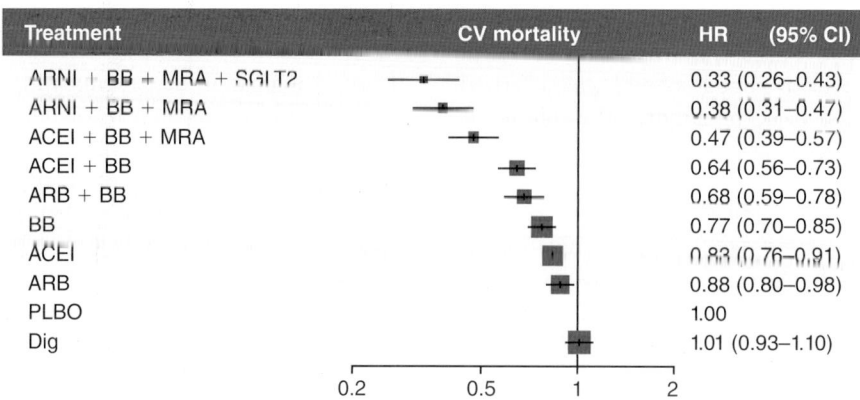

• **Fig. 53.3** Effect of various medications and combinations on cardiovascular mortality in adult heart failure studies. *ACEi,* Angiotensin-converting enzyme inhibitor; *ARNI,* angiotensin receptor blocker/neprilysin inhibitor; *BB,* beta-blocker; *CI,* confidence interval; *CV,* cardiovascular; *Dig,* digoxin; *HR,* hazard ratio; *MRA,* mineralocorticoid receptor antagonist; *PLBO,* placebo; *SGLT2i,* sodium-glucose cotransporter-2 inhibitor. (Adapted from Tromp J, Ouwerkerk W, Van Veldhuisen DJ, et al. A systematic review and network meta-analysis of pharmacological treatment of heart failure with reduced ejection fraction. *J Am Coll Cardiol.* 2022;10:73–84.)

additional consideration for a beta blocker and remodeling reversal therapy in stage C (angiotensin-converting enzyme inhibitors [ACEi], mineralocorticoid receptor antagonists [MRAs], beta-blockers, and sodium-glucose cotransporter inhibitors [SGLTi]), with additional drugs for symptom management, as indicated. Published guidelines for pediatric HF sponsored by the International Society for Heart and Lung Transplantation (ISHLT) have taken a similar approach while acknowledging that most of the recommendations are based on expert consensus and usually adopted from adult trials.[11,15]

Initial Management in Symptomatic Heart Failure

Children with pediatric HF are most often diagnosed in the setting of an acute or subacute decompensation. Since the majority of symptoms are not specific to HF and the disease is uncommon in this population, patients presenting with early symptoms are usually misdiagnosed as having recurrent respiratory infections, asthma, or feeding difficulties. As symptoms progress, children continue to present to care and fail to respond to initial therapies. Further diagnostics may reveal fluid overload, cardiomegaly on chest radiograph, or ventricular dysfunction which prompts referral to cardiology, often as part of or leading to inpatient admission. The initial treatment phase, after establishing the diagnosis of HF, is to stabilize the patient. Depending on the severity of hemodynamic derangement and end-organ dysfunction, this may require critical care for the initiation of vasoactive infusions, respiratory support, and potentially more invasive therapies, in addition to diuresis. These interventions are intended to improve cardiac output, decrease myocardial oxygen demand, decrease abnormally elevated filling pressures, and relieve congestion. These generally result in an improvement in end-organ function as well as symptoms. The second phase of treatment involves a methodical transition to oral HF therapies, typically beginning with ACEi while maintaining a favorable hemodynamic profile that may be continued long term during outpatient care. The third phase involves optimization of oral HF therapies that promote reverse remodeling and improved function. This is typically started during the hospital stay and continued with regular outpatient visits; this phase may be the initial management approach for mildly symptomatic patients.

Remodeling Reversal Therapy

ACEi are first line in the management of children with systolic ventricular dysfunction. By inhibiting angiotensin II production and thus RAAS activation, they reduce systemic vascular resistance and ventricular afterload. This leads to increased cardiac output and improvement in HF symptoms. Long-term use of ACEi in adult RCTs demonstrates improved survival in patients with symptomatic HF, reduced rate at which asymptomatic patients with severe LV dysfunction developed symptoms, and reversal of ventricular remodeling. The efficacy of ACEi is a class effect. RCT data in children are limited and difficult to interpret due to healthier baseline cohorts, smaller sample size, and shorter duration of follow-up compared with adult studies. In an RCT of 230 infants with single-ventricle anatomy and predominantly normal systemic ventricular function, somatic growth, ventricular function, HF severity, and 1-year mortality were similar in the enalapril and placebo groups.[16] In another RCT of perindopril in 57 children with Duchenne muscular dystrophy (DMD) with normal ejection fraction (EF), ventricular function was similar in both groups at 3 years.[17] However, fewer patients in the ACEi group had LV EF < 45% at 5 years (4% vs. 28%) with fewer deaths observed at 10 years (7% vs. 34%).[18] Despite the inconsistencies and limitations of the pediatric data, it is reasonable to believe that the well-established benefits of ACEi in adult

HF patients likely apply to pediatric patients. Potential side effects include hypotension, renal dysfunction, and hyperkalemia, particularly in neonates. A persistent dry cough or angioedema should prompt consideration of angiotensin receptor blocker (ARB) use.

ARB use is reserved for patients intolerant to ACEi. By blocking the angiotensin receptors, they also affect the RAAS thereby decreasing systemic vascular resistance and ventricular afterload, and increasing cardiac output. Long-term use of ARB leads to reverse remodeling, decreased fibrosis, and a reduction in HF mortality. The efficacy of ARB is considered a class effect. Common side effects are hypotension, renal dysfunction, and hyperkalemia. There is a paucity of data on the use of ARB in pediatric HF.

Sacubitril, a neprilysin inhibitor, prevents proteolytic degradation of the natriuretic peptides, bradykinin and adrenomedullin. When combined with valsartan, an ARB, it offers a newer, synergistic approach to afterload reduction therapy. An RCT of sacubitril-valsartan (200 mg twice a day) versus enalapril (10 mg twice a day) in 8442 adult HF patients with LV systolic dysfunction demonstrated lower rates of cardiovascular and all-cause mortality, as well as HF hospitalization among patients randomized to valsartan-sacubitril.[19] A pediatric RCT of sacubitril-valsartan versus enalapril is ongoing. Preliminary data have demonstrated efficacy in reducing (N-terminal) NT-proBNP in children. The Food and Drug Administration used these data in 2019 to approve use of sacubitril-valsartan for children 1 year of age and older.

Beta-blocker therapy is typically added to afterload reduction in patients with compensated systolic HF. Beta-blockers counteract the maladaptive effects of chronic myocardial sympathetic activation resulting in a gradual, time-dependent improvement in LV function. Three beta-blockers—carvedilol, metoprolol, and bisoprolol—have been shown to improve survival in adults with HF. An individual patient data meta-analysis of 11 RCTs of 13,833 adults with HF demonstrated beta-blockers to be equally effective across adult age in improving survival.[20] Studies of beta-blockers in pediatric HF have been limited by small sample size, short follow-up, and the use of surrogate endpoints. In a multicenter RCT of carvedilol versus placebo of 161 children, there were no significant differences between groups.[21] The study was considered underpowered, as the clinical course of all children enrolled was better than expected. There was a trend towards clinical improvement in children with a systemic LV, but not in those with a systemic RV, suggesting that the response to carvedilol may be affected by the morphology of the systemic ventricle. A subsequent randomized clinical trial in 89 pediatric HF patients also found no difference in clinical improvement with carvedilol compared with conventional treatment; however, improvements in echocardiographic parameters and serum BNP levels were noted with carvedilol.[22] Carvedilol therapy has also been shown to preserve LV function at 6 months follow-up after exposure to anthracyclines when compared with placebo in randomized patients.[23] Additionally, it can

improve LV function when added to ACEi therapy in patients with DMD and DCM.[24] Hemodynamically, beta-blockers have negative inotropic and chronotropic effects, may cause vasodilation (carvedilol), and are therefore initiated at low dose and advanced gradually. Common side effects include hypotension and bradycardia. A risk of hypoglycemia is also notable, particularly in infants with gastrointestinal illness or poor oral intake. Discontinuation or lowering the previously tolerated dose should be considered in patients with decompensated HF.

MRAs, spironolactone and eplerenone, reduce activation of the RAAS by competitively inhibiting the aldosterone receptor. Initially designed as potassium-sparing diuretics, MRAs were demonstrated to improve survival in adults with HF in large RCTs. This effect is mediated by inhibition of myocardial fibrosis and promotion of reverse remodeling.[25] Their potassium-sparing diuretic effect makes them suitable for use in conjunction with loop diuretics and thiazides. Side effects include hyperkalemia and gynecomastia (spironolactone). An RCT in 42 boys with DMD demonstrated that the addition of eplerenone to ACEi or ARB therapy attenuated the decline in LV systolic function.[26]

Sodium-glucose cotransporter-2 inhibitors (SGLT2i), also known as gliflozins, were recently added to adult GDMT for HF. They reduce glucose reabsorption in the proximal tubule and were developed as oral hypoglycemic drugs for type 2 diabetes. Recent RCTs in adults with HF have demonstrated significant reduction in major cardiovascular outcomes, including cardiovascular death. The proposed mechanisms of action include altered myocardial calcium handling, decreased inflammation, and improved cellular energy utilization.[27] No trials have been undertaken in pediatric HF. We have started using SGLT2i in adolescent patients with systolic and diastolic HF based on outcomes from adult studies. Side effects include diuresis, hypoglycemia, and increased risk of mycotic genitourinary infections.

Medications that Improve Heart Failure Symptoms

Diuretics are important in the management of vascular congestion in patients with symptomatic HF. Loop diuretics, such as furosemide, torsemide, and bumetanide, and thiazide diuretics help promote natriuresis; in conjunction with restriction of fluid intake, they relieve symptoms of congestion. In serial heart catheterization studies in patients with ventricular dysfunction presenting with fluid overload, normalizing filling pressures was not associated with a decrease in cardiac output. Patients on diuretics should be monitored for electrolyte imbalance, metabolic alkalosis, renal dysfunction, and with chronic use, nephrocalcinosis and bone health.

Digoxin is useful in patients with HF for improving symptoms. It works by inhibiting the myocardial sodium-potassium ATPase. This increases intracellular sodium which drives an influx of calcium into the myocardial cell, thereby increasing contractility. Digoxin toxicity can be life-threatening. With current dosing and low intended levels

(0.5–1 ng/mL), toxicity is rare. It is more common in the presence of renal dysfunction and with concurrent use of amiodarone, as both increase digoxin levels. Large RCTs of digoxin in adults with HF have demonstrated reduced hospitalization but no survival benefit. There are no RCTs of digoxin in children with HF.

Ivabradine has been demonstrated to reduce HF progression and hospitalization in adults, though no effect on all cause or cardiovascular mortality has been demonstrated, including in a meta-analysis.[28] Its negative chronotropic effect is mediated by blocking the inward rectifying funny channel on the sarcolemma, thus prolonging depolarization. Side effects are most notably bradycardia. For this reason, it should not be used in patients with decompensated HF where it may compromise cardiac output. Though not commonly used in children, it may be helpful in the management of hemodynamically stable patients with HF with inappropriate sinus tachycardia, particularly when intolerant of beta-blockade or digoxin. The use of ivabradine in children with DCM on stable oral therapy has been demonstrated to safely and effectively reduce resting heart rate when compared with placebo in an RCT of 116 children. At 1 year, patients on ivabradine had a small but significant improvement on LV EF (13.5% vs. 6.9%) with similar improvement in BNP.[29]

Additional Interventions

Cardiac resynchronization therapy (CRT) may improve ventricular function in patients with severe systolic dysfunction, mechanical dyssynchrony, and left bundle branch block. These findings are uncommon in children with HF, and no large RCTs are available. Some children with CHD with dyssynchrony and wide QRS duration have shown improvement in systemic ventricular function with CRT aimed at narrowing the QRS duration.

Maintenance of somatic growth is challenging in children with HF given increased metabolic demands, decreased appetite due to abdominal discomfort, and vomiting. The addition of supplemental nutrition under the guidance of a nutritionist is often necessary. Iron deficiency is common in HF and can exacerbate the physiologic effect of low cardiac output. Iron studies (serum iron level, transferrin saturation, and ferritin) are important to diagnose iron deficiency and should be performed periodically even with normal red cell morphology and count. Oral iron supplementation is poorly tolerated and is often ineffective. Intravenous iron supplementation is safe and known to improve functional class and exercise performance in adult patients. Small case series have reported safety and efficacy in improving iron levels in pediatric HF patients.

Safe return to physical activity is integral to successful HF management as deconditioning and obesity can exacerbate symptoms. Parental anxiety may contribute to the difficulty in reestablishing healthy levels of physical activity. Though physical activity is patient specific, a pediatric study of hospitalized children awaiting heart transplantation demonstrated safety even for children on inotropes.[30]

Pulmonary vasodilators may be useful in the management of HF in patients with single ventricle. Even modest elevations in PVR may affect pulmonary blood flow and increase venous pressures contributing to poor oxygenation and congestion. Adult randomized studies of pulmonary vasodilators (udenafil) in Fontan patients demonstrated improvement during exercise testing in ventilatory equivalents and work rate with a trend towards improved oxygen consumption.[31]

Advanced Heart Failure

Management of patients with HF refractory to oral HF therapy or those presenting with acute decompensated HF requires hospitalization. Inotropic agents are used to increase contractility in the setting of low cardiac output or poor organ perfusion. Milrinone, an inodilator that works by phosphodiesterase III inhibition and reduction in systemic vascular resistance and PVR, is the preferred agent in decompensated HF in the absence of significant hypotension. Patients who are stable but fail to wean from milrinone may be candidates for home infusion while awaiting heart transplantation or for end-of-life care. In addition to milrinone, dopamine is often chosen due to its effect on renal perfusion, though other catecholamines such as epinephrine and dobutamine are also used. Respiratory support is sometimes needed to manage respiratory failure, but also to mitigate myocardial oxygen demand by decreasing accessory and respiratory muscle work. Additional benefit is obtained by increasing blood oxygen content when hypoxemic. Furthermore, positive pressure ventilation decreases LV afterload by decreasing transmural wall stress. In patients at risk for cardiovascular collapse, myocardial oxygen consumption may be further decreased by intubation, sedation, and in extreme cases paralysis.

Mechanical Circulatory Support

For children in decompensated HF with low output refractory to medical therapy, mechanical circulatory support (MCS) can be lifesaving. MCS can help recover acute end-organ dysfunction and reduce myocardial oxygen demand. It may be used as a bridge to recovery, transplantation, or as destination therapy. In a report from the ISHLT, 30% of pediatric heart transplant recipients received MCS as a bridge to transplantation, including the majority of those with DCM older than 1 year of age.[32] The type of MCS chosen will depend on the rapidity of decompensation, expected time for support (temporary vs. durable MCS), anatomy, and patient age and size. Risks of MCS include high rate of hemocompatibility-related adverse events, such as stroke, and infection. Careful management of anticoagulation is critical. Analyses have demonstrated that pediatric patients bridged to heart transplant with a VAD have similar outcomes to children who did not require MCS, while those supported with extracorporeal membrane oxygenation (ECMO) have markedly increased peri-transplant morbidity and mortality.[32]

Heart Transplantation

Children with HF refractory to oral therapy, as well as those with severe HF and associated complications, such as growth failure, pulmonary hypertension, and refractory arrhythmias, are considered for heart transplantation. A formal evaluation for transplant candidacy elucidates risks and benefits of the procedure and provides families with sufficient knowledge to participate in informed consent. Associated end-organ dysfunction, sensitization, and the ability to manage the patient while on the transplant wait-list (including the potential need for mechanical support) are critical risks. The decision to pursue heart transplantation considers the expected survival with medical therapy, quality of life, alternative treatment options, and estimation of survival post-transplantation.

Outcomes

Outcomes for children with HF vary considerably depending on the underlying etiology and severity of disease. According to the Centers for Disease Control and Prevention and National Vital Statistics System, heart disease is the fifth leading cause of death for children aged 1–9 years, and sixth for those aged 10–14 years in the United States; HF mortality is the most prevalent diagnosis. Inpatient mortality for pediatric patients with acutely decompensated HF is high, especially for patients with complex CHD.[33] The proportion of patients admitted with pediatric HF who have CHD has continued to increase. For children with DCM, outcomes depend on the etiology, the degree of LV dysfunction, and the severity of symptoms. A retrospective study of 549 children with a dilated phenotype and ventricular dysfunction, including due to isolated DCM, neuromuscular cardiomyopathy, and myocarditis, demonstrated 27% ventricular functional recovery, 24% heart transplantation, and 9% mortality at a median follow-up of 1 year.[34] Notably, outcomes were significantly poorer for patients with neuromuscular disease than for those with isolated DCM, while those with myocarditis had the best reported outcomes. It is important to recognize that for children listed for heart transplantation, waitlist times have continued to increase. Pediatric patients undergoing heart transplantation have excellent outcomes, with 5-year and 10-year survival approaching 80% and 65%, respectively.[32] Additional details regarding MCS, cardiomyopathy, myocarditis, and heart transplantation are discussed elsewhere in this tome.

References

1. Bozkurt B, Coats A, Tsutsui H, et al. Universal definition and classification of heart failure. *J Card Fail.* 2021;27:387-413.
2. Shaddy RE, George AT, Jaecklin T, et al. Systematic literature review on the incidence and prevalence of heart failure in children and adolescents. *Pediatr Cardiol.* 2018;39:415-436.
3. Morales-Demori R, Motañes E, Erkonen G, et al. Epidemiology of pediatric heart failure in the USA: a 15-year multiinstitutional study. *Pediatr Cardiol.* 2021;42:1297-1307.
4. Lipshultz SE, Sleeper LA, Towbin JA, et al. The incidence of pediatric cardiomyopathy in two regions of the United States. *N Engl J Med.* 2003;348:1647-1655.
5. Rath A, Weintraub R. Overview of cardiomyopathies in childhood. *Front Pediatr.* 2021;9:708732.
6. Arola A, Pikkarainen E, Sipilä JO, et al. Occurrence and features of childhood myocarditis: a nationwide study in Finland. *J Am Heart Assoc.* 2017;18:e005306.
7. Alvarez JA, Orav EJ, Wilkinson JD, et al. Competing risks for death and cardiac transplantation in children with dilated cardiomyopathy: results from the Pediatric Cardiomyopathy Registry. *Circulation.* 2011;124:814-823.
8. Chow EJ, Leger KJ, Bhatt NS, et al. Paediatric cardio-oncology: epidemiology, screening, prevention, and treatment. *Cardiovasc Res.* 2019;115:922-934.
9. Mahle WT, Chenwei H, Trachtenberg F, et al. Heart failure after the Norwood procedure: an analysis of the Single Ventricle Reconstruction Trial. *J Heart Lung Transplant.* 2018;37:879-885.
10. Knudson JD, Cabrera AG. The pathophysiology of heart failure in children: the basics. *Curr Cardiol Rev.* 2016;12:99-103.
11. Kirk R, Dipchand AI, Rosenthal DN, et al. The International Society for Heart and Lung Transplantation Guidelines for the management of pediatric heart failure: executive summary. [Corrected]. *J Heart Lung Transplant.* 2014;33:888-909.
12. Kantor PF, Lougheed J, Dancea A, et al. Presentation, diagnosis, and medical management of heart failure in children: Canadian Cardiovascular Society Guidelines. *Can J Cardiol.* 2013;29:1535-1552.
13. Heidenreich PA, Bozkurt B, Aguilar D, et al. 2022 AHA/ACC/HFSA guideline for the management of heart failure: a report of the American College of Cardiology/American Heart Association Joint Committee on Clinical Practice Guidelines. *Circulation.* 2022;145:e895.
14. Tromp J, Ouwerkerk W, Van Veldhuisen DJ, et al. A systematic review and network meta-analysis of pharmacological treatment of heart failure with reduced ejection fraction. *J Am Coll Cardiol.* 2022;10:73-84.
15. Rosenthal DN, Chrisant MRK, Edens E, et al. International Society for Heart and Lung Transplantation: practice guidelines for management of heart failure in children. *J Heart Lung Transplant.* 2004;23:1313-1333.
16. Hsu DT, Zak V, Mahony L, et al. Enalapril in infants with single ventricle: results of a multicenter randomized trial. *Circulation.* 2010;122:333-340.
17. Duboc D, Meune C, Lerebours G, et al. Effect of perindopril on the onset and progression of left ventricular dysfunction in Duchenne muscular dystrophy. *J Am Coll Cardiol.* 2005;45:855-857.
18. Duboc D, Meune C, Pierre B, et al. Perindopril preventive treatment on mortality in Duchenne muscular dystrophy: 10 years' follow-up. *Am Heart J.* 2007;154:596-602.
19. McMurray JJ, Packer M, Desai AS, et al. Angiotensin–neprilysin inhibition versus enalapril in heart failure. *N Engl J Med.* 2014;371:993-1004.
20. Kotecha D, Manzano L, Krum H, et al. Effect of age and sex on efficacy and tolerability of β blockers in patients with heart failure with reduced ejection fraction: individual patient data meta-analysis. *BMJ.* 2016;353:i1855.
21. Shaddy RE, Boucek MM, Hsu DT, et al. Carvedilol for children and adolescents with heart failure: a randomized controlled trial. *JAMA.* 2007;298:1171-1179.

22. Huang M, Zhang X, Chen S, et al. The effect of carvedilol treatment on chronic heart failure in pediatric patients with dilated cardiomyopathy: a prospective, randomized-controlled study. *Pediatr Cardiol.* 2013;34:680-685.

23. Kalay N, Basar E, Ozdogru I, et al. Protective effects of carvedilol against anthracycline-induced cardiomyopathy. *J Am Coll Cardiol.* 2006;48:2258-2262.

24. Kajimoto H, Ishigaki K, Okumura K, et al. Beta-blocker therapy for cardiac dysfunction in patients with muscular dystrophy. *Circ J.* 2006;70:991-994.

25. Tsutamoto T, Wada A, Maeda K, et al. Effect of spironolactone on plasma brain natriuretic peptide and left ventricular remodeling in patients with congestive heart failure. *J Am Coll Cardiol.* 2001;37:1228-1233.

26. Raman SV, Hor KN, Mazur W, et al. Eplerenone for early cardiomyopathy in Duchenne muscular dystrophy: a randomised, double-blind, placebo-controlled trial. *Lancet Neurol.* 2015;14:153-161.

27. Braunwald E. Gliflozins in the management of cardiovascular disease. *N Engl J Med.* 2022;386:2024-2034.

28. Maagaard M, Nielsen EE, Sethi NJ, et al. Ivabradine added to usual care in patients with heart failure: a systematic review with meta-analysis and trial sequential analysis. *BMJ Evid Based Med.* 2022;27:224-234.

29. Bonnet D, Berger F, Jokinen E, et al. Ivabradine in children with dilated cardiomyopathy and symptomatic chronic heart failure. *J Am Coll Cardiol.* 2017;70:1262-1272.

30. McBride MG, Binder TJ, Paridon SM. Safety and feasibility of inpatient exercise training in pediatric heart failure: a preliminary report. *J Cardiopulm Rehabil Prev.* 2007;27:219-222.

31. Goldberg DJ, Zak V, Goldstein BH, et al. Results of the FUEL trial. *Circulation.* 2019;141:641-651.

32. Rossano JW, Singh TP, Cherikh WS, et al. The International Thoracic Organ Transplant Registry of the International Society for Heart and Lung Transplantation: twenty-second pediatric heart transplantation report – 2019. *J Heart Lung Transplant.* 2019;38:1028-1041.

33. Adebiyi EO, Edigin E, Shaka H, et al. Pediatric heart failure inpatient mortality: a cross-sectional analysis. *Cureus.* 2022;14:e26721.

34. Singh RK, Canter CE, Shi L, et al. Survival without cardiac transplantation among children with dilated cardiomyopathy. *J Am Coll Cardiol.* 2017;70:2663-2673.

54

Advanced Cardiac Therapies: Ventricular Assist Device and Heart Transplantation

CHRISTINA VANDERPLUYM, FRANCIS FYNN-THOMPSON, AND ELIZABETH D. BLUME

KEY LEARNING POINTS

- Use of ventricular assist devices has become the standard of care for children with acquired and congenital heart disease refractory to maximal medical management.
- Various types of mechanical circulatory support are now available to children of all sizes and types of anatomy, as bridge to recovery, bridge to transplant candidacy,

- bridge to transplant, or as an indefinite therapeutic option (destination therapy).
- Heart transplantation remains the gold standard for severe heart failure; improved survival over eras is related in part to advances in post-transplant immunosuppressive management and post-transplant surveillance and care.

Introduction

The population of patients requiring advanced cardiac therapies in the form of mechanical circulatory support (MCS) and transplantation is growing in both volume and complexity. Now, patients with complex congenital heart disease (CHD) who previously would have died in infancy are surviving into adolescence and adulthood due to tremendous advances in surgical and postsurgical care of CHD. Additional advancements in prenatal diagnosis, medical and surgical management, and expanding genetic investigations have transformed once fatal CHD and cardiomyopathy to a chronic disease state. While many of these patients require only surveillance cardiac care, some develop systolic and/or diastolic heart failure warranting a spectrum of heart therapies ranging from oral and intravenous medication to ventricular assist device (VAD) support and/or orthotopic heart transplantation (OHT). Given the overall rise in survival of children with congenital and acquired heart disease, there is constant growth in the number of children being considered for OHT, far surpassing growth in organ donation resulting in longer waitlist times. Longer waitlist times, in conjunction with pharmacological and technological innovation, has led to use of advanced cardiac therapies, namely VAD support, as the standard of

care for end-stage heart failure refractory to medical management.

Herein, we describe current utilization and outcomes of VAD support for children with cardiac disease, and how this advanced cardiac therapy interfaces with the evolving and improving outcomes of heart transplantation in children.

Mechanical Circulatory Support

Types of Support Strategies

MCS consists of an array of cardiac and pulmonary support devices that can be classified by the location of the circulatory "pump" to the thorax and the estimated duration of support. *Extracorporeal* denotes the pump is outside of the body and adjacent to the patient, as is seen in extracorporeal membrane oxygenation (ECMO), a modality of MCS that provides both cardiac and pulmonary support and is frequently used for acute cardiovascular collapse refractory to conventional resuscitative efforts. Historically, ECMO was the mainstay of support strategies as a bridge to transplantation (BTT), albeit with high waitlist mortality and morbidity. Since the 2012, the use of *paracorporeal* and *intracorporeal* VADs has dramatically increased the survival of patients awaiting transplantation and has now assumed the position of primary support modality for end-stage heart failure. *Paracorporeal* pumps are located outside the body and are connected to the heart and great vessels via tunneled cannulae, resting in close proximity to the patient's chest and/or abdomen. These pumps can be implanted to provide right ventricular support (RVAD) via right atrial and pulmonary artery cannula, and/or left ventricular support (LVAD) via left atrium or left ventricular apical and aortic cannula. *Paracorporeal* VADs can be further divided into the type of flow characteristics the pump provides: continuous as seen with PediMag, CentriMag, or Rotaflow pumps, or pulsatile as seen with the Berlin Heart EXCOR VAD. For close to a decade, the Berlin Heart was the most commonly used VAD in children worldwide, and the only VAD with Food and Drug Administration (FDA) labelling for use in children as a BTT.[1-3] However, the emergence of *intracorporeal* VADs in 2011 resulted in a tremendous growth in VADs for older children and adolescence, for whom the size of their ventricles and their thorax permitted implantation. *Intracorporeal* pumps are implanted directed into the ventricle or atrium with an outflow graft to the great vessels, and with externalization of the power source (batteries) and controller via driveline. The most commonly used *intracorporeal* pump is the HeartMate 3 Ventricular Assist System, which garnered pediatric labelling by the FDA in 2020.[3-5]

Role of VADs in Advanced Heart Failure and OHT

With the approval of the Berlin Heart EXCOR as a pediatric device in 2011, VAD has emerged as an accepted modality to support various types of heart disease in the pediatric population. Despite the increased use, the majority of pediatric centers implant fewer than 10 VADs in children per year.[6] To understand the larger scope of VAD use and outcomes in children has required the concerted efforts and collaboration of centers across North America, Europe, and elsewhere. In the United States, the Pedimacs registry evolved as the pediatric arm of Intermacs, a national prospective database of MCS devices. It has captured prospective data for all types of durable and temporary MCS devices implanted in children aged < 19 years.[7] These databases are a collaboration between the Society of Thoracic Surgery, National Heart, Lung, and Blood Institute, the United States FDA, the Centers for Medicare and Medicaid Services, industry, and implanting centers. In 2018, the Advanced Cardiac Therapies Improving Outcomes Network (ACTION) formed as a learning collaborative focused on improving the outcomes of children supported on VADs, namely stroke.[8,9] ACTION has collected prospective data on VAD utilization, outcomes, and adverse events in concert with Pedimacs, now allowing for robust understanding of the role of VADs advanced heart failure.

The Fifth Annual Pedimacs Report detailed the outcomes of 1011 patients supported on 1229 devices between September 19, 2012 and December 31, 2020.[3]

Cardiomyopathy remains the most common underlying diagnosis (58%) followed by CHD (25%) and myocarditis (10%). Intracorporeal devices were used at highest frequency (41%), followed by paracorporeal pulsatile device (Berlin Heart EXCOR; 27%) and paracorporeal continuous devices (PediMag, CentriMag, and Rotaflow; 26%). Percutaneous devices (namely the Impella, Abiomed) were used in 53 patients (5%). Overall survival at 6 months was 83% (transplanted, explanted, or alive on device), with intracorporeal VADs having the highest freedom from stroke (93%), followed by paracorporeal pulsatile VADs (85%) and paracorporeal continuous VADs (75%).[3]

In North America, the primary indication for VAD implantation is as a BTT, with over 55% of patients listed for transplantation at the time of implantation and 34% being assessed for candidacy.[10] Other reasons for VAD use include as a bridge to recovery (BTR) with the plan to explant the device once the heart has recovered sufficiently to support the patient's need. This strategy is still used infrequently at 6%, but there is ongoing it is an indication at way that BTR can be bolstered with investigational medical and gene therapies. Destination/chronic therapy is used when transplant is not considered a viable option, and is currently only used in approximately 2% of pediatric patients; it does, however, have expanding use in select patient populations, such as those with Duchenne muscular dystrophy.[11]

Given the rise in MCS use as BTT, many assume that its use affects the outcomes of transplantation. Edelson et al.[12] reported on a retrospective cohort of 5095 heart transplant recipients aged < 18 years in the International Society for Heart and Lung Transplantation Registry (ISHLT) between 2005 and 2017. Over a quarter of these patients required MCS prior to OHT (26%), with 4.7% on ECMO and 20.2% on VAD. A third of patients (29%) were less than one year old, and 44% had CHD. As seen in other studies, patients on ECMO had higher mortality than those requiring no MCS and those on VAD (OR 3.97 & 2.55; 95% CI 2.43–6.49 & 1.42–4.60), whereas patients on VAD had similar mortality to those patients who did not require MCS. Patients with CHD had highest mortality on ECMO compared with no MCS, but there was no difference in survival of patients with dilated cardiomyopathy (DCM) based on the need for VAD pretransplant.[12] This highlights the ongoing challenges of managing advanced heart failure in patients with CHD as compared with DCM, and also shows the remarkable improvement in VAD outcomes with comparable survival to patients transplanted without any form of MCS. Patient selection remains a paramount issue surrounding the VAD and OHT outcomes.

Pre-Implantation VAD Evaluation

Similar to evaluating for OHT candidacy, the determination of candidacy and risks for VAD implantation should include a multidisciplinary and multisystem approach.

Surgical Candidacy

For patients with DCM or acquired heart disease with normal biventricular anatomy, the placement of a VAD is a relatively simple surgical procedure. Surgical planning with computed tomography (CT) and magnetic resonance imaging (MRI) reconstruction may be useful in the setting of complex CHD, where multiple prior sternotomies and surgical palliations may have resulted in adhesions and distortion of the anatomy. As such, determination of surgical feasibility of VAD implantation is an important first step in the candidacy process. For determination of VAD types, measurement of patient size (weight, body surface area, and thoracic size) as well as ventricular size in systole, is necessary to assess candidacy for an intracorporeal device versus a paracorporeal device. Generally, intracorporeal devices are used in patients greater than 25 kg but are dependent on adequate ventricular size to accommodate the inflow cannula.[4]

Determination of support type, as well as need for right and/or left (biventricular) VAD, greatly affect the surgical complexity as well as post-VAD morbidity. RVAD alone can be considered in select cases of pure RV dysfunction, but is generally a rare occurrence, and not typically successful if RV failure is in the setting of pulmonary arterial hypertension; forcing blood across the pulmonary vascular bed with a VAD may result in significant hemolysis and acquired end-organ damage from hemolysis. Biventricular support can only be done with a biventricular circulation, while patients with single-ventricle anatomy will require systemic VAD. VAD outcomes in the Fontan population have improved significantly with comparable outcomes to those patients with LVAD without CHD. For the single-ventricle population as with all patients, it is paramount to ensure that end organ function remains preserved.

End-Organ Function

Operative risk and postoperative VAD management are significantly impacted by end-organ derangement. Determination of liver function, with liver enzymes, international normalized ratio (INR), and bilirubin, is important to predict the risk of acquired thrombophilic and bleeding disorders, as well as the risk of intraoperative liver induced vasoplegia. Elevated liver enzymes have been reported in a quarter of patients, and abnormal elevation in bilirubin is present in up to 45% of patients at the time of VAD.[13] This is usually related to congestive hepatopathy from right heart failure or failed single-ventricle circulation. Mortality is increased with elevated bilirubin and is most notable in patients < 10 kg (mortality 70%).[13]

Renal function is determined with blood urea nitrogen and creatinine, with variable definitions of renal dysfunction including serum creatinine > 1.6 mg/dL for patients aged > 10 years, or creatinine > 1.0 mg/dL for patients aged ≤ 10 years, or by estimated glomerular filtration rate using Schwartz formula of < 90 mL/min/1.73 m^2.[10] Post-VAD outcomes have been shown to be negatively impacted by renal dysfunction prior to VAD implantation.[14]

Ventilatory support is common at the time of VAD implantation, with reported use in 45–49% of patients. Determination of pulmonary function can be challenging in this setting, but accounting for ventilation settings, tidal volumes, and FiO_2 requirements can provide a reasonable assessment of ability of the lungs to ventilate and oxygenate.

Frailty is a term generally associated with adults and infrequently characterized in the pediatric population. However, the overall condition of a frail child is an important consideration and nutritional assessment is a good surrogate. Many children have poor oral intake due to abdominal angina related to inadequate perfusion of the mesentery. Chronic malnutrition impairs wound healing and negatively affects operative survival. The presence of tube feeding or total parental nutrition is reported in 64% of pediatric VAD recipients.[15]

Psychosocial Assessment

Beyond the physical manifestation of heart failure, there lies a much deeper impact of cardiac disease on the psychological well-being of the patient and the family. Chronic disease places families and patients at tremendous risk of financial challenges, mood and behavioral disorders, and interpersonal discord. As such, it is paramount to involve a dedicated social worker, psychologist, child life specialist, and psychiatrist to evaluate, support, guide, and treat the patient-family-care team complex. The goal of the pre-VAD evaluation is to ensure comprehensive understanding of the VAD procedure, post-VAD care requirements, and anticipated benefits of the VAD from the patient's and providers' perspectives. Aligning expectations for both positive and negative outcomes helps mitigate communication break down and establish goals of care early.

VAD Surgical Considerations

As with any cardiovascular surgery, an in-depth understanding of the anatomic and physiologic considerations, as well as the potential benefits, are critical in evaluation and preparation for VAD placement. To ensure proper functioning of the VAD, the inflow cannula must be sited in the optimal position to ensure no obstruction to flow or risk of hemolysis due to high shear stress of blood flowing into the cannula. Regardless of cannula type, generally the optimal inflow is directed toward the semilunar valve and parallel to the interventricular septum. This can be especially difficult in single-ventricle anatomy with morphological systemic RV. In patients with DCM, it is generally easy to determine optimal position utilizing echocardiographic guidance, but restrictive cardiomyopathy or mixed cardiomyopathy may prove much more challenging and warrant atrial cannulation. In the event where apical cannulation is still preferred, the ventricular cavity can be enlarged by extended LV myectomy and/or excision of mitral valve apparatus and leaflets. Having an adequate size capacitance chamber, be it ventricular or atrial, is necessary to ensure that adequate flow will be achieved through the pump; otherwise, there is the possibility of collapsing the chamber and risking "suction events" when the inflow cannula is obstructed by the internal structure of the heart.

Placement of the outflow graft or cannula can be challenging in select populations, namely those with past surgical interventions on the aorta. Modifications to outflow cannula placement, including interposition of a surgical graft between the outflow tip and aorta or innominate artery, has been described.[16]

Post-VAD Management

VAD Operating Parameters

Determination of the optimal settings for the device is variable over the course of VAD support. Hemodynamics and metabolic needs of the patient will vary between intraoperative, postoperative, and ambulatory conditions. As such, modification of the VAD operating parameters must consider whether a patient's metabolic needs are being met under the current clinical circumstances (i.e., positive pressure ventilation, trending of lactate and mixed venous saturation, blood pressure, central venous pressure, etc.).

Hemostasis and Antithrombosis Management

Historically, bleeding and thrombosis have been the most common adverse events related to VAD support, with paracorporeal devices having a higher adverse events profile than intracorporeal devices. Due to the predominance of ischemic strokes across paracorporeal VAD support, there has been a paradigm shift in antithrombosis practices, with the adoption of direct thrombin inhibitors (DTIs) as the primary anticoagulant agent.[17] DTIs are a class of intravenous medications that inhibit both clot-bound and circulating thrombin, have a linear dose response curve, and display predictable pharmacokinetics and pharmacodynamics. Unlike unfractionated heparin (UFH), DTIs do not require antithrombin III to potentiate the action of thrombin inhibition. This characteristic is particularly advantageous in the pediatric population where developmental hemostasis results in physiologic age-related differences in the quantity and quality of several hemostatic proteins, namely antithrombin III.

Our current approach for thromboprophylaxis at Boston Children's Hospital for paracorporeal devices is as follows:

Boston Bivalirudin Antithrombosis Guide

Pre-Implantation Workup

Prior to VAD implantation, all patients and families have a thorough history for past bleeding or thrombotic disorders suggestive of hemophilia or thrombophilia. A thrombophilia panel is sent on any patient with significant past or family history for thrombosis. Coagulation labs include activated partial thromboplastin time (aPTT), prothrombin time (PT)/INR, fibrinogen, complete blood count with differential, lactate dehydrogenase, plasma free hemoglobin, and C-reactive protein (CRP). A thrombophilia panel includes lupus anticoagulant (LA), antithrombin (AT), von Willebrand antigen (vWF), factor VIII, factor V Leiden, functional protein C and S, lipoprotein, homocysteine, beta-2 glycoprotein, immunoglobulins (IgG and IgM), and cardiolipin IgG, IgA, and IgM. Antiplatelet agents are held 5 days prior to VAD implantation.

Perioperative

All patients received UFH for cardiopulmonary bypass with full protamine reversal.

Postoperative and Maintenance

Within 1 hour of return from operating room, coagulation labs including aPTT, PT/INR, fibrinogen, and platelet count are drawn from a non-heparinized line (newly placed arterial line). The coagulation profile is normalized to goal aPTT < 35 msec, INR < 1.3, platelet count > 100,000 cells/μL and fibrinogen > 250 mg/dL with the replacement of blood products as needed. Coagulation labs are repeated every 4 hours until two sequential measurements are within target range. See Table 54.1 for dosing and monitoring of bivalirudin.

TABLE 54.1 **Boston Bivalirudin Antithrombosis Guide**

Bivalirudin initiated once:
1. Chest tube output <2 cc/kg/hour for 2 consecutive hours
2. Coagulation labs normalized (aPTT <35 msec, INR >1.3, platelet count >100,000 cells/uL, fibrinogen >250 mg/dl)

Bivalirudin infusion via peripheral IV or central line primed with bivalirudin to account for infusion rate:
- Normal renal function (>60ml/min/1.73 m²): 0.3 mg/kg/hour
- Mild-moderate renal dysfunction (30–60ml/min/1.73 m²): 0.2 mg/kg/hour
- Severe renal dysfunction (<30ml/min/1.73 m²): 0.15 mg/kg/hour

Monitoring via clinical report of bleeding (chest tube output) and appearance of pump, in addition to:
- Coagulation labs (aPTT and INR/PT) drawn 2 hours after dose adjustment, until 2 consecutive levels within target range then decrease frequency of monitoring to daily or every other day based on clinical status of patient/pump
- All values drawn from non heparinized line. If heparin infused through sampling line, then bivalirudin would be titrated to heparin absorbed aPTT values
- If INR values correlate to aPTT measurement, then INR would be used as secondary confirmatory variable for dosing. [Example: if aPTT 75–90 msec correlates to INR 2.2–2.6, then if aPTT>200 msec, and INR 2.2, no dose adjustment and repeat sample as needed]

Dosing bivalirudin would be done based on target aPTT/INR in conjunction with clinical exam of patient and pump:
- First 24–48 hours postoperative: target aPTT ~50–70 msec (~1.5-2x baseline aPTT)
- If no increase in bleeding, then goal aPTT 70–90 msec (~2-3x baseline) for duration of support
- Dose adjustment as follows:

% adjustment = (Target aPTT value)–(Current aPTT value)
[Example: increase 25% if target aPTT 80 msec, and current aPTT 55 msec)

aPTT, activated partial prothromboplastin time; *INR,* international normalized ratio

Antiplatelet Therapy

Antiplatelet therapy is initiated only after (1) therapeutic anticoagulation is established with no increase in bleeding; (2) thromboelastography (TEG) platelet mapping (PM) demonstrates arachidonic acid (AA) and adenosine diphosphate (ADP) inhibition less than 70% with clot strength greater than 55; and (3) patient is extubated. The appearance of the pump, specifically fibrin or thrombus formation, is the main factor determining the timing of antiplatelet therapy. We delay antiplatelet initiation until after extubation as this is a period of coughing, airway suctioning, and patient mobilization that appeared to be related to bleeding events in past patients. Aspirin is started at 5–10 mg/kg/day rounded to closest strength of 20.25 mg, 40.5 mg, or 81 mg daily. TEG with PM and VerifyNow for antiplatelet responsiveness is measured 3–5 days after initiation, with target AA inhibition < 70% and < 550RU, respectively on TEG and VerifyNow. Antiplatelet therapy is escalated based on appearance of the pump, with no escalation if pump remains clean on therapeutic anticoagulation, and escalation of dose to max 30 mg/kg/day only if pump develops clot in the setting of therapeutic anticoagulation.

Steroid Use for Acute Inflammation

Steroids are initiated in the setting of acute inflammation defined as: (1) fibrinogen > 500 mg/dL, and/or (2) rising CRP, and/or (3) rising erythrocyte sedimentation rate, and/or (4) acute rise in platelet count (>25%), **and** increased fibrin/platelet deposits in the pump or circuit. Methylprednisolone intravenous is started at 2 mg/kg/day divided twice daily. It is tapered once fibrinogen is < 500 mg/dL and other inflammatory markers are down trending, in conjunction with a stable appearance of the pump and therapeutic anticoagulation.

Driveline Care and Infection

Vigilant care of the cannulae or driveline is paramount in preventing infection and ensuring the longevity of the device at the skin interface. In young children, limited surface area may result in crowding of cannulae, which may be further complicated by the presence of surgical feeding tubes; this necessitates novel strategies to isolate areas at risk for infection while protecting skin integrity from breakdown associated with dressing materials.

Special Support Considerations: Single-Ventricle Anatomy

The single-ventricle patients pose multiple challenges when they require MCS. Ultimately, no two single-ventricle patients are the same, with variable age, size, anatomy, and prior palliative procedures complicating the ability to "standardize" VAD support.

The etiology and physiology of circulatory failure also require special attention and consideration when planning the optimal type of support. For the youngest single-ventricle patients, common modes of failure include primary ventricular systolic dysfunction with varying degrees of atrioventricular regurgitation. For patients already having undergone stage I procedure with RV-PA conduit (Sano), placement of a ventricular outflow cannula must be paired with transition to a modified Blalock-Thomas-Taussig shunt. MCS in the shunted neonate has been the most challenging population, with high mortality related to inadequate flows to support both the systemic and pulmonary circulations. Many of these patients have been placed on central ECMO circuits utilizing tunneled cannula that can later be transitioned to other types of paracorporeal VAD support, once they no longer require an oxygenator. Some centers have created innovative strategies including utilizing pharmacological therapies to maintain ductal patency and combining the stage 1 with VAD placement in a hybrid approach.[18]

Supporting the univentricular patient with Glenn physiology (bidirectional cavopulmonary shunt) has been done successfully, with multiple patients at our institution supported using EXCOR cannula to paracorporeal continuous flow devices, then transitioned to Berlin Heart. Cannulation generally involves the ventricular apex, with some coring of tissue to ensure there is no obstruction of the inflow cannula by valve apparatus or bands. The outflow is placed in the ascending aorta, with higher placement in the setting of a Damus-Kaye-Stansel anastomosis. It must be noted that these patients can still be cyanotic, with preferential flow from the lower venous system. Additionally, patients may develop aortopulmonary collaterals over time that may increase overall saturations but result in a systemic circulation steal, placing them at risk for hypoperfusion of end organs. As such, these patients require vigilant care, with frequent reassessment of VAD operating parameters and consideration for screening cardiac catheterization to assess hemodynamics and collateral burden.

Supporting the Fontan circulation with VAD is becoming more common as the population of patients with Fontan circulation continues to grow and age. Outcomes of primary systemic ventricular VAD support in this population are surprisingly good, with survival in adults with single-ventricle VAD equivalent to adults with non-CHD VADs. The underlying mode of failure is an important determinant of the type of VAD support and outcomes in this population. Systemic systolic ventricular dysfunction, with and without atrioventricular regurgitation, can be supported successfully with intracorporeal continuous flow VADs such as the HeartMate 3. Fontan failure, as defined by high transpulmonary gradient and/or predominance of systemic venous hypertension, often complicated further by hepatomegaly, ascites, and high central venous pressure, is much more challenging to support utilizing currently available VADs. There have been multiple attempts at exploring novel strategies and technologies to support the failed Fontan circulation; however, no device to date is readily available for clinical use.

Heart Transplantation

The field of heart transplantation in children has evolved dramatically since the surgery was first performed by Dr. Christian Bernard on December 3, 1967, with significant advancements in patient selection, donor selection, immune modulation, and post-transplant care. Today, pediatric heart transplantation is performed in over 210 centers worldwide as per the International Thoracic Organ Transplant (TTX) Registry, the largest global registry of data on pediatric heart transplantation with over 15,000 transplants reported in children. This registry, created in 1983, was intended to capture multicenter pediatric and adult transplant data with collection throughout the patients' and grafts' life. Detailed components are available on the registry website at https//ishlt.org/registries/ttx-registry. Increased volume and experience paired with improved surgical techniques, immune therapies, and transplant care have contributed to improved OHT outcomes. One-year post-transplant survival has improved to 92% during the most current era (2012–2017) compared with 87% from 2000 to 2005.[19] However, waitlist mortality remains high and varies between countries and centers within the Unites States; infants and patients with CHD are disproportionately affected.[20] This is in part related to an ongoing recipient to donor volume mismatch, with patients in need of OHT outpacing donors. As such, there has been more focus on optimizing donor utilization and expanding the donor pool. Herein, we will discuss the current landscape and innovations in pediatric heart transplantation.

Transplant Indications

Fundamentally, the indication for heart transplantation is an anticipated post-transplant survival and "natural history" superior to the sequelae of the underlying acquired or congenital heart disease. Given that heart transplantation is itself a chronic disease state that requires ongoing medical care and surveillance for associated medical conditions, the post-transplantation state must be viewed as one with ongoing risks that exceed those of a child with normal heart and immune system. At this time, heart transplantation is not a cure, it is yet another palliation, and as such, the indications for OHT remain a matter of judgement based on the individual's heart disease and projected course without transplantation.

Almost all forms of CHD are amenable to some form of non-transplantation intervention that will improve the patient's prospect for survival and functional status. Results with palliative and reparative procedures have continued to improve, and therefore institutional approaches to almost all forms of CHD has not included transplantation as primary therapy. In patients with CHD, the indication for heart transplantation is rarely the underlying structural abnormality, but rather failure of the prior intervention to establish a durable cardiovascular physiology to allow survival with a reasonable quality of life (QOL) in the patient.

CHD is the most common indication for heart transplantation in neonates and young children. Cardiomyopathy is a more frequent indication in older children and adolescents, of which DCM, restrictive, or mixed phenotypes are the most common.

Pre-Transplant Evaluation

The purpose of the pre-transplant evaluation is to identify patient-specific risk factors that will increase waitlist mortality, transplant procedure mortality, and post-transplant mortality and morbidity. It includes a multisystem evaluation by a multidisciplinary team to comprehensively understand the risks and prognosis of OHT for any given patient. At the most fundamental level, it involves a clear understanding of the anatomic and hemodynamic considerations in a patient, to ensure that placement of a new heart would result in the adequate functioning of the organ and favorable hemodynamics. As such, clear delineation of the cardiac and venous anatomy with assessment of pulmonary vascular resistance (PVR) and reactivity is necessary. One of the most important hemodynamic contraindications to transplantation is the presence of "fixed" pulmonary hypertension. In the presence of a significantly elevated PVR, the donor right ventricle, which has only been exposed to low PVR in the setting of normal circulation, is not physiologically prepared or preconditioned (hypertrophied) to overcome the afterload imposed by the recipient's elevated PVR. Therefore, evaluation of the potential recipient's PVR at cardiac catheterization is essential. This evaluation includes an assessment of reactivity to 100% oxygen, induced hypocarbia and respiratory alkalosis, and inhaled nitric oxide (iNO). A PVR of greater than 6 Woods units (PVR indexed to body surface area) despite one or more of these interventions significantly raises the risk for donor right ventricular failure and graft loss. Patients with restrictive cardiomyopathy who manifest with chronically elevated left atrial pressures and elevated PVR are a subgroup that has been at particular risk of donor right ventricular failure. There has been successful use of VAD support to unload the pulmonary venous system and reduce the PVR prior to OHT, which appears to be sustained post-transplant.

Other medical conditions serve as relative contraindications to transplantation. A history of prior malignancy is a relative contraindication depending on the disease-free interval from malignancy and the biology of the underlying neoplastic disease. Because immunosuppression is associated with an increased risk of new malignancy after transplantation, and because there is some evidence for a role of immune surveillance in the "prevention" of primary malignancies under normal conditions, it has been generally assumed that immunosuppression in the presence of an existing malignancy will lead to a worsening of the course of the primary malignancy.

Preexisting renal or hepatic dysfunction is an important consideration in the pre-transplant evaluation because of the important renal and hepatic toxicities of several of the immunosuppressive agents. Severe respiratory dysfunction with need for mechanical ventilation at the time of transplantation is a risk factor for post-transplant mortality. Pulmonary fibrosis with restrictive lung disease does occur in patients after certain chemotherapeutic regimens and exposure to radiation therapy. As such, pulmonary function tests are carried out as part of the pre-transplantation evaluation when possible.

Preexisting psychiatric, neurodevelopmental, and psychosocial conditions of both patients and their families are also considered during the pre-transplantation evaluation; the post-transplantation regimens for immunosuppression and surveillance for rejection require strict ongoing medical compliance. Assessments are made by a team of physicians, psychiatrists, nurse practitioners, and social workers. However, our ability to predict which patients and families will be able to comply and cope with the complex post-transplantation medical regimen remains imperfect. Ongoing support for patients and families throughout their lifetime is essential and often the most challenging to deliver effectively.

In summary, there are relatively few absolute contraindications to cardiac transplantation in children other than fixed severe elevation of PVR or progressive pulmonary vein disease (pulmonary veins remain native to the patient and are not transplanted). Decisions regarding the listing of patients for heart transplantation therefore rest on the development of a composite picture rather than considering each factor in isolation.

Waitlist Outcomes and Donor Utilization Strategies

The United States organ transplant community has collectively agreed on a set of donor organ-sharing criteria. An organization, United Network for Organ Sharing (UNOS), has been created to match potential donors and recipients and to allocate each donor organ according to these criteria. Patients receive priority for a potential donor based on several criteria including level of support (e.g., MCS, positive pressure ventilator support, inotropes), patient-specific factors (e.g., CHD), sensitization, distance from donor, and duration on the wait list.

The limited supply of donor organs for transplantation imposes another set of difficult considerations involving allocation of a scarce resource. In considering each individual recipient, the sometimes difficult question of whether transplantation of an organ or organs will do the "most good for the most patients" must be considered. The national allocation criteria that have been developed address this limited resource problem by giving priority to those patients who are judged to be at greatest risk for death in the short term. However, judgments regarding the impact of specific coexisting medical and psychosocial conditions on the likelihood of a successful transplantation for an individual patient remain with the individual transplantation program. The "allocation of a scarce resource" problem therefore imposes significant responsibilities on local clinicians when making the decision to list an individual patient for transplantation. We have adopted a shared responsibility/accountability approach to making these decisions involving all members of our transplant team, including physicians, surgeons, psychiatrists, nurse practitioners, and social workers.

As described in the previous section, the use of advanced cardiac therapies, namely MCS, has dramatically changed the outcomes of patients awaiting transplantation. As such, more critically ill children who previously would have died, are surviving to transplantation with the use of long-term support strategies. However, in populations where VAD options are more limited, such as infants and those with complex CHD, there remains significant waitlist mortality. In addition to finding support strategies for the smallest and most complex patients, there are improvements in waitlist outcomes by increasing the available donor pool. One such advancement that has revolutionized infant transplantation has been the widespread adoption of ABO-incompatible OHT.[21,22] Using ABO-incompatible donors (i.e., blood group-incompatible hearts), transplantation can be performed across a wider donor pool for the youngest patients (generally < 2 years of age before isohemagglutinins have developed across blood group types).

Pre-Transplantation Management

After the decision is reached that transplantation is the most appropriate therapy for an individual patient's cardiac condition, management involves optimizing the cardiovascular and end-organ function until a donor heart becomes available. Some patients can be managed on an outpatient basis with combinations of pharmacologic and pacing therapies. Many patients require pre-transplantation hospitalization for decompensated heart failure. If a patient fails optimization of an oral heart failure regime, intravenous milrinone is commonly used for its positive inotropic, lusitropic, and systemic and pulmonary vasodilatory properties. Additionally, we have extensive institutional experience with safe and effective management of home milrinone therapy while awaiting transplantation across a wide range of diagnoses, ages, developmental abilities, and psychosocial barriers. To reduce sensitization of the recipient to antigens expressed on the cell surface, transfusions are limited, and all blood products are leukocyte filtered. Optimizing nutritional status and maintaining overall conditioning are difficult in the end-stage cardiac population, but they remain important to the success of the pre- and post-transplantation course. Comorbid disorders, such as protein-losing enteropathy and chronic liver and renal disease, may contribute to ongoing nutritional disorders. Malnutrition and growth failure are common due to anorexia and vomiting from high venous pressures and low cardiac output and are worsened by malabsorption and the hypermetabolic state of heart failure. Because immunosuppressed patients have a less effective response to vaccines, immunizations should be given according to current recommendations.

Surgical Techniques

The fundamental techniques for implantation of a cardiac donor allograft were initially described by Lower and Shumway and have changed relatively little since this initial description.[23] Some modifications of the techniques of donor organ procurement and preservation and of implantation techniques in situations of venous and great arterial anomalies have been necessary.

Donor Selection and Procurement

The fundamental goal of the donor operation is to provide an organ that functions well after implantation. Donor selection is important in achieving this goal. Preexisting congenital or acquired cardiac disease (except for a secundum atrial septal defect) precludes heart donation in most situations. Other donor contraindications include active septicemia or malignancies outside the central nervous system. The remainder of the donor evaluation is centered on evaluation of the donor heart function. The circumstances under which donor brain death has occurred, particularly if there is a significant period of cardiac ischemia or a history of major blunt thoracic trauma, influence donor heart function. Measurement of markers of cardiac injury, including creatine phosphokinase MB and troponin, can indicate myocardial injury. Evaluation of cardiac function by echocardiogram, and hemodynamic measurements of central venous pressure, pulmonary capillary wedge pressure, and levels of inotropic support, are also important. The anticipated cardiac ischemic time between retrieval and implantation will affect donor heart function. We attempt to limit the ischemic time to fewer than 4 hours, but this limit has been exceeded, particularly when the condition of the recipient is critical and the condition of the donor is otherwise favorable.

The technique of organ procurement focuses on preservation of the donor heart for the period of ischemia required for transport, but also includes acquisition of sufficient lengths of great artery and systemic vein to meet the anatomic requirements imposed by the recipient's anatomy. Important aspects of the donor cardiectomy are the rapid induction of hypothermic cardiac arrest with cold cardioplegia solution and the avoidance of cardiac distention by adequate venting of the right and left heart. Once the heart is excised, it is placed in a sterile container filled with additional cardioplegia solution, and then it is transported to the recipient institution at temperatures maintained near 4°C.

Recipient Operation

The recipient operation involves excision of the recipient heart and then the sequential construction of anastomoses of the donor and recipient venous and arterial structures. Donor and recipient teams must remain in close communication so that the recipient operation proceeds to minimize donor ischemic time and recipient cardiopulmonary bypass times.

The heart is approached through a median sternotomy incision, and cannulae for bypass are placed in the distal ascending aorta, the superior vena cava, and the inferior vena cava. In certain anatomic situations, cannulation of the femoral artery and vein may be necessary, and in infants, the carotid artery and internal jugular vein may be used for cannulation.

After the removal of the recipient's heart, sequential anastomoses are constructed between the donor and recipient left atria, superior and inferior venae cavae, pulmonary arteries, and aortae. In situations in which there are significant stenoses in the recipient's central pulmonary arteries, the donor branch pulmonary arteries can be used as onlay patches to enlarge the stenotic areas. If the recipient's aortic arch is stenotic, the donor aortic arch can be used for arch augmentation using a period of deep hypothermia and circulatory arrest. The technique of direct anastomoses between the donor and recipient venae cavae was used initially only in patients with a prior atrial-level repair of transposition, but is now used in most cases.[7] Monitoring catheters to measure right atrial, left atrial, and (in some cases) pulmonary artery pressures, as well as temporary atrial and ventricular pacing wires, are placed. Pharmacologic support is used as necessary based on the hemodynamic parameters and on visual assessment of cardiac function. In certain situations, particularly those in which there is very marginal right ventricular function, primary closure of the sternotomy incision can be delayed. Closure of the sternotomy incision is typically accomplished within several days, after recovery of ventricular function and diuresis has occurred.

Postoperative Surgical Management

The immediate postoperative management of the cardiac transplant recipient closely resembles the management of other patients undergoing cardiac surgical procedures. Atrial filling pressures, pulmonary artery pressures, and systemic arterial pressure are monitored continuously using indwelling catheters. Assessment of cardiac output is made by monitoring of lactate clearance, mixed venous saturation from a central venous or pulmonary arterial line, and end-organ function. The most common cause for depressed cardiac output is the period of myocardial ischemia before implantation, although recipient immune responses to the donor organ must be considered. Generally, myocardial dysfunction is transient and can be managed with inotropic and vasodilatory support. Because the donor heart is denervated, the initial cardiac rhythm after transplantation may be slow, and atrial pacing with temporary epicardial pacing wires is used to enhance cardiac output. The most serious problem following cardiac transplantation is right ventricular dysfunction, particularly when the recipient has preexisting elevation of PVR. The diagnosis of right ventricular failure can be difficult. Echocardiography can provide a qualitative assessment of right ventricular distention and contractility. Right ventricular afterload should also be minimized in situations of right ventricular dysfunction through sophisticated management of mechanical ventilation and the use of iNO to minimize PVR. In severe cases, the circulation can be supported, and the right ventricle decompressed with a venoarterial ECMO system. In most situations of significant right ventricular failure after transplantation, function recovers.

Post-Transplantation Management Issues

Rejection

Modulation of the immune response remains the major challenge to organ transplantation, but the number of therapeutic agents available that alter the immune response has increased significantly in recent years. Aggressive monitoring for signs and symptoms of rejection is essential (Table 54.2). Rejection can be broadly classified into three categories of variable severity: (1) cellular rejection, (2) antibody-mediated rejection/humoral, or (3) mixed. Clinical presentation of rejection is variable and can range from hemodynamically significant impairment of systolic function and/or onset of atrial or ventricular arrhythmias, to more subtle changes in diastolic indices. Some patients may have no change in cardiac function, but laboratory data reveal the presence of donor-specific antibodies, elevated biomarkers, and/or other histopathological findings suggestive of rejection. Tissue for histologic examinations is obtained with a bioptome forceps introduced transvenously with right heart cardiac catheterization. Rejection identified by biopsy, particularly in the first year after transplantation, is aggressively treated with an increase in immunosuppression to minimize damage to the transplanted heart. Because acute rejection is most frequently seen in the first 3 to 6 months after transplantation, "surveillance" biopsies are carried out at frequent intervals during this period. However, any time there are indications that rejection may be occurring, the donor heart is biopsied immediately. Newer modalities for transplant rejection surveillance are actively being investigated, focusing on less invasive tests, that could be performed more routinely. Noninvasive imaging such as echocardiography for strain and cardiac MRI for myocardial edema as well as a multitude of biomarkers (troponins, brain natriuretic peptide, gene profiling of blood immune cell components, micro RNAs, and donor-derived cell free DNA) are promising alternatives.[24,25]

Immunosuppressive regimens are tailored to the specific immunogenicity of the patient (e.g., risk of rejection, time from transplantation, and degree of sensitization), as well as comorbid end-organ dysfunction (e.g., renal dysfunction, graft vasculopathy). The standard regimen includes use of antithymocyte globulin infusion for 5 days with concomitant steroids, as maintenance immunosuppression is being uptitrated. Maintenance immunosuppression includes the use of a calcineurin inhibitor (tacrolimus) to affect T-lymphocyte function, and mycophenolate mofetil or azathioprine to reduce the proliferation of immune responsive leukocytes. Calcineurin inhibitors are begun in the postoperative period once hemodynamic stability and renal function are reestablished. Alternative regimens have also been used in highly sensitized patients including the use of plasmapheresis, intravenous immunoglobulins, and rituximab and bortezomib, in variable intervals to reduce the burden of complement-fixing donor-specific antibodies.

Coronary Vasculopathy

A more insidious and difficult problem occurs in the later post-transplantation period, characterized by the development of progressive narrowing of the coronary arteries leading to myocardial ischemia, myocardial dysfunction, arrhythmias, and risk for sudden death. This post-transplantation coronary arteriopathy generally thought to represent the sequelae of antibody-mediated rejection is the leading cause of death among late survivors of OHT.

The diagnosis of coronary vasculopathy is difficult. Signs and symptoms are outlined in Table 54.3, although many patients are often asymptomatic. Surveillance for graft vasculopathy includes routine coronary angiography (yearly from 1 to 5 years post-transplant followed by alternating years with exercise stress tests assessing for segmental wall motion abnormalities), screening troponins, echocardiography strain testing for diastolic dysfunction, and MRI.

Infection

Infection is an important issue in the post-transplantation patient because of the immunosuppression required to prevent rejection of the transplanted heart. The availability of effective antibacterial, antiviral, and antifungal agents has allowed many of these post-transplantation infections to be treated, but this remains an important source of morbidity and potential mortality.

Viral infections represent a significant risk to the patient after transplantation but the emergence of several antiviral

TABLE 54.2	Signs and Symptoms of Acute Rejection in Children Following Heart Transplantation

Symptoms

- Fatigue
- Decreased appetite
- Nausea
- Abdominal pain
- Rapid increase in weight
- Fussiness, poor feeding (infants)

Signs

- Tachycardia
- Irregular rhythm, atrial flutter, ventricular tachycardia
- Fever
- Gallop (S3)
- Hepatomegaly

TABLE 54.3	Signs and Symptoms of Chronic Rejection Following Heart Transplantation in Children

- Ectopy/atrial flutter
- Presyncope
- Syncope
- Intermittent edema
- Exercise intolerance
- Chest pain (rare due to cardiac denervation)

therapies have, to some extent, mitigated these risks. Chronic early and late surveillance of cytomegalovirus and Epstein-Barr virus (EBV) is paramount, as each virus plays a role in graft vasculopathy and post-transplant lymphoproliferative disease (PTLD), respectively. In PTLD there is rapid proliferation of B lymphocytes, generally in a single anatomic area, and these proliferating lymphocytes frequently behave in a malignant fashion. The occurrence of PTLD has been significantly associated with the use of monoclonal or polyclonal antilymphocyte globulins (rabbit antithymocyte globulin or the murine antilymphocyte antibody OKT-3). Therefore, the use of these antilymphocyte globulins has been reserved for treatment of rejection refractory to other agents. The diagnosis is established by an excisional biopsy of the involved lymph nodes. The treatment of PTLD associated with EBV infection ranges from reductions in the dosages of immunosuppressive agents to the use of chemotherapeutic regimens depending on location, size, staging, and proliferation of the PTLD. Other infections, such as herpes zoster, parvovirus, and fungi, have been treated successfully but have a high risk for significant morbidity and mortality.

Long-Term Medical Management

Nephrotoxicity is common and may be exacerbated post transplantation from chronic calcineurin inhibitor therapy. As such, preservation of renal function pre-transplant is paramount followed by maintaining renal protective strategies post-transplant. Other long-term issues such as hypercholesterolemia, osteoporosis, insulin-dependent diabetes, and obesity must be followed closely and treated (Table 54.4).

Psychosocial Issues and Living With Chronic Disease

Heart transplantation is not a cure and requires lifelong medical intervention, adherence, and monitoring. As is seen in so many chronic medical conditions, there is a significant burden of anxiety, depression, patient and caregiver burnout, isolation, and a myriad of other underappreciated psychosocial stressors. Appreciation of the importance of QOL in these patients has increased over the last decades, with prolific research examining how to

TABLE 54.4 Optimizing Long-Term Health

- Cholesterol management
- Routine exercise
- Smoking cessation/counseling
- Aggressive blood pressure control
- Optimize bone health and prevention
- Family support and counseling
- Adolescent non-compliance issues
- Neurocognitive and neuropsychiatric support

study, report, and understand QOL in these patients. Patient-reported outcomes are one such strategy that allows patients and their families to report signs, symptoms, and feelings in a systematic fashion that allows for analyses. There is ongoing need for psychological assessment and support for patients and their families facing pediatric OHT; more than 25% will likely present with emotional adjustment difficulties.

Non-adherence to complicated and life-sustaining therapy is appreciated to be an important determinant of long-term outcomes. Normal adolescent development, combined with the complex psychological issues surrounding heart transplantation, creates a large population of recipients at risk. Non-adherence has been linked to late rejection, and higher mortality rates in the older adolescent group have been observed.

Conclusion

Overall outcomes continue to improve for children awaiting and following pediatric heart transplantation. Newer immunosuppressive agents with lower side-effect profiles, the possibility of immune tolerance, and close supervision of health maintenance issues allow for a promising future for many of these patients.

References

1. Rossano JW, Lorts A, Vanderpluym CJ, et al. Outcomes of pediatric patients supported with continuous-flow ventricular assist devices: a report from the Pediatric Interagency Registry for Mechanical Circulatory Support (PediMACS). *J Heart Lung Transplant.* 2016;35:585-590.
2. Lorts A, Conway J, Schweiger M, et al. ISHLT consensus statement for the selection and management of pediatric and congenital heart disease patients on ventricular assist devices Endorsed by the American Heart Association. *J Heart Lung Transplant.* 2021;40:709-732.
3. Rossano JW, VanderPluym CJ, Peng DM, et al. Fifth Annual Pediatric Interagency Registry for Mechanical Circulatory Support (Pedimacs) Report. *Ann Thorac Surg.* 2021;112:1763-1774.
4. O'Connor MJ, Lorts A, Davies RR, et al. Early experience with the HeartMate 3 continuous-flow ventricular assist device in pediatric patients and patients with congenital heart disease: a multicenter registry analysis. *J Heart Lung Transplant.* 2020;39:573-579.
5. Morales DLS, Adachi I, Peng DM, et al. Fourth Annual Pediatric Interagency Registry for Mechanical Circulatory Support (Pedimacs) Report. *Ann Thorac Surg.* 2020;110:1819-1831.
6. VanderPluym CJ, Blume ED. The role of continuous flow ventricular assist device for destination therapy in children: can it work or is it a bridge too far. *Prog Pediatr Cardiol.* 2016;40:25-27.
7. Blume ED, Rosenthal DN, Rossano JW, et al. Outcomes of children implanted with ventricular assist devices in the United States: first analysis of the Pediatric Interagency Registry for Mechanical Circulatory Support (PediMACS). *J Heart Lung Transplant.* 2016;35:578-584.
8. Peng DM, Rosenthal DN, Zafar F, et al. Collaboration and new data in ACTION: a learning health care system to improve

pediatric heart failure and ventricular assist device outcomes. *Transl Pediatr.* 2019;8(4):349-355. doi: 10.21037/tp.2019.07.12.

9. Lorts A, Smyth L, Gajarski RJ, et al. The creation of a pediatric health care learning network: the ACTION Quality Improvement Collaborative. *ASAIO J.* 2020;66:441-446.

10. Morales DLS, Rossano JW, VanderPluym C, et al. Third Annual Pediatric Interagency Registry for Mechanical Circulatory Support (Pedimacs) Report: preimplant characteristics and outcomes. *Ann Thorac Surg.* 2019;107:993-1004.

11. Villa CR, Lorts A. Cardiac destination therapy in pediatrics: are we there yet. *Pediatr Transplant.* 2016;20:738-739.

12. Edelson JB, Huang Y, Griffis H, et al. The influence of mechanical Circulatory support on post-transplant outcomes in pediatric patients: a multicenter study from the International Society for Heart and Lung Transplantation (ISHLT) Registry. *J Heart Lung Transplant.* 2021;40:1443-1453.

13. Conway J, St Louis J, Morales DLS, et al. Delineating survival outcomes in children. *JACC Heart Fail.* 2015;3:70-77.

14. Hollander SA, Cantor RS, Sutherland SM, et al. Renal injury and recovery in pediatric patients after ventricular assist device implantation and cardiac transplant. *Pediatr Transplant.* 2019;23:e13477.

15. Rossano JW, VanderPluym CJ, Peng DM, et al. Pedimacs Investigators. Fifth Annual Pediatric Interagency Registry for Mechanical Circulatory Support (Pedimacs) Report. *Ann Thorac Surg.* 2021;112(6):1763-1774.

16. Botha P, Hasan A, Perri G, et al. Modified technique for the implantation of berlin heart excor ventricular assist device in children. *World J Pediatr Congenit Heart Surg.* 2012;3:373-377.

17. Vanderpluym CJ, Cantor RS, MacHado D, et al. Utilization and outcomes of children treated with direct thrombin inhibitors on paracorporeal ventricular assist device support. *ASAIO J.* 2020; 66:939-945.

18. Bleiweis MS, Philip J, Peek GJ, et al. Palliation plus ventricular assist device insertion in 15 neonates and infants with functionally univentricular circulation. *Ann Thorac Surg.* 2022;114(4): 1412-1418. doi: 10.1016/j.athoracsur.2022.02.051.

19. Singh TP, Cherikh WS, Hsich E, et al. The international thoracic organ transplant registry of the international society for heart and lung transplantation: twenty-fifth pediatric heart transplantation report-2022; focus on infant heart transplantation. *J Heart Lung Transplant.* 2022;41(10):1357-1365.

20. Denfield SW, Azeka E, Das B, et al. Pediatric cardiac waitlist mortality: still too high. *Pediatr Transplant.* 2020;24(3):e13671.

21. West LJ, Pollock-Barziv SM, Dipchand AI, et al. ABO-incompatible heart transplantation in infants. *N Engl J Med.* 2001;344:793-800.

22. Urschel S, Ballweg JA, Cantor RS, et al. Clinical outcomes of children receiving ABO-incompatible versus ABO-compatible heart transplantation: a multicentre cohort study. *Lancet Child Adolesc Health.* 2021;5:341-349.

23. Lower RR, Shumway NE. Studies on orthotopic homotransplantation of the canine heart. *Surg Forum.* 1960;11:18-19. Available at: https://pubmed.ncbi.nlm.nih.gov/13763847/. Accessed August 25, 2022.

24. Agbor-Enoh S, Shah P, Tunc I, et al. Cell-Free DNA to detect heart allograft acute rejection. *Circulation.* 2021;143: 1184-1197.

25. Kittleson MM, Garg S. Solid gold, or liquid gold?: towards a new diagnostic standard for heart transplant rejection. *Circulation.* 2021;143:1198-1201.

55

Central Nervous System Sequelae of Congenital Heart Disease

MICHELLE GURVITZ AND JANE W. NEWBURGER

KEY LEARNING POINTS

- Patients with congenital heart disease have a high prevalence of neuropsychological and psychosocial impairments.
- Abnormalities in brain development in complex congenital heart disease begin *in utero*.
- Risk factors for neurological, cognitive, and behavioral morbidities are multifactorial, cumulative, and interactive.

- Neuropsychological and behavioral needs are dynamic throughout the life span, from fetus to adult.
- Early and regular neuropsychological and psychiatric screening are recommended to identify areas for intervention.

Introduction

With 85–90% of individuals born with congenital heart disease (CHD) now living to adulthood, neurological, neuropsychological, and behavioral disorders have emerged as among the most common and troubling morbidities that affect survivors.[1,2] Indeed, neuropsychological deficits occur in up to 50% of children with complex CHD, and brain MRIs in complex CHD commonly show disturbed development and injury even before the first surgical procedure.[1] Compared with the general population, individuals with CHD are more likely to have difficulties with processing speed, working memory, attention and impulsivity, executive function (EF), and social cognition, and they are more likely to require remedial services at school age. Over time, neurocognitive disabilities may adversely impact the highest level of education, employability, interpersonal relationships, and mental health.[3]

The causes of neurological and developmental impairments are interactive and cumulative over time. Established risk factors include genetic abnormalities, diminished cerebral oxygen delivery *in utero* and other maternal factors, brain immaturity at birth, perioperative and operative factors including prolonged hospital length of stay, and complications of heart disease itself, such as thromboembolic events. As in the general population, social determinants of health play a role in neuropsychological outcomes, and neurodevelopmental performance is generally worse among children of low socioeconomic status (Fig. 55.1).

Pathology

Autopsy studies of fetuses, infants, children, and adults with CHD reveal brain abnormalities at all stages of life, before and after surgical or catheter interventions. The most recent autopsy series, from fetal to adult age, showed ~60% of cases had acquired neuropathological injury, most commonly microscopic gray matter lesions and intracranial hemorrhages, as well as hippocampal injury and white matter gliosis; more severe focal lesions like periventricular leukomalacia were identified less commonly. While some cases had genetic abnormalities or extracardiac anomalies, most had isolated cyanotic CHD.[4] Clinical and autopsy studies have shown that 10–30% of patients with CHD have congenital anomalies of the brain, including microcephaly, absent corpus collosum, meningomyelocele, Dandy-Walker malformation, and lissencephaly.[4]

CNS Imaging and Monitoring

Brain magnetic resonance imaging (MRI) has been the mainstay for imaging central nervous system (CNS) structure, microstructure, and function in patients with CHD from fetal life through adulthood. Across a broad age range, 21–82% of patients with CHD, compared with < 7% in controls, have structural abnormalities, including focal infarcts, mineral and iron deposits, delayed myelination, ventriculomegaly, and congenital malformations. Other

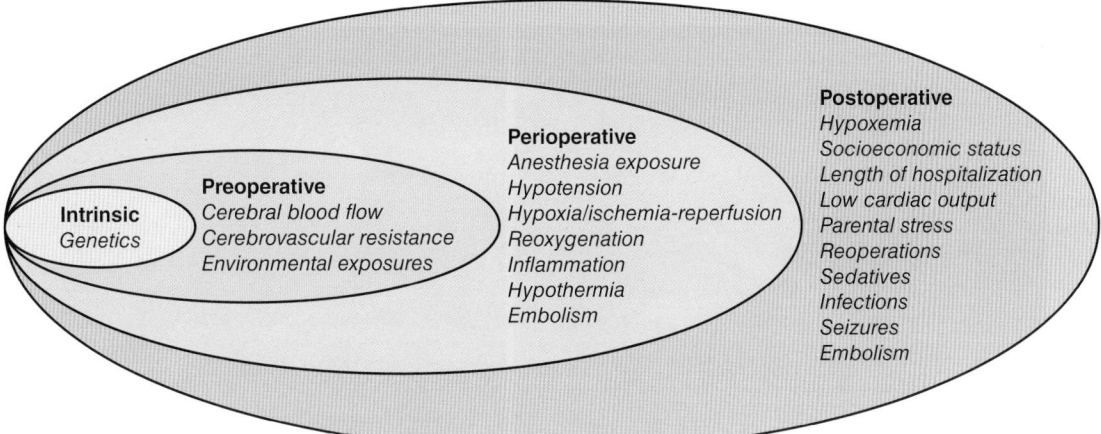

• **Fig. 55.1** Contributors to brain injury among patients with congenital heart disease. This diagram describes factors that can contribute to brain injury at different time points including intrinsic and pre-, peri-, and postoperative factors. (From Figure 3 in Morton PD, Ishibashi N, Jonas RA. Neurodevelopmental abnormalities and congenital heart disease: insights into altered brain maturation. *Circ Res.* 2017;120:960–977.)

common findings include the presence of T2-weighted hyperintensities produced by demyelination or axonal loss, and reduced cortical folding that limits the overall cortical surface area. Global hypoxic-ischemic brain injury may occur after cardiac arrest or a prolonged period of low perfusion.

Fetuses and newborns with CHD, particularly those with cyanotic CHD, have lower volumes of total brain volume, white, and gray matter, as well as reduced cortical thickness (Fig. 55.2). Brain structures involved in neurocognitive performance (e.g., hippocampus, cerebellum, caudate) are also affected.[5] In newborns, preoperative white matter injury (WMI) is present in ~20% of neonates with mixed forms of critical CHD, and is most highly related to brain immaturity, for example due to younger gestational age. Preoperative brain immaturity, in turn, is associated with new WMI after surgery and also with worse neurodevelopmental scores at age 2 years.[6] Some programs perform routine brain MRI to identify brain injury in neonates undergoing open heart surgery, but the cost benefit of this approach is uncertain.

Diffusion tensor imaging, with measurements of fractional anisotropy and diffusivity, in adolescents with critical CHD has shown widespread WMI that is correlated both with clinical risk factors and with concurrent neurocognitive function.[7] Such MRI techniques can be used to create a map of neural connections in the brain, called the connectome. Studies of the connectome in teens with complex CHD, compared with controls, have shown decreased global efficiency (network integration) and increased modularity (network segregation).[8]

Other forms of monitoring to detect brain injury in the immediate postoperative period include near-infrared spectroscopy (NIRS) and postoperative electroencephalogram (EEG) monitoring. NIRS uses near-infrared light to penetrate the outer layers of the scalp and skull to measure cerebral oxygen delivery and detect hypoxia. This allows early action to correct low oxygen delivery to the brain.[9] The EEG reflects cerebral function and can show both clinical

and subclinical seizures postoperatively. The occurrence of postoperative seizures in neonates after cardiac surgery is a powerful independent risk factor for adverse neurocognitive outcome in childhood and adolescence.[10]

Risk Factors for CNS Injury and Abnormality

Risk factors for CNS sequelae are multifactorial and include innate patient factors, medical risk factors, and environmental influences.

Innate Patient and Preoperative Risk Factors

Genetic abnormalities are present in ~50% of syndromic CHD and ~10% of non-syndromic CHD and include gross chromosomal abnormalities (e.g., trisomy 21), pathogenic copy number variants (e.g., DiGeorge syndrome), or single gene disorders (e.g., Noonan's syndrome).[11] The biological pathways that cause cardiac malformations in fetal life, for example those involved in chromatin or histone modification, transcription factors, cilia function, or calcium signaling, may also affect development of the fetal brain. This premise is supported by the finding from exome sequencing in > 1200 parent-offspring trios that damaging *de novo* mutations occur in only 2% of patients with isolated CHD, compared with 20% of those who have CHD, neurodevelopmental disability, and extracardiac anomalies.[12] Common genetic variants that moderate the brain's response to injury, such as apolipoprotein E (APOE), have also been implicated in CNS sequelae of CHD. APOE is involved in lipid transport and is important for neuronal repair after injury in ischemia, hemorrhage, and traumatic brain injury. Studies have shown associations between APOE genotypes and outcomes including worse psychomotor development at age 1 year and later behavior in

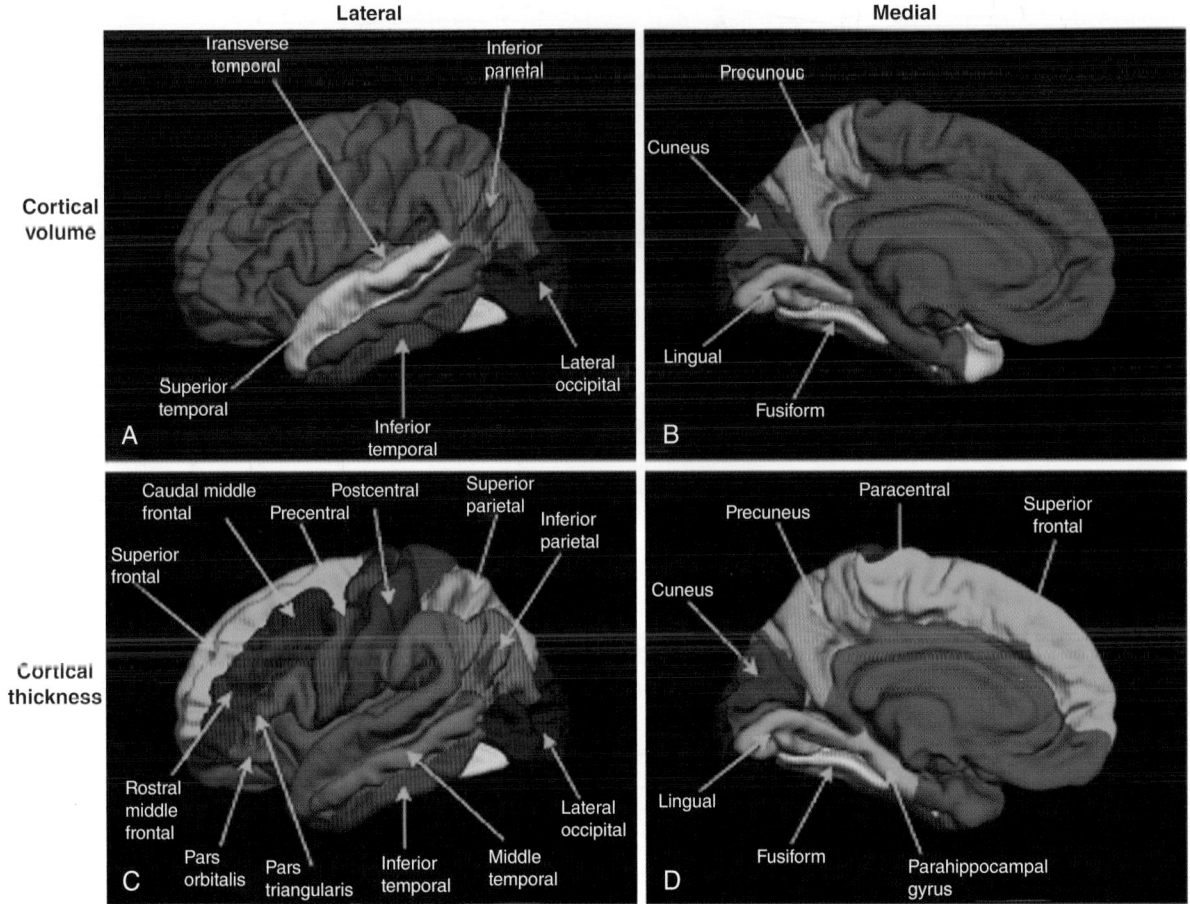

Lateral   **Medial**

Cortical volume

Transverse temporal   Inferior parietal
Superior temporal   Inferior temporal   Lateral occipital

Precuneus
Cuneus
Lingual   Fusiform

A   B

Cortical thickness

Caudal middle frontal   Postcentral   Superior parietal
Precentral   Inferior parietal
Superior frontal
Rostral middle frontal   Lateral occipital
Pars orbitalis   Pars triangularis   Inferior temporal   Middle temporal

Precuneus   Paracentral   Superior frontal
Cuneus
Lingual   Fusiform   Parahippocampal gyrus

C   D

• **Fig. 55.2** Areas of cerebral volume loss and decreased cortical thickness. Regions of cortical volume and thickness differences between Fontan and control groups. **(A)** Lateral and **(B)** medial views of the cortical surface showing locations of reduced mean regional volume in the Fontan group compared with the control group. **(C)** Lateral and **(D)** medial views of the cortical surface showing locations of reduced mean cortical thickness in the Fontan group compared with the control group. (From Figure 1 in Watson CG, Stopp C, Wypij D, Newburger JW, Rivkin MJ. Reduced cortical volume and thickness and their relationship to medical and operative features in post-Fontan children and adolescents. *Pediatr Res.* 2017;81:881–890.)

preschool children with CHD with the APOE2 allele.[13] The impact of APOE genotype appears to change with age; in adolescents, more frequent attention problems were identified in those with the APOE4 allele and those with APOE2 had better outcomes.[14]

In addition to genetics, the fetal environment and physiology also affect brain growth and development. The third trimester of pregnancy is an important time for advanced brain development and growth, with formation of neuronal connections. Complex CHDs, particularly those with single-ventricle physiology and transposition of the great arteries, may alter fetal cerebral hemodynamics and lower substrate delivery to the brain. This physiology has been associated with slowing of brain maturation, delayed cortical folding, decreased fetal brain volumes, and smaller head circumference at birth. A longitudinal fetal brain MRI study found smaller volumes in the subplate, intermediate, and ventricular zones in CHD fetuses than in control fetuses.[15] The greatest volume reduction was seen in fetuses with D-transposition of the great arteries and hypoplastic left

heart syndrome, presumably because these brain regions are populated by cell types, i.e., subplate neurons, premyelinating oligodendrocytes, and neural progenitor cells that are especially vulnerable to hypoxia-ischemia. Newborns with CHD show WMI and dysmaturation somewhat similar to findings in preterm neonates; indeed, brain total maturation scores in term infants with CHD are similar to those of children born 1 month premature.[16] Physiologic fetal adaptive responses, including cerebral autoregulation, that preserve cerebral blood flow may be impaired in some fetuses with CHD.

Other maternal factors also impact brain growth and development. Placental function may be impaired in pregnancies carrying complex CHD, lowering cerebral oxygen delivery with adverse effects on brain development and metabolism. A landmark report showed that elevated prenatal maternal psychological distress, prevalent in mothers anticipating the birth of a child with CHD, is associated with impaired development of the cerebellum and hippocampus in the second half of gestation.[17]

A growing body of literature supports the predictive validity of findings on fetal brain MRI for developmental outcomes. Sadhwani et al.[18] showed that fetal brain volume is a significant predictor of scores at age 2 years on cognitive, language, and motor domains of the Bayley III, as well as of adaptive function scores among individuals with CHD. In multivariable analysis including socioeconomic status, postnatal patient factors, and medical factors, fetal brain volume continued to explain a significant percentage of the variance in outcome across developmental domains. Another study showed that worse developmental performance metrics at age 18 months were associated both with greater stress during pregnancy and with particular anatomic findings on fetal brain MRI associated with greater maternal stress (gyrification index, sulcal depth).[19] These data highlight the importance of fetal brain development to future neurodevelopmental performance, as well as the importance of overall maternal well-being.

The postnatal, preoperative period also poses challenges for neurologic protection, particularly for the immature brain. With the decrease in oxygen delivery and increase in extraction, the brain is more susceptible to hypoxic-ischemic insult, which increases the risk for WMI.

Operative and Postoperative Factors

Cardiac surgery can be associated with neurologic complications including stroke, seizures, and hypoxic-ischemic encephalopathy in infants, children, and adults. CNS injury during cardiopulmonary bypass may result from thrombotic and gaseous macro- and microemboli, as well as hypoperfusion that causes global hypoxic-ischemic brain injury. Improvements in types of oxygenators and arterial filtration have lowered the risks of perioperative stroke since the early days of infant heart surgery. In recent years, starting with the Boston Circulatory Arrest Study evaluating bypass strategies in 1988,[20] much research has been dedicated to optimizing bypass techniques for protection of the brain and other vital organs. Randomized clinical trials have shown that independent risk factors for worse late neuropsychological function include longer duration of deep hypothermic circulatory arrest and lower hematocrit during the cooling phase of bypass. Observational studies have also suggested an adverse impact of rapid cooling as well as longer bypass and total support times. Despite early hopes, regional (antegrade) cerebral perfusion has not been shown to protect the brain during use of deep hypothermic circulatory arrest.

The type of intraoperative management strategy contributes less variance to long-term outcome than preoperative factors (e.g., genetic abnormalities, fetal cerebral hemodynamics, birth weight, brain maturity at surgery, maternal education, and social class) and postoperative morbidities. Indeed, the best surgical neuroprotection for the neonate with critical CHD is likely provided by a technically adequate operation that minimizes postoperative complications and shortens hospital course.

Postoperative complications, including hypotension, hypoxia, cardiac arrest, and extracorporeal membrane oxygenation (ECMO) support, may each cause brain injury. Postoperative seizures may not only be a sign of brain injury but have also been hypothesized to cause brain injury if prolonged and uncontrolled. Even when adjusting for postoperative complications like sepsis or seizures, however, longer hospital length of stay after infant heart surgery is one of the strongest independent risk factors for adverse late neuropsychological outcome. Underlying mechanisms for this relationship apart from cardiovascular instability may include alterations in the hormonal milieu and environmental toxicities, such as constant noise, pain, absence of stimulation (visual and touch), and exposure to plasticizers.[21]

Finally, repeated or prolonged exposure to anesthetic agents has caused neurotoxicity in animal models, resulting in black box warnings on many drugs commonly used for anesthesia during infant heart surgery. The association of volatile anesthetic agents with lower 1-year Bayley III scores in one study has suggested that alternative anesthetic and sedative drugs may be preferable.[22]

Other Risk Factors

Neurologic and developmental sequelae of CHD may result not only from innate patient factors and procedures but also from complications of heart disease itself. Longer years of severe cyanosis have been associated with lower IQ scores at age 5 years. Strokes are common, particularly in patients with single ventricle who had undergone the Fontan procedure, and they may be clinically silent or discovered only with brain imaging. Noncardiac factors also play a role in brain growth and development and neurodevelopmental outcomes for patients with CHD. Nutritional status is often poor in neonates, infants, and children with complex CHD due to increased metabolic needs, decreased gastric motility, reflux, and other GI conditions. In children with single ventricle heart disease, poorer nutritional status has been linked to worse neuropsychological outcomes. In addition, socioeconomic status has been related to neuropsychological outcomes in children with complex CHD, with those in the lowest tertile of neighborhood socioeconomic status and maternal education having worse outcomes and lower rates of specialty referrals than those in the upper tertiles.[16] Growing evidence suggests that parental mental health struggles and stress also play a significant role in worsening child neuropsychological outcomes, behavioral difficulties, and quality of life (QOL). One systematic review noted that over 80% of parents reported post-traumatic stress, psychological distress, depression, or anxiety. Helping to address these noncardiac, social, and parental conditions may optimize development and outcome for patients with CHD.[3]

Adults

As patients with CHD age, they are at risk for typical acquired conditions of adulthood including hypertension, diabetes, and coronary artery disease, each of which is a risk factor for CNS injury. Whereas the neurologic impact of these risk factors has not been assessed specifically in CHD patients, these conditions are known in the general population to confer a risk of cognitive impairment, including in language, attention, memory, and EFs. In addition, atrial fibrillation, hypertension, and coronary artery disease have been associated with stroke, dementia, and abnormal brain aging. Low cardiac output states in older adults have also been associated with smaller brain volumes, increased WMI, dementia, and decreased EF skills on cognitive testing.[2,23,24] CHD survivors thus are at risk for routine adult-onset CNS injury and sequelae that will be cumulative to CNS abnormalities incurred during childhood. Understanding the interaction of childhood neurologic and neuropsychological morbidities with routinely acquired forms of brain injury in adulthood is a critical knowledge gap that requires vigilance and further study. Because atherosclerosis begins in childhood, hyperlipidemia, hypertension, and other risk factors for adult-onset cardiovascular disease should be aggressively managed in all patients with CHD.

Neuropsychological Impairments

Concerns for neuropsychological impairment and social and emotional adjustment in children with CHD has been proposed since the 1960s. Neurocognitive disabilities are now recognized to affect over 50% of patients in infancy and childhood, creating a need for educational and social supports. Among those without genetic syndromes, neuropsychological deficits are most common in individuals born with cyanotic heart disease and complex lesions requiring early open heart surgery. Those with single ventricle heart disease are most affected. While individual intelligence is typically within the normal range, the average IQ of patients with CHD measures somewhat lower than peers without CHD. Areas of most pronounced deficits, however, include visuo-spatial skills, processing speed, nonverbal reasoning, language development, fine motor skills, socialization, attention, and EFs.[1] EFs include higher-order thinking including working memory, flexible thinking, organization, and inhibitory control and may not be recognized until patients are older and need to develop increased responsibility and independence.

While the neuropsychological phenotype described above among children with CHD is relatively consistent, performance varies widely among individuals. In larger studies, up to 50% of children with complex CHD require early interventional services or remedial help in school. Many patients have test results similar to those on the autism spectrum of disorders as they relate to social cognition (the ability to interpret social information and behave appropriately in a social environment) and other social interactions. This is also consistent with the potential genetic overlap identified between autism and CHD.

Neuropsychological impairments, particularly in the area of EFs, can also appear over time as children and adolescents are asked to take on more responsibility and independent roles. This may reveal areas of concern that were otherwise masked by support systems or parental assistance. There can be profound effects of such deficits as individuals grow into adulthood and take on additional responsibilities of employment, independent living, and intimate social relationships. Untreated, neuropsychological disabilities can lead to increased stress, anxiety, and depression. Some studies have shown that adults with CHD have lower rates of educational attainment, employment, and long-term relationships than peers.[3]

Only a small number of cross-sectional studies of cognitive deficits have explored outcomes in adult survivors of CHD. Small studies have identified challenges in EF, attention, visuo-spatial skills, and memory, areas of deficit similar to those identified in children and adolescents with CHD. Additional studies have suggested that adults with CHD may have cognitive impairment including memory difficulties and have an increased risk of dementia compared with the general population.[24,25] Because few studies have followed patients from childhood into adulthood, the tracking of deficits and the percentage of adult deficits attributable to antecedents in childhood are unknown and remains an important area for study.

Psychosocial Effects

Mental health and neuropsychological performance have a complex and bidirectional relationship. For example, anxiety and depression can affect neuropsychological functioning, including EFs, risk-taking behaviors, social relationships, and occupational opportunities. Conversely, neuropsychological deficits including executive dysfunction may predispose to life circumstances that, in turn, cause anxiety and depression.

QOL is worse in children with CHD than in age-matched peers. In school age, children with CHD have increased rates of social withdrawal, anxiety, depression, and aggressive behavior. Children with more complex heart disease, compared with the average child, may have an even greater increase in risk for anxiety, depression, and attention disorders.[3]

Adolescents with CHD must manage their heart condition and any learning impairments in addition to the routine challenges of psychosocial development. Challenges in this age group include increasingly difficult schoolwork, appearing different from others (e.g., scar, cyanosis), missing classes for appointments or hospitalizations, and parental overprotection. Social anxiety related to poorer social cognition skills can worsen the QOL at this age. Indeed, neuropsychological disorders have been shown to predict worse psychosocial health status in children and adolescents. Similarly, the prevalence of comorbid psychiatric disorders is three to four times higher among adults with neurocognitive impairment than in the general population. Adults with CHD have a high prevalence of depression and anxiety. Multiple studies have evaluated mood disorders in adults with CHD, with reported prevalence of up to 40% in self-report and surveys and up to 50% in studies using structured interviews.[3]

Paradoxically, studies of adults with CHD show QOL scores similar to or sometimes better than the general population. Worse scores in adults with CHD have occurred in domains of physical discomfort, anxiety, and depression. Older age, female sex, medications, and comorbid conditions have also been associated with lower QOL. Interestingly, severity of CHD does not necessarily correlate with QOL in adults, as those with relatively less complex CHDs, such as atrial septal defects, can have low QOL scores. Such mild defects may be diagnosed in adulthood, thus calling for a different psychosocial adjustment than in patients diagnosed in childhood who have likely adjusted their priorities, expectations, and coping mechanisms over time. In addition, whereas adults with CHD may have a relatively high prevalence of psychiatric impairments including anxiety and depression, these do not necessarily correlate with QOL or well-being.

Relationship of Imaging to Outcomes

While multiple CNS abnormalities have been identified on brain imaging and impaired neuropsychological and cognitive function is common in CHD, specific direct relationships between injury and outcome are few. Studies have generally shown a relationship between smaller brain volumes, abnormal topology, and evidence of injury with worse neuropsychological outcomes particularly in intelligence, memory, and EF. In patients with complex CHD, WMI has been associated with specific neuropsychological deficits in some studies. Smaller hippocampal and temporal volumes have been correlated with worse memory and worse verbal comprehension, and working memory was associated with impaired white matter tracts in the uncinate fasciculus, cingulum hippocampus, superior longitudinal fasciculus, and corticospinal tracts. Moreover, disruptions in neural networks or the connectome may mediate other neurocognitive disabilities, such as attention deficit and hyperactivity disorder.[14]

Recommended Screening, Follow-Up, and Potential Interventions

Given the high prevalence of neuropsychological and other CNS findings in infants and children with CHD, the American Heart Association (AHA) and American Academy of Pediatrics (AAP) published a scientific statement in 2012 outlining the evaluation and management of these conditions.[1] The statement recommends routine neurodevelopmental screening and testing of all high-risk children with CHD, as well as education of patients, families, and schools about neurodevelopmental morbidities. Individuals considered to be at higher risk include: (1) children who undergo open cardiac surgery in the first year of life; (2)

children with cyanotic heart lesions who did not undergo open heart surgery in the first year of life; (3) children with any type of CHD combined with at least one comorbidity that put them at risk for neurodevelopmental disability (e.g., prematurity < 37 weeks, developmental delay in the first year of life, genetic disorder, history of ECMO or ventricular assist device, heart transplantation, cardiopulmonary resuscitation, prolonger postoperative length of stay > 2 weeks in the hospital, perioperative seizures, significant neuroimaging abnormalities, or microcephaly); or (4) other conditions determined at the discretion of the medical home provider.

Because of the potential impact of neuropsychological and other CNS conditions on future development, education, relationships, and employment, their evaluation and treatment is a top priority for future well-being. Screening in the infant and early school age years allows for timely implementation of support and treatment strategies such as early intervention services, and individualized education plans (IEP). Because genetic abnormalities are common in CHD and affect neurodevelopmental outcome, early genetic testing can be helpful in guiding neurodevelopmental and other services and informing prognosis. Neuropsychological disabilities, such as executive dysfunction, may first become apparent at older ages, so routine surveillance for children with CHD is recommended throughout childhood and young adult years.[1] Depending on the area of residence, insurance status, and resources, screening may be performed by neurodevelopment programs, cardiology programs, or primary care providers.

Specific recommendations for high-risk children include: (1) early intervention or early childhood education services; (2) formal developmental and medical evaluation at ages 12–24 months, 3–5 years, and 11–12 years of age; (3) after age 12 years, an evaluation plan to be determined at the discretion of the medical home provider; and (4) referral of young adults for higher educational and/or vocational counseling. Adults with CHD also may benefit from cognitive and neuropsychological evaluation, as they often have not had prior screening, have an increased risk of disabilities and sometimes dementia, and may need social, neurocognitive, or psychological support. It is key for the healthcare team to be aware that these challenges are common and should be addressed as early as possible for the best outcomes.

Treatment strategies remain an area of great interest and research at this time. As the long-term effects of the CNS impairment in childhood remain unclear, it is hoped that optimization at younger ages would help prevent potential cognitive impairments at older ages. Current treatment strategies include referrals for early intervention programs, IEPs at school, and treatment for identified psychiatric disorders such as attention deficit and hyperactivity disorder. Interventions for memory and EF have been identified in other conditions such as traumatic brain injury and dementia, but it remains an area of active research as to whether such interventions will also benefit CHD patients as they age. Psychological interventions are also recommended for mental health conditions. Despite these recommendations and the screening recommendations from the AHA/AAP, many children and adults with CHD do not have access to screening or supportive services for multiple reasons. Even patients who participate in large trials have limited use of services, with only about one-third of patients receiving early intervention services. Challenges include a limited number of cardiac neurodevelopment programs, insurance status, and variations in public support available based on geographic location and other social determinants of health.

Summary

Neurologic and developmental sequelae are common among patients with CHD and require care from experts in genetics, imaging, neuropsychology, psychiatry, neurology, education, and social work. Moreover, neuropsychological and behavioral needs can be dynamic throughout the life span, from fetus to adult. Early and consistent screening to identify deficits and opportunities for intervention, as well as advocacy for broad access to optimal neuropsychological and psychiatric care, are critical to improving short- and long-term clinical and psychosocial outcomes of the burgeoning population of CHD survivors.

References

1. Marino BS, Lipkin PH, Newburger JW, et al. Neurodevelopmental outcomes in children with congenital heart disease: evaluation and management: a scientific statement from the American Heart Association. *Circulation.* 2012;126:1143-1172.
2. Marelli A, Miller SP, Marino BS, et al. Brain in congenital heart disease across the lifespan: the cumulative burden of injury. *Circulation.* 2016;133:1951-1962.
3. Kovacs AH, Brouillette J, Ibeziako P, et al. Psychological outcomes and interventions for individuals with congenital heart disease: a scientific statement from the American Heart Association. *Circ Cardiovasc Qual Outcomes.* 2022;15:e000110.
4. Rettenmaier LA, Kirby PA, Reinking BE, et al. Neuropathology of congenital heart disease in an inpatient autopsy cohort 2000-2017. *J Am Heart Assoc.* 2020;9:e013575.
5. Aleksonis HA, King TZ. Relationships among structural neuroimaging and neurocognitive outcomes in adolescents and young adults with congenital heart disease: a systematic review. *Neuropsychol Rev.* 2023;33:432-458.
6. Beca J, Gunn JK, Coleman L, et al. New white matter brain injury after infant heart surgery is associated with diagnostic group and the use of circulatory arrest. *Circulation.* 2013;127:971-979.
7. Rollins CK, Watson CG, Asaro LA, et al. White matter microstructure and cognition in adolescents with congenital heart disease. *J Pediatr.* 2014;165:936-944.e1-2.
8. Panigrahy A, Schmithorst VJ, Wisnowski JL, et al. Relationship of white matter network topology and cognitive outcome in adolescents with d-transposition of the great arteries. *Neuroimage Clin.* 2015;7:438-448.
9. Hansen JH, Rotermann I, Logoteta J, et al. Neurodevelopmental outcome in hypoplastic left heart syndrome: Impact of perioperative cerebral tissue oxygenation of the Norwood procedure. *J Thorac Cardiovasc Surg.* 2016;151:1358-1366.
10. Goldberg CS, Hu C, Brosig C, et al. Behavior and quality of life at 6 years for children with hypoplastic left heart syndrome. *Pediatrics.* 2019;144(5):e20191010.
11. Pierpont ME, Brueckner M, Chung WK, et al. Genetic basis for congenital heart disease: revisited: a scientific statement from the American Heart Association. *Circulation.* 2018;138:e653-e711.
12. Homsy J, Zaidi S, Shen Y, et al. De novo mutations in congenital heart disease with neurodevelopmental and other congenital anomalies. *Science.* 2015;350:1262-1266.
13. Gaynor JW, Kim DS, Arrington CB, et al. Validation of association of the apolipoprotein E epsilon2 allele with neurodevelopmental dysfunction after cardiac surgery in neonates and infants. *J Thorac Cardiovasc Surg.* 2014;148:2560-2566.
14. Schmithorst VJ, Panigrahy A, Gaynor JW, et al. Organizational topology of brain and its relationship to ADHD in adolescents with d-transposition of the great arteries. *Brain Behav.* 2016;6:e00504.
15. Rollins CK, Ortinau CM, Stopp C, et al. Regional brain growth trajectories in fetuses with congenital heart disease. *Ann Neurol.* 2021;89:143-157.
16. Howell HB, Zaccario M, Kazmi SH, et al. Neurodevelopmental outcomes of children with congenital heart disease: a review. *Curr Probl Pediatr Adolesc Health Care.* 2019;49:100685.
17. Wu Y, Kapse K, Jacobs M, et al. Association of maternal psychological distress with in utero brain development in fetuses with congenital heart disease. *JAMA Pediatr.* 2020;174:e195316.
18. Sadhwani A, Wypij D, Rofeberg V, et al. Fetal brain volume predicts neurodevelopment in congenital heart disease. *Circulation.* 2022;145:1108-1119.
19. Wu Y, Espinosa KM, Barnett SD, et al. Association of elevated maternal psychological distress, altered fetal brain, and offspring cognitive and social-emotional outcomes at 18 months. *JAMA Netw Open.* 2022;5:e229244.
20. Newburger JW, Jonas RA, Wernovsky G, et al. A comparison of the perioperative neurologic effects of hypothermic circulatory arrest versus low-flow cardiopulmonary bypass in infant heart surgery. *N Engl J Med.* 1993;329:1057-1064.
21. Gaynor JW, Ittenbach RF, Calafat AM, et al. Perioperative exposure to suspect neurotoxicants from medical devices in newborns with congenital heart defects. *Ann Thorac Surg.* 2019;107:567-572.
22. Andropoulos DB, Ahmad HB, Haq T, et al. The association between brain injury, perioperative anesthetic exposure, and 12-month neurodevelopmental outcomes after neonatal cardiac surgery: a retrospective cohort study. *Paediatr Anaesth.* 2014;24:266-274.
23. Ilardi D, Ono KE, McCartney R, et al. Neurocognitive functioning in adults with congenital heart disease. *Congenit Heart Dis.* 2017;12:166-173.
24. Bagge CN, Henderson VW, Laursen HB, et al. Risk of dementia in adults with congenital heart disease: population-based cohort study. *Circulation.* 2018;137:1912-1920.
25. Rodriguez CP, Clay E, Jakkam R, et al. Cognitive impairment in adult CHD survivors: a pilot study. *Int J Cardiol Congenit Heart Dis.* 2021;6:100290.

56

Pulmonary Hypertension

BRYAN D. SIEGEL AND MARY P. MULLEN

KEY LEARNING POINTS

- Pediatric pulmonary hypertension (PH) is a rare and heterogeneous disease associated with congenital heart disease, lung disease, and other systemic diseases.
- Pathophysiology is related to vasoconstriction, thrombus formation, and/or smooth muscle proliferation.

- Despite advancements, there is still significant morbidity and mortality associated with PH.
- Targeted PH drug therapies have improved long-term outcomes.
- Future advances involve collaborative multi-site registries and increasing identification of genetic causes of PH.

The pulmonary circulation, normally a site of low resistance to blood flow, is subject to physiologic changes as well as a variety of disease processes influencing pulmonary arterial pressures. Without therapy, sustained elevation in pulmonary vascular resistance may result in progressive right ventricular (RV) dysfunction and death. Recent advances in the understanding of molecular genetics, cell biology, pathophysiology, and treatment strategies have revolutionized the care of children with pulmonary vascular disease, resulting in improved survival and increased quality of life.[1] The pediatric cardiologist plays a critical role in the diagnosis and management of the child with pulmonary hypertension (PH). This chapter presents a general approach to PH and excludes specific management of lesions secondary to structural cardiac defects.

Pulmonary Vascular Development

The mechanisms involved in pulmonary vascular formation during lung development are complex and remain incompletely understood. It is known that vessel formation begins at the earliest stages of lung development and involves cell–extracellular matrix and cell–cell interactions.[2] Various growth factors have been implicated in the vascular development of the pulmonary circulation, including members of the vascular endothelial growth factor, angiopoietin, and ephrin families.

The pulmonary circulation undergoes important physiologic and anatomic changes in the first hours, weeks, and months of life. In utero, the pulmonary arteries are relatively thick walled, and pulmonary vascular resistance is very high, limiting pulmonary blood flow to less than 10% of combined RV and LV output. At birth, the combined effects of mechanical expansion of the lung, increased oxygen tension, and shear stress lead to an increase in prostacyclin and nitric oxide (NO) synthesis and to the release of humoral substances such as bradykinin and adenosine. This results in an acute decrease in pulmonary vascular resistance and allows the pulmonary circulation to accommodate 100% of cardiac output.[3]

Pathophysiology of Pulmonary Hypertension

Elevated pulmonary arterial pressure arises from well-characterized vascular changes: vasoconstriction, decreased vascular growth, thrombus formation, or proliferation of smooth muscle or endothelial cells in the pulmonary vessels. Thus, PH is associated with conditions causing chronic vasoconstriction, thrombosis, or abnormalities of vessel function.[4]

Recent advances in molecular biology have allowed for the identification of several key mediators of pulmonary vascular function. Arachidonic acid metabolites such as prostacyclin and thromboxane A_2 are active in the pulmonary vessels and associated with vasodilation and vasoconstriction, respectively. In addition, prostacyclin inhibits platelets and endothelial cell proliferation, whereas thromboxane A_2 is a platelet activator. NO is produced by endothelial cells through a cyclic guanosine monophosphate (cGMP)-dependent pathway; it induces vasodilation and inhibits platelet function as well as smooth vessel proliferation. Endothelin-1 is a vasoconstrictor that causes smooth muscle proliferation in pulmonary vessels.[5]

Clinical studies suggest patients with PH have imbalances in these potent vasoactive factors, as well as in other vasoactive compounds, such as vascular endothelial cell growth factor, adrenomedullin, serotonin, and vasoactive peptides. Altered homeostatic balances of these factors, tending toward prothrombotic, vasoconstrictive physiology, have been demonstrated consistently in patients with PH. These clinical findings suggest that acquired alterations in normal vascular physiology contribute to the onset of PH. Other conditions that promote chronic changes in the pulmonary vasculature include hypoxemia and small vessel thrombosis. Chronic hypoxemia contributes to pulmonary vasoconstriction. Thrombotic events in the microvasculature contribute to hypoxia and also release acute mediators that contribute to vasoconstriction.

The pathologic vascular changes were described by Heath and Edwards in patients with PH secondary to congenital septal defects.[6] Classic initial changes (Heath and Edwards grades 1 and 2) include medial hypertrophy, smooth muscle extension into non-muscular arteries, and intimal cell proliferation from smooth muscle thickening. Progressive changes include intimal fibrosis and eventual thinning of the media with dilation of the vessels (grades 3 and 4). Eventually, medial fibrosis and necrotizing arteritis changes (grades 5 and 6) arise in the pulmonary vessels (Fig. 56.1).

These observations suggest that the pathophysiology of PH is governed by alterations in the normal function of vascular tone, hemostatic activity, and vascular cell biology. Imbalances between vasodilators and vasoconstrictors, platelet activation and inhibition, and endothelial and smooth muscle cell proliferation and inhibition conspire to

cause chronic changes in pulmonary vessels and worsening clinical symptoms. Importantly, these contributing factors also serve as emerging targets for treatment; strategies that reverse their impact appear able to improve clinical function in patients.

Genetic Causes of Pulmonary Hypertension

Recent genetic studies led to the identification of numerous gene mutations that are associated with PH (Table 56.1).[7-9] Inheritance of these mutations is primarily autosomal dominant, although there is incomplete penetrance, meaning that the development of symptoms in affected individuals is highly variable. Bone morphogenetic protein receptor type 2 (BMPR2), a member of the transforming growth factor-β (TGF-β) receptor family and located on chromosome 2q33, was first linked to PH through familial studies and classic genetic linkage analyses. A variety of mutations in the receptor, including mutations in the extracellular, transmembrane, and intracellular kinase domains, have been characterized; all of these are associated with PH although different families possess unique mutations. Clinical studies of families with hereditary hemorrhagic telangiectasia (HHT) led to identification of additional genes in the TGF-β receptor family, ACVRL1 and endoglin (ENG), associated with both HHT and familial PH. HHT families with missense and nonsense mutations in ALK1 had cases of PH similar in clinical and pathologic appearance to those seen among patients with BMPR2 mutations. To date, it seems that about 10% of sporadic and between 55–80% of cases of heritable PH arise from mutations in BMPR2.[7,9] Among BMPR2 mutation carriers, the lifetime risk for PH is estimated to be between 15% and 20%.

One important outcome of these genetic findings has been the implication of the TGF-β signaling pathway in the pathogenesis of PH. Additional mutations in genes in this pathway including SMADs 1, 4, and 9 as well as GDF2 have been associated with PH. It is believed that changes in TGF-β receptor signaling contribute to endothelial and smooth muscle cell proliferation in the pulmonary vasculature. The low incidence of PH in individuals with known mutations in BMPR2 and ACVRL1 supports the concept that in addition to hereditary predisposition, additional triggers such as acquired events or environmental exposures are needed to give rise to the clinical syndrome.[10]

As genetic analysis has improved, the number of genes identified to play a role in the pathogenesis of PH has increased substantially. These include mutations in transcriptional regulatory genes T-box-4 (TBX4) and Sox 17, genes encoding potassium (KCNK3) and aquaporin channel proteins (AQP1) involved in regulation of vascular tone, and other regulatory processes including eukaryotic translation initiation factor 2-alpha kinase 4 (EIF2AK4) and caveolin-1 (CAV-1).[8] These advances continue to

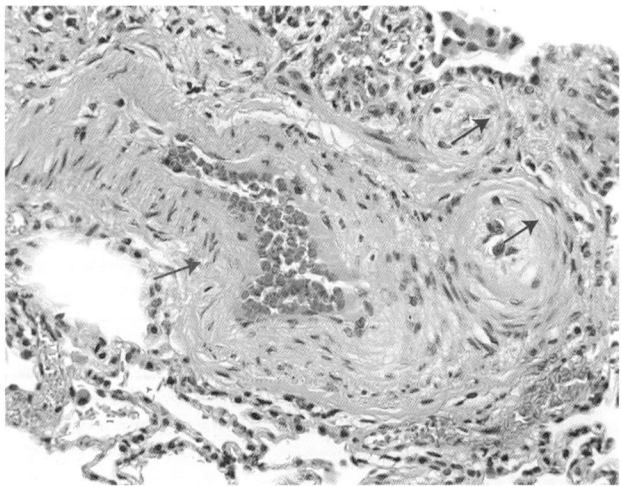

• **Fig. 56.1** Plexiform lesion demonstrates pulmonary arteries with medical muscular hypertrophy (*blue arrow*), and loss of internal elastic lamina and muscle with replacement by fibrous tissue (*red arrows*). The two small branches (*red arrows*) have fibrous walls and marked intimal thickening. (Courtesy of Harry Kozakewich, MD, Boston Childrens Hospital.)

TABLE 56.1	Genes with Known Associations to Pulmonary Hypertension			
Gene	Mode of Inheritance	Pathologic Pathway	Associations
BMPR2	AD	TGF-β	CHD, IPF, PVOD
TBX4	AD	Transcription factor	Developmental/parenchymal lung disease, small patella syndrome
ACVRL1	AD	TGF-β	HHT
EIF2AK4	AR/AD	Stress response	PVOD, PCH
ENG	AD	TGF-β	HHT, CHD
KCNK3	AD	Potassium channel	–
SMADS 1,4,9	AD	TGF-β	CHD
GDF2	AD/AR	TGF-β	HHT
SOX17	AD	Transcription factor	CHD
AQP1	AD	Aquaporin channel	–
CAV1	AD	TGF-β	CHD

AD, Autosomal dominant; AR, autosomal recessive; CHD, congenital heart disease; HHT, hereditary hemorrhagic telangiectasia; IPF, idiopathic pulmonary fibrosis; PCH, pulmonary capillary hemangiomatosis; PVOD, pulmonary veno-occlusive disease; TGF-β, transforming growth factor-β.
Adapted from Southgate L, Machado R, Graf S, et al. Molecular genetic framework underlying pulmonary arterial hypertension. *Nature Reviews: Cardiology.* 2020;17:85–95.

expand our understanding of the pathways involved in the pathogenesis of PH and may lead to future targeted therapies.

Patients diagnosed with PH merit a thorough family history to explore whether hereditary factors may contribute to disease risk. Genetic testing and professional counseling should be offered to patients diagnosed with idiopathic or heritable PH.

Definition and Clinical Classification of Pulmonary Hypertension

Pediatric PH encompasses heterogenous populations and disease processes. The definition for diagnosis has been updated by the World Symposium on Pulmonary Hypertension (WSPH) in 2018. Previously, it had been mean pulmonary artery pressure (mPAP) ≥ 25 after 3 months of age or an indexed pulmonary vascular resistance (PVRi) of ≥ 3 Wood units/m^2 (WU/m^2) as determined by cardiac catheterization. With the most recent modification, this definition for both adults and children has changed to a mPAP ≥ 20 *and* a PVRi ≥ 3 (WU). The WSPH has also updated the classification for various types of PH as it relates to the underlying etiology (Table 56.2). Briefly, this classification system breaks down etiologies into: (1) pulmonary arterial hypertension; (2) PH due to left heart disease; (3) PH due to lung disease and/or hypoxia; (4) PH due to pulmonary artery obstructions; and (5) PH with unclear or multifactorial mechanisms.[11] This classification provides a valuable differential diagnosis to the multifactorial problem of PH and guides the diagnostic workup of patients. A standardized classification system also supports multi-institutional registry studies in advancing the knowledge of a relatively rare disease.

Clinical Presentation and Evaluation of Patients with Pulmonary Hypertension

Symptoms

The pediatric patient with PH may be referred with symptoms including shortness of breath, exercise intolerance, and easy fatigability. Patients may experience chest pain, chronic cough, vomiting, and recurrent syncope. Children with right-to-left shunting in the setting of elevated right-sided pressures may appear intermittently cyanotic. Infants may be irritable, exhibit poor feeding, or display tachypnea. These findings are all non-specific and require thoughtful evaluation before a diagnosis of PH can be established. Based on the clinical history, the patient is assigned to a functional class (I to IV) according to World Health Organization Guidelines, which are a modification of the New York Heart Association heart failure classification (Table 56.3).[12] This classification scale allows prognosis of long-term outcomes and provides treatment recommendations.

Physical Examination

Initial examination of patients with PH may reveal tachypnea and cyanosis. Cardiac exam may reveal a RV heave and palpable second heart sound. Auscultation may disclose

TABLE 56.2 **World Symposium of Pulmonary Hypertension (WSPH) Classification of Pulmonary Hypertension (PH) (2019)**

1 Pulmonary arterial hypertension (PAH)
  1.1 Idiopathic PAH
  1.2 Heritable PAH
  1.3 Drug- and toxin-induced PAH
  1.4 PAH associated with:
    1.4.1 Connective tissue disorder
    1.4.2 HIV infection
    1.4.3 Portal hypertension
    1.4.4 Congenital heart disease
    1.4.5 Schistosomiasis
  1.5 PAH long-term responders to calcium channel blockers
  1.6 PAH with overt features of venous/capillaries (PVOD/PCH) involvement
  1.7 Persistent PH of the newborn syndrome

2 PH due to left heart disease
  2.1 PH due to heart failure with preserved LVEF
  2.2 PH due to heart failure with reduced LVEF
  2.3 Valvular heart disease
  2.4 Congenital/acquired cardiovascular conditions leading to post-capillary PH

3 PH due to lung disease and/or hypoxia
  3.1 Obstructive lung disease
  3.2 Restrictive lung disease
  3.3 Other lung disease with mixed restrictive/obstructive pattern
  3.4 Hypoxia without lung disease
  3.5 Developmental lung disease

4 PH due to pulmonary artery obstructions
  4.1 Chronic thromboembolism PH
  4.2 Other pulmonary artery obstructions

5 PH with unclear and/or multifactorial mechanisms
  5.1 Hematologic disorders
  5.2 Systemic and metabolic disorders
  5.3 Others
  5.4 Complex congenital heart disease

LVEF, Left ventricular ejection fraction; *PCH,* pulmonary capillary hemangiomatosis; *PVOD,* pulmonary veno-occlusive disease.
Adapted from Simonneau G, Montani D, Celermajer DS, et al. Haemodynamic definitions and updated clinical classification of pulmonary hypertension. *Eur Respir J.* 2019;53:1801913.

TABLE 56.3 **World Health Organization Classification of the Clinical Functional State in Patients With Pulmonary Hypertension**

I	Patients with pulmonary hypertension, but without resulting limitation of physical activity. Ordinary physical activity does not cause undue dyspnea or fatigue, chest pain, or near syncope.
II	Patients with pulmonary hypertension resulting in slight limitation of physical activity. They are comfortable at rest. Ordinary physical activity causes undue dyspnea or fatigue, chest pain, or near syncope.
III	Patients with pulmonary hypertension resulting in marked limitation of physical activity. They are comfortable at rest. Less than ordinary activity causes dyspnea or fatigue, chest pain, or near syncope.
IV	Patients with pulmonary hypertension with inability to carry out any physical activity without symptoms. These patients manifest signs of right heart failure. Dyspnea and/or fatigue may even be present at rest. Discomfort is increased by any physical activity.

Adapted from Rubin L. Diagnosis and management of pulmonary arterial hypertension: ACCP Evidence-based clinical practice guidelines. *Chest.* 2004;126:7S–10S.

and inverted T waves in the anterior and lateral chest leads consistent with increased RV strain (Fig. 56.2).

Chest Radiograph

The chest radiograph may show cardiac enlargement with a prominent main pulmonary artery segment. There may be decreased vasculature in the peripheral lung fields due to paucity of pulmonary blood flow (Fig. 56.3). Computed tomography (CT) is important in many patients with PH to exclude primary lung disease or along with CT angiography if chronic thromboembolic PH is suspected.

Cardiac Evaluation

When the diagnosis of PH is considered, a thorough initial cardiovascular evaluation is warranted to establish the diagnosis and to exclude structural cardiac lesions, as well as to characterize the patient's hemodynamics and potential response to therapy.

Echocardiography

The echocardiographic evaluation is essential to evaluate cardiac anatomy and rule out contributing causes such as left-sided structural heart disease, pulmonary vein stenosis, or shunt lesions. Patients with PH can have RV systolic pressure estimated through use of Doppler echocardiography if tricuspid regurgitation is present. Other imaging findings may include right atrial and ventricular enlargement, pulmonary artery dilation, and pulmonary valve regurgitation. Echocardiography also provides valuable information on RV

that the latter is single or narrowly split with an accentuated pulmonary component, reflecting elevated pulmonary artery pressure. There may be a soft blowing systolic murmur of tricuspid regurgitation along the left sternal border, and there may be an early high-frequency diastolic murmur of pulmonary regurgitation, both due to the elevated right-sided pressures. The child with right heart failure may have increased jugular venous pressure, hepatomegaly, ascites, and/or pedal edema.

Electrocardiogram

The electrocardiogram typically displays right-axis deviation and RV hypertrophy. There may be depressed S-T segments

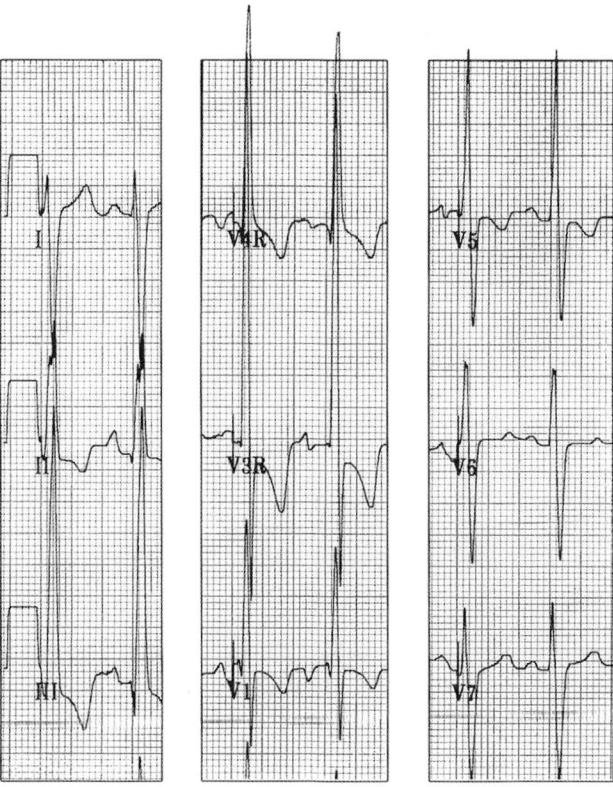

• **Fig. 56.2** Electrocardiogram from a 10-year-old patient with severe idiopathic pulmonary hypertension and systemic level pulmonary resistance unresponsive to vasodilators, showing marked right ventricular hypertrophy.

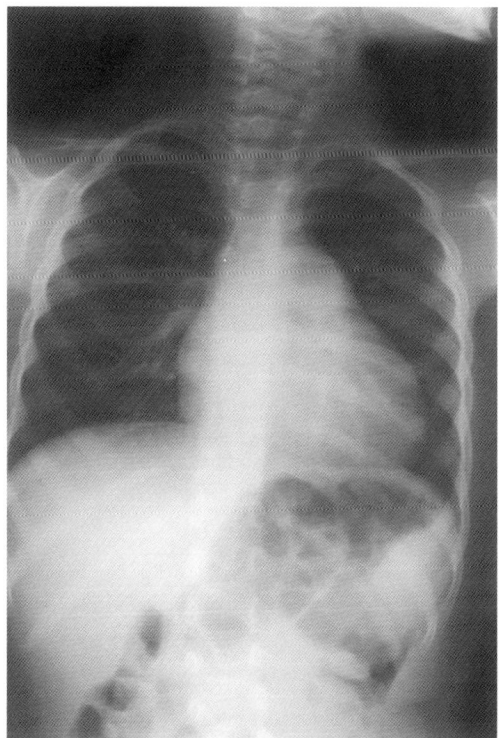

• **Fig. 56.3** Chest x-ray in a 3-year-old with idiopathic pulmonary hypertension. Note the prominent main pulmonary artery segment. (From Fyler DC [ed]. *Nadas' Pediatric Cardiology.* Philadelphia: Hanley and Belfus, 1992.)

performance which can be followed longitudinally to track disease progression or response to therapy. The RV performance can be evaluated by RV Tei index, 3D RV ejection fraction, tricuspid annular plane systolic excursion (TAPSE), and strain indices.[1]

Cardiac catheterization

Catheterization of the child with PH is essential for diagnosis and evaluation of therapeutic options, but must be planned carefully with coordinated interdisciplinary care before and after the procedure in order to minimize adverse outcomes in these high-risk patients. Scrupulous attention should be paid to the patient's hydration status before catheterization. Patients must be adequately sedated, oxygenated, and ventilated during the procedure. After cardiac catheterization, patients require careful observation for hypoventilation, which may contribute to acidosis and precipitate a pulmonary hypertensive crisis.

Cardiac output measurements are determined by thermodilution in patients without shunting or by the Fick method with measured oxygen consumption in those with a patent foramen ovale and minor shunting in either direction. It is imperative that in pediatric patients, all flow and resistance calculations are indexed to body surface area. Pulmonary vasodilator testing at the time of catheterization with a short-acting pulmonary vasodilator is critical to deciding on therapeutic options for the child with PH. Patients can be challenged with inhalation of 100% oxygen, use of short-acting agents such as inhaled nitric oxide (iNO), or by intravenous adenosine or prostacyclin to determine whether the pulmonary vasculature is responsive to vasodilator therapy. Response is defined as reduction in mPAP of at least 10 mm Hg to achieve mPAP of 40 mm Hg or less while maintaining normal or high cardiac output.[13] This subset of patients may benefit from long-term calcium channel blocker therapy and may have better outcomes overall. The rate of response in pediatric patients varies from 10% to 30% and children of younger age may be more likely to respond. Pulmonary vasodilator testing can also be used to evaluate for operability in patients with PH and shunt lesions (e.g., ventricular septal defects, patent ductus arteriosus, or atrial septal defect) although criteria for a positive response differs as change in mPAP would not be applicable.[1]

Angiography is performed after hemodynamic assessment, with great care being taken to avoid precipitating a pulmonary hypertensive crisis. Selective, preferably distal, pulmonary artery contrast injections are used to visualize the pulmonary vasculature. Distal stenotic lesions, whether congenital or acquired, are carefully balloon-dilated. In addition, an aortogram should be performed to exclude aortopulmonary connections.

Diagnostic Evaluation of Patients With Pulmonary Hypertension

When a diagnosis of PH has been made through echocardiography and cardiac catheterization, a thorough diagnostic investigation is mandatory; this includes all possible etiologies as in some instances there are reversible causes. The detailed diagnostic algorithm employed at Boston Children's Hospital is shown in Fig. 56.4. Testing is undertaken based on clinical history, family history, and presenting symptoms. Options for testing include ventilation-perfusion scans or high-resolution CT to rule out chronic thromboembolic disease, pulmonary function testing, exercise testing, sleep study, liver function tests and liver ultrasound, thyroid function tests, evaluation for collagen vascular disease, human immunodeficiency virus testing, hypercoagulability workup, and genetic and metabolic screening.[14] Given the increased morbidity and mortality risks associated with lung biopsy, this procedure is reserved for the diagnosis of diseases that may change therapy, including vasculitis, granulomatous lung disease, pulmonary veno-occlusive disease, pulmonary capillary hemangiomatosis, alveolar capillary dysplasia, and various interstitial lung diseases.

Cardiac magnetic resonance imaging (CMRI) is a reliable way to evaluate RV and LV performance, both of which can be important predictors of mortality in pediatric PH. CMRI also allows for characterization of the myocardial tissue; novel techniques are being investigated to allow noninvasive estimates of RV afterload, RV to PA afterload coupling, and strain which may, in the future, provide more prognostic information.

After the initial diagnostic workup, the data can be used to risk stratify patients into high or low risk (Table 56.4), inform prognostication, and guide therapy initiation and response.

The 6-minute walk test is used to evaluate adult patients and older children. Many of the parameters from baseline studies such as echocardiography and CMRI can be used to monitor the longitudinal cardiovascular health of these patients. Reevaluation through cardiac catheterization data is an important part of long-term evaluation and management. Recently, there has been promise in the utility of B-type natriuretic peptide (BNP) as a useful tool to correlate with severity of disease.

Natural History and Therapy for Pulmonary Hypertension

The true incidence of PH is not known. Estimates suggest 1 to 2 cases per 1 million people in the population with a slight predominance of cases in females.[15-17] Prior to the advent of target therapy, PH carried a grave prognosis in children. Recent advances in diagnosis and treatment have improved the natural history. Indeed, recent data suggest a median survival well in excess of 5 years in patients with access to vasodilator therapy; the prognosis is dependent on the specific classification of PH, with better outcomes in lung disease–related PH (Fig. 56.5). The most recent estimates of all pediatric PH 5-year survival are between 64% and 84%.[16-18] Prolonged survival is observed among those who respond favorably to vasodilator treatment. This finding places a premium on the correct classification of patients as responders or non-responders to acute vasodilator testing. Since the 1990s, pediatric PH hospitalization and

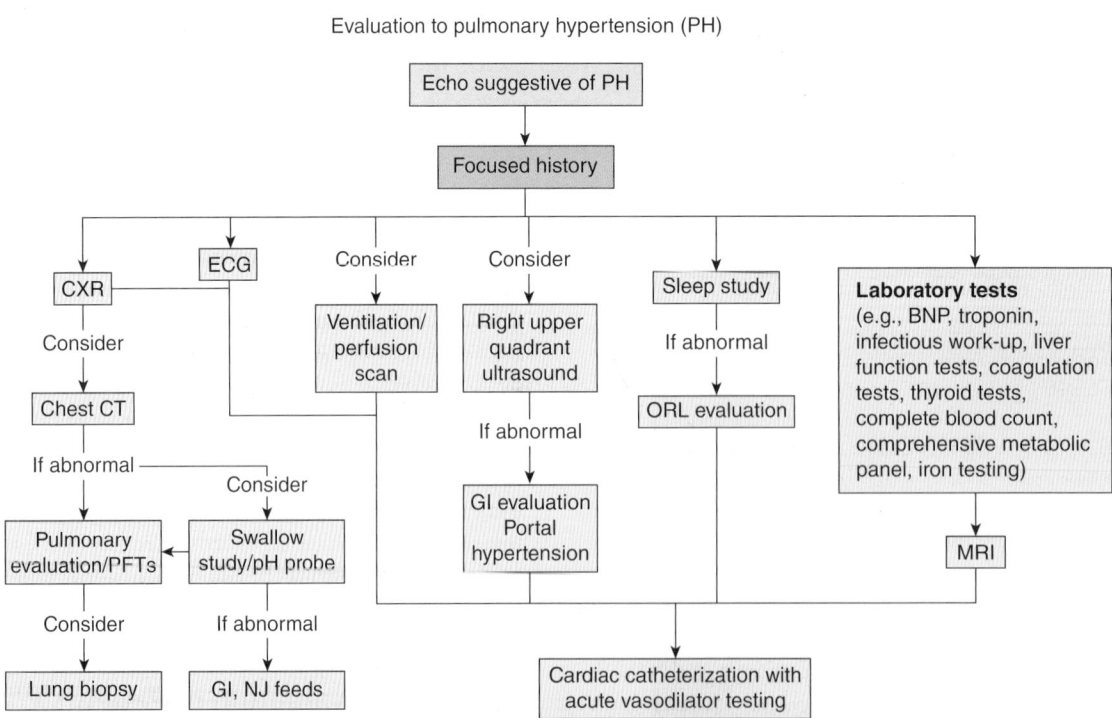

• **Fig. 56.4** Evaluation for pulmonary hypertension (PH). *BNP*, B-type natriuretic peptide; *CT*, computed tomography; *CXR*, chest x-ray; *GI*, gastrointestinal; *MRI*, magnetic resonance imaging; *NJ*, nasojejunal; *ORL*, otorhinolaryngology; *PFTs*, pulmonary function tests.

TABLE 56.4 Risk Stratification in Pediatric Pulmonary Hypertension		
Lower Risk	**Determinants of Risk**	**Higher Risk**
No	Evidence of RV failure	Yes
I-II	WHO functional class	III-IV
None	Syncope	Recurrent
Minimal RV dysfunction or dilation	Echocardiography	Significant RV dysfunction or dilation Pericardial effusion
PVR < 10 Wood units/m² CI > 3.0 L/min/m² PVR/SVR < 0.5	Hemodynamics	PVR > 20 Wood units/m² CI < 2.0 L/min/m² PVR/SVR > 1.0
Minimal elevation	B-type natriuretic peptide	Significantly elevated
Longer (>500 m)	6-minute walk test	Shorter (<300 m)
Peak VO₂ > 25 mL/kg/min	Cardiopulmonary exercise test	Peak VO₂ < 15 mL/kg/min

CI, Cardiac Index; *PVR*, Pulmonary Vascular Resistance; *RV*, Right Ventricle; *SVR*, Systemic Vascular Resistance; *VO₂*, Oxygen Consumption; *WHO*, World Health Organization.
Adapted from Abman S, Hansmann G, Archer S, et al. Pediatric pulmonary hypertension: guidelines from the American Heart Association and American Thoracic Society. *Circulation.* 2015;132:2037–2099.

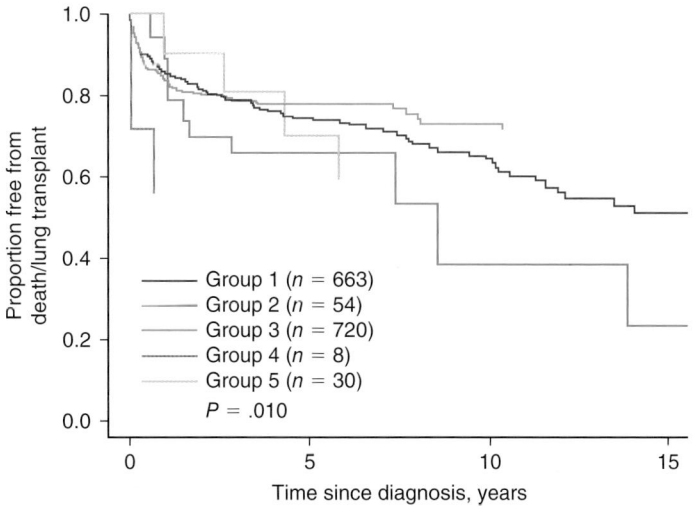

• **Fig. 56.5** Freedom from death/lung transplant by World Symposium on Pulmonary Hypertension classification. Group 1, pulmonary arterial hypertension (PAH); Group 2, PH associated with left heart disease; Group 3, PH associated with lung and hypoxia-related causes; Group 4, chronic thromboembolic PH (CTEPH); and Group 5, systemic and multifactorial disorders. (Reproduced with permission of the ERS 2023:European Respiratory Journal 59 (1) 2003337; DOI: 10.1183/13993003.03337-2020 Published 31 December 2021.)

resource utilization are increasing as the diagnostic and treatment possibilities are advancing. During this time period, morbidity and mortality have declined; however, patients and their families continue to suffer a significant decrease in quality of life, an increase in parental stress, and a significant burden of healthcare costs.[19,20]

There are several unique challenges when interpreting the treatment literature for PH. First, PH is a heterogeneous disorder, arising from many different etiologic factors, not all of which are known. This diversity complicates the understanding of the treatment and expected outcomes for

patients. Second, this disease, particularly in the pediatric population, is relatively rare. Thus, treatment principles for children are often derived from observations in adults, without large clinical experiences in pediatric patients to confirm applicability of the findings. There are reasons that data from adults may not be easily extrapolated to children, including the different natural life expectancy, different etiologies for PH, different intrinsic pulmonary vascular reactivity, and historically worse natural history of the disease in younger patients. Third, the critical end points for clinical trials are widely debated. Many trials have reported on mean changes in 6-minute walking distance or changes in hemodynamic parameters. Obtaining these data may be challenging in younger children. These limitations emphasize the importance of multi-site registries with standardized definitions of PH classification and clearly defined endpoints. Beyond these technical challenges, there are relatively few studies that have reported on long-term clinical outcomes such as survival, or on quality of life or functional status, which may be crucial measures for children and their families. For all these reasons, treatment of pediatric patients with PH remains individualized. Although many algorithms have been promulgated to guide treatment choices, the exact sequence, duration, combination, and timing of treatments have not been characterized.[1]

Therapy

The therapeutic approach to the child with PH begins with a thorough identification of underlying causes and initial treatments directed at these factors. These may include measures such as supplemental oxygen for patients with parenchymal lung disease, anti-inflammatory therapies for patients with collagen vascular disease, continuous positive airway pressure therapy and tonsillectomy for patients with obstructive sleep apnea, and anticoagulation and

potential thromboendarterectomy for chronic thromboembolic disease.[1] An example of a treatment algorithm for PH is presented in Fig. 56.6. Table 56.5 lists some of the agents commonly used with PH and includes mechanism of action and side effects. In those patients with PH due to an unrepaired systemic-to-pulmonary circulatory shunt (e.g., ventricular septal defect), treatment may involve determining operative candidacy based on pulmonary vascular resistance and pulmonary vasodilator testing (Fig. 56.7).[71] Complex cardiac disease with abnormal pulmonary vascular resistance, such as in tetralogy of Fallot with pulmonary atresia and multiple aortopulmonary collaterals, or with pulmonary venous hypertension due to complex left sided obstruction as in Shone's complex, is discussed elsewhere.

Acute Vasodilator Testing

The initial evaluation for treatment of PH is assessment of response to acute vasodilator therapy with iNO, intravenous prostacyclin, or other short-acting vasodilator. Patients with a significant hemodynamic response to acute vasodilator testing during cardiac catheterization (a decrease of at least 10 mm Hg in mPAP to 40 mm Hg or less, with no change or an increase in cardiac output) are defined as "responders" according to Sitbon criteria. They are likely to

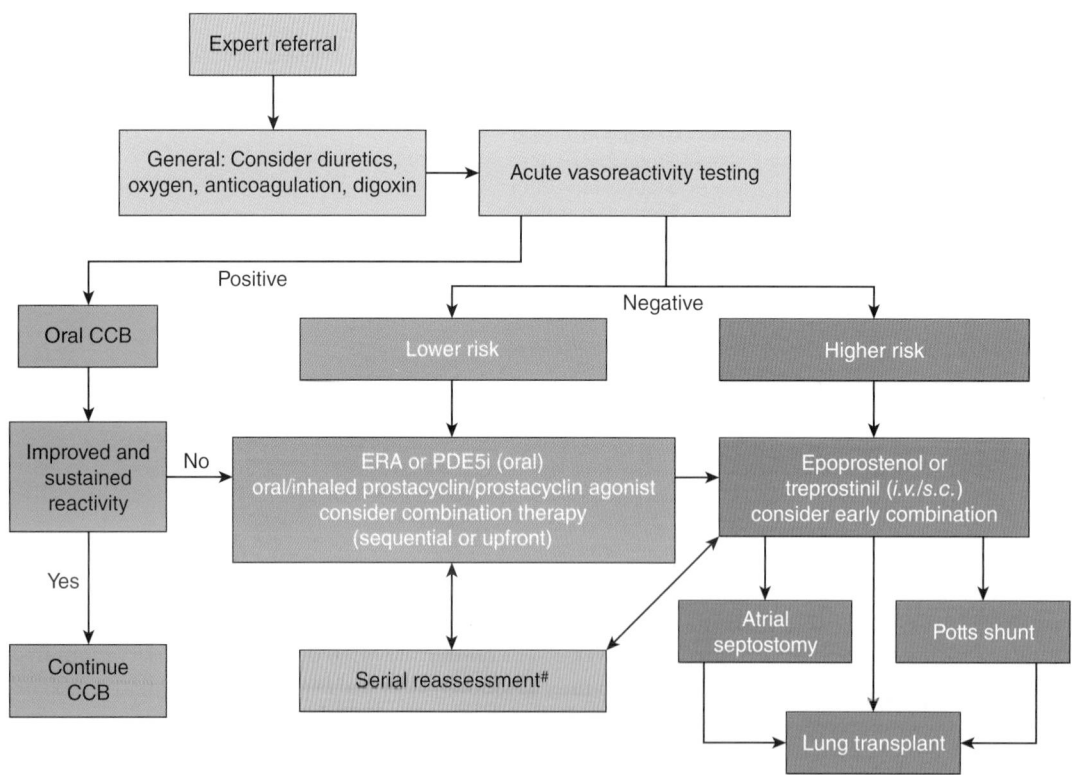

• **Fig. 56.6** Treatment algorithm for pediatric idiopathic/familial pulmonary hypertension. *CCB,* Calcium channel blocker; *ERA,* endothelin receptor antagonist; *PDE5i,* phosphodiesterase type 5 inhibitor; #, deterioration or not meeting treatment goals. (Reproduced with permission of the © ERS 2023: European Respiratory Journal 53 (1) 1801916; DOI: 10.1183/13993003.01916-2018 Published 24 January 2019.)

TABLE 56.5 Pharmacologic Therapy for Pulmonary Hypertension

		Route of Administration	Adverse Effects	Comments
Phosphodiesterase type 5 inhibitors	Sildenafil	Oral Intravenous	Headache, gastroesophageal reflux, irritability, flushing, rarely priapism, hypotension	May be used to prevent rebound pulmonary hypertension with inhaled nitric oxide discontinuation
	Tadalafil	Oral	Headache, flushing, rarely priapism, hypotension	Once-daily dosing
Endothelin Receptor Antagonist	Bosentan	Oral	Liver dysfunction, anemia, peripheral edema, hypotension	Requires long-term liver function test monitoring, teratogenic
	Ambrisentan	Oral	Anemia, peripheral edema, hypotension	Selective endothelin receptor A blockade Once-daily dosing Teratogenic
	Macitentan	Oral	Anemia, upper respiratory symptoms (nasal congestion, pharyngitis)	Dual endothelin receptor blockage Teratogenic
Prostacyclin	Treprostinil	Intravenous Inhaled Oral Subcutaneous	Flushing, hypotension, nausea, diarrhea, jaw pain, infusion site pain (subcutaneous), cough (inhalation)	Stable at room temperature Longer half-life (2–4 hours) Fewer side effects than epoprostenol
	Epoprostenol	Intravenous Inhaled	Nausea, diarrhea, jaw pain, bone pain, headaches	Short half-life (2–5 minutes) requiring continuous infusion and central catheter Required to be kept cold
	Iloprost	Inhaled	Airway reactivity, flushing, hypotension, nausea, diarrhea, jaw pain, cough	Nebulization 6 to 9 times daily, 10–15 minutes each Teratogenic
Non-Prostanoid IP Prostacyclin Receptor Agonist	Selexipag	Oral Intravenous	Flushing, diarrhea, nausea, headache, jaw pain, myalgias	Limited data in pediatrics
Soluble guanylate cyclase stimulant	Riociguat	Oral	Headaches, hypotension, nausea, diarrhea, vomiting, anemia	Limited data in pediatrics Embryo-fetal toxicity
Calcium channel Blockers	Nifedipine Diltiazem Amlodipine	Oral	Peripheral edema, bradycardia, hypotension, flushing, dizziness	Contraindicated in those < 1 year, those without vasoreactivity testing, non-responders, or right ventricular dysfunction

respond to calcium channel blockade and other vasodilator therapies, whereas in contrast, non-responders are unlikely to respond to calcium channel blocker therapy, and indeed their use in such patients is dangerous.[13]

Calcium Channel Blockers

Historical experience with use of calcium channel blockers as vasodilator therapy suggests that these drugs can prolong survival in patients deemed responders. Because of the potential for severe hemodynamic collapse during initial challenge with calcium channel blockers, these drugs are not appropriate for first-line diagnostic therapy. Instead, acute vasodilator testing is done with iNO (with or without oxygen), or prostacyclin.[1] Patients who respond to such therapies are candidates for initiation of calcium channel blocker treatment under close hemodynamic monitoring. Patients who tolerate initiation of calcium channel blockers and who have sustained hemodynamic benefit are continued on oral therapy. In patients without sustained benefit during initiation of therapy, calcium channel blockers should be discontinued. Dosage is cautiously titrated to optimize cardiac output and minimize PH. Fewer

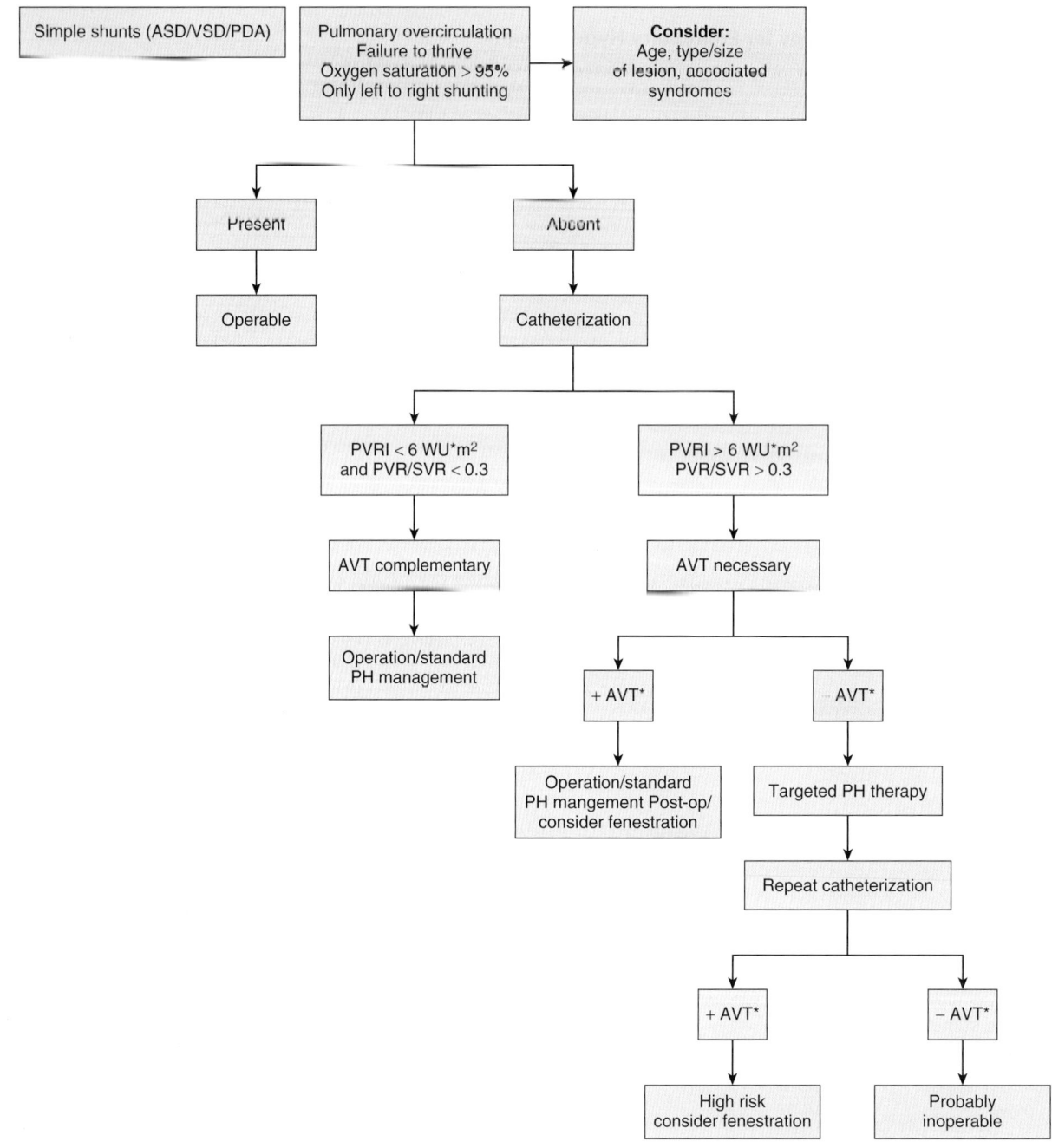

• **Fig. 56.7** Assessment of operability for shunt lesions in patients with congenital heart disease and pulmonary hypertension (PH). *ASD,* Atrial septal defect; *AVT,* acute vasoreactivity testing; *PDA,* patent ductus arteriosus; *PVR,* pulmonary vascular resistance; *PVRI,* pulmonary vascular resistance index; *SVR,* systemic vascular resistance; *VSD,* ventricular septal defect; *WU,* Wood units. *PVRI < 6 WU/m² and PVR/SVR < 0.3. (Used with permission from Antonio A. Lopes, Robin J. Barst and The Pulmonary Vascular Research Institute (pvrinstitute.org) and Abman S, Hansmann G, Archer S, Ivy D, et al. Pediatric Pulmonary Hypertension: Guidelines from the American Heart Association and American Thoracic Society. Circulation. 2015;132:2037-2099.)

than 20% of adults have a favorable clinical response compared with nearly 40% of children.[18]

Prostacyclin

Prostacyclin therapy has been widely studied in the treatment of PH. Although the precise mechanism of action is not known, it is a potent pulmonary vasodilator, and therefore a useful drug for these patients. It has been shown to improve hemodynamic function, exercise tolerance, quality of life, and survival for patients with primary PH.[1] Children can thrive on these medications over long periods of time. Prostacyclin and its analogues can be administered as intravenous medications, subcutaneous, inhaled, or oral.

These must be carefully titrated over time based on patient tolerance and response. They can be effective regardless of clinical response to acute pulmonary vasodilator testing. Intravenous therapy has the advantage of rapid titration but requires continuous long-term central venous access; patients are subject to a variety of complications including catheter-related bloodstream infections and, if treatment is interrupted inadvertently, significant hemodynamic changes. Treatment may be transitioned between administration routes but requires careful monitoring for efficacy and side effects. Resistance or tolerance to prostacyclin therapy can occur, the mechanisms of which are unknown. Selexipag is an oral non-prostanoid prostacyclin receptor agonist approved for adults with PH. Recent prospective observational experience showed promise as an add-on therapy to other targeted therapies.[22]

Endothelin Receptor Antagonists

Endothelin-1, a potent vasoconstrictor, mediates its activity through two types of endothelin receptors, ET_A and ET_B. Bosentan, a non-selective antagonist, has been shown in randomized clinical trials to improve functional capacity and hemodynamics in adults with PH, and similar proof of efficacy and safety have been found in children.[15] This drug may induce elevation of liver function tests and anemia, both of which are reversible. Thus, careful monitoring of transaminases and hemoglobin levels is necessary during treatment. Ambrisentan, with selective ETA antagonism, may reduce the risk of transaminitis. Macitentan with non-selective antagonism and improved pharmacodynamics may have decreased side effects, but pediatric specific studies are pending. All three endothelin receptor antagonists are potential teratogens. Young patients need to be counseled about these effects and to use effective forms of contraception.

Inhaled Nitric Oxide

iNO is a selective pulmonary vasodilator with a brief half-life and rapid inactivation by hemoglobin. Additional beneficial effects include improvement of oxygenation in the setting of ventilation-perfusion mismatch, inhibition of platelet aggregation, decreased proliferation of vascular smooth muscle, and promotion of vascular remodeling.[23] Treatment studies have demonstrated that iNO is effective in acute vasodilator testing in the catheterization laboratory, in treating persistent PH of the newborn,[24] and in managing postoperative PH after repair of congenital heart disease and after lung and heart transplantation.[23,25,26] Patients treated with iNO should be monitored for methemoglobin levels. They are at risk for rebound PH with abrupt discontinuation of therapy. Careful weaning of treatment is thus necessary to minimize this complication. Sildenafil can prolong the activity of NO and increase circulating cGMP levels; therefore, it has been used to aid in the discontinuation of iNO therapy.[27]

Type 5 Phosphodiesterase Inhibitors and Soluble Guanylate Cyclase Stimulators

Type 5 phosphodiesterase (PDE-5) breaks down cGMP and limits cGMP-mediated NO vasodilation. Inhibition of PDE-5 causes vasodilation and has anti-proliferative effects. Elevated amounts of PDE-5 are found in the pulmonary vasculature, making this class of drugs relatively specific for pulmonary vasodilation. Sildenafil is the best known and most studied of this class of drugs. Multiple observational and retrospective studies demonstrate improvements in oxygenation, exercise capacity, hemodynamic data, and incidence of PH crises with a low rate of adverse events. PDE-5 inhibitors are often the first-line agents used in initiating treatment for pediatric PH given their efficacy and overall safety profile. Randomized controlled trials, however, have yielded conflicting results, particularly the long-term extension study STARTS-2, which found an increase in mortality in high-dose sildenafil compared with medium- and low-dose regimens.[28] Review of data from this study prompted a Food and Drug Administration safety advisory for sildenafil usage in pediatric PH suggesting careful weighing of the risks and benefits of usage in each individual patient.[29] Tadalafil is another PDE-5 inhibitor with a longer half-life that has shown safety and efficacy in children. Riociguat, a novel agent, acts through the same pathway as phosphodiesterase inhibitors but directly stimulates soluble guanylate cyclase, increases sensitivity to NO, and augments cGMP activity.

Combination Therapy

Prostacyclins (and their analogues), endothelin antagonism, and PDE-5 inhibitors all have distinct pathways through which they act on the pulmonary vasculature. Given this, some advocate for use of these medicines in combination either at time of diagnosis or in a stepwise fashion. Randomized controlled trials in adults found starting with combination therapy (endothelin receptor antagonist and PDE-5 inhibitor) to be superior to monotherapy.[30] Retrospective data in pediatrics demonstrate that combination therapy was associated with improved survival, although timing of combination therapy was not evaluated.[31] Care must be taken when initiating multiple PH therapies as there may be some drug interactions affecting concentration levels.

General Supportive Care
Oxygen

Supplemental oxygen therapy can be valuable in certain patients with PH to alleviate chronic hypoxemia or to minimize nocturnal desaturation. Such patients include those with sleep apnea or other hypoventilation syndromes, patients with intrinsic lung disease or acute respiratory infection, and patients with exercise-induced hypoxia. Patients with advanced right heart failure and resting oxygen desaturation may also benefit from oxygen therapy.

Anticoagulation

Anticoagulation is considered helpful because microvessel thrombosis may contribute to the ongoing pathogenesis of PH. Microvessel thrombosis may be common in this population due to shear stress, endothelial dysfunction, and hypoxia causing thrombogenesis. Warfarin has been the anticoagulant studied most thoroughly in adults and has weak evidence towards improvement in survival; no pediatric trial data are available. It is known to be beneficial in those with chronic thromboembolism. Its usage is primarily in those with a known hypercoagulable state, severe idiopathic PH, and those with indwelling lines at risk for clot.[1] The optimal dose of warfarin in children is uncertain, but currently an international normalized ratio (INR) range of 1.5 to 2.0 is sought. For toddlers or patients at risk for bleeding, lower INR levels of less than 1.5 are used. In those with documented thromboembolism, hypercoagulable states such as positive cardiolipin or lupus anticoagulant tests, or known inherited thrombotic disorders, higher INR levels are targeted.

Management of right heart failure

Patients with PH and right heart failure may benefit from cardiac glycosides such as digoxin, and from diuretic therapy. Because these patients are vulnerable to reductions in cardiac preload, the initiation of diuretic therapy needs to be done cautiously to avoid excessive volume depletion and hypotension. Milrinone may be helpful in right heart failure for both inotropy and RV afterload reduction. Other vasoactives should be initiated as needed to maintain cardiac output in the context of decompensated heart failure.

Prophylactic measures

Because patients with PH are vulnerable to the effects of respiratory inflammation, they should be vaccinated against common viruses (e.g., influenza, COVID-19) and pneumococcal infections; respiratory infections should be managed aggressively. Patient with indwelling central lines should receive antibiotic prophylaxis according to standard guidelines.

Refractory Pulmonary Hypertension

Despite advances in medical management of PH, patients may be non-responsive to therapies or develop treatment-refractory disease. These patients, who often have marked symptoms of right heart failure or recurrent syncope reflecting severity of disease, have limited options. By facilitating right-to-left shunting, atrial septostomy may improve cardiac output, alleviate symptoms, improve functional class, and contribute to improved survival for patients with refractory PH.[1] Another consideration for those with refractory disease is a reverse Potts shunt. This procedure creates a connection between the descending aorta and the left pulmonary artery in an effort to decrease RV afterload and improve RV function. Recent retrospective evaluation has found long-term survival similar to lung transplantation with improvements in functional class and 6-minute walk test.[32] Mechanical circulatory support, specifically extracorporeal membrane oxygenation (ECMO), may be used in the setting of acute right heart failure and systemic hypoperfusion. This is a temporary circulatory support strategy, however, for use as a bridge to recovery or another more durable therapy. ECMO used as an extension of cardiopulmonary resuscitation (E-CPR) in patients with PH has guarded outcomes; these patients are poor CPR candidates given the challenges to creating effective pulmonary blood flow with compressions. Bilateral lung transplantation, as well as heart-lung transplantation, has been performed in patients with refractory PH. Results to date are highly variable with average 5-year survival of bilateral lung transplant nearing 50% and a high waitlist mortality.[33] Optimal transplantation procedure, timing of transplant, and patient selection criteria are not clearly established. In practice, patients with medically refractory PH should be referred for evaluation at a lung transplantation center.

Summary

Recent advances have illuminated the heterogeneous etiologies and pathophysiology of pediatric PH and enabled the development of more effective treatment options. As a consequence, children have experienced remarkable progress in both function and life expectancy. Because of the rarity of PH, complex physiology, and limited available treatment facilities, these patients merit evaluation and treatment at comprehensive medical centers with experience in the medical, interventional, and surgical management of this disease. Treatment recommendations are guided by the symptom profile of the patient, by identification of any etiologic factors, and by the response to various therapeutic options. With judicious management, patients can expect considerable improvement in their functional status and longevity. Future opportunities for advancement include the use of standardized classifications and endpoints for multisite registries, as well as ongoing clinical trials into new targeted therapeutics as the pathophysiology of pediatric PH is better understood.

References

1. Abman SH, Hansmann G, Archer SL, et al. Pediatric pulmonary hypertension: guidelines from the American Heart Association and American Thoracic Society. *Circulation.* 2015;132:2037-2099.

2. Copland I, Post M. Lung development and fetal lung growth. *Paediatr Respir Rev.* 2004;5:S259-S264.

3. Ghanayem NS, Gordon JB. Modulation of pulmonary vasomotor tone in the fetus and neonate. *Respir Res.* 2001;2:139-144.

4. Berkelhamer SK, Mestan KK, Steinhorn RH. Pulmonary hypertension in bronchopulmonary dysplasia. *Semin Perinatol.* 2013;37:124-131.

5. Black SM, Fineman JR. Oxidative and nitrosative stress in pediatric pulmonary hypertension: Roles of endothelin-1 and nitric oxide. *Vascul Pharmacol.* 2006;45:308-316.

6. Heath D, Edwards JE. The pathology of hypertensive pulmonary vascular disease; a description of six grades of structural changes in the pulmonary arteries with special reference to congenital cardiac septal defects. *Circulation.* 1958;18:533-547.

7. Haarman MG, Kerstjens-Frederikse WS, Vissia-Kazemier TR, et al. The genetic epidemiology of pediatric pulmonary arterial hypertension. *J Pediatr.* 2020;225:65-73.e5.

8. Southgate L, Machado RD, Gräf S, Morrell NW. Molecular genetic framework underlying pulmonary arterial hypertension. *Nat Rev Cardiol.* 2020;17:85-95.

9. Zhu N, Gonzaga-Jauregui C, Welch CL, et al. Exome sequencing in children with pulmonary arterial hypertension demonstrates differences compared with adults. *Circ Genomic Precis Med.* 2018;11:e001887.

10. Aldred MA, Morrell NW, Guignabert C. New mutations and pathogenesis of pulmonary hypertension: progress and puzzles in disease pathogenesis. *Circ Res.* 2022;130:1365-1381.

11. Simonneau G, Montani D, Celermajer DS, et al. Haemodynamic definitions and updated clinical classification of pulmonary hypertension. *Eur Respir J.* 2019;53:1801913.

12. Rubin LJ. Introduction: diagnosis and management of pulmonary arterial hypertension: ACCP evidence-based clinical practice guidelines. *Chest.* 2004;126:7S-10S.

13. Sitbon O, Humbert M, Jaïs X, et al. Long-term response to calcium channel blockers in idiopathic pulmonary arterial hypertension. *Circulation.* 2005;111:3105-3111.

14. Mullen MP. Diagnostic strategies for acute presentation of pulmonary hypertension in children: particular focus on use of echocardiography, cardiac catheterization, magnetic resonance imaging, chest computed tomography, and lung biopsy. *Pediatr Crit Care Med.* 2010;11:S23-S26.

15. Frank BS, Ivy DD. Pediatric pulmonary arterial hypertension. *Pediatr Clin North Am.* 2020;67:903-921.

16. Abman SH, Mullen MP, Sleeper LA, et al. Characterisation of paediatric pulmonary hypertensive vascular disease from the PPHNet Registry. *Eur Respir J.* 2022;59:2003337.

17. Constantine A, Dimopoulos K, Haworth SG, Muthurangu V, Moledina S. Twenty-year experience and outcomes in a National Pediatric Pulmonary Hypertension Service. *Am J Respir Crit Care Med.* 2022;206:758-766.

18. Barst RJ, McGoon MD, Elliott CG, Foreman AJ, Miller DP, Ivy DD. Survival in childhood pulmonary arterial hypertension: Insights from the registry to evaluate early and long-term pulmonary arterial hypertension disease management. *Circulation.* 2012;125:113-122.

19. Mullen MP, Andrus J, Labella MH, et al. Quality of life and parental adjustment in pediatric pulmonary hypertension. *Chest.* 2014;145:237-244.

20. Maxwell BG, Nies MK, Ajuba-iwuji CC, et al. Trends in hospitalization for pediatric pulmonary hypertension. *Pediatrics.* 2015;136:241-250.

21. Kozlik-Feldmann R, Hansmann G, Bonnet D, et al. Pulmonary hypertension in children with congenital heart disease (PAH-CHD, PPHVD-CHD). Expert consensus statement on the diagnosis and treatment of paediatric pulmonary hypertension. The European Paediatric Pulmonary Vascular Disease Network, endorsed by ISHLT and DGPK. *Heart.* 2016;102:ii42-ii48.

22. Hansmann G, Meinel K, Bukova M, et al. Selexipag for the treatment of children with pulmonary arterial hypertension: first multicenter experience in drug safety and efficacy. *J Heart Lung Transplant.* 2020;39:695-706.

23. Checchia PA, Bronicki RA. Review of inhaled nitric oxide in the pediatric cardiac surgery setting. *Pediatr Cardiol.* 2012;33:493-505.

24. Neonatal Inhaled Nitric Oxide Study Group. Inhaled nitric oxide in full-term and nearly full-term infants with hypoxic respiratory failure. *N Engl J Med.* 1997;336:597-604.

25. Wessel DL, Adatia I, Giglia TM, et al. Use of inhaled nitric oxide and acetylcholine in the evaluation of pulmonary hypertension and endothelial function after cardiopulmonary bypass. *Circulation.* 1993;88:2128-2138.

26. Wessel DL, Adatia I, Van Marter LJ, et al. Improved oxygenation in a randomized trial of inhaled nitric oxide for persistent pulmonary hypertension of the newborn. *Pediatrics.* 1997;100:e7.

27. Namachivayam P, Theilen U, Butt WW, et al. Sildenafil prevents rebound pulmonary hypertension after withdrawal of nitric oxide in children. *Am J Respir Crit Care Med.* 2006;174:1042-1047.

28. Barst RJ, Beghetti M, Pulido T, et al. STARTS-2: Long-term survival with oral sildenafil monotherapy in treatment-naive pediatric pulmonary arterial hypertension. *Circulation.* 2014;129:1914-1923.

29. Abman SH, Kinsella JP, Rosenzweig EB, et al. Implications of the US Food and Drug Administration warning against the use of sildenafil for the treatment of pediatric pulmonary hypertension. *Am J Respir Crit Care Med.* 2013;187:572-575.

30. Galiè N, Barberà JA, Frost AE, et al. Initial use of ambrisentan plus tadalafil in pulmonary arterial hypertension. *N Engl J Med.* 2015;373:834-844.

31. Zijlstra WMH, Douwes JM, Rosenzweig EB, et al. Survival differences in pediatric pulmonary arterial hypertension: clues to a better understanding of outcome and optimal treatment strategies. *J Am Coll Cardiol.* 2014;63:2159-2169.

32. Grady RM, Canter MW, Wan F, et al. Pulmonary-to-systemic arterial shunt to treat children with severe pulmonary hypertension. *J Am Coll Cardiol.* 2021;78:468-477.

33. Hayes D, Cherikh WS, Chambers DC, et al. The International Thoracic Organ Transplant Registry of the International Society for Heart and Lung Transplantation : Twenty-second pediatric lung and heart-lung transplantation report — 2019; Focus theme: Donor and recipient size match. *J Hear Lung Transplant.* 2019;38:1015-1027.

57

Adult Congenital Heart Disease

KERI M. SHAFER AND MICHAEL J. LANDZBERG

KEY LEARNING POINTS

- Care for adults with congenital heart disease (ACHD) is marked by clinical consequences of physiologies that change over their lifetime. With dynamic cardiovascular loading conditions, worsening myocardial performance, neurohormonal dysfunction, secondary systemic inflammation, and multiple organ system dysfunction, the approach to care must shift to meet these changing influences to prevent outcomes of importance.

- Heart failure has a multitude of presentations in patients with ACHD ranging from peripheral and pulmonary vascular disease to subpulmonary and subsystemic right and left heart dysfunction. These are key contributors to worsened functional capacity, and are associated with increased

morbidity and mortality; understanding and management remain core to ACHD care providers.

- ACC/AHA, European (ESC), and Canadian ACHD care guidelines provide a rich and current source of supportive data for clinicians providing both primary and collaborative care for ACHD.

- Optimal outcomes for ACHD hinge on patient-centered care planning that incorporates: (1) iterative review and understanding of patient priorities, and physical, social, psychological, and spiritual aspects of health and suffering; and (2) building and strengthening of adaptive coping skills over a lifetime.

Introduction

In the early to mid-1970s, the establishment of the first units (Los Angeles, London) specifically designed to care for adults with congenital cardiac disease (ACHD) paved the way for future recognition of issues in the management of congenital heart disease (CHD) that can be more apparent in, and at times unique to, adolescent and adult survivors with CHD. In the last 50 years, the care of patients with ACHD has changed seismically. Care for ACHD requires providers to integrate techniques pioneered by pediatric cardiologists in anatomic abnormalities and procedural management, as well as evidence-based practices of adult cardiologists in acquired heart disease, and apply these techniques to a unique population. ACHD is now a recognized field that carries unique aspects well beyond its parent fields. This chapter will highlight some of the fundamental aspects of ACHD beyond lesion management.

Over 90% of children born with CHD are now expected to survive to adulthood, resulting in more adults living with CHD than children.[1] Therefore, it is of utmost importance that providers have a framework for approach to care. Here we present a view that care of the patient with ACHD requires a holistic approach addressing all aspects of health while integrating complex physiology.

Despite their excellent survival into adulthood, patients with ACHD have residual and developing issues that require meticulous and lifelong care. Patients with ACHD are faced with premature mortality when compared with age-matched cohorts, as well as ongoing morbidity. Heart failure, pneumonia, sudden cardiac death, and cancer rank among the most common causes for death. Not surprisingly, patients with complex disease and poor physiologic status are at the highest risk for death.[2] Additionally, location of care impacts mortality. A recently published article showed a 22% lower risk for death in the referral centers almost entirely explained by care of the complex congenital patient.[3] Understanding the complex physiology is a key to providing holistic care to ACHD.

Physiology in Flux

Past assessment and review of the causes of physical incapacity in ACHD largely focused on measures of ventricular systolic performance, typically emphasizing relationship with the "old baggage" of long-standing alterations of volume and anatomic loading conditions on ventricular function. Heart failure, classically defined as the inability of the heart to functionally keep up with the demands of the body (with associated anatomic, serologic, and physiologic correlates), remains the primary source of morbidity and mortality for ACHD.[4,5] As described throughout this chapter, premature senescence and decrement of function appear to occur not only in the heart but in nearly every organ in ACHD. While such changes may appear sufficiently static at any one moment of measurement to allow description, physiologic organ performance (with associated abnormalities of markers of perfusion, inflammation, and injury) appears to be in flux over each ACHD's lifetime. Recognition of such potential for physiologic change, with associated effects on quality of life, physical performance, and mortality, contributed to a change in latest American College of Cardiology/American Heart Association (ACC/AHA) ACHD care guidelines, which now include a non static physiologic designation to patient classification specific to most recent patient encounter[6] (Fig. 57.1). This new global designation associates with differential recommendations regarding nature and frequency of patient surveillance, which appears to prognosticate and may ultimately affect outcomes.[7] The nature of optimal serologic, anatomic, hemodynamic, and performance measures to best define physiology-in-flux remains unspecified. At present, ACHD care providers are encouraged by care guidelines to consider testing modalities as complementary in understanding pathology and health potentials (Fig. 57.1). Examples of physiology that not uncommonly shifts over the lifetime of a patient with ACHD are included in the several vignettes discussed below.

Atrial septal defect (ASD): In the young person with ASD, magnitude and direction of intracardiac shunting is driven by combination of defect size (restriction) and mostly by the balance of resistance to flow between the right and left atrioventricular chambers. In youth, typically both sides of the heart have relatively compliant pressure-volume relationships, with the right atrioventricular chamber remaining more compliant than the left, allowing for left-to-right intra-atrial flow. As ACHD patients with ASD age, they witness an increasing left atrial and left ventricular noncompliance. This is driven by extraneous factors such as senescence of myocardium and greater peripheral arterial stiffness of aging, and potential development of additive risks for myocardial or peripheral arterial stiffness (including systemic arterial hypertension, diabetes, atherosclerosis, obesity, and hypercholesterolemia). Decreasing left atrioventricular compliance leads to greater left-to-right intracardiac shunting and associated consequences.[8] Defect closure in such circumstance, without addressing other contributing physiologies, might impact negatively on quality of life, function, and survival for affected ACHD.

Registry data have consistently suggested lesser survival for ACHD with prior ASD than for matched peers. This has remained perplexing given the "simple" nature of this congenital lesion. Explanation may in part lie in limits of pulmonary vascular resistance and capacitance reserve that accompany adverse remodeling due to left-to-right shunting, and which appear to exist in all aged persons with ASD. This lessening of pulmonary vascular reserve might be better tolerated in younger adults with healthier right ventricles and overall greater peripheral muscular adaptation to lesser cardiac output reserve to exercise. These changes have potential for being unmasked as adults age, have less adaptive peripheral muscular training effects, greater potential for additive insults to right ventricular performance (including

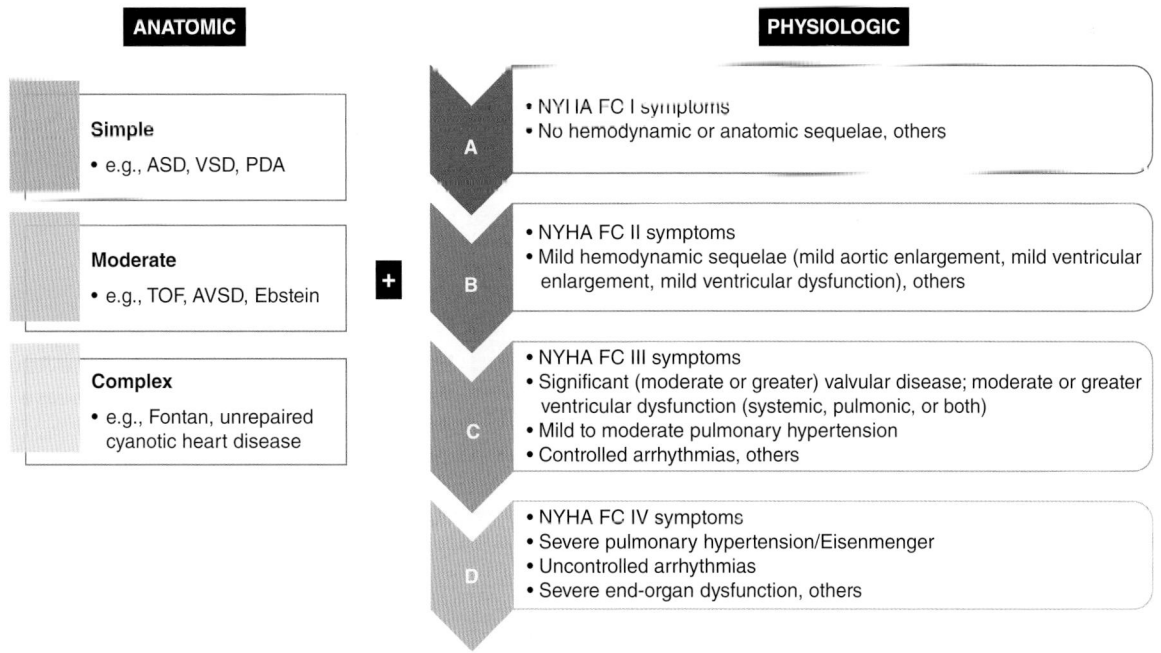

• **Fig. 57.1** Anatomic and physiologic classification of adult congenital heart disease. *ASD*, atrial septal defect; *VSD*, ventricular septal defect; *PDA*, patent ductus arteriosus; *TOF*, tetralogy of Fallot; *AVSD*, atrioventricular septal defect; *NYHA*, New York Heart Association; *FC*, functional class

obesity, sleep apnea, and toxin exposure including nicotine inhalation), and greater evolution of pulmonary vascular changes and increase in pulmonary vascular impedance.

Coarctation: In the younger person with aortic coarctation, a high intraventricular pressure is driven largely by late systolic loading of peripheral arterial vascular obstruction. This component of afterload (wall stress) tends to be balanced by concentric left ventricular hypertrophy and relatively normal ventricular chamber size, with preserved myocardial perfusion. Post intervention and restoration of normal aortic diameter, the aging patients with ACHD may typically have a mild (or pharmacologically controlled) pressure component of afterload (still driven by late systolic loading and more global peripheral arterial stiffness). Now, however, outcomes are largely impacted by what appears to be an inexorable peripheral vascular inflammation contributing to peripheral and coronary atherosclerosis, with associated effects on myocardial, cerebral, and renal blood flow and adverse outcomes.[9]

Single ventricle: In the younger person with single ventricle after Fontan palliation, normal systemic venous function and normal preload augmentation are observed. In addition, hemodynamic and cross-sectional imaging assessment tends to note normal volume component to preload and afterload, normal ventricular wall thickness, and normal systolic blood pressure components to preload and afterload, with normal, or at times elevated, systemic vascular resistance. In contradistinction, the symptomatic aging adult with Fontan palliation for single ventricle typically displays a panoply of abnormalities that create a physiology and imbalance in physical performance unique to the individual. Systemic venous dysfunction is common, with abnormal preload and pulmonary vascular reserve.[10,11] Atrial and ventricular resting volumes in such symptomatic patients tend to be increased and, combined with a hypertrophied ventricular wall and low-normal systolic pressure, contribute to increased wall stress and higher afterload.[12] Hepatic dysfunction and systemic arterial circulatory failure combine to create increasingly low systemic vascular resistance; together with elevated afterload, a physiology of hypoperfusion, injury, and abnormal performance ensues. Diagnostic mastery appears necessary to dissect out potentials that can be influenced to improve performance and outcomes.

Ventricular Vascular Coupling

Effective circulation within a ventricular-arterial system is designed as receipt of pulsatile flow and delivery of steady flow in a balance of forces that both preserves energy and minimizes stress relationships between ventricular myocardium and central and peripheral conduits, resistance vessels, and the microvasculature.[13] As well, balance of end-systolic and arterial elasticity allows for preservation of sensitivity to additional aspects of cardiac loading. Current understanding of ventricular-vascular coupling in health and disease suggests that determinants of systolic and diastolic ventricular performance and vascular function have

direct and profound effects on each other (including coronary perfusion).[13] Measures of the pulsatile hemodynamics of such coupling, including alterations in arterial stiffness and cushioning, pulse pressure, wave characteristics, and velocities, in both acquired systolic and nonsystolic heart failure, have been shown to correlate with changes in patient morbidity and mortality.[14] Demonstration of abnormal brachial arterial responsiveness to endothelium-dependent and -independent vasomediators in young adults after successful aortic coarctation repair led to investigation of conduit artery pulse wave velocity as a marker of arterial stiffness.

There is increasing recognition that patients with ACHD have additional cardiovascular abnormalities that directly affect key determinants of ventricular-vascular coupling. Changes in intrinsic heart rate (e.g., postoperative patients), stroke volume (e.g., patients with intracardiac mixing and volume loading), pulse pressure (e.g., patients with nonpulsatile pulmonary blood flow, patients with systemic arterial diastolic runoff), systemic arterial impedance (e.g., patients with aortic coarctation), neurohormonal or cardiac autonomic nervous system activity, or salt and water control (e.g., erythrocytotic patients with focal glomerular sclerosis), seen in such patients, may have real and substantive effects on health and functional capacity for affected individuals. As such, patients with ACHD may serve as prototypal models for evaluation of potential ventricular vascular coupling changes and their effects in health and disease.

Compromise of effective circulation may result from intrinsic factors not typically considered within the cardiopulmonary vascular tree (Table 57.1). For example, critical energy conservation within high-pressure nonpulsatile systemic venous inflow may be markedly diminished due to anatomic venous-atrial connections, jeopardizing forward output in atriopulmonary-type Fontan palliations. As well, impaired atrial-ventricular transport, due to intrinsic functional or anatomic baffle abnormalities, may be, in part, responsible for limits in stroke volume augmentation in patients with atrial-level repair for D-loop transposition of the great arteries[15] (Fig. 57.2).

TABLE 57.1	"Non-myocardial" Potential Cardiopulmonary Etiologies for "Heart Failure" in the Adult Patient With Congenital Heart Disease

Alteration in:
- Systemic venous-atrial transport
- Atrial-ventricular transport
- Ventricular transport
- Pulmonary vascular function
- Systemic arterial conduit function
- Pericardial constriction
- Residual anatomic obstruction

Shunting
Outflow tract aneurysm
Semilunar valve regurgitation
Intracardiac or vascular thrombosis

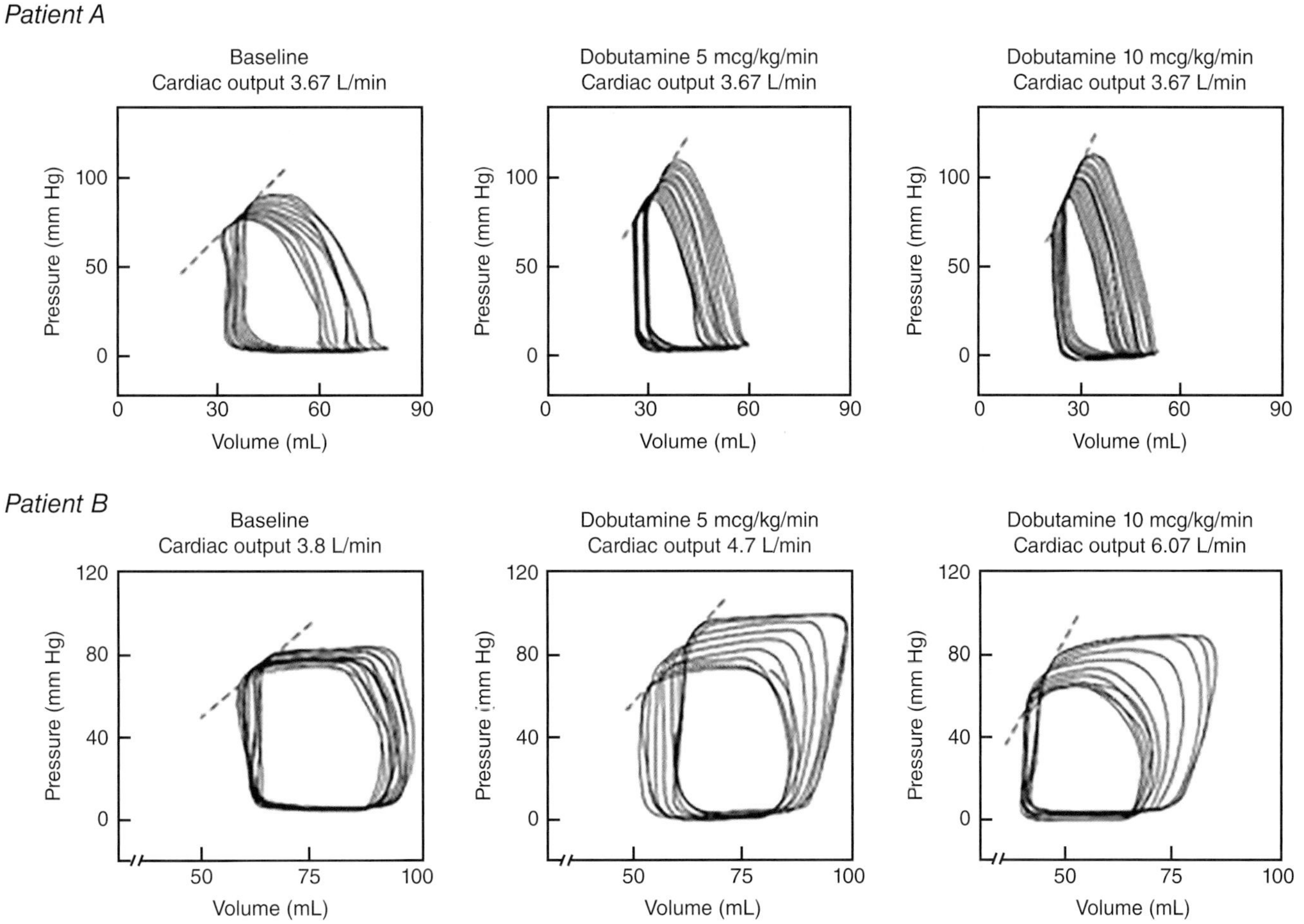

Patient A

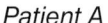

Patient B

• **Fig. 57.2** Flow volume loops during preload reduction in patients with (SDD) transposition of the great arteries. Patient A: Failure to increase cardiac output with dobutamine yet preservation of rise of contractile indices. Patient B: Increase in both cardiac output and contractility is seen. In both patients, however, fall in stroke volume occurs. (From Derrick GP, Narang I, White PA, et al. Failure of stroke volume augmentation during exercise and dobutamine stress is unrelated to load-independent indexes of right ventricular performance after the Mustard operation. *Circulation.* 2000;102:154.)

Pulmonary Vascular Disease

Pulmonary endothelial dysfunction, worse in nonpulsatile atriopulmonary connection-type repairs and in pulmonary arteriolar hypertension (PAH), contributes to an increase in nonanatomic pulmonary ventricular afterload. This results in reduction in transpulmonary flow in patients with intracardiac mixing or lower systemic output in patients with Fontan palliation.[12] Given that presence of pulmonary hypertension may not necessarily imply presence of PAH, but rather can be indicative of any of a number of additional triggers for such (e.g., pulmonary venous hypertension, restrictive or hypoventilatory lung disease, thromboembolic pulmonary vascular occlusion), catheter-based hemodynamic assessment remains critical as the hallmark of diagnosis of PAH associated with CHD (Fig. 57.3). Analyses of epidemiologic databases associated with patients with PAH have suggested similar untreated survival of patients with severe pulmonary hypertension, nearly universal regardless of etiology (with median survival between 2.8 and 3.4 years

for the affected adult patient). Correlation of survival with variables relating to right ventricular function (typically assessed by hemodynamic measure of systemic cardiac output and mixed venous oxygen saturation and right atrial pressure) and physical capacity (typically measured by 6-minute walking capacity), emphasizes the delicate balance and direct relationships between pulmonary afterload, cardiac function, physical capacity, and life.

For most affected patients, modern treatment centers on mediators of chemotaxis, cellular proliferation and differentiation, and regulation of vasoactive peptides and growth factors. These mediators currently include prostanoids (intravenous, inhaled, oral, subcutaneous), endothelin antagonists, nitroso compounds, and phosphodiesterase inhibitors. While large randomized controlled studies are still needed, smaller randomized studies have seen improvement in intermediate outcomes with phosphodiesterase inhibitors, endothelin receptor antagonists, and prostacyclins. While the optimal approach is still not defined, general consensus is that early treatment with pulmonary vascular resistance-lowering

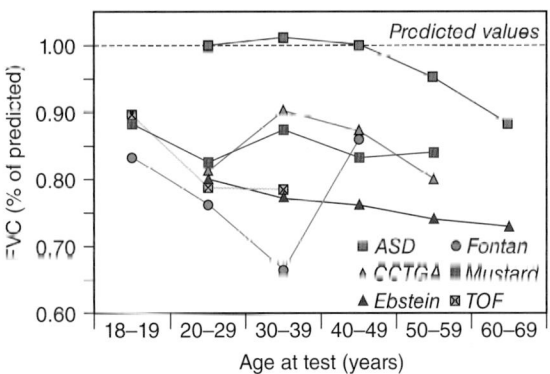

• **Fig. 57.3** Impaired vital capacity as a marker of restrictive lung disease in adult patients with congenital heart disease. *FVC,* forced vital capacity; *ASD,* atrial septal defect; *CCTGA,* congenitally corrected transposition of the great arteries; *TOF,* tetralogy of Fallot (From Fredriksen PM, Veldtman G, Hechter S, et al. Aerobic capacity in adults with various congenital heart diseases. *Am J Cardiol.* 2001;87: 310–314.)

medications can be helpful in preventing rapid progression of the disease[16] (see Chapter 56).

Heart Failure and Extracardiac Organ Dysfunction

Almost nowhere else in medicine does the categorization of a patient with "heart failure" carry so many pathophysiologic potentials as in the patient with ACHD. While ventricular function is assessed in many other chapters throughout this textbook, ACHD heart failure manifests with abnormalities and increased demand of nearly every organ system (Table 57.2). Increased potential for endocrinologic dysfunction, gas exchanging and non-parenchymal lung disease, abnormalities of renal or hepatic function, and altered skeleton and muscle metabolism highlight the multitude of extracardiac conditions contributing to abnormal functional capacity or performance. Not surprisingly, heart failure incidence increases with age and underlying complexity of heart disease and affects far beyond the patient's exercise capacity and quality of life.[5] The recent ACC/AHA guidelines works to characterize patients with the physiologic class heavily based on NYHA functional class (Fig. 57.1). On a recent evaluation of these guidelines, the classification did provide usefulness in the prediction of heart failure while reinforcing that age remains among the strongest predictors.[7] As the patient with ACHD ages, each organ system is affected resulting in dysfunction that requires understanding and consideration for treatment.

Neurohormonal: Abnormalities of cardiac autonomic nervous activity and elevations of neurohormones have been studied, recognized, and at times found to be predictive of outcomes (rehospitalization, functional capacity, mortality) in those with ACHD. These changes are in part related to recognized heart rate reduction after surgery, effects of prior thoracic operations, and subsequent surgery-mediated

TABLE 57.2	End-Organ Dysfunction

Endocrinologic
   Neurohormonal dysfunction
   Hypothyroidism
   Diabetes
   Loss of adrenergic and vagal responsiveness
Pulmonary
   Restrictive lung disease
   Hypoventilation, exercise induced oscillatory ventilation
   Obstructive sleep apnea
   Arteriovenous malformations
   Phrenic nerve injury, diaphragmatic paralysis
   Pulmonary vascular disease
   Chronic parenchymal infection
Liver
   Chronic hepatitis
   Portal hypertension
   Cirrhosis
Renal
   Altered glomerular filtration
   Altered water handling
   Hyperuricemia
Hematologic
   Iron deficiency
   Erythrocytosis
   Lymphopenia
Musculoskeletal
   Sarcopenia secondary to metabolic limitations,
     iatrogenic deconditioning, or lack of exercise
   Kyphosis and scoliosis, scoliosis
Infectious
   Immunodeficiencies (e.g., DiGeorge)
   Bioprosthetic valve infection (e.g., Melody)
Neurologic/Psychiatric
   Cerebrovascular injury
   Depression
   Anxiety
   Post-traumatic stress disorder

denervation, alterations in gas exchange, and aging. Abnormal neurohormonal axis contributes to exercise dysfunction which may respond to exercise training. Furthermore, it is a useful target of pharmacologic therapies in standard heart failure with potential in ACHD.[17,18] Moreover, significant adrenal dysfunction has been reported in chronically cyanotic patients.

Exercise capacity and pulmonary function: The adult with CHD objectively may be profoundly limited in aerobic functional capacity compared with normal controls.[19] Maximal achievable peak oxygen consumption (peak VO_2) in many patients is 30–50% of normal controls, with important reductions seen even in patients after repair of simple atrial level defects (Fig. 57.2). Restriction in ventilatory function (with respiratory volumes typically 75% to 85% normal predictions), whether due to developmental or acquired structural or physiologic changes, may contribute to fatigue and incapacity[20] (Fig. 57.4).

Hepatic and renal dysfunction: Hepatitis-induced and "cardiac" cirrhosis have found recapitulation in a patient population plagued by higher central venous pressures,

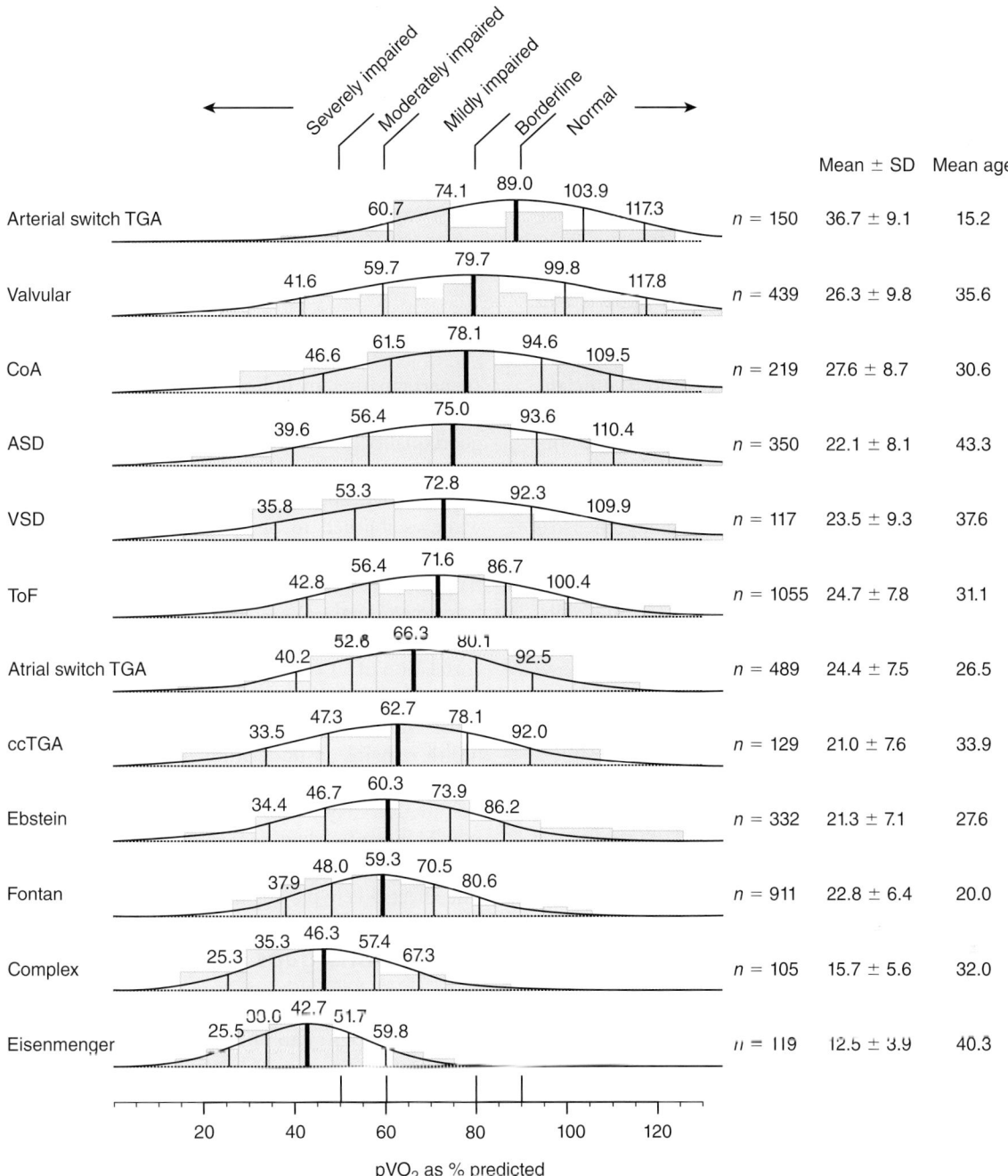

• **Fig. 57.4** Impaired maximal oxygen consumption in adult patients with congenital heart disease. *TGA*, transposition of the great arteries; *COA*, coarctation of the aorta; *ASD*, atrial septal defect; *VSD*, ventricular septal defect; *ToF*, tetralogy of Fallot; *ccTGA*, congenitally corrected transposition of the great arteries; *pVO2*, peak oxygen consumption; *SD*, standard deviation (From Kempny, A, Dimopoulos, K, Uebing, A, et al. Reference values for exercise limitations among adults with congenital heart disease. Relation to activities of daily life–single centre experience and review of published data. *Eur Heart J.* 2012;33:1386–1396.)

potential for low systemic cardiac index, and prior exposure to infected blood products (blood not screened for hepatitis C until 1992). The neurohormonal activation caused by portal hypertension may be profound, and it exacerbates volume retention and curbs functional ability. Fontan patients are among the best examples of multiorgan dysfunction due to CHD. As they age, Fontan patients develop significant liver and kidney dysfunction at least in part due to the persistent

elevation in venous pressures and decrease in perfusion pressure of these organs. This combined dysfunction may suggest why the MELD XI score (creatinine and bilirubin) was effective in predicting risk for adults with Fontan palliation. However, due to limitations in creatinine and particularly in the setting of variable muscle mass, alternative markers beyond creatinine such as cystatin C should be used in the assessment of patients with ACHD.[21]

Coping/lifelong Palliative Care

Transition from childhood living with CHD to young and older adult years optimally entails development and sustenance of a therapeutic relationship with a medical care provider team with knowledge and experience in ACHD care, together with a personal accrual, and use of adaptive coping skills (cognitive and behavioral efforts to manage stressful conditions or associated emotional distress). These life management skills, in part, may include information seeking and awareness of nonbinary medical options and outcomes, support acquisition, awareness of life priorities and outcomes deemed to be intolerable, compartmentalization of uncertainties and unloading those without sufficient data to act upon, forward thinking, planning and hope construction, and sustenance of life meaning despite surrounding stressors. Care providers may have limitations in their own ability to guide ACHD in their acquisition and refinement of adaptive coping tools. ACHD comprehensive care center accreditation mandates that ACHD have available to them palliative care specialists expert in serious illness communication, maintaining identity and meaning, and coping support.

LGBTQ+ adults, in aggregate, are more likely to have worse cardiovascular health than matched controls, based on retrospective review of cardiovascular risk profile (in particular cigarette smoking, and altered blood sugar profile). Such effects may be intensified by worsened sleep patterns, stress of discrimination, stigma, and fear of violence (in part contributing to greater self-medication with nicotine and alcohol products noted in LGBTQ+ populations). The ACHD population, in general, is well known to be vulnerable to prolonged absence from specialized care; LBGTQ+ adults have additive potential for health care avoidance due to fears regarding discrimination, and, in particularly underrepresented racial and ethnic groups, may have effects from insecure housing, less available health care, and higher poverty levels. Awareness of, and access to, reliable and expert-monitored health information and resources via national organizations and social media groups may assist in impacting such disparities as well as raising strength of identity and meaning.[22]

Despite progress that has been made with anatomic and pharmacologic interventions, as well as mechanical circulatory support and organ transplantation, patients with ACHD remain at lifelong risk for premature multiple-organ system morbidity and death. In retrospective studies of patients with ACHD who died during a hospital admission, only a minority had engaged in end-of-life discussions with their providers and most continued to receive aggressive treatment up until death.[4] Surveys of patients with ACHD confirm that up to 70% are willing to participate in advanced care planning and greater than 90% would choose to speak with a palliative care specialist.[23] By contrast, most ACHD providers worry that they are unable to reliably estimate prognosis and believe that patients are not ready for conversations regarding end-of-life care. Complicating symptom management of ACHD is a high rate of depression that is often undiagnosed and undertreated. Palliative care specialists that are aligned with ACHD and advanced heart disease teams can play an important role in addressing and supporting the unique needs of patients with ACHD, as discussed earlier, as well as regarding stressors particular to life-long serious medical disease, including younger age when experiencing frailty and vulnerability in health outcomes, "survivor" mentality, and complex relationship with aging parents and long-term medical providers.

Living a Meaningful Life

In participating in holistic care of patients with ACHD, understanding quality of life is crucial. Studies do show a good quality of life in these patients. Lower quality of life is found in those with older age, lack of employment, no marriage history, and worse NYHA class.[24] Exercise capacity, while established to be limited in patients with ACHD, does appropriately respond to exercise training.[25] Prior trials have shown an improvement in exercise capacity as defined by oxygen uptake (VO_2) and suggestion of improvement in quality of life in patients with ACHD. Given the strong correlation of VO_2 with survival, encouragement of routine physical activity is advised while cautioning patients to exercise within their limits and in a gradual fashion. Sexual health remains an understudied but critical component of the ACHD population. Initial studies suggest that sexual dysfunction may occur in up to ~25–30% of patients and at a higher rate than an age-matched cohort. Etiology is likely multifactorial with psychological health and medical side effects likely playing a large part.[26]

Conclusions/gaps and Future Directions

Care for patients with ACHD by the pediatric or general adult cardiologist can appear to be a natural extension of principle and practice. While such overlap in care provision appears both logical and necessary, a mastery of both an increasing body of unique scientific medical data as well as requisite skills in interdisciplinary care coordination and provision appears necessary for optimal outcomes for ACHD. Such awareness has led to both national board certification for ACHD cardiologists as well as accreditation for ACHD comprehensive care medical centers.

This chapter has largely reviewed salient principles in care that extend foundational knowledge for the pediatric or general adult cardiologist, as they apply to the ACHD. For greater specific information, readers are referred to any of the most recent national ACHD clinical care guidelines.[6,16]

Particular gaps in knowledge and future directions in optimization of care for ACHD, as highlighted by this chapter, include:

1. Development and refinement of patient- and disease-specific risk stratification tools so as to improve recognition of vulnerability and frailty in the adult (and pediatric) patients with CHD

2. Identification of optimal single- and multi-modality surveillance tools and strategy design for their implementation, with goals of greatest ability to identify aspects of both health and determinant risks

3. Creation, implementation, and outcome assessments of lifelong iterative patient-centered care planning that incorporate physical, social, psychological, and spiritual aspects of health and suffering

References

1. Moons P, Bovijn L, Budts W, et al. Temporal trends in survival to adulthood among patients born with congenital heart disease from 1970 to 1992 in Belgium. *Circulation.* 2010;122:2264-2272.

2. Diller GP, Kempny A, Alonso-Gonzalez R, et al. Survival prospects and circumstances of death in contemporary adult congenital heart disease patients under follow-up at a large tertiary centre. *Circulation.* 2015;132:2118-2125.

3. Mylotte D, Pilote L, Ionescu-Ittu R, et al. Specialized adult congenital heart disease care: the impact of policy on mortality. *Circulation.* 2014;129:1804-1812.

4. Van Bulck L, Goossens E, Morin L, et al. Last year of life of adults with congenital heart diseases: causes of death and patterns of care. *Eur Heart J.* 2022;43:4483-4492.

5. Lu CW, Wang JK, Yang HL, et al. Heart failure and patient-reported outcomes in adults with congenital heart disease from 15 countries. *JAMA.* 2022;11:e024993.

6. Stout KK, Daniels CJ, Aboulhosn JA, et al. 2018 AHA/ACC guideline for the management of adults with congenital heart disease: executive summary: a report of the American College of Cardiology/American Heart Association Task Force on Clinical Practice Guidelines. *J Am Coll Cardiol.* 2019;73:e81-e192.

7. Arnaert S, De Meester P, Troost E, et al. Heart failure related to adult congenital heart disease: prevalence, outcome and risk factors. *ESC Heart Fail.* 2021;8:2940-2950.

8. Martucci G, Landzberg M. Not just big kids: closing atrial septal defects in adults older than 60 years. *Circ Cardiovasc Interv.* 2009;2:83-84.

9. Roifman I, Therrien J, Ionescu-Ittu R, et al. Coarctation of the aorta and coronary artery disease: fact or fiction? *Circulation.* 2012;126:16-21.

10. Valente AM, Bhatt AB, Cook S, et al. The CALF (Congenital Heart Disease in Adults Lower Extremity Systemic Venous Health in Fontan Patients) study. *J Am Coll Cardiol.* 2010;56:144-150.

11. Shafer KM, Garcia JA, Babb TG, et al. The importance of the muscle and ventilatory blood pumps during exercise in patients without a subpulmonary ventricle (Fontan operation). *J Am Coll Cardiol.* 2012;60:2115-2121.

12. Gewillig M, Brown SC. The Fontan circulation after 45 years: update in physiology. *Heart.* 2016;102:1081-1086.

13. Monge García MI, Santos A. Understanding ventriculo-arterial coupling. *Ann Transl Med.* 2020;8:795.

14. Vasan RS, Pan S, Xanthakis V, et al. Arterial stiffness and long-term risk of health outcomes: The Framingham Heart Study. *Hypertension.* 2022;79:1045-1056.

15. Derrick GP, Narang I, White PA, et al. Failure of stroke volume augmentation during exercise and dobutamine stress is unrelated to load-independent indexes of right ventricular performance after the Mustard operation. *Circulation.* 2000;102:Iii154–Iii159.

16. Baumgartner H, De Backer J, Babu-Narayan SV, et al. 2020 ESC Guidelines for the management of adult congenital heart disease. *Eur Heart J.* 2021;42:563-645.

17. Bolger AP, Sharma R, Li W, et al. Neurohormonal activation and the chronic heart failure syndrome in adults with congenital heart disease. *Circulation.* 2002;106:92-99.

18. Zandstra TE, Nederend M, Jongbloed MRM, et al. Sacubitril/valsartan in the treatment of systemic right ventricular failure. *Heart.* 2021;107:1725-1730.

19. Kempny A, Dimopoulos K, Uebing A, et al. Reference values for exercise limitations among adults with congenital heart disease: relation to activities of daily life: single centre experience and review of published data. *Eur Heart J.* 2012;33:1386-1396.

20. Shafer KM, Opotowsky AR, Rhodes J. Exercise testing and spirometry as predictors of mortality in congenital heart disease: contrasting Fontan physiology with repaired tetralogy of Fallot. *Congenit Heart Dis.* 2018;13:903-910.

21. Opotowsky AR, Carazo M, Singh MN, et al. Creatinine versus cystatin C to estimate glomerular filtration rate in adults with congenital heart disease: results of the Boston Adult Congenital Heart Disease Biobank. *Am Heart J.* 2019;214:142-155.

22. Zipper Pride. In: @ZipperPrideCHD, #LGBTQ+ Adults with Congenital Heart Disease #CHD #ACHD #ZipperPride #CHDCare4Life Twitter; 2022.

23. Steiner JM, Oechslin EN, Veldtman G, et al. Advance care planning and palliative care in ACHD: the healthcare providers' perspective. *Cardiol Young.* 2020;30:402-408.

24. Apers S, Kovacs AH, Luyckx K, et al. Quality of life of adults with congenital heart disease in 15 countries: evaluating country-specific characteristics. *J Am Coll Cardiol.* 2016;67:2237-2245.

25. Opotowsky AR, Rhodes J, Landzberg MJ, et al. A randomized trial comparing cardiac rehabilitation to standard of care for adults with congenital heart disease. *World J Pediatr Congenit Heart Surg.* 2018;9:185-193.

26. Huang S, Cook SC. It is not taboo: addressing sexual function in adults with congenital heart disease. *Curr Cardiol Rep.* 2018;20:93.

58

Pregnancy and Reproductive Health in Patients with Congenital Heart Disease

CARLA P. RODRIGUEZ-MONSERRATE AND ANNE MARIE VALENTE

KEY LEARNING POINTS

- Pregnant persons with congenital heart disease should be cared for by a multidisciplinary team that understands the unique hemodynamic changes that occur and how these changes influence the underlying physiology.
- Pregnancy is associated with substantial increases in maternal plasma volume, cardiac output, and heart rate and a concurrent decrease in the systemic vascular resistance.
- High-risk features for adverse maternal cardiac outcomes include a prior cardiovascular event, baseline reduced

functional class, cyanosis, ventricular dysfunction, symptomatic left-sided obstructive lesions, pulmonary hypertension, and mechanical heart valves.
- The safety profile of cardiovascular medications used during pregnancy must include consideration of side effects for both mother and fetus.
- The majority of women with congenital heart disease may undergo successful pregnancy; however, they must recognize the increased risks to both themselves and their offspring.

Counseling Women With Congenital Heart Disease

The majority of women with congenital heart disease (CHD) experience pregnancy safely; however, there are potential risks to both mother and fetus. Some of the more common complications include heart failure, arrhythmias, premature birth, and postpartum hemorrhage.[1-4] Therefore, prenatal counseling and understanding of potential maternal and fetal risks are of great importance in this population. In addition, the hemodynamic impact of carrying a pregnancy on a mother with CHD should be discussed. Optimally, pregnant persons with CHD should be cared for by a multidisciplinary team with expertise in cardio-obstetrics to help guide them through the antenatal and postpartum periods, including discussions on the mode and timing of delivery as well as the potential of CHD in their offspring.[5-7]

Contraception

Every woman of childbearing age should be educated about contraception, with a thoughtful discussion of individualized risk and benefits recognizing their specific cardiac condition. Most commonly used contraceptives

are oral hormonal contraceptives (either combined estrogen and progesterone, or progesterone-only formulations), barrier methods, intrauterine device (IUD), or subdermal implants.[1,2,4,8] Combined oral contraceptives are highly effective but are associated with an increased risk of venous thrombosis, including deep vein thrombosis and pulmonary embolism. This is largely driven by estrogen, which increases the levels of circulating vitamin K-dependent clotting factors, plasminogen, and platelet adhesions and reduces antithrombin levels. Therefore, if oral contraceptives are utilized, formulations with the lowest dose of estrogen should be considered, and alternative forms of contraception should be offered to women at high risk for thromboembolic events (i.e., Fontan circulation, mechanical heart valves or residual shunts). For many women with CHD, an IUD is a reasonable option for contraception, yet caution must be taken in women with Fontan circulation or pulmonary hypertension (PH) undergoing implantation of an IUD to avoid vasovagal reactions and hypotension. Subdermal implants gradually release progesterone over a 3-month period providing a long-acting contraceptive alternative.[1] Women with extremely elevated risk of severe maternal complications or fatal events during pregnancy should be encouraged to undergo permanent sterilization, which includes discussion with their male partners about the potential for vasectomy.

Pregnancy-Related Cardiovascular Hemodynamic Changes

Dramatic hemodynamic changes occur during pregnancy and may have significant impact on women with CHD (Fig. 58.1). One of the most remarkable changes is the decrease in systemic vascular resistance (SVR) due to circulating hormones and effects of the placenta.[9] The drop in SVR is accompanied by an increase of the plasma volume, heart rate, and stroke volume. As a consequence, there is rise in the cardiac output (CO), which continues until the late second trimester, then plateaus, remaining elevated through delivery. These hemodynamic effects contribute to transitory left ventricular (LV) remodeling with increase in LV volumes. The LV ejection fraction does not change significantly; however, there may be alterations in LV strain late in pregnancy.[10,11] The anticipated electrocardiogram and echocardiogram findings are listed in Table 58.1.

Labor is a time of intense hemodynamic shifts. The CO increases with each contraction, and heart rate elevates further, often due to accompanying pain and anxiety. Immediately following delivery there is decompression of the inferior vena cava, which may further increase the CO as well as additional volume loading from the autotransfusion by delivery of the placenta.[1] Therefore, it is critical to monitor patients for the development of heart failure symptoms and pulmonary edema in the early postpartum period.

While the majority of women with CHD can tolerate the normal hemodynamic changes of pregnancy, they are at a higher risk of cardiovascular morbidity and mortality, and increased obstetric and neonatal complications.[3,12] The most common maternal cardiac complications include arrhythmias and heart failure. Arrhythmias are most

TABLE 58.1	Potential Electrocardiogram and Echocardiogram Changes in Pregnancy
Electrocardiogram Parameter	**Changes During Pregnancy**
Heart rate	↑ ~10% (may be blunted in women with repaired congenital heart disease and sinus node dysfunction)
Ventricular axis	May become leftward
Small q wave, inverted t or p wave	May appear, most likely in lead III
Non-specific t wave abnormalities	May appear
Qt interval	Lengthens
Premature atrial beats	May appear
Echocardiogram Parameter	**Changes During Pregnancy**
Left atrium	↑ 3–5 mm
Left ventricular end-diastolic dimension	↑ 2–4 mm
Left ventricular mass	↑ 5%–10%
Left ventricular ejection fraction	Unchanged or slightly ↑
E/A ratio	↓
E/e′ ratio	Unchanged
e′/a′ ratio	↓
Valve annulus diameter	↑ 1–2 cm
Valvar regurgitation	Physiologic ↑ in tricuspid, pulmonary, mitral valve regurgitation
Small pericardial effusion	Reported in up to 25%

commonly supraventricular in nature. Heart failure usually occurs during the late second or third trimester or in the early postpartum period. Table 58.2 summarizes some of the concerning signs and symptoms to be aware of in pregnant persons with CHD as well as potential interventions.

Maternal Risk Stratification Variables

Risk Scores

The risk of adverse outcomes during pregnancy in patients with cardiovascular disease has been studied extensively. Risk stratification of women with CHD who desire pregnancy requires an extensive medical history, physical exam, and careful evaluation of the recent diagnostic tests as well as multidisciplinary input from cardiologists, anesthesiologists, and maternal-fetal medicine specialists. Several risk

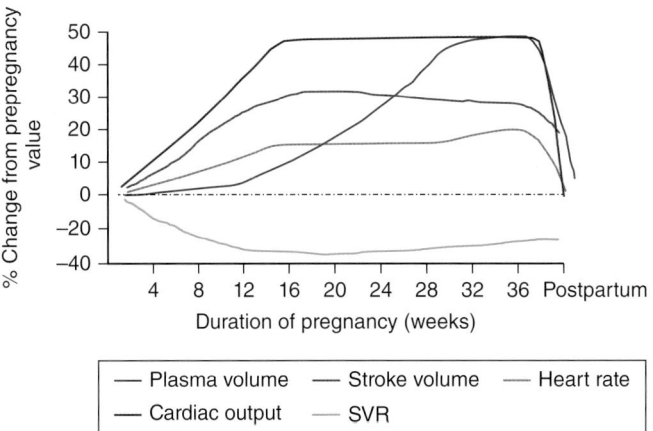

• **Fig. 58.1** Hemodynamic changes throughout pregnancy. *SVR*, Systemic vascular resistance.

TABLE 58.2	Concerning Signs and Symptoms During Pregnancy and Potential Interventions
Maternal Red Flags	**Potential Interventions**
• Oxygen saturation < 90%	• Supplemental oxygen
• Sustained or symptomatic arrhythmias, hemodynamically stable	• Beta-blocker therapy • Vagal maneuver, adenosine administration for supraventricular tachycardia
• Sustained or symptomatic arrhythmias, hemodynamically unstable	• Immediate direct current cardioversion
• Symptoms of heart failure, confirmed by physical exam and/or biomarkers	• Lower extremity compression stockings • Diuretics
• Significant ventricular dysfunction	• Diuretics • Afterload reduction with hydralazine, nitrates • Plan for advanced mechanical support if hemodynamic collapse
• Symptoms in the setting of underlying outflow tract obstruction	• Consider transcatheter therapies if refractory symptoms with medical management • Consider cardiac surgery in refractory cases
• Elevated pulmonary vascular resistance	• Discussion regarding risks of continuing pregnancy in the setting of significant pulmonary hypertension
• Valve thrombosis	• Thrombolytic therapy • Consider urgent catheter or surgical intervention

scores, including the modified World Health Organization (WHO), Cardiac Disease in Pregnancy Study (CARPREG), and Zwangerschap bij Aangeboren HARtAfwijkingen (ZA-HARA) scores, have been developed to predict adverse maternal cardiovascular events.[13] Fig. 58.2 illustrates the modified WHO risk classification and the CARPREG-II risk score.

Natriuretic Peptide Levels

As in other cardiovascular diseases, increased levels of natriuretic peptide or pro-natriuretic peptide during pregnancy correlate with adverse cardiovascular outcomes in women with heart disease. A threshold of less than 100 pg/mL has been identified in some studies as the cutoff for normalcy.[14,15]

Cardiopulmonary Exercise Test

Cardiopulmonary exercise testing is often used to evaluate exercise capacity, chronotropic incompetence, and blood pressure (BP) response in adults with CHD including women who are considering pregnancy. Several guidelines have recommended exercise test evaluation before pregnancy or in the early stages of pregnancy. A blunted heart rate response to exercise in women with CHD is associated with a higher risk for maternal cardiac and neonatal adverse events.[16]

Medications During Pregnancy and Postpartum

Many women with CHD of childbearing age are taking cardiovascular medications. It is important to review and counsel patients about medications' potential effects on the fetus and the need for discontinuation or adjustment during pregnancy. The pharmacokinetics are affected by several factors unique to pregnancy such as delayed gastric emptying, increased plasma volume, increased volume of distribution, decreased albumin, and increased hepatic and renal clearance.[1,8,9,13] In 2015, the Federal Drug Administration has developed a pregnancy and lactation labeling rule to provide relevant information for critical decision-making when treating pregnant or lactating women, and clinicians should use this resource when considering medication choices.

Supraventricular tachycardia (SVT) is the most common sustained arrhythmia during pregnancy, and *adenosine* is considered safe in pregnancy. For patients in stable SVT, *beta-blockers* (preferably B1-selective agents) may be utilized. In fact, patients with CHD are frequently on beta-blockers pre-pregnancy and one of the largest concerns during pregnancy is the potential for intrauterine growth restriction (IUGR). The growth of the fetus should be closely monitored, and discontinuation or adjustment of this medication should be done only if fetal risk outweighs maternal benefits. In the early postpartum period, neonatal

Modified world health organization (mWHO) classification

	mWHO I	mWHO II	mWHO II–III	mWHO III	mWHO IV
Diagnosis (if otherwise well and uncomplicated)	Small or mild – pulmonary stenosis – patent ductus arteriosus – mitral valve prolapse Successfully repaired simple lesions (atrial or ventricular septal defect, patent ductus arteriosus, anomalous pulmonary venous drainage) Atrial or ventricular ectopic beats, isolated	Unoperated atrial or ventricular septal defect Repaired tetralogy of Fallot Most arrhythmias (supraventricular arrhythmias) Turner syndrome without aortic dilatation	Mild left ventricular impairment (EF >45%) Hypertrophic cardiomyopathy Native or tissue valve disease not considered WHO I or IV (mild mitral stenosis, moderate aortic stenosis) Marfan or other HTAD syndrome without aortic dilatation Aorta <45 mm in bicuspid aortic valve pathology Repaired coarctation Atrioventricular septal defect	Moderate left ventricular impairment (EF 30–45%) Previous peripartum cardiomyopathy without any residual left ventricular impairment Mechanical valve Systemic right ventricle with good or mildly decreased ventricular function Fontan circulation. If otherwise the patient is well and the cardiac condition uncomplicated Unrepaired cyanotic heart disease Other complex heart disease Moderate mitral stenosis Severe asymptomatic aortic stenosis Moderate aortic dilatation (40–45 mm in Marfan syndrome or other HTAD; 45–50 mm in bicuspid aortic valve, Tumer syndrome ASI 20–25 mm/m^2, tetralogy of Fallot <50 mm) Ventricular tachycardia	Pulmonary arterial hypertension Severe systemic ventricular dysfunction (EF <30% or NYHA class III–IV) Previous peripartum cardiomyopathy with any residual left ventricular impairment Severe mitral stenosis Severe symptomatic aortic stenosis Systemic right ventricle with moderate or severely decreased ventricular function Severe aortic dilatation (>45 mm in Marfan syndrome or other HTAD, >50 mm in bicuspid aortic valve, Turner syndrome ASI >25 mm/m^2, tetralogy of Fallot >50 mm) Vascular Ehlers–Danlos Severe (re) coarctation Fontan with any complication
Risk	No detectable increased risk of maternal mortality and no/mild increased risk in morbidity	Small increased risk of maternal mortality or moderate increase in morbidity	Intermediate increased risk of maternal mortality or moderate to severe increase in morbidity	Significantly increased risk of maternal mortality or severe morbidity	Extremely high-risk of maternal mortality or severe morbidity

CARPREG-II Risk model

Predictor	Points
Prior cardiac events or arrhythmias	3
Baseline NYHA III–IV or cyanosis	3
Mechanical valve	3
Ventricular dysfunction	2
High-risk left-sided valve disease	2
Pulmonary hypertension	2
Coronary artery disease	2
High-risk aortopathy	2
No prior cardiac intervention	1
Late pregnancy assessment	1

Maternal cardiac risk: 3 points ~15%, 4 points ~22%, >4 points ~41%

• **Fig. 58.2** Maternal risk stratification scores. *ASI,* aortic size index; *EF,* Ejection Fraction; *HTAD,* Hereditable Thoracic Aortic Disease; *NYHA,* New York Heart Association class (Modified from Regitz-Zagrosek V, Roos-Hesselink JW, Bauersachs J, et al. 2018 ESC Guidelines for the management of cardiovascular diseases during pregnancy. *Eur Heart J.* 2018;39:3165–3241; Silversides CK, Grewal J, Mason J, et al. Pregnancy outcomes in women with heart disease: the CARPREG II study. *J AmColl Cardiol.* 2018;71:2419–2430.)

hypoglycemia may occur. The most common beta-blockers use during pregnancy are labetalol and metoprolol; historical evidence would recommend avoidance of atenolol. Of note, pregnant individuals with SVT and unstable hemodynamics should undergo urgent direct current cardioversion, which is safe for both mother and fetus.

Calcium channel blockers may also be used as third-line therapy for atrial arrhythmias. Flecainide or propafenone are safe for pregnant patients with pre-excitation syndromes. Amiodarone should be use as a last resource when other therapies have failed, due to high risk of fetal thyroid and neurodevelopmental complications. Digoxin can be used for atrial flutter or atrial fibrillation; however, serum levels are unreliable throughout pregnancy, and dose adjustments may be needed. Another class of medications used occasionally in pregnant CHD patients is *diuretics* (such as furosemide). Rare side effects include placenta hypoperfusion and oligohydramnios. There have been rare reports of neonatal thrombocytopenia and jaundice with maternal use of diuretics. *Angiotensin-converting enzyme inhibitors, angiotensin receptor blockers, aldosterone antagonists, direct renin inhibitors*, and *angiotensin receptor-neprilysin inhibitors* are contraindicated due to their teratogenic potential. The most common side effects include oligohydramnios, renal dysgenesis, and IUGR.

Women needing anticoagulation during pregnancy are particularly challenging to manage. Pregnancy is a hypercoagulable state due to the enhanced production of hypercoagulable factors VII, VIII, X, von Willebrand Factor, and fibrinogen and decreased levels of protein S, resulting in increased risk of thrombotic events, which are highest in the early postpartum period.[17] Indications for anticoagulation during pregnancy include treatment of venous thromboembolism, inherited thrombophilia, antiphospholipid syndrome, and mechanical heart valves. *Vitamin K antagonists* (VKA, i.e., warfarin) are safest for the mother, yet doses greater than 5 mg daily must be avoided in the first trimester due to potential effects to the fetus, including facial dysmorphisms, central nervous system abnormalities, and cardiac defects. Current guidelines for the management of pregnant patients with mechanical valves recommend switching to low-molecular-weight heparin (LMWH) or unfractionated heparin during the first trimester if warfarin doses more than 5 mg are required to achieve therapeutic anticoagulation. The highest risk of thrombosis of mechanical valves are during this time of transition from one anticoagulant to another. Patients on LMWH should be followed by anti-Xa levels (peak and trough) with a goal of 0.8–1.2 during the pregnancy.[18]

Women who received VKA during pregnancy should be transitioned to LMWH or unfractionated heparin by the 36th week of gestation to avoid hemorrhagic complications. Low-dose aspirin is recommended for patients with mechanical and bioprosthetic valves. There is no evidence that the use of this increases the risk of maternal or fetal bleeding. There is insufficient safety data on clopidogrel, ticagrelor, prasugrel, eptifibatide, or the novel oral anticoagulants, thus their use during pregnancy is not recommended.[9]

Cardiovascular Care During Pregnancy

Optimal care of pregnant patients with CHD requires a multidisciplinary approach, with representation from maternal-fetal medicine, adult CHD, and obstetric anesthesia teams.[2] Pregnant patients with moderate or greater risk should be followed closely each trimester or more if necessary, and discussed at a multidisciplinary meeting that includes decisions on methods and timing of delivery, anesthesia, and any necessary cardiac monitoring.

Diagnostic Studies

The echocardiographic dimensions of all four cardiac chambers increase during pregnancy. There is also an increase in the LV wall thickness and mass. The systemic ventricular diastolic dimensions tend to increase 7–12% during pregnancy, although systolic dimensions remain about the same to pre-pregnancy dimensions. This type of remodeling may last up to 12 months postpartum. There is limited data on ventricular mechanics in pregnant persons with CHD; however, one small series in women with repaired tetralogy of Fallot (TOF) demonstrated a decrease in LV longitudinal strain during pregnancy.[11]

Cardiac Interventions

The number of women with CHD who require urgent cardiac interventions during pregnancy is low; however, in developing countries, cardiac interventions due to valvular disease are as high as 5%.[19] Invasive interventions are associated with increased maternal and fetal risk and should only be performed when noninvasive measures have failed. Cardiac catheterization should be performed with limited fluoroscopy time and radiation exposure, utilizing transesophageal echocardiography or 3D mapping when needed. In cases of symptomatic severe aortic stenosis, transcatheter aortic valve replacement (TAVR) may avoid the complications associated with cardiopulmonary bypass.[20]

Rarely, cardiac surgery may be necessary in pregnant individuals with heart disease, which poses an increased risk of fetal demise. Strategies to improve outcomes include higher pump flow rate, higher perfusion pressure, normothermia, and reduced cardiopulmonary bypass and aortic cross-clamp time. If the fetus is viable, it is often preferable to perform a caesarian delivery prior to maternal cardiac surgery.[19,21]

Cardiovascular Care During Delivery and Postpartum

The peripartum period is a critical time where the cardiac work is maximal and major changes in blood volume can occur. Many problems can be anticipated in the antenatal period, and by the third trimester every pregnant person with CHD should have a plan about mode of delivery, including second and third stages of labor management. During labor, CO is maximal during the second stage, and studies have suggested the benefits of pain control in cardiac patients during labor to mitigate further surges in CO. In some cases, an assisted second stage of delivery may be useful, particularly in patients with significant aortopathies or severe left-sided obstructive lesions.[4]

There is no maternal benefit of planned cesarean delivery over attempted vaginal delivery in women with CHD.[6] The incidence of subacute bacterial endocarditis (SBE) is extremely rare, and the same criteria for non-pregnant CHD patients applies for pregnancy. In the current era, there are no recommendations for the use of antibiotics for SBE prophylaxis before vaginal or cesarean delivery.[8] Major cardiovascular changes occur in the immediate postpartum period, including autotransfusion from the placenta further increasing CO and increased vascular resistance, both in the systemic and pulmonary circulations. Women with high-risk features for thromboembolic events should be continued on anticoagulation for at least 6 weeks postpartum. Patients with CHD should have a clinical visit between 6 and 12 weeks, at which time counseling about future pregnancies should be discussed.

Specific Congenital Heart Conditions

Shunt Lesions

Despite the drop in SVR, and the increase in pulmonary blood flow, patients with unrepaired atrial septal defect (ASD) usually tolerate the hemodynamics impact of pregnancy well.[22] Closure of an isolated ASD during pregnancy is rarely necessary. Studies have demonstrated that the most common complications of patients with ASD during pregnancy are atrial arrhythmias and thromboembolic complications, the latter in unrepaired patients.[23] Patients who underwent ASD repair in childhood have similar outcomes to the general population. Patients with ventricular septal defect (VSD) are usually diagnosed and repaired during childhood. For those who are not repaired, in the absence of PH, the main concern is volume overload. Pregnant patients with small or repaired VSD generally do well if they have preserved ventricular function. The major maternal and fetal complications found in several studies is preeclampsia and small for gestational age (SGA).[24] Patients with unrepaired atrioventricular septal defect (AVSD) without pulmonary stenosis usually have PH and are at a very high risk for maternal mortality. Retrospective studies on patients with repaired AVSD have shown NYHA class deterioration and worsening of preexisting atrioventricular valvular regurgitation.[25] AVSD has a higher risk of transmission up to 8%, for which genetic counseling and testing should be recommended. Patent ductus arteriosus (PDA) is rarely encountered in adults without PH or Eisenmenger

syndrome (ES). Patients with small PDAs without PH usually do well. In the postpartum period, patients can be referred for closure if indications are met.[26]

Right-Sided Heart Lesions

Tetralogy of Fallot

TOF is one of the most common maternal repaired congenital cardiac conditions. In general, pregnancy is low risk for those who do not have any significant residual lesions and good biventricular function. Pulmonary regurgitation is the most common consequence of repaired TOF and is generally tolerated well as long as right ventricular (RV) function is preserved.[27] The combination of pulmonary regurgitation and increased stroke volume in the setting of pregnancy may cause worsening RV function and predispose patients to arrhythmias and volume overload.[11,28] In small studies, pregnancy outcomes did not differ in patients with repaired TOF who have undergone a pulmonary valve replacement (PVR), although persistent RV dilation was seen more commonly in those without PVR.[29]

In cases of residual pulmonary stenosis or right ventricular outflow tract obstruction, valvar gradients may increase during pregnancy, which may result in symptoms of heart failure, worsening RV function, and arrhythmia. Intractable symptomatic cases are considered for balloon valvuloplasty.[4] Patients with RV or LV dysfunction may be at risk for pulmonary edema and require close follow-up in the postpartum period.

Ebstein Anomaly

Patients with Ebstein anomaly with good RV dysfunction and without evidence of cyanosis tend to do well during pregnancy. Those with RV dysfunction are at higher risk of arrhythmias or heart failure symptoms.[30,31] Some expected changes that occur are worsening tricuspid regurgitation in the setting of increased volume and RV dilation. In the presence of an interatrial shunt, there can be worsening cyanosis as the SVR decreases and the CO rises. It is important to discuss anesthetic considerations, as certain agents cause a rapid decrease in preload. Oxytocin use in the postpartum setting can increase the pulmonary artery pressures and right-to-left shunt resulting in worsening cyanosis and RV function.

Left-Sided Heart Lesions

Coarctation of the Aorta

Hormonal alterations and systemic hypertension can affect the aortic wall during pregnancy and predispose patients with coarctation of the aorta (CoA) to risks such as aortic dissection or rupture. During pregnancy, it is important to follow BP carefully, as a crucial balance between BP control and placental perfusion must be achieved during the pregnancy. In unrepaired CoA or restenosis of a prior CoA site, patients with hypertension can be treated conservatively with medications; however, in cases of placenta hypoperfusion, surgical or catheter intervention should be considered.[8] There is also a higher rate of preeclampsia and miscarriage in this population.[32] Patients with aortic dilation greater than 4.5 cm or those with rapid growth should be advised against pregnancy and considered for repair prior to pregnancy.[2]

Left-Sided Valvular Stenosis

Severe left-sided valve stenosis or LV outflow tract obstruction are considered some of the highest maternal cardiac risk factors for adverse outcomes. Patients with stenotic valvular lesions may have limited ability to increase the CO during pregnancy. Patients who are asymptomatic prior to pregnancy may become symptomatic during pregnancy as SVR drops and they cannot meet the demands of increasing CO and become at risk for myocardial ischemia. Patients with severe, symptomatic aortic stenosis require hospitalization more frequently during pregnancy and have greater chance of SGA infants.[33] Subvalvular and supravalvular stenosis associated with other medical conditions such as William syndrome and hypertrophic cardiomyopathy are fixed lesions that behave in a similar fashion to aortic valvular stenosis. In the cases of mitral stenosis, mild stenosis is usually tolerated during pregnancy. Higher degrees of stenosis are associated with worsening NYHA class as pregnancy progresses due to decreased diastolic filling time, increased pulmonary artery pressures, and maternal complications such as arrhythmias or thromboembolic events.

It is common to see an increased transvalvular gradients on echocardiogram during pregnancy, although the valve area should remain constant. Symptomatic patients should be monitored closely and receive medications such as diuretics and beta-blockers to increase the diastolic filling time. If symptoms do not improve with medications, invasive procedures such as balloon valvuloplasty or TAVR should be considered.[20] In terms of mode of delivery, asymptomatic patients with aortic or mitral stenosis often will tolerate vaginal delivery which is associated with lower degrees of fluid shifts, blood loss, thrombogenic risk, and infections than cesarean birth. In the postpartum period, it is important to monitor signs and symptoms of heart failure as hemodynamic changes will take several weeks to normalize.[1]

Left-Sided Regurgitant Lesions

Mitral regurgitation is commonly encountered during pregnancy due to mitral valve prolapse. Chronic mitral regurgitation with normal ventricular systolic function is well tolerated during pregnancy. The decrease in SVR and systolic BP is favorable in patients with regurgitant valve lesions.[19,27] Similarly, aortic regurgitation is often well tolerated during pregnancy due to the decrease in afterload. If there is LV dysfunction, patients may present with symptoms of heart failure and pulmonary congestion and benefit from diuretics during pregnancy and in the postpartum period.

Mechanical Heart Valves

Thrombotic events are more common during pregnancy due to the physiologic prothrombotic changes associated with pregnancy. Patients with mechanical heart valves pose particular challenging management decisions during pregnancy. Mechanical valve thrombosis has been reported in up to 4.7% of maternal deaths. The most appropriate management strategy during pregnancy in a patient with mechanical valve must be individualized based on patient-specific factors and local expertise. In cases of acute valve thrombosis with large thrombus burden, thrombolysis is less likely to have favorable outcomes with higher risks of embolization in the systemic circulation. Although streptokinase and tissue plasminogen activator do not cross the placenta and are the most commonly used in practice, they are associated with higher risk of maternal bleeding.[17]

Complex Lesions

Transposition of the Great Arteries s/p Atrial Switch

Patients with transposition of the great arteries (D-loop TGA) who have undergone atrial switch procedures (Mustard, Senning) are usually categorized as moderate or high risk for pregnancy (WHO III or WHO IV). Those who have undergone an arterial switch procedure without complications are usually categorized as WHO II.[34] The most common cardiac complications reported in different meta-analyses of pregnant persons with D-loop TGA and atrial switch are arrhythmias, heart failure, and thromboembolic events.[35,36] These patients should have evaluations during each trimester including echocardiographic assessment of ventricular function and measurement of serial NT-pro BNP. Continuous electrocardiographic monitoring during delivery and in the postpartum period is recommended for patients with history of prior arrhythmias or arrhythmias during pregnancy. Patients with systemic right ventricle with moderate to severe ventricular dysfunction and severe tricuspid regurgitation should be counseled against pregnancy. Additionally, patients with systemic right ventricle should be counseled that RV function could get worse during pregnancy with the possibility of non-complete recovery following delivery.[4]

Single Ventricular Circulation

Despite the anatomic complexity of a mother with Fontan circulation, pregnant persons with a well-functioning Fontan may have successful pregnancies. Preconception counseling is very important, as these patients are at higher risk for cardiac, obstetric, and neonatal complications. Patients with Fontan circulation should be cared for in tertiary centers by a multidisciplinary cardio-obstetric team. Fontan patients are at a high risk for arrhythmias, especially if they have history of arrhythmias and/or heart failure symptoms and in those with systemic right ventricles.[37] Serial echocardiograms, oxygen supplementation in the setting of worsening cyanosis, and diuretics may be considered during pregnancy. For labor, vaginal delivery is preferable, as it is associated with less bleeding and thromboembolic complications, less risk of infection, and faster recovery. Obstetric complications are common in this population, such as first-trimester miscarriages, prematurity, SGA infants, and postpartum hemorrhage.[4]

Cyanotic Lesions Without Eisenmenger Syndrome

The prevalence of patients with cyanotic CHD has decreased with improved fetal diagnosis and surgical approaches. Women with cyanotic CHD are more likely to have delayed onset of menstruation, abnormal menstrual patterns, and higher risk of infertility.[35,38] Rarely, pregnant CHD patients may present with cyanosis due to systemic-to-pulmonary venous collaterals in those with Fontan circulation, or due to increased right-to-left shunting across and atrial level defect in others. Due to the vascular wall stiffness in pregnant patients with cyanosis and any elevation in pulmonary resistance, heart failure is more common due to the inability to accommodate the increase in CO during pregnancy. This is particularly important in labor where the CO can increase up to 80% from baseline.

Patients with cyanotic heart disease during pregnancy are at higher risk of arrhythmias, heart failure symptoms, and thromboembolic complications from right-to-left shunting. They are also a higher risk of fetal and obstetric complications such as spontaneous abortion, IUGR, and preterm delivery.[38,39] Most of the obstetric complications are secondary to poor oxygen delivery to the placenta and limited utero placenta perfusion. There is a higher risk of CHD defects in fetuses from cyanotic mothers.[40] Pregnant patients with resting oxygen saturations less than 90% should be encouraged to wear supplemental oxygen throughout pregnancy.

Eisenmenger Syndrome

Women with unrepaired large shunts are at high risk of having irreversible PH or ES by childbearing age. Please refer to Chapter 56 for more details of PH and ES. In patients with PH and ES, the risk of spontaneous abortion is as high as 85%.[1,8] This group of patients have an extremely high risk of maternal mortality, which is highest in the postpartum period, as the RV cannot meet the demands of increased CO against a fixed pulmonary vascular resistance, and these patients should be counseled strongly against pregnancy. If they decide to continue with pregnancy, targeted medical therapy should continue, except for endothelin receptor antagonists such as bosentan which are teratogenic.

Summary

The number of patients with CHD desiring pregnancy continues to increase. Discussion of potential risks should begin in the preconception period with careful planning and anticipation of the possible complications that may arise during the antepartum, intrapartum, and the postpartum periods. Pregnant persons with CHD should be cared for by a multidisciplinary team that understands the unique hemodynamic changes that occur and how these changes affect women and their offspring both during pregnancy and beyond.

References

1. Roos-Hesselink JW, Johnson MR. *Pregnancy and Congenital Heart Disease. Congenital Heart Disease in Adolescents and Adults.* Switzerland: Springer International Publishing; 2017.
2. Stout KK, Daniels CJ, Aboulhosn JA, et al. 2018 AHA/ACC guideline for the management of adults with congenital heart disease: a report of the American College of Cardiology/American Heart Association Task Force on Clinical Practice Guidelines. *J Am Coll Cardiol.* 2019;73:e81-e192.
3. Silversides CK, Grewal J, Mason J, et al. Pregnancy outcomes in women with heart disease: the CARPREG II study. *J Am Coll Cardiol.* 2018;71:2419-2430.
4. Canobbio MM, Warnes CA, Aboulhosn J, et al. Management of pregnancy in patients with complex congenital heart disease: a scientific statement for healthcare professionals from the American Heart Association. *Circulation.* 2017;135:e50-e87.
5. Davis MB, Walsh MN. Cardio-obstetrics. *Circ Cardiovasc Qual Outcomes.* 2019;12:e005417.
6. Easter SR, Rouse CE, Duarte V, et al. Planned vaginal delivery and cardiovascular morbidity in pregnant women with heart disease. *Am J Obstet Gynecol.* 2020;222:77.e1-77.e11.
7. Rouse CE, Easter SR, Duarte VE, et al. Timing of delivery in women with cardiac disease. *Am J Perinatol.* 2022;39:1196-1203.
8. Regitz-Zagrosek V, Roos-Hesselink JW, Bauersachs J, et al. 2018 ESC Guidelines for the management of cardiovascular diseases during pregnancy. *Eur Heart J.* 2018;39:3165-3241.
9. Halpern DG, Weinberg CR, Pinnelas R, et al. Use of medication for cardiovascular disease during pregnancy: JACC state-of-the-art review. *J Am Coll Cardiol.* 2019;73:457-476.
10. Stout KK. Chapter 32, Role of Echocardiography in the Diagnosis and Management of Heart Disease in Pregnancy. In: Otto CM, ed. *The Practice of Clinical Echocardiography.* 3rd ed. Philadelphia: WB Saunders; 2007:755-790.
11. Duarte VE, Graf JA, Gauvreau K, et al. Impact of pregnancy on ventricular strain in women with repaired tetralogy of Fallot. *Pediatr Cardiol.* 2020;41:1795-1799.
12. Valente AM, Landzberg MJ, Gauvreau K, et al. Standardized outcomes in reproductive cardiovascular care: The STORCC initiative. *Am Heart J.* 2019;217:112-120.
13. van Hagen IM, Roos-Hesselink JW. Pregnancy in congenital heart disease: risk prediction and counselling. *Heart.* 2020;106:1853-1861.
14. Dockree S, Brook J, Shine B, et al. Pregnancy-specific reference intervals for BNP and NT-pro BNP-changes in natriuretic peptides related to pregnancy. *J Endocr Soc.* 2021;5:bvab091.
15. Sheikh M, Ostadrahimi P, Salarzaei M, et al. Cardiac complications in pregnancy: a systematic review and meta-analysis of

diagnostic accuracy of BNP and N-terminal pro-BNP. *Cardiol Ther.* 2021;10:501-514.

16. Lui GK, Silversides CK, Khairy P, et al. Heart rate response during exercise and pregnancy outcome in women with congenital heart disease. *Circulation.* 2011;123:242-248.

17. Rutz T, Eggel-Hort B, Alberio L, et al. Anticoagulation of women with congenital heart disease during pregnancy. *Int J Cardiol Congenit Heart Dis.* 2021;5:100210.

18. Otto CM, Nishimura RA, Bonow RO, et al. 2020 ACC/AHA guideline for the management of patients with valvular heart disease: a report of the American College of Cardiology/American Heart Association Joint Committee on Clinical Practice Guidelines. *Circulation.* 2021;143:e72-e227.

19. Cauldwell M, Johnson M, Jahangiri M, et al. Cardiac interventions and cardiac surgery and pregnancy. *Int J Cardiol.* 2019;276:43-47.

20. Berry N, Sawlani N, Economy K, et al. Transcatheter aortic valve replacement for bioprosthetic aortic stenosis in pregnancy. *JACC Cardiovasc Interv.* 2018;11:e161-e162.

21. Jha N, Jha AK, Chauhan RC, et al. Maternal and fetal outcome after cardiac operations during pregnancy: a meta-analysis. *Ann Thorac Surg.* 2018;106:618-626.

22. Zuber M, Gautschi N, Oechslin E, et al. Outcome of pregnancy in women with congenital shunt lesions. *Heart.* 1999;81:271-275.

23. Bredy C, Mongeon FP, Leduc L, et al. Pregnancy in adults with repaired/unrepaired atrial septal defect. *J Thorac Dis.* 2018;10: S2945-S2952.

24. Yap SC, Drenthen W, Pieper PG, et al. Pregnancy outcome in women with repaired versus unrepaired isolated ventricular septal defect. *BJOG.* 2010;117:683-689.

25. Drenthen W, Pieper PG, van der Tuuk K, et al. Cardiac complications relating to pregnancy and recurrence of disease in the offspring of women with atrioventricular septal defects. *Eur Heart J.* 2005;26:2581-2587.

26. Zhang Z, Wengrofsky A, Wolfe DS, et al. Patent ductus arteriosus in pregnancy: cardio-obstetrics management in a late presentation. *CASE (Phila).* 2021;5:119-122.

27. Khairy P, Ouyang DW, Fernandes SM, et al. Pregnancy outcomes in women with congenital heart disease. *Circulation.* 2006;113: 517-524.

28. Assenza GE, Cassater D, Landzberg M, et al. The effects of pregnancy on right ventricular remodeling in women with repaired tetralogy of Fallot. *Int J Cardiol.* 2012;168:1847-1852.

29. Yamamura K, Duarte V, Karur GR, et al. The impact of pulmonary valve replacement on pregnancy outcomes in women with tetralogy of Fallot. *Int J Cardiol.* 2021;330:43-49.

30. Connolly HM, Warnes CA. Ebstein's anomaly: outcome of pregnancy. *J Am Coll Cardiol.* 1994;23:1194-1198.

31. Lima FV, Koutrolou-Sotiropoulou P, Yen TY, et al. Clinical characteristics and outcomes in pregnant women with Ebstein anomaly at the time of delivery in the USA: 2003–2012. *Arch Cardiovasc Dis.* 2016;109:390-398.

32. Vriend JW, Drenthen W, Pieper PG, et al. Outcome of pregnancy in patients after repair of aortic coarctation. *Eur Heart J.* 2005;26:2173-2178.

33. Orwat S, Diller GP, van Hagen IM, et al. Risk of pregnancy in moderate and severe aortic stenosis: from the multinational ROPAC registry. *J Am Coll Cardiol.* 2016;68:1727-1737.

34. Tutarel O, Baris L, Budts W, et al. Pregnancy outcomes in women with a systemic right ventricle and transposition of the great arteries results from the ESC-EORP Registry of Pregnancy and Cardiac disease (ROPAC). *Heart.* 2022;108:117-123.

35. Canobbio MM, Morris CD, Graham TP, et al. Pregnancy outcomes after atrial repair for transposition of the great arteries. *Am J Cardiol.* 2006;98:668-672.

36. Cataldo S, Doohan M, Rice K, et al. Pregnancy following Mustard or Senning correction of transposition of the great arteries: a retrospective study. *BJOG.* 2016;123:807-813.

37. Garcia Ropero A, Baskar S, Roos Hesselink JW, et al. Pregnancy in women with a Fontan circulation: a systematic review of the literature. *Circ Cardiovasc Qual Outcomes.* 2018;11:e004575.

38. Ladouceur M, Nizard J. Challenges and management of pregnancy in cyanotic congenital heart disease. *Int J Cardiol Congenit Heart Dis.* 2021;5:100231.

39. Ladouceur M, Benoit L, Basquin A, et al. How pregnancy impacts adult cyanotic congenital heart disease: a multicenter observational study. *Circulation.* 2017;135:2444-2447.

40. Patton DE, Lee W, Cotton DB, et al. Cyanotic maternal heart disease in pregnancy. *Obstet Gynecol Surv.* 1990;45:594-600.

59

The Fontan Circulation

FRED M. WU, JOHN E. MAYER JR., AND RAHUL H. RATHOD

KEY LEARNING POINTS

- The Fontan procedure has undergone numerous modifications and improvements since its introduction in 1971.
- The primary physiologic consequences of the Fontan circulation is obligatory systemic venous hypertension and reduced ability to increase cardiac output.
- While current survival outcomes are improving, there remain considerable and increasing cardiac comorbidities as these patients age in postoperative follow-up.

- A multidisciplinary approach to Fontan care can help manage the noncardiac complications and create localized center expertise.
- Multi-institutional collaboration (randomized controlled trials, registries) may be an important way to accelerate our learning and impact the care of Fontan patients.

Introduction

The final stage of surgical palliation in patients with functional single ventricle heart disease is a total cavopulmonary connection where all systemic venous return flows directly to the pulmonary arteries (PAs) without a subpulmonary ventricle. This inherently unnatural "Fontan" circulation has undergone numerous surgical and medical modifications and advancements in care. While survival is highly dependent on the type of Fontan and era of care,[1] survival is improving with modern care models showing 10-, 20-, and 30-year survival approaching 80–90%.[2] This finding is reinforced by the fact that the number of surviving patients continues to increase each year with current worldwide estimates at 50,000 to 70,000 living patients added per year.[3] These improved outcomes have appropriately recentered the focus on active postoperative management to minimize the incidence of morbidities that increases as these patients age. This chapter will review the history that brought us to this current state, describe the nuances of the Fontan physiology, and detail some of the more common complications secondary to the Fontan circulation.

History of the Fontan and Its Modifications

The original publication (in English) by Francis Fontan of the procedure to bypass the right heart and direct systemic venous return directly into the PAs was in 1971.[4] A description of a very similar approach was provided by Kreutzer at

the Argentinian Society of Cardiology in the same year, and the procedure has thereafter often been referred to as the Fontan-Kreutzer or Fontan procedure. The original procedure involved a direct connection between the right atrium and the PAs, a superior vena cava (SVC) to right PA anastomosis (classical Glenn procedure), and closure of the atrial septal defect (ASD). Fontan believed that contraction of the hypertrophied right atrium in tricuspid atresia patients would help overcome pulmonary resistance, and also thought that it was indispensable to provide the right atrium with homograft valves in the atriopulmonary (AP) connection and at the inferior vena cava–right atrial junction to maintain forward flow.[4] Kreutzer reported closure of the ASD and use of either a homograft or the disconnected native pulmonary valve in the right atrial to PA connection and did not employ the additional SVC-to-PA anastomosis.[5] Another variation of the Fontan principle of right heart bypass for tricuspid atresia was the Bjork modification in which the right atrium was directly connected to the infundibular chamber below a normal-sized pulmonary valve with closure of the interventricular communication and the ASD.[6] By 1984, follow-up hemodynamic evaluations showed that the valves in these AP connections remained continuously open throughout the cardiac cycle and thus did not contribute to forward pulmonary blood flow (PBF).[7] The Fontan-Kreutzer concept of right heart bypass was extended further to other forms of functional single ventricle,[8] and the techniques for right heart bypass evolved to include the lateral tunnel technique, the use of a fenestration between systemic and pulmonary venous return, and the extracardiac tube graft.[9] The lateral tunnel and extracardiac tube modifications were developed as techniques to avoid intracardiac obstructions to pulmonary venous blood reaching the systemic atrioventricular valve(s) and the single ventricle, particularly for those with left heart hypoplasia.

Patients who are born with a single functional ventricle (including those with tricuspid atresia) have a dismal prognosis without surgical intervention, and the immediate outcomes of the Fontan operation, which is currently the "definitive" procedure for these patients, are now quite good.[10] Although the focus of this chapter is on the Fontan operation, the critical importance of beginning management from the time of birth should be recognized, as early management sets the stage for subsequent Fontan candidacy. Critical considerations involve creating conditions that lead to low pulmonary vascular resistance (PVR), avoidance of PA distortions, avoidance or relief of lesions resulting in pulmonary venous obstruction, and preservation of both systolic and diastolic ventricular function and atrioventricular valve function. In the current era, most single ventricle patients undergo staged management that begins with neonatal procedures directed at relieving systemic ventricular outflow and/or aortic obstruction (to minimize the development of concentric ventricular hypertrophy and depressed systolic and/or diastolic function), providing a controlled source of PBF to achieve adequate oxygenation but low PVR, and ensuring unobstructed pulmonary venous return. The second stage of management typically involves the creation of a bidirectional SVC-to-PA anastomosis, which serves to reduce the volume load on the functional single ventricle. The final stage is the "Fontan" procedure in which the remainder of the systemic venous return from the inferior vena cava is directed into the pulmonary circulation.

The effect of the Fontan procedure is to separate the systemic venous return from the pulmonary venous return and to direct the systemic venous return directly into the PAs. By doing so the patient's oxygen saturation is raised to near normal levels. A variety of techniques are employed to accomplish this goal of separation of the systemic and pulmonary venous return, including the lateral tunnel technique and the extracardiac Fontan procedure (Fig. 59.1). The clearest advantage of the lateral tunnel technique is that it minimizes the likelihood of obstruction of the pulmonary venous return when the pulmonary venous return must reach the right atrioventricular valve (as in cases with mitral atresia or hypoplastic left heart syndrome). This problem of the systemic venous pathway causing pulmonary venous obstruction was a common cause of mortality in our early experience with Fontan operations for hypoplastic left heart syndrome.[8] A second advantage of the lateral tunnel technique is that it avoids the marked right atrial enlargement, which frequently occurs when the entire right atrium is exposed to elevated venous pressure. This "giant" right atrium can lead to turbulence and consequent energy losses in the systemic venous return reaching the right atrium, although the magnitude of these energy losses is difficult to evaluate.

The distended right atrium can also cause compression of the right pulmonary veins that lie immediately behind the right atrium and can also serve as a predisposing factor for atrial arrhythmias. Any of these consequences of a giant right atrium will be disadvantageous for the patient with a Fontan circulation.

The institutional practice at Boston Children's Hospital is to use a "fenestration" in the lateral tunnel baffle in virtually all patients since there is reasonably good evidence to suggest that both mortality and morbidity are reduced.[11] A 4-mm coronary punch is typically used to create the fenestration. Many patients will spontaneously close their fenestrations with time, and those that do not close can be closed in the catheterization laboratory with ASD devices. Cavopulmonary anastomoses are preferable to AP connections because there is less likelihood of kinking or obstruction at these anastomoses.

Less common anatomic situations may require different approaches to achieve the goals of an unobstructed systemic venous pathway from the superior and inferior vena cavae to the PAs and an unobstructed pathway for pulmonary venous blood to reach the atrioventricular valves and systemic ventricle. In patients with a left SVC, the operation is modified by adding a left SVC to left PA anastomosis using the same technique as for a right SVC. In patients with the heterotaxy syndromes, there are frequent anomalies of systemic and pulmonary venous connections, and these may require the use of extracardiac polytetrafluoroethylene (PTFE) tube grafts to avoid complex intracardiac baffling, which increases the risk of creating pulmonary venous obstruction. The use of an extracardiac tube graft to convey inferior vena cava blood to the PAs has been more commonly employed for all Fontan patients in recent years due to its technical simplicity and ability to perform this procedure without aortic cross-clamping. Creation of a fenestration is possible but may be associated with higher early closure rates. All communications between the single ventricle and the pulmonary arterial circulation must be closed, and if there is a semilunar valve in this pathway to be closed, the leaflets should be resected to remove potential sources of stasis, which can result in thrombus formation and embolization. It is essential to achieve unobstructed pathways from the systemic veins to the PAs and to avoid any pulmonary venous obstruction, as this is very poorly tolerated when the only driving force for PBF is the systemic venous pressure.

Physiology of the Fontan Circulation

The Fontan operation can improve oxygenation in the systemic arterial system, but the resulting physiology is clearly abnormal due to the absence of a ventricle to provide forward flow into the pulmonary circulation. PBF therefore depends on the systemic venous pressure to overcome both the PVR and filling of the single ventricle. In terms of hydrodynamics, essentially all of the energy imparted to the circulating blood is provided by the contraction of the single ventricle, although there are additional contributions from the skeletal muscles, which compress the systemic

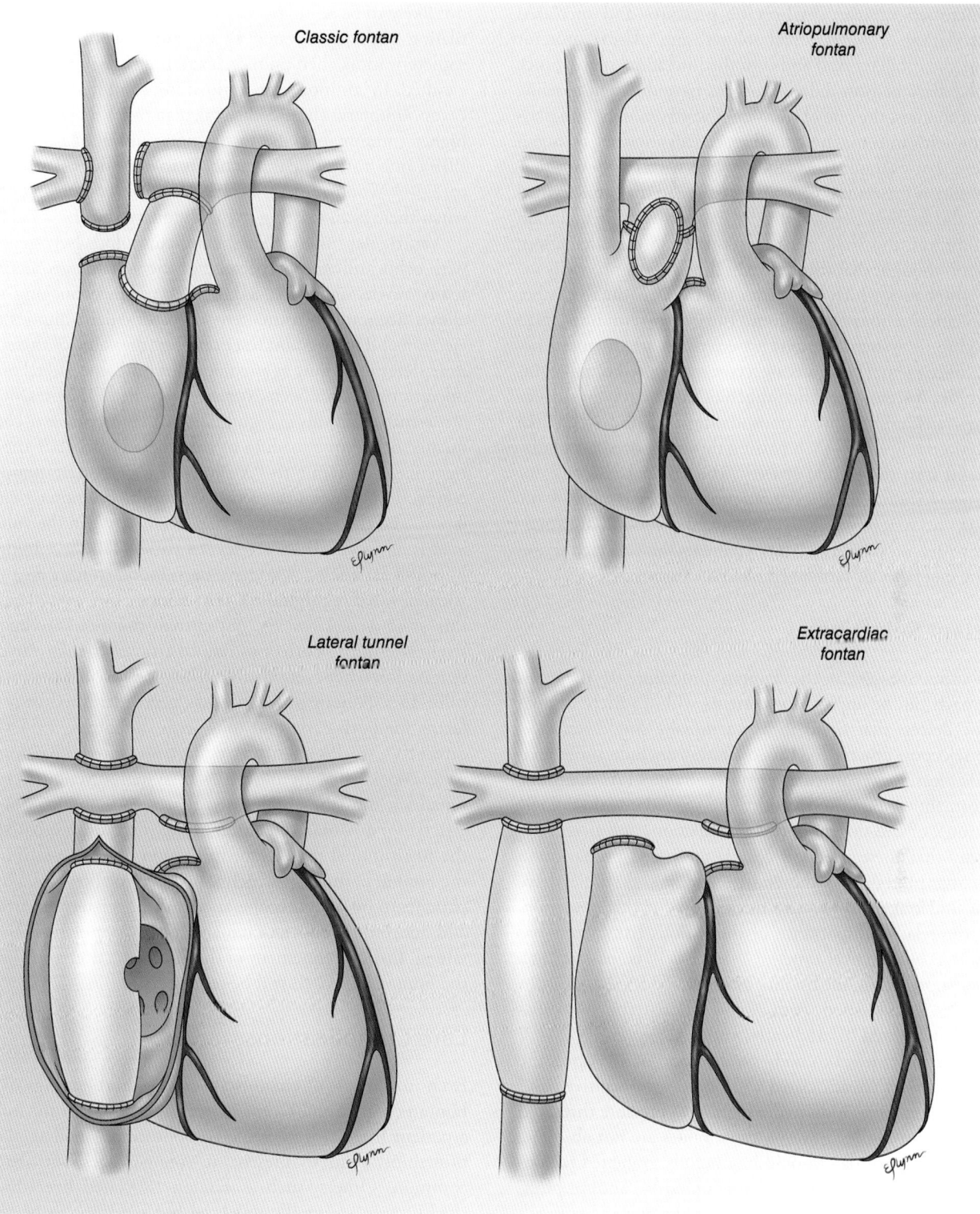

Classic fontan

Atriopulmonary fontan

Lateral tunnel fontan

Extracardiac fontan

• **Fig. 59.1** Most common types of Fontan modifications. Most modern surgical approaches involve the use of the lateral tunnel and extracardiac Fontan techniques.

veins, and from the respiratory muscles which create negative intrathoracic pressure during spontaneous inspiration and thus contribute to systemic venous return. Thus, from an energetics perspective, the blood leaving the single ventricle must have enough total energy (kinetic + potential/

pressure) to overcome both systemic and PVRs and then fill the same single ventricle during diastole.

The primary adverse physiologic effect of having a Fontan circulation is obligatory systemic venous hypertension. At the microvascular level, the elevated venous pressure results in increased capillary hydrostatic pressures and increased transudation of water, small solutes, and plasma proteins across the capillary wall and into the interstitial space. Since the capillary beds in different organs have different baseline permeabilities, the rate of transfer of water, solutes, and plasma proteins into the interstitial space will also vary by organ system. For example, the capillary bed with the lowest permeability is the central nervous system, and the capillary bed with the highest permeability is in the liver. To maintain equilibrium, this fluid must be returned to the circulation, and it is thought that this return of fluid occurs primarily via the lymphatics which drain into the thoracic duct or other lymphatico-venous connections. The longer-term impacts of this chronic systemic venous hypertension are discussed below. Since pleural effusions are a common post-Fontan complication, it seems likely that much of this pleural fluid arises from transcapillary fluid transudating into the interstitial space in the liver and then passing through pores in the diaphragm into the pleural space.[12] The original rationale for adding a fenestration to a Fontan procedure is to mitigate the rise in the systemic venous pressure, and the initial experience with fenestration in Fontan patients showed a reduction in the incidence of prolonged pleural effusions.[11]

Patient Selection

The attractiveness of the Fontan procedure is that this approach can be applied for patients with a variety of anatomic defects that result in a functionally single ventricle. The selection criteria for this operation include some anatomic features, particularly unrepairable PA anatomic abnormalities, but the majority are related to physiologic measures of the single ventricle circulation, and it is noteworthy that these selection criteria are based primarily on operative mortality as the end point. Several studies have been undertaken to identify risk factors for this operation, and the relative importance of the various risk factors has been in evolution over time.[8,13,14] Since PBF is "passive" in a Fontan circulation, the finding that elevated PVR and/or PA pressure is associated with worse short-term outcomes is not unexpected,[8,13] and early studies suggest a PVR > 2 Wood units (indexed to body surface area) or a PA pressure >15 mm Hg were associated with increased operative risk.[8] Subsequent studies indicated a higher PA pressure threshold of < 19 mm Hg.[13] However, these values are not absolute, and each piece of data should be carefully evaluated for potential measurement errors, calculation errors, and for physiologic conditions that might temporarily alter the patient's physiology and thereby convey an erroneous impression of the patient's ability to tolerate a Fontan operation. For example, the calculation of PVR requires knowledge of both PA mean pressure and calculation of PBF. Calculation of PBF by the Fick method depends on measurement of oxygen uptake and on accurate measurement of PA and pulmonary venous oxygen content. If there is more than one source of PBF, and if the two sources do not have the same oxygen content, then calculation of PBF and resistance is

not likely to be accurate. Similarly, if the patient is hypoventilating with an elevated PCO_2 and low pH during the catheterization, then pulmonary resistance will be artificially elevated. In addition, due to the impression that after a prior cavopulmonary shunt, the calculated PVR tends to be higher (presumably due to the non-pulsatile nature of the PBF), our institutional practice is to consider a PVR of up to 2.5–3 Wood units as acceptable for a Fontan operation when there is an existing cavopulmonary shunt.

Ventricular function can be difficult to precisely quantify with echocardiography because of the variable geometry of many single ventricles. Magnetic resonance imaging now allows accurate measurement of ventricular volumes and ejection and regurgitant fractions, but the value of these volume determinations as predictors of outcome after Fontan operations has not been extensively studied. The presence of atrioventricular valvar regurgitation may occur as a consequence of volume loading of the single ventricle if the patient has a systemic-to-PA shunt or a persistent anatomic connection between the ventricle and the pulmonary circulation, and the regurgitation may improve when the volume load is removed. There are several patients in the Children's Hospital experience who have been found to have atrioventricular valve regurgitation post-Fontan but are tolerating this quite well. However, our current practice is to aggressively attempt to correct or reduce atrioventricular valve regurgitation whenever possible. The presence of a pacemaker prior to a Fontan procedure has been identified as a risk factor for both early and long-term outcomes.[13,14] Use of direct SVC-to-PA anastomoses have mitigated the risks that were associated with anomalies of systemic venous return. Finally, it must be emphasized that the "loosening" of the criteria for a Fontan operation in this institution is based on the institutional practice of utilization of a fenestration in the Fontan pathway,[11] which is believed to allow less "ideal" patients to tolerate this operation. As longer-term mortality and morbidity information about this population is obtained, further refinement of the selection criteria for use of the Fontan approach will be required.

Late Complications

Even in the best of circumstances, the shortcomings of the Fontan circulation become increasingly apparent the longer a patient lives with it. Some complications, such as plastic bronchitis, tend to present at younger ages but are less common. Others, such as Fontan-associated liver disease (FALD), are essentially universal but tend not to be clinically apparent until patients reach adulthood.

Plastic Bronchitis

Plastic bronchitis is a rare but dreaded complication of the Fontan circulation with an estimated prevalence of 4–14% of Fontan patients and a reported mortality of about 33%. The disease is characterized by production of rubbery, fibrin casts of the bronchial tree that cause airway obstruction and, if unable to be expectorated, potentially death from asphyxia. Plastic bronchitis typically occurs within 4–5 years of Fontan, but it can present initially as late as 15 years post-Fontan.

An improved understanding of the lymphatic abnormalities associated with Fontan circulation has shed new light on the likely pathophysiologic mechanisms leading to plastic bronchitis in this population. Dori et al.[15] described a high prevalence of abnormal lymphatic drainage into the peribronchial lymphatic vessels in patients presenting with plastic bronchitis, believed to be driven by increased central venous pressures that create an impedance to normal lymphatic drainage via the thoracic duct. At the same time, limitations in cardiac output result in mucosal injury, permitting leakage of lymph proteins into the airways where they solidify into airway casts. Because cast formation is commonly described in the context of respiratory infections, airway inflammation and resultant increased capillary permeability likely play a role as well.

The immediate priority of treatment is to relieve airway obstruction; next, to reduce cast formation. Reported strategies include inhaled tissue plasminogen activator, inhaled corticosteroids, bronchodilators, mucolytics, and aggressive pulmonary toilet. In cases of acute respiratory compromise, bronchoscopy for manual extraction of casts may be needed.

Careful evaluation for conditions exacerbating venous hypertension or limiting cardiac output may identify targets for catheter-based or surgical interventions. In the absence of specific targets, creation of a Fontan fenestration may allow for improved cardiac output and decreased venous congestion. Alternatively, pulmonary vasodilators such as phosphodiesterase type 5 (PDE5) inhibitors and endothelin antagonists have been reported to reverse plastic bronchitis. More recently, selective embolization of lymphatic branches feeding into the lung parenchyma has shown great promise.[16] Diversion of the innominate vein (into which the thoracic duct drains) to the atria has been described as well.

Protein-Losing Enteropathy

Similar to plastic bronchitis, protein-losing enteropathy (PLE) is an uncommon complication of Fontan circulation affecting 5–12% of Fontan patients with a mortality of 12% within 5 years. PLE could be described as a gastrointestinal analogue to plastic bronchitis, characterized by excessive gastrointestinal loss of proteins into the intestinal lumen from the intestinal lymphatics. Unlike plastic bronchitis, PLE tends to occur later after Fontan surgery, as much as 25+ years afterward. Its clinical manifestations are generally due to hypoproteinemia, with younger patients presenting with malnutrition and failure to thrive and older patients presenting with edema, pleural effusions, and diarrhea. Death related to PLE is typically due to heart failure, thromboembolism, arrhythmia, or sepsis.[17]

The increased protein losses that are characteristic of PLE are believed to be a result of increased venous pressures and decreased perfusion compromising the integrity of the gut epithelium. Inflammation may also be a factor, as budesonide has been shown to improve serum albumin levels, but similar to plastic bronchitis, newer imaging techniques have revealed abnormal lymphatic vessels to be a key factor causing drainage of protein-rich lymph into the intestinal lumen.

Proposed treatment algorithms for PLE include low-fat/high-protein diet, medium-chain triglycerides, subcutaneous heparin, octreotide, diuresis, and albumin infusion. Patients who develop PLE earlier seem to respond better to oral budesonide than those who present later. A careful search for conditions that may be exacerbating venous hypertension or limiting cardiac output should be undertaken. Fenestration of the Fontan pathway and use of PDE5 inhibitors or endothelin antagonists have been used in this setting with some success as well. The role of lymphatic interventions seems to be less effective in PLE than in plastic bronchitis.[16] Due to the poor prognosis, PLE that fails to respond to the above treatments is considered an indication for transplant.

Arrhythmias

Atrial arrhythmias are the most common cardiac complication affecting individuals after Fontan operation. Driven by atrial distension, extensive suture lines, and atrial fibrosis, the prevalence of atrial arrhythmias increases steadily with time after Fontan completion. Among patients with AP connection Fontan, roughly half develop atrial arrhythmias by 15 years post-Fontan, and this is associated with a sixfold increase in death or transplantation. The prevalence observed among patients with a lateral tunnel or extracardiac conduit Fontan is demonstrably lower compared with AP Fontan patients of similar age.[16]

The loss of atrial systole or the increased ventricular rate resulting from atrial arrhythmias can each lead to hemodynamic compromise, stroke and other embolic complications, and progressive ventricular dysfunction. Therefore, as in patients without congenital heart disease (CHD), the principal objectives of treating atrial arrhythmias are to reduce the risk of embolic events, to control heart rate, and to prevent symptoms.

The appearance of atrial arrhythmias is often the impetus to switch a patient from aspirin to warfarin. However, it should be noted that no studies have yet demonstrated a clear benefit of vitamin K antagonists over aspirin only for preventing thromboembolic events in Fontan patients. There is even less evidence to support the use of direct oral anticoagulants for this purpose in Fontan circulation, although small studies seem to suggest that they are safe in short-term follow-up studies.[16]

While "rate control" is often a preferred treatment strategy among non-CHD patients with long-standing atrial arrhythmias, patients with Fontan physiology generally do not tolerate atrial arrhythmias persisting for more than a few days. In the short term, cardioversion should be considered for persistent atrial tachycardia, especially if patients are symptomatic. In the longer term, various strategies can be considered to prevent future arrhythmia episodes.

Treatment strategies should be dictated by the patient's arrhythmia burden and how well they tolerate their arrhythmia.

For patients with short, infrequent episodes of arrhythmia, beta-blockers may be a reasonable starting point to reduce the likelihood of recurrence. For more frequent and/or more persistent arrhythmias, a class III antiarrhythmic agent may be appropriate. However, depending on local expertise, radio-frequency ablation can be a valuable tool for controlling arrhythmias in the Fontan population.

Fontan conversion may be considered for patients with an AP connection and persistent atrial arrhythmias. This conversion procedure generally consists of partial resection of a dilated right atrium, placement of an intra- or extracardiac cavopulmonary conduit, and performance of an atrial maze operation. A competing option for patients being considered for a Fontan conversion is a referral for heart transplant.

The converse to atrial arrhythmias as discussed above is sinus node dysfunction and chronotropic incompetence. The occurrence of sinus node dysfunction in patients with Fontan circulation is likely related to injury of the sinus node or its arterial supply at the time of surgery or to post-operative atrial remodeling. In such cases, placement of a pacemaker may be indicated, but due to the unique Fontan anatomy, the involvement of an electrophysiologist with expertise in complex CHD is mandatory.

Stroke/Thromboembolic Risk

Thromboembolic complications are an important contributor to Fontan mortality, being responsible for as many as 10% of late Fontan deaths. Even if not fatal, thromboembolic events can have a major adverse impact on quality of life. Thrombosis occurs in 8% to 33% of patients with Fontan physiology, and commonly affected sites include the systemic veins, the PAs, the pulmonary venous atrium (particularly in the setting of atrial arrhythmias), and, when present, the right atrium in patients with AP Fontan and the residual PA stump. Thrombus is most common in the first several years after surgery with a second peak in later adulthood, likely related to late Fontan circulatory failure.

The high rate of thromboembolic events in Fontan patients has been attributed to several factors. First, the Fontan circulation's absence of a right-sided pumping chamber results in decreased pulsatility and areas of relatively sluggish or stagnant flow within the Fontan pathway. This is especially true in people with AP Fontan connections in whom blood can often be seen slowly swirling within a massively dilated right atrium on echocardiography. Similarly, the high prevalence of lower extremity venous insufficiency in Fontan patients increases the risk of deep venous thrombosis. Second, abnormalities in coagulation factors can be demonstrated in most patients with Fontan physiology, factor VIII deficiency and protein C deficiency being the most common, although alterations in nearly every coagulation factor have been described. Third, enhanced platelet activation and thrombin formation and reduced fibrinolysis are common. Finally, as noted in the section above, the atrial arrhythmias that are commonly seen among Fontan patients also predispose them to thrombus formation in the absence of anticoagulation.

Recognizing coagulation abnormalities using standard laboratory testing is difficult. Prothrombin time and partial thromboplastin time are often prolonged despite an overall procoagulant state. Testing of individual clotting factors and natural anticoagulant factors is not routinely practiced. Similarly, diagnosis of thromboembolism in patients with Fontan physiology poses a clinical challenge as well.

While deep vein thrombosis of the upper or lower extremities can be relatively easily confirmed or excluded with compression ultrasound, thrombus in the Fontan pathway including pulmonary embolism are much more difficult to diagnose. Because there is no subpulmonary ventricle to aid in the even mixing of contrast and venous blood, CT pulmonary angiograms following the standard pulmonary embolism protocol are almost invariably marred by streaming and swirling artifacts and a high rate of false-positive results. Nuclear lung perfusion scans can be similarly unreliable because of asymmetric PBF patterns at baseline. Multidetector CT angiography with simultaneous contrast injection into upper and lower extremity veins with early- and late-phase image acquisition can improve diagnostic accuracy.

Given the high rate of thrombotic complications in patients with Fontan physiology, lifelong thromboprophylaxis is advised, but there is no consensus regarding whether to use antiplatelet therapy or anticoagulation. Studies show a significant increase in the risk of thromboembolic death among Fontan patients not taking aspirin or warfarin. However, studies have yet to show a clear benefit of warfarin over aspirin alone.[16] The relative safety and efficacy of non–vitamin K antagonist oral anticoagulants in adults with CHD have not been established, but many centers are already using them as first- or second-line options for thromboprophylaxis.

Kidney Disease

Studies have reported a 10% to 50% prevalence of glomerular filtration rate (GFR) < 90 mL/min/1.73 m^2 in Fontan patients.[16] Since individuals with Fontan circulation tend to have lower muscle mass, GFR calculation based on creatinine may underestimate kidney disease. Cystatin C is not impacted by body composition and tends to better reflect true kidney function.

The exact mechanisms for such a high rate of kidney disease is not completely understood but may be due to multiple factors including number of cardiopulmonary bypass runs, reduced renal perfusion pressure due to increased venous pressure and decreased cardiac output, and hypoxemia. Even a modest reduction in renal function is an important predictor of adverse outcomes.

Kidney disease is important to recognize from a practical management standpoint. Many cardiac medications have the potential to cause or exacerbate kidney injury, particularly angiotensin-converting enzyme inhibitors, nonsteroidal anti-inflammatory agents, diuretics, and some antiarrhythmic medications. Use of such medications in patients with Fontan circulation warrants regular surveillance of renal function.

Additionally, interventional procedures and imaging studies requiring contrast must be approached mindfully to avoid additional kidney injury.

Liver Disease

FALD appears to be virtually inevitable in patients with Fontan physiology and may begin immediately after Fontan completion, if not earlier. Manifestations range from asymptomatic hepatic congestion, as seen in most cases, to cirrhosis and hepatic dysfunction in advanced cases. Findings associated with portal hypertension such as esophageal varices, ascites, thrombocytopenia, and splenomegaly predict adverse outcomes. Perhaps most importantly, the presence of liver disease can be a barrier to eventual heart transplant in many patients with Fontan physiology. Additionally, hepatocellular carcinoma (HCC) among older patients with Fontan physiology is a growing concern associated with a very poor prognosis.[18]

Hepatic fibrosis resulting from congestive heart failure is primarily a sinusoidal process with portal tract involvement seen in more advanced cases. The factors associated with more advanced liver disease in individuals with Fontan circulation remain incompletely understood. The fibrosis stage appears be correlated with poorer hemodynamics and increased time after Fontan, but these findings have been inconsistent.[19] This fibrosis is thought to be mediated primarily by increased central venous pressure, which induces hepatic injury through sinusoidal stasis, stromal stretch, and compression of adjacent hepatocytic plates.

The optimal strategy for surveillance and diagnosis of liver health in Fontan patients remains an area of debate. Commonly ordered blood tests are known to be insensitive for detecting liver disease. Biopsy is still considered to be the gold standard for diagnosis and staging of liver disease, but the patchy nature of FALD may limit reproducibility in this cohort. In many centers, elastography is becoming the primary noninvasive strategy for assessing liver fibrosis, but standard cutoffs for liver stiffness measurements can overestimate fibrosis due to underlying hepatic congestion. Thus, liver imaging with CT or MRI may be the best method for routine hepatic surveillance.[18]

In cases where advanced liver disease is demonstrated or suspected, potential sources of Fontan pathway obstruction that may be exacerbating hepatic congestion should be sought and intervention considered if present. HCC is a relatively uncommon but devastating complication of FALD associated with a mortality of ~50% within 2 years of diagnosis. Specific risk factors for HCC within the Fontan population are unclear, making consensus on screening protocols difficult.[16]

Transplant after Fontan

Cardiac transplantation is necessary for a small but slowly increasing number of patients after the Fontan operation. The mechanisms of Fontan failure requiring cardiac transplant include ventricular systolic or diastolic dysfunction and the manifestations of chronic systemic venous hypertension, particularly PLE and plastic bronchitis. A sizable percentage of patients seem to have preserved ventricular systolic function but low cardiac output and elevated PVR.

Particularly in older patients, comorbidities such as liver disease and kidney disease can be an important barrier to transplant as both of these are associated with poor posttransplant outcomes. In Fontan patients with significant hepatic dysfunction or in those with HCC, combined heart-liver transplantation (CHLT) is considered the treatment of choice.[18] However, it is less clear how to identify those patients who have less severe liver disease but who are at high risk for fulminant hepatic failure after heart transplantation alone.

Advantages to proceeding with CHLT include posttransplant outcomes at least as good as, if not better than, outcomes after heart transplant alone, and lower rates of rejection, potentially requiring lower levels of immunosuppression. However, performing a CHLT when a heart transplant alone might be appropriate does put an additional strain on the allocation of an already scarce resource. In addition, relatively few centers offer CHLT, especially in the setting of complex CHD, making it infeasible for some patients.[18]

Ultimately, decisions regarding CHLT versus heart transplant alone should be made by a multidisciplinary transplantation team based on individual patient factors and local resources and expertise.

Risk Factors and Outcome Prediction

There are numerous papers that identify important potential risk factors associated with adverse outcomes, often focusing on death and/or transplant as a composite endpoint. Some of these risk factors for death and/or transplant include a history of PLE, decreased peak VO_2, having an AP Fontan, ventricular dilation, heart failure symptoms or need for diuretic use, arrhythmias, ventricular dysfunction, or > moderate atrioventricular valvar regurgitation.[20-22] While these data are promising, the risk models remain incomplete as most of these papers are single-center retrospective studies of less than 500 patients. Larger, multi-institutional studies are needed to create more robust risk prediction models that can be integrated into clinical care paradigms and potentially used for early listing for heart transplantation.

Longitudinal Fontan Surveillance

There is considerable historical practice variation for longitudinal Fontan evaluation and testing. In 2019, an expert consensus panel proposed a construct for cardiovascular surveillance testing tailed for children (<12 years), adolescents (12–18 years), and adults (>18 years) with a Fontan circulation.[16] Taken from the same consensus document, Table 59.1 details the frequency of outpatient evaluation and surveillance testing in this population.

TABLE 59.1	Fontan Cardiovascular System Surveillance Frequency and Testing[16]		
Test	Child	Adolescent	Adult
Outpatient visit, including physical examination	Every 6–12 mo	Every 6–12 mo	Every 6–12 mo
ECG	Every 6–12 mo	Every 6–12 mo	Every 6–12 mo
Echocardiogram	Yearly	Yearly	Yearly
Holter 24-hour monitor	Every 2–3 y	Every 1–2 y	Every 1–2 y
Exercise stress test	Every 2–3 y	Every 1–3 y	Every 1–2 y
Serum BNP or NT-proBNP	Once in childhood	Every 1–3 y	Every 1–2 y
Cardiac MRI	Once every 3 y	Every 2–3 y	Every 2–3 y
CT angiography	As clinically indicated	As clinically indicated	As clinically indicated
Cardiac catheterization	As clinically indicated	Once every 10 y	Once every 10 y

Our understanding of the late complications of Fontan physiology has recently brought crisp attention to the fact that a purely cardiac-centric view of Fontan care may be a disservice to this vulnerable patient population. In fact, a holistic approach is warranted with the engagement of providers across numerous specialties. At some centers, this is done informally with tailored referrals to non-cardiology subspecialists with an identified interest or expertise in Fontan patients. In a growing number of centers, this takes the form of a multidisciplinary Fontan clinic, where a comprehensive evaluation is done over 1–2 days. Regardless of the implementation strategy, the identification and cultivation of individuals across the following domains may, in fact, improve our care paradigm.

Hepatology

As detailed above, FALD is a universal complication of the Fontan circulation. While the optimum surveillance and intervention strategies are still not yet known, there is general consensus that every Fontan patient should be periodically evaluated by a hepatologist with specific expertise in FALD, especially as patients enter the second decade of life. Basic tenants of surveillance include laboratory serum testing, liver ultrasounds, and potentially ultrasound or MRI elastography. Serum α-fetoprotein is a sensitive screening biomarker for potential HCC.

Exercise Assessment and Exercise Prescriptions

Cardiopulmonary exercise testing is a core tool in the quantitation of Fontan physiology and exercise capacity. This testing should be coupled with additional assessment of core strength and lower body muscle mass. Data has shown that lower extremity resistance training can increase systemic venous return, increase cardiac output, and improve peak exercise testing parameters.[23] Using "exercise as a prescription" is a potentially powerful tool and may have a greater long-term impact than many pharmacological interventions.

Endocrinology

As patients age, there is an increasing frequency of vitamin D deficiency and secondary hyperparathyroidism. This often affects somatic growth and can be associated with decreased lean muscle mass and exercise intolerance. Osteopenia can lead to increased fractures as well. Serial measurement of serum calcium and vitamin D every 2–3 years can help lead to early identification of imbalances. Consultation with an endocrinologist can provide triaging for additional testing (e.g., bone densitometry scans) and facilitate medical management.

Nutrition

Maintaining a heart healthy dietary pattern is essential for long-term health following the Fontan, including but not limited to supporting a healthy weight and BMI, a normal lipid profile, liver function, and cardiac function. Foundations of this dietary pattern includes fiber-rich fresh fruit and vegetables, whole grains, legumes, lean proteins like fish and skinless poultry, low-fat dairy products, and unsaturated fats like olive oil, avocado, nuts, and seeds. Ideally, patients are encouraged to limit foods high in saturated fat (red meat, processed meats, fried foods, baked goods, and fast food), refined grains, added sugar (including sugar-sweetened beverages), and salt. The early incorporation of a nutritionist into the Fontan care model can reinforce these concepts and help patients make healthy dietary choices.

Neurodevelopmental

Neurodevelopmental and behavioral abnormalities in single-ventricle patients have been well described. The etiologies for these findings are complex and multifactorial but include potentially unfavorable *in utero* circulation, numerous cardiopulmonary bypass operations, hemodynamic alterations associated with perioperative care, and the inherent concerns of the Fontan physiology itself. Studies have shown that Fontan patients have lower reading and mathematics scores, impaired memory, and poor visual-spatial skills.[24] Attention-deficit/hyperactivity disorder, executive functioning problems, and anxiety are also more common than in the general population. Any of these potential issues can have a profound impact on quality of life, social adjustment, or employment. Screening by behavioral health specialists who understand the unique challenges of Fontan patients can lead to early identification of potential problems, increased school support services, and initiation of pharmacological interventions.

A Collaborative Approach to Discovery

While there has been considerable discovery and optimization of care models for Fontan patients, historically much of this progress has occurred through single-center studies. Significant progress towards collaboration through large consortiums, such as the Pediatric Heart Network (PHN), has resulted in numerous organized prospective trials (including randomized control trials) in single ventricle and Fontan patients.[25] These types of more rigorous scientific efforts are a significant step forward in the maturation of our field. However, unlike adult cardiology studies, these studies are relatively small with less than 600 patients.

Emboldened by the success of the PHN, parallel efforts toward creating larger Fontan datasets have also taken the form of multi-institutional Fontan registries. These registries are potentially powerful datasets given their size and number of patients. The first of these Fontan registries is the Australia and New Zealand Fontan Registry of 1700 patients.[2] Newer registries include the Fontan Outcomes Registry using CMR Examinations (FORCE) and the Fontan Outcomes Network (FON). As of 2023, FORCE already has >3500 patients captured, and FON just recently launched in 2023. These types of collaborative, multi-institutional efforts have significant potential to transform modern Fontan care paradigms by accelerating our learnings and discoveries.

References

1. Pundi KN, Johnson JN, Dearani JA, et al. 40-year follow-up after the Fontan operation: long-term outcomes of 1,052 patients. *J Am Coll Cardiol.* 2015;66:1700-1710.
2. d'Udekem Y, Iyengar AJ, Galati JC, et al. Redefining expectations of long-term survival after the Fontan procedure: twenty-five years of follow-up from the entire population of Australia and New Zealand. *Circulation.* 2014;130:S32-S38.
3. Schilling C, Dalziel K, Nunn R, et al. The Fontan epidemic: population projections from the Australia and New Zealand Fontan Registry. *Int J Cardiol.* 2016;219:14-19.
4. Fontan F, Baudet E. Surgical repair of tricuspid atresia. *Thorax.* 1971;26:240-248.
5. Kreutzer G, Galíndez E, Bono H, et al. An operation for the correction of tricuspid atresia. *J Thorac Cardiovasc Surg.* 1973; 66:613-621.
6. Björk VO, Olin CL, Bjarke BB, et al. Right atrial-right ventricular anastomosis for correction of tricuspid atresia. *J Thorac Cardiovasc Surg.* 1979;77:452-458.
7. Ishikawa T, Neutze JM, Brandt PW, et al. Hemodynamics following the Kreutzer procedure for tricuspid atresia in patients under two years of age. *J Thorac Cardiovasc Surg.* 1984;88: 373-379.
8. Mayer Jr JE, Helgason H, Jonas RA, et al. Extending the limits for modified Fontan procedures. *J Thorac Cardiovasc Surg.* 1986; 92:1021-1028.
9. Castaneda AR. From Glenn to Fontan: a continuing evolution. *Circulation.* 1992;86:II80-II84.
10. Jacobs ML, Jacobs JP, Thibault D, et al. Updating an empirically based tool for analyzing congenital heart surgery mortality. *World J Pediatr Congenit Heart Surg.* 2021;12:246-281.
11. Bridges ND, Mayer Jr JE, Lock JE, et al. Effect of baffle fenestration on outcome of the modified Fontan operation. *Circulation.* 1992;86:1762-1769.
12. Jacobs ML, Norwood Jr WI. Fontan operation: influence of modifications on morbidity and mortality. *Ann Thorac Surg.* 1994;58:945-951; discussion 951-952.
13. Gentles TL, Mayer Jr JE, Gauvreau K, et al. Fontan operation in five hundred consecutive patients: factors influencing early and late outcome. *J Thorac Cardiovasc Surg.* 1997;114:376-391.
14. Poh CL, Cordina RL, Iyengar AJ, et al. Pre- and post-operative determinants of transplantation-free survival after Fontan: the Australia and New Zealand experience. *Int J Cardiol Heart Vasc.* 2021;35:100825.
15. Dori Y, Keller MS, Rome JJ, et al. Percutaneous lymphatic embolization of abnormal pulmonary lymphatic flow as treatment of plastic bronchitis in patients with congenital heart disease. *Circulation.* 2016;133:1160-1170.
16. Rychik J, Atz AM, Celermajer DS, et al. Evaluation and management of the child and adult With Fontan circulation: a scientific statement from the American Heart Association. *Circulation.* 2019;140:e234-e284.
17. John AS, Johnson JA, Khan M, et al. Clinical outcomes and improved survival in patients with protein-losing enteropathy after the Fontan operation. *J Am Coll Cardiol.* 2014;64:54-62.
18. Emamaullee J, Zaidi AN, Schiano T, et al. Fontan-associated liver disease: screening, management, and transplant considerations. *Circulation.* 2020;142:591-604.
19. Wu FM, Kogon B, Earing MG, et al. Liver health in adults with Fontan circulation: a multicenter cross-sectional study. *J Thorac Cardiovasc Surg.* 2017;153:656-664.
20. Alsaied T, Bokma JP, Engel ME, et al. Predicting long-term mortality after Fontan procedures: A risk score based on 6707 patients from 28 studies. *Congenit Heart Dis.* 2017;12:393-398.
21. Cunningham JW, Nathan AS, Rhodes J, et al. Decline in peak oxygen consumption over time predicts death or transplantation in adults with a Fontan circulation. *Am Heart J.* 2017;189:184-192.
22. Meyer SL, St. Clair N, Powell AJ, et al. Integrated clinical and magnetic resonance imaging assessments late after Fontan operation. *J Am Coll Cardiol.* 2021;77:2480-2489.

23. Cordina RL, O'Meagher S, Karmali A, et al. Resistance training improves cardiac output, exercise capacity and tolerance to positive airway pressure in Fontan physiology. *Int J Cardiol.* 2013;168:780-788.

24. Bellinger DC, Watson CG, Rivkin MJ, et al. Neuropsychological status and structural brain imaging in adolescents with single ventricle who underwent the Fontan procedure. *J Am Heart Assoc.* 2015;4:e002302.

25. Goldberg DJ, Zak V, Goldstein BH, et al. Results of the FUEL trial. *Circulation.* 2020;141:641-651.

60

Fundamentals of Cardiopulmonary Bypass for Congenital Heart Surgery

GREGORY S. MATTE, MICHAEL KWON, AND JOHN E. MAYER JR.

KEY LEARNING POINTS

- Cardiopulmonary bypass (CPB) is a form of extracorporeal circulation that diverts a patient's venous blood away from the heart and lungs into a series of devices that oxygenate, ventilate, filter, and pump the blood back to the patient's arterial circulation in order to make a variety of cardiac surgical procedures possible.
- A CPB strategy is selected based on anticipated cardiac output/pump flow requirements and patient anatomy.

- The coronary circulation is often isolated and the heart is arrested with cardioplegia solution to allow the surgeon to safely and accurately perform intracardiac repairs.
- Anticoagulation is required as blood contacts numerous artificial surfaces during CPB; this anticoagulation is reversed after the surgical repair is completed and the bypass support is discontinued.

Background/Introduction

Cardiopulmonary bypass (CPB) is an essential tool for the surgical repair and palliation of congenital heart disease (CHD). The first operations utilizing CPB for repair of CHD are credited to Dr. John Gibbon in the 1950s with Drs. James Kirklin and C. Walton Lillehei adding significant modifications soon after. The techniques and technologies utilized for CPB have evolved significantly over the ensuing decades and today, the perfusionist is tasked with operating the heart-lung machine during procedures requiring CPB. The perfusionist works under the direction of the cardiac surgeon and cardiac anesthesiologist in the cardiovascular operating room (CVOR) to develop and execute a patient-specific CPB plan for each procedure.

CPB by definition is the condition in which a patient is connected to an artificial extracorporeal cardiopulmonary support circuit so that blood flow can be diverted away from the heart, lungs, and great vessels, thereby allowing the surgeon to more safely operate on or around those organs. Fundamentally, the purpose of CPB is to *take over the function of the heart and lungs* so that systemic perfusion is preserved during periods when the native heart and lungs are not contributing meaningfully to cardiac output and gas exchange, respectively. This is accomplished by placing one or more venous cannulae to drain systemic venous blood that would otherwise return to the right heart and divert it instead into an extracorporeal reservoir from which blood is then actively pumped into an oxygenator and then subsequently into a return cannula connected to the systemic arterial circulation (most commonly at the level of the distal ascending aorta). In this manner, the native heart and lungs are effectively bypassed, but systemic perfusion with adequately oxygenated blood is preserved since it is being provided by the CPB circuit and heart-lung machine.

In this chapter, we will first introduce the basic physical components of the CPB circuit, and then provide a framework for how these components are used to create a tailored CPB strategy that addresses the specific needs of a patient undergoing a specific type of cardiac repair. We will then describe some of the fundamental considerations in the management of CPB with regard to ensuring safety from thromboembolism, hypoperfusion, systemic venous hypertension, and improper gas exchange. Finally, we will briefly discuss two important adjuncts to CPB (ventricular fibrillatory arrest and circulatory arrest/regional perfusion) insofar as their roles and implications.

Basic Components of the Cardiopulmonary Bypass Circuit

The basic components of a CPB circuit are shown in Fig. 60.1 schematic. Key components are described below.

1. **Venous reservoir:** The venous reservoir in modern CPB circuits has several key features that increase the safety of cardiac operations done on bypass. The reservoir houses

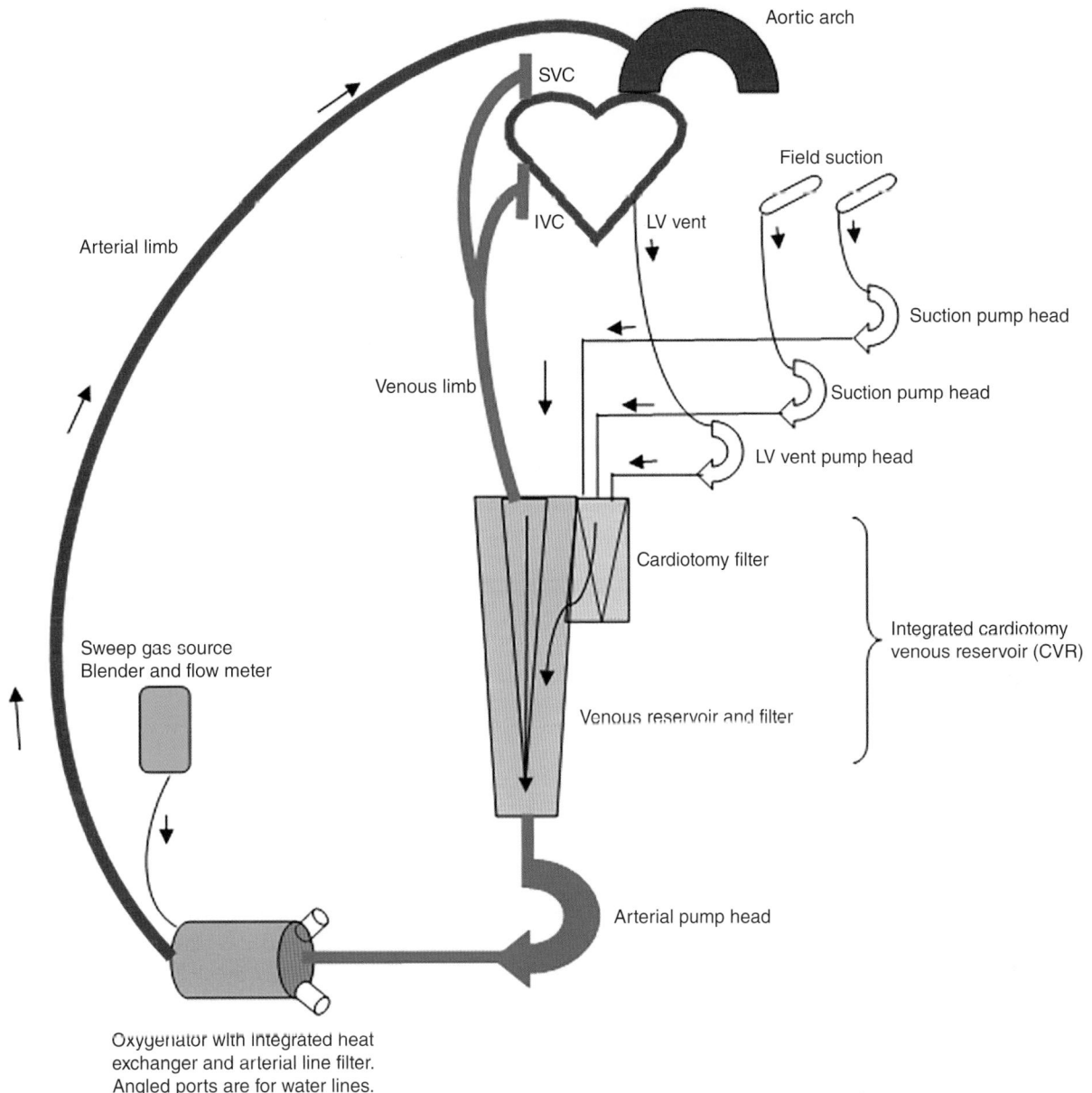

• **Fig. 60.1** Cardiopulmonary bypass circuit schematic. *IVC*, Inferior vena cava; *SVC*, superior vena cava.

the cardiotomy filter for blood suctioned from the operative field and vent return as well as the venous filter for blood draining directly from the cavae or other sources. Blood flow from the patient to the reservoir generally occurs by a siphonage mechanism, with the height difference between the venous reservoir fluid level and the venous cannulae insertion sites determining the amount of siphonage force that results from the effect of gravity on the blood draining from the patient to the reservoir. A greater vertical distance between the patient and the reservoir will therefore increase the venous drainage. Approximately 90–95% of the blood returning to the heart should be captured by the cannulae. If drainage is poor, one can either raise the height of the patient (the reservoir is typically placed at ground level to maximize

the gravitational force for drainage from the patient to the reservoir), or add a vacuum force to the circuit (vacuum assist) as is done in many centers. If assisted venous drainage is used by the perfusionist, the need for a height differential between the patient and the reservoir decreases as the application of negative pressure to the venous side of the circuit enhances venous drainage.

A noteworthy consideration is that because blood exits from the bottom of the reservoir, it is acceptable to have air in the upper portion of the reservoir as long as the reservoir remains at least partially filled, in order to prevent the delivery of air into the arterial side of the CPB circuit and then to the patient. This is termed an "open system" because the circulating volume is open-to-atmosphere within the venous reservoir. In contrast, a veno-arterial extracorporeal membrane oxygenation (ECMO) system requires a completely air-free circuit since there is no reservoir. ECMO circuits are thus "closed" systems. Closed systems do not provide the ability to scavenge blood from the operative field and return it to the reservoir. The reservoir in a standard CPB circuit allows for the incorporation of multiple sources of inflow into the reservoir, including and especially additional suction devices (cardiotomy suction). Cardiotomy suction tubing returns blood from intracardiac and aortic vents and field suction attachments, all of which return blood to the same common reservoir. Thus, for example, in the course of a reoperative sternotomy, if a major vascular structure is injured, as long as an arterial cannula is in place and the patient is heparinized, one can scavenge all the blood in the field to the venous reservoir using cardiotomy (field) suction, provide gas exchange, and then return that volume to the patient to effectively prevent exsanguination. The venous reservoir may also be termed a cardiotomy-venous-reservoir considering this integration of components. Fig. 60.2 shows three blue-colored ports on the upper right which lead to the cardiotomy filter, which is positioned to allow it to drain to the lower venous outlet.

2. **Oxygenators:** The oxygenator design that is most commonly used in modern CPB circuits is a hollow fiber

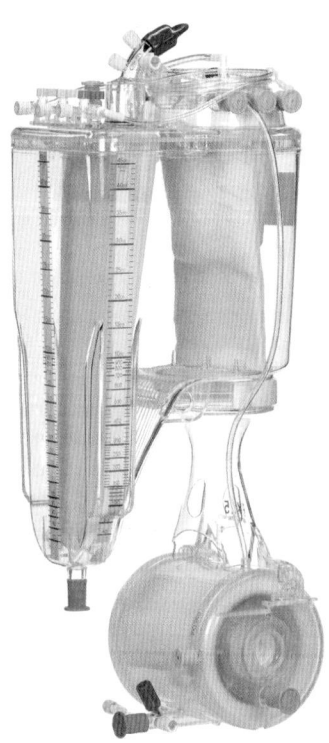

• **Fig. 60.2** Cardiotomoy venous reservoir on top for Terumo's Capiox FX25 Advance Oxygenator with Integrated Arterial Filter. (Terumo's® Capiox™ FX25 Advance Oxygenator with Integrated Arterial Filter. Photo is courtesy of Terumo Corporation.)

membrane oxygenator which contains a high surface area membrane that acts as the blood-gas interface. The overall surface area of the membrane is only about 10% of the overall surface area of the capillary bed of the native pulmonary circulation in an adult, but due to overall slower transit time ("dwell time"), the efficiency of gas exchange is generally sufficient to achieve a PaO_2 over 400 mm Hg and a normal $PaCO_2$. Fig. 60.3 shows the primary components of an oxygenator device.

The "oxygenator" portion of the circuit actually includes several integrated components including the microporous membrane oxygenator, cardiotomy venous reservoir, heat-exchanger and very commonly, an integrated 20–40 µ arterial line filter. The oxygenator component is rated by the manufacturer for a maximum flow, which takes into account oxygen and carbon dioxide transfer, venous drainage, and heat-exchange capacity, among other considerations. The perfusionist selects the oxygenator with the smallest priming volume that still safely meets the anticipated patient requirements for flow, gas exchange, and heat exchange. Typically, the pediatric perfusion team has access to as many as five sizes of oxygenators which allows them to customize the bypass circuit for different patient sizes and flow requirements. Smaller oxygenators typically have smaller prime volumes which helps control hemodilution.

3. **Roller pump and tubing:** The pump portion of the circuit most commonly uses a roller pump which is arranged so that the tubing of the circuit is placed in a semicircular shaped structure called the "raceway" and a spinning rotor with rollers that nearly or completely occlude the tubing and thus move the point of tubing occlusion progressively further along the tubing in the raceway, thereby providing the energy to displace the blood within the tubing in a forward direction (toward the patient), as shown in Fig. 60.4. Increasing the revolutions per minute of the rollers increases forward flow. This flow becomes the equivalent of the patient's cardiac output, which may or may not be supported with native heart flow, depending on the time period in an operation.

Tubing for CPB is provided in sterile packaging in various calibers; in congenital cases, the aim is to use the smallest sized tubing which will safely allow for the anticipated pump flow requirements during support. Avoiding unnecessarily large tubing minimizes transfusion requirements since the fluid used to fill ("prime") the tubing in the circuit will mix with and dilute the patient's blood. The internal diameter of the arterial, venous, pump header, field suction and cardioplegia circuit tubing commonly ranges from 1/8 in to 1/2 in. Smaller tubing decreases "prime" volume and the resulting hemodilution during the period when the patient is on extracorporeal support, but there are limitations to the flow capacities for each size. Tubing connects

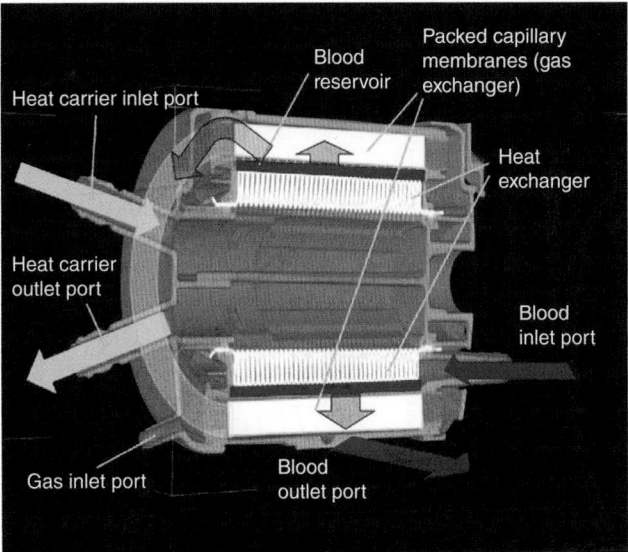

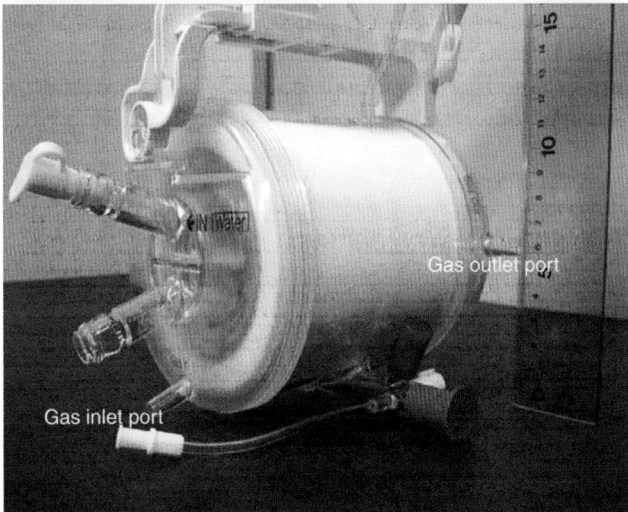

• **Fig. 60.3** Detailed image of an oxygenator device. (Figure 4 in Newly Developed Pediatric Membrane Oxygenator that Suppresses Excessive Pressure Drop in Cardiopulmonary Bypass and Extracorporeal Membrane Oxygenation (ECMO), by Makoto Fukuda, Asako Tokumine, Kyohei Noda and Kiyotaka Sakai. https://doi.org/10.3390/membranes10110362.)

the surgically inserted cannulae to the disposable components on the heart-lung machine. The prime volume for the bypass circuit, including the tubing and oxygenator, commonly ranges 200–1200 mL with circuits in the 200 mL range serving neonates and infants and circuits in the 1200 mL range reserved for adults. The CPB circuit is arranged on the heart-lung machine which includes several roller head pumps and may also include one or more centrifugal pumps. The pumps allow for independent flow control for the arterial pump (cardiac output), cardioplegia (direct coronary delivery), field suckers, left atrial or left ventricle vent, aortic root vent, active and modified ultrafiltration (MUF), and more.

4. **Cannulae:** The connection between the CPB machine disposable components and the patient is made using cannulae that the surgeon temporarily implants. The cannulae come in a variety of types and sizes to accommodate the wide range of patient and vessel sizes the congenital heart surgeon encounters. Arterial, venous, aortic root, vent, and other types of cannulae are placed as needed. Sizing is dependent on both patient size, vessel size, and specific anatomy which may vary with cardiac disease (i.e., left superior vena cava [SVC], interrupted inferior vena cava [IVC] with azygous continuation, etc.) in consideration of anticipated flow requirements on CPB. The chosen cannulae must be sufficient to provide a cardiac index of greater than 2.2 L/min/m² of body surface area at minimum in order to ensure adequate systemic perfusion on bypass although it is common for congenital heart surgery cases to plan for an index flow of 3.0 L/min/m² or more. Cannulae for CPB applications have flow and pressure drop ratings which the perfusionist references when assisting the surgeon in selecting appropriate sizes. Venous drainage on bypass is carefully monitored to ensure blood is not "backing up" in the brain/upper body (SVC) or liver/kidneys/lower body (IVC). Typically, an operation does not proceed until the surgeon and perfusionist confirm that venous drainage and arterial return are at expected levels through the provided cannulae. Cerebral and somatic near-infrared spectroscopy (NIRS), central venous pressure, venous blood saturation, arterial and venous lab panels, visual inspection of the head, heart and abdomen, and volume monitoring in the venous reservoir are among the parameters that are continuously monitored to ensure the adequacy of perfusion during CPB.

Essential Elements of the Conduct of Cardiopulmonary Bypass

With this basic schema as a foundation for understanding the building blocks of the CPB circuit, there are multiple variations that are employed in a manner tailored to patient-specific anatomy and the goals of the operation. These variations take into account the following fundamental considerations:

1. **Cannulation strategy:** The optimal cannulation strategy (number and location of venous and arterial cannulae) depends upon both the availability of structures that are candidates for/require cannulation and the objectives of the operation. For example, for an intracardiac repair of an atrial septal defect (ASD), in which a right atrial incision is employed to expose the ASD, cannulating both the SVC and IVC is imperative so that those vessels can be snared to achieve complete vascular control of the systemic venous return into the heart and provide for a well-drained atrial cavity for exposure of the defect. By contrast, during an aortic valve repair in a patient

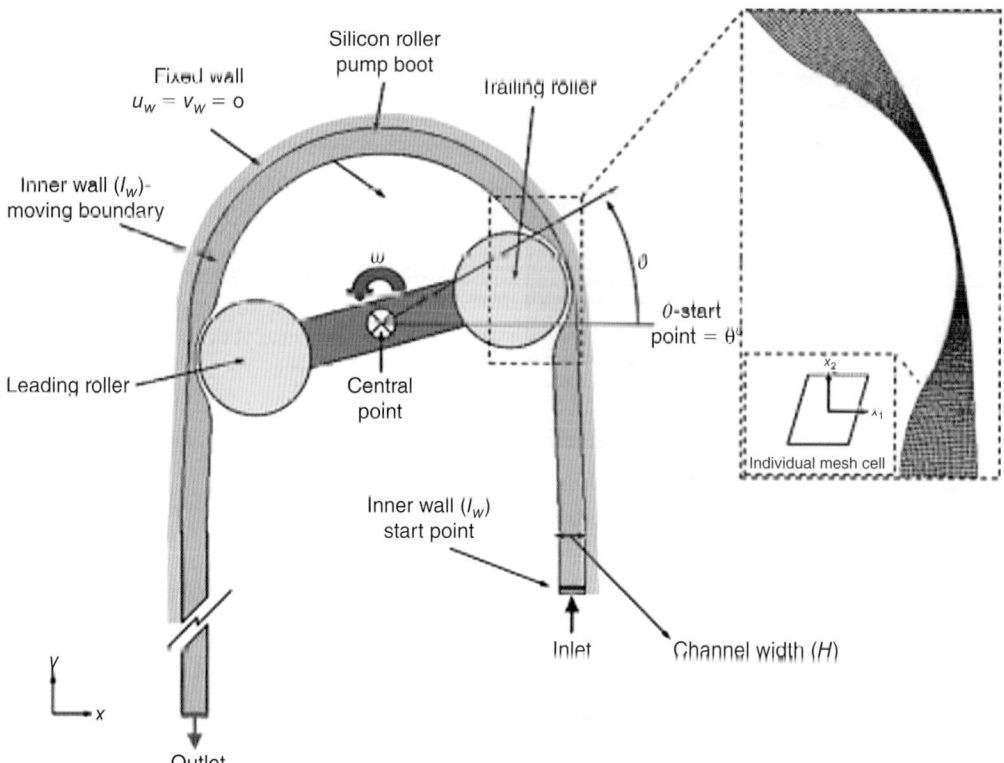

• **Fig. 60.4** Detailed image of a roller head pump. (From Fig. 5.4 in Mulholland JW, Shelton J, Luo X. Blood flow and damage by the roller pumps during cardiopulmonary bypass. *J Fluids Struct.* 2005;20:129–140.)

without intracardiac shunts, a single venous cannula can be placed directly into the right atrium since the exposure to the aortic valve is typically accomplished via an aortic incision rather than an atrial one. In certain instances in which a patient has a left SVC in addition to the right SVC without a bridging vein, a third venous cannula is required, i.e., tricaval cannulation.

Caval cannulation (separate venous cannulae to drain the SVC and IVC, respectively) is most often utilized because it affords the surgeon the ability to place snares around the SVC and IVC to achieve complete vascular control of the systemic venous return to the heart and thereby open the systemic venous atrium without having blood flooding the field. The placement of caval snares approximates the caval walls to the outside of the cannulae, and this is necessary to avoid entraining air into the venous cannulas and tubing as the entrained air will disrupt the cohesive fluid viscous forces that are necessary to maintain gravity venous drainage (i.e., prevent air lock). CPB with caval snares applied is commonly termed "complete" CPB since no blood is returning to the heart and lungs. When the caval snares are off, it is referred to as "partial" CPB since at least a portion of the venous return is allowed to transit the cardiac and pulmonary circulation.

With respect to the arterial cannula, a single cannula is usually placed into the distal ascending aorta or the proximal arch for non-arch reconstruction cases, whereas if the arch requires repair, a cannula can be placed in the innominate artery to facilitate regional perfusion to the brain during arch repair. In the setting of a reoperative sternotomy in older children and adult patients, a femoral artery and vein can be cannulated prior to opening the chest to minimize the blood loss from vascular structures such as the aorta or a conduit that are at risk for injury during re-entry into the mediastinum. Alternatively, in cases such as a neonatal interrupted aortic arch repair, dual arterial cannulae (one in the ascending aorta and one perfusing the descending aorta) are often required to adequately perfuse the systemic circulation both proximal and distal to the arch interruption.

2. **Prevention of systemic air embolism:** Aside from cardiac operations performed exclusively on the right side of the heart in the setting of no intracardiac shunts, operations in which the pulmonary venous atrium, systemic ventricle, or proximal aorta are opened to ambient air expose the patient to the risk that this air could potentially embolize into the systemic circulation. Therefore, these operations are generally performed with an ascending aortic cross-clamp that separates the systemic

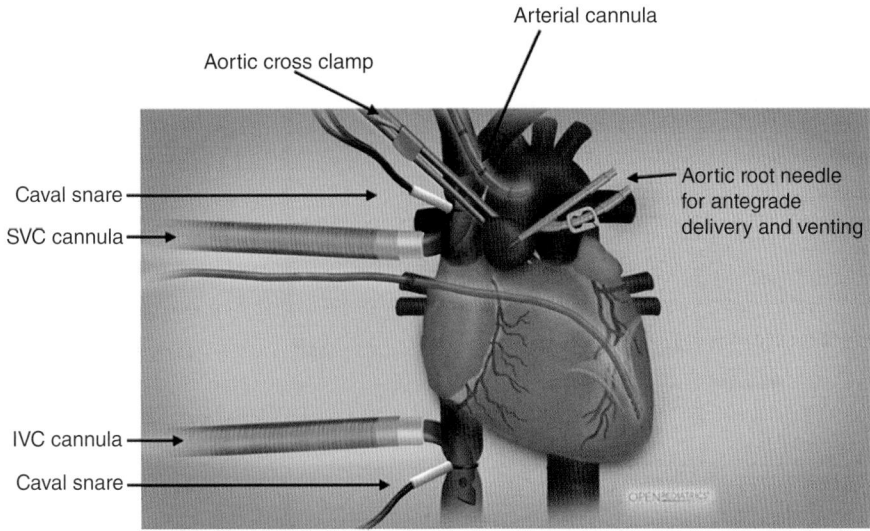

• **Fig. 60.5** Bicaval venous cannulation with a single arterial cannula in the distal ascending aorta, aortic cross clamp in pace, aortic root needle for cardioplegia delivery in place, and placement of the left ventricular vent through the right superior pulmonary vein and then across the mitral valve. *IVC,* Inferior vena cava; *SVC,* superior vena cava. (Image used with permission from OPENediatrics.)

arterial compartment that is perfused by the arterial cannula (exclusive of the coronary circulation which is proximal to the level of cross-clamp placement) and the intravascular/intracardiac compartment that is being opened surgically to perform the operation as shown in Fig. 60.5. The effect of this separation of the heart from the circulation is to minimize the risk of systemic air embolization and stroke as well as to improve surgical exposure.

3. **Cardioplegia and myocardial protection strategy:** Cardioplegia is delivered immediately after placement of the aortic cross-clamp, as this is the moment when coronary blood flow ceases and therefore marks the beginning of the ischemic period of the operation. It is typically delivered by one of three routes; antegrade, retrograde, and/or direct ostial delivery. Most commonly, antegrade delivery into the aortic root is achieved via a dedicated cardioplegia catheter that is placed into the ascending aorta above the sinotubular junction but proximal to the level of the aortic cross-clamp. As long as the aortic valve is competent, all of the delivered cardioplegia perfuses the coronary arteries exclusively. Retrograde cardioplegia is an option in which cardioplegia is delivered via a trans-right atrial catheter placed into the coronary sinus. Finally, direct ostial cardioplegia delivery may be employed in the setting of an open aortic root or ascending aorta. In virtually all cases, an applied cross-clamp eliminates coronary perfusion from the heart-lung machine and results in myocardial ischemia. To minimize myocardial metabolic demand and resulting ischemic injury, the heart is pharmacologically arrested with a solution (cardioplegia) that eliminates

the normal electrical potential difference across the cell membrane, preventing the myocardial depolarization cycle and mechanical activity. The addition of extracellular potassium reduces the membrane potential from −85 mV to −50 mV, which then decreases the availability of open sodium channels for sodium influx into the cell, which is what is otherwise required to start phase 1 of the cardiomyocyte action potential, as shown in Fig. 60.6. This prevents the ability of the calcium-sodium exchanger to allow an influx of calcium into the cell, and thereby prevents the contraction of the myocyte, which is dependent on this calcium influx. In addition, the absence of the action potential prevents release of calcium from the sarcoplasmic reticulum. In order to further reduce myocardial metabolic demand during this induced ischemia, the cardioplegia solution is significantly cooled (4-12 degrees C) at most centers. By virtue of both cessation of myocardial contraction and electrical conduction, and the induction of hypothermia, cardioplegia markedly reduces myocardial oxygen demand in the setting of the reduced supply created by the application of the aortic cross-clamp and cessation of myocardial blood flow. Minimizing ischemic injury is well understood to protect the ability of the myocardium to resume function when the heart is reperfused by releasing the aortic cross-clamp.

The diastolic arrest of the heart is also beneficial for the surgeon, since the heart is decompressed and motionless, but also is flaccid, so that one can easily manipulate it in three dimensions to gain the optimal exposure necessary to perform a safe and effective operation.

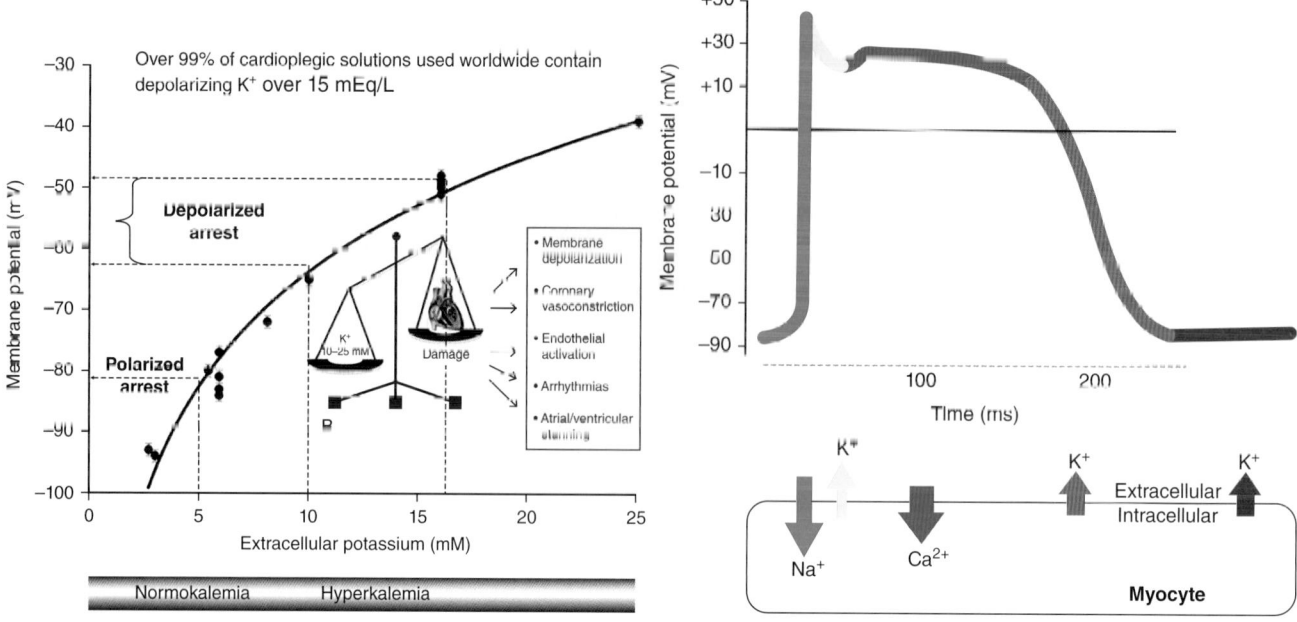

• **Fig. 60.6** The cardiomyocyte action potential, primary electrolyte flows, and the impact of extracellular hyperkalemia during cardioplegia delivery. (Left figure is from Fig. 3 in Dobson GP, Faggian G, Onorati F, Vinten Johansen J. Hyperkalemic cardioplegia for adult and pediatric surgery: end of an era?. *Front Physiol.* 2013;4:228.)

While some types of cardioplegia are given at specific intervals, such as every 20–40 minutes, one of the more widely used forms of myocardial protection for congenital heart surgery patients is given much less frequently. This formulation is referred to as del Nido cardioplegia and it is a mixture of 20% patient whole blood and 80% crystalloid solution with specific additives including potassium, bicarbonate, mannitol, magnesium, and lidocaine. It is delivered at 8–12°C.[1] This solution is typically given in a single-dose strategy especially in neonates and infants, but there are centers which administer it every 45–90 minutes, particularly for larger patients.

4. **Venting strategy:** Although venous cannulation is able to remove 90–95% of systemic venous return to the heart, the ongoing contributions of pulmonary venous return from blood originating from the bronchial arterial circulation (and aortopulmonary collaterals, if present) often leads to significant filling of the pulmonary venous atrium and systemic ventricle in many patients. With the primary intent of providing enough drainage to allow the surgeon to visualize the structures requiring repair without having the exposure compromised by blood in the field, additional vent cannulas are placed in various positions in the heart to further empty the heart and thereby facilitate the operation. These vents are generally smaller cannulae that are connected by separate tubing to the cardiotomy-venous reservoir. The most commonly employed vents in most centers are an aortic root vent placed in the proximal ascending aorta and a left ventricular vent placed through the right superior pulmonary vein, as shown in

Fig. 60.5. Such vents, for example, keep the left ventricle empty during a ventricular septal defect repair so that the surgeon can better visualize the defect, and more generally can also assist with de-airing of the heart prior to releasing the aortic cross-clamp. Finally, vents are instrumental in protecting the ventricles from distention, particularly during the period of early reperfusion after aortic cross-clamp removal but before the heart regains spontaneous ventricular activity.

5. **Systemic hypothermia:** Systemic hypothermia can be an important adjunct while employing CPB. Its primary purpose is to decrease the overall metabolic activity of not only the heart in between doses of cold cardioplegia but to also protect the brain and visceral organs from warm ischemic injury, particularly during periods of reduced flow rates on CPB or complete interruptions in pump flow (circulatory arrest with or without regional cerebral perfusion), which may be required to adequately perform certain technical aspects of an operation (e.g., aortic arch repair).

Efficiently decreasing the patient's temperature can be accomplished through the heat-exchanger located within the oxygenator. The oxygenator device has a sealed membrane with blood flow on one side and temperature-controlled water flow on the other. The blood flow through the bypass circuit allows the perfusionist to precisely control core temperature through central cooling. Hypothermia decreases the metabolic rate which decreases the cardiac output/ pump flow requirements during bypass. It is not uncommon for congenital cardiac operations to be performed at target temperatures of 28–32°C. Lower pump flows also aid the surgeon's visualization during surgery and also add a margin of safety for central neurologic and visceral organ injury, in particular, during planned (or unplanned) periods of low flow. A lower metabolic rate gives the team more time to react to surgical and heart-lung machine issues which require a significant reduction or interruption in the pump flow. Deep hypothermia to 18–22°C is less commonly used since the advent of selective cerebral perfusion, with or without direct lower body perfusion.[2,3] These techniques are typical for Norwood stage 1 procedures and aortic arch repair cases. Innovative perfusion strategies that perfuse the majority of the patient's circulation instead of allowing for selective or total circulatory arrest have reduced the need for significant hypothermia during cardiac surgery.[3] Regardless of the target temperature during surgery, the patient is always rewarmed utilizing established temperature gradients which have been shown to help preserve neurologic function.[4,5] Additionally, the patient should never be rewarmed beyond 37°C as this has been shown to add risk for worse neurologic and renal outcomes.[4-6]

Physiologic Management During Cardiopulmonary Bypass

1. **Anticoagulation:** Due to the universal thrombogenic effect of foreign (non-endothelial) surfaces on the circulating blood, both the tubing but more importantly the oxygenator in CPB circuits require a high level of anticoagulation, most often with heparin. While other forms of anticoagulation including direct thrombin inhibitors such as argatroban and bivalirudin have been used for cardiac surgery, heparin remains the most common anticoagulant. An activated clotting time (ACT) is used in the operating room to monitor the anticoagulant effect with most centers utilizing an ACT of > 400–480 seconds during CPB as an indicator of adequate anticoagulation.[7] This ACT level is much higher than the level of anticoagulation used in ECMO, but is essential during CPB because of the "open" nature of the system where blood is regularly exposed to air in the operative field returned to the venous reservoir via cardiotomy suction, and in the venous reservoir itself. ECMO utilizes a closed system without the field suction which activates the blood coagulation system to a lesser degree. The perfusionist monitors the effect of heparin after the initial bolus before CPB and then throughout the bypass period as heparin levels decrease over time due to renal excretion and loss through bleeding or washing of shed blood in an autologous cell salvage device. Repeat dosing on bypass is utilized as needed to maintain a therapeutic ACT. While all centers utilize the ACT to monitor heparin's effect, some centers also monitor the actual

level of heparin in the blood. In theory, this practice may better maintain an antithrombin effect since other factors may increase the ACT including thrombocytopenia, platelet dysfunction, hemodilution, and hypothermia.[8] Regardless of technique, proper anticoagulation to prevent thrombin formation is essential to provide safe cardiopulmonary support. The perfusionist is vigilant to prevent thrombosis in the bypass circuit. Anticoagulation is reversed after bypass once the cardiologist and surgeon verify the surgical repair with transesophageal or epicardial echocardiography.

2. **Bypass circuit prime and hematocrit management:** The CPB circuit is always initially "primed" with a crystalloid solution. A clear balanced-electrolyte solution prime allows the perfusionist to ensure the circuit is free of unwanted air, to check for leaks in the system, and to wet the filters in the system to help rid the circuit of micro air bubbles. Once the circuit integrity is confirmed and the patient hematocrit is checked, the perfusionist calculates the dilutional hematocrit if the patient were to receive a crystalloid-only prime, which is calculated based on the patient's circulating red blood cell volume and the circuit prime volume. The care team typically has protocols for minimum hematocrit levels on bypass and for separating from bypass. If the calculated dilutional hematocrit warrants, red blood cells are added to the prime to displace some of the clear solution so that the hematocrit on bypass will be at an acceptable level. Plasma may also be added. While there is not definitive evidence for a minimal hematocrit on bypass, a metanalysis of studies conducted at Boston Children's Hospital in the 1990s and 2000s found that in two-ventricle patients presenting for cardiac surgery utilizing bypass, there were more favorable outcome measures at a hematocrit > 23.5%.[9] Primary outcome differences were that lactate levels were lower and 1 year postoperative psychomotor development scores were higher in this group with hematocrit levels > 23.5%. Patients with single-ventricle physiology are typically maintained with a higher hematocrit on bypass, commonly in the ≥ 30%–35% range. The risk-benefit ratio for transfusion will vary by patient diagnosis, type and state of surgery, and numerous other factors the care team must consider during CPB for congenital heart patients. Adjunct techniques such as modified ultra filtration (MUF) and the use of autologous red blood cell salvage (cell savers) are very commonly utilized to help return as much blood as possible to the patient after separation from bypass.[10,11]

3. **Blood gas management:** The tensions of oxygen and carbon dioxide in a patient's blood, along with pH, may be managed in different ways during CPB. These are critically important considerations for patients with CHD. While it is widely understood that the oxygen content in the blood does not increase significantly with a PaO_2 above 100 mm Hg (as the hemoglobin is fully saturated and provides >95% of the oxygen carrying capacity),

there are some theoretical advantages to a hyperoxic strategy during CPB. First and foremost, CPB is not truly physiologic. The patient on CPB generally experiences non-pulsatile pump flow, regular changes in overall flow and perfused capillary density, changes in temperature, circulating gaseous microemboli, and many other perturbations.[10,12] For these and other reasons, hyperoxia on bypass is preferred by many institutions during the CPB period. Other institutions utilize normoxemia or a PaO_2 in the 200–300 mm Hg range to reduce the theoretical risks of oxygen free radical formation during CPB. Numerous studies have shown evidence of oxidative stress with a hyperoxic strategy, but differences in clinical outcomes are lacking.[13]

Management of $PaCO_2$ and pH during hypothermic bypass is important in congenital heart surgery, and there are two common strategies, pH stat and alpha stat. The pH-stat technique maintains the $PaCO_2$ at 40 mm Hg at the patient's actual temperature. It should be kept in mind that all blood gas machines warm the blood sample to 37°C, and the $PaCO_2$ that the patient is experiencing at temperatures <37°C is then extrapolated back to the patient's actual temperature for the pH-stat technique. Since the partial pressure of a dissolved gas decreases as temperature decreases (gas solubility increases), to maintain a $PaCO_2 = 40$ mm Hg at 20°C, it will be measured in the blood gas analyzer as 74 mm Hg at 37°C (~2 mm Hg/°C). The alternate technique of alpha-stat management maintains the $PaCO_2$ at 40 mm Hg as it is measured at the standardized temperature of 37°C. The pH-stat technique most often requires supplemental carbon dioxide in the oxygenator sweep gas as gases are more soluble at colder temperatures. A higher $PaCO_2$ with pH-stat (if corrected to 37°C and compared to the alpha-stat technique) offers the benefits of cerebral vasodilation (extra or luxurious cerebral blood flow), pulmonary vasoconstriction, better oxygen off-loading with a right shift of the oxyhemoglobin dissociation curve due to lower pH, which opposes the leftward shift of the oxyhemoglobin dissociation curve resulting from hypothermia, and more homogeneous cooling and rewarming.[10] Alpha-stat management utilizes a lower $PaCO_2$ than pH-stat, and this helps to preserve cerebral autoregulation. The alpha-stat technique may be particularly beneficial for adults who are at a higher risk of embolic phenomenon from calcified great vessel plaques and vascular disease as cerebral blood flow is maintained at the autoregulatory rate which limits cerebral embolic exposure, if present.

4. **Blood pressure management:** The cerebral, cardiac, and other vital organs have some ability to autoregulate blood flow through vasodilation or vasoconstriction, although the ability to autoregulate is reduced with hypothermia. The perfusionist works with the surgeon and anesthesiologist to establish a target safe mean arterial blood pressure during CPB. The mean arterial pressure during CPB is often referred to as the perfusion pressure. The on-bypass target value takes into consideration preoperative values, NIRS values, electrocardiogram values, and surgical needs. There are generalized target ranges for different age patients, but these values must be cautiously considered against specific patient diagnoses, changing operative needs, variable pump flows (cardiac output), temperature, oxygen delivery, and oxygen consumption.[10] Vasoconstrictors and vasodilators are administered through the bypass circuit as needed to maintain the target perfusion pressure during the CPB period.

5. **Checklists and time-outs for patient safety:** The perfusionist utilizes several checklists to help ensure patient safety.[10] The most extensive checklist is performed well before bypass to verify all circuit components are set up properly and ready for patient care. Shorter checklists may also be used before commencing bypass, before terminating bypass, and for unique perfusion strategies. Perfusion checklists are performed by the primary perfusionist and may also incorporate a challenge format with assistance from another clinician. Time-outs for patient safety are often guided by the operating room nurse and include participation by the entire CVOR team. These may be performed upon patient entry into the operating suite, before surgical incision, upon closing the chest, and before the patient is transported to the intensive care unit.[14-16]

Alternate CPB schema: Most operations using CPB are performed in such a manner as to avoid interruptions in systemic perfusion as the source of circulation is transitioned from the patient's native cardiopulmonary circulation to that of the CPB circuit, and then back. However, in certain types of operations, including and especially in aortic arch repair, partial or complete cessation of CPB flow during the bypass period is required to facilitate the goals of the operation itself. For a patient requiring aortic arch reconstruction, since the aortic arch has to be opened, arterial flow from the arterial cannula in the ascending aorta or innominate artery cannot continue to provide systemic perfusion to the lower body. Therefore, such operations are performed under a period of circulatory arrest, with the patient cooled to deep hypothermic levels to protect the brain and viscera from warm ischemic injury. In deep hypothermic circulatory arrest (DHCA), the flow from the CPB circuit is completely halted for a period of time to allow the surgeon to perform the arch repair. The safe time interval for DHCA that avoids undue risk of neurologic injury is determined by the level of deep hypothermia. A DHCA period of 30–40 minutes is generally thought to be safe at a core temperature of 18°C (Fig. 60.7).

Recognizing that the risk of neurologic injury is higher than the risk of visceral organ injury during DHCA at a given temperature, techniques were developed to provide ongoing perfusion to the brain during periods of circulatory arrest to the body during arch repair. Antegrade cerebral perfusion is a form of regional perfusion in which an arterial cannula usually connected to the right brachiocephalic artery via a tube graft or via direct cannulation, provides ongoing flow at 20–50 cc/kg/min to the brain (assuming an intact circle of Willis) during periods of circulatory arrest to the rest of the body (Fig. 60.7B). The use of antegrade cerebral perfusion has not, however, been shown, even in randomized controlled trials of arch reconstruction in neonates, to be associated with improved neurologic outcomes in comparison with DHCA.[17]

Ventricular fibrillatory arrest/Induced ventricular fibrillation: An additional form of myocardial protection is the use of induced ventricular fibrillation which may be used alone or as an adjunct to cardioplegia delivery. A surgeon may elect to fibrillate the heart using epicardial fibrillator pads connected to a fibrillator device in situations in which cross-clamping is technically not feasible, for shorter intracardiac repairs, or to limit a subsequent myocardial arrest/ischemic period. The success of induced fibrillation is predicated on the heart being empty without wall stress, at least mildly hypothermic, and with excellent coronary perfusion while on CPB.[18,19] The systemic ventricle can entrain air but since the ventricle is not contracting, air will not be ejected

across the aortic valve to the systemic circulation. In general, successful use of fibrillatory arrest requires a competent aortic valve so that the left ventricle does not become distended by blood passing retrograde through the aortic valve, which would also compromise coronary perfusion. One point of caution to consider in the use of this technique is that although it does have the advantage of limiting overall ischemic time (since the coronaries are still being perfused during this period), fibrillation does increase myocardial oxygen consumption by $\geq$ 10% compared to the beating non-working heart at normothermia. For this reason, it is important for the surgeon to ensure the heart is empty, without wall stress, and at least mildly hypothermic for optimal myocardial protection with induced fibrillation.

Summary

CPB is a significant but necessary undertaking for many congenital cardiac operations. Understanding the capabilities and limitations of the equipment that comprises the modern CPB circuit, along with a keen understanding of the specific needs of a patient and the goals of the operation, allows for the creation of a sound CPB strategy so that a patient can be adequately supported and then weaned off of CPB in order to accomplish the goals of the operation while protecting the heart, brain, and organ systems from injury.

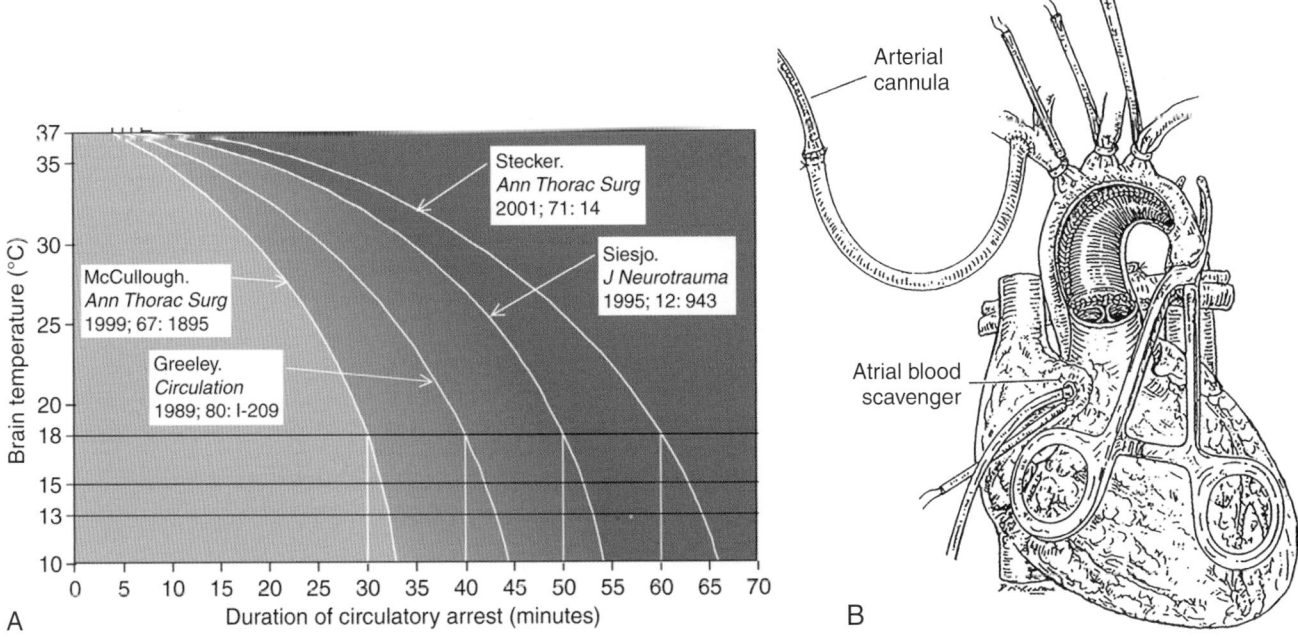

• **Fig. 60.7** (A) Brain temperature and likely safe duration of circulatory arrest. (B) Arterial cannulation for aortic arch repair with head vessels from arch snared to prevent air entrainment during antegrade cerebral perfusion. (A, From Arrowsmith JA, Hogue CW. Deep hypothermic circulatory arrest. In: Ghosh S, Falter F, Cook D. *Cardiopulmonary Bypass.* Cambridge University Press, Cambridge 2009: 125–139; B, Pigula FA, Nemoto EM, Griffith BP, Siewers RD. Regional low-flow perfusion provides cerebral circulatory support during neonatal aortic arch reconstruction. J Thorac Cardiovasc Surg. 2000;119(2):331-339.)

References

1. Matte GS, del Nido PJ. History and use of del Nido cardioplegia at Boston Children's Hospital. *J Extra Corpor Technol*. 2012;43: 98-103.

2. Pigula FA, Nemoto EM, Griffith BP, et al. Regional low-flow perfusion provides cerebral circulatory support during neonatal aortic arch reconstruction. *J Thorac Cardiovasc Surg* 2000;119: 331-339.

3. Sittring I, Prabhu N, Evans A, et al. Sustained total all region (STAR) perfusion: an optimized perfusion strategy for Norwood reconstruction. *J Extra Corpor Technol*. 2020;52:332-336.

4. Motshabi-Chakane P, Mogane P, Moutlana J, et al. Contemporary neuroprotection strategies during cardiac surgery: state of the art review. *Int J Environ Res Public Health* 2021;18:12747.

5. Shann KG, Likosky DS, Murkin JM, et al. An evidence-based review of the practice of cardiopulmonary bypass in adults: a focus on neurologic injury, glycemic control, hemodilution, and the inflammatory response. *J Thorac Cardiovasc Surg*. 2006;132: 283-290.

6. Newland RF, Tully PJ, Baker RA. Hyperthermic perfusion during cardiopulmonary bypass and postoperative temperature are independent predictors of acute kidney injury following cardiac surgery. *Perfusion*. 2013;28:223-231.

7. Matte GS, Howe RJ, Ibla J, et al. Transition from Hemochron Response to Hemochron Signature Elite activated clotting time devices in a congenital cardiac surgery practice. *J Extra Corpor Technol*. 2019;51:221-226.

8. Gruenwald CE, Manlhiot C, Crawford-Lean L, et al. Management and monitoring of anticoagulation for children undergoing cardiopulmonary bypass in cardiac surgery. *J Extra Corpor Technol*. 2010;42:9-19.

9. Wypij D, Jonas RA, Bellinger DC, et al. The effect of hematocrit during hypothermic cardiopulmonary bypass in infant heart surgery: results from the combined Boston hematocrit trials. *J Thorac Cardiovasc Surg*. 2008;135:355-360.

10. The Bypass Plan, In: Matte GS, ed. *Perfusion for Congenital Heart Surgery: Notes on Cardiopulmonary Bypass for a Complex Patient Population*. Oxford: Wiley Blackwell; 2015:53-71.

11. Nathan M, Tishler B, Gauvreau K, et al. A red cell preservation strategy reduces postoperative transfusions in pediatric heart surgery patients. *Ped Anesth*. 2018;28:450-457.

12. Matte GS, Connor KR, Liu H, et al. Arterial limb microemboli during cardiopulmonary bypass: observations from a congenital cardiac surgery practice. *J Extra Corpor Technol*. 2016;48:5-10.

13. Caputo M, Mokhtari A, Rogers CA, et al. The effects of normoxic versus hyperoxic cardiopulmonary bypass on oxidative stress and inflammatory response in cyanotic pediatric patients undergoing open cardiac surgery: a randomized control trial. *J Thorac Cardiovasc Surg*. 2009;138:206-214.

14. Croti UA, Jenkins KJ, Braile DM. Checklist in pediatric cardiac surgery in Brazil: a useful and necessary adaptation of the Quality Improvement Collaborative International Congenital Heart Surgery in Developing Countries. *Rev Bras Cir Cardiovasc*. 2011;26: 511-515.

15. Guy IA, Kerstein RL, Brennan PA. How to WHO: lessons from aviation in checklists and debriefs. *Ann R Coll Surg Engl*. 2022; 104:510-516.

16. Konfirst C, Preston S, Yeh T. Checklists and safety in pediatric cardiac surgery. *Semin Thorac Cardiovasc Surg Pediatr Card Surg Annu*. 2015;18:43-50.

17. Algra SO, Jansen NJ, van der Tweel I, et al. Neurological injury after neonatal cardiac surgery: a randomized, controlled trial of 2 perfusion techniques. *Circulation*. 2014;129:224-233.

18. Buckberg GD, Brazier JR, Nelson RL, et al. Cooper N. Studies of the effects of hypothermia on regional myocardial blood flow and metabolism during cardiopulmonary bypass I: the adequately perfused beating, fibrillating and arrested heart. *J Thorac Cardiovasc Surg*. 1977;73:87-94.

19. Jessen ME, Abd-Elfattah AS, Wechsler AS. Neonatal myocardial oxygen consumption during ventricular fibrillation, hypothermia, and potassium arrest. *Ann Thorac Surg*. 1996;61:82-87.

61

Ventricular Recruitment in Patients with Borderline Ventricles

ERIC N. FEINS, MEENA NATHAN, REBECCA BEROUKHIM, AND SITARAM M. EMANI

KEY LEARNING POINTS

- Traditional decision-making for patients with borderline left or right heart was binary: single ventricle palliation versus primary biventricular repair.
- Patients with moderate left or right heart hypoplasia may be candidates for eventual biventricular repair, even if primary creation of a biventricular circulation is not feasible.
- Staged ventricular recruitment involves one or more surgical procedures to "grow" the hypoplastic left or right ventricle so that it can ultimately support a full cardiac output.

- Staged recruitment allows for gradual volume loading of the hypoplastic right or left ventricle and allows for repeated assessment of candidacy for biventricular conversion utilizing echocardiography, cardiac catheterization, and cardiac MRI.
- Management during the staging phase of left heart recruitment requires careful monitoring of left atrial/pulmonary artery pressures so that single ventricle palliation is kept open as a long-term alternative.

Introduction

Certain patients with congenital heart disease may manifest right or left heart hypoplasia ranging from mild to severe. Traditionally, treatment of such patients was dichotomous—single ventricle palliation or biventricular repair. Importantly, the decision to undergo single ventricle palliation versus primary biventricular repair is often made during the neonatal period, committing the child to the chosen circulation. Although results of single ventricular palliation have improved over the years, long-term complications of Fontan circulation are concerning.[1] On the other hand, survival is poor in patients undergoing high-risk primary biventricular repair.[2-4] Furthermore, anatomy of the hypoplastic left or right heart may be variable, even though the treatment options appear binary. At either end of the spectrum, the choice of strategy is obvious—biventricular repair for mild hypoplasia of the left or right heart, and single ventricle palliation for severe hypoplasia. However, appropriate strategies for management of patients with "borderline" left or right heart structures is more nuanced. This chapter describes recent attempts to perform biventricular repair or 1½ ventricle repair in patients with borderline left or right heart hypoplasia in attempts to avoid terminal single ventricle palliation as the definitive therapy.

Definition of Borderline Left or Right Heart

A borderline heart may be characterized by the small size of the ventricular chamber or of the inlet or outlet valves. Size of left and right heart structures can be measured in absolute dimensions (end-diastolic volume, annular dimensions), normalized size (dimension indexed to body surface area [BSA; m²]), or as normative Z scores. The latter methodology accounts for age and BSA and is the most commonly utilized metric for assessing borderline left or right hearts. Ventricular or valvular dimension Z scores < –2.0 indicate hypoplasia, with Z scores < –5.0 considered severe hypoplasia, and Z scores between –2 and –5 constituting borderline hypoplasia. A patient may be considered to have a borderline left heart due to left ventricular (LV) hypoplasia, LV dysfunction, complex left-sided valvular disease, or complex intracardiac anatomy. Diagnoses associated with borderline left heart include hypoplastic left heart syndrome (HLHS), Shone's complex, right-dominant unbalanced atrioventricular (AV) canal defect, double-outlet right ventricle, interrupted aortic arch with ventricular septal defect (VSD), straddling AV valves, and complex forms of transposition of the great arteries with LV hypoplasia. A borderline right heart maybe defined as hypoplasia of the right ventricle (RV), tricuspid valve, and pulmonary valve. Diagnoses associated with borderline right heart include tricuspid atresia or stenosis, pulmonary atresia with intact ventricular septum (PA/IVS), critical pulmonary stenosis, left-dominant AV canal defect, and complex transposition of the great arteries or straddling valves with RV hypoplasia.

The Borderline Left Heart

Numerous studies have focused on utilizing morphologic and physiologic characteristics of the left heart at the time of presentation to determine probability of successful biventricular repair in a single operation (primary biventricular repair).[5,6] Scoring tools have been developed to assist with this decision-making that estimate the probability of successful repair, but these tools are difficult to implement clinically. Frequently, the decision for primary biventricular repair must be made during infancy, when complex repairs may yield suboptimal results. Physiologically the patient may not be ready for a biventricular circulation if multiple left-sided lesions present in tandem (i.e., valvular disease and LV hypoplasia). Forced into a corner, the team is faced with a very challenging choice to attempt a "high-risk" biventricular repair or "bail" to single ventricle palliation.

The current trend toward primary biventricular repair over single ventricle palliation; however, frequently leads to inappropriate choice of biventricular repair, and resultant high mortality.[7,8] Frequently when a primary biventricular repair is performed for the borderline left heart, the systemic circulation must depend upon a left heart that is suboptimal in size and function and valves that are imperfect, resulting in left atrial and pulmonary hypertension. Centers that aggressively pursue primary biventricular repair must develop thresholds for takedown to single ventricle palliation in case of circulatory insufficiency. It is no surprise that inappropriate primary biventricular repair leads to dire consequences, including prolonged ventilation, prolonged ICU and hospital lengths of stay, and not infrequently, death.

An alternative strategy to single ventricle palliation and primary biventricular repair in patients with various forms of borderline left heart is staged left ventricular recruitment (SLVR).[9-11] Recent experience with this strategy is summarized below.

Staged Left Ventricular Recruitment

SLVR refers to the strategy in which single ventricle palliation is initially pursued and adjunctive procedures are performed at interstage operations in order to "rehabilitate" the left heart.[12] Rehabilitation procedures include valve repair, removal of obstructing lesions within the LV (e.g., outflow tract obstruction or endocardial fibroelastosis [EFE]), and restriction of the atrial septal defect (ASD) to promote blood flow through the left heart.[13] The underlying principle is that increasing flow through a valve or chamber will promote growth of these structures. The goal is to encourage growth of left heart structures gradually, thus optimizing

chances of eventual successful biventricular conversion. In patients with complex intracardiac anatomy, staged repair may include distributing components of the repair over a series of separate operative procedures to reduce the risk of each procedure. Throughout the interstages, suitability of single ventricle palliation is ensured by close monitoring of atrial trans-septal gradient by echocardiography (as a surrogate for left atrial pressure). If adequate growth and function of left heart structures can be achieved, then the patient is converted to biventricular circulation by separation of right and left heart circulations with takedown of the aortopulmonary amalgamation and/or cavopulmonary anastomoses, and closure of intracardiac shunts.

Candidates For SLVR

Diagnoses that are traditionally treated with single ventricle palliation but in whom staged ventricular recruitment may be feasible include HLHS, Shone's variants, unbalanced AV canal defect, double-outlet right ventricle or complex forms of transposition of the great arteries with LV hypoplasia, and interrupted aortic arch with VSD. These patients all share several features in common: hypoplastic LV with mitral valve and/or aortic valve stenosis, without atresia of valves. There are often straddling AV valves in those defects with a VSD. A contraindication to SLVR is complete atresia of inflow or outflow valves to/from the LV. The success of SLVR depends upon promotion of growth of the left heart structures by increased flow through the left heart. Patients with atresia of the mitral or aortic valves do not have the opportunity for flow through the valves with current technology.

Rationale For SLVR

In various forms of congenital heart disease, the left heart structures demonstrate growth in the first few years of life if exposed to the appropriate flow stimulus. A notable example is total anomalous pulmonary venous connection. In this lesion, reduced volume loading of the LV is known to occur *in utero* and results in a smaller volume LV. However, following complete repair of this lesion, with redirection of pulmonary venous flow into the left heart, LV volumes normalize within months. A similar observation has been made in patients with critical aortic stenosis and borderline LV following balloon aortic valve dilation.[14,15] The growth potential of the neonatal and infant heart is not surprising, even though the underlying biochemical and molecular mechanisms of growth are not well understood. Yet, sudden volume loading of a hypoplastic and unprepared ventricle can lead to disastrous hemodynamic consequences. Since the remodeling process can take months to years, the goal of SLVR is gradual loading of the left heart while the systemic circulation is supported by the RV. Underlying SLVR is the premise that surgical relief of inflow and outflow obstructions and gradual volume loading of the hypoplastic ventricle will lead to sufficient growth that the rehabilitated ventricle will ultimately be able to handle a full cardiac output. Another assumption is that biventricular circulation is superior to single ventricle circulation; however, this assumption holds true only if the left heart can sustain a full cardiac output with low filling pressures and functional valves. In patients with risk factors for single ventricle circulation (e.g., pulmonary vein stenosis, systemic RV dysfunction, single lung, pulmonary artery stenosis, AV valve regurgitation) or failing single ventricle circulation, biventricular circulation or transplantation may be the only options for survival.[16]

Theoretically, recruitment of the left heart may also augment the total cardiac output in patients with single ventricle circulation. Although this hypothesis has not been rigorously proven by prospective randomized controlled trials, comparison of cardiac index prior to and following recruitment has shown improvement in total cardiac output in interstage patients.

Advantages of SLVR Over Primary Biventricular Repair

SLVR may be considered as an alternative to a high-risk biventricular repair in patients with borderline left heart. SLVR allows one to:

1. *Delay making a decision about ultimate long-term circulation*: SLVR allows one to delay commitment to either single ventricle or biventricular circulation for several years while the left heart is being rehabilitated. During this period, the circulation is supported with single ventricle palliation, but maneuvers are performed to relieve obstructions and promote flow through the left heart. During the phase of left heart rehabilitation, one does not "burn bridges" for terminal single ventricle palliation if the transitional circulation is managed properly. It is critical that significant left atrial hypertension be avoided since this can cause irreversible pulmonary vascular changes, which can preclude a single ventricle strategy.
2. *Gradually and gently increase the load on the left heart*: A common mode of failure of primary biventricular repair is the sudden increase in demands placed upon a borderline left heart. The ventricle may be ill-prepared to handle the acute burden of a full cardiac output, resulting in elevated end-diastolic, left atrial, and RV pressures. On the other hand, the left heart may be better able to handle a systemic circulation if it has been gradually loaded rather than acutely burdened with a full cardiac output, as occurs in primary biventricular repair. The success of SLVR hinges upon a gradual increase in preload, allowing time for the left heart to remodel and accommodate the increased workload. The gradual loading may reduce the risk of early cardiac failure following biventricular conversion. In patients with complex anatomy, distributing components of repair over a series of operations attenuates the risk associated with a single long, complex, multicomponent biventricular repair. Moreover, surgical modifications to the complex repair

of aortic or AV valves can be safely performed over a series of operations since the systemic circulation is not dependent solely upon the left heart. Optimization of valve function prior to biventricular conversion increases the likelihood of favorable hemodynamics following conversion and reduces risk of early reintervention.
3. *Provide clarity regarding choice of ultimate strategy by examining response of the left heart to increased load*: Despite volume loading and relief of obstructions, some ventricles simply do not grow, or demonstrate persistent diastolic dysfunction. If ventricular response is unfavorable despite rehabilitation, single ventricle palliation is pursued. Adequacy of the intracardiac baffles and valve repair can be assessed and factored into decision-making regarding biventricular conversion or ongoing single ventricle management.

Timeline of Events

A patient with borderline left heart presents for consideration of surgical intervention typically as a neonate or infant. Initial single ventricle palliation is pursued by either stage I palliation or pulmonary artery banding. At the time of second stage palliation (4–6 months), surgical rehabilitation procedures are performed while essentially maintaining a palliated single ventricle circulation. Hybrid stage 1 palliation as initial palliation may allow delay of biventricular repair by several months and is best suited for patients with only mild hypoplasia of the left heart in whom staged surgical rehabilitation of intracardiac structures is not necessary.[17] For most patients, we prefer traditional stage 1 palliation as it allows more opportunities for staged intracardiac reconstruction. Typically, an interval of 1–2 years is necessary to determine response of the left heart structures to loading maneuvers. Thus, by the time a patient is ready for the Fontan procedure, a decision can be made about whether to convert to biventricular circulation or perform definitive single ventricle palliation.

SLVR Diagnosis-Specific Strategies and Considerations

Hypoplastic Left Heart Syndrome Variants/ Shone's Syndrome

SLVR involves resection of EFE, repair of mitral and aortic valves, and restriction of the ASD with a fenestration. Neonatal stage I palliation (traditional or hybrid) is performed once the diagnosis of borderline left heart is established.[11,17] At this stage, the ASD is left unrestrictive to avoid left atrial hypertension, except in patients with mild forms of hypoplasia.

At 4–6 months of age, when the child returns for the second stage procedure, magnetic resonance imaging (MRI) and cardiac catheterization are performed to assess the left heart structures and function. Mechanism and degree of mitral stenosis, aortic stenosis, and LV EFE are assessed. At the second stage procedure, a bidirectional Glenn (BDG) or upsizing of the systemic to pulmonary artery shunt is performed to increase pulmonary blood flow. The ASD is restricted to promote blood flow into the LV. Mitral valve stenosis is addressed, and EFE is resected from the LV. Mitral valve pathology in patients with HLHS includes fusion of papillary muscles, single papillary muscle, and shortened chordal attachments that are often basally displaced. Surgical maneuvers include division of fused papillary muscles, splitting of a single papillary muscle, and division of chordal attachments. Aortic valve stenosis is addressed, usually with a commissurotomy. If a BDG is performed, augmentation of pulmonary blood flow by maintaining or replacement of the systemic-to-pulmonary shunt should be considered as a means of volume loading the left heart. Banding the PA between the BDG anastomosis and the systemic-to-pulmonary shunt prevents retrograde/pulsatile flow from the shunt into the BDG/superior vena cava (SVC), which is often observed when antegrade (systemic to pulmonary) blood flow is maintained in addition to the BDG circulation. In a study reviewing 1½ ventricle repair at Boston Children's Hospital, Prasanna et al.[18] demonstrated that children without restriction between the BDG and antegrade pulmonary blood flow were at significantly higher risk of developing SVC hypertension than those who had septation of their pulmonary artery between the BDG and antegrade pulmonary blood flow (44% vs. 10%; P = .04).

Additional operations for rehabilitation may be necessary over the next 6–24 months to optimize left heart function. Increase in the size of the left heart structures including LV, mitral, and aortic valves can be demonstrated. An analysis by Emani et al.[11] of left heart structures following SLVR demonstrated significant size increase when compared with children who underwent traditional single ventricle palliation (Fig. 61.1). Flow measurements across the mitral and aortic valves should be obtained by MRI and correlated with intracardiac pressures measured by catheterization. If the flow across the LV approximates a full cardiac output with LV end-diastolic pressures < 13 mm Hg, then conversion to anatomic biventricular circulation can be performed. Biventricular conversion consists of takedown of the aortopulmonary connection and BDG, re-anastomosis of the main pulmonary artery to the branch pulmonary arteries, and removal of any existing shunts. Factors associated with successful biventricular repair are summarized in the Table 61.1.

After LV recruitment has been performed, if the LV has not yet responded to recruitment maneuvers, further surgery for recruitment can be performed to relieve residual valvular lesions or resect residual EFE. Importantly, EFE is not always limited to the endocardial surface and can involve deeper fibrosis of the myocardium leading to a restrictive cardiomyopathy-type picture. Alternatively, the LV and left heart can be used as a subpulmonary ventricle by performing a reverse double switch operation, in which an atrial switch and arterial switch are performed, thus using the RV as a systemic ventricle and the LV as a pulmonary ventricle.[19]

Biventricular conversion is generally performed between 2 and 4 years of age if adequate left heart growth and function is achieved. However, diastolic dysfunction with ongoing LV non-compliance is not an uncommon characteristic of these patients and can contribute to left atrial and pulmonary hypertension following biventricular conversion despite adequate growth in the volume of left heart structures. In a study evaluating preoperative hemodynamic parameters predictive of adverse outcomes, Herrin et al.[20] found pre-repair LV end-diastolic pressure > 13 mm Hg to be a risk factor for failure of biventricular circulation (Fig. 61.2A) Adjunctive strategies to alleviate ventricular non compliance are being developed to optimize results in this patient population.

Unbalanced Atrioventricular Canal Defect

Patients with right-dominant AV canal defect (primum ASD, VSD, varying degree of left AV valve hypoplasia, abnormality of subvalvar structures, and LV hypoplasia) can undergo recruitment of the hypoplastic LV simply by closing the ASD while leaving the VSD open. This approach was reported in a study by Kwak et al.,[21] who showed significant increase in end-diastolic volume (as measured by MRI) following restriction of the ASD at the time of recruitment procedure (Fig. 61.2B). During the neonatal period, initial palliation may be performed either by stage I palliation (traditional or hybrid) or pulmonary artery banding (Fig. 61.3A and B). At the second stage operation (4–6 months old) recruitment of the left heart is undertaken, during which the atrial septum is closed with a fenestration to promote pulmonary venous return into the hypoplastic LV, and the VSD is left open[22] (Fig. 61.3C). Closure of the VSD during staged recruitment may detrimentally restrict cardiac output and is unnecessary to achieve left heart growth. It is counterintuitive and interesting to note that ASD restriction alone without VSD closure leads to growth of the left heart in most patients with a VSD. This observation suggests that transvalvular flow patterns, not end-diastolic pressure, stimulate left heart growth. Concomitant procedures to improve inflow into the LV are crucial. This includes deviation of the atrial patch onto the right side of the AV valve when dividing a common AV valve into right and left components. This approach effectively steals right AV valve tissue onto the hypoplastic left side. Additionally, a single left-sided papillary muscle is split to encourage left AV valve inflow into the LV. Addition of accessory pulmonary blood flow at the time of the BDG may augment left heart throughput. In patients with significant AV valve regurgitation, a favorable by-product of the SLVR strategy is stabilization of the common AV valve and more durable AV valve function during the interstage period. Growth of the hypoplastic ventricle should be observed over a period of 10–12 months. If ventricular growth is not observed, additional intervention on the left AV valve may be necessary to improve inflow. In some situations, despite atrial septation with a fenestrated patch, left AV valve inflow is directed into the RV through the VSD. Since ventricular growth is

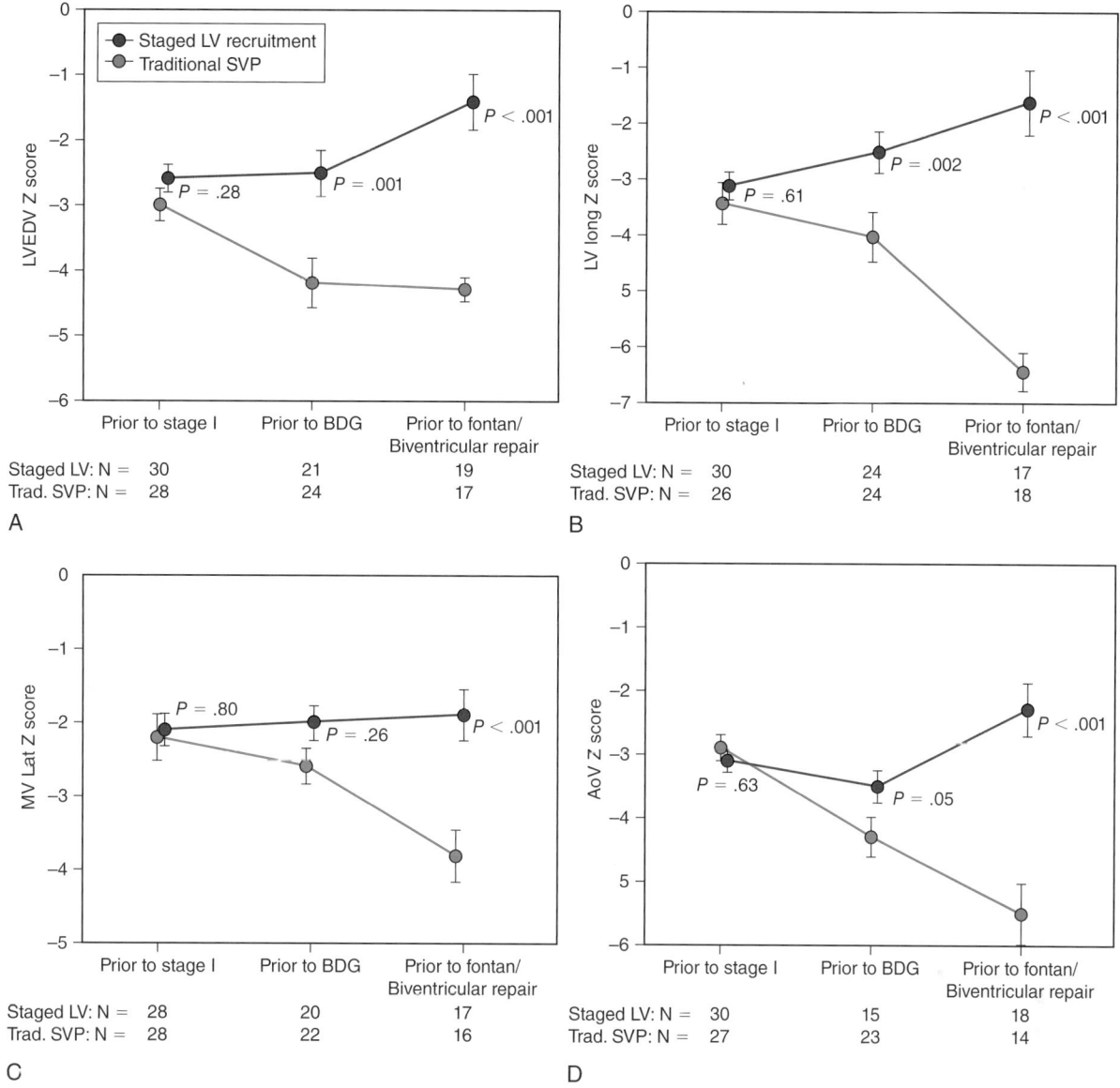

• **Fig. 61.1** Left heart dimensions at various palliative stages in patients undergoing staged left ventricular *(LV)* recruitment *(blue circles)* versus traditional single ventricle palliation *(SVP)* *(green circles)*. (A) Increase in LV end-diastolic volume (LVEDV) Z score in recruitment patients versus traditional SVP patients. (B) Increase in LV long-axis dimension Z score in recruitment patients versus SVP patients. (C) and (D) Larger mitral valve *(MV)* and aortic valve *(AoV)* Z scores in recruitment patients versus traditional SVP patients. *BDG,* Bidirectional Glenn. (Credit: Emani SM, McElhinney DB, Tworetzky W, et al. Staged left ventricular recruitment after single-ventricle palliation in patients with borderline left heart hypoplasia. *J Am Coll Cardiol.* 2012;60:1966–1974.)

<table>
<tr><td>TABLE
61.1</td><td>**Predictors of Successful Biventricular Repair for Borderline Left Ventricle**</td></tr>
</table>

- Valves (size/function) and outflow tracts
- Morphology, size, and function of left ventricle
- Minimum left ventricular end-diastolic volume 35 mL/m² (patients with ventral septal defect)[22]
- Healthy myocardium (absence of endocardial fibroelastosis/intact ventricular septum)
- Preoperative left ventricular end-diastolic pressure < 13 mm Hg[20]
- Absence of endocardial fibroelastosis
- Comorbidities

influenced by fluid shear forces on the endocardium of the ventricle, left AV valve inflow into the RV does not provide the necessary stimulus for LV growth. In this situation, partial or complete closure of the VSD may be useful to encourage left AV valve inflow into the LV.

If adequate growth of the left heart is demonstrated, repeat MRI and catheterization are performed, and determination of ventricular adequacy is made. As in patients with HLHS, flow through the left AV valve and end-diastolic pressures are the chief metrics in determining adequacy of the LV to serve as the systemic ventricle. Biventricular repair/conversion can be performed if the LV end-diastolic

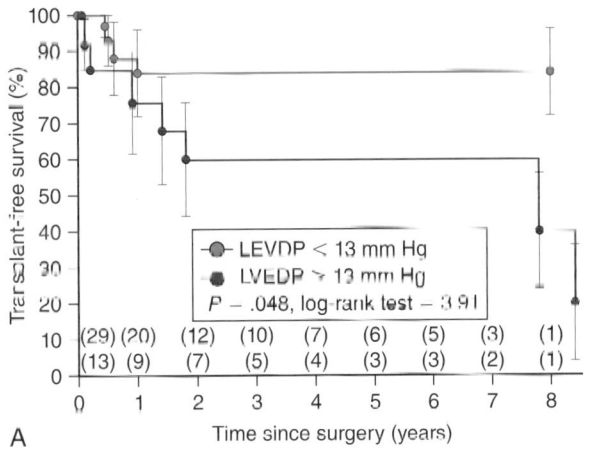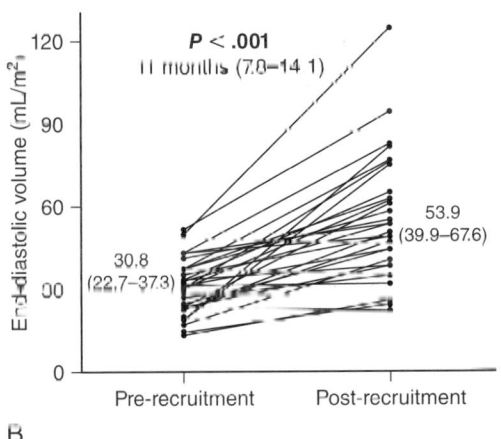

• **Fig. 61.2** Ventricular recruitment outcomes. (A) Outcomes in patients with left ventricular end-diastolic pressure *(LVEDP)* < 13 mm Hg *(green circles)* versus patients with LVEDP ≥ 13 mm Hg *(red circles)*. Improved transplant-free survival in patients with lower LVEDP. (B) Impact of atrial septal defect (ASD) restriction on ventricular growth in patients with a hypoplastic ventricle and ventricular septal defect who undergo ASD restriction. Pre- versus post-recruitment indexed end-diastolic volume on magnetic resonance imaging shows significant ventricular growth following ASD restriction. (Credit: *A,* Herrin MA, Zurakowski D, Baird CW, et al. Hemodynamic parameters predict adverse outcomes following biventricular conversion with single-ventricle palliation takedown. *J Thorac Cardiovasc Surg.* 2017;154:572–582; *B,* Kwak JG, Del Nido PJ, Piekarski B, Marx G, Emani SM. Restriction of atrial septal defect leads to growth of hypoplastic ventricle in patients with borderline right or left heart. *Semin Thorac Cardiovasc Surg.* 2022;34:215–223.)

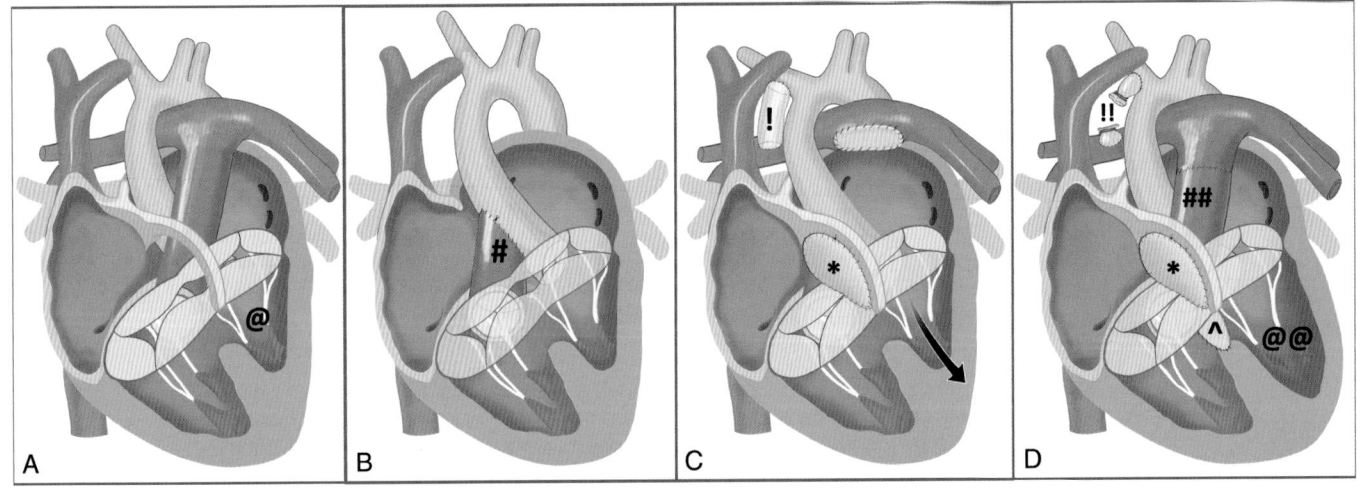

• **Fig. 61.3** Schematic of staged ventricular recruitment for right-dominant atrioventricular canal defect with left ventricular (LV) hypoplasia. (A) Anatomy shows hypoplastic, non-apex forming LV *(@)*. (B) Initial single ventricle palliation: neonatal stage 1 operation with atrial septectomy and Damus-Kaye-Stansel (DKS) procedure *(#)*; right ventricle-to-pulmonary artery conduit not shown. (C) Staging procedure at 4–6 months old: atrial septal defect patch with fenestration *(*)*, ventricular septal defect (VSD) left open, aortopulmonary shunt created *(!)* to augment pulmonary blood flow and left heart return; bidirectional Glenn (BDG) not depicted but often performed at this operation. (D) Completion of biventricular conversion after achieving LV growth *(@@)*: VSD closed *(^)*, DKS taken down with main pulmonary artery reconnection *(##)*, aortopulmonary shunt *(!!)* and BDG taken down.

pressure remains < 13 mm Hg when the LV sustains a full cardiac output (Fig. 61.3D). However, if ongoing ventricular noncompliance and/or persistent valvular dysfunction are present, a reverse double switch operation may be an option with the hypoplastic left heart serving as a subpulmonary ventricle.[19] In their study of predictors of successful biventricular conversion, Kwak et al.[21] found that when

compared with patients with HLHS, patients with unbalanced AV canal defect are more likely to achieve successful biventricular conversion. Thirty percent of patients with HLHS experienced the primary outcome of death, transplant, or biventricular takedown, whereas only 6% of patients with unbalanced AV canal defect experienced this outcome ($P = .03$).[20] Long-term outcomes following biventricular conversion are similar to those of less complex patients undergoing primary biventricular repair.[23] The lack of EFE and myocardial fibrosis likely contributes to this favorable outcome.

Double-Outlet Right Ventricle/Complex Transposition of the Great Arteries

Primary biventricular repair may be high risk if these lesions are associated with complex anatomy (i.e., complete AV canal defect with single papillary muscle, straddling AV valve, uncommitted VSDs with longer distance between LV and aorta, transposition of the great arteries with multiple VSDs and/or LV outflow tract obstruction), younger age at surgery, or borderline LV size.[8,16] In such patients, the staged approach may be applied for either growth of the ventricle or to distribute repair components over several operations in patients with complex anatomy. If the principal deficit is hypoplasia of the LV, mitral valve and/or LV outflow tract, then the staging procedure includes placement of a fenestrated ASD patch with partial repair of the left AV valve, LV outflow tract resection, and placement of an aortopulmonary shunt.[24] Growth of the borderline LV and left AV valve has been demonstrated to occur over time, and the response to left heart loading helps to determine suitability for eventual biventricular conversion (Fig. 61.4).

In patients with complex anatomy (straddling AV valves, AV discordance, elongated LV-aorta pathway) but normal-sized ventricles, a staged approach to repair is performed to avoid a single prolonged duration of cardiopulmonary bypass and aortic cross-clamp which can impair LV compliance and function in the early postoperative period. The presence of residual lesions impairs recovery and increases risk of mortality with biventricular conversion. The advantage of staged repair in patients with complex anatomy is serial assessment of the anatomic result and correction of any residual valvular lesions prior to biventricular conversion.[25]

Disadvantages of Staged Ventricular Recruitment

The most obvious disadvantage of the SLVR approach is the inherent need for multiple operations performed solely for left heart rehabilitation. Reoperation exposes a patient to additional risks associated with redo-sternotomy, cardiopulmonary bypass, and aortic cross-clamp. Surgical manipulation of the left heart adds the risk of valvular insufficiency and need for permanent pacemaker in a patient who might otherwise not incur such risks if undergoing standard single ventricle palliation. If the transitional circulation is not appropriately managed, suboptimal hemodynamics for single ventricle palliation may result. Specifically, left atrial and pulmonary hypertension from atrial septal restriction and valvular insufficiency may jeopardize the patient's candidacy for terminal single ventricle palliation or cardiac transplantation.

Much of the morbidity and mortality associated with single ventricle palliation are incurred in the first few months of life, following the stage I palliation. The early hazard associated with single ventricle palliation is not altered by staged ventricular recruitment. Since biventricular conversion is performed at 2–4 years of age, only the long-term risks of Fontan may be mitigated by SLVR strategy. Importantly, there are no data that demonstrate superiority of SLVR biventricular circulation over Fontan circulation.

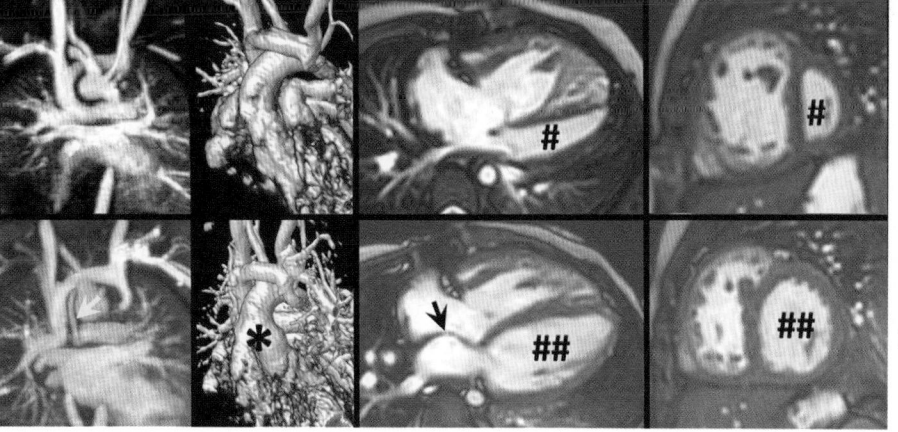

| Before LV recruitment | | LVEDVI 22 mL/m² MV flow 1.5 L/min/m² |

| After LV recruitment | | LVEDVi 85 mL/m² MV flow 4.4 L/min/m² |

• **Fig. 61.4** Before and after left ventricular (LV) recruitment. An 18-month-old child with transposition of the great arteries, LV outflow tract obstruction, and LV hypoplasia (#) had previously undergone atrial septectomy and bidirectional Glenn shunt (top row). The LV was moderately hypoplastic (22 mL/m²), and the mitral valve (MV) inflow volume was low (1.5 L/min/m²). Approximately 8 months after staged LV recruitment (bottom row) with addition of right Blalock-Taussig-Thomas shunt (yellow arrow) and fenestrated patch separating the branch pulmonary arteries, Damus-Kaye-Stansel (*), and atrial septal restriction (black arrow), the LV size increased (##) to 82 mL/m² and MV inflow volume increased to 4.4 L/min/m². The child subsequently underwent an uncomplicated biventricular repair. *LVEDVi,* Left ventricular end-diastolic volume index.

Who Should Be Considered Candidates for SLVR?

A patient should be considered for SLVR if the risk of primary biventricular repair is high and there are reasons to avoid sequelae of long-term single ventricle circulation. The risk assessment is institution-dependent. For example, a neonate with severe congenital mitral regurgitation may be deemed acceptable risk for primary repair at centers with experience in neonatal valve surgery but considered high risk at most other institutions. SLVR "takes the pressure off" of the surgeon to perform a high-risk primary biventricular repair by providing an option for gradual repair and eventual biventricular conversion.

In patients with risk factors for Fontan circulation (e.g., tricuspid regurgitation, RV dysfunction, pulmonary vein stenosis, pulmonary artery stenosis, elevated pulmonary vascular resistance, lung disease, Down syndrome), SLVR with biventricular conversion may be preferable to a high-risk Fontan circulation. At Boston Children's Hospital, patients with borderline left heart are candidates for SLVR even if they lack risk factors for Fontan. However, since patients without risk factors may demonstrate excellent outcomes for 10–20 years after Fontan, long-term data regarding success of SLVR-biventricular conversion are necessary to demonstrate benefit in this population. Patients who undergo salvage single ventricle palliation following unsuccessful biventricular repair should also be considered candidates for SLVR. With gradual left heart rehabilitation, patients who failed primary biventricular repair may become suitable candidates for eventual biventricular conversion.

When to Convert to Biventricular Circulation?

Between 2 and 4 years of age, the decision regarding ultimate circulation is made. Catheterization and MRI are used to inform this decision. Flow through the left heart as measured by MRI combined with the hemodynamics measured at catheterization help to determine ventricular compliance. Test occlusion of the residual ASD with simultaneous measurement of LV end-diastolic or left atrial pressure adds additional information regarding LV compliance. Biventricular conversion is reasonable for a patient with an LV end-diastolic volume > 30 mL/m^2, ejection fraction $> 45\%$, and end-diastolic pressures < 13 mm Hg with at least 50% of a full cardiac output crossing the left heart. Patients who do not meet these criteria are best managed along the single ventricle palliation pathway (Fontan).

The Borderline Right Heart

A borderline right heart involves hypoplasia of the tricuspid valve, RV, and pulmonary valve, and includes diagnoses such as tricuspid atresia or stenosis, PA/IVS, critical pulmonary valvar stenosis, left-dominant AV canal defect, and straddling valves with RV hypoplasia. As with the borderline left heart, the right heart structures typically have varying degrees of hypoplasia, which is likely related to flow-mediated growth and development. Tricuspid valve annular size is a good predictor of RV size and morphology. In patients with PA/IVS, severe tricuspid valve hypoplasia (i.e., annular Z score < -4) is associated with a severely hypoplastic, unipartite RV, frequently along with RV-dependent coronary circulation. In contrast, a tricuspid valve in the low-normal to mildly hypoplastic range (i.e., annular Z score -2 or greater) predicts a tripartite RV that is more amenable to biventricular repair.

As with the borderline left heart, it is typically wise to pursue initial single ventricle palliation in the newborn with a severely hypoplastic right heart. In these children, the right heart complex is not able to provide enough antegrade pulmonary blood flow to maintain acceptable saturations. Obligate right-to-left shunting at the atrial level supports systemic cardiac output (i.e., LV preload), but at the expense of reduced systemic oxygen saturations. A stable source of pulmonary blood flow is required in the form of a Blalock-Taussig-Thomas shunt or ductal stent. In the absence of RV-dependent coronary circulation, attempts to decompress the RV can be pursued in the newborn period for patients with PA/IVS. This can be done surgically with a transannular RV outflow tract patch, although transcatheter approaches are frequently used as well, including perforation of membranous or platelike pulmonary atresia and/or balloon dilation of stenotic pulmonary valves. In patients with critical pulmonary stenosis, catheter-based balloon dilation is the conventional therapy for the newborn. Decompressing the RV lowers the RV pressure and can improve ventricular compliance over time. Additionally, induced pulmonary regurgitation, either with a transannular patch or pulmonary valve balloon dilation, enables some retrograde flow in the RV that can help promote ventricular growth.

RV recruitment procedures are most commonly undertaken when a child is 4–6 months old, which is also around the time when a BDG would be performed. At this stage, evaluation of the right heart complex includes echocardiography and MRI to characterize right heart size and morphology, and to quantify flow across the tricuspid valve, ASD, and RV outflow tract. Catheterization and intracardiac pressure measurements can provide some measures for RV compliance. RV EFE can be seen in patients with PA/IVS, which can impact ventricular compliance. Test occlusion of an ASD can determine how reliant a child is on right-to-left atrial shunting and whether the right heart can handle a full cardiac output.

Ventricular recruitment addresses the three components of the right heart: tricuspid valve, RV, and RV outflow tract. Tricuspid valve intervention can involve annular enlargement with "relaxing" incisions on the annulus to enable annular expansion in response to increased transvalvular blood flow. In patients with PA/IVS, tethering attachments of the tricuspid valve leaflets to the ventricular wall are usually found and can be divided to improve leaflet mobility. Papillary muscles can also be split to improve tricuspid inflow. A critical component of RV recruitment is trabecular muscle bundle division and resection out towards the RV apex to improve chamber size. Preoperative echo and MRI are important for understanding ventricular wall thickness/hypertrophy when planning ventricular muscle division/resection. Transannular RV outflow tract reconstruction is also performed to provide an unobstructed egress of blood. In milder forms of right heart hypoplasia, where it is felt that the right heart can support a full (or nearly full) cardiac output, a fenestrated ASD patch is placed to partially offload the right heart (via right-to-left ASD shunting) and protect systemic cardiac output. In more severe forms of right heart hypoplasia, the recruitment procedure should include a BDG. This helps improve oxygen saturations and lessens the reliance on the right heart, which now need only support/pump IVC blood to the lungs. Right heart recruitment with a BDG creates a "1½ ventricular" circulation: the LV supports a full cardiac output, and the RV supports only about half of the cardiac output. Interval follow-up to assess right heart growth can be done with echocardiography and MRI. Repeat recruitment procedures, including re-intervention on the tricuspid valve, additional RV muscle division/resection, and RV outflow tract reconstruction, are sometimes required. In this regard, right heart recruitment is staged/gradual, in a way that is analogous to left heart recruitment, thereby

allowing for reassessment of right heart growth and adequacy. In cases where the right heart grows in response to recruitment, consideration can be given to complete biventricular conversion. This involves taking down the BDG so that the right heart complex supports the full cardiac output.

In patients with left-dominant AV canal defects, recruitment can involve "cheating" onto the left side of the common AV valve when partitioning the valve, analogous to what is done for right-dominant AV canal defects with LV hypoplasia. Importantly, unlike the borderline left heart, where an aortopulmonary shunt can be added to augment pulmonary blood flow and left heart preload, there is no way to augment right heart inflow using an aortopulmonary shunt. As such, recruitment relies on direct valvular work, "excavation" of the muscle bundles in the hypoplastic RV to increase cavity size, and RV decompression by opening the outflow tract. Furthermore, fenestrated ASD closure plays an important role by directing caval blood flow across the right heart. Fenestration size must be appropriate to promote trans-tricuspid flow without causing excessively high right atrial pressures (Fig. 61.5).

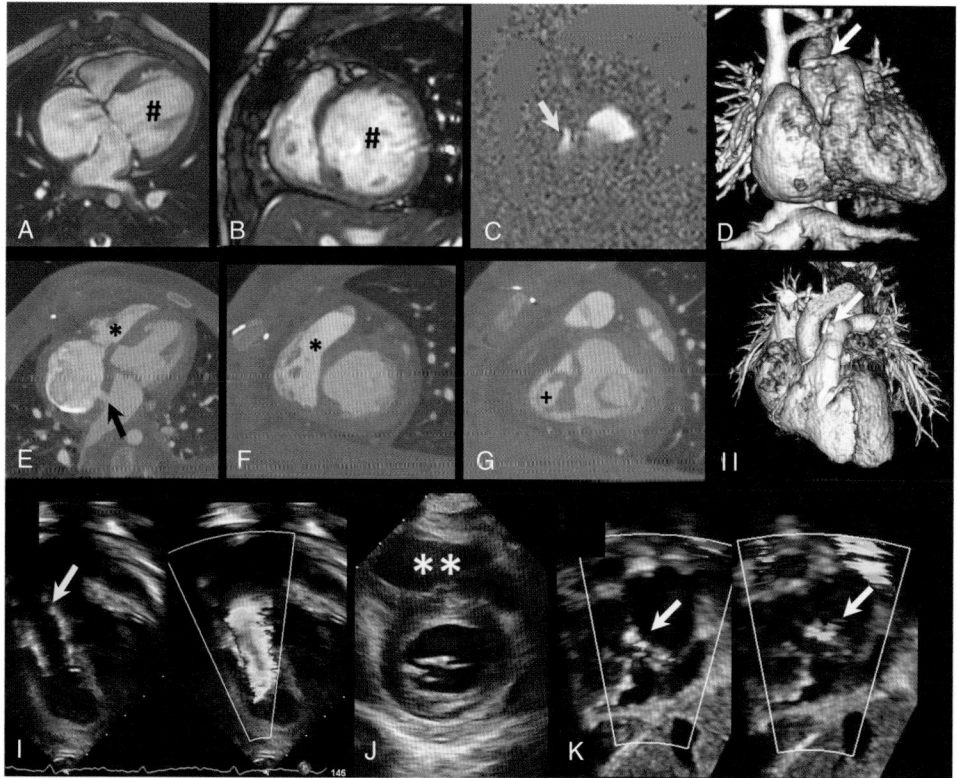

15 mo
S/P modified starnes with central shunt
RVEDVi 29 mL/m²
LVEDVi 107 mL/m²

34 mo
S/P BIV repair with 4 mm atrial fenestration
O₂ sats high 00's
RVEDVi 30 mL/m²
LVEDVi 56 mL/m²

5 yo
S/P melody in TV position
O₂ sat 97%
Mild RV hypoplasia with normal function

• **Fig. 61.5** Right ventricular (RV) recruitment to a biventricular (BIV) circulation. A 15-month-old child with trisomy 21 and left-dominant atrioventricular canal defect had undergone a modified Starnes procedure with central shunt. Top row: (A) and (B) There is notable ventricular size discrepancy (L > R) with dilation of the left ventricle (#) from atrioventricular valve regurgitation. (C) Tricuspid inflow is severely reduced (yellow arrow). (D) A central shunt provides the majority of pulmonary blood flow (white arrow). Middle row: (E) Following a BIV repair with central shunt takedown and a 4-mm atrial fenestration (black arrow). (F) and (G) The right ventricle (*) remains hypoplastic with a small tricuspid valve orifice (+). (H) A clip is visualized at the site of central shunt takedown (white arrow). Bottom row: (I) At 5 years old following tricuspid valve (TV) replacement with a Melody valve (yellow arrow). (J) The RV volume has improved (**). (K) There is bidirectional flow across the atrial fenestration (white arrows) and higher oxygen saturations. LVEDVi, Left ventricular end-diastolic volume index; RVEDVi, right ventricular end-diastolic volume index.

Conclusion

Staged rehabilitation of the borderline left or right heart provides an alternative to high-risk primary biventricular repair and terminal single ventricle palliation. In a patient with borderline left or right heart that is considered high-risk for repair, the ventricular recruitment strategy avoids "rolling the dice" early in life. The ventricular recruitment approach takes the predictable risk of initial single ventricle palliation, and the planned staged repair with gradual loading of the hypoplastic left or right heart allows serial assessments of the individual patient's candidacy for single vs. biventricular treatment pathway. If the left or right heart responds well, then one can feel more confident pursuing biventricular conversion in a controlled manner when hemodynamics are appropriate. Importantly, initial single ventricle palliation does not irreversibly commit a patient to long-term single ventricle circulation. When presented with a patient with a borderline left or right heart who has undergone previous single ventricle palliation, the current approach is to consider the possibility of rehabilitating the hypoplastic left or right heart at the time of BDG. It has been surprising in some cases as to how well the left and right heart can remodel if provided a gentle hemodynamic nudge. In conclusion, the current approach of *"Don't give up on the borderline left or right heart"* has been demonstrated to allow significant numbers of patients to achieve a biventricular circulation.

References

1. Alsaied T, Bokma JP, Engel ME, et al. Factors associated with long-term mortality after Fontan procedures: a systematic review. *Heart.* 2017;103:104-110.
2. Corno AF. Borderline left ventricle. *Eur J Cardiothorac Surg.* 2005;27:67-73.
3. Serraf A, Piot JD, Bonnet N, et al. Biventricular repair approach in ducto-dependent neonates with hypoplastic but morphologically normal left ventricle. *J Am Coll Cardiol.* 1999;33:827-834.
4. Tchervenkov CI, Tahta SA, Jutras LC, et al. Biventricular repair in neonates with hypoplastic left heart complex. *Ann Thorac Surg.* 1998;66:1350-1357.
5. Lofland GK, McCrindle BW, Williams WG, et al. Critical aortic stenosis in the neonate: a multi-institutional study of management, outcomes, and risk factors. Congenital Heart Surgeons Society. *J Thorac Cardiovasc Surg.* 2001;121:10-27.
6. Schwartz ML, Gauvreau K, Geva T. Predictors of outcome of biventricular repair in infants with multiple left heart obstructive lesions. *Circulation.* 2001;104:682-687.
7. Hickey EJ, Caldarone CA, Blackstone EH, et al. Critical left ventricular outflow tract obstruction: The disproportionate impact of biventricular repair in borderline cases. *J Thorac Cardiovasc Surg.* 2007;134:1429-1436; discussion 1436-1437.
8. Bradley TJ, Karamlou T, Kulik A, et al. Determinants of repair type, reintervention, and mortality in 393 children with double-outlet right ventricle. *J Thorac Cardiovasc Surg.* 2007;134:967-973.e6.
9. Erez E, Tam VK, Kanter KR, et al. Successful biventricular repair after initial Norwood operation for interrupted aortic arch with severe left ventricular outflow tract obstruction. *Ann Thorac Surg* 2001;71:1974-1977.
10. Pearl JM, Cripe LW, Manning PB. Biventricular repair after Norwood palliation. *Ann Thorac Surg.* 2003;75:132-136; discussion 136-137.
11. Emani SM, McElhinney DB, Tworetzky W, et al. Staged left ventricular recruitment after single-ventricle palliation in patients with borderline left heart hypoplasia. *J Am Coll Cardiol.* 2012; 60:1966-1974.
12. Emani SM, del Nido PJ. Strategies to maintain biventricular circulation in patients with high-risk anatomy. *Semin Thorac Cardiovasc Surg.* 2013;16:37-42.
13. Kalish BT, Banka P, Lafranchi T, et al. Biventricular conversion after single ventricle palliation in patients with small left heart structures: short-term outcomes. *Ann Thorac Surg.* 2013;96: 1406-1412.
14. McElhinney DB, Lock JE, Keane JF, et al. Left heart growth, function, and reintervention after balloon aortic valvuloplasty for neonatal aortic stenosis. *Circulation.* 2005;111:451-458.
15. Han RK, Gurofsky RC, Lee KJ, et al. Outcome and growth potential of left heart structures after neonatal intervention for aortic valve stenosis. *J Am Coll Cardiol.* 2007;50:2406-2414.
16. Takeuchi K, McGowan Jr FX, Bacha EA, et al. Analysis of surgical outcome in complex double-outlet right ventricle with heterotaxy syndrome or complete atrioventricular canal defect. *Ann Thorac Surg.* 2006,82:146-152.
17. Yerebakan C, Murray J, Valeske K, et al. Long-term results of biventricular repair after initial Giessen hybrid approach for hypoplastic left heart variants. *J Thorac Cardiovasc Surg.* 2015;149: 1112-1120; discussion 1120-1122.e2.
18. Prasanna A, Tan CW, Anastasopoulos A, et al. One and one-half ventricle repair: role for restricting antegrade pulmonary blood flow. *Ann Thorac Surg.* 2022;114:176-183.
19. Scully BB, Feins EN, Tworetzky W, et al. Early experience with reverse double switch operation for the borderline left heart. *Semin Thorac Cardiovasc Surg.* 2022.
20. Herrin MA, Zurakowski D, Baird CW, et al. Hemodynamic parameters predict adverse outcomes following biventricular conversion with single-ventricle palliation takedown. *J Thorac Cardiovasc Surg.* 2017;154:572-582.
21. Kwak JG, Del Nido PJ, Piekarski B, et al. Restriction of atrial septal defect leads to growth of hypoplastic ventricle in patients with borderline right or left heart. *Semin Thorac Cardiovasc Surg.* 2022;34:215-223.
22. Oladunjoye OO, Piekarski B, Banka P, et al. Staged ventricular recruitment in patients with borderline ventricles and large ventricular septal defects. *J Thorac Cardiovasc Surg.* 2018;156:254-264.
23. Nathan M, Liu H, Pigula FA, et al. Biventricular conversion after single-ventricle palliation in unbalanced atrioventricular canal defects. *Ann Thorac Surg.* 2013;95:2086-2095; discussion 2095-2096.
24. Oladunjoye OO, Piekarski B, Banka P, et al. Staged ventricular recruitment in patients with borderline ventricles and large ventricular septal defects. *J Thorac Cardiovasc Surg.* 2018;156: 254-264.
25. Nathan M, Karamichalis J, Liu H, et al. Technical performance scores are strongly associated with early mortality, postoperative adverse events, and intensive care unit length of stay-analysis of consecutive discharges for 2 years. *J Thorac Cardiovasc Surg.* 2014;147:389-394, 396.e1-396.e3.

62

Emerging Techniques in Cardiac Surgery

PEDRO J. DEL NIDO, ADITYA K. KAZA, AND DAVID HOGANSON

KEY LEARNING POINTS

- Congenital cardiac surgery continues to evolve through the decades. The chapter illustrates some of the innovative techniques that have been incorporated in the care of this patient cohort.
- There are emerging data with regards to the use of catheter-based palliation to stabilize neonates with congenital cardiac defects.

- Three-dimensional and flow modeling techniques can help us deliver more personalized care for patients with congenital cardiac defects.
- There are emerging techniques that can help surgeons determine location of conduction system inside the heart during open heart surgery.

Over the past 10 years, the field of pediatric cardiac surgery has been greatly impacted by the emerging late results of procedures that initially were felt to be definitive but, in fact, have turned out to be palliative. The long-term impact of hemodynamic and likely genetic factors on the progression of structural heart disease has resulted in development of new complications that were not readily apparent 20 years ago. An example is the management of single ventricle heart defects where direct cavopulmonary connections, which initially were deemed an excellent solution, are now recognized as resulting in progressive end-organ damage that is not readily reversed. At the same time, catheter interventions have advanced at a rapid pace to the point that many surgical palliative procedures aimed at balancing circulation pending more definitive repair are being replaced by minimally invasive catheter-based procedures. In parallel, diagnostic imaging has become less invasive and more precise and has evolved as not only a diagnostic tool but also an indispensable technique for surgical procedure planning and simulation, long before the patient enters the operating room (OR). These advances have led to the development of complex reconstructive techniques in cardiac surgery to address valvular heart disease, complex atrioventricular (AV) and ventriculoarterial connections, and techniques to optimize hemodynamics in ways that were not feasible in the past. Fetal imaging has also had an impact on neonatal procedures as the surgeon now has much more precise diagnostic and hemodynamic information than was available in the past, and this has permitted refinement of neonatal procedures with consequent improvement in operative

survival and frequency and severity of complications. We will address each one of these areas and describe the surgical techniques that are being developed.

Neonatal and Infant Surgery

Over the past 15 years, the practice of pediatric cardiac surgery has matured as a specialty. Among the most important changes that have occurred are those related to the surgical management of complex forms of congenital heart disease (CHD) in the neonate and infant. There have been significant advances in our understanding of the physiology of CHD, particularly with respect to the management of the single ventricle circulation. While neonatal corrections of most lesions where there are two ventricles has now become the standard, timing of the surgical correction has focused on optimizing the child's physiology and noncardiac status in order to reduce surgical risk and optimize late outcomes. The most significant impact has occurred as a consequence of new transcatheter interventions to stabilize physiology that can provide palliation often for days to weeks before surgical correction. Interventions such as ductal stenting for ductal dependent pulmonary circulation[1] and for ductal dependent systemic circulation offer alternatives to urgent surgical interventions for palliation, which are now being increasingly adopted. Catheter techniques still in development, such as blood flow restrictors to control pulmonary blood flow[2] and balance the circulation, will likely have an equally important impact on neonatal stabilization prior to definitive surgical intervention.

Biventricular Repair

To avoid the ongoing burden of an abnormal circulation, early anatomic correction is pursued whenever possible. Justification for early repair includes avoiding the chronic hemodynamic burden that palliation imposes on the developing myocardium, protection of the pulmonary vascular bed, and providing optimal support for the developing central nervous system. Furthermore, the palliated circulation is precarious and is associated with significant morbidity and measurable mortality, particularly during the early interstage period while the infant is awaiting definitive establishment of biventricular physiology. Examples of lesions that undergo definitive biventricular repair in the neonatal period include: transposition of the great arteries, with or without ventricular septal defect (VSD); aortic arch anomalies including coarctation and interrupted aortic arch (IAA); truncus arteriosus; and pulmonary atresia with VSD. In these lesions, symptoms of severe cyanosis or restricted systemic circulation are the major indications for intervention. In lesions where neonates are usually asymptomatic, definitive repair is usually deferred for several weeks to months, particularly if intervention on the AV valves is required as the surgical techniques for valve reconstruction in neonates and young infants still carry significant risk of residual defects and need for reintervention. Examples of these types of lesions include isolated VSDs and common AV canal defects.

Arterial Switch Operation for D-transposition of the Great Arteries

The surgical treatment of neonates with transposition of the great arteries has undergone a dramatic shift during the past 40 years. Before the introduction of the arterial switch operation (ASO) by Jatene et al. in 1975,[3] atrial-level repairs were the usual treatment. However, because late failure of the right ventricle and tricuspid valve in the systemic circulation was common, the ASO has become the procedure of choice in neonates with D-transposition, with or without ventricular septal defect. Whereas the atrial level switch was once reserved for difficult coronary artery patterns, even this indication has disappeared. In fact, the boundaries for the ASO are continuing to be defined. Because of concerns about left ventricular deconditioning for transposition of the great arteries/intact ventricular septum (IVS), early operation (before 3 weeks of age) has been considered mandatory. Patients presenting later have been considered for atrial-level switch operation, or two-stage repair. The latter entails an initial operation to perform pulmonary artery banding (often in conjunction with a Blalock-Taussig shunt) followed by ASO 7 to 10 days later. Although this approach has been successful, it has the disadvantage of two procedures, with an increased risk. Recent data suggest that primary ASO/IVS can be performed, supplanting the two-stage approach, even in older children with a poorly prepared left ventricle. In a report by Kang et al.,[4] 105

patients older than 3 weeks of age undergoing ASO, the mortality rate was 3.8%, and not different from the early (age younger than 3 weeks) group. Postoperative extracorporeal membrane oxygenation requirements were the same for both groups. These data would suggest that primary repair can be considered even for late presenting children with D-transposition of the great arteries/IVS. A VSD is present in about 25% of children with D-transposition. When unrestrictive, deconditioning of the left ventricle does not occur. However, prompt repair of D-transposition of the great arteries/VSD is recommended because these patients tend to develop early pulmonary vascular occlusive disease.

Surgery for Interrupted Aortic Arch

There has been a progressive improvement in the outcomes for children born with IAA complex. A recent review[5] of 472 neonates presenting with IAA between 1987 and 1997 was reported by McCrindle et al. and the Congenital Heart Surgeons Society. They reported an overall survival rate of 59% at 16 years, but noted improving survival over the time course of the study. Low birth weight, type B IAA, and associated major cardiac anomalies place the patient at higher risk for death. The incidence of subsequent interventions remains high. Thirty-four percent of survivors required later left ventricular outflow tract (LVOT) intervention, whereas 29% required intervention for arch obstruction. Some authors have advocated staged repair of IAA complex with severe subaortic LVOT. In these cases, Norwood palliation is performed, followed by subsequent VSD closure and the insertion of a right ventricle-to-pulmonary artery (RVPA) homograft. Although this is possible, we prefer to perform primary repair in the neonatal period. This approach has the advantage of comparable survival, with the additional benefit of a biventricular circulation in the perioperative period. Staged approaches (establishment of aortic continuity with a synthetic or tissue conduit, followed by later VSD closure) are largely of historic interest.

Tetralogy of Fallot

The goal of surgical treatment for tetralogy of Fallot is separation of the pulmonary and systemic circulations and relief of right ventricular outflow tract obstruction. Achievement of this goal depends on patient-specific anatomic substrate. Adopting the philosophy that early anatomic repair normalizes the circulation, early single-stage repairs of tetralogy of Fallot have been advocated by many groups. The major determinant of the suitability for primary single-stage repair rests on adequate development and distribution of the pulmonary vasculature. Asymptomatic patients ("pink tetralogy") are analogous to VSD patients with a pulmonary artery band, and primary repair is deferred until 4 to 6 months of age. For symptomatic (desaturated) patients presenting with adequate pulmonary arteries, prompt primary repair is performed. In these patients, complete repair includes VSD closure and relief of RVPA obstruction (usually with a transannular patch).

An atrial-level communication is intentionally left behind to allow right-to-left shunting at the atrial level during the postoperative period. This strategy has proven successful. In our review of 99 neonates and infants with tetralogy of Fallot with or without pulmonary atresia,[6] early mortality was 3%. Patients with pulmonary atresia were found to require reintervention more frequently as a consequence of the homograft repair. Although the long-term impact of early repair on right ventricular function remains unclear, this is our preferred approach to the symptomatic neonate or infant with suitable pulmonary artery anatomy. Palliation with a Blalock-Taussig-Thomas shunt is reserved for patients with significant comorbidities and contraindications to open heart surgery. More recently, we are able to palliate a majority of these patients in the catheterization laboratory with either a ductal stent or stenting of the right ventricular outflow tract. Although primary repair is suitable for patients with adequate pulmonary arteries, these vessels may be diminutive, discontinuous, or even absent in some. Whenever possible, we attempt to recruit the true pulmonary arteries by establishing antegrade flow from the right ventricle. Insertion of small aortic homografts (6 to 8 mm) into even very small pulmonary arteries (1 to 2 mm) is effective in stimulating pulmonary artery growth. In addition, this provides the interventional cardiologist access to the pulmonary circulation for the further rehabilitation of the pulmonary arteries. If these pulmonary arteries have adequate intraparenchymal distribution, the aortopulmonary (AP) collaterals become redundant and can be coil-occluded or ligated at surgery. For patients dependent on AP collaterals for pulmonary blood flow, the true pulmonary arteries are inadequate by virtue of their development, distribution, or both. In these cases, staged reconstruction of the pulmonary vasculature is often required. This involves the unifocalization of the AP collaterals into continuity with the available true pulmonary arteries, with connection to the right ventricle. In these cases, interventional rehabilitation of the pulmonary vasculature is indispensable in recruiting pulmonary vascular segments.

Because the approach for both scenarios must maintain and preserve right ventricular function, the VSD is closed when the pulmonary vasculature is deemed suitable and able to accept a full cardiac output with PA pressures that are <65-75% of systemic arterial pressures. In questionable cases, we have found it helpful to fenestrate the VSD patch. In the case of inadequate pulmonary vascular bed, this allows the shunting of blood from the right ventricle to the left ventricle, avoiding suprasystemic right ventricular pressures. With further pulmonary artery rehabilitation, the fenestration can be closed electively with a device during catheterization. This approach has been successful in managing this difficult group of patients.

Complete Atrioventricular Septal Defect

The endocardial cushion defects, frequently associated with trisomy 21, result from lack of development of the central portion of the heart. Anatomically, this results in characteristic defects in the atrial septum and ventricular septum. As a consequence, these patients have one large (common) AV valve spanning the AV connection. The surgical goal is the removal of all significant intracardiac shunts, and conversion of the single large AV valve into two separate AV valves, each dedicated to one ventricle. This is accomplished using one of three techniques that have been well described elsewhere. Briefly, the one-patch technique, the two-patch technique, and the so-called Australian technique have been used to repair these defects. After initial repair, 15% of children have required reoperation to address left AV valve repair. Valve re-repair was accomplished 75% of the time with the remainder requiring valve replacement. These children typically present for surgery after a period of medical management, and surgical repair is usually performed within the first 3 months of life. Children demonstrating important or intractable congestive heart failure before this should undergo prompt repair. For the occasional patient who appears to thrive during early infancy, persistent elevation in the pulmonary vascular resistance should be suspected, and early operation is likewise recommended.

Management of the Neonate and Infant With Single Ventricle Physiology

About 1 child in 5000 is born with CHD consisting of anatomy suitable initially for only single ventricle circulations. These lesions include hypoplastic left heart syndrome (HLHS), unbalanced atrioventricular canal defects (uCAVCs), double-inlet left ventricle, complex forms of double-outlet right ventricle (remote VSD or straddling or hypoplastic inlet valves), tricuspid atresia, and pulmonary atresia/IVS with right ventricle–dependent coronary circulation. The unifying theme of these lesions is a circulation supported by a single pumping chamber. While the list of lesions treated as single ventricle via staged palliative procedures is decreasing as new techniques for achieving biventricular circulation evolve, the basic concepts of initial management in the neonatal period remain. HLHS is characterized by a generalized underdevelopment of the left ventricle and its closely related structures: the mitral valve, the aortic valve, and the preductal/ductal aorta. In HLHS, the right ventricle must support both the systemic and pulmonary circulation. Pulmonary venous return must have unrestricted access to the right atrium, through an atrial septal defect (ASD), patent foramen ovale, or, rarely, anomalous pulmonary venous connections to the systemic veins. Systemic output, delivered through the ductus arteriosus, is entirely dependent on ductal patency. The treatment of HLHS has dramatically evolved since the 1980s. With little to offer before Norwood's introduction of stage 1 palliation in 1983,[7] treatment has developed into a three-stage progression to the Fontan operation. Although the 1-month mortality rate for untreated patients is 95%, the current 1-month survival rate among specialized centers approaches 80% to 90%. The "standard" Norwood operation involves incorporation of the pulmonary valve into the systemic circulation (Stansel connection), with patch augmentation of the hypoplastic aortic arch. Because the pulmonary valve is now committed to the systemic circulation, an alternative source of pulmonary blood flow is required. There have been systematic improvements in the surgical management of neonates with HLHS over the decades. The goals of the stage 1 surgical procedure have remained unchanged; these include preserving systemic perfusion, providing a calibrated source of pulmonary blood flow to protect the pulmonary vasculature, and creating an unrestrictive ASD. The goal of preserving systemic perfusion is achieved by aortic arch augmentation and the Stansel connection to combine the aortic and pulmonary roots. We routinely use regional cerebral and/or cardiac perfusion during the arch repairs, thus avoiding prolonged periods of deep hypothermic circulatory arrest.[8] We routinely excise the ductal tissue from the aorta circumferentially and augment the arch with either pulmonary allograft or autologous pericardium. An additional change that we have adopted for the Stansel connection is to surgically enlarge the diminutive aortic root in patients with aortic atresia to prevent any restriction to coronary blood flow.[9] There have been numerous iterations of providing calibrated pulmonary blood flow, which is done to both maintain adequate systemic saturations and protect the pulmonary vasculature for future palliations such as cavopulmonary connection. The most widely used source of pulmonary blood flow is the AP shunts. These AP shunts provide reliable pulmonary blood flow for the first few months of life until the child is an acceptable candidate for cavopulmonary connection. The significant diastolic runoff in patients with this type of shunt and adverse outcomes in patients with aortic atresia had prompted development of the RVPA shunts.[10] The current iteration of the shunt we utilize consists of a calibrated ringed GORE-TEX graft "dunked" into the right ventricle proximally and a piece of cryopreserved femoral vein with its valve distally which is anastomosed to the branch pulmonary arteries.[11] The theoretical advantage of this composite shunt is that the presence of venous valve prevents the diastolic runoff into the right ventricle and thus reduces the volume load on the systemic right ventricle. Atrial septectomy is performed using a brief period of circulatory arrest or low flow bypass. We routinely perform epicardial echocardiography at the conclusion of the procedure to ensure an unobstructed arch, good flow in the proximal coronary arteries, unobstructed branch pulmonary arteries, and an unrestrictive ASD. If there are any concerns for hemodynamic lability or hemostasis, we elect to perform temporary chest closure. In certain newborns with other comorbidities, such as extreme prematurity, severe growth restriction, an intra-cerebral bleed, or restrictive atrial septum, we have palliated them with a hybrid approach. The traditional hybrid approach consisted of branch pulmonary artery bands placed surgically and patent ductus arteriosus (PDA) stent and atrial septostomy performed in the catheterization laboratory.[12] We have since evolved into a nonsurgical hybrid done entirely in the catheterization laboratory. This entails placing flow restrictors within the branch pulmonary arteries, an atrial septostomy, and PDA stent versus continuing PGE infusion.[13] This approach has allowed us to achieve hemodynamic stability and overcome the additional comorbidities without an open surgical insult. These patients then subsequently undergo the stage 1 procedure. More recently, an alternative approach, one that targets manipulation of the systemic vascular resistance to maintain the balance between the pulmonary and systemic circulations, has been shown to be effective.[14]

Congenital Heart Valve Disease

Structural abnormalities of the cardiac valves are present in about a quarter of all congenital heart defects. Any of the four heart valves can be abnormal with a wide range of defects from hypoplasia and stenosis to malformations of the entire valve and subvalvular apparatus. In general, the surgical approach to malformed heart valves in children is to reconstruct the valves whenever possible with the recognition that repairs frequently do not result in long-term durability; however, the options for valve replacement carry a similar, or at times worse, late outcomes due to the added complexity of re-replacement later in life.

Aortic Valve Surgery

One of the more common valve defects involving the left side of the heart is malformation of the aortic valve cusps with leaflet fusion, often associated with annular hypoplasia resulting in stenosis. Since these lesions are present *in utero*, they can impact left heart growth and development with extreme forms resulting in HLHS. When the aortic valve lesion is the primary pathology, valvotomy to increase the effective orifice of the valve is the initial intervention, either by catheter balloon dilation, which is usually very effective,[15] or surgical valvotomy,[16] which achieves a similar result. Reintervention in the first 5 years of life is common, at times with repeat balloon dilation; however, if aortic valve regurgitation is present, then surgical intervention is usually recommended.[17]

Surgical repair of a dysplastic and poorly functioning aortic valve aims to improve mobility of valve leaflets that are reasonably well formed but fused and replace the leaflet segment that is either damaged or very deficient. A variety of techniques have been described, including leaflet augmentation with autologous pericardium, usually treated with glutaraldehyde to cross-link the collagen and prevent early deterioration.[18] Other tissue substitutes have been tried such as bovine pericardium, and porcine intestinal submucosa. Durability of these latter materials is also poor with rapid deterioration and calcification such that return of valve dysfunction requiring reintervention is seen on average 5 to 6 years after surgery. For this reason, some centers advocate valve replacement as the primary therapy with the pulmonary root autograft as the replacement valve of choice (Ross procedure). Since the native pulmonary root is used for aortic valve replacement, then usually a human allograft is used for pulmonary valve replacement. Late dilation of the autograft, now neo-aorta, is one complication of this procedure along with the technical challenges with performing the operation in a young infant. For this reason, many centers prefer to reconstruct the valve as the initial step, deferring the Ross operation to an older age. Valve replacement with bioprosthetic valves in children is uncommon due to the very poor durability of these bioprostheses with rapid deterioration and calcification. Mechanical valves offer better durability, although in a growing child, valve re-replacement will be necessary before reaching adult age, with the added disadvantage of needing systemic anticoagulation therapy as long as the mechanical valve is in place.

Mitral Valve Surgery

Congenital mitral valve disease poses some of the greatest management challenges faced by cardiac surgeons and cardiologists. The wide range of structural defects that can present as stenosis, regurgitation, or mixed disease along with the lack of viable replacement options, particularly for young infants, can at times lead clinicians to treat severe mitral disease with single ventricle reconstruction strategies used for HLHS. Despite the challenges, advances in reconstructive techniques and innovative use of off-label devices have yielded improved outcomes.

One of the more common presentations for mitral valve dysfunction is following repair of complete AV canal defects. Numerous repair techniques have been described for this indication, as often the problem is related to residual or re-opened cleft anteriorly. Reconstructive techniques for mitral valve in children have begun to borrow methods used in adult repairs, such as artificial chords made of expanded polytetrafluoroethylene (PTFE) to replace absent or torn native chords.[19] While early results are promising, reoperation rates of nearly 30% within 5 years are to be expected. For mitral valve replacement, small size mechanical valves down to 15 mm in diameter have been available since 2018 with approval of the SJM Master's series valve. While experience is limited, recent reports have shown improved mortality even in very young infants compared to previous reports with bioprosthetic devices, although median time to reoperation and explant was only 3.5 years.[1,20] Reports of implantation of a stented bovine jugular vein valve (Melody valve) have shown even more promising results with the added ability to catheter balloon expand the valves as the child grows.[21]

Pulmonary Valve Replacement

Pulmonary valve dysfunction is most commonly seen with tetralogy of Fallot, although isolated pulmonary valve disease, usually stenosis, is the second most common pathology. While catheter balloon dilation is an effective long-term, though not permanent, treatment, for isolated pulmonary stenosis, the associated lesions in tetralogy of Fallot require surgical intervention for definitive repair. Pulmonary valve-sparing techniques have been described with repair surgery for tetralogy, although late follow-up has often shown

progressive pulmonary regurgitation and right ventricular dilation similar to transannular patch relief of right ventricular outflow obstruction. Indications for pulmonary valve insertion for chronic pulmonary regurgitation continue to evolve as the consequences of chronic right ventricular dilation have been better understood.[22] Current options for pulmonary valve insertion are surgical prosthetic valve placement and, in selected cases, transcatheter implantation of expandable or self-expanding valves. The vast majority of valves implanted are bioprosthetic, either bovine pericardial or porcine glutaraldehyde-preserved valves. The results with these valves, however, have been disappointing in the structural deterioration with calcification with associated stenosis and/or regurgitation occurring in the majority of patients within 6–7 years following initial implant.[23] Valve-in-valve catheter placement of a new bioprosthetic valve is now common, although durability is still limited.[24]

Tricuspid Valve Surgery

Isolated tricuspid valve disease as seen in Ebstein anomaly or in congenital dysplastic or tethered valve is rare but can present in early infancy in the more severe forms. Usually surgical intervention is performed in children and young adults. Reconstructive surgery is the most common approach with excellent long-term results in experienced centers.[25] The most common indication for surgery in the tricuspid valve is when regurgitation is present and the tricuspid valve is the systemic AV valve, such as in HLHS. Large series place the incidence of moderate or worse tricuspid regurgitation in patients with HLHS at around 20%, persisting through all the stages of single ventricle reconstruction and a risk factor for survival following staged surgery.[26] Results with tricuspid valve plasty suggest a significant survival advantage when the repair reduced regurgitation by at least one grade. Preoperative right ventricular dilation and dysfunction were significant risk factors for reintervention and overall survival.

New Techniques

Electrophysiologic Mapping During Cardiac Surgery

Using techniques developed in the electrophysiology laboratory, our group has been able to use multielectrode catheters during open heart surgery. The patient is placed on cardiopulmonary bypass and fibrillated, the heart chamber is then opened, and after ensuring that there is no ejection the heart is defibrillated back into sinus rhythm. The multielectrode catheter array is utilized to provide an electrocardiographic road map of the HIS bundle and HIS purkinje system. This information is utilized to plan surgery and avoid injury to these conduction regions during surgery. Our group has successfully used this technique to decrease system conduction injuries in patients undergoing surgery for complex congenital heart defects.[27]

Fiberoptic Confocal Microscopy Mapping

Optical imaging using fiberoptic confocal microscopy (FCM) has been developed for use in congenital heart surgery. The process entails the use of a small fiberoptic probe and a topical dye, which enhances the autofluorescence of extracellular space. With this imaging technique, there are distinct features of the conduction system that can help distinguish this tissue from the adjacent normal myocardium (Fig. 62.1). Preliminary data have shown significant differences in the tissue architecture of normal myocardium compared with the tissue of the conduction system. The methodology has been found to be safe for use in humans.[28] Preliminary studies with this imaging modality has shown that there is considerable variability in the location of conduction tissue (Fig. 62.2) in hearts with simple defects such as VSD, tetralogy of Fallot, and AV canal.[29] Currently, a clinical trial is in progress to evaluate the role of FCM imaging in preserving conduction health in patients with complex CHD undergoing surgery.

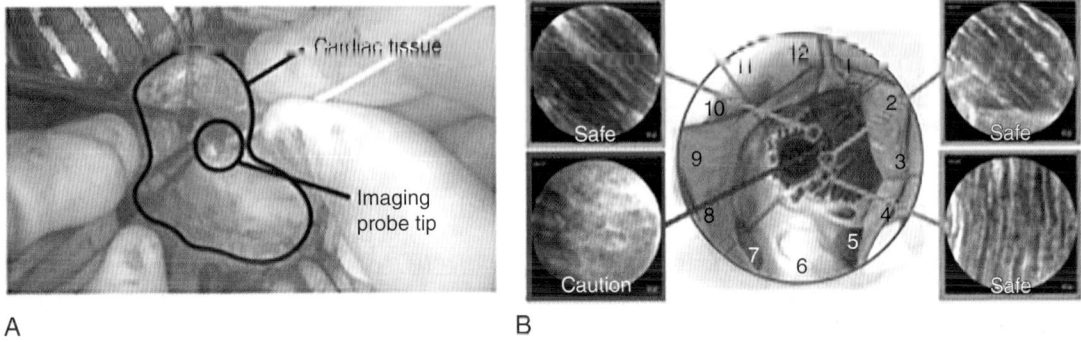

• **Fig. 62.1** Intraoperative identification of conduction tissue regions using fiberoptic confocal microscopy. (A) View of the pediatric heart surgical site from the surgeon's head camera. The imaging probe is held by the surgeon's fingers, stabilized with forceps, and placed on the region of interest. The faint blue coloration at the probe tip is light from the laser. (B) Clockface schematic with sites marked for imaging with example images taken from clockface regions 1 to 4 o'clock. Striated patterns at 1, 3, and 4 o'clock indicate the tissue in this region is working myocardium and the region safe for operative procedures. The pattern taken at the 2 o'clock position is irregular and reticulated, indicating a nodal tissue region, which should be avoided in surgical procedures. (Adapted from Kaza AK, Hitchcock R, Mondal A, et al. Systematic mapping of conduction tissue regions during congenital heart surgery. *Ann Thorac Surg*. 2022;114:1500–1504.)

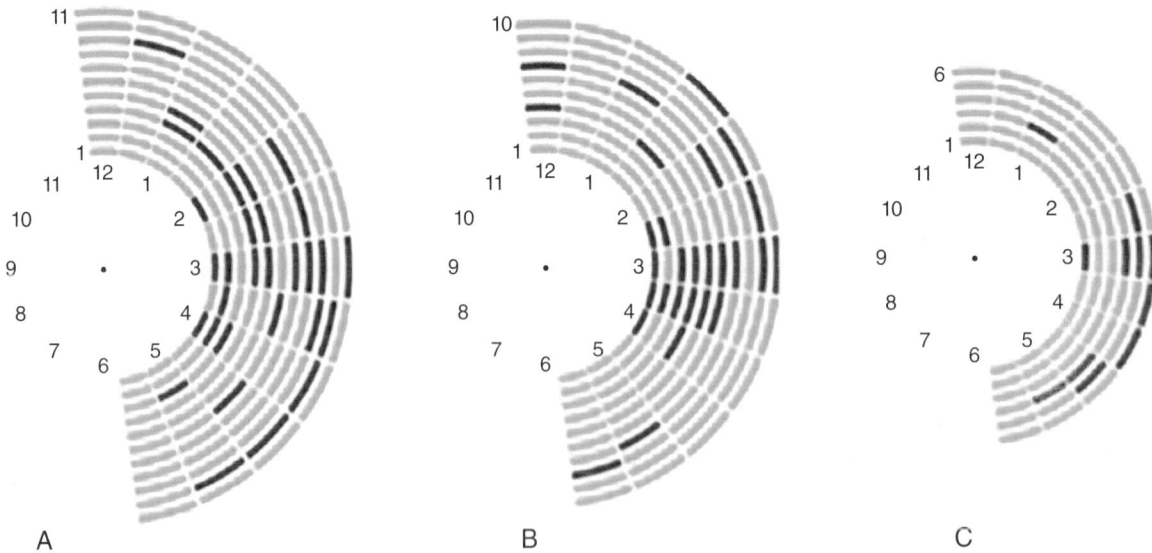

• **Fig. 62.2** Tissue type mapping on the clockface schematic during surgical repair of (A) ventricular septal defects, (B) atrioventricular canal, and (C) tetralogy of Fallot for 11, 10, and 6 patients, respectively. Each patient's mapping is stacked radially in concentric rings in increasing order of patient number. Mapping of the working myocardium and the conduction tissue region is indicated in green and red, respectively. Each arc describes the mapping for a single patient. (Adapted from Kaza AK, Hitchcock R, Mondal A, et al. Systematic mapping of conduction tissue regions during congenital heart surgery. *Ann Thorac Surg*. 2022;114:1500–1504.)

Clinical 3D Modeling and Surgical Simulation

The anatomic and physiologic complexities of patients with CHD demand intricate planning and consideration ahead of any surgical or interventional procedure. The more complex the case, the harder it is for the surgeon to visualize a complex, intracardiac reconstruction or the precise location relationships of all the cardiac structures during repair. The creation of 3D models from cardiac CT and MRI scans has become a mainstay technology for preoperative planning and intraoperative guidance of patients with complex CHD.

At Boston Children's Hospital, we have established workflows for creation and utilization of 3D models (Fig. 62.3). Segmentation software (Mimics, Materialize, Leuven, Belgium) is utilized by a trained team of engineers to create a precise surface 3D model of the patient's anatomy. The digital 3D model is employed in one of three workflows. The models are used as a digital model shared with the cardiologist, surgeon, and other members of the heart center team for preoperative planning and intraoperative guidance. In an additional workflow, the models can be used to virtually perform surgery for the purposes of quantitative reconstructive planning such as planning a patch reconstruction or a complex aortic valve repair. The final workflow involves virtual surgery, typically for single ventricle heart disease, and then flow simulation utilizing models to test different operative techniques using computational fluid dynamics software.

The 3D models created are shared across the heart center on an all-digital platform (Mimics Viewer, Materialize). During the segmentation process, the models are made with each of the different components of the anatomy constructed as different colored parts. Utilizing the Mimics Viewer (Fig. 62.4A), any combination of anatomical features from any view, including cut planes to look inside the structures are possible. This gives the clinician truly unlimited options to view the anatomy and plan an intervention. Shown in Fig. 62.4B is a 3D model of a patient with tetralogy of Fallot with pulmonary atresia and major aortopulmonary collateral arteries (MAPCAs), with the MAPCAs highlighted in different colors with two MAPCAs coursing behind the esophagus. The relationship between the MAPCAs and the airway (Fig. 62.4C) can be clearly visualized. In our center, over 800 3D models have been created for individual patients. Highlighted in Fig. 62.4D is a patient with multiple muscular VSDs visualized by looking into the right ventricle where the VSDs are outlined in green by the segmentation engineering team and the orange left ventricle can be seen through the VSDs. Fig 62.4E shows the same ventricular septum now visualized from the left ventricle where further anatomical details of the significant VSD burden can be appreciated. Patients with biventricular repair are among the most challenging intracardiac repairs. Fig 62.4F highlights a patient with d-TGA and multiple VSDs being considered for 1½ ventricle repair. The 3D model enables for visualization of the anatomy to plan baffling of the left ventricle to the aorta and the right ventricle to the posterior pulmonary valve. Before the release of the web-based digital viewer, 3D printing of cardiac models were the mainstay (and only means) of sharing the 3D models in our program. Given the fidelity of the digital 3D models and the unlimited views and combination of views with 3D viewer, 3D models are now only communicated through digital models. This includes the virtual surgery and flow modeling workflows. The models are utilized

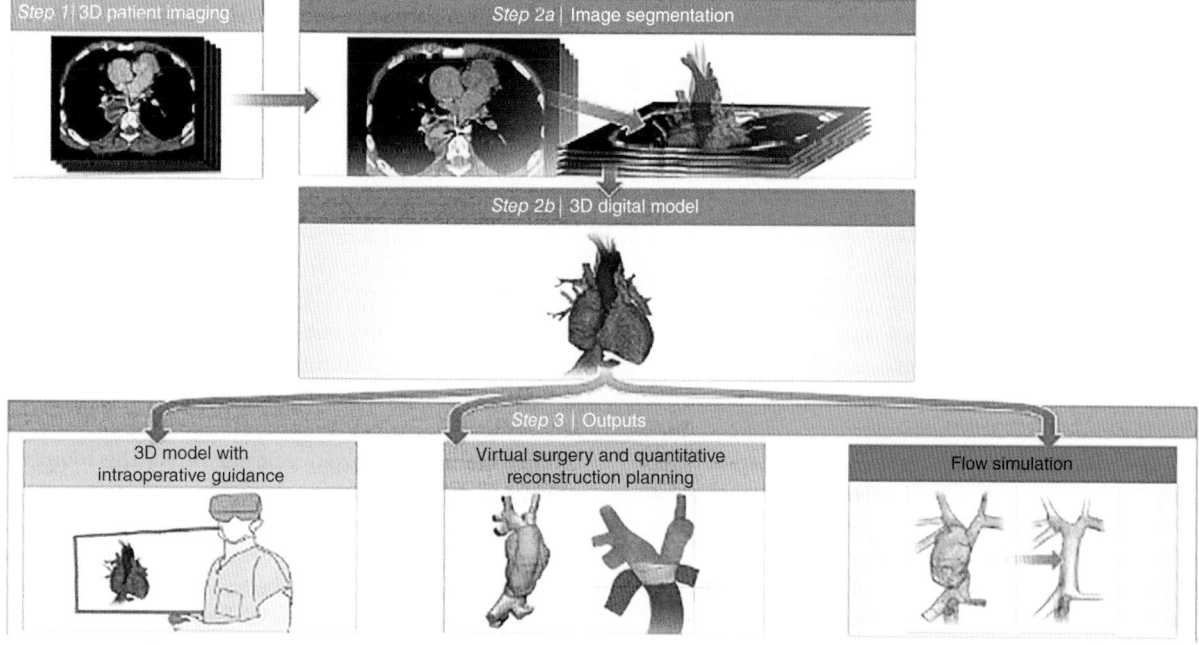

• **Fig. 62.3** Workflow to create patient-specific 3D digital models and utilize them for preoperative planning and intraoperative guidance, virtual surgery, and quantitative reconstructive planning and flow simulation.

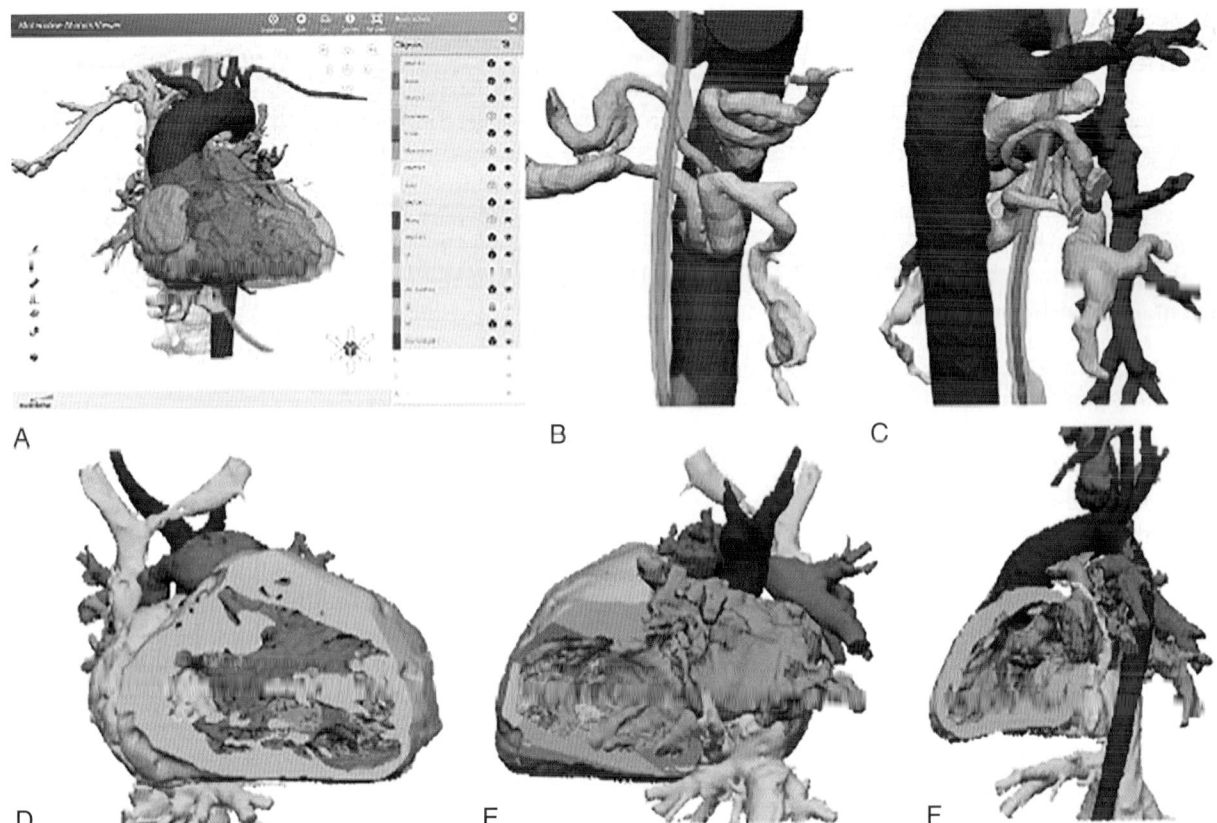

• **Fig. 62.4** Patient-specific 3D models (A) visualized on a digital web-based platform. (B) and (C) Model of a patient with tetralogy of Fallot with pulmonary valve atresia and major aortopulmonary collateral arteries (MAPCAs) where the MAPCAs (pink, light blue, brown, and green) are visualized arising from the descending aorta and coursing around the esophagus *(green)* and airway *(blue)*. (D) and (E) Model of a patient with multiple muscular ventricular septal defects (VSDs) visualized from the right ventricle (RV) (D) with the RV cavity shown *(blue)* and VSDs outlined *(green)* with left ventricle (LV) (orange) visualized through the VSDs. The same patient viewed from the LV (E) provides additional information on location and features of the VSDs. (F) Model of a patient with D-transposition of the great arteries and multiple VSDs viewed into LV *(orange)* with VSDs outlined *(green)* for planning of 1½ ventricle repair.

at our medical-surgical planning conference and many other clinical conferences every week. The 3D printed hearts are no longer utilized at our center. The cost and time savings of this digital-only platform have been enormous. Although the 3D models are exquisitely useful to better understand the anatomy and visualize repair options, virtual surgery and quantitative reconstruction planning can provide the surgeon with incredibly detailed information, which often cannot be reproduced only by intraoperative assessment of the anatomy of the arrested heart. The 3D models are created with hearts in a pressurized and active state, and depending upon the features of the scan, systole, diastole, or both states can be modeled. This capability is essentially important, as it allows dimensioning of patches, baffles, or other repairs to match the working state of the heart, not its flaccid state during reconstruction.

An example of the value of quantitative planning is shown in Fig. 62.5A. This is a teenage patient with complex single ventricle heart disease who underwent a lateral tunnel Fontan as a child. He has developed the markedly dilated lateral portion of his right atrium with tremendous flow recirculation and energy loss as a result. In planning a Fontan revision, the complexities of his PA anatomy made a simple extracardiac Fontan revision not feasible. The Fontan and graft would need connection to the branch pulmonary arteries that came off the top of the atria and in a Y-shape fashion. A custom "transition cuff" was required between the branch pulmonary arteries and the PTFE Fontan graft. Utilizing 3DEXPERIENCE modeling software (Dassault Systèmes, Vélizy-Villacoublay, France), this custom cuff design was created as a complex 3D shape (Fig. 62.5B and C) and then that shape digitally flattened (Fig. 62.5D) to provide a template for cutting the shape from a flat patch material to reconstruct the desired 3D cuff geometry. This template was utilized in the OR where a bovine pericardial cuff was created with excellent geometric fit to anastomose to the PTFE extracardiac Fontan conduit. Another example of quantitative preoperative planning is precise patch planning for neonatal arch reconstruction. This is a workflow in development that highlights the opportunity of 3D modeling to precisely plan surgical reconstruction and carry dimensioned plans for patches, baffles, and other interventions into the OR.

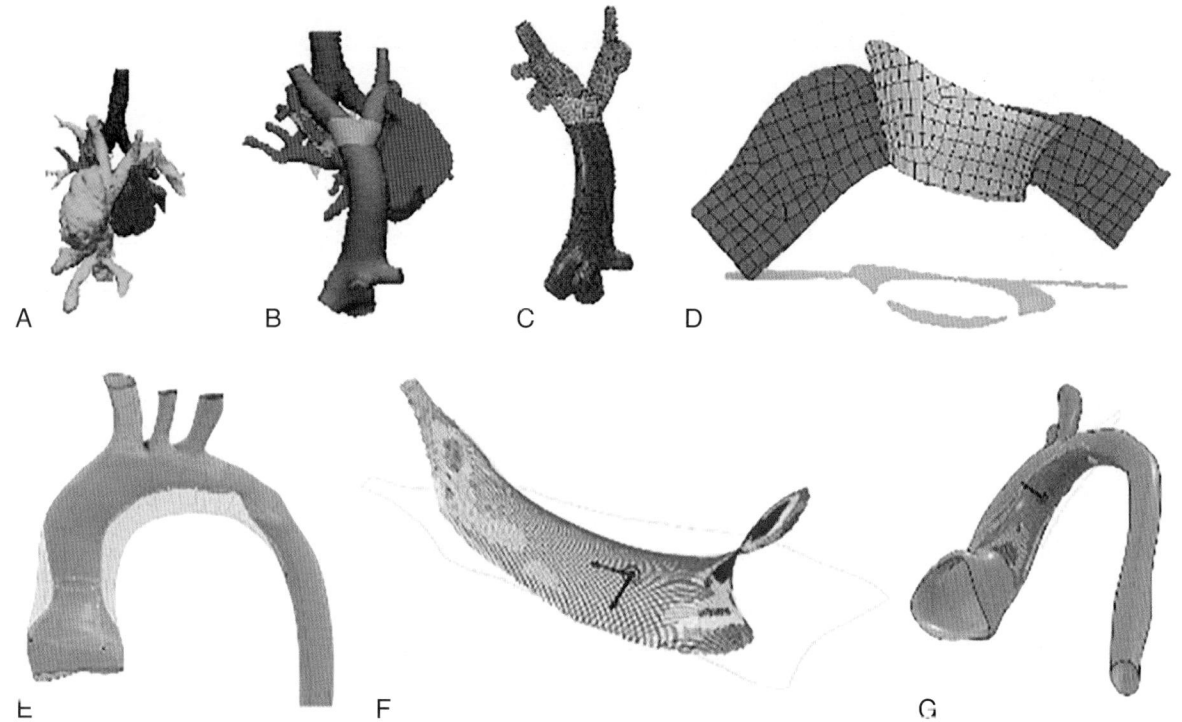

• **Fig. 62.5** (A) A 3D model of a Fontan patient with dilated right atrium *(teal)*. (B) Planned reconstruction with extracardiac Fontan conduit and transition cuff *(gray)*. (C) Engineering modeling of transition cuff *(gray)* to join conduit *(dark gray)* and pulmonary arteries *(pink)*. (D) Transition cuff design *(gray)* with flattened pattern equivalent that was used in the operating room to create the transition cuff from a flat patch material. (E) 3D model of hypoplastic aortic arch *(dark grey)* with planned arch reconstruction *(light grey)*. (F) Prospectively planned arch reconstruction patch with colors representing the stretch in the patch. (G) Planned aortic arch patch *(blue)* in digitally reconstructed aorta *(dark grey)*.

Shown in Fig. 62.5E is a hypoplastic aorta segmented from a CT scan with the native aorta in dark gray and the plan reconstructed aorta shown in light gray. This workflow for patch planning takes into account the mechanical properties of the native aorta and patch materials. The intended patch size is planned for the pressurized aorta and then that size adjusted according to the mechanical properties of the patch to a smaller size, which reflects the patch size at zero pressure. This is the state where the patches are cut out and sewn into the aorta. The 3D patch with the degree of curvature across the patch is highlighted by the color map (Fig. 62.5F). The maximal curvature of the patch is calculated and compared against the known maximal curvature of the patch material to ensure the patch will not kink when pressurized. The patch then undergoes a flattening algorithm with the flattened shape shown as a yellow outline (Fig. 62.5F). Fig. 62.5G shows the position of the patch on the underside of the aorta that accomplishes the desired reconstruction. Similarly, workflows are being developed for intercardiac patches including complex VSD closures and baffling of the left ventricle to the aorta in biventricular repairs. Pulmonary artery reconstruction will also benefit from this type of workflow as similar to the aorta, these are often multi-curve patches that have to be shaped from a planar patch material and the opportunities for patch kinking, residual narrowing, or oversizing the patch remain an everyday challenge.

Flow simulation of single ventricle patients have been demonstrated by several groups to have utility in accurate prediction of flow distribution and energy loss after Fontan reconstruction. Although seemingly straightforward in most patients, many nuances of the Fontan reconstruction deserve optimization. Given the lifelong impact of elevated Fontan pressures, small changes in resistance through the Fontana pathway can be very impactful. Single ventricle patients with complex systemic venous anatomy are at high risk for imbalance of hepatic venous return after Fontan completion. Our current clinical workflow (Fig. 62.6) begins with creation of the patient-specific 3D model, then virtual surgeries are performed to create models of the surgical options. These may include extracardiac Fontan, lateral tunnel Fontan, a hepatoazygous shunt for interrupted inferior vena cava (IVC) patients, or additional surgical maneuvers such as creation of a neo-innominate vein. Boundary conditions for the computational fluid dynamics problem are acquired from preoperative catheterization data and flows from 4D flow MRI. Flow simulation through the different surgical options are not only performed under the anesthetized condition that the catheterization and MRI data was acquired but also scaled up to predict normal resting physiology, postprandial state, and exercise state. These flow simulations for multiple physiologic states give a more holistic picture of the robustness of the surgical solution to deliver balanced hepatic venous return to the lungs in real-life conditions. Shown in Fig. 62.7A

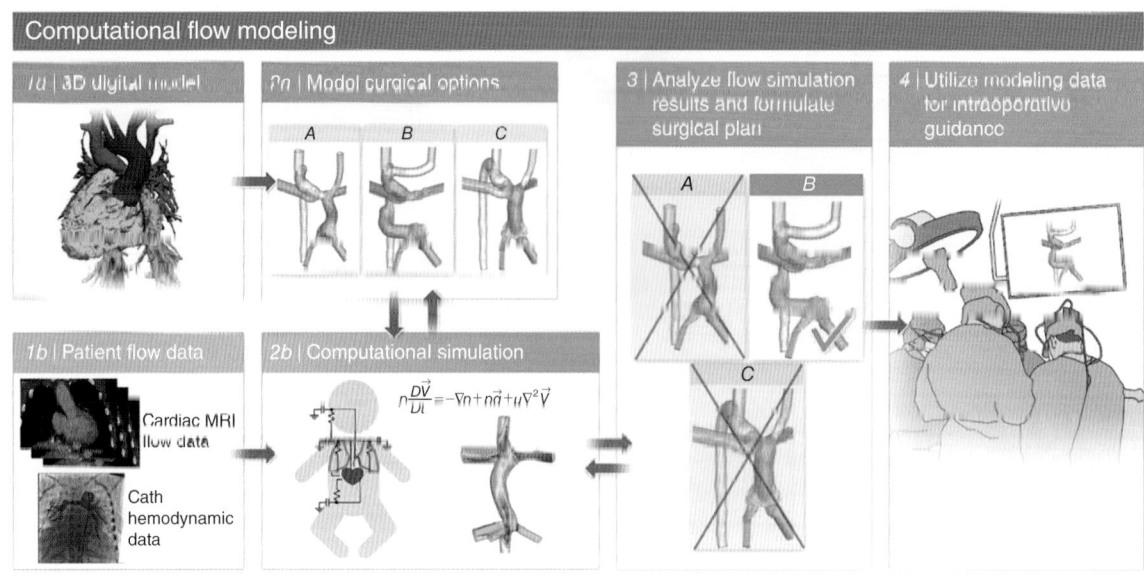

• **Fig. 62.6** Computational flow modeling workflow.

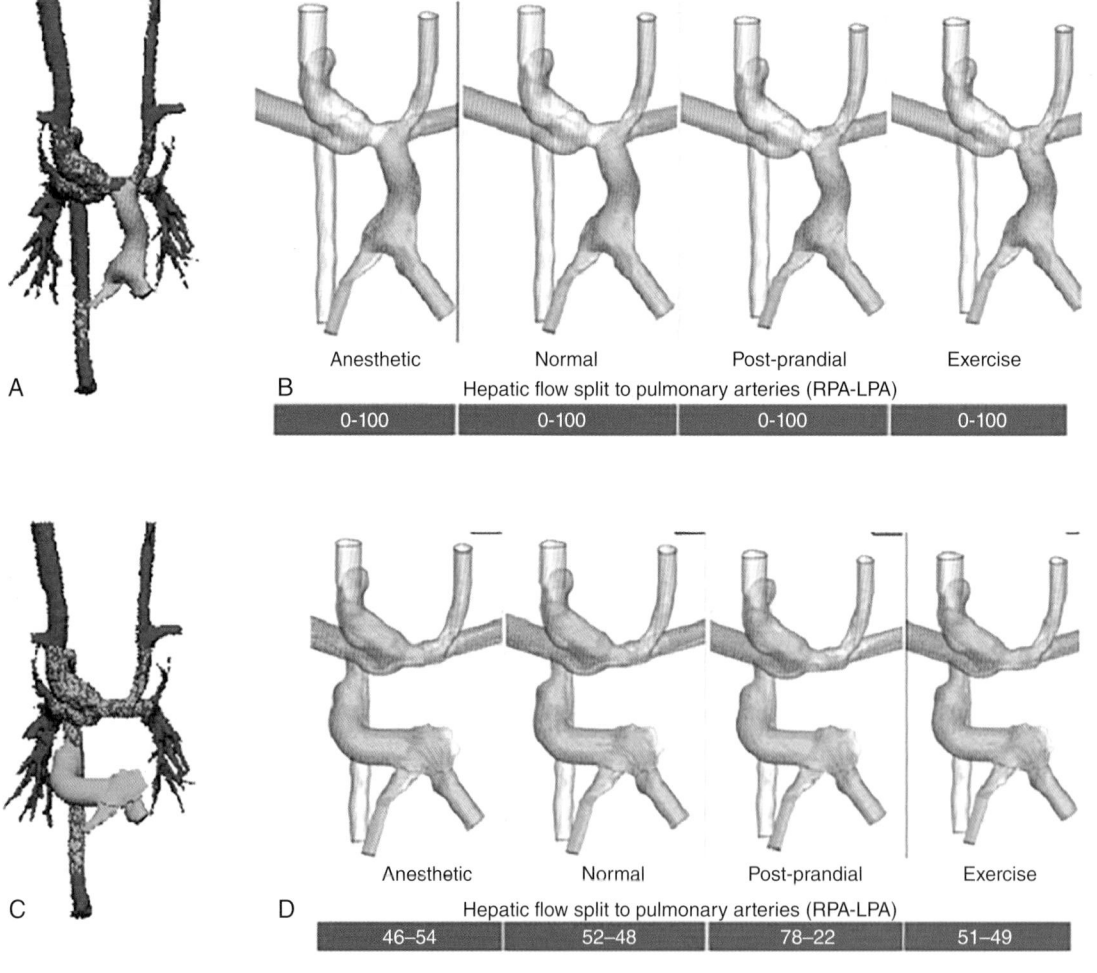

• **Fig. 62.7** (A) A 3D model of patient with interrupted inferior vena cava and azygous continuation with surgical option of extracardiac Fontan completion modeled with virtual surgery. (B) Flow simulation results of extracardiac Fontan over four physiologic states demonstrating all of the flow from the hepatic veins to the left lung. (C) Virtual surgery model of hepatoazygous shunt *(green)*. (D) Flow simulation results of hepatoazygous shunt over four physiologic states demonstrating good balance of hepatic venous return to both lungs.

is the anatomy of a complex patient with heterotaxy and interrupted IVC with azygos continuation on the right that had undergone a right-sided Kawashima procedure. The hepatic veins enter the mediastinum on the left. The initial proposed surgical approach was a completion extracardiac Fontan from the hepatic veins up to the pulmonary arteries. Flow simulation of this approach across the four physiologic states (Fig. 62.7B) demonstrate that the flow from the hepatic veins through the extracardiac Fontan graft would go only to the left lung. The child would have surely developed arteriovenous malformations in the right lung over time and required a Fontan revision. Given these results, flow simulations were performed for a hepatoazygous shunt (Fig. 62.7C). Flow simulation results across the four physiologic states (Fig. 62.7D) demonstrated good balance of hepatic venous flow to both lungs across. This child underwent a hepatoazygous shunt placement for Fontan completion and is doing well with no development of arteriovenous malformation. This workflow highlights the value of flow simulation in complex Fontan patients. This value can be extended to bilateral bidirectional Glenn procedures and even in a standard Fontan operation where there the placement options of the Fontan graft onto the pulmonary arteries relative to the Glenn connection may be optimized. These patients are at substantial risk for unbalanced hepatic venous flow to the lungs after the Fontan operation. Workflows for clinical 3D modeling and simulation have been developed that enhance preoperative planning and intraoperative guidance. Virtual surgery techniques using advanced modeling software by a trained engineering team in conjunction with the clinicians can result in computational preoperative planning for patches, baffles, and valve reconstructions. Single ventricle patients have benefited from virtual surgery plus additional flow simulation to understand hepatic venous flow balance and energy loss in different single ventricle reconstruction options. This flow simulation is also now being developed for pulmonary and arterial circulation with many opportunities to further optimize reconstructions that are performed. Given the tremendous complexities in congenital heart surgery, these workflows have been transformational in understanding and planning reconstructions.

References

1. Michel-Behnke I, Akintuerk H, Thul J, Bauer J, Hagel KJ, Schranz D. Stent implantation in the ductus arteriosus for pulmonary blood supply in congenital heart disease. *Catheter Cardiovasc Interv*. 2004;61:242-252.
2. Schranz D, Esmaeili A, Akintuerk H. Hypoplastic left heart: stage-I will be performed interventionally, soon. *Pediatr Cardiol*. 2021;42:727-735.
3. Jatene AD, Fontes VF, Paulista PP, et al. Successful anatomic correction of transposition of the great vessels: a preliminary report. *Arq Bras Cardiol*. 1975;28:461-464.
4. Kang N, de Leval MR, Elliott M, et al. Extending the boundaries of the primary arterial switch operation in patients with transposition of the great arteries and intact ventricular septum. *Circulation*. 2004;110:II123-II127.
5. McCrindle BW, Tchervenkov CI, Konstantinov IE, et al. Risk factors associated with mortality and interventions in 472 neonates with interrupted aortic arch: a Congenital Heart Surgeons Society study. *J Thorac Cardiovasc Surg*. 2005;129:343-350.
6. Pigula FA, Khalil PN, Mayer JE, del Nido PJ, Jonas RA. Repair of tetralogy of Fallot in neonates and young infants. *Circulation*. 1999;100:II157-II161.
7. Norwood WI, Lang P, Castaneda AR, Campbell DN. Experience with operations for hypoplastic left heart syndrome. *J Thorac Cardiovasc Surg*. 1981;82:511-519.
8. Tchervenkov CI, Chu VF, Shum-Tim D, Laliberte E, Reyes TU. Norwood operation without circulatory arrest: a new surgical technique. *Ann Thorac Surg*. 2000;70:1730-1733.
9. Hoganson DM, Piekarski BL, Quinonez LG, et al. Patch augmentation of small ascending aorta during stage I procedure reduces the risk of morbidity and mortality. *Eur J Cardiothorac Surg*. 2022;61:555-561.
10. Sano S, Ishino K, Kawada M, et al. Right ventricle-pulmonary artery shunt in first-stage palliation of hypoplastic left heart syndrome. *J Thorac Cardiovasc Surg*. 2003;126:504-509.
11. Hoganson DM, Cigarroa CL, van den Bosch SJ, et al. Impact of a composite valved RV-PA graft after stage 1 palliation. *Ann Thorac Surg*. 2018;106:1452-1459.
12. Schranz D, Bauer A, Reich B, et al. Fifteen-year single center experience with the "Giessen Hybrid" approach for hypoplastic left heart and variants: current strategies and outcomes. *Pediatr Cardiol*. 2015;36:365-373.
13. Kurtz JD, Alsoufi B, Wilkens SJ, Kim E. Modified microvascular plug as a flow restrictor in hypoplastic left heart syndrome with dysplastic tricuspid and pulmonary valves. *Pediatr Cardiol*. 2021;42:1653-1657.
14. Mills KI, Kaza AK, Walsh BK, et al. Phosphodiesterase inhibitor-based vasodilation improves oxygen delivery and clinical outcomes following stage 1 palliation. *J Am Heart Assoc*. 2016;5:e003554.
15. McElhinney DB, Lock JE, Keane JF, Moran AM, Colan SD. Left heart growth, function, and reintervention after balloon aortic valvuloplasty for neonatal aortic stenosis. *Circulation*. 2005;111:451-458.
16. Buratto E, Konstantinov IE. Aortic valve surgery in children. *J Thorac Cardiovasc Surg*. 2021;161:244-250.
17. Kido T, Guariento A, Doulamis IP, et al. Aortic valve surgery after neonatal balloon aortic valvuloplasty in congenital aortic stenosis. *Circ Cardiovasc Interv*. 2021;14:e009933.
18. Baird CW, Cooney B, Chávez M, Sleeper LA, Marx GR, Del Nido PJ. Congenital aortic and truncal valve reconstruction using the Ozaki technique: short-term clinical results. *J Thorac Cardiovasc Surg*. 2021;161:1567-1577.
19. Oda S, Nakano T, Tatewaki H, Hinokiyama K, Machida D, Kado H. A 17-year experience with mitral valve repair with artificial chordae in infants and children. *Eur J Cardiothorac Surg*. 2013;44:e40-e45.
20. Isselhof RJ, Slieker MG, Hazekamp MG, et al. Mitral valve replacement with the 15-mm mechanical valve: a 20-year multicenter experience. *Ann Thorac Surg*. 2020;110:956-961.
21. Pluchinotta FR, Piekarski BL, Milani V, et al. Surgical atrioventricular valve replacement with Melody valve in infants and children: a multicenter study. *Circ Cardiovasc Interv*. 2018;11:e007145.
22. Fuller S. Tetralogy of Fallot and pulmonary valve replacement: timing and techniques in the asymptomatic patient. *Semin Thorac Cardiovasc Surg Pediatr Card Surg Annu*. 2014;17:30-37.

23. Nomoto R, Sleeper LA, Borisuk MJ, et al. Outcome and performance of bioprosthetic pulmonary valve replacement in patients with congenital heart disease. *J Thorac Cardiovasc Surg*. 2016;152:1333-1342.

24. McElhinney DB, Zhang Y, Levi DS, et al. Reintervention and survival after transcatheter pulmonary valve replacement. *J Am Coll Cardiol*. 2022;79:18-32.

25. Da Silva JP, Viegas M, Castro Medina M, Da Silva LD. The Da Silva cone operation after the Starnes procedure for Ebstein's anomaly: new surgical strategy and initial results. *JTCVS Tech*. 2020;3:281-283.

26. Wamala I, Friedman KG, Saeed MI, et al. Tricuspid valve repair concomitant with the Norwood operation among babies with hypoplastic left heart syndrome. *Eur J Cardiothorac Surg*. 2022; 62:ezac033.

27. Feins EN, O'Leary ET, Hoganson DM, et al. Intraoperative conduction mapping in complex congenital heart surgery. *JTCVS Tech*. 2022;12:159-163.

28. Kaza AK, Mondal A, Piekarski B, Sachse FB, Hitchcock R. Intraoperative localization of cardiac conduction tissue regions using real-time fibre-optic confocal microscopy: first in human trial. *Eur J Cardiothorac Surg*. 2020;58:261-268.

29. Kaza AK, Hitchcock R, Mondal A, et al. Systematic mapping of conduction tissue regions during congenital heart surgery. *Ann Thorac Surg*. 2022;114:1500-1504.

63

Sedation and Anesthesia in Cardiac Procedures

VIVIANE G. NASR AND JAMES DINARDO

KEY LEARNING POINTS

- There is substantial diversity and variation in severity and pathophysiology of each lesion in patients with congenital and acquired heart disease. Individualized sedation/anesthetic management is critical and should be based on the known effects of sedative and anesthetic agents in patients with variable hemodynamic reserve.
- The American Society of Anesthesiologists has clearly defined the continuum of sedation and anesthesia including: Anxiolysis, Conscious sedation, Deep Sedation/Analgesia, and General Anesthesia.
- There are a variety of inhaled and non-inhaled agents that can be effectively utilized, alone or in combination with other agents, to provide premedication, sedation, induction, and maintenance of general anesthesia. Understanding

the mechanisms of action, pharmacokinetics, and potential adverse events is a must when caring for patients with congenital heart disease.

- Important considerations when caring for patients with sedation/general anesthesia include location, procedure, temperature management, radiation safety, patient positioning, and mechanical support devices.
- Through interactions with receptors and ion channels in the myocardium, commonly used anesthetics and sedatives have varying degrees of direct effect on normal cardiac conduction and on the three primary mechanisms of arrhythmogenesis. In addition, these agents may indirectly affect cardiac electrophysiology through modulation of sympathetic and parasympathetic tone.

Introduction

Comprehensive care of patients with congenital heart disease (CHD) lesions is often dependent upon meticulous planning and execution of catheter-based and surgical procedures. Essential to this process is information obtained from advanced imaging techniques. While general anesthesia (GA) is a necessity for performance of virtually all surgical procedures, sedation or GA may also be necessary to facilitate performance of imaging and catheter-based procedures in neonates, infants, young children, and some adults. There is substantial diversity and variation in severity and pathophysiology of each lesion in patients with CHD and acquired heart disease. Individualized sedation/anesthetic management is critical and should be based on the known effects of sedative and anesthetic agents in patients with variable hemodynamic reserve. This chapter will review the most common sedative and anesthetic agents and highlight specific considerations during surgical procedures, cardiac catheterizations, electrophysiologic studies, and imaging.

Defining Levels of Sedation and General Anesthesia

The American Society of Anesthesiologists has clearly defined the continuum of sedation and anesthesia, and this is summarized in Table 63.1.[1] From a practical point of view, all pediatric patients require moderate to deep sedation or GA to facilitate successful performance of surgical and interventional procedures. In some instances, deep sedation or GA may be necessary to allow performance of diagnostic and noninvasive imaging procedures. Ideally the sedation or anesthesia plan should ensure patient comfort and safety, and limit movement. In infants and young children, or older children and young adults with psychological or behavioral limitations, the anesthetic plan generally requires GA. Moderate to deep sedation may be appropriate for older, more cooperative patients and procedures where a GA is not needed. In instances where the indication for intervention relies on physiology that is significantly affected by the level of sedation, such as obtaining a valvar gradient for balloon aortic valvuloplasty, minimal sedation

TABLE 63.1	Continuum of Depth of Sedation: Definition of General Anesthesia and Levels of Sedation/Analgesia			
	Minimal sedation (Anxiolysis)	Moderate sedation/analgesia (conscious sedation)	Deep sedation/analgesia	General anesthesia
Responsiveness	Normal response to verbal stimulation	Purposeful response to verbal or tactile stimulation*	Purposeful response after repeated or painful stimulation	Unarousable, even with painful stimulus
Airway	Unaffected	No intervention required	Intervention may be required	Intervention often required
Spontaneous ventilation	Unaffected	Adequate	May be inadequate	Frequently inadequate
Cardiovascular function	Unaffected	Usually maintained	Usually maintained	May be impaired

*Reflex withdrawal from a painful stimulus is not considered a purposeful response.
From the Report by the American Society of Anesthesiologists Task Force on Moderate Procedural Sedation and Analgesia. (Anesthesiology 2018)[1]

with local anesthetic may be desirable prior to initiation of deep sedation or GA for the actual intervention. GA may be necessary during long procedures to facilitate patient comfort or during procedures where difficult vascular access or complex catheter manipulations are anticipated. Because individual responses to the sedative medications are not predictable, the practitioner must be adequately qualified to manage the airway and the hemodynamic alterations associated with deeper levels of sedation than initially planned.

Non-inhaled Sedative and Anesthetic Agents

There are a variety of non-inhaled agents which can be effectively utilized, alone or in combination with other agents, to provide premedication, sedation, and induction and maintenance of GA. These are summarized in Table 63.2.

Benzodiazepines

Midazolam is the most commonly used benzodiazepine in anesthesia practice. It has a rapid onset of action, a short duration of action, and a short half-life. It can be administered via intravenous (IV), oral, intranasal, intramuscular (IM), and rectal routes. Midazolam is metabolized in the liver by the cytochrome p450 isoenzyme 3A4 and is highly protein bound. An increase in free fraction can occur in patients receiving other highly protein-bound medications, and in patients with liver and renal failure. Midazolam's pharmacokinetic profile makes it suitable for continuous infusion without excessive accumulation.[2] Remimazolam, like midazolam, inhibits neural activity by enhancing γ-amino-butyric acid A receptor activity. It is a "soft drug" with a carboxylic ester moiety incorporated into its core. Consequently, similar to remifentanil, remimazolam is rapidly hydrolyzed to a pharmacologically inactive metabolite

via non-specific tissue esterase activity; this leads to the fast onset and offset of sedation and predictable duration of action. As with other benzodiazepines, flumazenil can be used to reverse the sedation effect of remimazolam.[3]

Intravenous Anesthetics

Ketamine is a phencyclidine derivative, classified as a dissociative anesthetic agent. It effectively dissociates the thalamic and limbic systems and provides intense analgesia. An IV dose of 2 to 3 mg/kg has a rapid onset, short duration of action between 10 and 15 minutes, and elimination half-life between 2 and 3 hours. Ketamine typically provides hemodynamic stability because both heart rate and blood pressure usually increase through sympathomimetic actions resulting from central stimulation and diminished postganglionic catecholamine uptake. There are conflicting reports about the effect of ketamine on pulmonary vascular resistance.[4] Although patients predisposed to pulmonary hypertension may demonstrate an increase in pulmonary artery pressure after ketamine administration, the response is usually minimal. On balance, therefore, ketamine can be used in patients with pulmonary hypertension, provided events such as hypoventilation and airway obstruction are avoided.

Etomidate is an IV agent that provides loss of consciousness and analgesia with the advantage of minimal cardiovascular and respiratory depression.[5] An IV dose of 0.3 mg/kg induces a rapid loss of consciousness with a duration of 3 to 5 minutes. It may cause pain on injection and is associated with spontaneous movements, hiccupping, and myoclonus. It is primarily used as an alternative to the synthetic opioids for induction of GA in patients with limited myocardial reserve. It is not approved for continuous infusion because of depression to adrenal steroidogenesis.[6]

Propofol is an IV hypnotic drug that is used for induction and maintenance of sedation and GA. It exerts its effects through potentiation of the inhibitory neurotransmitter

TABLE 63.2	Route of Administration, Pharmacokinetic Properties, and Adverse Effects of Commonly Used Sedatives and Analgesics				
Drugs	**Route**	**Bolus**	**Infusion**	**Pharmacokinetic properties**	**Adverse effects**
Benzodiazepine					
Midazolam	Oral Intramuscular Intravenous Intranasal Rectal	Yes	Yes	Onset 1–5 minutes Duration of action 10–30 minutes Half life varies with patient age 2.5–10 hours	Increased accumulation in hepatic and renal impairment
Remimazolam	Intravenous	Yes	No	Peak effect 3–3.5 minutes Duration of action 11–14 minutes after last dose Half life 37–53 minutes	Not studied in children
Anesthetics/Sedatives					
Propofol	Intravenous	Yes	Yes	Onset 30 seconds Half-life 30–60 minutes	Respiratory depression, apnea, propofol infusion syndrome (PRIS), cardiovascular depressant
Dexmedetomidine	Intravenous Intranasal	Yes	Yes	Intravenous: onset 5–10 minutes Intranasal: onset 45–60 minutes Half-life varies with patient age	Intravenous bolus associated with bradycardia and hypo/ hypertension
Ketamine	Oral Intramuscular Intravenous	Yes	Yes	Onset 30 seconds Half-life 2.5 hours	Nausea, salivation, bronchospasm, hypotension in patients with depleted catecholamine
Etomidate	Intravenous	Yes	No	Onset 30–60 seconds Half-life 2.6–3.5 hours	
Opioids					
Fentanyl	Intravenous	Yes	Yes	Onset 30 seconds Short duration of action Half-life 2 hours, context-sensitive half-life 21 hours	Nausea, constipation, respiratory depression
Remifentanil	Intravenous	Yes	Yes	Very quick onset Half-life 5–10 minutes Steady state 10–15 minutes after administration of a continuous infusion	Bradycardia, respiratory depression
Morphine	Intravenous	Yes	Yes	Peak at 20 minutes Half-life 1–3 hours in infants and children, 10–20 hours in preterm neonates	Nausea, constipation, respiratory depression, bronchospasm, vasodilation, hypotension, pruritus
Methadone	Intravenous	Yes	No	Peak at 1–2 hours Half-life 19 hours	Bradycardia, hypotension, arrhythmias (prolonged QT interval)

γ-aminobutyric acid (GABA) at the GABA A receptor. Propofol is known to affect mitochondrial metabolism via multiple mechanisms; uncoupling oxidative phosphorylation and inhibiting complexes I, II, and IV. Perhaps more importantly, it inhibits the transport of long-chain acylcarnitine esters via an inhibition of acylcarnitine transferase. This effect has been implicated as the mechanism behind propofol infusion syndrome (PRIS), a potentially fatal complication of long-term propofol infusions. Given the multiple mitochondrial effect sites of propofol, propofol-based anesthetic techniques should be avoided in patients with known or suspected mitochondrial disorder.[7]

Therapeutic plasma concentrations of propofol result in a decrease in mean arterial blood pressure due to the interaction of decreased stressed venous volume (venodilation), reduced systemic vascular resistance, reduced resistance to venous return, and maintained cardiac output.[8] Propofol is a phenol derivative supplied in a soy emulsion and egg phospholipid to make an injectable substance. Because propofol has a short duration of action and rapid clearance, it has been used by infusion or repeated bolus doses with patients awakening rapidly when it is discontinued. Titrated doses of propofol 1 to 2 mg/kg can be used to induce loss of consciousness for short procedures such as cardioversion in hemodynamically stable patients. A major disadvantage is pain on injection. Perhaps more important is propofol's narrow therapeutic index. It is not uncommon for a dose of propofol intended to induce sedation to result in apnea, hypotension, and the need for advanced airway and hemodynamic management skills to rescue the patient.

Dexmedetomidine is a potent and highly selective central α-2 adrenergic receptor agonist with sedative, anxiolytic, sympatholytic, and analgesic properties. The use of a background infusion of dexmedetomidine (0.2–1.0 ug/kg/h) during sedation and GA has become increasingly popular as a method to reduce opioid and benzodiazepine requirements. While useful for sedation for non-painful procedures, it has been largely unsuccessful in providing adequate analgesia when used alone for painful procedures. There is some enthusiasm for its use because it reduces neuroapoptosis and ameliorates the longer-term neurobehavioral effects caused by volatile anesthetics in neonatal animal models.[9] Bradycardia or a decrease in resting heart rate (up to a 30% decrease from baseline) is expected and should be considered as a predictable physiological response. A dose-related biphasic response on blood pressure is observed with mild hypotension at lower dosages and hypertension at higher dosages.[10]

Opioids

High-dose synthetic opioid anesthesia with fentanyl (10–50 μg/kg total dose) provides excellent cardiovascular stability in children with CHD. In practice, fentanyl, either as intermittent boluses or as a continuous infusion, is used in conjunction with an amnestic agent and a neuromuscular blocking agent (NMBA). An opioid anesthetic technique is generally preferred for patients with limited cardiorespiratory reserve; when the surgical procedure is extensive and complex; when the cardiopulmonary technique includes deep hypothermia with circulatory arrest or selective antegrade cerebral perfusion; when there are anticipated postcardiotomy complications such as bleeding from high-pressure suture lines, dysrhythmias, or residual lesions such as atrioventricular valve insufficiency; or when the anticipated postoperative course in the intensive care unit (ICU) is prolonged.[11,12] It may also be employed for catheter-based techniques where the need for post-procedure mechanical ventilation or when hemodynamic instability is anticipated.

Remifentanil is a synthetic ultra-short-acting opioid, rapidly metabolized by nonspecific tissue esterases.[13] It is unique among the currently available opioids because of its extremely short context-sensitive half-life (3–5 minutes), which is largely independent of the duration of infusion. As with all opioids, remifentanil may cause respiratory depression. It may be useful for patients with limited cardiorespiratory reserve undergoing procedures such as cardiac catheterization or pacemaker placement, because intense analgesia is provided without significant hemodynamic compromise. It may also be used to maintain anesthesia during cardiopulmonary bypass (CPB) for patients who are candidates for early extubation either immediately in the operating room (OR) or after 1–2 hours in the ICU (e.g., isolated atrial septal defect [ASD] repair).[11]

Muscle Relaxants

Rocuronium is an aminosteroid non-depolarizing muscle relaxant with a rapid onset, intermediate duration of action, and is the most commonly used NMBA. Time to complete neuromuscular blockade for an intubating dose of 0.6 mg/kg ranges from 30 to 180 seconds, although adequate intubating conditions are usually achieved within 60 seconds. It is therefore a suitable alternative to succinylcholine during rapid-sequence induction. The duration of action averages 25 minutes although recovery is slower in infants. It is a safe drug to administer to patients with limited hemodynamic reserve and does not cause histamine release. For patients in whom a short-acting, non-depolarizing muscle relaxant is desirable (i.e., duration of action 30 minutes), cisatracurium and vecuronium are ideal agents with few cardiovascular side effects. Succinylcholine is a rapid-onset, short-duration, depolarizing muscle relaxant that is used primarily during a rapid sequence induction in patients with a full stomach to facilitate intubation and control of the airway. Succinylcholine acts on nicotinic and muscarinic parasympathetic receptors, and atropine or glycopyrrolate should also be administered to avoid associated bradycardia or even sinus arrest.

In regard to use of all of these medications during CPB procedures, it should be noted that drug pharmacokinetics may be substantially altered by hypothermia, hemodilution, reduced protein binding, binding of drugs to the bypass circuit and oxygenator membrane, sequestration of drugs within the pulmonary vascular bed, and reduced hepatic and renal clearance. Drug pharmacodynamics may also be altered due to CPB variables such as flow rate and perfusion pressure as well as the use of vasoactive drugs.[14]

Inhaled Anesthetic Agents

The volatile agents most commonly used during pediatric anesthesia are isoflurane and sevoflurane. Increased sensitivity of the immature cardiovascular system and decreased cardiovascular reserves reduce the margin of safety in infants and younger children with severe CHD. Volatile anesthetics cause dose-dependent direct myocardial depression primarily by limiting calcium availability within the myocyte. Given the immaturity of the neonatal and infant myocardium, the potential for systolic dysfunction in these patients may be increased when volatile agents are used. They also have a direct vasodilating effect on arteriole smooth muscle. These agents must therefore be titrated with caution because of their ability to cause hypotension. Nonetheless, sevoflurane at a concentration of 1 mean alveolar concentration (MAC) has been shown to have no effect on the myocardial performance index of infants with single ventricle physiology.[15] Both sevoflurane and isoflurane at 1.5 MAC have a minimal effect on ejection fraction or Qp:Qs in children with isolated ASD or ventricular septal defect (VSD).[16]

Isoflurane causes less direct myocardial depression, has a faster uptake and emergence, has no effect on intracardiac conduction, and causes much less sensitization of the myocardium to catecholamines compared with halothane. It is a very useful agent to maintain anesthesia throughout cardiac surgery and CPB. It may be used as a sole agent for patients in whom extubation in the immediate postoperative period is planned. Because of peripheral vasodilating properties, isoflurane is a useful adjunct during high-dose opioid anesthesia, particularly if the patient is hypertensive. During bypass, isoflurane 0.5% to 1.0% can be delivered into the fresh gas flow of the bypass circuit and titrated to hemodynamic response.

Sevoflurane, due to its lack of pungency and minimal airway irritant effects, is the only volatile anesthetic agent suitable for inhalation induction of anesthesia in children and can be safely used for most patients with CHD.[17] Its low solubility contributes to faster onset of action and subsequent emergence from anesthesia. As with isoflurane, it causes less myocardial depression and has a low risk for arrhythmias in children compared with halothane. However, because of cost and rapid emergence, there appears little advantage to continue sevoflurane during maintenance of anesthesia.

The use of nitrous oxide in children with CHD and shunts is limited because of its potential for enlarging systemic air emboli and for potentially increasing pulmonary vascular resistance.

Preoperative Assessment and Preparation

Complete and accurate preoperative assessment is essential for the successful anesthetic management of patients with CHD. The appropriate organization of preoperative patient data, preparation of the patient, and decisions about monitoring, anesthetic agents, and postoperative care are best accomplished by focusing on the pathophysiology of the lesion. This guides discussion of sedation and anesthesia techniques, expectations of patient and families, and postoperative management considerations.

Fasting guidelines are summarized in Table 63.3. Although more than 90% of elective patients are suitable for same day admission for cardiac surgical and catheterization procedures, admission to the hospital before the procedure is recommended when hydration with IV fluids is necessary due to erythrocytosis, to initiate vasoactive or inotropic support if the patient has a significant low cardiac output state, and for monitoring of heart rate and rhythm.

Premedication

The immediate preprocedure period is an anxious time for patients and parents. Many patients may have undergone

TABLE 63.3	Nil per os (NPO) guidelines

NPO Guidelines for Elective Surgical and Nonsurgical Procedures[A]	
Type of intake	NPO time prior to procedure
Clear liquids (e.g., water, apple juice, Pedialyte, carbonated beverages)	1 hour
Breast milk	4 hours
Formula, fortified breast milk and thickened fluids, G-tube/J-tube feeding	6 hours
Light meal (e.g., toast)	6 hours
Solid food	8 hours (stop before midnight)

*For emergency procedures, appropriate NPO status may be determined by the attending anesthesiologist in consideration of a patient's acuity and urgency of procedure.

prior surgery or other procedures, and separation from parents may be difficult. The most commonly employed premedication agents are midazolam, ketamine, and dexmedetomidine. The routes of administration of these agents, the dosages, the onset and duration of action, and the hemodynamic effects are summarized in Table 63.2.

Oral midazolam alone is often an effective anxiolytic, and although it may not produce hypnosis, it will enable separation from the family. In young children who are particularly anxious and for those who have undergone previous procedures, oral ketamine may be added to provide a reliable state of hypnosis and dissociation. In circumstances where premedication is deemed important because of the extreme separation anxiety and limited hemodynamic reserve, an IM premedication with ketamine and midazolam is effective. Intranasal dexmedetomidine doses of 2 to 4 μg/kg in children 2 to 6 years of age is also being used with increased frequency to provide premedication and minimal to moderate sedation.[18] It is characterized by a relatively fast onset of sedative properties paralleling natural sleep, suppression of airway reflexes with minimal respiratory depression, and an opioid- and benzodiazepine-sparing effect.

Induction of Sedation/Anesthesia

Whatever the method of anesthesia or sedation, it is essential the procedure is discussed with staff prior to starting, and that the potential complications during the procedure are appreciated. The choice of induction technique is influenced by the response to premedication and the anesthetic management plan. IV induction is simple and rapid; however, establishing IV access may be difficult in children. To facilitate IV access, a heavy premedication may be necessary, but the use of a topical local anesthetic cream or the combination with inhaled nitrous oxide may simplify placement of an IV catheter. If IV access is difficult and stressful in infants, IM induction can be considered. In the absence of IV access, inhalational induction with sevoflurane in an FiO_2 of 30% can be used safely in patients with cyanotic heart disease, although initial uptake may be slower in the presence of a significant physiologic right-to-left shunt.[19] Peripheral oxygen saturations will generally increase provided cardiac output is maintained and airway obstruction avoided. In children with CHD, it is generally advised to limit the inhaled concentration of sevoflurane to 4% to avoid excessive myocardial depression and vasodilation. Once the child's alveolar concentration of sevoflurane equilibrates at 4%, IV access can be obtained and IV agents can be utilized to complete the induction.

Monitoring

Because of the potential for rapid and dramatic hemodynamic changes in young patients with CHD, especially infants, complete preparation of anesthetic and monitoring equipment and resuscitation drugs is essential. Assistance should be immediately available during the induction of anesthesia in case problems develop.

Routine monitoring for any pediatric patient undergoing anesthesia includes pulse oximetry, electrocardiogram, non-invasive blood pressure, and end-tidal carbon dioxide (CO_2) monitoring. Pulse oximetry may reflect the adequacy of gas exchange, cardiac output, pulmonary blood flow, and intracardiac shunting, although its accuracy at low oxygen saturations (75–80%) is limited.[20] Direct arterial pressure monitoring yields important beat-to-beat information in cardiac patients. In general, radial arterial lines are preferred, but caution is required in flushing radial artery catheters because volumes as small as 0.3 mL force microbubbles and small thrombi retrograde into the carotid arteries.[21] Although femoral arterial lines are an excellent alternative to radial arterial lines, they may be associated with a higher complication rate in neonates. Femoral artery catheters should be removed as soon as practical after surgery to reduce the risk for nosocomial infection and to prevent occlusion from thrombus, which may affect limb growth and access for cardiac catheterization if later studies are necessary. An alternative location in neonates is the axillary artery. Arterial lines in the foot may not accurately reflect the central aortic pressure of hypothermic children, especially during CPB and deep hypothermia.

Systemic air emboli are a constant risk in patients with CHD, regardless of their usual shunting pattern, because of the dynamic nature of shunts during anesthesia and surgery. Air traps are advisable for all IV lines but are not a substitute for meticulous attention and constant vigilance concerning the purging of air bubbles.

End-tidal CO_2 monitoring should be used for all patients who are intubated to monitor for misplacement or obstruction of the endotracheal tube (ETT) and as guide to the effectiveness of mechanical ventilation and the amount of pulmonary blood flow. The gradient between the $Paco_2$ and end-tidal CO_2 should be determined soon after intubation once arterial access has been established; the normal $Paco_2$ minus end-tidal CO_2 difference is 5 to 10 mm Hg. An increase in the arterial to end-tidal CO_2 difference may occur with altered ventilation/perfusion matching in the lung. Conversely, a sudden decrease in pulmonary blood flow will cause a sudden fall in end-tidal CO_2; specific clinical circumstances include a fall in cardiac output, an increase in right-to-left intracardiac shunt, air embolism, and occlusion of a systemic-to-pulmonary artery shunt or restriction of pulmonary blood flow such as from a vessel loop or during balloon dilation.

Cerebral oximetry measured with non-invasive near-infrared spectroscopy (NIRS) is used to monitor brain oxygenation in patients undergoing cardiac surgical and catheterization procedures. The most commonly used NIRS technology utilizes continuous wave near-infrared light (700–1000 nm) with transmitters and receivers that are placed on the patient's forehead in order to obtain information non-invasively regarding regional cerebral oxygenation. Analysis of the differential absorption spectra of the oxygen-dependent chromophores in the near-infrared range allows the measurement of tissue oxygenation and blood flow. As regards to neuromonitoring modalities, NIRS offers several advantages over jugular bulb oximetry, transcranial Doppler sonography, and electroencephalography in that it is non-invasive, portable, provides continuous measurements, easy to use, and relatively inexpensive. However, because forehead NIRS only interrogates the frontal lobes supplied by the superficial branches of the anterior and middle cerebral arteries, it is possible to have hypoxia/ischemia in the territories supplied by the deeper branches of the anterior and middle cerebral arteries or the vertebrobasilar system without any change in the measured frontal cerebral oxygen saturation.[22,23]

Intracardiac Pressure Measurement

Placement of a percutaneous central venous catheter is not necessary for all patients undergoing cardiac surgery. They are indicated in situations where large blood loss may be anticipated and when inotrope support is necessary before bypass. Measurement of the superior vena cava (SVC) oxygen (O_2) saturation and the arterial minus SVC O_2 saturation difference (normally 20–30%) provides information as to the adequacy of the cardiac output. During surgery and bypass, the central venous pressure may be a useful monitor for adequate cerebral venous drainage after placement of the SVC venous cannula. Postoperative complications of transvenous central venous lines (CVL) include venous thrombus and infection. This is particularly true in neonates and infants and may cause SVC syndrome and/or persistent pleural effusions and will significantly affect the success of later surgical procedures in patients undergoing staged repairs. The CVL should therefore be removed as soon as practical following the procedure. Transthoracic right, left, or common atrial and pulmonary artery catheters (either directly into the pulmonary artery or across the tricuspid valve) may be placed by the surgeon before discontinuing CPB. These lines are generally not of sufficient caliber to accommodate rapid volume replacement but can be utilized for bolus and continuous administration of medications.[24] Atrial pressure gives useful information about the adequacy of circulating blood volume, ventricular and atrioventricular valve function, and can be used to assess preload recruitable stroke work. Oxygen saturation data from pulmonary arterial catheters provide reliable data for determination of Qp:Qs, while pressure data may reflect pulmonary vascular reactivity. Changes in pressure recorded when the pulmonary artery catheter is pulled back from the pulmonary artery to the right ventricle provide useful information about the adequacy of the right ventricular outflow tract repair.[21] Transcutaneous pulmonary artery balloon catheters may be difficult to place, and measurement of the thermodilution cardiac output is inaccurate in patients with intracardiac shunting.

Intraoperative Echocardiography

Intraoperative echocardiography, both epicardial and transesophageal, has an established role in monitoring, diagnosis, and comprehensive assessment of the adequacy of technical repair in children undergoing repair of CHD.[25,26] Placement of a transesophageal probe after the induction of anesthesia in the OR provides the opportunity to reevaluate the anatomy before surgical intervention but, more importantly, the adequacy of surgical repair can be evaluated as soon as the patient is weaned from CPB. Interference of the airway by the probe and the impact on hemodynamics before and after CPB must be carefully evaluated to avoid complications.

Anesthesia for Cardiac Surgery

Management During Cardiopulmonary Bypass

Once the patient is on CPB, anesthesia can be maintained using different strategies, including bolus dosing, continuous infusions of opioids and/or benzodiazepines, and/or use of isoflurane via a vaporizer connected to the sweep gas to the bypass circuit. The depth of hypothermia is an important variable affecting anesthesia level; in general, as the core and brain temperature decreases and reaches deep hypothermic levels, the electroencephalogram (EEG) in effect becomes isoelectric and anesthetic agents or drugs are generally not necessary during this phase. However, at mild to moderate hypothermic levels, cerebral metabolic rate and EEG activity increase and loss of consciousness cannot be guaranteed. This is particularly a concern for patients undergoing surgical repair at mild hypothermic levels and during the rewarming phase of CPB.

Anesthesia during CPB is associated with an increased risk of patient awareness.[27] Although these studies have been performed in adults, there is no reason to suspect that infants and children do not have the same potential risk. Monitoring the adequacy of anesthetic depth during CPB is difficult, but possible indices include changes in autonomic responses such as an increase in perfusion pressure for a given flow rate, tearing and diaphoresis, and metabolic responses such as a fall in mixed venous oxygen saturation and a rise in lactate level. Monitoring the depth of anesthesia during a procedure is critically important to ensure patients are adequately anesthetized, and devices such as the Bispectral Index which monitor a processed EEG signal may be used.[28-32]

Management After Cardiopulmonary Bypass

Chest closure is a time of particular potential physiologic instability after operations for CHD. If there are concerns for ventricular dysfunction or inadequate hemostasis, it is common for the chest to be left open and covered with a silastic membrane after surgery. Delayed closure of the sternum can be undertaken in the cardiovascular ICU once the patient is in a stable condition. We have previously demonstrated that this approach is associated with improved outcome and low risk for morbidity and infection.[33]

Transfer from the operating table and to the ICU from the OR can be associated with substantial hemodynamic instability. All monitoring must continue uninterrupted. A full oxygen cylinder must be used and the breathing circuit checked for leaks. Equipment for reintubation and resuscitation drugs must be taken with the patient in case of inadvertent problems during transport. The ETT should be secure and the airway suctioned to remove secretions to reduce the risk for obstruction. Additional anesthesia and muscle relaxants may be necessary if the patient becomes hypertensive or tachycardic when moved. If there is unexpected hypotension or dysrhythmia before the patient leaves the OR, immediate evaluation is essential to determine the cause and establish stability.

Anesthesia for Cardiac Catheterization

Although the underlying cardiac status or physiologic status of a patient may increase the risk for adverse events during catheterization, in many circumstances complications are sudden, occur without warning, and reflect the inherent risk for specific procedures.[34,35] Hence, all staff, including catheterizers, anesthesiologists, nurses, and technicians, must be vigilant and prepared for immediate intervention.

Placement of catheters in the heart increases the risk for dysrhythmias, perforation of the myocardium, damage to valve leaflets and chordae, cerebral vascular accidents, and air embolism. The use of radiopaque contrast material may cause an acute allergic reaction (although this is rare in children with nonionic contrast media), pulmonary hypertension, and myocardial depression. Blood loss may be sudden and unexpected when using large-bore catheters, vessels are ruptured, or vessel entry sites are inadvertently beyond the pubic ramus in the pelvis and cannot be compressed following catheter removal. More insidious blood loss may occur over several hours in heparinized small children or neonates owing to bleeding around the catheter site or multiple aspirations and flushes of catheters. Transfusion requirements and appropriate vascular access should be continually assessed. Arrhythmias, albeit often transient, may be recurrent and fatal if not promptly treated. On most occasions, removal of the wire or catheter is sufficient for the arrhythmia to resolve, but when this does not happen, it is important that full resuscitation and cardioversion equipment be available.

Ergonomics

Because the catheterization and electrophysiology (EP) laboratories are by necessity configured differently than a standard OR, and because they are usually located in an area remote from central anesthesia supplies and equipment, the environment can be challenging. The location of apparatus such as a C-arm limits access to the patient, and anesthesia equipment must often be moved to facilitate positioning of the imaging tools. Routine tasks such as managing the airway or starting additional IV lines can be compromised or impossible once the procedure has started. Conversion from sedation to GA with an ETT or supraglottic airway (SGA) is substantially more complicated given the limited access to the patient's head and neck. With this in mind, control of the airway with an ETT or SGA from the outset should be considered in patients with a known or suspected difficult airway, particularly if they are undergoing a long, complicated procedure. Rotation of the imaging equipment is not controlled by the anesthesiologist, and movement around the patient can disrupt the breathing circuit, IV tubing, and monitoring cables. Care must be taken to assure that these items are positioned safely and have the extra length to allow full camera mobility.

Radiation Safety

Radiation exposure is a continuous risk to sedation and anesthesia providers during catheterization procedures.[36-38] The principle of as low as reasonably achievable (ALARA) emphasizes that there is no specific amount of radiation that can be considered safe and makes reduction of radiation exposure an ethical priority. Practical considerations, however, dictate that clinicians take personal responsibility for minimizing their exposure by recognizing the importance of time, distance, and shielding. Reducing time and increasing distance to exposure directly reduces radiation dose. Shielding oneself from the radiation source with lead aprons and thyroid shields, mobile lead shields, lead glasses with temple shields, and lead barriers should be routine.

Temperature Regulation

Ambient temperatures in the catheterization and EP laboratories are kept near 15°C for the comfort of the personnel wearing heavy lead and surgical gowns. In addition, infused crystalloid (including irrigation for catheters) is delivered at room temperature. The combination can lower the patient's core temperature, especially in infants. Consequently, meticulous attention must be paid to keeping the patient normothermic (e.g., warm air blankets and fluid warmers).

Positioning

Minimizing patient movement is important for interventional procedures (e.g., balloon dilations, stenting of vascular structures), accurate EP mapping, and successful ablation. Care must be taken when positioning a patient on the catheterization table because of the risk for pressure areas and nerve traction injury. In particular, brachial plexus injury may occur when patients have their arms positioned above their heads for a prolonged period of time to make room for the lateral cameras. As the patient is lying immobile for many hours, elbows and all bony prominences should be padded appropriately. For sedated patients, soft restraints are applied to limit potential body and arm movement. In case of need for external cardioversion, special attention should be directed toward protecting the patient from excessive body movement and arm swinging. The tongue should be protected with a soft bite block. To facilitate femoral vein and arterial access, the pelvis is commonly elevated from the catheterization table. This may displace abdominal contents cephalad, restrict diaphragm excursion, and increase the risk for respiratory depression in a sedated patient.

Sedation for Cardiac Catheterization

Many diagnostic, non-interventional hemodynamic catheterization studies can be performed with the patient sedated and breathing room air. This allows meaningful hemodynamic data and oxygen saturations to be measured, together with accurate calculations of cardiac output, shunt fraction, and vascular resistances. It is important that adequate local anesthetic be used at vascular access sites in order to limit the amount of sedation. In older children and adults, interventional procedures that cause minimal or transient hemodynamic perturbations and minimal discomfort (e.g., patent ductus arteriosus and ASD device occlusion, coil embolization of vessels) can be performed using sedation techniques.

General Anesthesia for Cardiac Catheterization

Patient and procedural factors are considerations when planning GA. Patients who have limited cardiorespiratory reserve may not tolerate prolonged procedures under IV sedation, particularly if respiratory depression or airway obstruction occurs concurrently. Respiratory distress may occur in some patients when positioned supine, particularly if they have significant left atrial hypertension from any cause, pulmonary hypertension, or limited diaphragm excursion secondary to paralysis/paresis or due to an enlarged liver or ascites. It should be recognized that hemodynamic changes induced by anesthetic agents can influence interpretation of catheterization data. For example, an anesthetic technique that reduces systemic vascular resistance may cause a significant underestimation of the severity of atrial valve regurgitation that would be present in the awake state. Likewise, the reduced cardiac output present in an anesthetized patient can lead to a significant underestimation of the severity of aortic stenosis.

GA may be indicated due to the risks and possible complications associated with certain procedures. At critical phases during some interventions such as device and stent placement, it is essential that patients remain absolutely still; sudden patient movement induced by discomfort may dislodge the device or alter stent position. In addition, GA is usually recommended for procedures predictably associated with hemodynamic compromise such as placement of a VSD occlusion device, dilation of multiple peripheral pulmonary artery stenoses, or balloon dilation of a stenotic mitral valve.

Patients may breathe spontaneously or have assisted ventilation during GA which can be achieved with IV anesthetic agents such as ketamine and propofol, or with inhalation anesthetic agents and airway protection using a SGA. For the most part, however, GA will require controlled ventilation following paralysis with a neuromuscular blocking drug and endotracheal intubation.

Special Considerations During Electrophysiology Ablations

An anesthesiologist should be present for the entire procedure and should be part of the entire perioperative planning and evaluation process of ventricular tachycardia (VT) ablation. Some electrophysiologists advocate for very little sedation, or no sedation, be administered during the mapping phase for idiopathic VT.[39] This is particularly important because some electrophysiologists feel strongly that anesthetic agents can suppress spontaneous ventricular ectopy or VT, although this has not been conclusively demonstrated.[40] Consequently, these cases require a meticulous evaluation of the patient's physical status as well as psychological disposition and cooperation level when mild to moderate sedation is considered. A detailed preoperative discussion of the plan with the treating team members and a discussion of that plan with the patient and/or parents is necessary. It must be recognized that the initial sedation/anesthesia plan may need to be modified during the procedure as dictated by the technical constraints of the procedure, hemodynamics, and patient comfort.

An additional concern is that sustained VT can lead to the development of myopathy and can have severe hemodynamic consequences in patients with already limited cardiac reserve.[39,40] In the instances where ventricular function is very poor, the procedure may need to be performed with mechanical support including extracorporeal membrane oxygenation, percutaneous left ventricular assist devices, or

an intra-aortic balloon pump in place. If a general anesthetic is administered to these patients, it must be anticipated that significant hemodynamic decompensation is a very real possibility.

When sustained VT is hemodynamically unstable, rapid termination by pacing is attempted first. If unsuccessful, cardioversion is performed after ensuring an adequate level of sedation and amnesia to minimize the chances of causing a traumatizing experience. For VT originating from the left ventricle, access to the left ventricle is commonly achieved in a retrograde fashion through the aortic valve which may cause some degree of aortic regurgitation and further hemodynamic instability. In some circumstances, a percutaneous epicardial approach to the arrhythmic focus is necessary. Particular concerns with this approach are the development of intrapericardial bleeding and tamponade, as well as coronary artery injury. The epicardial catheter is introduced through a subxiphoid puncture and generally requires moderate to deep sedation or GA.[38] When phrenic nerve stimulation is needed, muscle relaxants are contraindicated.[39]

Not infrequently, patients undergoing VT ablation require some inotropic or vasopressor support to maintain acceptable hemodynamics during mapping. The electrophysiologist should be made aware of administration of any medications that can influence hemodynamics or suppress or provoke the arrhythmia.

Postoperative Nausea and Vomiting

The incidence of nausea and vomiting in patients undergoing catheter ablation under GA has been reported to be as high as 60%.[41] The risk factors have been identified as longer duration of anesthesia, previous history of postoperative nausea and vomiting, prolonged use of nitrous oxide, and use of inhalation agent-based technique as opposed to a propofol-based technique for maintenance of anesthesia. Administration of antiemetics (most studied being ondansetron) appears to decrease the incidence of this complication.[41,42] An infusion of a sub-hypnotic dose of propofol during the procedure decreases the risk of vomiting postoperatively but not the occurrence of nausea. The infusion range of propofol used for that purpose varies widely in the literature, with a median of 25 mcg/kg/min in one study in the EP laboratory, but a dose-effect relationship could not be determined.[42]

Electrophysiologic Effects of Anesthetic and Sedative Agents

Through interactions with receptors and ion channels in the myocardium, commonly used anesthetics and sedatives have varying degrees of direct effect on normal cardiac conduction and on the three primary mechanisms of arrhythmogenesis. In addition, these agents may indirectly affect cardiac electrophysiology through modulation of sympathetic and parasympathetic tone.[38] It has been difficult to directly assess the electrophysiologic effects of anesthetic agents because multiple agents are administered concomitantly in the

TABLE 63.4   Electrophysiologic effects of anesthetic and sedative agents

Common anesthetic agents	Effect on				Inducibility of arrhythmia and other comments
	SA node conduction	AV node conduction	AP conduction	QTc	
Isoflurane		↑ refractory period	↑ refractory period	Prolongs QTc	No significant clinical effect for SVT ablation in adolescents. Insufficient data in adults
Sevoflurane	↑ but not clinically significant	No effect	No effect	Prolongs QTc	No significant clinical effect for SVT ablation. Insufficient data in adults
Desflurane	No effect	No effect	↑ refractory period	Prolongs QTc	Impaired SVT inducibility in some patients
Propofol	No effect	No effect/few reports of ↓ AV node conduction	No effect	No effect on QTc (can reverse sevoflurane QTc prolongation)	No significant clinical effect for SVT ablation. Report of reduced inducibility of EAT in children
Fentanyl/ Alfentanil/ Sufentanil	No effect	No effect/minimal effect	No effect	Fentanyl: no effect. Sufentanil: prolongs QT	No significant clinical effect for SVT ablation (in moderate doses). Can enhance vagal tone and cause bradycardia
Remifentanil	↓	↓/no effect			Controversial: discussion with electrophysiologist recommended
Midazolam	No effect	No effect	No effect	No effect/ anxiolysis effect can shorten QT	No effect
Ketamine	No effect	No effect or ↑		No effect (but sympathomimetic, better avoid)	Could promote inducibility of SVT
Dexmedetomidine	↓	↓		Controversial/ conflicting data	Caution and discussion with electrophysiologist recommended
Non-depolarizing muscle relaxants	No effect	No effect	No effect	No effect	No effect, but caution in phrenic nerve monitoring needed
Succinylcholine				Prolongs QT (avoid)	

AP, Action potential; *AV,* atrioventricular; *EAT,* ectopic atrial tachycardia; *SA,* sinoatrial; *SVT,* supraventricular tachycardia.

clinical setting. That being said, the major electrophysiologic effects of the most commonly used anesthetics and sedatives are summarized in Table 63.4.

Magnetic Resonance Imaging and Angiography

The claustrophobic small bore of the magnetic resonance imaging (MRI) machine and noise during imaging mean that sedation is necessary for most children undergoing cardiac MRI and magnetic resonance angiography procedures. To allow three-dimensional magnetic resonance angiography and gradient echo sequences for images of blood flow, breath holding is necessary during image acquisition; therefore, GA is frequently required for neonates, infants, and young children. As in the catheterization laboratory, administering GA amid the MRI equipment is often difficult and hemodynamic monitoring may be limited.[43]

References

1. Practice Guidelines for Moderate Procedural Sedation and Analgesia 2018: A Report by the American Society of Anesthesiologists Task Force on Moderate Procedural Sedation and Analgesia, the American Association of Oral and Maxillofacial Surgeons, American College of Radiology, American Dental Association, American Society of Dentist Anesthesiologists, and Society of Interventional Radiology. *Anesthesiology.* 2018;128:437-479.

2. Nasr VG, DiNardo JA. Sedation and analgesia in pediatric cardiac critical care. *Pediatr Crit Care Med.* 2016;17:S225-S231.

3. Kim KM. Remimazolam: pharmacological characteristics and clinical applications in anesthesiology. *Anesth Pain Med (Seoul).* 2022;17:1-11.

4. Hickey PR, Hansen DD, Cramolini GM, et al. Pulmonary and systemic hemodynamic responses to ketamine in infants with normal and elevated pulmonary vascular resistance. *Anesthesiology.* 1985;62:287-293.

5. Sarkar M, Laussen PC, Zurakowski D, et al. Hemodynamic responses to etomidate on induction of anesthesia in pediatric patients. *Anesth Analg.* 2005;101:645-650.

6. Ostwald P, Doenicke AW. Etomidate revisited. *Curr Opin Anaesthesiol.* 1990;11:391-390.

7. Hsieh VC, Krane EJ, Morgan PG. Mitochondrial disease and anesthesia. *J Inborn Errors Metab Screen.* 2017;5:1-5.

8. de Wit F, van Vliet AL, de Wilde RB, et al. The effect of propofol on haemodynamics: cardiac output, venous return, mean systemic filling pressure, and vascular resistances. *Br J Anaesth.* 2016;116:784-789.

9. Zuppa AF, Nicolson SC, Wilder NS, et al. Pediatric Heart Network Investigators. Results of a phase 1 multicentre investigation of dexmedetomidine bolus and infusion in corrective infant cardiac surgery. *Br J Anaesth.* 2019;123:839-852.

10. Mahmoud M, Mason KP. Dexmedetomidine: review, update, and future considerations of paediatric perioperative and periprocedural applications and limitations. *Br J Anaesth.* 2015;115:171-182.

11. Roy N, Parra MF, Brown ML, et al. Enhancing recovery in congenital cardiac surgery. *Ann Thorac Surg.* 2022;114:1754-1761.

12. Hansen DD, Hickey PR. Anesthesia for hypoplastic left heart syndrome: high dose fentanyl in 30 neonates. *Anesth Analg.* 1986;65:127-132.

13. Lynn AM. Editorial. Remifentanil. The paediatric anaesthetist's opiate? *Paediatr Anaesth.* 1996;6:433-435.

14. Kuntz MT, Pereira LM, Matte GS, et al. Sequestration of midazolam, fentanyl, and morphine by an ex vivo cardiopulmonary bypass circuit. *ASAIO J.* 2021;67:1342-1348.

15. Ikemba CM, Su JT, Stayer SA, et al. Myocardial performance index with sevoflurane-pancuronium versus fentanyl-midazolam-pancuronium in infants with a functional single ventricle. *Anesthesiology.* 2004;101:1298-1305.

16. Laird TH, Stayer SA, Rivenes SM, et al. Pulmonary-to-systemic blood flow ratio effects of sevoflurane, isoflurane, halothane, and fentanyl/midazolam with 100% oxygen in children with congenital heart disease. *Anesth Analg.* 2002;95:1200-1206.

17. Holzman RS, van der Velde ME, Kaus SJ, et al. Sevoflurane depresses myocardial contractility less than halothane during induction of anesthesia in children. *Anesthesiology.* 1996;85:1260-1267.

18. Grogan K, Thibault C, Moorthy G, et al. Dose escalation pharmacokinetic study of intranasal atomized dexmedetomidine in pediatric patients with congenital heart disease. *Anesth Analg.* 2022;136:152-162.

19. Tanner GE, Angers DG, Barash PG, et al. Effect of left-to-right, mixed left-to-right, and right-to-left shunts on inhalational anesthetic induction in children: a computer model. *Anesth Analg.* 1985;64:101-107.

20. Gold JP, Jonas RA, Lang P, et al. Transthoracic intracardiac monitoring lines in pediatric surgical patients: a ten-year experience. *Ann Thorac Surg.* 1986;42:185-191.

21. Lang P, Chipman CW, Siden H, et al. Early assessment of hemodynamic status after repair of tetralogy of Fallot: a comparison of 24 hour (intensive care unit) and 1 year postoperative data in 98 patients. *Am J Cardiol.* 1982;50:795-799.

22. Zaleski KL, Kussman BD. Near-infrared spectroscopy in pediatric congenital heart disease. *J Cardiothorac Vasc Anesth.* 2020;34:489-500.

23. Olbrecht VA, Skowno J, Marchesini V, et al. An international, multicenter, observational study of cerebral oxygenation during infant and neonatal anesthesia. *Anesthesiology.* 2018;128:85-96.

24. Stein ML, Quinonez LG, DiNardo JA, et al. Complications of transthoracic intracardiac and central venous lines in neonates undergoing cardiac surgery. *Pediatr Cardiol.* 2019;40:733-737.

25. Stern KWD, Emani SM, Peek GJ, et al. Epicardial echocardiography in pediatric and congenital heart surgery. *World J Pediatr Congenit Heart Surg.* 2019;10:343-350.

26. Puchalski MD, Lui GK, Miller-Hance WC, et al. Guidelines for performing a comprehensive transesophageal echocardiographic examination in children and all patients with congenital heart disease: recommendations from the American Society of Echocardiography. *J Am Soc Echocardiogr.* 2019;32:173-215. [Erratum in: J Am Soc Echocardiogr. 2019;32(5):681. Erratum in: J Am Soc Echocardiogr. 2019 Oct;32(10):1373-1378].

27. Dowd NP, Cheng DC, Karski JM, et al. Intraoperative awareness in fast-track cardiac anesthesia. *Anesthesiology.* 1998;89:1068-1073.

28. Davidson AJ, McCann ME, Devavaram P, et al. The differences in the bispectral index between infants and children during emergence from anesthesia after circumcision surgery. *Anesth Analg.* 2001;93:326-330.

29. McCann ME, Brustowicz RM, Bacsik J, et al. The bispectral index and explicit recall during the intraoperative wake-up test for scoliosis surgery. *Anesth Analg.* 2002;94:1474-1478.

30. McCann ME, Bacsik J, Davidson A, et al. The correlation of bispectral index with endtidal sevoflurane concentration and haemodynamic parameters in preschoolers. *Paediatr Anaesth.* 2002;12:519-525.

31. Laussen PC, Murphy JA, Zurakowski D, et al. Bispectral index monitoring in children undergoing mild hypothermic cardiopulmonary bypass. *Paediatr Anaesth.* 2001;11:567-573.

32. Kussman BD, Gruber EM, Zurakowski D, et al. Bispectral index monitoring during infant cardiac surgery: relationship of BIS to the stress response and plasma fentanyl levels. *Paediatr Anaesth.* 2001;11:663-669.

33. Tabbutt S, Duncan BW, McLaughlin D, et al. Delayed sternal closure after cardiac operations in a pediatric population. *J Thorac Cardiovasc Surg.* 1997;113:886-893.

34. Odegard KC, Bergersen L, Thiagarajan R, et al. The frequency of cardiac arrests in patients with congenital heart disease undergoing cardiac catheterization. *Anesth Analg.* 2014;118:175-182.

35. Allan CK, Thiagarajan RR, Armsby LR, et al. Emergent use of extracorporeal membrane oxygenation during pediatric cardiac catheterization. *Pediatr Crit Care Med.* 2006;7:212-219.

36. Haines DE, Beheiry S, Akar JG, et al. Heart Rhythm Society expert consensus statement on electrophysiology laboratory

standards: process, protocols, equipment, personnel, and safety. *Heart Rhythm.* 2014;11:e9-e51.

37. Nicoara A, Holmquist F, Raggains C, et al. Anesthesia for catheter ablation procedures. *J Cardiothorac Vasc Anesth.* 2014;28:1589-1603.

38. Saul PJ, Kanter RJ, Writing Committee, et al. PACES/HRS expert consensus statement on the use of catheter ablation in children and patients with congenital heart disease: Developed in partnership with the Pediatric and Congenital Electrophysiology Society (PACES) and the Heart Rhythm Society (HRS). Endorsed by the governing bodies of PACES, HRS, the American Academy of Pediatrics (AAP), the American Heart Association (AHA), and the Association for European Pediatric and Congenital Cardiology (AEPC). *Heart Rhythm.* 2016;13:e251-e289.

39. Price A, Santucci P. Electrophysiology procedures: weighing the factors affecting choice of anesthesia. *Semin Cardiothorac Vasc Anesth.* 2013;17:203-211.

40. Gerstein NS, Young A, Schulman PM, et al. Sedation in the electrophysiology laboratory: a multidisciplinary review. *J Am Heart Assoc.* 2016;5:e003629.

41. Erb TO, Hall JM, Ing RJ, et al. Postoperative nausea and vomiting in children and adolescents undergoing radiofrequency catheter ablation: a randomized comparison of propofol- and isoflurane-based anesthetics. *Anesth Analg.* 2002;95:1577-1581.

42. Lee Y, Banooni A, Yuki K, et al. Incidence and predictors of postoperative nausea and vomiting in children undergoing electrophysiology ablation procedures. *Paediatr Anaesth.* 2020;30:147-152.

43. Odegard KC, DiNardo JA, Tsai-Goodman B, et al. Anaesthesia considerations for cardiac MRI in infants and small children. *Paediatr Anaesth.* 2004;14:471-476.

64

Cardiac Intensive Care Unit

SARAH A. TEELE, JOAN M. LAROVERE, AND RAVI R. THIAGARAJAN

KEY LEARNING POINTS

- Expert cardiac intensive care teams have a pivotal role in short- and long-term outcomes for pediatric patients with congenital and acquired heart disease.
- Care of specialized populations of patients such as neonates requires knowledge of their unique physiologic characteristics to guide management strategies.
- Cardiac intensive care clinicians should recognize clinical exam findings consistent with a low cardiac output state

- and be well versed in the range of therapies available to treat patients, including pharmacologic agents, mechanical ventilation, and mechanical circulatory support.
- Multidisciplinary collaborative teams are needed to meet the diverse and challenging needs of these complex, high-acuity patients.
- Multi-institutional collaborative research can inform local and national initiatives to improve quality of life outcomes.

Since the last edition of this textbook, there have been exponential advances in imaging, medical therapies, procedural techniques, bedside care, supportive technologies, and outcomes research in patients with congenital (CHD) and acquired heart disease. This growth has occurred in parallel with the dramatically expanding field of pediatric critical care medicine. Evolving at the intersection of the two subspecialties, pediatric cardiac intensive care medicine has benefited from developments in both spheres. As a consequence, optimal management of patients requires clinicians to synthesize efficiently a tremendous volume of up-to-date interdisciplinary knowledge. Furthermore, supervising the dynamic interprofessional teams essential for delivery of complex care requires expertise in communication, collaboration, and leadership. The need for these diverse competencies has impacted training models and led to the development of more formal curricula by experts in the field.

History

The value of a hospital ward dedicated to patients requiring intensive care was appreciated during the polio epidemic of the 1950s. The need to mechanically ventilate dozens of patients simultaneously demanded a reorganization of hospital-based care. The modern era of continuous invasive monitoring, pharmacologic manipulation of blood pressure and cardiac output, and resuscitation of critically ill patients of all types arose in large part with the advent of cardiopulmonary bypass (CPB) techniques in the 1950s; the ability to conduct open heart surgery established a need for specialized postoperative care. Soon thereafter, younger

children and infants became appropriate candidates for hemodynamic and interventional cardiac catheterization (e.g., atrial septostomy) in addition to surgical palliation. At the same time, pediatric critical care emerged as a specialized discipline attracting subspecialists primarily from pediatric cardiology and pediatric anesthesia.

As of 2016, there were 48 dedicated pediatric cardiac critical units in the United States alone.[1] Survival into adulthood for children born with CHD is now > 90% and clinicians' focus has turned to optimizing quality of life metrics (Fig. 64.1). Care delivery in the cardiac intensive care unit (CICU) plays a pivotal role in short- and long-term outcomes for many patients with complex CHD. In addition to bedside nursing, respiratory therapists, physician trainees, advanced practice providers, and physician faculty, CICU teams of the 21st century frequently include diverse specialists such as nutritionists, pharmacists, physical and occupational therapists, social workers, spiritual care providers, and consulting sub-specialty teams. Interprofessional teams support the multifaceted requirements of patients in the acute setting and play a critical role in long-term considerations such as neurodevelopment. Care of the neonate with CHD is a prime example of this need for sophisticated care delivery in a rapidly expanding field of research and quality improvement (QI) initiatives.

Newborn Considerations

Intensive care management of the critically ill neonate requires an appreciation of the special structural and functional features of immature organs, the physiology of the

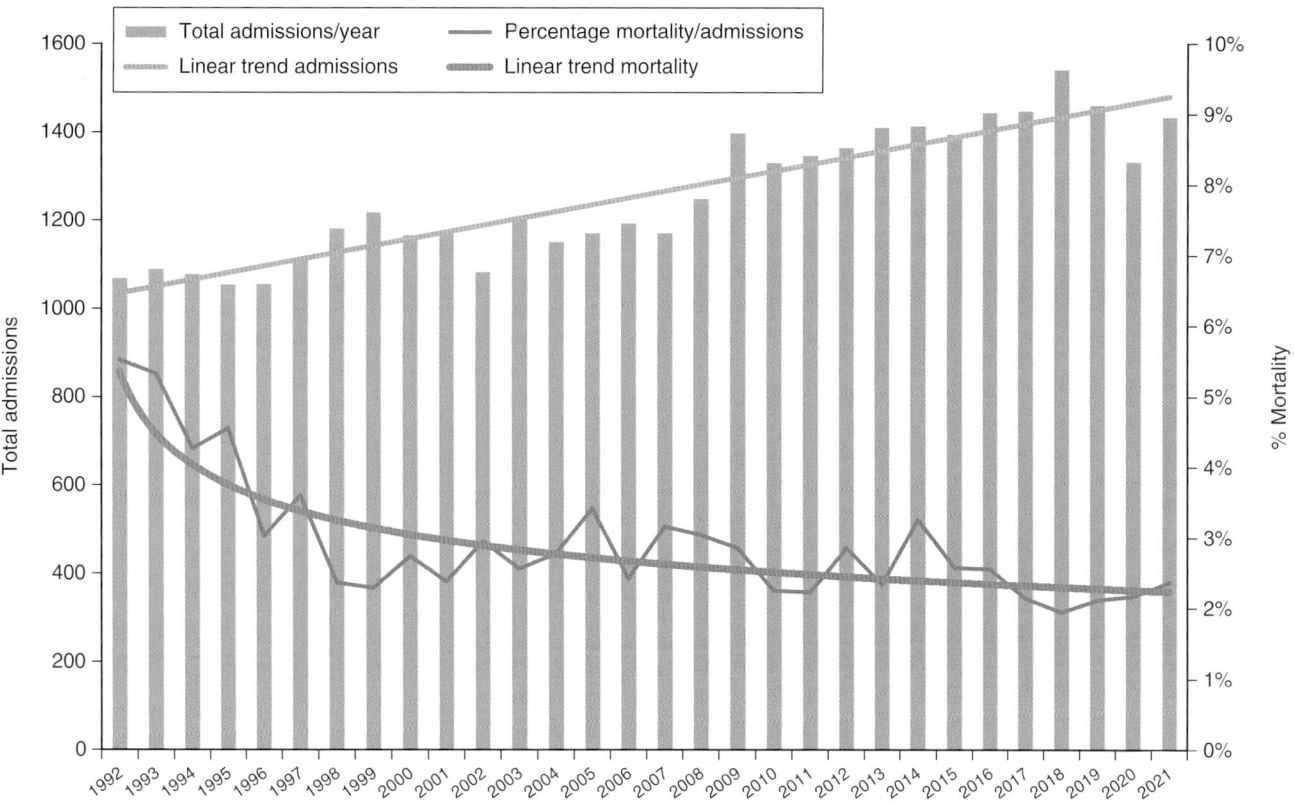

• **Fig. 64.1** Trends in admissions and mortality for patients admitted to the cardiac intensive care unit at Boston Children's Hospital. Percentage of deaths to admissions represented by year and by trend over time.

transitional neonatal circulation, and the secondary effects of the congenital heart lesion on other organ systems.[2] The neonate appears to respond more quickly and profoundly to physiologically stressful circumstances, which may be expressed in terms of rapid changes in pH, lactic acid, glucose, and temperature. Neonates have diminished fat and carbohydrate reserves. The higher metabolic rate and oxygen consumption of the neonate account for the rapid appearance of hypoxia when these patients become apneic. Immaturity of the liver and kidney may be associated with reduced protein synthesis and glomerular filtration such that drug metabolism is altered and hepatic synthetic function is reduced. These issues may be compounded by the normal increased total body water of the neonate compared with that of the older patient, along with the propensity of the immature capillary system to leak fluid from the intravascular space. This is especially prominent in the lung of the neonate where the pulmonary vascular bed is nearly fully recruited at rest; lymphatic recruitment required to handle increased mean capillary pressures associated with increases in pulmonary blood flow may be unavailable.[3] The neonatal myocardium is less compliant than in the older child, less tolerant of increases in afterload and less responsive to increases in preload. Younger age also predisposes the myocardium to the adverse effects of CPB and hypothermic ischemia surgical support techniques used frequently for reparative operations. These factors do not preclude intervention in the neonate, they simply dictate that extraordinary vigilance be applied to the

care of these children and intensive care management plans emerge to account for the immature physiology.

The number of infants born with critical CHD and the observed benefits of neonatal reparative operations demand that care of the neonate with complex CHD after CPB is a central feature of cardiac intensive care (Fig. 64.2). This includes premature infants, who represent approximately 10% of newborns.[4] Acknowledging the potential positive and negative impacts of early-life decision-making and care to short- and long-term outcomes is critical. Factors to consider include optimal timing of surgical repair versus staged repair, early recognition and response to residual cardiac lesions, early diagnosis and management of comorbidities such as tracheobronchomalacia, and a team-based focus on issues specific to the neonate and premature infant. These issues include adequate growth and nutrition, neurodevelopment and cerebral protection, and vigilant attention to vascular access points given the need for life-long access and the particular risks of thrombus, infection, and chylothorax. To optimize the care of this particularly fragile cohort, the Boston Children's Hospital (BCH) Cardiovascular Program created a multidisciplinary neonatal working group to track data specific to this patient population and to systematically discuss in detail each intensive care inpatient neonate with CHD or acquired heart disease.

As outcomes continue to improve, pediatric cardiac intensivists find themselves responsible for the care of a growing number of adults with CHD. As with neonates,

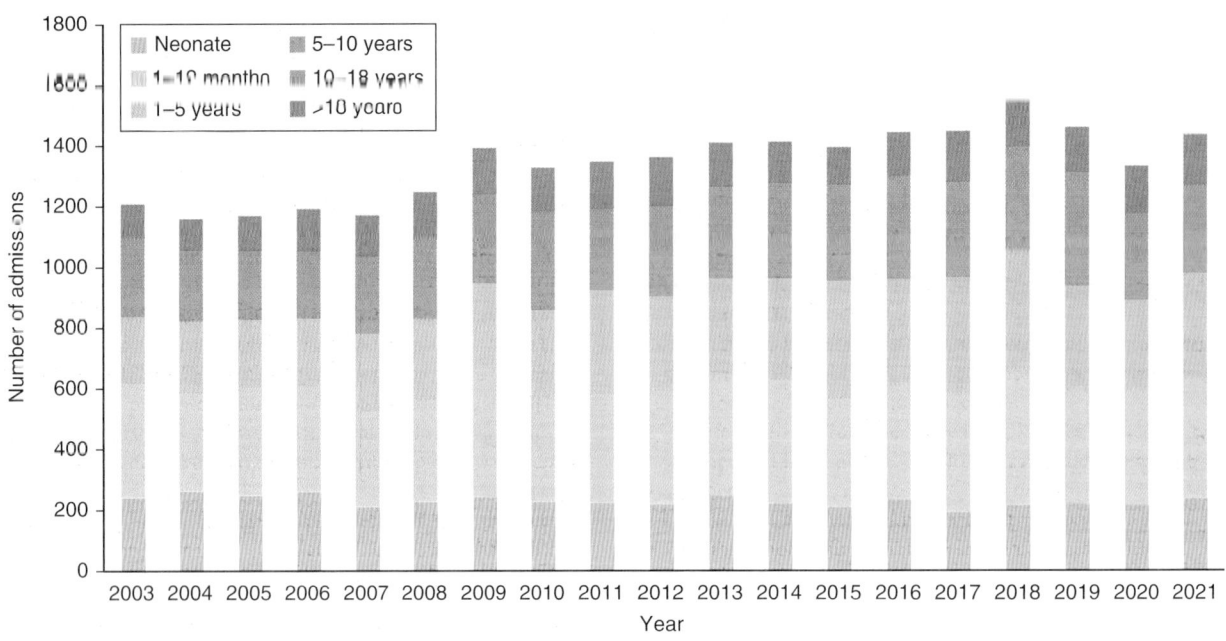

Fig. 64.2 Annual admissions to the cardiac intensive care unit at Boston Children's Hospital by age.

this population demands sophisticated and coordinated care delivery. Management should consider the multiorgan system impacts of longstanding pathophysiology, implications of prior interventions including cardiac catheterization(s) and cardiac surgery, and establishing transparent goals of care. Please see Chapters 57, 58, and 59 for more details.

Preoperative Care

The increasing frequency of fetal diagnoses provides opportunities for proactive counseling of families, adjustments in maternal care, and delivery planning. Once admitted to CICU, optimal care for all patients may involve (1) initial stabilization including airway management and establishment of vascular access; (2) a complete and thorough non-invasive delineation of the anatomic defect(s); (3) resuscitation with evaluation and treatment of secondary organ dysfunction, particularly the brain, kidneys, and liver; (4) cardiac catheterization and/or additional cross-sectional imaging if necessary—typically for physiologic assessment, interventional procedures, or anatomic definition not visible by echocardiography; and (5) surgical management when cardiac, pulmonary, renal, and central nervous systems (CNS) are optimized. Crucial in this process is ongoing multidisciplinary consultation and communication.

Postoperative Care

Assessment

Recognizing the vulnerabilities inherent in handovers of patients from the operative team to the intensive care team, BCH embraces the Formula 1 approach for patients following cardiac surgical procedures. This sequenced set of tasks and explicit communication strategies have been found to reduce errors and omissions.[5] First, the patient's history and indications for surgery are reported by the surgical team. The anesthesia team follows with pre-CPB airway, vascular access, and anesthetic strategies, being sure to note expected or unexpected clinical findings. The surgeon then addresses the operative repair including cardiovascular support strategy, concerns for adequacy of myocardial protection, details of the procedure, recovery of myocardial contractility, postoperative hemodynamics, and findings from intraoperative imaging. The anesthesia team reports on how the patient separated from CPB, offers additional commentary on the patient's current hemodynamics and whether they have changed over the course of transport, and acknowledges vasoactive medication and mechanical ventilation requirements. Finally, the CICU team asks clarifying questions, briefly summarizes the information that has just been relayed highlighting both reassuring and concerning findings, and presents a management plan for postoperative care. The complex information relayed in this handover guides subsequent examinations and expected clinical course which should focus on the quality of the repair or palliation plus ongoing assessment of cardiac output and recovery (Table 64.1).

When the clinical course of patients after cardiac surgery deviates from expectations, a clinician's first responsibility is to verify the accuracy of the preoperative diagnosis and the adequacy of the surgical repair. Significant residual lesions can lead to serious adverse outcomes including irreversible multiorgan injury. Getting the right postoperative assessment is therefore imperative and treatment follows accordingly. Evaluation of the postoperative patient relies

TABLE 64.1	Intensive Care Strategies to Diagnose And Support Low Cardiac Output States

Know the cardiac anatomy in detail and its physiologic consequences

Understand the specialized considerations of the newborn and implications of reparative rather than palliative surgery

Diversify personnel to include expertise in neonatal and adult congenital heart disease

Monitor, measure, and image the heart to rule out residual disease as a cause of postoperative hemodynamic instability or low cardiac output, then maintain aortic perfusion and improve the contractile state

Optimize preload (including atrial shunting)

Reduce afterload

Control heart rate, rhythm and synchrony

Optimize heart lung interactions

Provide mechanical support when needed

on physical examination, continuous monitoring with active interpretation of vital signs and trends, and integration with additional bedside data and imaging (Table 64.2). Postoperative cardiac catheterization may be indicated and should be considered early in the postoperative course if the patient is not progressing as predicted. Once the accuracy of the diagnosis and adequacy of the repair are established, then a low cardiac output state can be presumed, and treatment optimized. Treating low cardiac output states and preventing cardiovascular collapse are often the central features of pediatric cardiac intensive care.[6] This topic will be the focus of this chapter, without detailing the specific considerations for each lesion, which instead are presented in their respective chapters.

Monitoring

The level of bedside monitoring that is appropriate for each patient depends upon the individual's diagnosis, the type of

TABLE 64.2	Signs of Heart Failure or Low Cardiac Output States

Signs:

Cool extremities/poor perfusion

Oliguria and other end organ failure

Tachycardia

Hypotension

Acidosis

Cardiomegaly

Pleural effusions

Monitor and measure:

Heart rate, blood pressure, intracardiac pressure

Extremity temperature, central temperature

Urine output

Mixed venous oxygen saturation

Arterial blood gas pH and lactate

Laboratory measures of end-organ function

Echocardiography

repair or palliation if a procedure was performed, and anticipated requirements for real-time data (e.g., hemodynamic, respiratory, neurologic). Continuous monitoring of heart rate and rhythm by electrocardiogram, systemic arterial blood pressure, oxygen saturation by pulse oximetry, and respiratory rate should be considered in all patients. The CICU team should identify the least invasive monitoring needed for an individual patient's safety which includes assessment of clinical status and the impact of interventions. As a patient progresses to recovery, the need for invasive monitoring, if present, should be addressed at regular intervals to encourage discontinuation and avoid unnecessary complications.

Central venous pressure (CVP) measurement is routine for many patients following cardiac surgery and commonly used in medical CICU patients, for example, those presenting in acute heart failure. If the tip of an intravascular catheter is in the superior vena cava, one can obtain a mixed venous saturation (MVS) to assess cardiac output and, in single ventricle patients, calculate an estimated Qp/Qs. An arteriovenous oxygen difference of 25% is normal and reflects appropriate oxygen delivery and extraction. Following reparative surgery, patients with no intracardiac shunts and an adequate cardiac output may have a mild reduction in MVS to approximately 60%. A lower MVS does not necessarily indicate low cardiac output if a patient has arterial desaturation (e.g., common mixing lesions, lung diseases). A higher-than-expected MVS requires attention as it may reflect a potentially pathological state such as generous left-to-right shunting at the atrial level, significant tricuspid valve regurgitation, partial anomalous pulmonary venous return, cerebral arteriovenous malformation, or decreased extraction from neurological injury or sepsis.

Intracardiac or transthoracic right (RA) and left atrial (LA) catheters may be used to monitor patients after complex surgical procedures. Atrial pressure data reflect several factors including volume status, atrioventricular valve function, ventricular compliance and afterload, heart rate and rhythm, and pleural pressure. In addition, atrial pressure waveforms offer insight into residual disease and atrioventricular synchrony. RA catheters should not be used to measure MVS as the sample may be contaminated by the tip's source including left-to-right shunting at the atrial septum, blood from the coronary sinus, or a specific organ's venous systems in cases where the catheter tip ends in the inferior vena cava. Blood in the LA is normally fully saturated with oxygen (i.e., approximately 100%). The two chief causes of reduced LA oxygen saturation are an atrial level right-to-left shunt and pulmonary venous desaturation from abnormal gas exchange. LA pressure data are especially helpful in the management of patients with left ventricular (LV) systolic or diastolic dysfunction, those at risk for coronary artery perfusion abnormalities resulting in ischemia (e.g., patients following arterial switch operations), and mitral valve disease (Table 64.3). Interpretation of RA and LA data, therefore, requires consideration of the patient's status, trends over time, and identified vulnerabilities in underlying

TABLE 64.3 Common Causes of Elevated Left Atrial Pressure After Cardiotomy

Decreased ventricular systolic or diastolic function
Myocardial ischemia
Dilated cardiomyopathy
Systemic ventricular hypertrophy
Left atrioventricular valve disease
Large left-to-right intracardiac shunt
Chamber hypoplasia
Intravascular or ventricular volume overload
Cardiac tamponade
Arrhythmia:
    Tachyarrhythmia, junctional rhythm
    Complete heart block

physiology and/or surgical interventions (Table 64.4). In the current era, pulmonary artery (PA) catheters are seldom used but may help guide management in patients with or at risk for pulmonary hypertension (PHT).

Additional monitoring data are available in mechanically ventilated patients. Breath-to-breath end-tidal carbon dioxide ($ETCO_2$) monitoring is routine, and trends can be helpful in interpreting a patient's physiology, especially when paired with a simultaneous arterial blood gas. Acute changes in $ETCO_2$ are cause for concern as the data may reflect abrupt changes in pulmonary blood flow and/or cardiac output, or mechanical issues with the ventilator circuit including the endotracheal tube and patient's native airway.

The voluminous amount of real-time data available to CICU clinicians can quickly lead to cognitive overload and alarm fatigue. Predictive analytics is a growing area of research with diverse goals including support of complex

decision-making and early warning systems in patients at risk for clinical decompensation.[7] In addition to offering real-time assistance for clinicians, predictive analytics offer opportunities to understand practice patterns, the impact of the systems on care delivery, and resource allocation. Consistent integration of this technology into clinical practice, however, is yet to be achieved.

Low Cardiac Output State

Although some causes of low cardiac output after CPB are attributable to residual or undiagnosed structural lesions, progressive low cardiac output states do occur. Several factors have been implicated in the development of myocardial dysfunction following CPB including (1) the inflammatory response associated with CPB; (2) the effects of myocardial ischemia from aortic cross clamping; (3) hypothermia; (4) reperfusion injury; (5) inadequate myocardial protection; and (6) ventriculotomy (when performed). A typical and predictable decrease in cardiac index in newborns following cardiac surgery has been reported (Fig 64.1).[8] Appropriate anticipation and intervention for low cardiac output can do much to avert morbidity or the need for mechanical support. Signs of low cardiac output are listed in Table 64.2.

Volume adjustments

After CPB, the factors that influence cardiac output such as preload, afterload, myocardial contractility, heart rate, and rhythm must be assessed and manipulated. Volume therapy (increasing preload) is often necessary, followed by appropriate use of inotropic and afterload-reducing agents. Atrial pressure and the ventricular response to these interventions

TABLE 64.4 Causes of Abnormal Right Atrial, Left Atrial, or Pulmonary Artery Oxygen Saturation

Location	Elevated	Reduced
RA	Atrial level left-to-right shunt	↑ VO_2 (e.g., low CO, fever)
	Anomalous pulmonary venous return	↓ SaO_2 saturation with a normal A-V O_2 difference
	Left ventricular-to-right atrial shunt	Anemia
	↑ dissolved O_2 content	Catheter tip position (e.g., near CS)
	↓ O_2 extraction	
	Catheter tip position (e.g., near renal veins)	
LA	Does not occur	Atrial level right-to-left shunt
		↓ PvO_2 (e.g., parenchymal lung disease)
PA	Significant left-to-right shunt	↑ O_2 extraction (e.g., low CO, fever)
	Small left-to-right shunt with incomplete mixing of blood	↓SaO_2 saturation with a normal A-V O_2 difference
	Catheter tip position (e.g., PA "wedge")	Anemia

A-V, Arteriovenous; *CO*, cardiac output; *CS*, coronary sinus; *LA*, left atrium; *PA*, pulmonary artery; *PvO2*, pulmonary vein oxygen tension; *RA*, right atrium; *SaO2*, arterial oxygen saturation; *VO2*, oxygenation consumption.

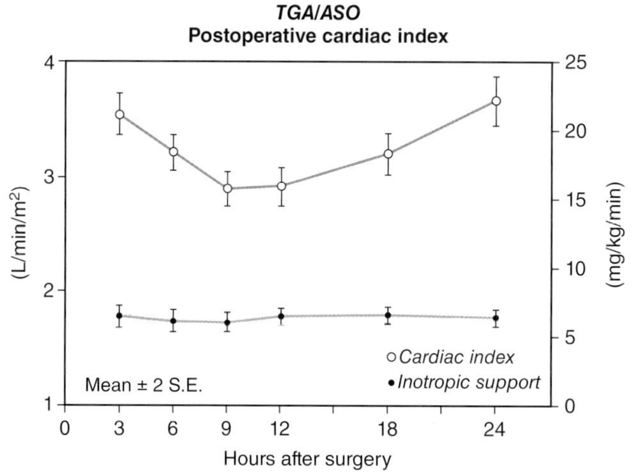

• **Fig. 64.3** Cardiac index measured in infants following the arterial switch operation declines during the first 12 hours. A fourth of the patients reach a value less than 2.0 L/min/m^2. The median reduction in cardiac index the first night is 33%. *TGA*, transposition of the great arteries; *ASO*, arterial switch operation. (See Wernovsky G, Wypij D, Jonas RA, et al. Postoperative course and hemodynamic profile after the arterial switch operation in neonates and infants. A comparison of low-flow cardiopulmonary bypass and circulatory arrest. *Circulation.* 1995;92:2226–2235, with permission.)

must be evaluated continuously. Ventricular response is judged by observing systemic arterial pressure and waveform, heart rate, skin color, core versus peripheral extremity temperature gradient, peripheral pulse magnitude, urine flow, and acid-base balance.

Preserving and creating right-to-left shunts

Select children with low cardiac output may benefit from strategies that allow right-to-left shunting at the atrial level in the face of postoperative right ventricular (RV) dysfunction. Without this "pop-off" a patient will have high oxygen saturations, but the stunned RV is unable to maintain cardiac output leading to inadequate LV filling and hypotension. A typical example is early repair of tetralogy of Fallot, when the moderately hypertrophied, non-compliant RV has undergone a ventriculotomy. It may be further compromised by an increased volume load from pulmonary regurgitation secondary to a transannular patch on the RV outflow tract. In these patients, it is very useful to leave an appropriately sized atrial level communication to permit right-to-left shunting of blood; one accepts a level of cyanosis in exchange for adequate LV filling and cardiac output. This concept has been extended to older patients undergoing the Fontan operation for single ventricle physiology.[9] The Fontan circulation relies on passive flow of blood through the pulmonary circulation without the benefit of a pulmonary ventricle. If a fenestration is created at the time of the Fontan procedure, the resulting right-to-left shunt helps preserve cardiac output.

Pharmacologic Support

Pharmacologic support of the circulation with inotrope, inodilator, or pure vasodilators to support cardiovascular function is commonplace in the CICU. In general, these agents are used after optimizing preload. Table 64.5 provides a list of commonly used agents in the CICU, dose range, and mechanisms of action.[10]

Catecholamines

Catecholamines increase heart rate, blood pressure, and myocardial contractility. Dopamine and epinephrine are

TABLE 64.5 Summary Of selected Vasoactive Active Agents

Non-catecholamines

Agent	Dose (IV)*	Effects		
		Peripheral	*Cardiac*	*Conduction System*
Calcium Chloride Gluconate	 10–20 mg/kg 60–200 mg/kg	Variable; age dependent, vasoconstrictor	Inotropic effect; depends on ionized calcium levels	Slows sinus node; decreases atrioventricular conduction
Nitroprusside	0.5–5 mcg/kg/min	Systemic and pulmonary vasodilator; donates nitric oxide group to relax smooth muscle	Increases cardiac output by reducing afterload	Reflex tachycardia
Nitroglycerin	0.25–10 mcg/kg/min	Primarily venodilator; as a nitric oxide donor may cause pulmonary vasodilation; enhances coronary vasoreactivity after aortic cross-clamping	Decreases preload, may decrease afterload, reduces myocardial work related to change in wall stress	Minimal
Milrinone	Loading dose 25-50 mcg/kg Maintenance 0.25–1.0 mcg/kg/min	Systemic and pulmonary vasodilator	Diastolic relaxation (lusitropy)	Minimal tachycardia

Continued

TABLE 64.5	Summary of Selected Vasoactive Active Agents—cont'd

Non-catecholamines

Agent	Dose (IV)*	Effects		
		Peripheral	Cardiac	Conduction System
Nicardipine	Initial dose 0.5–1 mcg/kg/min, titrate every 15–30 min up to 5 mcg/kg/min	Peripheral arterial vasodilator	Decreased afterload from peripheral vasodilation	Reflex tachycardia
Vasopressin	0.05–2 milli-units/kg/min	Potent systemic arterial vasoconstrictor	No direct effect	None known

Catecholamines

Agent	Dose	Receptor effects				Cardiac effects
		Alpha$_1$	Beta$_1$	Beta$_2$	Dopa	
Dobutamine	2–20 mcg/kg/min	+	+++	+	0	Increases cardiac output (CO); higher dose can cause tachyarrhythmias
Dopamine	< 5 mcg/kg/min	0	0	0	++++	Splanchnic and renal vasodilator
	5–10 mcg/kg/min	+	+++	+	++	Increased contractility and CO
	>10 mcg/kg/min	++++	+++	+	+	Increased contractility and CO; vasoconstriction and increased systemic vascular resistance (SVR)
Epinephrine	0.01–1 mcg/kg/min	++	+++	++	0	Low doses increase contractility and CO; higher doses increase SVR; can induce arrhythmias
Norepinephrine	0.05–1 mcg/kg/min	++++	++	0	0	Increases SVR; may cause renal ischemia; can induce tachyarrhythmias; extravasation can produce ischemic necrosis
Phenylephrine	0.04–2 mcg/kg/min	++++	0	0	0	Increases SVR; can cause reflex bradycardia; may cause renal ischemia; extravasation can produce ischemic necrosis
Isoproterenol	0.05–0.5 mcg/kg/min	0	++++	++++	0	Inotropic and chronotropic agent; peripheral vasodilation; reduces preload; can cause tachycardia, increasing myocardial oxygen consumption

*Appropriateness of use and dosing range for an individual patient will vary.

commonly used agents in CICUs. Dopamine has inotropic effects seen at doses of 5–10 mcg/kg/min and vasoconstrictor effects at doses > 10 mcg/kg/min. Dopamine increases myocardial oxygen consumption and heart rate in a dose-dependent manner. Epinephrine is used as a first-line agent or concurrently with other agents like dopamine. Epinephrine at lower doses predominantly increases myocardial contractility, while higher doses cause vasoconstriction. Bolus-dose epinephrine is the drug of choice for cardiopulmonary resuscitation. Dobutamine has inotropic and vasodilatory properties that can be useful in the management of children with decompensated systolic heart failure. Dobutamine is more commonly used in adults with systolic heart failure. Norepinephrine has predominantly vasoconstrictor effects and is useful in patients with vasodilatory shock unresponsive to dopamine or epinephrine. Norepinephrine can increase coronary blood flow by increasing diastolic blood pressure. Isoproterenol has chronotropic and inotropic properties in addition to being a systemic and pulmonary vasodilator. Its use in children is limited and primarily to affect a temporary increase in ventricular escape rate in patients with complete heart block while other definitive therapies are being arranged.

Although catecholamine infusions can be lifesaving in critically ill children, they should be used with caution and thoughtful consideration of potential side effects. Postoperative arrhythmias can be caused or exacerbated by use of catecholamines which may contribute to morbidity and mortality. Increasing perioperative experience in neonates and children provides insight into the adverse effects of catecholamine infusions in this population. Myocardial necrosis caused by high doses of epinephrine infusions has been identified in neonatal animal models after CPB.[11] During high-dose dopamine infusion, less compliant neonatal myocardium, like the ischemic adult heart, will develop increased end-diastolic pressure which can present clinically as extreme non-compliance. Although catecholamines increase cardiac output, concomitant increase in ventricular filling pressure is less well tolerated by the immature neonatal myocardium than it is in older children. In patients with single ventricle CHD, catecholamine-induced diastolic function may be very poorly tolerated. Nevertheless, the predictable and often significant decrease in cardiac output in patients following CPB continues to justify the practice of judiciously using catecholamines to support the heart and circulation in the immediate postoperative period.

Phosphodiesterase III inhibitors

Phosphodiesterase III inhibitors are used extensively in patients with heart failure. Milrinone has emerged as an important inotropic agent for use in children after open heart surgery. It is a non-glycosidic, non-catecholamine inotropic agent with additional vasodilatory and lusitropic properties. This class of drugs exerts its principal effects by inhibiting phosphodiesterase III, the enzyme that metabolizes cyclic adenosine monophosphate (cAMP). By increasing intracellular cAMP, calcium transport into the cell is favored, and the increased intracellular calcium stores enhance the contractile state of the myocyte. In addition, the reuptake of calcium is a cAMP-dependent process, and these agents may therefore enhance diastolic relaxation of the myocardium by increasing the rate of calcium reuptake after systole (lusitropy). The drug also appears to work synergistically with low doses of β-agonists and has fewer side effects than other catecholamine vasodilators, such as dobutamine or isoproterenol. In studies of critically ill postoperative newborns, milrinone increased cardiac output, lowered filling pressures, and reduced PA pressures.[12] Phosphodiesterase III inhibitors are often used in combination with catecholamines to achieve increased cardiac output, maintain arterial perfusion pressure, and potentially improve diastolic function.

Other vasoactive agents

When systemic blood pressure is elevated and cardiac output appears low or normal, a primary vasodilator is indicated to normalize blood pressure and decrease afterload on the LV. This is especially true for the newborn myocardium, which is especially sensitive to changes in afterload and tolerates elevated systemic resistance poorly. Although nitroprusside has no known direct inotropic effects, this potent vasodilator has the advantage of being readily titratable with a short biologic half-life. Use of nitroglycerin avoids the toxic metabolites, cyanide and thiocyanate, associated with nitroprusside use (especially in hepatic and renal insufficiency), but its potency as a vasodilator is less than that of nitroprusside. Inhibitors of angiotensin-converting enzyme have proven to be important adjuvants to chronic anti-congestive therapy in pediatric patients. Intravenous forms are available and may be useful in treatment of systemic hypertension immediately after coarctation repair or when afterload reduction with these inhibitors would benefit patients unable to receive oral medications. Sudden hypotension with the intravenous forms may limit use among infants. Nicardipine, a smooth muscle selective calcium channel blocker, that causes selective peripheral arterial vasodilation is used for management of hypertension, especially in children post-coarctectomy. Nicardipine can cause reflex tachycardia and thus increase myocardial oxygen consumption.

Fenoldopam is a dopaminergic agent useful in the treatment of systemic hypertension and may have beneficial effects on renal blood flow. It has no known chronotropic or inotropic effects on the heart but reduces afterload and may augment urine output in critically ill patients. Levosimendan is a calcium sensitizer that enhances the contractile state of the ventricle by increasing myocyte sensitivity to calcium and inducing vasodilation; this increases cardiac output by increasing stroke volume. It is independent of cAMP pathways that characterize the mechanism of action of both the catecholamines and the type III phosphodiesterase inhibitors. With its positive inotropic effects, levosimendan may be of value as adjunctive therapy to other inotropic drugs in patients who are refractory or tachyphylactic to other forms of inotropic support. The hemodynamic effect of levosimendan in children is uncertain, but its pharmacokinetic profile seems similar to that in adults. Arginine vasopressin improves blood pressure by increasing systemic vascular resistance and some have advocated for its use in catecholamine refractory vasodilatory shock following cardiac surgery with CPB.

Other Strategies

Additional strategies to support low cardiac output associated with cardiac surgery in children include the use of atrioventricular pacing for patients with complete heart block, prolonged interventricular conduction delays, or asynchronous contraction. The hemodynamic effects of positive and negative pressure mechanical ventilation may be used to facilitate cardiac output. Avoidance of hyperthermia and even inducing modest hypothermia may decrease oxygen demand and provide end-organ protection during periods of low cardiac output.

Management of the Cyanotic Patient

Cyanosis is a common presenting feature in critically ill children with CHD. A disciplined approach to the differential diagnosis is helpful in guiding next steps and focusing diagnostic studies. Potential etiologies of cyanosis in this patient population include low inspired oxygen fraction, pulmonary vein desaturation, decreased pulmonary blood flow, decreased dissolved oxygen content, or a combination of the above factors. A low fraction of inspired oxygen may be secondary to inadequate delivery or failure of an oxygen delivery device. Pulmonary vein desaturation may be secondary to impaired diffusion as seen in an alveolar process (e.g., edema) or restrictive process (e.g., effusion, atelectasis). Pulmonary vein desaturation may also be seen with an intrapulmonary shunt (e.g., collaterals, arteriovenous malformation, respiratory distress syndrome). The etiology of decreased pulmonary blood flow includes anatomic obstruction, increased pulmonary vascular resistance (PVR) or intracardiac right-to-left shunt. Dissolved oxygen content may exist in patients with a low hemoglobin concentration or a low mixed venous saturation from a low cardiac output state. The contribution of the latter is often underappreciated in CHD and reinforces the need for adequate and accurate monitoring of a patient's hemodynamic state A wide difference in arterial to end-expired carbon dioxide supports significant dead space ventilation and may represent right-to-left shunting and reduced pulmonary blood flow. Diagnosis includes obtaining a chest radiograph to rule out lung pathology and an echocardiogram to evaluate adequacy of pulmonary blood flow and cardiac output. Cardiac catheterization, and in some cases surgical intervention, may be indicated in patients with clinically significant cyanosis refractory to medical management.

Diastolic Dysfunction

The management of diastolic dysfunction and its sequelae remains one of the biggest challenges for clinicians in the CICU. Current echocardiographic technology does not provide the same visceral sense of impaired ventricular compliance the way one can immediately visualize systolic dysfunction. Hemodynamic data obtained during cardiac catheterization may represent one moment in time and not the physiologic reality of changing intravascular preload and afterload. Pressure-volume-loop data from conductance catheters may offer critical insight but are still early in development. These limitations can make the diagnosis of diastolic dysfunction difficult to recognize. In some cases, such as myocardial edema following CPB, it may be reversible with time and diuresis. In many patients with CHD, however, decreased ventricular compliance appears fixed and therefore may reflect developmental abnormalities of the myocardium or irreversible remodeling from chronic pathophysiology.

Despite initial optimism with a handful of pharmacological agents over the past few decades, few options exist for the cardiac intensivist to meaningfully improve diastolic function in the most severely affected patients. Avoiding exacerbating factors such as residual outflow tract obstruction or excessive use of exogenous catecholamines (e.g., dopamine or epinephrine) is a critical first step. A gradual increase in intravascular volume to augment ventricular capacity, in addition to the use of low doses of inotropic agents, has proven to provide modest benefit. Tachycardia should be avoided to optimize diastolic filling time and to decrease myocardial oxygen demands. If low cardiac output continues despite the above-outlined treatment, therapy with vasodilators can be carefully attempted to alter systolic wall tension (afterload) and thus decrease the work of the ventricle. Because the capacity of the vascular bed increases after vasodilation, simultaneous volume replacement is often indicated. Phosphodiesterase inhibitors are useful under these circumstances, since, in contrast to other inotropes, these agents are non-catecholamine inodilators with vasodilating and lusitropic properties. It is important to recognize the negative impact of elevated end-diastolic pressure on coronary perfusion pressure, especially when pharmacologically decreasing mean arterial pressure and/or increasing intravascular volume.

Diastolic dysfunction continues to be poorly understood and characterized, negatively impacts the outcomes of pediatric patients with CHD and acquired heart disease, and has limited treatment options.[13] It therefore presents ample opportunities for research and innovation.

Cardiovascular Interactions with other Organs

Cardiopulmonary Interactions

Altered respiratory mechanics and positive pressure ventilation may significantly influence a patient's hemodynamics after congenital heart surgery and in acute decompensated heart failure. Approaches to mechanical ventilation should therefore target desired gas exchange while simultaneously acknowledging the potential positive or negative cardiorespiratory interactions for an individual patient. Frequent modifications to the mode and pattern of ventilation may be necessary during a patient's recovery with attention to changes in lung volume and mean airway pressure.

Positive pressure ventilation influences preload and afterload on the heart (Table 64.6).[14] Afterload on the subpulmonary ventricle is increased during a positive pressure breath secondary to the increase in mean intrathoracic pressure and changes in lung volume. Changes in lung volume have a major effect on PVR which is lowest at the lung's functional residual capacity (FRC). Hypo- or hyperinflation may result in a significant increase in PVR because of altered traction on alveolar septa and extra-alveolar vessels. Increasing intrathoracic pressure decreases preload to the RA and LA. If this is significant, or there is limited functional

	Afterload	Preload
TABLE 64.6 Cardiorespiratory Interactions of a Positive Pressure Mechanical Breath		
Pulmonary Ventricle	Elevated Effect: ↑ RVEDp ↑ RVp ↓ Antegrade PBF ↑ PR and/or TR	Reduced Effect: ↓ RVEDV ↓ RAp
Systemic Ventricle	Reduced Effect: ↓LVEDp ↓ LAp ↓ Pulmonary edema ↑ Increase cardiac output	Reduced Effect: ↓LVEDV ↓ LAp

LAp, Left atrial pressure; *LVEDp,* left ventricle end-diastolic pressure; *LVEDV,* left ventricle end-diastolic volume; *PBF,* pulmonary blood flow; *PR,* pulmonary regurgitation; *RAp,* right atrial pressure; *RVEDp,* right ventricle end-diastolic pressure; *RVEDV,* right ventricle end-diastolic volume; *RVp,* right ventricle pressure; *TR,* tricuspid regurgitation. Please note that in some cases the morphologic ventricle in the systemic and/or pulmonary position may be different than what is indicated above. The physiologic implications remain consistent.

reserve, RV stroke volume may be reduced and end-diastolic pressure increased. This in turn may contribute to a low cardiac output state with evidence of RV dysfunction including tricuspid regurgitation, hepatomegaly, ascites, and pleural effusions. It is therefore important to actively manage the ventilator settings to obtain ideal lung volumes (targeting FRC to achieve lowest PVR) with simultaneous consideration of the impact of mean airway pressure on the circulation.

In contrast to the RV, the afterload on the systemic ventricle is decreased during a positive pressure breath secondary to a fall in the ventricle transmural pressure. LV dysfunction, including increased end-diastolic volume and pressure, may lead to impaired pulmonary mechanics such as increased lung water, decreased lung compliance, and increased airway resistance. A significant proportion of total body oxygen consumption may be needed to support the increased work of breathing associated with these sequelae; this results in poor feeding and failure to thrive. Therefore, positive pressure ventilation has an additional benefit in patients with significant volume overload and systemic ventricular dysfunction by reducing the work of breathing and oxygen demand.

The use of positive end-expiratory pressure (PEEP) in patients with CHD and acquired heart disease can be challenging. PEEP increases FRC, enables lung recruitment, and redistributes lung water from alveolar septal regions to the more compliant perihilar regions. These actions will improve gas exchange and reduce PVR. Usually, 3 to 5 cm H_2O of PEEP will help maintain FRC and redistribute lung water without causing hemodynamic compromise. Excessive levels of PEEP, however, can be detrimental by increasing afterload on the right side of the circulation; this is especially true in circulations with passive pulmonary blood flow such as the Glenn and Fontan. The optimal condition for these circulations occurs when the patient can breathe spontaneously, thereby generating negative pleural and

intrathoracic pressures and facilitating systemic venous return. Early transition to a pressure-support mode of breathing with the goal of extubation during the first few postoperative hours is the goal. Sedation strategies that support spontaneous respiratory effort and therefore minimize mean airway pressure may serve to optimize a patient's hemodynamics.

Pulmonary edema, atelectasis, and inflammation are the most common causes of lower airway and alveolar abnormalities that interfere with gas exchange. If the cause is pulmonary edema, therapy is aimed toward lowering the left atrial pressure through diuresis as well as pharmacologic means to reduce afterload and improve the lusitropic state of the heart. For infants, fluid restriction is frequently incompatible with adequate nutrition and, therefore, an aggressive diuretic regimen is preferable to restriction of caloric intake. Adjustment of end-expiratory pressure and mechanical ventilation serve as supportive therapies until the alveoli and pulmonary interstitium are cleared of the fluid that interferes with gas exchange. Patients who have secretions from the tracheal aspirate with many visible organisms and polymorphonuclear cells on microscopy, together with fever and an elevated white blood cell count, require treatment with appropriate antibiotics and pulmonary toilet. This may require more nuanced care in at-risk patients such as those with ciliary dysfunction (e.g., heterotaxy syndrome).

Pleural effusions and ascites may occur in patients with elevated CVPs, for example, following Fontan operation, reparative procedures requiring a right ventriculotomy, or as a consequence of RV systolic or diastolic dysfunction. Evacuation of the pleural space and/or decompression of the abdomen will support gas exchange at lower mean airway pressures and should be considered early in the course of a hemodynamically vulnerable patient, especially in a challenging Fontan circulation. Testing pleural fluid for evidence of chyle should be considered in patients with elevated CVP, at risk for clot in the central venous system of the head and neck (e.g., central venous line *in situ*), or in whom there may have been trauma to the thoracic lymphatics. It is important to note that chylous effusions will not always appear "milky"; the fluids characteristics will reflect an individual patient's nutritional status. Furthermore, low lymphocyte counts in pleural fluid may reflect overall lymphopenia in the patient. It is therefore recommended that pleural fluid is sampled for both triglycerides and lymphocyte count, and that the diagnostic criteria are evaluated in the context of the patient's overall status.

Diaphragmatic paresis (reduced motion) or paralysis (paradoxical movement) may precipitate and promote respiratory failure, particularly in the neonate or young infant who relies on diaphragmatic function for breathing more than older patients. Injury to the phrenic nerve, usually the left, may occur during operations that require dissection of the branch pulmonary arteries well out to the hilum (e.g., tetralogy of Fallot, arterial switch operation), arch reconstruction from the midline (e.g., Norwood operation), manipulation of the superior vena cava (e.g., Glenn shunts), takedown of previous systemic-to-pulmonary shunts, or after percutaneous subclavian or internal jugular central venous access. Phrenic injury may occur more frequently at reoperation, when adhesions and scarring may obscure landmarks. Topical cooling with ice during deep hypothermia may also cause transient phrenic palsy. Increased work of breathing on low ventilator settings, increased Pco_2, and a chest radiograph revealing an elevated hemidiaphragm are suggestive of diaphragmatic dysfunction. The chest radiograph may be misleading if taken during peak positive pressure ventilation. Ultrasonography or fluoroscopy is useful for identifying diaphragmatic motion or paradoxical excursion. Recovery of diaphragmatic contraction usually occurs but may require substantial time that is not justified by the risks of a prolonged CICU course. If a patient fails to tolerate repeat extubation attempts despite optimizing cardiovascular and nutritional status, and diaphragmatic dysfunction persists with volume loss in the affected lung, then the diaphragm may need to be surgically plicated. Although only a temporary effect is gained, mitigating collapse and volume loss in the affected lung may provide the critical advantage.

There are multiple etiologies for extubation failures in this patient population. Post-extubation stridor may be due to mucosal swelling of the large airway and a nebulized, inhaled alpha agonist such as racemic epinephrine may promote vasoconstriction and decreases hyperemia and edema. If reintubation is necessary, a smaller endotracheal tube should be used, if possible, along with diuresis and consideration of a short-term course of steroids, prior to a subsequent attempt at extubation in 24–36 hours. The prevalence of vocal cord dysfunction, notably in patients who have undergone aortic arch reconstruction with risk of injury to the recurrent laryngeal nerve, is a growing area of research. Patients with a weak cry or persistent upper airway obstruction should be evaluated, as findings may impact not only a patient's cardiopulmonary status but the ability to successfully feed by mouth without risk of aspiration. Bronchospasm may be treated by inhaled or systemically administered bronchodilators but must be used with caution considering their chronotropic and tachyarrhythmic potential. In addition, wheezing on exam may be a consequence of primary or secondary PHT in which case cardiovascular interventions should be prioritized over pulmonary therapies. Patients with CHD are at increased risk of airways disease such as tracheobronchomalacia.[15] Dependence on positive pressure ventilation beyond expected timeframes should prompt consideration of additional airway evaluation.

Central Nervous System

The dramatic reduction in surgical mortality since the mid-20th century has been accompanied by a growing recognition of adverse neurologic sequelae in some survivors. CNS abnormalities may be a function of coexisting brain abnormalities or acquired events unrelated to surgical management (e.g., paradoxical embolus, effects of chronic cyanosis), but CNS insults appear to occur most frequently during or immediately after surgery. Support techniques used during neonatal and infant cardiac surgery including CPB, profound

hypothermia, and circulatory arrest, have been implicated as important causes of brain injury.[16]

Our patient population is also at risk of micro- and macro-embolic events from cardiac catheterization procedures, long-term maintenance of central access—particularly in those with residual right-to-left shunts, and mechanical circulatory support. During hypothermic CPB, there are multiple perfusion variables that might influence the risk of brain injury. These include (but are probably not limited to) (1) the total duration of CPB and the duration and rate of core cooling; (2) pH management during core cooling; (3) duration of circulatory arrest; (4) type of oxygenator; (5) presence of arterial filtration; and (6) depth of hypothermia. Undoubtedly, there is interaction between these various elements, and CNS injury following CPB is likely multifactorial. Early postoperative studies reveal a higher incidence of neurologic perturbation in patients undergoing circulatory arrest including a higher incidence of clinical and electroencephalographic (EEG) seizures, a longer recovery time to the first reappearance of EEG activity, and greater release of the brain isoenzyme of creatine kinase (see Chapter 55).

Seizures are the most frequently observed neurologic consequence of cardiac surgery using CPB with an incidence in older studies of 4% to 25%. Benzodiazepine-refractory seizures are treated aggressively in the BCH CICU using antiseizure medications such as levetiracetam, phenobarbital, fosphenytoin, or valproic acid.[17] Reducing or eliminating, where possible, practices that may be associated with brain injury after CPB is a priority. Avoiding fever, maintaining temperature <37.5°C in the early postoperative period, and treating any metabolic derangements promptly is thought to be protective.[18] Continuous EEG monitoring is increasingly used for routine screening following CPB and for seizure detection in patients with limited clinical exams (e.g., patients who are muscle relaxed).

Intraventricular hemorrhage may occur as a consequence of perinatal events or circulatory collapse in the first few days of life, and it is commonly associated with prematurity. At this time there is not universal agreement regarding the best approach to pre-CPB screening of infants.[19] Head ultrasound and head MRI should be considered, especially in high-risk patients. Each modality requires resources, however, and varies in sensitivity and specificity. It is important to acknowledge circumstances that may put patients at risk which exceeds potential benefit. In cases where intraventricular bleeding is documented, surgical intervention is delayed for several days. Our strategy of deferring operations in very premature newborns for several days to weeks after birth is associated with a lower incidence of intraventricular hemorrhage in these high risk patients despite use of CPB.[20]

The BCH CICU benefits from a neurocritical care consult service and stroke team that aids in the management of acute brain injury. Neurological surveillance of our patients includes neuroimaging and non-invasive neuromonitoring with continuous bedside EEG and near-infrared spectroscopy (NIRS) to trend cerebral perfusion. Attention is paid to monitoring and addressing withdrawal from sedatives and analgesics, preventing delirium, and establishing a proper day-night cycle to optimize adequate sleep time.

An overarching goal of care for children with CHD, particularly those who have suffered acute brain injury (e.g., stroke, seizures) is to optimize neuromotor development and trajectory. We have incorporated input from physical medicine rehabilitation faculty and specialty rehabilitative services such as physical therapy, occupational therapy, speech and language, feeding team services, child life and behavioral services with a goal of maximizing patients' function and successful re-entry back into home life (e.g., social interactions, school, sports).

Renal Function and Postoperative Fluid Management

Risk factors for postoperative renal failure include preoperative renal dysfunction, prolonged bypass time, low cardiac output, cardiac arrest, and venoarterial extracorporeal membrane oxygenation (VA ECMO). Medical and surgical factors including pre-existing pathophysiology, nephrotoxic agents, and complications such as sepsis may cause injury to the kidneys independent of the postoperative state.

There is an inflammatory response to bypass leading to significant increase in total body water; therefore, fluid management in the immediate postoperative period is critical. During CPB, optimizing the circuit prime, hematocrit, and oncotic pressure, attenuating the inflammatory response with steroids and protease inhibitors such as aprotinin, and using modified ultrafiltration techniques have all been recommended to limit interstitial fluid accumulation. During the first 24 hours after surgery, maintenance fluids should be used judiciously. Volume replacement should be thoughtfully titrated to an individual patient's appropriate filling pressures and hemodynamic response accounting for anatomy, anticipated physiology, and surgical history. Oliguria in the first 24 hours after complex surgery and CPB is common in neonates and infants until cardiac output recovers and neurohumoral mechanisms abate. Capillary leak and interstitial fluid accumulation may continue beyond 24 hours postoperatively necessitating ongoing volume replacement with colloid or blood products. A fall in cardiac output and increased antidiuretic hormone secretion contribute to delayed water clearance and potential prerenal dysfunction; this can progress to acute tubular necrosis and renal failure if a low cardiac output state persists. Although diuretics are commonly prescribed in the immediate postoperative period, the neurohumoral influence on urine output is powerful. Time after CPB and enhancement of cardiac output through volume and pharmacologic adjustments are the most important factors in promoting diuresis.

Peritoneal dialysis, intermittent hemodialysis, and continuous veno-venous hemofiltration (CVVH) provide alternate renal support in patients with severe oliguria and renal failure. Indications for, and timing of initiation of renal replacement therapy (RRT), remain an area of debate and an

opportunity for future research. It is reasonable to include blood urea nitrogen level above 100 mg/dL, life-threatening electrolyte imbalance such as severe hyperkalemia, ongoing metabolic acidosis, fluid restrictions limiting nutrition, and increased mechanical ventilation requirements secondary to persistent pulmonary edema or ascites. Some advocate for earlier or even preemptive dialysis in at-risk populations as a longer duration of acute kidney injury prior to initiating RRT has been associated with mortality in this patient population. The impact of residual lesions on renal failure and the success of RRT is yet to be fully elucidated; however, the potential to improve renal pathophysiology by improving the systemic circulation through catheter-based or surgical interventions (including re-interventions) should be considered early in a patient's course.

Gastrointestinal Issues

Adequate nutrition is exceedingly important for all age groups following cardiac surgery. Oftentimes, these critically ill patients have decreased caloric intake and increased energy demand; in particular, the neonate has limited metabolic and fat reserves. Research and QI initiatives in this field are increasing exponentially as clinicians focus on optimizing short-term strategies to achieve better long-term outcomes.

Upper gastrointestinal bleeding and ulcer formation may occur following the stress of cardiac surgery in children and adults. There are limited reports of the efficacy of histamine H2-receptor antagonists, sucralfate, or oral antacids in pediatric cardiac patients, although their use is common in many intensive care units. Drawbacks include a negative impact on the microbiome with potential to increase risk of necrotizing enterocolitis and hospital-acquired infections.

Hepatic failure may occur after cardiac surgery if there is inadequate arterial perfusion, acutely elevated CVP leading to hepatic congestion, or both. Patients presenting with elevated lactate burden in the setting of a reassuring clinical exam should be screened for liver dysfunction. Patients at risk for congestive hepatopathy with changes in mental status should have a serum ammonia level checked. Please see Chapter 59 for discussion of liver disease in patients with Fontan circulation.

Necrotizing enterocolitis, although typically a disease of premature infants, is seen with considerable frequency in neonates with CHD. Risk factors include (1) left-sided obstructive lesions, (2) umbilical or femoral arterial catheterization/angiography, (3) hypoxemia, and (4) "run-off" lesions with retrograde flow in the mesenteric vessels during diastole manifesting as wide aortic pulse pressures (e.g., patent ductus arteriosus, surgical systemic-to-pulmonary vascular bed shunts, severe aortic regurgitation). Frequently, multiple risk factors exist in the same patient, making a specific etiology difficult to establish. Treatment includes continuous nasogastric suction, parenteral nutrition, and broad-spectrum antibiotics. Bowel exploration or resection may be necessary in severe cases.

Infection

Low-grade (<38.5°C) fever during the immediate postoperative period is common and may be present for 3 to 4 days, even without a demonstrable infectious etiology. A centrally mediated etiology of fever following CPB has been postulated. There are, however, several reports of increased susceptibility to infection after CPB. CPB may activate complement and other mediators of inflammation but can also lead to derangements of the immune system and increase the likelihood of infection. Sepsis and nosocomial infection after cardiac surgery contribute substantially to overall morbidity. Meticulous procedural hygiene and daily care routines which emphasize early removal of invasive lines and catheters may improve outcomes. Collaborative QI initiatives with surgical, nursing, and respiratory colleagues are critical for success.

Mediastinitis occurs in a small percentage of patients undergoing cardiac surgery; risk factors include delayed sternal closure, early re-exploration for bleeding, and reoperation. Mediastinitis is characterized by persistent fever, purulent drainage from the sternotomy wound, instability of the sternum, and leukocytosis. Treatment usually involves debridement and antibiotic therapy.

Managing Acute Pulmonary Hypertension in the Intensive Care Unit

Elevation in PVR is common in many forms of CHD and may be evident in both preoperative and postoperative setting. The etiology relates to many different and often interacting factors including the underlying physiology, pulmonary vascular endothelial dysfunction, micro emboli, an imbalance of various endogenous vasoactive agents favoring vasoconstriction, atelectasis, edema, and hypoxia. A more detailed description of PHT can be found in Chapter 56 and the cited guideline.[21] Evaluation of postoperative PVR should include exclusion of residual left-to-right shunts and anatomic causes such as left atrial hypertension, pulmonary venous obstruction, and postoperative anatomical anomalies of the pulmonary vasculature. The duration of CPB may also influence PVR, but the prevalence of pulmonary hypertensive crises has been markedly reduced by surgery at earlier ages, pharmacologic intervention, and other postoperative management strategies (Table 64.7). Adequate ventilation around the FRC should be employed in all patients to minimize the hypoxic and mechanical effects on PVR.

Pulmonary Vasodilators

Many intravenous vasodilators have been used with variable success in patients with postoperative PHT. Prostacyclin (PGI2), a prostanoid mediating inflammation with vasodilatory and potent platelet aggregation inhibition effects, increases levels of cellular cAMP by stimulation of adenylate cyclase and appears to have some selectivity for the pulmonary circulation but at high doses can precipitate a hypotensive crisis in unstable postoperative patients with refractory PHT. It is best suited for chronic outpatient therapy in severe forms of primary PHT. Agents that improve ventricular function in addition to reducing afterload (e.g., type III phosphodiesterase inhibitors, such as milrinone, which inhibit breakdown of cAMP) are more appealing when cardiac output is low. The pulmonary vasoconstrictor endothelin, which acts via both endothelin-A (ET-A) and endothelin-B (ET-B) receptors, which have differing effects on PVR, is elevated in various pulmonary hypertensive states which may be further exacerbated following CPB. Endothelin receptor agonists (ERA) may help alleviate acute and chronic PHT. Phosphodiesterase 5 inhibitors (PDE5i), such as sildenafil and tadalafil, exert a pulmonary vasodilatory effect via cGMP pathways, and have also been used with significant benefit in differing

TABLE 64.7	Critical Care Strategies for Postoperative Treatment of Pulmonary Hypertension	
Encourage	**Avoid**
1. Anatomic investigation	1. Residual anatomic disease
2. Opportunities for atrial shunting as "pop-off"	2. Intact atrial septum
3. Sedation/anesthesia	3. Agitation/pain
4. Moderate hyperventilation	4. Respiratory acidosis
5. Moderate alkalosis	5. Metabolic acidosis
6. Adequate inspired oxygen	6. Alveolar hypoxia
7. Normal lung volumes	7. Atelectasis or overdistention
8. Optimal hematocrit	8. Excessive hematocrit
9. Inotropic support	9. Low output and/or inadequate coronary perfusion
10. Vasodilators	10. Vasoconstrictors/increased afterload

forms of PHT. Given the complex and multifactorial nature of PHT, synergistic effects may be seen with multiple agents used simultaneously, although the vasoactive nature may lead to significant hemodynamic side effects which may be exacerbated in the precarious postoperative circulation.

Endogenous nitric oxide (NO) is derived from L-arginine and oxygen catalyzed by NO synthase, and acts via cGMP pathways to cause pulmonary vasodilation of pulmonary vascular smooth muscle. Therapeutic NO can be delivered as an inhaled agent in a ventilatory circuit, and due to its rapid inactivation by hemoglobin, has a selective effect on the pulmonary vascular bed. This makes it an especially effective agent in the postoperative management of PHT in various forms of CHD where deleterious effects on cardiac output are minimal.[22] Inhaled NO can be highly effective in anatomic lesions associated with pulmonary venous hypertension such as mitral stenosis, repaired total anomalous pulmonary venous connection, and pulmonary veno-occlusive disorders but should be used with caution as it may exacerbate underlying pathophysiology. Inhaled NO can also be used to distinguish PHT secondary to vasoactive disease as opposed to anatomic lesions, where the latter may require surgical intervention.[23] As both PDE5i and NO cause pulmonary vasodilation via the cGMP pathway, PDE5i, in particular sildenafil, has been used successfully to limit rebound PHT and wean inhaled NO and ventilatory support following cardiac surgery.[24]

Mechanical Support of the Circulation

Aggressive identification and treatment of low cardiac output conditions after cardiac surgery is central to the critical care of children with CHD. Successful application of these strategies and thoughtful use of pharmacologic intervention has undoubtedly contributed to the remarkable decline in mortality associated with congenital heart surgery since the latter half of the 20th century. Despite these interventions, however, some preoperative and postoperative children cannot be adequately stabilized with medical management alone. In these situations, mechanical support strategies have important roles in enabling myocardial recovery and in some situations, providing longer-term support while awaiting cardiac transplantation.[25] Although a variety of assist devices are available, ECMO is the predominant temporary mode of mechanical circulatory support for children when recovery of myocardial function is expected in the short-term. ECMO adverse events increase with ECMO duration; therefore, ECMO is not a suitable mechanical circulatory support device for children who require transplantation. Durable mechanical circulatory support devices such as ventricular assist devices (VADs) have largely replaced ECMO for this indication. VADs are discussed in more detail in Chapter 54.

Indications and contraindications for ECMO in patients with CHD are summarized in Tables 64.8 and 64.9. VA ECMO provides both cardiac and respiratory support and is the most common approach in children with CHD or

TABLE 64.8	Indications for Cardiac ECMO

Inadequate Oxygen Delivery

A. Low cardiac output
   Preoperative stabilization
   Failure to wean from cardiopulmonary bypass
   Progressive postoperative failure
   Pulmonary hypertensive crisis
   Refractory arrhythmias
   Severe sepsis
   Acute decompensated heart failure
   Cardiac arrest

B. Profound cyanosis
   Intracardiac shunting and cardiovascular collapse
   Acute respiratory failure
   Acute systemic-to-pulmonary artery shunt thrombosis

C. Procedural support

TABLE 64.9	Relative Contraindications for ECMO

End-stage, irreversible, or inoperable disease
Extreme size (weight < 2 kg) and prematurity (gestational age < 34 weeks)
Severe neurological injury
Irreversible end-organ dysfunction
Uncontrollable bleeding
Family or patient goals of care to limit resuscitation

acquired heart disease. Ideally, recovery for children requiring ECMO following surgery for CHD is 5–7 days; however, there is a significant incidence of residual structural lesions when ECMO is needed in the postoperative period.[26] These lesions should be promptly diagnosed and corrected so that ECMO can be weaned and discontinued efficiently. Inability to wean off ECMO should prompt discussions about need for additional surgical interventions or candidacy for heart transplantation. Patients supported with VA ECMO beyond 14 days have increased risks for irreversible end-organ injury and death. It is therefore imperative that the CICU team proactively address any anatomic or physiologic challenges that may prevent a patient's successful separation from ECMO.

There is substantial institutional variability in patient selection and delivery of care for ECMO patients. Centers with an efficient and well-established ECMO service are more likely to use this form of support in patients with low cardiac output. This form of mechanical support had been demonstrated to be lifesaving, and it can be argued that it should be available when needed for selected patients following congenital heart surgery.[27] Immediate referral to centers with ECMO capabilities should be considered in patients at risk for acute hemodynamic collapse (e.g., acute fulminant myocarditis, refractory arrhythmias). ECMO for pediatric resuscitation (rapid deployment during active cardiopulmonary resuscitation [E-CPR]) in a pulseless circulation remains a controversial issue but is a commonly used rescue mechanism in centers where such resources exist.

The Extracorporeal Life Support Organization (ELSO) is an organization that collects ECMO-related information from nearly 400 centers around the world. Its data reflect increasing use of ECMO in children with cardiac disease and 40% survival to hospital discharge in this patient population (www.ELSO.org). Neonates, those suffering a cardiac arrest prior to ECMO, and patients with single ventricle CHD have lower survival outcomes and should be considered high-risk ECMO patients.

Summary

It is important to recognize that almost every treatment approach has its own set of adverse effects that may contribute to morbidity and mortality. Supporting cardiac output in a vulnerable circulation is a balance between the promise and poison of therapy. Optimizing preload involves more than just giving volume to a hypotensive patient. Fluid itself can be detrimental if excess extravascular water results in interstitial edema and end-organ dysfunction of vital organs like the heart, lungs, and brain. Maintaining aortic perfusion, after CPB or in a patient with acute decompensated heart failure, is a reasonable goal but exogenous catecholamines may have deleterious consequences in some situations. The benefits of afterload reduction are well known, but in excess there may be hypotension leading to end-organ injury, coronary insufficiency, and cardiovascular collapse. Cardiopulmonary interactions are magnified by positive pressure ventilation, which may serve to benefit a struggling patient (e.g., decreasing afterload in the patient with LV dysfunction) or offer additional challenges to the intensivist managing a suboptimal circulation (e.g., negatively impacting venous return and pulmonary blood flow in a Fontan patient). Finally, mechanical support of the failing myocardium in the form of mechanical support strategies like ECMO, while lifesaving in many instances, presents its own set of time limitations and potential negative consequences.

Future Directions

CICUs exist at the crux of care delivery in high-volume pediatric cardiology programs; as such, they play a crucial role in short- and long-term patient outcomes and the success of cardiovascular centers as a whole. Well-trained intensivists with extensive experience in pediatric cardiology and pediatric critical care medicine must also have the capacity to lead diverse teams and navigate the complexities of high-acuity care delivery. A better understanding of the human factors involved in routine decision-making, as well as in high stakes situations, is needed.

Although survival has improved dramatically for patients with CHD and pediatric acquired heart disease, there is increasing recognition that long-term outcomes such as quality of life and neurodevelopment are not optimal. Critical self-reflection that guides change and inspires innovation is

necessary. Multi-institutional collaborative research offers opportunities for insight. This approach has been demonstrated successfully with national initiatives to reduce narcotic and sedative exposure, routinely implement delirium screening, and encourage early mobilization. Ideally this endeavor will inspire others to challenge our established practice patterns with fresh perspectives.

Disparities in healthcare delivery and resource allocation are a harsh reality that demands our attention. Patients and families increasingly desire direct participation in decision-making with a focus on quality of life. Palliative care, spiritual care, and ethics teams are growing to meet this need. Nowhere are multidisciplinary skills and collaborative practices more valued or necessary. As we look to the future of healthcare delivery in the pediatric CICU, we must find ways to adequately prepare the next generation of cardiac intensivists, actively sustain the clinicians navigating this challenging environment, and constantly scrutinize our standards of care. A thoughtful combination of critical thinking anchored in first principles, informed technology, and humanistic care delivery forms the path towards the future of this exciting subspecialty.

Acknowledgment

It is with immense gratitude that the authors acknowledge the foundational work of David L. Wessel, MD, and Peter C. Laussen, MBBS, on the original version of this chapter, as well as their impact as role models, mentors, and friends to countless clinicians, patients, and families around the world.

References

1. Horak RV, Alexander PM, Amirnovin R, et al. Pediatric cardiac intensive care distribution, service delivery, and staffing in the United States in 2018. *Pediatr Crit Care Med*. 2020;21:797-803.
2. Friedman WF. The intrinsic physiologic properties of the developing heart. *Prog Cardiovasc Dis*. 1972;15:87-111.
3. Mills AN, Haworth SG. Greater permeability of the neonatal lung: postnatal changes in surface charge and biochemistry of porcine pulmonary capillary endothelium. *J Thorac Cardiovasc Surg*. 1991;101:909-916.
4. Available at: https://www.cdc.gov/reproductivehealth/maternalinfanthealth/pretermbirth.htm.
5. Catchpole KR, de Leval MR, McEwan A, et al. Patient handover from surgery to intensive care: using Formula 1 pit-stop and aviation models to improve safety and quality. *Paediatr Anaesth*. 2007;17:470-478.
6. Wessel DL. Managing low cardiac output syndrome after congenital heart surgery. *Crit Care Med*. 2001;29:S220-S230.
7. Hames DL, Sleeper LA, Bullock KJ, et al. Associations with extubation failure and predictive value of risk analytics algorithms with extubation readiness tests following congenital cardiac surgery. *Pediatr Crit Care Med*. 2022;23:e208-e218.
8. Wernovsky G, Wypij D, Jonas RA, et al. Postoperative course and hemodynamic profile after the arterial switch operation in neonates and infants: a comparison of low-flow cardiopulmonary bypass and circulatory arrest. *Circulation*. 1995;92:2226-2235.

9. Bridges ND, Mayer Jr JE, Lock JE, et al. Effect of baffle fenestration on outcome of the modified Fontan operation. *Circulation*. 1992;86:1762-1769.

10. Procaccini DA, Sawyer JE Watt KM. Chapter 19: pharmacology of cardiovascular drugs. In: Ungerleider RE, Meliones JN, McMillan KN, Cooper DS, Jacobs JP, eds. *Critical Heart Disease in Infants and Children*. 3rd ed. Philadelphia: Elsevier; 2006.

11. Capsi J Coles JG Benson LN, et al. Age-related response to epinephrine-induced myocardial stress: a functional and ultrasound study. *Circulation*. 1991;84:III394-III399.

12. Chang AC, Atz AM, Wernovsky G, et al. Milrinone: systemic and pulmonary hemodynamic effects in neonates after cardiac surgery. *Crit Care Med*. 1995;23:1907-1914.

13. Kantor PF, Redington AN. Pathophysiology and management of heart failure in repaired congenital heart disease. *Heart Fail Clin*. 2010;6:497-506, ix.

14. Jenkins J, Lynn A, Edmonds J, et al. Effects of mechanical ventilation on cardiopulmonary function in children after open-heart surgery. *Crit Care Med*. 1985;13:77-80.

15. Rapp JB, White AM, Otero HJ, et al. Computed tomography of the airways and lungs in congenital heart disease. *Pediatr Radiol*. 2022;52:2529-2537.

16. Newburger JW, Jonas RA, Wernovsky G, et al. Perioperative neurologic effects of hypothermic arrest during infant heart surgery: the Boston Circulatory Arrest Study. The Boston Circulatory Arrest Study. *N Engl J Med*. 1993;329:1057-1064.

17. Kapur J, Elm J, Chamberlain JM, et al. Randomized trial of three anticonvulsant medications for status epilepticus. *N Engl J Med*. 2019;381:2103-2113.

18. Moler F, Silverstein F, Holubkov R, et al. Therapeutic hypothermia after in-hospital cardiac arrest in children. *N Engl J Med*. 2017;376:318-329.

19. Rios DR, Welty SE, Gunn JK, et al. Usefulness of routine head ultrasound scans before surgery for congenital heart disease. *Pediatrics*. 2013;131:e1765-e1770.

20. Reddy VM, McElhinney DB, Sagrado T, et al. Results of 102 cases of complete repair of congenital heart defects in patients weighing 700 to 2500 grams. *J Thorac Cardiovasc Surg*. 1999;117:324.

21. Abman SH, Hansmann G, Archer SL, et al. Pediatric pulmonary hypertension: guidelines from the American Heart Association and American Thoracic Society. *Circulation*. 2015;132:2037-2099.

22. Miller OI, Tang SF, Keech A, et al. Inhaled nitric oxide and prevention of pulmonary hypertension after congenital heart surgery: a randomized double-blind study. *Lancet*. 2000;356:1464-1469.

23. Adatia I, Atz AM, Jonas RA, et al. Diagnostic use of inhaled nitric oxide after neonatal cardiac operations. *J Thorac Cardiovasc Surg*. 1996;112:1403-1405.

24. Atz AM, Wessel DL. Sildenafil ameliorates effects of inhaled nitric oxide withdrawal. *Anesthesiology*. 1999;91:307-310.

25. Hoskote A, Stiller B, Thiagarajan RR. What's new in mechanical support strategies for the intensivist in children with severe cardiac failure. *Intensive Care Med*. 2021;47:1152-1155.

26. Howard TS, Kalish BT, Wigmore D, et al. Association of extracorporeal membrane oxygenation support adequacy and residual lesions with outcomes in neonates supported after cardiac surgery. *Pediatr Crit Care Med*. 2016;17:1045-1054.

27. Bratton SL, Chan T, Barrett CS, et al. Metrics to assess extracorporeal membrane oxygenation utilization in pediatric cardiac surgery programs. *Pediatr Crit Care Med*. 2017;18:779-786.

65

Contemporary Pediatric Cardiovascular Nursing

THERESA SAIA, PATRICIA O'BRIEN, AND PATRICIA HICKEY

KEY LEARNING POINTS

- A culture of safety, quality improvement, and research science supports the achievement of exemplary cardiovascular nursing practice.
- Evidence-based, interdisciplinary team-based care, and a higher nurse practitioner and registered nurse (RN) to bed ratio is linked to improved outcomes. These include lower mortality, shorter length of stay, reduced cost of care, and reduced readmissions, as well as staff reports of better care quality, lower burnout, higher job satisfaction, and greater intention of remaining in current position.
- The Complexity Assessment and Monitoring to Ensure Optimal Outcomes (CAMEO) inpatient nursing workload tool can be utilized to inform staffing plans.

- Assessment of patient status and acuity is effectively guided via nurse developed tools such as red flags of Home Monitoring Program in the ambulatory setting and via Children's Hospital Early Warning System (CHEWS) in the inpatient setting.
- Innovation will continue to foster RN and advanced practice nurse role refinement/expansion, the acquisition of new knowledge and technical skills, and a reliance on nursing leaders and nurse educators to transform care from the time of fetal diagnosis through the adulthood in collaboration with the interdisciplinary team.

Introduction

The field of pediatric cardiovascular and critical care nursing continues to mature and innovate in alignment with the fields of pediatric cardiology, cardiac surgery, and cardiac anesthesia. Advancements in diagnostic imaging, medical therapies, and surgical techniques have improved outcomes and overall quality of life for patients with congenital and acquired heart disease. In parallel, registered nurses (RNs) and advanced practice nurses (APNs) acquire, create, and apply new clinical knowledge and technical skills to support the Institute of Medicine's goal to provide safe, timely, effective, efficient, and equitable patient-centered care.[1] Innovation requires role expansion and the creation of new structures and processes, all of which necessitate rigorous assessment of outcomes. Interdisciplinary, evidence-based care is the gold standard in the Boston Children's Hospital (BCH) Heart Center (HC). Effective collaboration is fundamental to patient safety. Successful programs leverage collective expertise and understand the entire team's impact is greater than that of any single individual or discipline.

Within this team of professionals, cardiovascular RNs and APNs facilitate access, coordinate treatment, perform complex procedures, provide education, and participate in research and quality improvement (QI) activities to enhance the safety and quality of care provided. A healthy work environment (HWE) provides a strong foundation to support this collaborative work; the six HWE standards include authentic leadership, skilled communication, true collaboration, effective decision-making, appropriate staffing, and meaningful recognition.[2] The HC surveys all staff annually to assess the health of the work environment and subsequent action plans target opportunities for improvement.

This chapter describes contemporary pediatric cardiovascular nursing practice with examples drawn from the HC. Themes include leadership and organizational structure, patient safety, care coordination, and staff development and support.

Nursing Leadership and Organizational Structure

The Senior Vice President (SVP) and Associate Chief Nurse Officer of Nursing and Patient Care Operations (ACNO-PCO) maintain accountability for nursing and patient care services within the five patient care areas of the HC: (1) the cardiovascular intensive care unit (CICU), (2) acute care cardiology unit (ACCU), (3) cardiac catheterization laboratories and adjacent procedure and recovery rooms, (4) cardiac operating rooms, and (5) ambulatory cardiovascular clinics. The HC Oversight Committee includes the SVP/ACNO and the Chiefs of Cardiology, Cardiac Surgery, Cardiac Anesthesia, and the Senior Director of Finance. The HC Oversight Committee is accountable for the daily operations of each patient care area. Nurse leaders have shared accountability for regulatory readiness, fiscal oversight, human resource management, and the safety and quality of nursing care provided on each unit.

As of May 2022, the HC employed 350 specialized cardiovascular nurses and 80 APNs who provide care at the bedside or in the clinics. Among this group, 97% of RNs possess a Bachelor of Science in Nursing (BSN) or higher. The Synergy Model provides the theoretical foundation of nursing practice at BCH.[3] The eight dimensions of nursing practice within this model include clinical judgment, clinical inquiry, caring practices, response to diversity, advocacy/moral agency, facilitation of learning, collaboration, and systems thinking. The goal of this theoretical model is to match the knowledge, skills, experience, and attitudes needed for individualized patient care requirements. RNs and APNs in all HC settings undergo a competency-based orientation (Table 65.1).

Experience and education of nursing staff impacts outcomes in pediatric patients; higher levels of RN experience and education have been associated with fewer deaths in patients undergoing cardiac surgery.[4] These findings highlight the importance of retention strategies to maintain experienced nursing staff. The presence of APNs with advanced education is also associated with positive patient outcomes. Hospitals with a higher nurse practitioner (NP)-to-bed ratios have a lower 30-day mortality, lower 7-day readmission rate, shorter average length of stay, and lower costs. In addition, patients and RNs in these hospitals were more likely to report better quality of care and safety. RNs reported lower burnout, higher job satisfaction, and greater intention to remain in current job.[5]

Cardiovascular nurses care for a spectrum of patients with congenital heart disease, from prenatally diagnosed neonates to adults. The individual needs of the patients ultimately determine nursing staffing. Researchers in the HC developed and validated a unique pediatric critical care nursing productivity tool that assesses cognitive workload associated with patient assignments.[6] While other instruments focus on patient acuity measures or on required nursing tasks, this tool added important indirect care activities such as patient and parent education, psychosocial

TABLE 65.1	Registered Nurse and Advanced Practice Nursing Responsibilities

Possess knowledge of anatomy, physiology, and treatment of congenital and acquired heart disease
Recognize arrhythmias and knowledge of drug and device therapies
Provide preoperative and postoperative care, assess for, and manage complications
Manage complex therapies: vasoactive drugs, mechanical ventilation, ECMO/VAD
Interpret hemodynamic, diagnostic testing, and laboratory data
Practice safe medication administration
Assess pain and provide comfort
Assess and optimize nutrition
Maintain skin integrity and prevention of pressure ulcers
Infection prevention
Foster mobility
Provide patient- and family-centered, culturally competent, and developmentally appropriate care
Patient and family education and anticipatory guidance
Interprofessional collaboration and communication

ECMO, Extracorporeal membrane oxygenation; *VAD,* ventricular assist device.

support, and care coordination with other disciplines. The Complexity Assessment and Monitoring to Ensure Optimal Outcomes (CAMEO) tool includes 14 domains of clinical activities, each of which is divided into levels of complexity from 1 to 5. A composite score reflects the cognitive complexity of care from low (class I) to high (class V). Most CICU patients fall into class III or IV, reflecting complex nursing actions (e.g., maintenance of hemodynamic stability and care coordination for infants and children following cardiac surgery). The tool underwent validation, modification, and was renamed the ICU CAMEO III; its use has subsequently expanded to non-cardiac ICUs (Fig. 65.1).[7] Similar methodology supported the development of an inpatient CAMEO tool for patients on the ACCU and utilized to allocate nursing resources.[8,9]

Over the past several decades, volume and complexity of care has expanded in the ambulatory setting as well. This has led to the creation of subspecialty clinics and a reorganization of clinic staff into physician and nurse teams who support safe, timely, efficient, and effective patient and family-centered care. This model improves patient flow, resource utilization, continuity, and follow-up. It has been associated with high patient and staff satisfaction on annual surveys. Future work will focus on tools to understand and measure complexity of care in the ambulatory setting in both pediatric and adult age groups.

Patient Safety and Quality

BCH is committed to being a high-reliability organization whose objective is to reduce the probability that an error occurs within our systems or processes; this is achieved through attention to detail, clear communication, and speaking up for safety.[10] Examples Include "time-out" prior to procedures, closed loop communication, structured hand-offs with all transitions using the I-PASS model (Illness severity, Patient summary, Action list, Situation awareness and contingency planning, Synthesis by receiver),[11] daily clinical huddles in all areas of the IIC, and a HC centralized leadership huddle. Infection control strategies are expanded via new protocols that address placement and maintenance of central lines through approaches designed to reduce infection.

ICU CAMEO III©

Total Score: 54+ _____

Unit: _____

Complexity: _____

Date at Start of Shift: _____ Shift: AM / PM Patient: Medical / Surgical/ Cardiac
# of patients at start of shift: _____ # of transfers/admissions: _____ # of discharges: _____ # of patients at end of shift: _____
RN Years of Experience: 0-2 years 3-5 years 6-10 years 11-15 years 16+ years

Form Instructions: Circle answer items as applicable. Item points are in parentheses.

Nursing Management Trend Throughout Shift (circle all that apply)

Pt. Behavioral: Escalation of care(2) Maintenance of care De-escalation of care (2)
Pt. Clinical: Escalation of care(2) Maintenance of care De-escalation of care (2)
Resuscitation: (CPR, defibrillation, bag mask, cardioversion, emergency medicine) (5)
Family/Caregiver: Escalation of care(2) Maintenance of care De-escalation of care (2) Parent Absence (2)
Time to support family:
Standard (0-30 min) (1); **Intermediate (31-60 min) (2);** **Complex (>60 min) (3)**

Monitoring (circle all that apply)

Fluid balance (UO, CTs, PD, CVVH, drains): Q 30 min (1), Q 15 min (2), Q < 15 min (3)
Noninvasive VS (HR, RR, BP, temp, O2 sat, vent settings, pupils, LOC, pain):Q 30 min (1); Q 15 min (2); Q < 15 min (3)
Invasive (CVP, UAP/UVP, art BP, intracardiac pressures, ICP, IAP): Q 1 hour (1); Q 30 min (2); Q 15 min (3); Q < 15 min (4)

Medications (circle all that apply)

Intermittent Medications. 1-10 (1), 11-20 (2); 21 30 (3); 31 40 (4); >41 (5)
Vasoactive Infusion : 1 drip (1); 2 drips (2); 3 drips (3); 4 drips (4); 5+ drips (5)
Continuous IV Fluids/Meds:1 drip (1); 2 drips (2); 3 drips (3); 4 drips (4); 5+ drips (5)

Respiratory Support (circle all that apply)

Non-invasive support (5)
Conventional ventilation (14)
Conventional ventilation + JET/HVOF (19)
Continuous respiratory medications (heliox/iNO/albuterol) (3) isoflurane (5)

Nursing Assessment, Monitoring & Intervention (circle all that apply)

CVL/ART/Intracardiac/PICC Line (mgt/infusion/line change, lab draw, specimen mgt, lab data interpretation) (13)	
ECMO (4)	Assisted device (VAD, Impella, Quadrox) (5)
External ventricular device (EVD)/intracranial bolt management (4)	Arrhythmia management (5)
Seizures (4)	End of life/post mortem care (5)
CT/drains (3)	Wound care/dressing change: simple (2); complex (3)
Enhanced Contact Precautions (2)	Full PPE (3)

ADLs/Self/Assisted Care & Developmental Considerations (Reference on back page)

Number of ADLs performed: 0-2 (1); 3-5 (4); ≥6 (6)
Patient Age: Premature (< 38 weeks) (2) >18 years old (2)
Developmental Age : Age Appropriate ; Delayed (2)

Procedures/ Testing in the ICU (Reference on back page)

1 procedure (3); >1 procedure (5)
Time to complete procedure:
0-1 hour (3); >1 hour (6); > 2 hours (9)

Transfers/Admissions/Transport (circle all that apply)

1 event (3); >1 event (5)
Time to complete event:
0-1 hour (3); >1 hour (6); > 2 hours (9)

Coordination of Care/Teaching/Anticipatory Guidance/Discharge Planning/Education (Reference on back page)

Number: 0-5 (3); 6 – 10 (9); 11 – 15 (13); 16 – 20 (18); > 20 (22)
Time to complete coordination of care/teaching/discharge planning:
0-1 hour (1); >1 hour (3); > 2 hours (5)

Professional/Environmental Management (Reference on back page)

0-2 (1); 3-5 (4); 6-8 (7); 9-12 (10)
Time to complete professional management:
Standard (0-30 min) (1); Intermediate (30-60 min) (2); Complex (>60 min) (3)

CAMEO III©: 06/08/2016

• **Fig. 65.1** Complexity Assessment and Monitoring to Ensure Optimal Outcomes (CAMEO), renamed as ICU CAMEO III, intensive care unit tool.

ADLs /Self/Assisted Care	
PO feeding with assistance	Linen changes with patient in bed/crib
Bottle feeding	Skin care, complex
NG/NJ/GT/JT feeds	Ambulation with assistance
Diaper change	Isolette change
Out of bed complex	

Procedures/Testing in the ICU	
Intubation	X-Ray (chest, KUB)
Extubation	US (head, abdomen, etc.)
Bronchoscopy	EEG
Cardioversion	Head CT
CT/drain: placement / removal	Lumbar puncture
EKG	Plasmapheresis
ECHO Echo requiring hands-on asst.	Hemofiltration
ECMO cannulation/decannulation/circuit change CVVH	Peripheral stick for lab draw
VAD pump head change	PIV insertion/removal
Balloon atrial septostomy (BAS)	
Chest exploration/opening/closure	
Abdominal exploration	
Vacuum Assisted Wound (VAC) dressing: insertion / change	
CVL/ intracardiac/art/umbilical/PICC line: insertion / removal	

Transfers/Admissions/Transport		
Floor	MRI	Interventional radiology
Home	Cath lab	Outside facility
OR	Radiology (CT scan, US, xray) ED	

Coordination of Care/Teaching/Anticipatory Guidance		
Case manager consult	Disease process education	CAMP team consult
Social work consult	Medication education	Volunteer consult
Child life consult	Procedure/treatment	Med/Surg consult
Resource specialist consult	Family presence facilitation	
Psychology consult	Preop/Postoperative education	
PT/OT consult	Clergy Consult	
Lactation/feeding team	Multidisciplinary care meeting/family meeting	
Interpreter services	Organ donation	
Nutritionist	Ethics consult	
Admission/discharge	PACT	
Orientation to the unit/floor Other:		

Discharge Planning/Education	
Medications/prescription review	CPR training
Immunizations (scheduled/seasonal)	Car seat challenge
Ventilator or noninvasive ventilation	Eye exam (ROP)
Enteral feeding (formula review/teaching)	Hearing screen
G tube, GJ tube, J tube, or PEG teaching	PKU/state screen
Equipment/supplies	"All Babies Cry"/shaken baby guide
Tracheostomy/suctioning	Other:

Professional/Environmental Management	
Management plans	Shift report - complex
Incident reporting (SERS)	Staff development (side by sides/resource)
Precept: employee	Care Companion
Precept: student	Security
Research data collection	Unit/institution meetings
Assisted outside current assignment; In unit/Outside unit	
Absence of CA/Resource nurse	

• **Fig. 65.1, cont'd**

Inpatient care bundles target inventions to reduce pneumonias, urinary tract infections, gastric ulcers, and skin breakdown. Patient safety initiatives embedded in the environment exert a constant effort to reduce harm while nursing staff provide a pivotal role since they practice closest to the patient. Two important safety initiatives include the Children's Hospital Early Warning System (CHEWS) and the Randomized Evaluation of Sedation Titration for Respiratory Failure (RESTORE) ICU Pain Management Algorithm.

Children's Hospital Early Warning System (CHEWS)

The development and validation of an early warning score assessment tool was an important patient safety initiative within the HC. Historically, cardiopulmonary arrests occurred in 1–2% of all inpatient pediatric admissions, and survival to discharge was poor. While respiratory failure was the most common cause of cardiac arrest in the general pediatric population, arrhythmias occurred in about 40% of arrests in the cardiac population. Symptoms of clinical deterioration were often present for 6–12 hours prior to an arrest, providing a window of opportunity to identify clinical decline and intervene.[12]

CHEWS was adapted from an existing tool that scored patients on three domains (behavior/neurologic, cardiovascular, and respiratory) in addition to four categories from "normal" to "significant" severity of illness. The HC added two additional categories, family concern and staff concern, and later modified the tool to include age-discriminating vital sign ranges, oxygen saturations, and physiologic changes including seizures, apnea, and arrhythmias. The updated

tool proved to be a better predictor of clinical deterioration in the cardiac population. After validation among the general pediatric population, BCH adopted CHEWS. Fig. 65.2 notes the current BCH CHEWS domains.

Nurses calculate a CHEWS score based on bedside assessments of patients every 4 hours, concurrently with vital signs, and document it in the medical record. A three-tiered escalation of care algorithm, graded 0–5, identifies patients with signs of clinical deterioration. Level 3 or 4 results in increased monitoring and notification of the primary team, while level 5 requires prompt treatment and possible activation of the rapid response team. CHEWS has increased the warning time to identify unstable patients.[13] All units within BCH implemented the CHEWS tool; some children's hospitals across the United States have since done the same.

Randomized Evaluation of Sedation Titration for Respiratory Failure (RESTORE) ICU Pain Management

Management of pain and sedation are important aspects of nursing care of the hospitalized child with heart disease,

Children's Hospital Early Warning Score (CHEWS) Reference Tool

Children's Hospital Boston

Children's Hospital Early Warning Score					
	0	1	2	3	Score
Behavior/Neuro	• Playing/sleeping appropriately • Alert at patient's baseline	• Sleepy, somnolent when not disturbed	• Irritable, difficult to console • Increase in patient's baseline seizure activity	• Lethargic, confused, floppy • Reduced response to pain • Prolonged or frequent seizures • Pupils asymmetric or sluggish	
Cardiovascular	• Skin tone appropriate for patient • Capillary refill ≤ 2 seconds	• Pale • Capillary refill 3–4 seconds • Mild* tachycardia • Intermittent ectopy or irregular heart rhythm (not new)	• Grey • Capillary refill 4–5 seconds • Moderate* tachycardia	• Grey and mottled • Capillary refill >5 seconds • Severe* tachycardia • New onset bradycardia • New onset/increase in ectopy, irregular heart rhythm or heart block	
Respiratory	• Within normal parameters • No retractions	• Mild* tachypnea/ • Mild increased WOB (flaring, retracting) • Up to 40% supplemental oxygen via mask • Up to 1L NC > patient's baseline need • Mild* desaturation (< 5 below patient's baseline) • Intermittent apnea self-resolving	• Moderate* tachypnea • Moderate increased WOB (flaring, retracting, grunting, use of accessory muscles) • 40–60 % oxygen via mask • 1–2 L NC > patient's baseline need • Nebs q 1-2 hr • Moderate* desaturation (< 10 below patient's baseline) • Apnea requiring repositioning or stimulation	• Severe* tachypnea • RR below normal for age* • Severe increased WOB (i.e. head bobbing, paradoxical breathing) • >60 % oxygen via mask • > 2 L NC > patient's baseline need • Nebs q 30 minutes–1 hr • Severe* desaturation (<15 below patient's baseline) • Apnea requiring interventions other than repositioning or stimulation	
Staff Concern		Concerned			
Family Concern		Concerned or absent			
				Total Score	

*Please refer to Vital Sign Reference Tool, the CHEWS Heart Rate and Respiratory Rate Reference Tool, and the Electronic Physiological Bedside Monitoring Policy

		Mild	Moderate	Severe
Respiratory Rate and Heart Rate	Infant	≥ 10% ↑ for age	≥ 15% ↑ for age	≥ 25% ↑ for age
	Toddler and Older	≥ 10% ↑ for age	≥ 25% ↑ for age	≥ 50% ↑ for age
Desaturation from patient's baseline O₂ saturation	All ages	5 points	10 points	15 points

• **Fig. 65.2** Children's Hospital Early Warning System (CHEWS) tool.

especially following surgery. Various pharmacologic and non-pharmacologic methods provide comfort and maintain hemodynamic stability. Lincoln et al.[14] studied the impact of a nurse-implemented goal-directed strategy to improve pain and sedation management in the cardiac ICU. The goal of this QI project was to decrease practice variation through reduced use of opioid and sedation medications without an increase in pain, agitation, or withdrawal symptoms. Phased in over several weeks in 2015, the cardiac iteration of the RESTORE protocol included daily team discussion during bedside rounds of the patient's trajectory of illness (acute, titration, or weaning phase) and a target sedation score, arousal assessments, and an opioid and/or sedation titration plan. Nurses assessed withdrawal symptoms via the Withdrawal Assessment Tool (WAT) scores.[15] Baseline and post-protocol implementation data, examined at three intervals each 3–6 months apart, assessed outcomes and the sustainability of this approach in a busy ICU. The RESTORE protocol resulted in a 50% reduction in opioid and benzodiazepine use without an increase in use of other sedatives. Fewer patients required methadone for withdrawal after leaving the ICU. A decrease in duration of mechanical ventilation and reduced ICU length of stay and hospital length of stay was demonstrated.[16]

Care Coordination and APN-managed Clinical Programs

The value of APN/MD teams to provide complex, comprehensive care to vulnerable populations of children with heart disease remains well established across the HC (see Table 65.2). Many of these roles provide critical continuity for patients and staff by providing care across the continuum from hospital to home. In 2009, in response to long wait times for outpatient clinic visits, APN managed general cardiology clinics were established.[17] Expert senior NPs see a variety of general cardiology and subspecialty patients in the outpatient setting for evaluation of murmurs, chest pain, syncope, hypertension, and palpitations, as well as ongoing management of congenital heart defects. NP clinics are highly productive, performing more than 3000 independent clinic visits in 2021, while their practice, accessibility, and community presence strengthen the community referral network.

In addition, the HC has integrated APNs to the care team of specific populations, fostering the development of expertise and continuity of care for patients and families. Table 65.2 notes other examples of population health NP-managed programs.

Cardiac Anticoagulation Monitoring Program

Responding to the 2008 Joint Commission National Patient Safety Goal to reduce patient harm associated with anticoagulation therapy, BCH implemented a monitoring program supported by the Hematology and Cardiology Departments at BCH. The Cardiac Anticoagulation Monitoring Program (CAMP) multidisciplinary team includes NPs who provide clinical management in collaboration with a medical director, as well as a pharmacist, RN, and a dietitian. Institution-wide protocols for anticoagulation assessment, dosing guidelines, and drug monitoring inform practice and education programs for patients and staff through contemporary evidence-based care.

While initially designed for outpatient management of patients primarily treated with warfarin, CAMP rapidly expanded with the development of new medications, new technologies, and changing clinical requirements. CAMP added an inpatient role for NPs to provide assessment and education for patients beginning anticoagulation therapy which has since expanded into a consultative role providing expertise for all patients requiring the use of antithrombotic therapy. Novel anticoagulants, such as apixaban in the pediatric population, have come into clinical use in the last decade. A growing number of patients undergoing interventional catheterization procedures involving stents or valves require anticoagulation management post-procedure, and the use of anticoagulants post-cardiac surgery has increased. New technologies that carry a high risk of thrombosis such as ventricular assist devices require sophisticated anticoagulation management individualized to each patient. The CAMP team plays a vital role patient management, especially for those managed at home.

Home Monitoring Program

The Single Ventricle Home Monitoring Program (HMP), started in 2009, follows infants with single ventricle heart disease between their newborn first stage procedure and a later second stage procedure at approximately 4–6 months of age.

TABLE 65.2	**Population Health Nurse Practitioner Roles**		
Advanced cardiac therapies	**Cardiac preadmission**	**Electrophysiology**	**Preventive cardiology**
Adult congenital heart	Consult service	Fontan	Pulmonary hypertension
Advanced fetal care	Coronary artery	Heterotaxy	Pulmonary vein stenosis
Regional referrals	Home monitoring	Anticoagulation monitoring	Ventricular assist device
Cardiac catheterization	Cardiac ICU	Acute care: medical	Acute care: cardiac surgery

It is modeled on a program developed to reduce interstage mortality for infants with hypoplastic left heart syndrome (HLHS), implemented at a time when mortality averaged 15% in the early 2000s.[18] Parents receive extensive pre-discharge education about their infant's heart disease and warning signs or "red flags" of clinical deterioration. Parents learn to use a pulse oximeter and a baby scale to monitor their child at home. They are supported by weekly phone calls from a RN or NP, close follow-up with a dietitian, and coordinated follow-up with local visiting nurse agencies, primary care providers, and pediatric cardiologists. Management of the HMP is by a NP who coordinates all aspects of the program, provides extensive education to parents prior to discharge, and follows most of the infants. Two outpatient NPs, a part time RN, a dietitian, an administrative assistant, and case managers are integral to the team and provide support.

Though designed for infants with HLHS during the interstage period, the HMP population quickly expanded to all single ventricle infants including all infants dependent on a modified Blalock-Thomas-Taussig shunt (mBTTS), and, more recently, all infants dependent on a patent ductus arteriosus stent for pulmonary blood flow. The HMP has been very successful in reducing interstage mortality. From 2010 to 2021, the program followed 444 infants. The yearly volume of patients averaged 35–40 patients over the years 2010–2020 with an increase in 2021 to 57 patients. At the inception of HMP, interstage mortality in the HC was 12%. Since then, there has been a notable reduction in mortality (3.4% over the years 2010–2021) and there were no interstage deaths in 2021.[19]

Cardiac Preadmission Clinic

The Cardiac Preadmission Clinic, begun in 1995, is the largest NP-managed clinical program in the HC. It is currently staffed by five NP full-time equivalents, two administrative assistants, and the support of a child life specialist and social worker. The clinic oversees all preprocedural assessments, testing, documentation, and patient and parent education, for patients coming for same-day admission surgical procedures, catheterizations, and outpatient imaging procedures requiring anesthesia. The team completes a pre-anesthesia assessment and collaborates with the anesthesia staff, cardiologists, surgeons, and others to plan procedural care. Inpatient teams receive a clinical summary via email communication and documentation is kept in the medical record. Most visits occur within 1–2 days of the planned procedure and average 4–5 hours. The clinic manages 10–12 patients a day. Since inception in 2010, the program has expanded from 1500 to 2000 pre-procedural patients in 2022

Professional Development, Advancement, and Staff Support

Staff nurses gain promotion via a clinical ladder within the department as they demonstrate advancement in their clinical skills and expertise. Level I staff nurses are entry-level competent nurses. Level II staff nurses are members of the leadership group with responsibility to support unit operations such as orientation of new staff and special projects. Level III, attained by a small number of staff nurses, requires clinical expertise and successful leadership experience. A three-tiered Professional Advancement Model (PAM) for APNs at BCH launched in 2017 with three domains: clinical practice and outcomes, impact, and leadership.[20] In 2022, the PAM added a level IV status which allows expert senior NPs to assume formal leadership roles as Lead NP on subspecialty teams and units.

Nurse Practitioner Fellowship

Responding to the 2010 Institute for Medicine *Future of Nursing Report* that highlighted the need for "Transition to Practice Programs" and recognizing the future need for NPs with cardiovascular expertise, HC leadership prioritized the development of an NP Fellowship program in 2019.[21] The NP Fellowship provides robust didactic content and direct clinical care opportunities in several care environments (ICU, acute care ward, and ambulatory), high fidelity simulation, and formal mentorship. This supports mastery of knowledge and clinical skills essential to a cardiovascular NP role and allows for the cultivation of leadership and clinical inquiry skills. The length of training is 9 months with an additional 3 months of formal orientation onto the unit of hire. To date, the fellowship has graduated nine NP Fellows all of whom are practicing successfully since hire. The NP Fellows oriented on their unit of hire more quickly and possessed baseline competencies that exceeded those of new graduate NPs hired prior to the fellowship's inception. There is a high level of satisfaction for all key stakeholders, including NP Fellows, preceptors, collaborating MDs, and unit nurse leaders.

Nursing Research – Clinical Inquiry

Recognizing that clinical inquiry is vital to providing a scientific basis for nursing care, the HC leadership supports clinical nursing research. In 2003, a PhD educated nurse assumed the role of Nurse Scientist; she led research efforts and implemented several programs aimed at involving staff in nursing inquiry. The Nursing Science Fellowship is a 2-year structured program consisting of didactic sessions and mentorship with a nurse scientist; nursing staff choose a topic of interest and pursue a QI or nursing research project. Initially piloted in the HC, the program later expanded to the broader institution. From 2011 to 2020, 84 fellows completed the program, more than half of the graduates received grant funding, and 78 external disseminations have resulted from their work.[22]

Another effort is an institution-wide Evidenced-Based Practice Mentorship program, which is a 1-year self-directed experience to allow staff nurses to experience the evidenced-based practice process under the guidance of an experienced mentor.[23] These programs have had a positive impact on scholarship. HC nurses have been first or last authors on nine peer-reviewed publications annually for the last 3 years and more than 25 publications a year included nurses.

Staff Support

Several innovative initiatives provide staff support. The Program to Enhance Relational and Communication Skills (PERCS) Rounds was created as a "just-in-time" learning format to support and mentor interdisciplinary staff. The program provides a supportive milieu where staff can develop relational skills by exploring highly sensitive topics not otherwise covered in traditional venues. PERCS Rounds has provided consistently 1-hour offerings to staff within the HC and BCH critical care units for over 12 years. A newer program, the Nursing Education and Support Team (NEST), created in 2017, provides peer-to-peer coaching support to guide front-line critical care nurses through morally and ethically challenging situations. From 2017 to 2019, NEST coaches completed greater than 6000 consults with 85% of staff surveyed ranking satisfaction as high and 80% indicating they would seek NEST support again.[23]

Conclusion

Cardiovascular nurses have made significant contributions to the outstanding family-centered patient care and excellent patient outcomes in the HC. They continue to play a major role in patient safety initiatives. APNs manage several clinical programs with expanding patient volume. Cardiovascular nurses have advanced the science of pediatric cardiovascular nursing through their leadership and national research efforts. Innovation, interprofessional collaboration, a healthy work environment, opportunities for professional development and career advancement, and innovative staff support programs provide a solid foundation to recruit, retain, and develop exceptional nurses and nurse leaders across the care continuum of the HC. Nursing collaborates effectively with the interprofessional team to assure the best possible patient care outcomes and the operational success of the HC.

References

1. Institute of Medicine. *Crossing the Quality Chasm: A New Health System for the 21st Century.* Washington, DC: National Academy Press, 2001.
2. AACN. Available at: https://www.aacn.org/nursing-excellence/healthy-work-environments.
3. Curley MAQ. Patient-nurse synergy, optimizing patient outcomes. *Am J Crit Care.* 1998;7:64.
4. Hickey PA, Gauvreau K, Curley MAQ, et al. Effect of critical care nursing and organizational characteristics on pediatric cardiac surgery mortality in the United States. *J Nurs Admin.* 2013;43:637-644.
5. Aiken LH, Sloane DM, Brom HM, et al. Value of nurse practitioner inpatient hospital staffing. *Med Care.* 2021;39:857-863.
6. Connor JA, LaGrasta C, Hickey PA. Complexity assessment and monitoring to ensure optimal outcomes tool for measuring pediatric critical care nursing. *Am J Crit Care.* 2015;24:297-308.
7. Connor JA, LaGrasta C, Cerrato B, et al. Measuring acuity and pediatric critical care nursing workload by using ICU CAMEO III. *Am J Crit Care.* 2022;31:119-126.
8. Connor JA, LaGrasta C, Porter C, et al. Measurement of pediatric inpatient nursing using the complexity assessment and monitoring to ensure optimal outcomes (CAMEO) tool. *J Pediatr Nurs.* 2020;51:42-48.
9. Hurtig M, Liseno S, McLellan MC, et al. Development and implementation of an inpatient CAMEO staffing algorithm to inform nurse-patient assignments in a pediatric cardiac inpatient unit. *J Pediatr Nurs.* 2021;60:275-280.
10. AHRQ. *High Reliability.* 2019. Available at: https://psnet.ahrq.gov/primer/high-reliability.
11. Starmer AJ, Spector ND, Srivastava R, et al. Changes in medical errors after implementation of a handoff program. *N Eng J Med.* 2014;371:1803-1812.
12. McLellan MC, Connor JA. The Cardiac Children's Hospital early warning score (C-CHEWS). *J Pediatr Nurs.* 2013;28:171-178.
13. McLellan MC, Gauvreau K, Connor JA. Validation of the Children's Hospital early warning system for critical deterioration recognition. J Pediatr Nurs. 2017;32:52-58.
14. Lincoln PA, Whelan K, Hartwell LP, et al. Nurse-implemented goal-directed strategy to improve pain and sedation management in a pediatric cardiac ICU. *Pediatr Crit Care Med.* 2020;21:1064-1070.
15. Franck LS, Harris SK, Soetenga DJ, et al. Withdrawal Assessment Tool-1 (WAT-1): an assessment instrument for monitoring opioid and benzodiazepine withdrawal symptoms in pediatric patients. *Pediatr Crit Care Med.* 2008;9:573-580.
16. Evangelista, JK, Connor JA, Pintz C, et al. Paediatric nurse practitioner managed cardiology clinics: patient satisfaction and appointment access. J Adv Nurs. 2011;68:2165-2174.
17. Ghanayem NS, Hoffman GM, Mussatto KA, et al. Home surveillance program prevents interstage mortality after the Norwood procedure. *J Thor Cardiovasc Surg.* 2003;126:1367-1375.
18. Schroeder M. Personal Communication, 2022.
19. Paul F, Abecassis L, Freiberger D, et al. Competency-based professional advancement model for advanced practice RN's. *J Nurs Admin.* 2019;49:66-72.
20. Institute of Medicine. *Future of Nursing: Leading Change, Advancing Health.* Washington DC: National Academy Press; 2010.
21. Connor JA, Mott S, DeGrazzia M, et al. Nursing science fellowship at Boston Children's Hospital. *Appl Nurs Res.* 2020;55:151292.
22. Schuler E, Paul F, Connor L, et al. Cultivating evidenced-based practice through mentorship. *Appl Nurs Res.* 2020;55:151295.
23. DeGrazia M, Porter C, Sheehan A, et al. Building moral resiliency through the nurse education and support initiative. *Am J Crit Care.* 2021;30:95-102.

66

Translational Research in Pediatric Cardiology

VASSILIOS J. BEZZERIDES AND WILLIAM T. PU

KEY LEARNING POINTS

- Technical advances are leading to the development of models of human heart diseases and to new insights into heart disease pathogenesis
- Improved understanding of the impact of genetics and molecular mechanisms on outcomes promise to enhance patient management and enable precision medicine approaches.
- Molecularly targeted therapies are poised to revolutionize treatment of a subset of cardiovascular disorder.

In the coming decades, we anticipate that major improvements in the outcomes of pediatric heart disease patients will come from enhanced understanding of biological disease mechanisms and the application of novel therapies that target underlying molecular and cellular mechanisms. Innovations in human disease modeling, next-generation sequencing, high-throughput screening, stem cell biology, and novel therapeutic development are poised to revolutionize the field of pediatric cardiology. In this chapter, we outline the state-of-the-art techniques and in-depth biological insights that will drive innovative care of pediatric and congenital cardiac patients for the next 50 years.

Introduction

The past several decades have seen remarkable improvements in outcomes for patients with congenital heart disease (CHD). For example, patients with hypoplastic left heart syndrome had no available therapy until the advent of the Norwood procedure in 1979, and in the subsequent four decades the 5-year survival has increased to approximately 70%. These remarkable improvements in pediatric cardiology outcomes have largely come from clinical improvements in cardiac surgery, cardiopulmonary bypass, cardiac imaging, and postoperative management.

With advances in these areas yielding such rapid improvements in outcomes, they have naturally been the focal point of pediatric cardiology programs, and relatively less resources have been committed towards basic and translational research. At the same time, industry investment in cardiac disease has been relatively low compared with other disease areas, at least in part because of the high cost and long timelines for clinical trials for heart disease. These factors have led to few advances in the medical management of most conditions (with some notable exceptions). For example, while the management of structural heart disease achieved these remarkable improvements, outcomes for pediatric patients with myocardial dysfunction have improved incrementally, with the major therapy available continuing to be heart transplantation.

It is the authors' opinion that we are at a turning point, when gains that come from further optimization of technical performance and from improved hemodynamics will become more incremental, and that advances stemming from enhanced biological insight will drive the most transformative advances. Basic research over the past decades has provided a rich knowledge base, and an exploding array of molecular and cellular tools have emerged that will provide more knowledge about disease pathophysiology and more ways to intervene to alter disease trajectories based on that knowledge. Now more than ever pediatric cardiology needs physician-scientists and scientists who understand the major challenges faced by patients and have the scientific skills to surmount these challenges using the growing armamentarium available to modern cardiovascular biologists.

The goal of this chapter is to introduce pediatric cardiologists, particularly those who are in training, to translational research in pediatric cardiology and convey the wealth of opportunities in this field. We will examine some of the model systems relevant for translational cardiovascular research, provide examples of approaches to understand disease mechanisms, and discuss some ways in which translational research can improve patient management.

Model Systems

For more than 100 years, animal models of cardiovascular disease (CVD) have provided tremendous insights into cardiac development, physiology, disease progression, and therapeutic development. The relative ease of genetic manipulation, low cost, and short breeding cycles of mice have made them the main animal model for cardiovascular research, despite differences with humans in size and some aspects of cardiovascular physiology. Mouse models have been complemented by a host of other models, including zebrafish, large animals, and human induced pluripotent stem cells (iPSCs), providing a wealth of experimental systems to model human development and disease.

The creation of mouse models for CVD can be generally divided into three categories: genetic, surgical, and environmental.

Genetically Modified Mouse Models

Gene ablation directly interrogates the requirement of a gene for a biological process. Since the 1990s, genetic loss-of-function (LoF) mouse lines have ushered in a revolution of insight into cardiac development, cardiomyocyte biology, disease mechanisms, and gene regulation.[1] For example, knock-out models for cardiac transcription factor genes including *Tbx5*,[2] *Nkx2-5*,[3] and *Gata4*[4] demonstrated their essential roles in cardiac development and their contribution to CHD. To pinpoint the function of genes in specific cell types and to circumvent lethality that can be caused by whole body gene ablation, researchers have used conditional ablation strategies. A gene targeted for ablation is flanked by short DNA recognition sequences (loxP sites). Expression of a recombinase (Cre) excises sequences between these recognition sequences, resulting in gene inactivation in cells expressing Cre and their descendants (Fig. 66.1A). The precision of this conditional inactivation strategy can be further enhanced by temporally controlling the activity or expression of Cre,

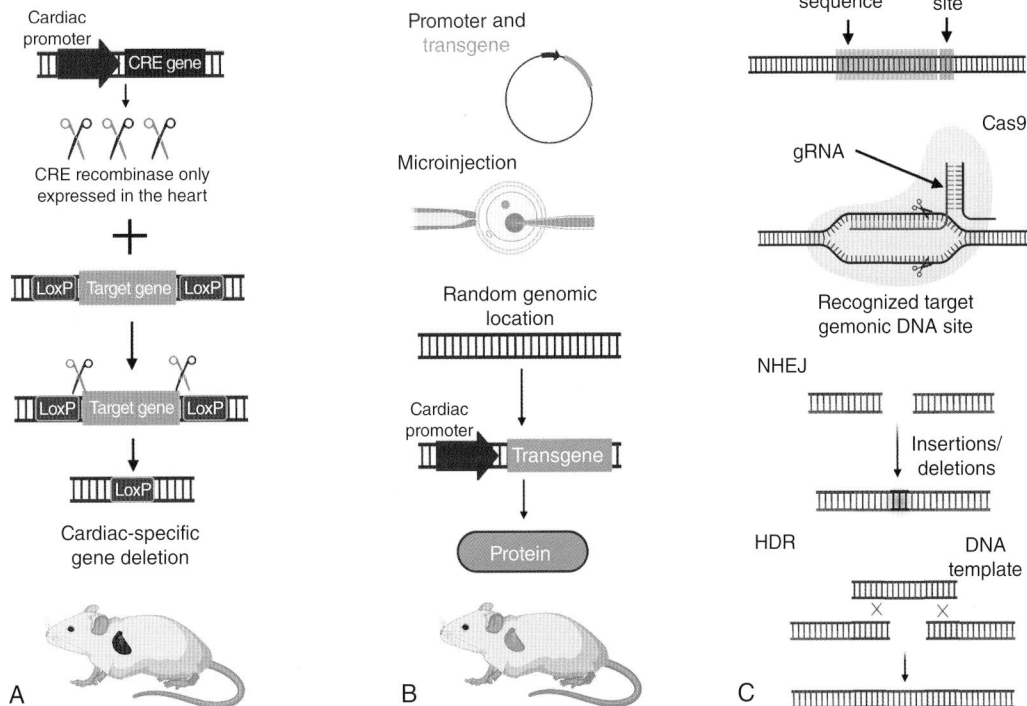

• **Fig. 66.1** Genetically modified mouse models. **(A)** The mouse genome is modified so that LoxP sites flank the gene targeted for ablation. Cre protein expression driven by a cell type specific (e.g., cardiac) promoter induces excision of the target gene and loss of function (LoF) only in the Cre-expressing cell type and its descendants. **(B)** To create a transgenic model, a DNA construct containing an appropriate promoter (e.g., cardiac promoter to target transgene expression to cardiomyocytes) and the gene of interest are microinjected into murine zygotes, which are then implanted into a recipient pseudopregnant female. The DNA construct is randomly inserted into the host genome and the protein is expressed in cells as directed by the promoter. **(C)** The recognition sequence for CRISPR/Cas9 consists of a 20 nucleotide (nt) sequence adjacent to a 3 nt protospacer adjacent motif (PAM) site. Introducing Cas9 protein with a target guide RNA *(gRNA)* into a host cell will induce a double-stranded DNA (dsDNA) break within the target sequence. Repair of the dsDNA break occurs through two mechanisms, non-homologous end-joining *(NHEJ)* or homologous-directed repair *(HDR)*. *Figure created with Biorender.com.*

e.g., studies of gene function in the adult heart without disrupting heart development.[5,6] In addition to illuminating the genes that regulate heart development, LoF models have also been instrumental in mechanistic understanding of cardiomyopathies, including dilated cardiomyopathy caused by mutation of the splicing regulator *Rbm20*[7] and many others.

To complement gene inactivation, researchers have developed methods to overexpress genes and thereby study their sufficiency for modifying a biological process. An important gain-of-function (GoF) method is to insert a transgene into the genome (Fig. 66.1B). The transgene typically contains a promoter that drives the exogenous gene's expression in a cell type of interest, such as cardiomyocytes. For example, transgenic overexpression of the gene YAP1 illustrated its key role in promoting embryonic heart growth and in stimulating heart regeneration.[8] In postnatal mice, genes can be efficiently overexpressed in cardiomyocytes using adeno-associated virus (AAV), which circumvents the need to create genetically modified mouse lines but is constrained by the ~4.7 kb packaging limit of AAV.

In 2012, Jennifer Doudna and Emmanuelle Charpentier reported the discovery of a bacterial system, Clustered Regularly Interspaced Short Palindromic Repeats (CRISPR), in which a nuclease was targeted to specific sequences by an RNA guide.[9] While this system evolved for bacterial defense against viruses, it has been exploited by biologists to enable highly efficient and flexible targeting of nearly any site within the mammalian genome for cleavage. Expression of the nuclease (Cas9) and an engineered guide RNA (gRNA) in a host cell results in selective cleavage of the cell's genomic DNA at the site matching the gRNA (Fig. 66.1C). The cleaved DNA is repaired by one of two pathways, nonhomologous end-joining (NHEJ) or homology-directed repair (HDR). Repair by NHEJ yields random insertions or deletions (Indels) that can disrupt gene expression. When a DNA template matching sequences adjacent to the cut site is provided, repair by HDR allows the targeted introduction of new genetic information contained within the DNA template. This technique has revolutionized experimental biology, and Doudna and Charpentier were awarded the Nobel Prize in Chemistry in 2021 for their discovery. The advent of highly efficient and precise genomic engineering has transformed human disease modeling by markedly expediting the creation of mouse and cell models with human disease-causing point mutations.[10] This method of rapid model development is rapidly expanding our understanding of cardiac disease mechanisms and development of novel therapies. Combining the Cas9 system with the cardiotropic properties of AAV also enables LoF studies that circumvent the laborious step of creating genetically modified mice.[11] Moreover, reducing the AAV dose allows creation of "genetic mosaics" in which only a small percentage of cells harbor a LoF mutation, allowing the study of cell-autonomous effects of gene disruption without confounding effects of cardiac dysfunction.

Surgical Models

Surgical models are used to model pathological conditions. Often surgical models are superimposed on genetic modifications to dissect gene function in pathological responses.

To model myocardial hypertrophy and pressure-overload induced heart failure, a ligature is tied around the aorta and a sizing needle, most commonly just distal to the take-off of the first brachiocephalic artery.[12] The sizing needle is then removed, resulting in a surgical band that obstructs aortic blood flow and results in left ventricular hypertrophy, dilation, dysfunction, and fibrosis. Responses in this transverse aortic constriction (TAC) model depend on ligature tightness, age and size, sex, mouse strain, and surgical technique. This model is widely used to dissect pathways that regulate cardiac hypertrophy and the progression to myocardial dysfunction, and to test novel therapies for the treatment of ventricular dysfunction.

To model the effects of myocardial ischemia, researchers ligate the left anterior descending artery (LAD) to cause myocardial infarction (MI), resulting in a transmural infarct with associated wall motion abnormalities and myocardial dysfunction.[13] To mimic acute coronary occlusion followed by revascularization, now a common clinical scenario in the era of percutaneous coronary intervention, or to create myocardial injury without irreversible damage to the vascular system, short-term ischemia and reperfusion (IR) models have been developed, in which the surgical ligature is removed after 30–60 minutes. These models have been critical in informing our mechanistic understanding of the signaling pathways involved both immediately following myocardial injury and the subsequent adverse neurohumoral-mediated remodeling leading to cardiac dysfunction. These models are also being used to test regenerative therapies designed to replace lost cardiomyocytes with exogenous cardiomyocytes (e.g., stem-cell derived cardiomyocytes[14]), with cardiomyocytes generated from existing endogenous cardiomyocytes (cardiomyocyte proliferation[15]), or with cardiomyocytes transdifferentiated from other cell types (e.g., fibroblast to cardiomyocyte reprogramming[16]).

While TAC, MI, and IR recapitulate conditions commonly observed in adult cardiology, hemodynamic conditions predominantly seen in pediatric cardiology have less established models. Right ventricle (RV) pressure overload has been modeled with pulmonary artery banding,[17] and RV volume overload by pulmonary regurgitation caused by a transpulmonary valve surgical ligature.[18] Volume overload caused by left-to-right shunts have been infrequently studied, usually by creation of a fistula between the aorta and the inferior vena cava.[19] Postnatal right-to-left shunting has not, to our knowledge, been experimentally modeled in small mammals, although a short-term ovine model using an interposition graft between the pulmonary artery and the left atrium has been used to study its effects on ischemia/reperfusion.[20] Interestingly, surgical amputation or LAD ligation of the newborn mouse heart has shown that it has substantial regenerative capabilities that are lost by the end of the first postnatal week.[21] This exciting observation has potential implications for clinical observations in infants with anomalous left coronary artery, for potential advantages of neonatal surgical repair of congenital heart lesions, and for potential regenerative strategies for conditions with deficient myocardium, such as single ventricle heart disease.

Environmental Models

Neurohormonal Dysregulation

Systemic hypertension is a common risk factor for many acquired CVDs. The combination of increased afterload and dysregulation of neurohormonal signaling can negatively impact the heart, causing end-organ damage through a variety of mechanisms. Elevated levels of the peptide hormone angiotensin II (ANG II) cause heart failure, and inhibiting this signaling pathway is a mainstay of cardiac disease management.[22] ANG II and other stable compounds can be continuously infused into mice for several weeks from small subcutaneous "osmotic minipumps," in which a drug reservoir is gradually compressed by expansion of a surrounding water absorbent layer. ANG II primarily binds to the angiotensin 1 receptor (AT_1R), activating multiple signaling pathways within cardiomyocytes, cardiac fibroblasts, and endothelial cells. Prolonged exposure to ANG II causes cardiomyocyte hypertrophy, adverse cardiac remodeling, activation/survival of myofibroblasts, and smooth muscle cell contraction. Osmotic minipumps have also been used for chronic infusion of isoproterenol. The resulting chronic stimulation of β-adrenergic receptors induces cardiac remodeling, ventricular dysfunction, and cardiac fibrosis without systemic hypertension.

Obesity, type II diabetes, hypertension, and a sedentary lifestyle are significant risk factors for the development of coronary artery disease and for "heart failure with preserved ejection fraction" (HFpEF), which accounts for more than half of adult heart failure cases. Understanding how metabolic disease contributes to CVD has been a focus of cardiovascular research for the last several decades. However, no single model entirely encompasses all of the metabolic and cardiovascular effects seen in humans with metabolic syndrome-mediated CVD. While mice fed chow enriched in dietary fats, animal protein, and processed sugars will have increased serum glucose levels, insulin resistance, and steatohepatitis, the effects on cardiovascular function are limited. The pro-atherosclerotic effects of high-fat diet on mice can be augmented by overlaying this dietary challenge on top of genetic ablation of ApoE.

Researchers have long sought to model HFpEF in mice. Recently, a two-hit model was reported in which concurrent metabolic (high-fat diet) and hypertensive (inhibition of nitric oxide signaling by a small molecule, L-NAME, added to drinking water) stress yielded mice with diastolic dysfunction and pulmonary edema.[23] Further study of the molecular mechanisms underlying development of HFpEF promises to yield new mechanistic insights and therapeutic targets.

Zebrafish

Zebrafish (*Danio rerio*) are small, freshwater, tropical fish that are a robust research model for cardiovascular development and genetics. While zebrafish have only a single atria and a single ventricle, they share many of the same well-conversed genetic pathways that govern cardiac development and physiology as other amniotes. Compared with mammalian species, zebrafish are easily and economically maintained in a laboratory environment, and CRISPR/Cas9 has enabled the creation of zebrafish with targeted genetic modifications. Embryos develop rapidly *ex vivo* and are transparent during the critical aspects of cardiovascular system development. The embryos' small size and rapid cardiac development enable their use in high-throughput screening in 384-well plates with biologically active small molecules.[24] The discovery by Poss et al. in 2002 that adult zebrafish could completely regenerate their hearts after apical amputation established zebrafish as a unique model system to study heart regeneration.[25] Subsequent research using this system has identified critical regulators of cardiac regeneration.

Induced Pluripotent Stem Cells

In 2006, Shinya Yamanaka published a landmark paper demonstrating that somatic cells such as skin fibroblasts could be converted into pluripotent stem cells (PSCs) using just four transcription factors: Sox2, Oct4, c-Myc, and Klf4.[26] These iPSCs circumvented the ethical concerns with human embryonic stem cells and ushered in a new era of human disease modeling in which a patient's somatic cells could be reprogrammed to iPSCs, resulting in perpetual disease models harboring the patients' genetic information. These patient-derived iPSCs could be differentiated into any cell type, including cardiomyocytes (iPSC-CMs), and studied as single cells or as part of bioengineered tissues or organoids. Genome editing with CRISPR/Cas9 enabled creation of isogenic iPSC lines with and without human disease mutations and permitted genetic dissection of disease mechanisms in human cardiac cells. Enabling these studies in human cardiac cells was a substantial advance because human cardiomyocytes are rarely available for experimental studies and rodent cardiomyocytes have notable differences in cardiac physiology from human cardiomyocytes. For example, patient-derived and genome-edited iPSC-CMs have been advantageous in assessing arrhythmogenic risk in both congenital and acquired long QT syndromes, because of electrophysiologic disparities between rodents and humans. Preclinical therapeutic development programs use iPSC-CMs for drug screening, assessment of cardiovascular toxicity, and for cell-based therapies.

In comparison with other cardiovascular models, iPSC-CMs are limited by relative immaturity compared with adult cardiomyocytes, high costs for large-scale production, and the inability to phenotypically model structural heart disease. Despite these limitations, iPSC-CMs are an invaluable and increasingly used model system for translational cardiovascular research.

Understanding Disease Mechanisms

The starting point for improved patient management and development of novel therapeutics is improved understanding of disease pathophysiological mechanisms. The past decades have seen tremendous advances in our basic understanding of cardiovascular development and disease. Space limitations preclude a detailed review; instead, we provide some illustrative examples.

Congenital Heart Disease Genetics

The genetic basis for CHD has been recognized for several decades.[27] Chromosomal abnormalities are associated with CHD, and some specific chromosomal anomalies have provided insight into the underlying developmental mechanism (e.g., Williams syndrome and DiGeorge syndrome). For non-syndromic forms of CHD, the relative recurrence risk in related family members is substantially greater than the general population, demonstrating a genetic basis, but the absolute recurrence risk is less than 5%, suggesting incomplete penetrance, polygenic inheritance, or interactions between genetic and environmental factors. To gain insight into the underlying genetic basis for CHD, the National Heart, Lung, and Blood Institute established the Pediatric Cardiac Genomics Consortium (PCGC) to better understand the genetic basis of CHD. Currently more than 13,000 patients and 18,000 relatives have been enrolled in the study. Analyses include whole exome and whole genome sequencing, determination of copy number variation, and detailed clinical and phenotypic data collection.

Initial analysis focused on sequencing of CHD probands and parents to identify *de novo* coding mutations and recessive genes associated with CHD. Patients with CHD were found to have an excessive burden of truncating and predicted protein damaging mutations in genes robustly expressed in the embryonic heart.[28,29] Genes involved in chromatin remodeling were enriched among the affected genes. Patients with both CHD and neurodevelopmental disabilities were 10-fold more likely to have protein-damaging *de novo* mutations compared with patients with isolated CHD, suggesting a shared etiology for these disorders and arguing that genetic factors, in addition to cardiopulmonary bypass, contribute to neurodevelopmental disabilities in CHD patients.[29,30] Overall, *de novo* protein-damaging variants contribute to ~8% of CHD, rare inherited variants ~1.8%, copy number variants ~10%, and aneuploidies ~13%.[29] The majority of CHD cases remain unexplained. WGS of CHD patients and parents found that CHD patients had an increased burden of *de novo* non-coding variants in predicted cardiac transcriptional regulatory regions, suggesting that non-coding *de novo* variants contribute to CHD by altering the regulation of key heart development genes.[31]

The contribution of genetic variation to CHD outcomes is a major area of ongoing research that requires multidisciplinary efforts to link genetic factors to clinical outcomes.

Cardiovascular Development

Human genetics has identified over 200 genes that cause CHD. Intense study of cardiac development in murine, zebrafish, and other systems has revealed the intricate steps that transform a linear muscular tube into a four-chambered, valved heart and has delineated the functions of many of these CHD genes. One important experimental technique that has improved the understanding of heart development and cardiac malformations is "lineage tracing," which provides information on the origins and fates of cell populations in the developing heart. In models in which direct embryo manipulation is possible (zebrafish and chick), lineage tracing can be performed by marking specific cell populations with dyes or integrating viruses. In mice, lineage tracing is achieved by driving Cre recombinase in the population to be marked. By excising a transcriptional stop signal, Cre irreversibly activates expression of an easily monitored reporter gene in Cre-expressing cells and their progeny (Fig. 66.2A and B).

Lineage tracing in both chick and mice was used to show that a distinct cardiac progenitor population "second heart field (SHF) progenitors" gave rise to most of the RV, the RV outflow tract, and portions of both atria.[32,33] These progenitors are initially located adjacent to the cardiac crescent (Fig. 66.2C and D, E7), which contains the first heart field cells that form the initial heart tube and ultimately much of the left ventricle. SHF progenitors persist at either pole of the heart tube and contribute to heart tube growth by adding cardiac cells at either end (Fig. 66.2C and D, E8.5). SHF progenitors express distinct markers, such as *Isl1* and *Tbx1*, and participate in distinct gene-regulatory networks that contribute to morphologic specificity of RV and the outflow tract. Several right-sided congenital heart defects are associated with abnormalities of the SHF and can be directly linked to dysregulation of SHF-specific signaling pathways. For example, patients with DiGeorge syndrome display a range of conotruncal defects including tetralogy of Fallot and are haplo-insufficient for a multigene deletion on chromosome 22 (22q11) including the SHF-associated transcription factor gene *Tbx1*.

Lineage tracing further revealed that a portion of the SHF near the venous pole forms the dorsal mesenchymal protrusion (DMP), which projects into the cavity of the common atrium (Fig. 66.2E).[34] Fusion of the DMP with the mesenchymal cap of the primary atrial septum and with the atrioventricular endocardial cushions is required to close the ostium primum and form the crux of the heart. While atrioventricular septal defects were previously thought to be due to abnormal development of the endocardial cushions, it is now known that defects in DMP, such as those caused by *Tbx5*,[35] *Gata4*,[36] or hedgehog pathway mutations,[35] also contribute to atrioventricular septal defects (Fig. 66.2F and G).

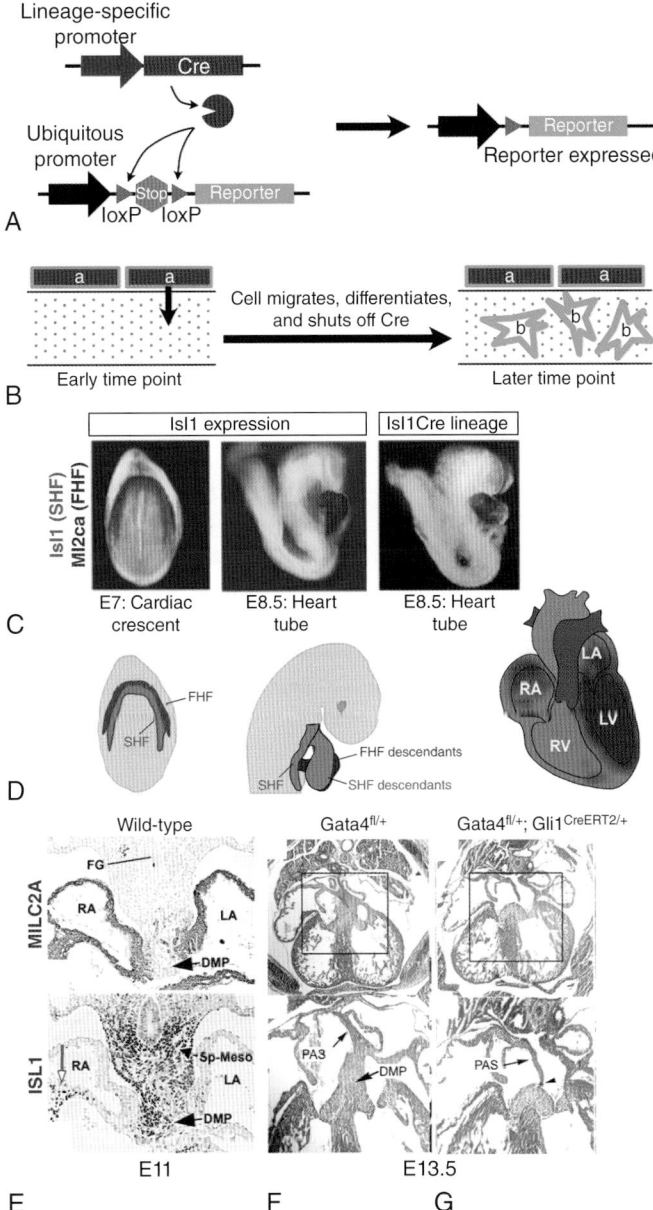

• **Fig. 66.2** Genetic lineage tracing of second heart field progenitors illuminates development of the right ventricle, outflow tract, and atrioventricular septum. **(A)** Genetic lineage tracing using Cre-LoxP. A lineage-specific promoter drives expression of Cre, which indelibly excises a Cre reporter gene stop cassette so that the reporter is expressed in the cell and its progeny. **(B)** Schematic of a lineage tracing experiment. Cre is expressed only in cell type a, resulting in activation of the Cre-dependent reporter in "a" cells. Later in development, if the reporter is expressed in "b" cells, then it suggests that "b" cells develop from "a" cells. **(C)** to **(E)** Lineage tracing establishes the contribution of second heart field *(SHF)* cells to the developing heart. Data from embryos are shown in **(C)**, and summarized in cartoons in **(D)**. At E7, SHF progenitors expressing *Isl1* are located adjacent to FHF cells in the cardiac crescent, marked by *Mlc2a*. At E8, the heart tube has formed and continues to express *Mlc2a*. The SHF, marked by *Isl1*, is present in the mesoderm dorsal to the heart. Cells within the heart tube do not express *Isl1*. The Isl1^Cre lineage, shown in blue in the right image, includes both the SHF and derivatives located in the atria, outflow tract, and right ventricle. This indicates SHF located at either pole of the heart contributes to heart tube growth by supplying cardiac cells at either end. Contributions of SHF and FHF to the four-chambered heart are shown in **(D, rightmost panel)**. **(E)** to **(G)** SHF contributes to formation of the atrioventricular septum. **(E)** E11 heart sections stained for cardiomyocyte marker MLC2A (top) and SHF progenitor marker ISL1 (bottom). ISL1+ SHF progenitors are located within the dorsal mesenchymal protrusion (DMP) that extends into the common atrium. **(F)** and **(G)** H&E stained E13.5 control (f) and mutant (g) heart sections. Boxed areas are enlarged in the lower panels. Mutation of *Gata4* within a subpopulation of the SHF that receives hedgehog signals (marked by Gli^CreERT2) results in primum atrial septal defects and abnormal development of the DMP *(arrowhead*, h, lower panel). *PAS*, Primary atrial septum. (*C, F, G,* and *H*, Adapted with permission from: Cai et al., 2003;[32] Snarr et al, 2007;[34] Zhou et al., 2017,[36] respectively.)

Improving Patient Management

The ultimate goal of translational research is to improve patient outcomes through application of scientific discoveries and innovation. One way that scientific advances can improve patient management is by enhancing the selection of patients for specific therapies. A second way is through the development of novel therapies that directly target disease mechanisms. The following sections provide illustrative examples of how the products of basic and translational research are being deployed to improve patient management.

Patient-Specific Models and Precision Medicine

Facile reprogramming of patient-derived cells to pluripotency has made creation of patient-specific disease models a reality. Since these cells share the patient's genetic information, conceptually it should be possible to use the cells to help stratify patient risk, evaluate response to specific therapies, and study

disease mechanisms (Fig. 66.3). In one proof-of-concept study, iPSC-CMs from patients with breast cancer were compared for toxic effects of the chemotherapy drug doxorubicin. Cells derived from patients with doxorubicin-induced cardiomyopathy showed greater toxic effects than those derived from patients who did not develop doxorubicin-induced cardiomyopathy.[37] A second study investigated the ability of iPSC CMs to predict the QT-prolonging effect of sotalol on individual patients. Patients were challenged with sotalol, and iPSC-CMs were generated from those with the greatest and least QT prolongation. The response of each patient's iPSC-CMs to sotalol was found to correlate with their clinical responses,[38] and candidate genes responsible for these differences were identified. Studies such as these point to the promise of patient-derived iPSCs to fulfill the goal of precision medicine, to allow rational individualization of each patient's therapy. However, widespread use of iPSCs for this goal requires additional validation of their predictive value. Bioengineering approaches will yield more physiological, tissue-level models and expand the range of quantifiable phenotypes.[39,40] Furthermore, the creation of a single iPSC line

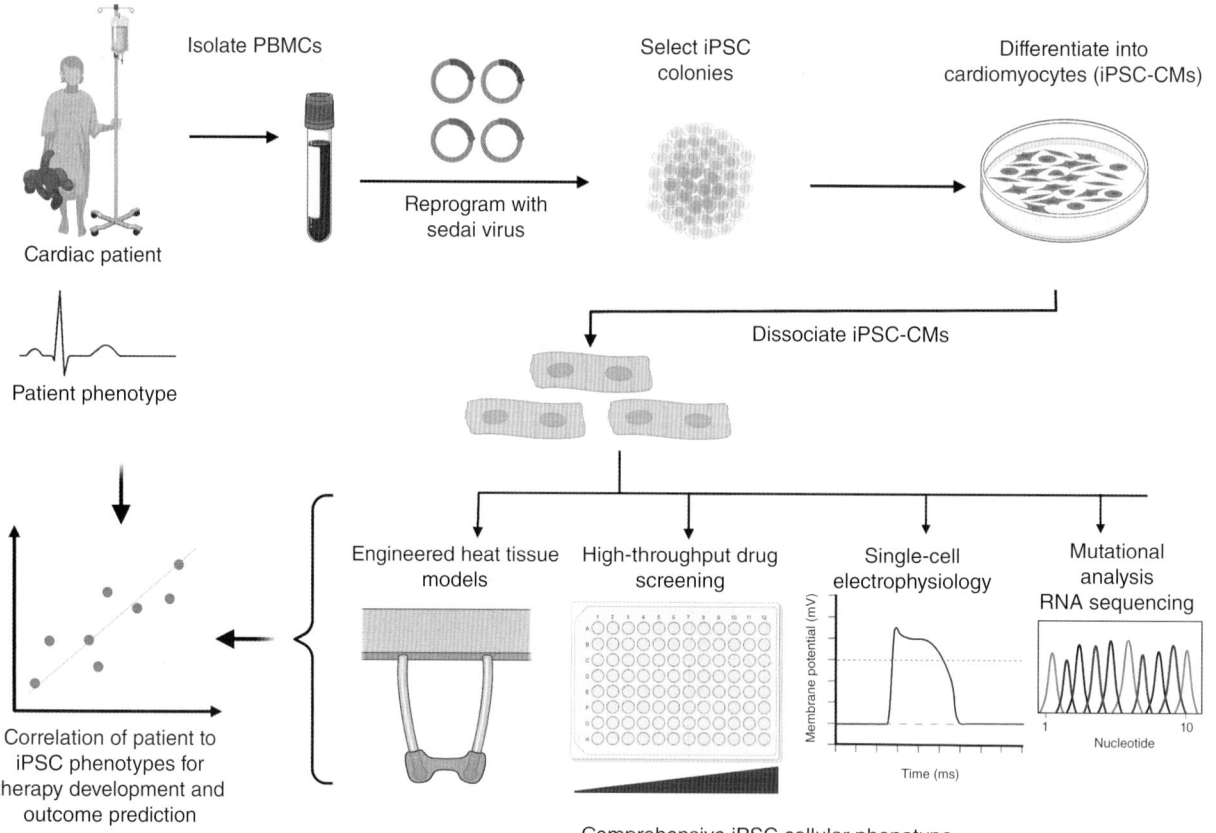

• **Fig. 66.3** Induced pluripotent stem cells *(iPSCs)* as models of cardiac disease. Overview of using iPSCs for modeling cardiac disorders. After isolation of somatic cells from an identified patient, transduction with Sedai viruses expressing *Sox2, c-Myc, Klf4,* and *Oct3/4* induces cellular reprogramming to iPSCs. Exposure to small molecules differentiate iPSCs to cardiomyocytes *(iPSC-CMs)* that can be functionally characterized by multiple assays. Quantitative cellular phenotypic data from cellular and engineered tissue assays is then correlated to patient outcomes to refine patient management and develop new therapeutics. *Figure created with Biorender.com.*

from a patient typically requires at least 2–3 months and can cost as much as $17,000, limiting the universal production of iPSC lines for each patient. Improvements in reprogramming and differentiation techniques and advances in genome-editing technology will be necessary to create cohorts of patient-derived iPSC models for large-scale correlative studies.

Individualization of therapy also extends to interventional cardiology, electrophysiology, and CHD surgery. With the widespread use of MRI and CT for cardiac patients, there has been an explosion of high-resolution and multidimensional data available to researchers. These data, combined with high-powered computing and machine learning techniques, enable the development of computational models for the extraction of relevant physiologic parameters or building three-dimensional (3D) models. At Boston Children's Hospital, CHD patients with complex anatomy routinely undergo high-resolution cross-sectional imaging that is used to generate 3D segmented models for surgical planning and visualization. One translational research use of these models is to optimize surgical planning. For instance, application of fluid dynamics has been used to minimize energy loss in planned Fontan circulations.[41] Another is surgical lead placement in multisite pacing strategies for cardiac resynchronization therapy. Using high-resolution imaging to create computational models from cohorts of ischemic and non-ischemic cardiomyopathy patients, researchers identified optimal locations for LV pacing leads, depending on the location and extent of the residual scar.[42] It is likely that these types of modeling techniques could also be used for more complex anatomies such as patients with L-loop transposition (L-TGA) or single ventricle physiology, where optimal placement of pacing leads may be nonstandard.

Genetics strongly contribute to the pathogenesis of CHD, cardiomyopathies, and some arrhythmias. However, our understanding of how genotype impacts clinical outcomes for the majority of CHD remains in its infancy. In some cases, knowledge about the involvement of specific genes may guide management beyond assessment of recurrence risk. For example, awareness of TBX5 or NKX2-5 mutation leads to careful surveillance for progressive heart block; discovery of a de novo damaging mutation in a patient with CHD may lead to proactive guidance and testing for neurodevelopmental delay. But in most cases, additional studies are needed to identify genotype-phenotype relationships strong enough to guide patient management and to develop targeted therapies, which will likely have greatest efficacy on specific genotypes. We anticipate that this will be fertile ground for translational research in the coming years.

Development of Targeted Drug Therapy

In oncology, current drug development is increasingly focused on therapy that targets pathogenic genes or signaling pathways. As our knowledge of CVD pathogenic mechanisms increases, we can anticipate the development of mechanistically targeted therapies. While safe and effective, β-blockers or ACE inhibitors—current mainstays of heart disease management—modulate maladaptive neurohumoral pathways rather than direct disease-driving mechanisms.

In 2003, a novel GoF was identified in proprotein convertase subtilisin/kexin type 9 (PCSK9) in two French families with autosomal dominant hypercholesterolemia.[42a] Within the next 2–3 years, missense variants were identified in a small percentage of patients of African descent with very low low-density lipoprotein-cholesterol (LDL-C) levels conferring protection from coronary artery disease without other health problems.[43] Mouse models of PCSK9 overexpression and genetic deletion confirmed the hypothesis that PCSK9 modulated plasma cholesterol levels with correlative effects on the development of atherosclerosis.[44] Given the well-known correlation between serum lipid levels and coronary artery disease risk, a search for inhibitors of PCSK9 was pursued with vigor and within less than a decade, the first inhibitor, alirocumab, was approved by the Food and Drug Administration (FDA). Subsequently, additional PCSK9 inhibitors have been approved and have entered clinical practice in the treatment of severe hypercholesterolemia and coronary artery disease. This story illustrates the critical application of human genetics, disease modeling, and focused drug development to create a novel targeted therapy.

Recently, mavacamten was approved by the FDA for treatment of hypertrophic cardiomyopathy (HCM), the first new medication for HCM approved in over 30 years. In HCM, mutations in myosin and other thick filament proteins cause excessive actin-myosin cross-bridge cycling and hyper-contractility. Mavacamten was developed by selection of compounds that inhibit myosin ATPase activity and normalize myocardial energetics.[45] In preclinical and clinical trials, mavacamten reduced LV outflow tract obstruction observed in HCM, and improved LV filling.[46] Other small molecules targeting myosin ATPase activity through distinct mechanisms are under development.

Nucleic Acid Therapy

The delivery of bioactive molecules to the heart promises to open avenues for therapies targeting molecules not "druggable" through conventional small molecules. Among the leading modalities for cardiac gene therapy is AAV (Fig. 66.4). Other modalities under development are antisense oligonucleotides and modified mRNA.

AAV is a small DNA virus that is not known to naturally cause human disease. AAV has been extensively engineered so that current AAV vectors contain no viral host genes and only ~300 nucleotides of viral DNA. AAV cargo is retained in target cells for at least several years as a stable episome. The types of cells that AAV can transduce are determined by its surface proteins (capsid). AAV9 is a naturally occurring serotype that robustly transduces cardiac muscle, as well as skeletal muscle, liver, and many other tissues. An important limitation of AAV is that its cargo capacity is limited to

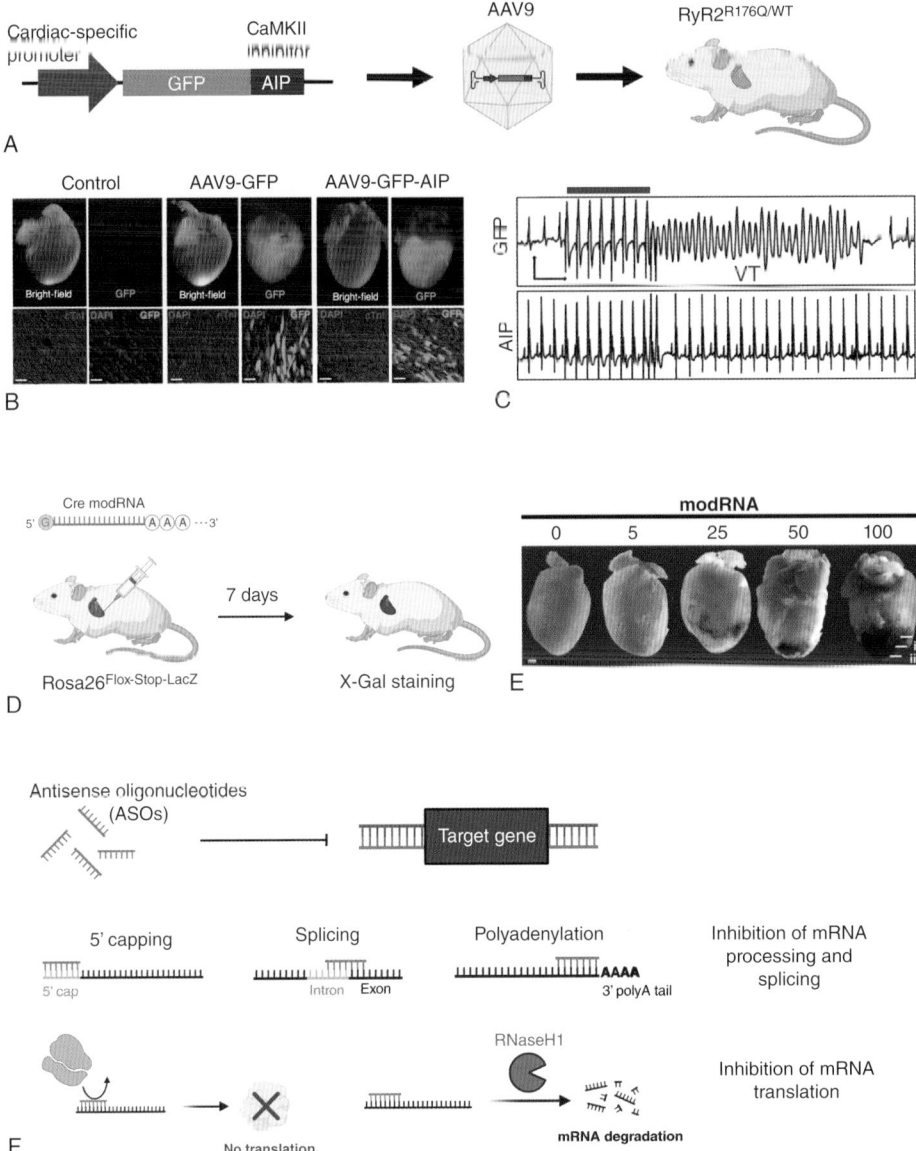

• **Fig. 66.4** Methods for using nucleic acids as targeted cardiac therapeutics. **(A)** The CaMKII inhibitor AIP was fused to GFP and packaged into AAV9 particles under the control of a cardiac-specific promoter. AAV9 was injected into RyR2$^{R176Q/WT}$ mice, a model of catecholaminergic polymorphic ventricular tachycardia (CPVT). **(B)** Whole-heart and histologic imaging demonstrated high-efficiency heart transduction. **(C)** Electrophysiologic testing revealed suppression of induced ventricular arrhythmias in the AAV9-GFP-AIP animals, demonstrating that AAV9-mediated CaMKII inhibition effectively treats CPVT in mice. **(D)** Modified RNA gene delivery to the heart. Modified RNA encoding Cre was synthesized and directly injected into Rosa26$^{Flox-Stop-LacZ}$ Cre-reporter mouse hearts. Translation of the modified mRNA produces Cre recombinase, which activates expression of the reporter gene LacZ. LacZ is conveniently visualized by histochemical staining with X-gal. **(E)** Whole heart X-gal staining revealed dose-dependent modRNA Cre expression after 7 days. **(F)** Antisense oligonucleotides (ASOs) are designed to inhibit mRNA translation by multiple mechanisms. Gene-specific ASO can interfere with mRNA splicing or mRNA processing, effectively inhibiting mRNA maturation. Alternatively, ASOs can directly inhibit translation or induce mRNA degradation. All these methods are exploited for suppression of the target gene. (b and c, e, were adapted with permission from: Bezzerides et. al 2019[50] and Zangi et. al. 2013,[57] respectively. *Figure created in part with Biorender.com.*)

~4.7 kb, which precludes its use for some lengthy cardiac genes such as dystrophin. A second limitation is that high doses of AAV must be delivered systemically to adequately transduce skeletal muscle. At these doses, acute toxicity is being observed in some patients, which has led to suspension or delays of several muscle-targeted gene therapy programs. Engineered variants are now emerging that markedly enhance AAV's ability to transduce specific cell types,[47] including cardiomyocytes and skeletal muscle cells, and these enhanced variants may address this hurdle.

One application of AAV is to deliver normal copies of genes to replace endogenous copies that contain inactivating mutations. For example, Danon disease, which affects the heart, skeletal muscle, and liver, is caused by inactivating mutations in LAMP2. AAV9-LAMP2B improved phenotypes in LAMP2 knockout mice.[48] Clinical trials are currently underway. Several AAV gene therapy trials are also underway for Duchenne muscular dystrophy, in which progressive dilated cardiomyopathy and skeletal myopathy are caused by inactivating mutations in dystrophin (DMD). AAV's cargo is insufficient to carry full length DMD, so smaller DMD variants (microdystrophins) were engineered that provide functional improvement over complete lack of DMD. In animal DMD knockout models, AAV-microdystrophin improved muscle pathology and dystrophic cardiomyopathy.[49] Several AAV-microdystrophin clinical gene therapy trials are currently underway.

For dominant mutations or other conditions involving large genes, gene replacement therapy may not be effective or feasible. An alternative strategy is to use AAV to target essential disease signaling pathways. The autosomal dominant form of the inherited arrhythmia, catecholaminergic polymorphic ventricular tachycardia (CPVT), is predominantly caused by GoF mutations in the cardiac ryanodine receptor (RYR2), the major intracellular Ca^{2+} release channel of cardiomyocytes. Arrhythmias in patients with CPVT are triggered by adrenergic stimuli. Adrenergic stimuli activate Ca^{2+}-calmodulin-dependent kinase II (CaMKII), which phosphorylates and activates RYR2. This event is critical to precipitate arrhythmias in CPVT. CaMKII has been a major pharmaceutical target for decades, because it has been implicated in the pathogenesis of heart failure and arrhythmia in multiple conditions. However, small molecule inhibitors have not progressed into clinical trials because of CaMKII's essential function in other tissues, most notably the brain. Using a cardiac-specific promoter and the cardiotropic properties of AAV9, it was possible to safely inhibit CaMKII and block CPVT arrhythmias in a mouse and human iPSC-CM models of CPVT.[50]

AAV gene delivery is also being combined with Cas9 genome editing. Perhaps the most successful example of this is genome editing for Duchenne muscular dystrophy. Many patients with Duchenne muscular dystrophy harbor frameshift mutations within a limited number of exons, which lie within a protein region containing repeated protein domains. Cas9-targeted mutations can cause the skipping of specific exons, such that the reading frame is restored. This restores protein expression, albeit with a small, well-tolerated deletion. This strategy was effective in mouse and dog Duchenne muscular dystrophy models.[51] While the risk of genotoxicity is higher than for microdystrophin replacement, the Cas9 exon skipping strategy results in a more complete protein, and the genomic correction will not be lost over time, as may occur with AAV episomes, especially in the face of repeated cycles of injury and repair by satellite cells.

Antisense oligonucleotides are short RNA or DNA sequences that alter gene expression by promoting transcript degradation, altering splicing, or inhibiting translation.[52]

For example, antisense oligonucleotides that promote exon skipping in Duchenne muscle dystrophy have been approved for clinical use.[53] However, current delivery methods used in the clinic are inefficient for muscle cells, limiting efficacy. In contrast, delivery of oligonucleotides modified by N-acetylgalactosamine (GalNAc) to hepatocytes is highly efficient. As a result, oligonucleotides directed at hepatic targets are becoming increasingly used in the clinic. For example, a GalNAc-siRNA targeting PCSK9, inclisiran, was approved by the FDA in 2021, and oligonucleotides targeting transthyretin, have been effective for treating transthyretin-mediated cardiomyopathy, caused by accumulation of transthyretin aggregates in the heart and other tissues. Antisense oligonucleotides targeting cardiomyocytes are under development, spurred by new technologies that enhance cardiomyocyte delivery.[54] For example, oligonucleotide knockdown of phospholamban has shown efficacy in a mouse model of cardiomyopathy caused by phospholamban mutation (PLN-R14del).[55] An exciting aspect of oligonucleotide therapies are that their targeting and toxicity profiles are suitable for the development of individualized, N-of-1 therapies, as recently exemplified by the development of such a therapy for Batten disease.[56]

Modified mRNA has now been administered to millions of humans as a vaccine for COVID-19. Modified mRNA offers the possibility of delivering long coding sequences to cells without the challenges or potential genotoxicity of viral vectors. Myocardial injection of modified mRNA encoding the angiogenic factor VEGFA was demonstrated to improve outcome in mice and larger animals after MI,[57] and this therapy is currently in clinical trials. More widespread application of modified mRNA for cardiac indications awaits more effective delivery mechanisms, such as lipid nanoparticles, which do not require direct myocardial injection.

Conclusion

We are in an exciting era of translational research in pediatric cardiology. Advances in our understanding of disease pathogenesis are yielding new therapeutic targets and strategies. At the same time, technologies have been developed to enable molecular and cellular therapeutic interventions to enter the clinic and inform patient care. We anticipate that the coming years will see an ever growing array of molecular and cellular therapies making the jump from bench to bedside to transform the lives of our patients.

References

1. Bruneau BG. Signaling and transcriptional networks in heart development and regeneration. *Cold Spring Harb Perspect Biol.* 2013;5:a008292. Available at: http://cshperspectives.cshlp.org/content/5/3/a008292.abstract.
2. Bruneau BG, Nemer G, Schmitt JP, et al. A murine model of Holt-Oram syndrome defines roles of the T-box transcription factor Tbx5 in cardiogenesis and disease. *Cell.* 2001;106:709-721.

3. Lyons I, Parsons LM, Hartley L, et al. Myogenic and morphogenetic defects in the heart tubes of murine embryos lacking the homeo box gene Nkx2-5. *Genes Dev*. 1995;9:1654-1666.

4. Molkentin JD, Lin Q, Duncan SA, Olson EN. Requirement of the transcription factor GATA4 for heart tube formation and ventral morphogenesis. *Genes Dev*. 1997;11:1061-1072.

5. Sohal DS, Nghiem M, Crackower MA, et al. Temporally regulated and tissue-specific gene manipulations in the adult and embryonic heart using a tamoxifen-inducible Cre protein. *Circ Res*. 2001;89:20-25.

6. Prendiville TW, Guo H, Lin Z, et al. Novel roles of GATA4/6 in the postnatal heart identified through temporally controlled, cardiomyocyte-specific gene inactivation by adeno-associated virus delivery of Cre recombinase. *PLoS One*. 2015;10:e0128105

7. Guo W, Schafer S, Greaser ML, et al. RBM20, a gene for hereditary cardiomyopathy, regulates titin splicing. *Nat Med*. 2012;18:766-773.

8. von Gise A, Lin Z, Schlegelmilch K, et al. YAP1, the nuclear target of Hippo signaling, stimulates heart growth through cardiomyocyte proliferation but not hypertrophy. *Proc Natl Acad Sci U S A*. 2012;109:2394-2399.

9. Jinek M, Chylinski K, Fonfara I, et al. A Programmable dual-RNA–guided DNA endonuclease in adaptive bacterial immunity. *Science*. 2012;337:816-821.

10. Yang H, Wang H, Shivalila CS, et al. One-step generation of mice carrying reporter and conditional alleles by CRISPR/Cas-mediated genome engineering. *Cell*. 2013;154:1370-1379.

11. Guo Y, VanDusen NJ, Zhang L, et al. Analysis of cardiac myocyte maturation using CASAAV, a platform for rapid dissection of cardiac myocyte gene function in vivo. *Circ Res*. 2017;120:1874-1888.

12. Rockman HA, Ross RS, Harris AN, et al. Segregation of atrial-specific and inducible expression of an atrial natriuretic factor transgene in an in vivo murine model of cardiac hypertrophy. *Proc Natl Acad Sci U S A*. 1991;88:8277-8281.

13. McMullen JR, Shioi T, Huang WY, et al. The insulin-like growth factor 1 receptor induces physiological heart growth via the phosphoinositide 3-kinase(p110alpha) pathway. *J Biol Chem*. 2004;279:4782-4793.

14. Laflamme MA, Chen KY, Naumova AV, et al. Cardiomyocytes derived from human embryonic stem cells in pro-survival factors enhance function of infarcted rat hearts. *Nat Biotechnol*. 2007;25:1015-1024.

15. Liu S, Li K, Wagner Florencio L, et al. Gene therapy knockdown of Hippo signaling induces cardiomyocyte renewal in pigs after myocardial infarction. *Sci Transl Med*. 2021;13:eabd6892.

16. Qian L, Huang Y, Spencer CI, et al. In vivo reprogramming of murine cardiac fibroblasts into induced cardiomyocytes. *Nature*. 2012;485:593-598.

17. Hwang HV, Sandeep N, Nair RV, et al. Transcriptomic and functional analyses of mitochondrial dysfunction in pressure overload-induced right ventricular failure. *J Am Heart Assoc*. 2021;10:e017835.

18. Reddy S, Hu DQ, Zhao M, et al. miR-21 is associated with fibrosis and right ventricular failure. *JCI Insight*. 2017;2:e91625.

19. Hu Y, Li D, Zhou C, et al. Molecular changes in prepubertal left ventricular development under experimental volume overload. *Front Cardiovasc Med*. 2022;9:850248.

20. Fujiwara T, Kurtts T, Anderson W, Heinle J, Mayer Jr JE. Myocardial protection in cyanotic neonatal lambs. *J Thorac Cardiovasc Surg*. 1988;96(5):700-710.

21. Porrello ER, Mahmoud AI, Simpson E, et al. Transient regenerative potential of the neonatal mouse heart. *Science*. 2011;331:1078-1080.

22. Solomon SD, McMurray JJV, Anand IS, et al. Angiotensin–neprilysin inhibition in heart failure with preserved ejection fraction. *N Engl J Med*. 2019;381:1609-1620.

23. Schiattarella GG, Altamirano F, Tong D, et al. Nitrosative stress drives heart failure with preserved ejection fraction. *Nature*. 2019;568:351-356.

24. Asimaki A, Kapoor S, Plovie E, et al. Identification of a new modulator of the intercalated disc in a zebrafish model of arrhythmogenic cardiomyopathy. *Sci Transl Med*. 2014;6:240ra74.

25. Poss KD, Wilson LG, Keating MT. Heart regeneration in zebrafish. *Science*. 2002;298:2188-2190.

26. Takahashi K, Yamanaka S. Induction of pluripotent stem cells from mouse embryonic and adult fibroblast cultures by defined factors. *Cell*. 2006;126:663-676.

27. Pierpont ME, Brueckner M, Chung WK, et al. Genetic basis for congenital heart disease: revisited: a scientific statement from the American Heart Association. *Circulation*. 2018;138:e653-e711.

28. Zaidi S, Choi M, Wakimoto H, et al. De novo mutations in histone-modifying genes in congenital heart disease. *Nature*. 2013;498:220-223.

29. Zaidi S, Brueckner M. Genetics and genomics of congenital heart disease. *Circ Res*. 2017;120:923-940.

30. Homsy J, Zaidi S, Shen Y, et al. De novo mutations in congenital heart disease with neurodevelopmental and other congenital anomalies. *Science*. 2015;350:1262-1266.

31. Richter F, Morton SU, Kim SW, et al. Genomic analyses implicate noncoding de novo variants in congenital heart disease. *Nat Genet*. 2020;52:769-777.

32. Cai CL, Liang X, Shi Y, et al. Isl1 identifies a cardiac progenitor population that proliferates prior to differentiation and contributes a majority of cells to the heart. *Dev Cell*. 2003;5:877-889.

33. Santini MP, Forte E, Harvey RP, et al. Developmental origin and lineage plasticity of endogenous cardiac stem cells. *Development*. 2016;143:1242-1258.

34. Snarr BS, O'Neal JL, Chintalapudi MR, et al. Isl1 expression at the venous pole identifies a novel role for the second heart field in cardiac development. *Circ Res*. 2007;101:971-974.

35. Xie L, Hoffmann AD, Burnicka-Turek O, et al. Tbx5-hedgehog molecular networks are essential in the second heart field for atrial septation. *Dev Cell*. 2012;23:280-291.

36. Zhou L, Liu J, Xiang M, et al. Gata4 potentiates second heart field proliferation and Hedgehog signaling for cardiac septation. *Proc Natl Acad Sci U S A*. 2017;114:E1422-E1431.

37. Burridge PW, Li YF, Matsa E, et al. Human induced pluripotent stem cell-derived cardiomyocytes recapitulate the predilection of breast cancer patients to doxorubicin-induced cardiotoxicity. *Nat Med*. 2016;22(5):547-556.

38. Stillitano F, Hansen J, Kong CW, et al. Modeling susceptibility to drug-induced long QT with a panel of subject-specific induced pluripotent stem cells. *Elife*. 2017;6:e19406.

39. Wang G, McCain ML, Yang L, et al. Modeling the mitochondrial cardiomyopathy of Barth syndrome with induced pluripotent stem cell and heart-on-chip technologies. *Nat Med*. 2014;20:616-623.

40. Park SJ, Zhang D, Qi Y, et al. Insights into the pathogenesis of catecholaminergic polymorphic ventricular tachycardia from engineered human heart tissue. *Circulation*. 2019;140:390-404.

41. Hammer PE, Hoganson DM, Del Nido PJ. A Tribute to Ajit Yoganathan's cardiovascular fluid mechanics lab: a survey of its contributions to our understanding of the physiology and management of single-ventricle patients. *Cardiovasc Eng Technol*. 2021;12:631-639.

42. Niederer SA, Lumens J, Trayanova NA. Computational models in cardiology. *Nat Rev Cardiol.* 2019;16:100-111.

42a. Abifadel M, Varret M, Rabès JP, et al. Mutations in PCSK9 cause autosomal dominant hypercholesterolemia. *Nat Genet.* 2003;34(2):154-156. doi:10.1038/ng1161.

43. Cohen JC, Boerwinkle E, Mosley Jr TH, et al. Sequence variations in PCSK9, low LDL, and protection against coronary heart disease. *N Engl J Med.* 2006;354:1264-1272.

44. Dot C, Guigay J, Adamus G. Anti-alpha-enolase antibodies in cancer-associated retinopathy with small cell carcinoma of the lung. *Am J Ophthalmol.* 2005;139:746-747.

45. Green EM, Wakimoto H, Anderson RL, et al. A small-molecule inhibitor of sarcomere contractility suppresses hypertrophic cardiomyopathy in mice. *Science.* 2016;351:617-621.

46. Olivotto I, Oreziak A, Barriales-Villa R, et al. Mavacamten for treatment of symptomatic obstructive hypertrophic cardiomyopathy (EXPLORER-HCM): a randomised, double-blind, placebo-controlled, phase 3 trial. *Lancet.* 2020;396:759-769.

47. Tabebordbar M, Lagerborg KA, Stanton A, et al. Directed evolution of a family of AAV capsid variants enabling potent muscle-directed gene delivery across species. *Cell.* 2021;184:4919-4938.e22.

48. Manso AM, Hashem SI, Nelson BC, et al. Systemic AAV9. LAMP2B injection reverses metabolic and physiologic multiorgan dysfunction in a murine model of Danon disease. *Sci Transl Med.* 2020;12:eaax1744.

49. Duan D. Systemic AAV micro-dystrophin gene therapy for duchenne muscular dystrophy. *Mol Ther.* 2018;26:2337-2356.

50. Bezzerides VJ, Caballero A, Wang S, et al. Gene therapy for catecholaminergic polymorphic ventricular tachycardia by inhibition of Ca2+/calmodulin-dependent kinase II. *Circulation.* 2019;140:405-419.

51. Long C, Amoasii L, Mireault AA, et al. Postnatal genome editing partially restores dystrophin expression in a mouse model of muscular dystrophy. *Science.* 2016;351:400-403.

52. Jay PY, Maier MA, Saltonstall L, et al. Gene silencing therapeutics in cardiology: a review article. *Int J Cardiovasc Sci.* 2021;35:665-675.

53. Matsuo M. Antisense oligonucleotide-mediated exon-skipping therapies: precision medicine spreading from duchenne muscular dystrophy. *JMAJ.* 2021;4:232-240.

54. Prakash TP, Mullick AE, Lee RG, et al. Fatty acid conjugation enhances potency of antisense oligonucleotides in muscle. *Nucleic Acids Res.* 2019;47:6029-6044.

55. Grote Beverborg N, Später D, Knöll R, et al. Phospholamban antisense oligonucleotides improve cardiac function in murine cardiomyopathy. *Nat Commun.* 2021;12:5180.

56. Kim J, Hu C, Moufawad El Achkar C, et al. Patient-customized oligonucleotide therapy for a rare genetic disease. *N Engl J Med.* 2019;381:1644-1652.

57. Zangi L, Lui KO, von Gise A, et al. Modified mRNA directs the fate of heart progenitor cells and induces vascular regeneration after myocardial infarction. *Nat Biotechnol.* 2013;31:898-907.

Future Direction

67

Innovation and Areas for Future Research

EDWARD P. WALSH, JOHN E. MAYER JR., SARAH A. TEELE, AND DAVID W. BROWN

The preceding chapters provided a practical survey of modern clinical practice in pediatric cardiology and congenital cardiac surgery. Although it is clear that the field has progressed dramatically, nobody should be satisfied with the status quo. There are still far too many areas where our knowledge is incomplete and our therapeutic options are limited. This final chapter sets out to highlight such areas and serve as a challenge to the next generation entering this dynamic field.

Table 67.1 lists just a few of the worthy topics for future research and development. Some of these involve basic science, some focus on clinical care, and some center on sociologic and cultural hurdles to optimal care delivery. We have chosen five of these items for brief discussion here.

Hepatic Factor and Pulmonary Arteriovenous Malformations

It is difficult to fathom how such a consequential item in cardiopulmonary biology has managed to escape detection for so long. The development of pulmonary arteriovenous malformations in the absence of pulmonary blood flow from the inferior vena cava has been recognized since the 1970s,[1] and even today remains a serious problem for patients with long-standing Glenn shunts, the Kawashima operation, and certain forms of heterotaxy. Moreover, it is now well known that the problem can be reversed in most cases with restoration of hepatic flow,[2] yet we still do not completely understand why.

Many investigators have tried to close this embarrassing knowledge gap. None have been entirely successful to date, though clever experiments are ongoing comparing protein profiles in superior caval blood with inferior caval blood from both normal and congenitally abnormal hearts. Several angiogenically active candidate proteins have recently been identified as differing between the two cavae, including angiopoietin-1, CXC motif chemokine ligand 16, leukemia inhibitory factor, sVEGFR1, and hepatocyte growth factor.[3-5] Among these, circulating sVEGFR1 (an inhibitor of sorts in the vascular endothelial growth factor system) seems to hold promise. Experiments using various models of angiogenesis are now being performed to study effects of these candidate proteins. No firm conclusions can yet be reached, but the work has profound implications, not only for pediatric cardiology but for many other disease conditions that involve abnormal angiogenesis, including tumor growth. This is undoubtedly a riddle that demands an expeditious solution.

Improved Localization of the Conduction Tissues During Cardiac Surgery

Acquired complete heart block remains an unfortunate complication of surgical repair for certain congenital heart defects. The 1-year mortality is very high unless paced,[6] but despite all advances in pacemaker technology, artificial pacing (even with chronic resynchronization devices) is never as efficient as an intact atrioventricular (AV) node and His-Purkinje system. Chronic pacing can be associated with long-term ventricular dysfunction even in a structurally normal heart, but is especially problematic in complex anatomy such as single ventricle and systemic right ventricle.

Because specialized conduction tissues do not stand apart from working myocardium by simple visual inspection in the operating room, our understanding of location for the compact AV node and His-Purkinje tissue in complex hearts has largely depended upon catheter mapping in the electrophysiology laboratory and elegant pathologic studies involving careful microscopy of serial sections in various congenital malformations.[7] These efforts have generated useful patterns to help guide placement of sutures and incisions to reduce the risk of inadvertent conduction block. However, the volume of pathologic material that has been properly examined is understandably limited, exceptions to the rules are not uncommon (especially in heterotaxy), and even

804

TABLE 67.1   Potential Areas for Future Innovation and Research

Topic	Relevant Chapters in this Textbook
Use of artificial intelligence and the role of algorithms to inform complex decisions	64, 65
Critical look at ethical considerations with advanced medical technologies	54, 64, 65
Better tools to evaluate diastolic function	11, 12, 13, 53
Improved understanding of hepatic factor and its role in the pulmonary vasculature	53, 54, 56, 59
Development of more durable and physiologic valves and conduits (transcatheter and/or surgical)	14, 33, 45, 50, 62
Better solutions for pulmonary vein stenosis	39, 40, 62
Improved risk-analysis to protect against sudden cardiac death in adult congenital heart disease	17, 18, 19, 57
Improved risk-analysis to protect against sudden cardiac death in cardiomyopathies	17, 18, 19, 20, 48
Improved understanding of lymphatics and the effects of Fontan physiology	15, 59
Improved understanding of hepatic damage from Fontan physiology	57, 59
Better understanding of the hypertrophic response to pressure and volume loads	2, 4, 11, 12, 13, 48, 53, 54, 62
Improved localization of conduction tissue during cardiac surgery	17, 18, 62
Improved neuroprotection during surgery and convalescence	55, 60, 63
Improved understanding of cellular electrophysiology and abnormal automaticity	8, 17, 20, 66
Gene therapy and molecular therapy for channelopathies	17, 20, 66
Gene therapy and molecular therapy for hereditary cardiomyopathies	48, 66
Better understanding of outcomes for bi-ventricular repair of functional single ventricle	61, 62
Improved risk-analysis for right coronary artery from left sinus of Valsalva	9, 10, 12, 42, 52
Improved understanding and therapy for failing myocardium	53, 54, 62, 66
Improved understanding of etiology for Kawasaki disease and prevention of coronary aneurysms	42, 46, 47
Optimizing medical care delivery across age, racial, economic, geographic lines	57, 64, 65
More efficient medical education in the 21st century	67

when the expected pattern holds true, the difference of just a few millimeters during surgery can make all the difference between intact conduction and permanent block. It is therefore desirable to trace the precise location of the conduction tissues in real time during congenital heart repairs. This is not a new concept. Dick et al.[8] were performing this sort of mapping in the operating room in the mid-1970s, but the technique was never widely adapted. Now, there is a renaissance in intraoperative mapping of conduction tissue in response to the demands of increasingly complex surgical repairs in patients with heterotaxy and borderline single ventricle undergoing biventricular repairs. The challenge is being met on two fronts. First, intraoperative mapping of His-Purkinje signals by the surgeon and an electrophysiologist has become a fairly standard maneuver during complex repairs at our center,[9] and the technique has begun to spread to a growing number of other institutions as well. Second, a method of fiberoptic microscopy that can distinguish conduction tissue from myocardium has now been developed,[10] which can serve in conjunction with electrogram mapping to refine localization. Data obtained by these two methods are being carefully catalogued and analyzed to uncover potential new patterns. Using such techniques, it is anticipated that the incidence of surgical heart block can be further reduced, with an ultimate goal of preventing all surgically acquired conduction disorders.

Ideal Cardiovascular Replacement Devices for Congenital Heart Disease

The ideal device for use in repairing the defects associated with congenital heart disease (CHD) requires that these devices reproduce the characteristics of normal cardiovascular tissues, including immediate, normal valve or blood vessel function, durability (for a lifetime), elasticity with resistance to excess deformation, responsiveness to changes in hemodynamic conditions, resistance to infection, non-immunogenicity, non-thrombogenicity, and the ability to grow.[11] These are the characteristics of normal living cardiovascular tissue, and no currently available cardiovascular devices possesses more than one or two of these characteristics, and none have shown biological growth. The obvious challenge going forward remains the creation of replacement valves and conduits that function as normal human tissues would in the same hemodynamic and biologic environments, particularly the ability to grow with the patient. Despite the pursuit of this holy grail for patients with CHD for over 25 years, and despite promising advances in knowledge, this goal of the development of the ideal replacement devices remains as a challenge.

The shortcomings of existing materials and devices are well known.[12] Current mechanical heart valves are functional at implant and durable but are thrombogenic, are more easily infected than a normal valve, and do not have growth potential. The durability of current generation prosthetic valves is related to the materials (pyrolytic carbon approaches the hardness of a diamond) and the absence of any flexion or stretching of the prosthetic materials during the cardiac cycle. Bioprosthetic heart valves, constructed as a composite of prosthetic valve frames and chemically cross-linked animal valve or pericardial tissues attached to these frames seem to be less thrombogenic but are also significantly less durable, subject to calcification with resulting loss of leaflet mobility, and again, lack growth potential. Human tissue used for valve replacement (homografts) also have limited durability and can evoke immune responses to donor antigens, although the immunogenicity can be partially mitigated with chemical decellularization. Similar problems exist for prosthetic or biological tissues used for blood vessel repair or replacement.

At a conceptual level, many questions remain unsolved and are the subject of ongoing investigations. To achieve the characteristics necessary for an ideal cardiovascular device, is it necessary to employ living tissue? There have been some creative approaches to provide growth potential for replacement devices constructed from prosthetic materials,[13] but the durability of non-biologic flexible materials that must undergo millions of cycles of flexion and stretch each year remains unknown. An alternative approach utilizing a tissue engineering approach to create living, cellularized cardiovascular tissues has been pursued for both cardiac valves and conduit arteries,[14] but an additional series of important conceptual questions remain for this approach. The initial challenge is how to populate these devices with cells. Should the device be prepopulated with cells prior to the time of the implant into the circulation, or can the host be induced to populate the implant with appropriate cell types after it is inserted? What cell type or types should be part of the device at implant or after in situ repopulation? A very important consideration for both cardiac valves and blood vessels is the composition of the extracellular matrix (ECM). There is an increasing understanding that this ECM serves as not only a determinant of the biomechanical characteristics of the tissue but also provides both micromechanical and biochemical signals to the cells that are attached to the ECM. The ability to reproduce this biomechanical and biochemical environment with either human-made or biologic scaffolds are almost certainly a major determinant of cell phenotype and behavior in engineered tissues. Finally, there is increasing appreciation of the host immune response to the implanted materials as a major determinant of the function of implanted materials.[15]

The phenomenon of a wider impact of research beyond the initial narrow goal has marked much of CHD research, reminiscent of the advances in knowledge of CHD anatomy that followed the early attempts at the repair of congenital heart defects. In this context, pursuit of the development of such ideal cardiovascular devices remains an extremely important clinical goal, in and of itself, but it should be kept in mind that research in pursuit of this goal will continue to yield important insights into the structure and function of both normal and abnormal cardiovascular structures.

Healthcare Delivery

When the first edition of this textbook was published in 1957, the 1-year survival rate for patients with complex forms of CHD was 20%. Pediatric cardiology experienced a medical and surgical renaissance in the latter half of the 20th century with major advances in diagnostic capabilities, management, and procedural techniques. Mortality from CHD has continued to decrease over the first quarter of the 21st century such that today greater than 80% of infants in the United States with critical CHD survive to 1 year.[16] When we look to the future of this specialty, our focus therefore shifts to early identification of disease, prevention of progression, targeting higher-risk populations, mitigation of morbidity, and optimizing quality of life for our patients. The way in which we deliver healthcare influences all these foci and consequently is one of the most important areas for improvement. Research and innovation in healthcare delivery offer tremendous opportunities for the next generation of pediatric cardiologists to positively impact patients, families, healthcare teams, and society.

The outcomes of patients with CHD have differed by ethnicity since the inception of the field.[16] Identifying and advocating for healthcare delivery that meets the needs of patients and families from underserved and marginalized populations is a global priority. Timely and targeted medical care informed by medical advances may dramatically alter an individual's long-term prognosis; this is true whether in outpatient clinic or in the intensive care unit with multiorgan considerations. Improved healthcare delivery models may result in fewer invasive procedures over an individual's lifetime. Identifying opportunities to decrease in-hospital length of stay are critical for mitigating patient morbidity, negative socioeconomic impact on families, and hospitals' capacity constraints.

Continuing to characterize quality-of-life outcomes for our patients is crucial.[17] Health professionals can direct interventions informed by these insights to enhance a patient's and family's experience with CHD. Delivering care with a holistic approach that considers the challenges of living with CHD may improve patient and family education and meaningfully inform life choices.[18]

Comprehensive and up-to-date care delivery to our patients and families requires interprofessional teams who provide diverse clinical expertise, patient and staff education, and psychosocial support. Advanced practice providers are an increasing presence in outpatient and inpatient settings, providing an opportunity to expand high-quality care delivery, and facilitate initiatives.[19] In addition, the presence of non-physician experts such as pharmacists, nutritionists, and physical and occupational therapists is now common on care teams, as are dedicated clinics that include specialists in multiorgan disease states. The growing population of adults with CHD requires the support of experts in all facets of internal medicine, including obstetrics.[20]

Teams are complex entities, however. Understanding and successfully navigating the decision-making and healthcare delivery that occurs within them requires leadership skills anchored in collaboration. Furthermore, multifaceted teams thrive in systems that support clear communication. These needs offer opportunities for mixed methods research, interdisciplinary quality improvement, and clinician education initiatives.[21]

As this book goes to publication, we are wrestling with methods to incorporate technology into our clinical practice and systems of healthcare delivery. In many circumstances, clinicians criticize technologic tools for impeding workflow and negatively impacting providers' experience. Exploring ways to improve healthcare delivery that works in concert with technology to augment the patient, family, and provider experience is needed. This includes the growing field of ethical considerations with advanced medical technologies.[22] Anchoring ourselves in humanistic healthcare while simultaneously embracing state-of-the art therapeutics is a daunting task that demands accountability.

Although COVID-19 caused substantial challenges to healthcare delivery, it also forced an accelerated rate of innovation, especially with regards to technology. At this time, it remains unclear how acute solutions to the pandemic, such as virtual clinical visits, will remain common practice. On the other hand, the widespread adoption of technology as a valid educational tool has supported faster and broader dissemination of knowledge. Providers from specialized pediatric cardiac care centers like Boston Children's Hospital can contribute to provide quality care for those in less physically accessible communities nationally and internationally. This field has exponential potential for growth and worldwide impact.

Artificial intelligence–driven interventions in diagnosis, mortality and morbidity risk assessment, surveillance, and health policy and planning already impact healthcare delivery.[23] Predictive analytics, for example, may improve decision-making and mitigate cognitive load in complex patients and systems common in CHD. These advanced tools, however, remain vulnerable to the biases and limitations of their creators. As we look to the next generation of pediatric cardiologists raised as digital natives, we are inspired by their potential to utilize technology in ways we have not yet conceived while simultaneously recognizing its shortcomings.

Training in Pediatric Cardiology for the 21st Century

With the remarkable changes in the landscape of delivery of care to patients with CHD and acquired cardiovascular disease, the education and training of the next generation of physicians must similarly evolve. A recent paradigm shift in training toward competency-based objectives is one example. While prior guidelines were based on the assumption that competency for given activities, tasks, or procedures would naturally follow from proscriptions of months of exposure and numeric targets, the 2015 training guidelines for Pediatric Cardiology[24] reflect the reality that it is competence that is the goal of training, and that there is wide variation in how and when this develops among learners. In addition, the American College of Graduate Medical Education has delineated six core competency categories that should be included in training paradigms. However, the accurate and continuous measurement of competence in our trainees remains a challenge.

A major barrier to the assessment of trainees in pediatric cardiology is the lack of appropriate tools and instruments with which to evaluate competence. While in-service examinations and board examination scores may be reliable and reproducible in assessing medical knowledge, these only address one domain of competence and fall short of assessing overall clinical performance. Current iterations of the 360-degree evaluation, including direct faculty observation and self-assessment, are important but remain subjective and dependent upon "time and chance" encounters in the clinical environment. Competency assessment tools modeled after the objective, structured clinical examination (OSCE), such as one recently described assessment exercise in the performance and interpretation of pediatric echocardiography,[25] are promising in providing both trainees and mentors valuable information on competence. The development of entrustable professional activities (EPAs) in congenital cardiology care may provide additional tools for competency assessment. EPAs are work descriptors that outline the essential tasks necessary for professional practice, with the level of supervision required to perform those work tasks reflecting increasing entrustment as trainees progress from novice to expert. EPAs have recently been developed for pediatric cardiology[26] (no small task!) and are currently in the process of being implemented; if properly constructed, EPAs offer not only assessment tools but also targets for curricular development as educational need gaps are identified to produce capable, independent practitioners.

The current cardiovascular training environment relative to prior eras is notable for the increased complexity of cardiac care and corresponding patient acuity, decreased trainee autonomy, increased work hour restrictions, and across-the-board expansion of in-house attending coverage. The rise of the patient safety movement and the increasing focus of hospitals and payors on healthcare quality over the past decade have dramatically improved the delivery of medical care and patient outcomes, but with considerable impact on training. The overall balance of trainee autonomy has shifted toward increased supervision, which has positive aspects—improved opportunities for teachers/mentor interaction, direct observation, evaluation and feedback, and modeling of professional behaviors. However, increased supervision is at tension with the development of graduated responsibility, increasing entrustment, and potential lack of readiness in the fellow-to-faculty transition that can result in increased stress during initial years of clinical practice. Training programs of the future will need to continue to innovate to develop forms of graduated responsibility and independent practice in the context of a medical environment of increasing complexity and acuity.

Dedicated early instructional periods offer one method to meet the needs of trainees attempting to acclimate to the highly technical clinical environment we work in. So-called "boot camps" allow the rapid introduction of key knowledge and skills in order for trainees to become rapidly functional and safe in the clinical setting.[27] Such dedicated instructional time has also been advocated as a way to mitigate the "July effect," a decrease in efficiency and increase in adverse outcomes seen in some hospital settings at the onset of the academic year. As our field continues to advance in technical and therapeutic complexity, the future of cardiovascular training will likely involve increasing expansion of these types of early instructional periods. Similarly, simulation training offers the ability to learn and practice key procedural skills in an environment free of risk to patient harm. Simulation training has been successfully employed to address high-risk procedures or clinical scenarios that have been traditionally taught by the "see one, do one, teach one" approach. The simulation environment has also been associated with positive instructional behaviors, particularly in procedural fields, where high acuity, time pressure, and task fixation in the live setting may impair instructional technique; importantly, simulation-based education has been associated with improved patient outcomes from procedural care. Training programs of the future will benefit from the further expansion of simulation training to teach catheterization skills such as vascular access, catheter manipulation, balloon atrial septostomy; imaging skills such as learning appropriate transthoracic and transesophageal views; and intensive care unit skills such as airway management and crisis resource management (e.g., code blue) drills.

Electronic medical records (EMRs) are now an integral component of inpatient and outpatient training environments, and interaction with the EMR seems to consume an ever-increasing portion of our clinical time. However, the EMR can be harnessed to help track the exposure and progress of trainees with unprecedented functionality. Most EMRs now have the ability to generate the age, diagnoses, site of care, even treatment codes for patients encountered in various settings; this offers the remarkable opportunity to move beyond accidental time-and-chance encounter education to intentional education, to create truly individualized education plans for our trainees. Training programs in the future will be able to integrate robust informatics tools to harness the EMR for such intentional training and evaluation.

Flexible Training Periods and Pathways

As the concept of competency-based training becomes more fully embraced, the traditional concept of a fixed 3-year categorical training with optional additional fourth-year subspecialty training should evolve into more flexible approaches. Training programs will need to be able to shorten and/or lengthen individuals' training programs to meet their needs based upon their progress toward independent practice; this will require the buy-in by regulatory bodies such as the American Board of Pediatrics. The development and application of EPAs will likely help push this issue forward, as well as the development of certification standards for advanced training in fields such as imaging and catheterization. Furthermore, as the field of pediatric cardiology has grown and matured, the number and shape of possible career paths have broadened considerably. In addition to a subspecialty area of focus, trainees today may contemplate an academic career as a basic investigator, a clinical investigator, clinician-educator, clinician-scholar, quality improvement specialist, or administrator. Each of these requires additional focused training and skill sets that are well beyond the focus of the traditional categorical training program. Training programs in the future will continue to need to revisit the definition of what constitutes that minimum core training required for every pediatric cardiologist, and what types of supporting activities could be selected to prepare trainees for their particular focus of choice.

References

1. McFaul RC, Tajik AJ, Mair DD, et al. Development of pulmonary arteriovenous shunt after superior vena cava-right pulmonary artery (Glenn) anastomosis. Report of four cases. *Circulation*. 1977;55:212-216.
2. Srivastava D, Preminger T, Lock JE. Hepatic venous blood and the development of pulmonary arteriovenous malformations in congenital heart disease. *Circulation*. 1995;92:1217-1222.
3. Vettukattil JJ. Is the hepatic factor a miRNA that maintains the integrity of pulmonary microvasculature by inhibiting the vascular endothelial growth factor? *Curr Cardiol Rev*. 2017;13:244-250.
4. Spearman AD, Gupta A, Pan AY, et al. sVEGFR1 is enriched in hepatic vein blood: evidence for a provisional hepatic factor candidate? *Front Pediatr*. 2021;9:679572.
5. Bartoli CR, Hennessy-Strahs S, Dowling RD, et al. Abnormalities in the Von Willebrand-angiopoietin axis contribute to dysregulated angiogenesis and angiodysplasia in children with a Glenn circulation. *JACC Basic Transl Sci*. 2021;6:222-235.

6. Lillehei CW, Sellers RD, Bonnabeau RC, et al. Chronic postsurgical complete heart block: with particular reference to prognosis, management, and a new P-wave pacemaker. *J Thorac Cardiovasc Surg.* 1963;46:436-456.

7. Anderson RH, Ho SY. The disposition of the conduction tissues in congenitally malformed hearts with reference to their embryological development. *J Perinat Med.* 1991;19:201-206.

8. Dick M II, Norwood WI, Chipman C, et al. Intraoperative recording of specialized atrioventricular conduction tissue electrograms in 47 patients. *Circulation.* 1979;59:150-160.

9. Feins EN, O'Leary ET, Hoganson DM, et al. Intraoperative conduction mapping in complex congenital heart surgery. *JTCVS Tech.* 2022;12:159-163.

10. Kaza AK, Mondal A, Piekarski B, et al. Intraoperative localization of cardiac conduction tissue regions using real-time fibreoptic confocal microscopy: first in human trial. *Eur J Cardiothorac Surg.* 2020;58:261-268.

11. Henaine R, Roubertie F, Vergnat M, et al. Valve replacement in children: a challenge for a whole life. *Arch Cardiovasc Dis.* 2012;105:517-528.

12. Singh M, Sporn ZA, Schaff HV, et al. ACC/AHA versus ESC guidelines on prosthetic heart valve management. *JACC.* 2019;73:1707-1718.

13. Hofferberth SC, Said MY, Tomholt L, et al. A geometrically adaptable heart valve replacement. *Sci Transl Med.* 2020;12:1-23.

14. Fioretta ES, Motta SE, Lintas V, et al. Next-generation tissue-engineered heart valves with repair, remodeling and regeneration capacity. *Nat Rev.* 2021;18:92-116.

15. Franz S, Rammelt S, Scharnweber D, et al. Immune response to implants: a review of the implications for the design of immunomodulatory biomaterials. *Biomaterials.* 2011;22:6692-6709.

16. Lopez KN, Morris SA, Sexson Tejtel SK, et al. US mortality attributable to congenital heart disease across the lifespan from 1999 through 2017 exposes persistent racial/ethnic disparities. *Circulation.* 2020;142:1132-1147.

17. Moons P, Luyckx K. Quality-of-life research in adult patients with congenital heart disease: current status and the way forward. *Acta Paediatr.* 2019;108:1765-1772.

18. Reid GJ, Webb GD, Barzel M, et al. Estimates of life expectancy by adolescents and young adults with congenital heart disease. *J Am Coll Cardiol.* 2006;48:349-355.

19. Gilliland J, Donnellan A, Justice L, et al. Establishment of pediatric cardiac intensive care advanced practice provider services. *World J Pediatr Congenit Heart Surg.* 2016;7:72-80.

20. Gilboa SM, Devine OJ, Kucik JE, et al. Congenital heart defects in the United States: estimating the magnitude of the affected population in 2010. *Circulation.* 2016;134:101-109.

21. Rosen MA, DiazGranados D, Dietz AS, et al. Teamwork in healthcare: key discoveries enabling safer, high-quality care. *Am Psychol.* 2018;73:433-450.

22. Moynihan KM, Dorste A, Siegel BD, et al. Decision-making, ethics, and end-of-life care in pediatric extracorporeal membrane oxygenation: a comprehensive narrative review. *Pediatr Crit Care Med.* 2021;22:806-812.

23. Topol EJ. High-performance medicine: the convergence of human and artificial intelligence. *Nat Med.* 2019;25:44-56.

24. Ross RD, Brook M, Feinstein JA, et al. 2015 SPCTPD/ACC/AAP/AHA training guidelines for pediatric cardiology fellowship programs (Revision of the 2005 Training Guidelines for Pediatric Cardiology Fellowship Programs). *J Am Coll Cardiol.* 2015;66:672-676.

25. Levine JC, Geva T, Brown DW. Competency testing for pediatric cardiology fellows learning transthoracic echocardiography: implementation, fellow experience, and lessons learned. *Pediatr Cardiol.* 2015;36:1700-1711.

26. Srivastava S, Braunlin E, Brown DW, et al. Curricula components for entrustable professional activities for the subspecialty of pediatric cardiology. *Prog Pediatr Cardiol.* 2017;44:17-32.

27. Allan CK, Tannous P, DeWitt E, et al. A Pediatric Cardiology Fellowship Boot Camp improves trainee confidence. *Cardiol Young.* 2016;26:1514-1521.

Glossary of Epononymous Cardiac Procedures

Eponymous Procedure Terminology

Cardiac Catheterization and Surgery

Alfieri procedure: A procedure for treatment of mitral valvar regurgitation in which the central segment of the anterior and posterior mitral valve leaflet are sewn together.

Baffes procedure: A procedure for D-transposition of the great arteries (D-TGA) originally described by Lillehei in which the right pulmonary veins were translocated into the right atrium and the inferior vena cava was translocated into the left atrium. Baffes' modification was to use homografts as interposition grafts to accomplish the same partial rerouting of the systemic and pulmonary venous drainage into the opposite atria to improve oxygenation in D-TGA with intact ventricular septum.

Bentall procedure: A procedure to replace the aortic root, ascending aorta, and aortic valve with a prosthetic conduit that contains a prosthetic aortic valve. The coronary arteries are explanted from the native aortic root and re-implanted into the wall of the conduit.

Blalock-Hanlon procedure: An early procedure for D-TGA to create an atrial septal defect (ASD) to improve mixing of pulmonary venous and systemic venous return without the use of cardiopulmonary bypass, typically carried out through a right thoracotomy.

Blalock-Thomas-Taussig shunt (classic): Anastomosis of right subclavian artery to right pulmonary artery to augment pulmonary blood flow. This terminology with the addition of *"modified"* is used for systemic-to-pulmonary shunts using a synthetic graft interposed between the subclavian or innominate artery and the ipsilateral pulmonary artery.

Brock procedure: A procedure performed for pulmonary valvar stenosis involves introduction of a tenotomy knife through a purse-string suture in the free wall of the infundibulum to incise the stenotic or atretic pulmonary valve.

Brockenbrough procedure: A procedure to puncture the atrial septum for access to left atrium and other left-sided heart structures from the femoral vein using a long needle/sheath/dilator.

Damus-Kaye-Stansel procedure: This procedure was described nearly simultaneously by all three of the named surgeons, and involves anastomosis of divided pulmonary artery to the ascending aorta, typically combined with a systemic-to-pulmonary artery shunt to restore pulmonary blood flow. This procedure has been used to treat subaortic or valvar aortic stenosis, particularly in single ventricle patients.

Fontan procedure: A procedure originally used to treat tricuspid atresia in which all of the systemic venous return is diverted directly into the pulmonary arteries without any contribution by a ventricle. A similar procedure was reported by Guillermo Kreutzer, and in some descriptions the operations based on this principle are referred to as Fontan-Kreutzer procedures. Currently, the same term is used to describe a number of technical variations that accomplish the same goal of separating the systemic venous return from the pulmonary venous return and directing the systemic venous return into the pulmonary arteries to achieve normal systemic arterial oxygen saturation.

Glenn procedure: This was originally described as a procedure to direct all of the superior vena cava (SVC) blood flow to the right pulmonary artery. The right pulmonary artery is divided and sewn into the posterior aspect of the SVC with occlusion of the SVC junction with the right atrium. Currently, a *"bidirectional" Glenn shunt* involves division of the SVC and anastomosis into the superior aspect of the right pulmonary artery. As the right pulmonary artery is not divided, the SVC blood flows to both the right and left pulmonary arteries and is thus "bidirectional." The correct physiologic description of the resulting circulatory state is a "bidirectional cavopulmonary shunt."

Hemi-Fontan procedure: This is a technical variation of a bidirectional cavopulmonary shunt in which a patch is used to enlarge the central pulmonary arteries and this patch is continued through the roof of the right atrium to separate the superior part of the right atrium that receives the SVC from the remainder of the right atrium and thus diverts SVC blood into both pulmonary arteries.

Jatene procedure: Arterial switch procedure typically carried out for D-TGA, which includes division of both the native aorta and pulmonary artery above the semilunar valves and reversal (switching) of their proximal connections. The proximal vessel arising from the left ventricle (neo-aorta) is anastomosed to the distal native aorta, and the proximal vessel arising from the right ventricle (neo-pulmonary artery) is anastomosed to the distal native pulmonary artery. The procedure also involves translocation of the coronary arteries from the original aorta into the proximal segment of the "neo-aorta" (original proximal pulmonary artery).

Kawashima procedure: This procedure refers to a bidirectional cavopulmonary shunt procedure when it is carried out in a patient with an interrupted inferior vena cava such that all of the venous return from the lower body, except from the liver and mesenteric circulation, reaches the SVC via an azygous vein.

Konno procedure: An aortic valve replacement procedure in which the aortic annulus is enlarged with an incision in the ventricular septum in the area of the right-left aortic valve commissure, creating a ventricular septal defect (VSD), and then closing the created VSD with a prosthetic patch to enlarge the aortic annulus. Typically, the right ventricular outflow tract is also enlarged with a patch.

LeCompte maneuver: This term refers to an element of the arterial switch operation (Jatene procedure) for D-TGA in which the distal pulmonary arteries are translocated anterior to the native ascending aorta in order to reduce tension on the anastomosis of the proximal neo-pulmonary artery to the distal true pulmonary arteries.

Manougian procedure: An aortic valve procedure in which the aortic annulus is enlarged by making an incision across the aortic annulus in the area of the commissure between the non-coronary sinus and the left coronary sinus which is then patched to enlarge the aortic annulus.

Mustard procedure: Atrial baffling (or atrial switching) procedure using pericardium or prosthetic patch material to direct systemic venous return to the left atrioventricular valve and the pulmonary venous return to the right atrioventricular valve. Originally used for treatment of D-transposition, currently more frequently used as a component of a "double switch" procedure for L-transposition.

Nicks procedure: An aortic valve procedure in which the aortic annulus is enlarged by making an incision across the aortic annulus in the non-coronary sinus which is then patched to enlarge the aortic annulus.

Nikaidoh procedure: This procedure is typically carried out for patients with D-TGA, a conoventricular VSD, and subvalvar or valvar pulmonary stenosis. It differs from the Rastelli procedure for this anatomy in that the native aortic valve and root excised from their native infundibular origin and translocated into the native pulmonary root that arises from the left ventricle. This native pulmonary root is enlarged with an incision through the annulus into the VSD, and the root is then enlarged with a patch that baffles the LV outflow to this neo-aortic root and also becomes part of the neo-aortic annulus. Right ventricle to pulmonary artery continuity is restored by anastomosis of the distal pulmonary arteries to the infundibulotomy.

Norwood procedure: This procedure is performed for the first-stage surgical treatment of hypoplastic left heart syndrome, but this terminology is also used for other forms of single ventricle with obstruction to systemic blood from the heart and associated aortic arch obstruction. In this procedure, the main pulmonary artery is divided and is directly connected to the ascending aorta, the aortic arch is augmented with patch material, the atrial septum is resected, and a modified Blalock-Thomas-Taussig shunt is used to provide pulmonary blood flow.

Ozaki procedure: An aortic valve procedure involving resection of one or more diseased native leaflets and replacement with new leaflets, typically constructed from glutaraldehyde cross-linked autologous pericardium or other biologic materials.

Potts procedure: A procedure to increase pulmonary blood flow in which an anastomosis is created between the descending aorta and the proximal left pulmonary artery.

Rashkind procedure: Transcatheter balloon atrial septostomy.

Rastelli procedure: This procedure is typically performed for D-TGA with associated VSD and obstruction of left ventricle to the pulmonary artery pathway. The VSD is used as the outflow from the left ventricle, and a baffle from the VSD to the aortic valve is placed within the right ventricle. The remaining right ventricle is then connected to the distal pulmonary arteries with a conduit, typically a homograft or other valved conduit.

Ross procedure: A procedure for aortic valve disease in which the pulmonary valve, typically with the surrounding cylinder of the pulmonary artery wall, is transferred into the aortic root as an aortic valve replacement. The original pulmonary valve is replaced, typically with a homograft or other valved conduit.

Ross-Konno procedure: In this procedure, the Konno technique for aortic annulus enlargement is combined with the Ross procedure using the native pulmonary valve autograft for the aortic valve replacement.

Sano procedure: This procedure is performed for the first-stage surgical treatment of hypoplastic left heart syndrome, but this terminology is also used for other forms of single ventricle with obstruction to systemic blood from the heart and associated aortic arch obstruction. In this procedure, the main pulmonary artery is divided and is directly connected to the ascending aorta, the aortic arch is augmented with patch material, the atrial septum is resected, and a small, restrictive conduit is placed between the right ventricle and the distal pulmonary arteries to provide pulmonary blood flow.

Seldinger technique: A method for vascular access using a flexible wire advanced through a hollow needle, with the wire then used as a rail for advancing a vascular sheath.

Senning procedure: An atrial baffling procedure using flaps of atrial septum and right atrial free wall to direct systemic venous return to the left atrioventricular valve and the pulmonary venous return to the right atrioventricular valve. Originally used for treatment of D-transposition, currently more frequently used as a component of a "double switch" procedure for L-transposition.

Starnes procedure: A procedure used for neonatal patients with the combination of Ebstein anomaly of the tricuspid valve with severe tricuspid regurgitation and low right ventricular pressures, pulmonary valve atresia, and severe cardiomegaly. In this procedure, the tricuspid orifice is covered with a fenestrated patch (to allow egress of Thebesian vein flow from the right ventricle), most of the right atrial free wall is resected, and a systemic-to-pulmonary artery shunt is constructed.

Takeuchi procedure: This procedure is carried out for anomalous origin of the left coronary artery from the pulmonary artery and involves use of a flap of anterior main pulmonary artery wall as a baffle across the posterior wall of the pulmonary artery in conjunction with creation of an aorto-pulmonary anastomosis "behind" the baffle to allow flow from the aorta to the left coronary artery.

Warden procedure: Procedure for correction of a superior sinus venosus ASD with anomalous drainage in which the SVC is divided above the entrance site of the anomalously draining right pulmonary veins and anastomosed to the right atrial appendage. The anomalous pulmonary right pulmonary veins are baffled to the left atrium with a patch that covers the original SVC orifice and the sinus venosus ASD.

Waterston-Cooley shunt: Creation of a direct anastomosis between the ascending aorta and the right pulmonary artery to augment pulmonary blood flow.

Yasui procedure: Procedure utilized for patients with a relatively normal-sized mitral valve and left ventricle but severe left ventricular outflow tract obstruction and a conoventricular VSD. The VSD is used as the outflow from the LV and a baffle is placed in the right ventricle to direct LV output to the native pulmonary valve. The proximal main pulmonary artery is divided and anastomosed to the aorta, and a right ventricle to pulmonary artery conduit is placed to provide a pathway from the right ventricle to the pulmonary circulation. In the neonatal period, reconstruction of a hypoplastic aortic arch is also required.

It is noteworthy that many of the operations and interventional catheterization techniques that were first described by a particular surgeon or cardiologist did not become known by an eponym relating that surgeon or cardiologist to the procedure. A few specific examples include the following: C. Walton Lillehei, who performed the first open cardiac repairs of VSD, tetralogy of Fallot, and atrioventricular canal defect with Richard Varco; Robert Gross, who performed the first successful ligation of a patent ductus arteriosus and the first successful repair of aorto-pulmonary window; F. John Lewis and Richard Varco, who performed the first successful closure of an ASD under inflow occlusion with moderate hypothermia; and John Gibbon, who performed the first successful closure of an ASD using cardiopulmonary bypass.

Index

Note: Page numbers followed by 'f' represent figures, by 't' represent tables, and by 'b' represent boxes.